The Comprehensive
Respiratory Therapist
Exam Review

The Comprehensive
Respiratory Therapist
Exam Review

6th Edition

JAMES R. SILLS, MEd, CPFT, RRT

Professor Emeritus
Former Director, Respiratory Care Program
Rock Valley College
Rockford, Illinois

ELSEVIER

ELSEVIER

3251 Riverport Lane
St. Louis, Missouri 63043

Previous editions copyrighted 2010, 2006, 2002, and 1995.

Library of Congress Cataloging-in-Publication Data

Sills, James R., author.
 The comprehensive respiratory therapist exam review / James R. Sills. --Sixth edition.
     p. ; cm.
 Includes bibliographical references and index.
 ISBN 978-0-323-24134-2 (pbk. : alk. paper)
 I. Title.
 [DNLM: 1. Respiratory Therapy--methods--Examination Questions. WF 18.2]
 RC735.I5
 615.836076--dc23

2014049890

Executive Content Strategist: Sonya Seigafuse
Content Development Manager: Billie Sharp
Senior Content Development Specialist: Rae L. Robertson
Publishing Services Manager: Jeff Patterson
Project Manager: Bill Drone
Senior Designer: Amy Buxton
Selected Illustrations: Sandra Hogan and Jeanne Robertson

Printed in the United States of America

Last digit is the print number: 9 8 7 6 5 4 3 2 1

 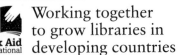

This book is dedicated to my wife,
Deb,
and our children, **Rachael** *and* **David,**
who make my life full and complete;
the memory of my **Mom,** *who always showed her love and support for me,*
and **Dad,** *who taught me through his actions;*
our dogs, **Amber** *and* **Abby,** *who took me for long walks in the woods and on the Lake Michigan beach;*
and
Carl Hammond,
who taught me respiratory care.

Words to live by:
The journey of 1000 miles begins with a single step.
Confucius

Hope for the best but plan against the worst.

Reviewers

Gayle A. Carr, MS, RRT

Adjunct Faculty
Illinois Central College
East Peoria, Illinois

Christopher Cox, BS, RRT

Clinical Education Specialist
Mercy Hospital Joplin
Joplin, Missouri

Erin E. Davis, MS, MEd, RRT-NPS, CPFT

Staff Therapist, Intensive Care
Ochsner Medical Center
New Orleans, Louisiana

Cynthia A. Duncan, BS, RRT

Clinical Coordinator
St. Luke's College—UnityPoint Health
Sioux City, Iowa

Lindsay Fox, MEd, RRT-NPS

Program Coordinator
Southwestern Illinois College
Belleville, Illinois

Kathryn Wirt Grahn, RRT, BSRT, RCP

Formerly Respiratory Care Faculty
Midlands Technical College
Columbia, South Carolina

Sharon L. Hatfield, PhD, RRT, RPFT, AE-C

Chair of Community Health Sciences
Jefferson College of Health Sciences
Roanoke, Virginia

Chris E. Kallus, MEd, RRT

Professor and Program Chair
Respiratory Care Program
Victoria College
Victoria, Texas

Amber L. Magers, BS, RRT-NPS, RPSGT

Director, Respiratory Therapy and Polysomnography
  Programs
Concorde Career College
San Bernardino, California

Jacki Moss, MEd, RRT, RCP

Clinical Coordinator, Respiratory Care
Rock Valley College
Rockford, Illinois

Paula Denise Silver, BS, PharmD

Medical Instructor
College of Technology and Health Sciences
ECPI University
Newport News, Virginia

Kenneth A. Wyka, MS, RRT, AE-C, FAARC

Adjunct Professor, Respiratory Therapy Program
Independence University
Salt Lake City, Utah

Foreword

Again, Jim Sills nailed it! The sixth edition of the *Comprehensive Respiratory Therapist Exam Review* continues to provide the most comprehensive—and important—resource for all respiratory therapists preparing for the **National Board for Respiratory Care (NBRC) Therapist Multiple Choice (TMC) Examination and Clinical Simulation Examination (CSE)**. In addition to the author's superb ability to provide the reader with the essential components required to be a safe and competent respiratory therapist—i.e., the knowledge, skills, and professional characteristics fundamental to respiratory therapy—in a straightforward, easy to read—and, importantly, clear—manner, the sixth edition of this textbook now provides the following new and critical features:

All of the content throughout the textbook has been completely updated—it covers every item identified as testable on the **NBRC's TMC Examination Detailed Content Outline**. Furthermore, all the content throughout the textbook has been updated to the most current standards and clinical practice guidelines. In addition, the new 160 item *pretest* (practice mode) **TMC Exam** and the new 160 item *posttest* (exam mode) **TMC Exam** both parallel the question mix on the new **NBRC TMC Exam**. These two exams are on the book's website. The two exams also include rationales and scoring feedback. The posttest exam mode version runs like the actual NBRC TMC exam.

The website also includes 22 clinical simulation scenarios that match the number and mix of scenarios on the new **NBRC CSE**. Importantly, the 22 clinical simulation scenarios also parallel the new, shorter CSE format. Every option has a rationale and scoring feedback. Finally, each of the 22 clinical simulations can be taken individually in the practice mode or in one sitting, similar to the actual NBRC CSE. The exam version runs like the actual NBRC CSE. All of the scenarios are on the book's website.

For the reader preparing to successfully navigate through the NBRC's TMC Examination and CSE system, the sixth edition of *Comprehensive Respiratory Therapist Exam Review* is the essential textbook. Jim Sills continues to provide future respiratory therapists—and the patients they treat—a valuable and important resource. Enjoy, and welcome to the profession of respiratory care.

Terry Des Jardins, MEd, RRT
Former Director, Professor Emeritus
Department of Respiratory Care
Parkland College
Champaign, Illinois;
Faculty/Staff Member
University of Illinois
College of Medicine
Urbana–Champaign, Illinois

Preface

The sixth edition of *The Comprehensive Respiratory Therapist Exam Review* has been completely revised while holding true to its core principles. The revisions relate to the content and expectations specified by the National Board for Respiratory Care (NBRC) in the *Therapist Multiple-Choice (TMC) Examination Detailed Content Outline* that was released in July 2013. The new TMC Exam starts in January 2015. For the first time, a single multiple-choice exam will be used to determine the minimum passing threshold to earn the Certified Respiratory Therapist (CRT) credential and a higher passing threshold for permission to take the restructured Clinical Simulation Examination (CSE). The candidate who passes the expanded 20 patient scenarios on the CSE will be awarded the Registered Respiratory Therapist (RRT) credential.

Holding to the core principles of this book from its first edition, every item listed as testable by the NBRC will be presented and the practice exams will present a realistic preview of what to expect when taking the TMC and CSE. To help prepare students and graduates for the NBRC exams, these updates have been made: (1) new testable items have been added and discussed, (2) new untested items have been deleted, (3) chapter "Exam Hints" have been updated for the most commonly seen question areas, (4) the end-of-chapter Self-Study Questions have been updated and revised as necessary, (5) the TMC study mode (pretest) and exam mode (posttest) have been updated to reflect current exam content, and (6) the clinical simulation scenarios have been extensively revised. These two TMC exams, the practice CSE, and other supporting documents can be accessed online at http://evolve.elsevier.com/Sills/respiratorycare. To create a realistic NBRC exam experience, the two TMC exams are 160 questions in length and the CSE contains 22 patient scenarios. The CSE scenarios match the mix specifications for the actual CSE. As with previous editions, all end-of-chapter questions, TMC questions, and CSE options will have a rationale to explain the correct or incorrect responses.

It is my sincere hope that this new edition will help the educator, student, and graduate understand the full scope of respiratory care practice and prepare for the NBRC exams to earn the CRT and RRT credentials.

James R. Sills, MEd, CPFT, RRT

Acknowledgments

Every author hopes for great editorial support from the publisher. I have been fortunate to have two such groups. I want to first thank Kathy Sartori and Billie Sharp, who worked with me through the fifth edition of this book, the *Case Studies and Clinical Simulations for Respiratory Care* web-based learning project, and the start of this sixth edition. Their suggestions, input, and contributions have been greatly appreciated. But, as George Harrison sang, "All things must pass." When informed that Kathy and Billie could not work with me to the conclusion of this sixth edition, I was concerned about our successful "team" being broken up. Fortunately, my concerns were unwarranted. My new team of Rae Robertson and Sonya Seigafuse has provided a near seamless transition. Because of the hard work of Rae and Sonya, this book, its e-book, and website have all been completed to my great satisfaction. Again, it has been my good fortune to work with two great teams of Elsevier professionals. My heartfelt thanks go out to Kathy, Billie, Rae, and Sonya!

I am most grateful for the feedback provided by the reviewers of the manuscript, clinical simulation scenarios, and practice Therapist Multiple-Choice Exams. Your careful, professional proofreading; helpful suggestions; and thought-provoking questions have made this a better book and learning package.

Lastly, I need to thank Terry Des Jardins for being such a good friend and mentor for over 30 years. When I first had the idea of writing a respiratory care textbook, I sought Terry's advice. He gave me great input then, and I still seek his counsel when pondering a challenging topic. Terry, thanks in so many ways.

Jim Sills

Introduction

Introduction and Recommendations for Exam Success

The National Board for Respiratory Care (NBRC) released the following documents in July 2013 to help guide test takers:

1. Therapist Multiple-Choice Examination Detailed Content Outline. This provides details on the testable items and difficulty level of questions found on the new Therapist Multiple-Choice (TMC) Examination. This exam reflects the most recent survey by the NBRC on the range and importance of activities performed by entry level and advanced respiratory therapists. The results show that their clinical skills are matched to the point of having only one multiple-choice examination. So, the new TMC Examination replaces the previous Entry Level Examination (to earn the Certified Respiratory Therapist, CRT, credential) and the Written Registry Examination. With this major change comes a change in exam scoring. The TMC will have two threshold (cut) scores. The exam taker who passed the lower threshold score will be awarded the CRT credential. In all but one state with a licensure law, a person must have earned the CRT credential to get a state license to practice and be hired as a respiratory therapist. The exam taker who passes the higher threshold score will be awarded the CRT credential and will be permitted to sit for the Clinical Simulation Examination (CSE). After the CSE is passed, the Registered Respiratory Therapist (RRT) credential will be awarded. Ohio requires the RRT credential to gain a state license to practice as a respiratory therapist.

2. Clinical Simulation Examination Detailed Content Outline. This provides details on the testable items found on the CSE. The listed content is identical to the TMC Examination Detailed Content Outline but no difficulty levels are provided. Only the exam taker who hits the higher threshold score on the TMC can take the CSE. After passing the CSE, the exam taker will be awarded the RRT credential.

These two documents can be accessed online at www.NBRC.org. The *Therapist Multiple-Choice Examination Detailed Content Outline* and the *Clinical Simulation Examination Detailed Content Outline* are also included on the Evolve site for this book.

The purpose of this book is to help you prepare to take and pass the TMC Examination and CSE.

There are several assets that will assist you as you prepare:

- Exam hints within the chapters are matched to the TMC. These will point out commonly tested item areas.
- Self-assessment questions appear at the end of each chapter. Answering these questions will allow you to see what you have retained while reading the content of the chapter. To a lesser extent, there will be some added content from other chapters. (Rationales will be found in the appendix to this book.)
- The online practice TMC exams, both in study mode (pretest) and exam mode (posttest), will help you analyze your strengths and weaknesses. The exam mode (posttest) will run like the actual TMC Examination. Every question on both exams has a rationale for the correct and incorrect answers. (These two exams, the CSE, and all rationales can be found on the Evolve website.)

It is recommended that the TMC pretest be taken and analyzed before beginning the text and studying. After studying, take the TMC posttest to identify your improvement and find any areas still needing remediation. Both TMC sample tests are designed to follow the format, question styles, difficulty levels, and relative weight of the tested areas on the real TMC Examination. The 22 CSE problems are the same mix of patient scenarios that will be seen on the actual exam.

The text includes **boldface** topic headings followed by two codes. The first code (in parentheses) is the NBRC code for that subject taken from the *Therapist Multiple-Choice Examination Detailed Content Outline*. Remember that the CSE is comprehensive and includes everything testable on the TMC Examination. My choice of words for topic headings is either the NBRC's or a paraphrasing of it. Occasionally a heading appears without an NBRC code after it. These headings were added to help you understand what the NBRC is testing for. Some discussion of pathologic processes is included in the general discussion of each chapter as they relate to the treatment or procedure that the respiratory therapist performs. It is recommended that you study the major types of adult and infant disease states and abnormal conditions.

The second code [in brackets] is the NBRC code for the difficulty level of the questions that will be used to test your understanding of the material. *R* stands for *Recall*,

Ap stands for *Ap*plication, and *An* stands for *An*alysis. You will find that the NBRC asks questions at these three different levels of difficulty. See below for more discussion on the difficulty levels. The NBRC does not provide a difficulty code for items tested on the CSE. Be prepared for any difficulty level in the 22 patient scenarios.

Therapist Multiple-Choice Examination

Critical points to remember:

- The TMC Examination consists of 160 total questions; 140 are actual tested questions. The NBRC also includes 20 extra questions being pretested for future versions of the examination. These pretested questions are not scored as part of your exam. Because it is not possible to tell the actual from the pretested questions, take each question seriously. The examination is offered in a computer-based testing format through the Internet. Make sure to follow all commands listed on the computer screens so that you do not make any mistakes. You cannot bring a calculator or any other type of test aid device with you. A pencil and blank piece of paper are provided for making notes and calculations.
- You will have 3 hours to complete the examination. Do not leave any questions unanswered. There is no penalty for guessing.
- The TMC Examination is replacing the Entry Level Examination and the Written Registry Examination. The NBRC will be calculating two threshold (cut) scores for the TMC Examination. Those who pass the first, lower threshold score will be awarded the CRT credential. Those who pass the second, higher threshold score will be awarded the CRT credential and be eligible to take the CSE. The NBRC has not announced what the two threshold scores will be. They may vary depending on which version of the TMC Examination is taken. (Those who pass the CSE will be awarded the RRT credential. See below for more information on the CSE.)

The TMC Examination has three difficulty levels to its questions. Despite the different levels of difficulty, each question has the same point value. At the end of the exam, the candidate will receive a raw score for correct answers and the high and low threshold scores. There will be no scaled scores as seen on the previous Entry Level Examination and Written Registry Examination.

Recall (R)

Recall refers to remembering factual information that was previously learned. "Identify" is a commonly used action verb in this type of question. You may be asked to identify specific facts, terms, methods, procedures, principles, or concepts. Prepare for this type of question by studying the full range of factual information, equations, and so on that are seen in respiratory care practice. These types of questions are on the lowest order of difficulty. You either know the answer or you do not; there is little to ponder more deeply. It is very important to have a solid

understanding of the factual basis of respiratory care to do well in this and the next two categories of questions.

Application (Ap)

Application refers to being able to use factual information in real clinical situations that may be new to you. "Apply," "classify," and "calculate" are commonly used action verbs in this type of question. You may be asked to apply laws, theories, concepts, and/or principles to new, practical clinical situations. Calculations may have to be performed. Charts and graphs, such as seen in pulmonary function testing or ventilator graphics, may need to be used. This type of question is on a higher order of difficulty than the Recall (R) type. Critical thinking must be applied to the factual information to answer these questions.

Analysis (An)

Analysis refers to being able to separate a patient care problem into its component parts or elements to evaluate the relationship of the parts or elements to the whole problem. "Evaluate," "compare," "contrast," "revise," and "select" are commonly used action verbs in this type of question. You may be questioned about revising a patient care plan or evaluating therapy. This type of question requires the highest level of critical thinking. You may have to recall previously learned information, apply it to a patient care situation, and make a judgment as to the best way to care for the patient. Frequently you must analyze cross-connections between subject areas to make a patient care decision, for example, interpreting arterial blood gas results and bedside spirometry data to determine a patient's readiness to wean from the mechanical ventilator. The key element that makes an analysis level question is the need to make a clinical change based on the assessment of patient care data.

You will find that the NBRC uses two different types of questions on the exam in the following three ways:

One best answer (the NBRC calls this "one best response" multiple choice)

This type of question has a stem (the question) followed by four possible answers coded A, B, C, and D. You must select the best answer from among those presented. Only one is clearly best, even though other possible answers may be good. Carefully read the stem to make sure that you do not misunderstand the clear intent of the question. Controversial issues may be questioned. The use of SHOULD in the stem will clue you in to the need to select the answer that would be selected by the majority of practitioners. The large majority of questions on the exam will be One Best Response type.

Multiple true–false (the NBRC calls this "complex" multiple choice)

This type of question has a stem (the question) followed by four (or five possible) answers numbered 1, 2, 3, and 4. Following this are four combinations of the answers listed by letters A, B, C, and D. The stem may ask you to include all true statements or all false statements in the final answer. You must select the letter that represents the correct combination of answers.

No controversial answers should be offered. They are all either clearly correct or incorrect. That is the key to selecting the best answer. Read each possible answer as separate from the others. It is suggested that you mark each possible answer as true or false. Even if you are not sure of every option, you should be able to determine the best answer.

Qualifying words

Qualifying words give direction to the focus of any type of question. They really direct how you should answer the question. Examples of qualifying words include, but are not limited to, INITIALLY, SHOULD, FIRST, MOST, LEAST. Phrases using qualifying words include "What would be the INITIAL thing to do...," "What is the FIRST thing…," "What is the MOST important thing…," and "What is the LEAST important thing…"

In the past, the NBRC has included some questions with three correct answers and one incorrect answer. The incorrect answer is the one that needs to be selected. The use of "except" will clue you in to this type of question. For example: "The colors of the American flag include all of the following colors EXCEPT: red, white, blue, green." Obviously, the correct answer is the incorrect color, green. The NBRC is phasing out, but has not eliminated, this type of question. Some are included within the chapter questions and NBRC style exams because of past practice, so that the test taker is familiar with this style of question.

Situational sets

Anticipate one or two Situational Sets at the end of the exam. The Situation Sets involve the use of a patient care scenario that may include such information as the patient's history, vital signs, blood gas values, or pulmonary function results. Three to five questions follow that ask you about patient or equipment management. These questions are the "one best answer" or "multiple true-false" types, as discussed above. However, because of the amount of information offered and the critical thinking required, these questions are categorized as being at the Application or Analysis level of difficulty. Carefully read the scenario to fully understand the information. After reading the related question, refer back to the scenario for information that can help you pick the best answer. Do this for each question and also refer to the prior questions for information that may help you with the current one.

Suggestions for preparing for the therapist multiple-choice examination

1. Pace yourself so that you have enough time to get through all of the questions. A good pace is about 50-55 questions per hour. Make a note on your blank paper on any difficult questions that you skip or want to go back to.

You can also computer "bookmark" any questions you want to come back to later. The computer-based test will prompt you if any questions have been skipped. Come back to them at the end of the test time. Do not leave any blank questions. You will not be penalized for guessing on the last few questions if you are running out of time.

2. Completely read each question. Determine what it is that you are really being asked. Look for qualifying words as discussed above.

3. Separate the important information from that which is not important. Many questions contain patient information and data on blood gases, pulmonary function, hemodynamics, ventilator settings, and so on. Disregard what does not pertain to the question being asked. Interpret the important data.

4. Do not read beyond the question. Resist the temptation to "psych out" what you think the question writer wants. Use only what is given to you.

5. Carefully read every answer that is offered.

6. Pick the best answer that is offered. The answer that you might like best may not be offered. Regardless, you must pick from among those that are offered.

7. In multiple true-false questions, use the following strategy: (1) Find an option that you know to be incorrect and cross off any of the answers that contain it; (2) find an option that you know to be correct and cross off any answers that do not contain it; (3) find the remaining answer, which must be correct.

8. Again, answer every question. There is no penalty for guessing incorrectly.

9. Take practice exams. They are available on the NBRC website (listed on p. xxii) and accompany this text on the online Evolve Learning System (http://evolve.elsevier.com/Sills/respiratorycare/). Evaluate your strengths and weaknesses and spend more time studying your weak areas. The online tests with this book contain an interactive pretest (study mode) and posttest (exam mode) formatted like the actual examination.

Relative weights of the various tested areas on the therapist multiple-choice examination

I have attempted to analyze the content of each of the questions on the TMC Validation Study Examination and the available past Entry Level Examinations and Written Registry Examinations. Each question has been matched to one of the chapters in this book, listed in Table 1 below. The numbers of questions and percentages are averages and may not be followed exactly on all versions of the examination. However, the relative weights can offer solid guidance as to what content is relatively more important or less important. Study time can be spent accordingly.

Suggestions for maximizing exam preparation time.

1. Spend the majority of your time studying the most heavily tested areas: Chapter 15: Mechanical Ventilation of the Adult; Chapter 1: Patient Assessment; Chapter 3: Blood Gas Sampling, Analysis, Monitoring,

TABLE 1	Anticipated Average Examination Content Found in Each Chapter*		
Chapter		**Number of Questions**	**Percentage of Exam Content (%)**
1. Patient Assessment		12	9
2. Infection Control		4	3
3. Blood Gas Sampling, Analysis, Monitoring, and Interpretation		10	7
4. Pulmonary Function Testing		6	4
5. Advanced Cardiopulmonary Monitoring		4	3
6. Oxygen and Medical Gas Therapy		10	7
7. Hyperinflation Therapy		2	1
8. Humidity and Aerosol Therapy		8	6
9. Pharmacology		10	7
10. Airway Clearance Therapy		3	2
11. Cardiac Monitoring and Cardiopulmonary Resuscitation		5	4
12. Airway Management		10	7
13. Suctioning the Airway		4	3
14. Intermittent Positive-Pressure Breathing		3	2
15. Mechanical Ventilation of the Adult		36	26
16. Mechanical Ventilation of the Neonate		2	1
17. Home Care and Pulmonary Rehabilitation		4	3
18. Special Procedures		5	4
Pathologic conditions, such as those listed in Table 2, should be studied from a clinical medicine textbook.		2	1
Total		140	100

*The number of questions shown reflects the average found on past NBRC exams. While individual Therapist Multiple Choice Examinations may vary somewhat in question mix, it can be anticipated that the importance of broad content areas will correlate with this table.

and Interpretation; Chapter 6: Oxygen and Medical Gas Therapy; Chapter 9: Pharmacology; and Chapter 12: Airway Management. As time permits, study all remaining chapters.

2. Review the Exam Hint topics in all chapters.
3. Thoroughly understand bedside and advanced patient assessment by studying Chapters 1, 3, 4, and 5. This content is important by itself and is also incorporated into questions covering all therapeutic procedures.
4. Arterial blood gas interpretation must be understood to answer questions related to oxygen administration and mechanical ventilation.
5. Pulmonary function testing must be understood to understand how to interpret the results of bronchodilator therapy and assess a patient's need for mechanical ventilation.
6. Bedside patient assessment, blood gas interpretation, and pulmonary function testing must be understood to assess a patient to make the correct mechanical ventilator adjustments.
7. Chapter 15: Mechanical Ventilation of the Adult has the most heavily questioned content of all the chapters. You *must* understand mechanical ventilation to do well on the TMC Examination and CSE.

CLINICAL SIMULATION EXAMINATION

Critical points to remember:
- The CSE is composed of 22 broad-based patient scenarios; 20 are actual tested scenarios. The NBRC also includes two extra scenarios being pretested for future versions of the examination. Because you cannot tell which scenario is being pretested, approach each one seriously.
- These patient cases are designed to evaluate how well the exam taker is able to gather information, evaluate it, and make clinical decisions that relate to simulated real patient situations. The CSE tests well beyond the recollection of simple facts. Table 2 lists the typical types of patient care problems that will be seen. The computer-based examination process is unique. Each clinical simulation problem is designed to flow in the same manner in which actual patient data are delivered and care decisions are made. In most scenarios, patient care progresses in a straight ideal path to completion. However, some scenarios are designed in a branching logic format. This means that in addition to the ideal path, there will be an alternate, less ideal side path. To some extent, you choose your own path; however, only one path is best. Choosing the best path will result in the highest score.

TABLE 2 The Specifications for Each Clinical Simulation Examination Form	
Problem Type	**Specifications**
A1. COPD**, conservative management These patients could have chronic bronchitis and/or emphysema (COPD), bronchiectasis, and/or asthma. Areas of focus on the simulation could include, but are not limited to, pulmonary function testing, oxygen therapy, inhaled medications, home care, rehabilitation, and infection control.	2
A2. COPD**, critical care management These patients could have chronic bronchitis and/or emphysema (COPD), bronchiectasis, and/or asthma. Areas of focus on the simulation could include, but are not limited to, pre- and postoperative evaluation, critical care management, and mechanical ventilation.	2
B. Adult trauma Trauma could include, but is not limited to, chest, head, or skeletal injuries, pneumothorax, surface burns, smoke inhalation, carbon monoxide poisoning, drowning, and hypothermia.	3
C. Adult cardiovascular These patients could have congestive heart failure, pulmonary edema, coronary artery disease, myocardial infarction, valvular heart disease, or cardiac surgery.	3
D. Adult neurological or neuromuscular These patients could have myasthenia gravis, Guillain-Barré syndrome, tetanus, muscular dystrophy, cerebrovascular accident (stroke), or drug overdosage.	2
E. Pediatric These patients could have epiglottitis, laryngotracheobronchitis (croup), bronchiolitis, asthma, cystic fibrosis, foreign body aspiration, toxic substance ingestion, or bronchopulmonary dysplasia.	2
F. Neonatal These patients could require care in the delivery room, need resuscitation, have infant apnea, meconium aspiration syndrome, respiratory distress syndrome, persistent pulmonary hypertension of the neonate, or a congenital heart defect.	2
F. Adult medical or surgical Examples of possible scenarios could include, but are not limited to, head, neck, or thoracic surgery; obesity-hypoventilation syndrome, pneumonia, sleep apnea, pulmonary hypertension, and acquired immune deficiency syndrome (AIDS).	4
Total tested scenarios	20
Pretested problems*	2
Total of all scenarios taken	22

Note: The two pretested scenarios included on the website for this text will be in categories A1 and A2. They will be scored the same as the other scenarios to provide you with useful feedback.

*Pretested problems are being evaluated for validity for inclusion in later versions of the Clinical Simulation Examination. They do not count toward the actual final score of the exam. There is no way to differentiate between actual scored scenarios and pretested scenarios and all must be completed to finish the exam.

**COPD, chronic obstructive pulmonary disease

- The exam taker is allowed 4 hours to complete the exam, which works out to about 11 minutes per problem. (The previous version of the CSE had 10 tested and 1 pretested scenarios to complete in 4 hours. These older scenarios were about twice as long as the newer scenarios.)
- The clinical simulation scenarios have between four and six correct steps on the ideal path. If an alternate path is taken, there will be more than four to six steps.

There are three components to the clinical simulation problem: (1) the scenario, (2) the information gathering (IG) sections, and (3) the decision-making (DM) sections. Each is discussed in turn.

Scenario

The scenario establishes the setting for the patient, and for you, as the respiratory therapist. Typically, it includes the setting such as home or hospital, where the patient is within the hospital, and the time of day. General information about the patient, such as name, age, and sex; some general presenting conditions; and a brief history of the illness or event are given. Your role as a respiratory therapist is described. You will have to either initially gather more information or make a clinical decision. Determine if the situation is an emergency. If it is, you will have to take immediate steps to help the patient. (The exam taker should assume that any and all services needed to give optimal care are available in any of the patient scenarios.)

Information gathering (IG) sections

Usually, the respiratory therapist is first directed to an IG section to find out more about the patient. There is a list of about 15 parameters from which to choose. These could include, for example, vital signs, blood gases, pulmonary function tests, and various laboratory studies. You will be instructed to select as many as you believe are important based on what you know at that point in time. Obviously, you should not select information that is unnecessarily risky or irrelevant or that delays important care. Select the desired information. The computer screen will then reveal the data. Interpret the data to make the proper decisions in the next section. When you have finished gathering and interpreting the data, you will be directed to go to a decision making (DM) section. Usually there are about two IG steps in each clinical simulation problem.

Decision making (DM) sections

After the selected patient data are analyzed, the test taker is directed to a DM section. It is now required that you make a decision on the best care for the patient based on the information that you have at this point in time. Usually you are instructed to "choose only one" from about four or five options. One of the choices is best, one or two others may be acceptable, and the others are not acceptable. Select the option and the computer will reveal the answer. Usually, it will say "Physician agrees. Done" or something to that effect. One or more of the available answers will reveal "Physician disagrees. Make another selection in this section" when it is exposed. This may or may not mean that a bad choice was made. It is possible that the author of the scenario simply does not want to follow that particular course of action. Proceed to select another option.

Occasionally, you will be directed to "select as many as indicated" for the situation with which you are dealing. This involves a scenario in which proper care includes several procedures being done simultaneously with a patient. Again, select the options, and the computer will reveal the answer.

When your DM is finished, you will be taken to the next step in the scenario. Often this includes an update on the patient's condition with the need for more DM. At some point, the next step will involve another IG section. You will now need to evaluate how the patient responded to your earlier decision(s). This pattern of DM and IG repeats itself until the scenario is ended. Typically, there are about four decision-making steps in each clinical simulation scenario. When these have been completed, you will go on to the next scenario until all 22 have been completed. See Table 3 for how this unique examination is scored.

Scoring of the clinical simulation problem and examination

All of the selected options are scored as shown in Table 3. Each option's score is based on how appropriate it is to the condition of the patient at the time it was selected.

Exam scoring

Each of the 20 actual scenarios and the 2 pretested scenarios are individually scored for IG and DM based on the judgment of the NBRC examination committee. The scores in these two areas on all 20 actual scenarios are

TABLE 3	Clinical Simulation Scoring
Score	**Score Rationale**
+3	Critically important for good patient care. It is necessary for prompt, proper care. Omitting it would result in the patient being seriously harmed from delays in care, pain, cost, and increased chance of morbidity and/or mortality.
+2	Very important for good patient care.
+1	Helpful for good patient care.
0	Neither helpful nor harmful to patient care.
−1	Somewhat counterproductive to good patient care.
−2	Quite counterproductive to good patient care.
−3	Extremely counterproductive to good patient care. Detrimental to prompt, proper care. Its inclusion will result in the patient being seriously harmed from delays in care, pain, cost, and increased chance of morbidity and/or mortality.

then totaled for a final score. The examination committee determines the minimum passing level (MLP, also called "cut score") for each clinical simulation test form. The general guidelines used by the NBRC for constructing a CSE and scoring its MLP are as follows:

1. More than half of the points on a test form will come from IG sections.
2. DM cut score range is 60%-70%. An average difficulty test form DM cut score would be 65%.
3. IG cut score range is 77%-81%. An average difficulty test form IG cut score would be 79%.

Even though each clinical simulation test form will be different, all will be similar in content and difficulty and scored using these guidelines. For example, an average difficulty test form would have an MLP of about 72% of the total points (65% + 79% = 144%; 144% ÷ 2 = 72%).

As stated above, the NBRC will add the exam taker's DM and IG points for a final score. If the exam taker's final score meets the MLP, the exam will have been passed. The NBRC will also provide the exam taker with the earned DM points and MLP for DM, and the earned IG points and MLP for IG. This is provided for learning purposes to help the exam taker evaluate strengths and weaknesses.

Note to Users of This Book's Clinical Simulations: The NBRC's above-stated scoring principles will be applied to each of the 22 clinical simulations when taken individually and to the whole group when the user takes the Clinical Simulation Practice Examination. An MLP of 72% will be applied for each individual clinical simulation and for the Clinical Simulation Practice Examination.

Suggestions for preparing for the clinical simulation examination

Things you should do:

1. Carefully follow all directions. If instructed to make only one choice, make only one.

2. Read the scenario carefully to understand the patient's situation and what you are required to do. Is this an emergency? If it is, you will want to gather only the most vital information needed to make a patient care decision. Quick action will be required to decide on the best care to give. If it is not an emergency, more complete IG is called for. Then a more well-considered decision for patient care can be made.

3. Know the rules for the initiation and changing of mechanical ventilation parameters. In general, the initial tidal volume setting should be about 7 mL/kg of ideal body weight. As discussed in Chapter 15, there may be clinical circumstances when a smaller tidal volume is justified. Make adjustments from there based on arterial blood gas results.

4. Thoroughly read all options. For IG sections, it may be helpful to make a list of each desirable option on your paper before making your choices. Choose all the options that will give you important information. You will be penalized for skipping over important data and also for making dangerous or wasteful choices. When you are sure of your selections, reveal them all and then review and interpret them. Avoid the temptation to reveal and interpret one piece of data at a time. You may mistakenly decide to not gather some important information later.

5. Try to visualize yourself in the real situation as described. Do what you would do on the job. Make the best choice(s) that you can based on what you know at this point. This is true for both IG and DM sections. It may be necessary to go back over past information or choices.

6. It may be helpful to make a map on your paper of where you have been for each of the 22 problems. This will help you keep track of past choices. However, the software allows you to go back in the scenario history to review previous selections.

7. Pace yourself to get through all 22 problems in the 4-hour time limit. That gives you about 11 minutes per scenario. For example, you should be finishing your fifth problem after 1 hour. Unlike the TMC Examination, you should not rush ahead at the end and pick just anything. You *will* be penalized for incorrect choices.

8. Take a practice Clinical Simulation Examination. Twenty-two practice patient simulations are offered on the Evolve website (http://evolve.elsevier.com/Sills/respiratorycare/). Others are available from the NBRC at www.NRBC.org.

Things you should avoid:

1. Do not try to jump ahead in the scenario or try to guess what the author is leading to. With the branching logic format, there are alternate pathways. Work only with what you know now and from the past.

2. Try not to become flustered if you are faced with a scenario you have never experienced at work. Imagine what you would do if faced with this problem and go from there. Also, do not become frustrated if the choice that you prefer is not available. There may be more than one way to take care of a patient's problems. Make your next best choice and move on.

3. Do not make changes in patient care unless they are needed. If a patient is stable with acceptable arterial blood gas values and vital signs, be content to leave the patient as he or she is.

4. Do not get flustered by patient complications or equipment problems. They do not necessarily mean that you did anything wrong! They are meant to test your ability to solve problems.

5. Do not select everything in the IG sections. You will lose points by choosing unimportant, time-consuming, unnecessarily expensive, or dangerous procedures.

6. Avoid selecting new or unusual procedures that you are not familiar with—high-frequency jet ventilation, for example. You will lower your score if you do not know how to operate the equipment properly.

7. Do not misinterpret the data you are given. Avoid assumptions about things that are not spelled out for you.

SUMMARY—GENERAL SUGGESTIONS

1. Take the NBRC's free TMC Examination and CSE and the practice tests available online with this text. Evaluate your results to find your strengths and weaknesses.

2. Begin studying about 2 months before the exam. Pace yourself so that everything can be covered in the time that you have. Avoid "cramming" a few days before the examination; these tests demand more than the simple recall of facts.

3. Study the most important and heavily tested areas first (see Tables 1 and 2). Spend any remaining time studying less heavily tested topics or disease conditions.

4. Focus on the areas where you are weakest, especially if they are heavily tested.

5. If it is necessary to travel out of your hometown to take the exam, arrive at the city where the test will be given the evening before the exam. Make a practice drive from your motel to the test site and determine where you will park. Check the time required to get there and add more for traffic congestion.

6. Have a good dinner. Avoid alcohol, even if you are nervous, to keep a clear head in the morning.

7. Do not "cram" for the exam back at the motel. Unfortunately, if you are not prepared by now, a few more hours will not really help. If necessary, brush up on only a few test areas.

8. Set the alarm to get you up in plenty of time to be ready. Get a good night's sleep. Avoid sleeping pills.

9. Eat a good meal before the exam. Minimize caffeine. You will have plenty of adrenaline running through your system to keep you awake while taking the test!

10. You must be on time for your scheduled exam. Bring your scheduling information and a photo ID such as a driver's license to prove who you are.
11. Attempt to relax with the self-confidence that comes from knowing that you are well prepared.

IMPORTANT ADDRESSES AND PHONE NUMBERS

For information on applying for an exam, scheduling an exam date and location (linking to Applied Measurement Professionals), exam processes, taking free practice exams, purchasing other practice exams, and getting a copy of the exam detailed content outlines, contact:

National Board for Respiratory Care
18000 W. 105th Street
Olanthe, Kansas 66061-7543
Toll free: 888-341-4811
Telephone: (913) 895-4900
Fax: (913) 895-4650
Internet address: http://www.nbrc.org

For information on exam sites and to schedule an exam, purchasing practice exams, and getting a copy of exam content outlines, contact:

Applied Measurement Professionals
18000 W. 105th Street
Olanthe, Kansas 66061-7543
Telephone: (913) 895-4600
Fax: (913) 895-4650
Internet address: http://www.goamp.com

For information on accredited respiratory care educational programs, contact:

Commission on Accreditation for Respiratory Care
1248 Harwood Road
Bedford, Texas 76021-4244
Telephone: (817) 283-2835
Fax: (817) 354-8519
Internet address: http://www.coarc.com

For information on professional activities and resources, including Clinical Practice Guidelines, and links to state societies, contact:

American Association for Respiratory Care
9425 N. MacArthur Boulevard
Suite 100
Irving, Texas 75063-4706
Telephone: (972) 243-AARC (2272)
Fax: (972) 484-2720
E-mail: info@aarc.org
Internet address: http://www.aarc.org

Contents

1 Patient Assessment

Note: It can be anticipated that the Therapist Multiple-Choice Examination (TMC) will include an *average of 12 of 140 actual questions* (9% of the exam) on patient assessment. (This is based on the question mix typically found on the National Board of Respiratory Care's (NBRC's) previous Entry Level Examinations and Written Registry Examinations.)

Remember that the TMC version you take will include 20 additional questions being evaluated for possible inclusion in other versions of the TMC. So, there will be a total of 160 questions taken. There is no way to differentiate between the 140 actual questions and the 20 questions being evaluated for future use. Please go to the Introduction for detailed information on the Therapist Multiple-Choice Examination and the Clinical Simulation Examination.

MODULE A

Evaluate data in the patient record.

Note: The following discussion involves noninvasive, bedside activities that apply to adults in most respiratory care settings. Some assessment items have been placed in later chapters, because they are procedure specific. Topics that relate to neonates and children are included in Module H.

1. Review the patient's history: history, admission data, progress notes, diagnosis, respiratory care orders, medication history, do not resuscitate (DNR) status and advance directives, and social history (code: IA1) [difficulty: R, Ap]

a. Patient history

Review the complete initial patient history and note the following:

1. Date of history taking
2. Patient data: name, age, gender, race, and occupation
3. Primary complaints
4. Secondary complaints
5. Present illness history and symptoms
6. Family history
7. Medical history of cardiopulmonary disease(s), including smoking history, cough, sputum production, allergies, and activities of daily living
8. Review of body systems

It is important that the respiratory therapist obtain a *brief* history before beginning therapeutic procedures. Determine how the patient has been doing since the last treatment. Has there been a change in dyspnea, cough and secretions, chest pain, and so on? This will help guide therapy as effectively as possible.

b. Admission data

The attending physician writes up his or her key findings and how they are related to the reason the patient was admitted to the hospital.

c. Progress notes

Review the physician's, nurse's, and respiratory therapist's patient progress notes before seeing the patient and beginning the therapeutic procedure. Look for any cardiopulmonary or other organ-system changes that will have an impact on the patient's ability to take the treatment. You may need to revise the therapy, get different equipment, or seek help. Check for new patient care orders if the physician notes a change in the patient's care plan.

d. Diagnosis

After the medical history, physical exam, and laboratory tests are completed, the patient will be placed into one of the following four diagnostic categories. Refer to Table 1-1 for examples of each category:
- Crisis/acute onset of illness
- Intermittent but repeated illness
- Progressive worsening
- Mixed patterns/multiple problems

e. Current respiratory care orders

Physician orders must have the patient's name, the date, the time, complete and proper orders for each therapeutic procedure, and the physician's signature. Verbal orders from the physician to the nurse or respiratory therapist must follow hospital guidelines and include the preceding information. Incomplete, improper, or questionable orders must be confirmed by calling the physician for clarification or correction.

f. Medication history

Note the respiratory medications that the patient is currently taking. In addition, note any medications used to help manage cardiovascular, renal, or neurological problems that may also affect the patient's respiratory status.

TABLE 1-1	Patient Illness Categories
Category	**Examples**
Crisis/acute onset of illness	Trauma, myocardial infarction, allergic reaction, aspiration of a foreign body, pneumothorax, pulmonary embolism, and some pneumonias
Intermittent but repeated illness	Asthma, chronic bronchitis, congestive heart failure, angina pectoris, myasthenia gravis, and some pneumonias
Progressive worsening	Congestive heart failure, chronic bronchitis, emphysema, and upper respiratory tract infection leading to bronchitis or pneumonia
Mixed patterns/ multiple problems	Chronic obstructive pulmonary disease and cystic fibrosis complicated by multiple problems, mucous plugging, or infection; mix of congestive heart failure and chronic lung disease; mix of neuromuscular and lung disease; mix of renal failure and congestive heart failure with chronic lung disease

g. DNR status and advance directives

The physician, patient, and family should determine the patient's cardiopulmonary resuscitation status. A patient with a terminal condition, such as end-stage chronic obstructive pulmonary disease (COPD), often will choose not to be resuscitated. If it has been determined that the patient does not want to be resuscitated, his or her DNR status should be clearly posted in the electronic medical record, in the patient's room, and on a wrist bracelet. All members of the health care team should be aware of the patient's decision.

An advance directive is an advance declaration by a patient regarding the type and level of care to be provided. This is a particularly important document for a patient who is so hopelessly and terminally ill that he or she does not wish to be connected to life-support equipment. This statement could preclude the use of a mechanical ventilator, kidney dialysis equipment, cardiac pacemaker, or other means of artificially prolonging life. The advance directive also can declare that the patient does not want to be resuscitated if a cardiac arrest should occur. This is commonly called a *do not resuscitate (DNR) order*, and it should be clearly noted in the electronic medical record. The advance directive legal document should be part of the patient's medical record. The document may also be known as a *living will* in some states. A related legal document is the Durable Power of Attorney for Health Care. This document assigns another person, such as a relative or close friend, the right to make medical decisions when the patient is unable to do so. This can include stopping or withdrawal of medical treatment and the DNR order. Always be sensitive to a patient's feelings about such a personal and difficult decision. The patient's emotional state

may very well determine his or her readiness for an advance directive. A related issue is the patient's ability to cooperate based on his or her emotional and physical condition.

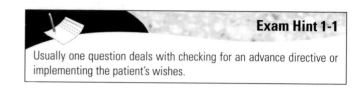

Exam Hint 1-1

Usually one question deals with checking for an advance directive or implementing the patient's wishes.

h. Social history

Social history can involve many aspects of a patient's life. Your ability to assess the patient and provide needed care can be influenced positively or negatively by the patient's and your social backgrounds. Review the patient's record for information on the following:

Language. What language does the patient and family speak? If the patient does not speak English, a medical translator will be needed to continue with an interview or to provide medical care.

Ethnicity/culture. What is the patient's ethnic heritage? Are there any cultural practices that would present a barrier to the patient's needed medical care?

Home environment and family members. Does the patient have strong or weak family connections? Is there a stable home environment?

Education. What is the patient's education level? Any medical education materials must be suited to the patient's ability to understand them.

Economic status. What is the patient's economic/socioeconomic status? Is the patient receiving state or federal assistance for food, medicine, and medical care? Is the patient homeless?

Disability. Does the patient have a mental disability, illness, or condition that would require an accommodation for care? Does the patient have a physical disability or limitation that would require an accommodation for care?

2. Review the results of the physical examination related to the cardiopulmonary system (code: IA2) [difficulty: R, Ap]

Review the results of the physical examinations performed by physicians, physician assistants, nurses, and respiratory therapists. Review the following organ systems:

- Pulmonary
- Cardiovascular
- Neuromuscular/neurological
- Renal

3. Evaluate data in the patient's record for trends in vital signs (code: IA13b) [difficulty: R, Ap]

a. Current vital signs

Review the current vital signs in the patient's chart. Compare them with the admission vital signs and what you observe in the patient now. Look for a change in pattern that suggests either worsening or improvement in the patient.

b. Temperature

The textbook "normal" oral body temperature is 98.6° F (37° C). However, some range from 96.5° F-99.5° F (35.8-37.4° C) is normal. Make sure the patient has not eaten any hot or cold foods recently and has not been smoking before taking an oral temperature.

A rectal or core temperature is commonly taken in very sick patients, because it is more accurate and reliable. The normal rectal temperature is 97.5-100.4° F (36.4-38° C). Some variance is normal, but less so than with oral temperatures. Axillary temperatures are used as a last resort in stable adult patients. These run 1° F lower than oral temperatures and are less accurate and reliable.

The variations in temperature noted depend on the time of day, activity level, and, in women, stage of the menstrual cycle. For example, a lower body temperature is normal when a person is in a deep sleep. An oral temperature higher than 99.4° F (37.4° C) in a patient with a history of respiratory disease indicates a fever. Typically, it can be caused by atelectasis or a pulmonary or systemic infection. Patients commonly are treated to keep their temperature below 103° F, if possible. In general, a rectal temperature below 97° F (36° C) is considered hypothermic. In some procedures, such as open-heart surgery, a patient's temperature is lowered to reduce metabolism and oxygen needs. The rectal temperature must be kept above 90° F (32° C) to prevent cardiac dysrhythmias caused by the cold.

c. Respiratory rate

The respiratory rate (*f* for frequency) is the number of breaths the patient takes in 1 minute. The number is counted by looking at or feeling the chest or abdominal movements, or both. The normal rate varies with age (Table 1-2). It is assumed that the patient is resting but awake and has a normal temperature and metabolic rate. A respiratory rate above or below normal is cause for alarm.

Hyperthermia (fever), acidosis, hypoxemia, fear, anxiety, and pain cause a patient to breathe more rapidly. Hypothermia, alkalosis, and hyperoxia in a patient breathing on hypoxic drive, sedation, and coma cause a patient to breathe more slowly.

Remember that even in healthy people, considerable variation is found in the respiratory rate. It is best to consider the respiratory rate and the patient's tidal volume and minute volume to get a more complete impression of how the patient is breathing. Carefully measure the respiratory rate of any patient with cardiopulmonary disease or with a respiratory rate outside the normal range. The rate should be checked as often as needed to monitor the patient's condition.

TABLE 1-2	Normal Resting Respiratory Rates	
Age (Years)	**Male**	**Female**
0	31 ± 8	30 ± 6
1-2	26 ± 4	27 ± 4
2-4	25 ± 4	25 ± 3
5-7	22 ± 2	21 ± 2
8-11	19 ± 2	19 ± 2
12-14	19 ± 2	18 ± 2
15-16	17 ± 3	18 ± 3
17-18	16 ± 3	17 ± 3
Older	16 ± 3	17 ± 3

Modified from Eubanks DH, Bone RC: Comprehensive respiratory care, ed 2, St Louis, 1990, Mosby.

d. Blood pressure

The blood pressure (BP) is the result of the pumping ability of the left ventricle (made up of the heart rate and stroke volume), arterial resistance, and blood volume. Normal BP results when all three factors are in balance with one another. If one factor is abnormal, the other two have some ability to compensate. For example, if the patient has lost a lot of blood, the body attempts to maintain BP by increasing both arterial resistance and the heart rate.

Normal Blood Pressures

- Adults: lower than 120/80 mm Hg
- Infants and children younger than 10 years of age: 60-100/20-70 mm Hg

As with the other vital signs, some variation in BP is noted among individuals. It is important to know the patient's normal BP to compare it with the current value. Carefully measure the BP in any patient who has cardiopulmonary disease or a history of hypotension or hypertension.

Hypotension in the adult is a systolic BP of less than 90 mm Hg. Recommend a BP measurement for any patient who has a history of hypotension, appears to be in shock, has lost a lot of blood, has a weak pulse, shows mental confusion, is unconscious, or has low urine output.

Hypertension in the adult is a systolic BP of 140 mm Hg or greater or a diastolic BP of 90 mm Hg or greater, or both. Carefully measure the BP of any patient with a history of hypertension, bounding pulse, or symptoms of a stroke (mental confusion, headache, and sudden weakness or partial paralysis). Fear, anxiety, and pain also cause the patient's BP to increase temporarily.

e. Heart/pulse rate

The heart/pulse rate (HR) is the number of heartbeats per minute. It can be counted by listening to the heart tones with a stethoscope or by feeling any of the common sites where an artery is easy to locate. Table 1-3 shows the normal pulse rates based on age. It is assumed that the patient is alert but resting when the pulse is counted. Carefully measure the heart/pulse rate in any patient with cardiopulmonary disease or any of the aforementioned conditions for hypotension or hypertension.

4. Serum electrolytes and other blood chemistries

a. Evaluate data in the patient record (code: IA4) [difficulty: R, Ap]

See below.

b. Recommend a serum electrolyte blood test (code: IE2) [difficulty: R, Ap, An]

The serum (blood) electrolytes are measured in most patients when they are admitted to the hospital and as needed thereafter. This is to determine whether the values are within the normal ranges listed in Table 1-4. Diet and a number of medications can affect the various electrolytes.

1. Potassium (K+)

Potassium is the most important electrolyte to monitor because of its effect on general nerve function and cardiac function. Hyperkalemia is a high blood level of potassium. It causes the following electrocardiographic changes: high, peaked T waves and depressed ST segments; widening QRS complex; and bradycardia. Hypokalemia is a low blood level of potassium. It causes the following electrocardiographic changes: flat or inverted T waves, depression of the ST segments, premature ventricular contractions, and ventricular fibrillation (if severe enough). Chapter 11 offers a more complete discussion of electrocardiogram (ECG) interpretation.

Exam Hint 1-2

Hypokalemia can be caused by the use of diuretic medications such as furosemide (Lasix). Signs of hypokalemia include the cardiac rhythm disturbances noted previously and muscle weakness. In addition, a metabolic alkalosis is found when the results of an arterial blood gas analysis are interpreted. Be prepared to recommend the administration of potassium if the serum level is low.

2. Chloride (Cl−)

Hyperchloremia is a high blood level of chloride, which causes significant prolongation of the ST segment and the QT interval on the ECG. Hypochloremia is a low blood level of chloride, which shortens the QT interval and perhaps widens and rounds off the T waves on the ECG.

3. Sodium (Na+)

Hypernatremia is a high blood level of sodium. It might be seen in a patient who is dehydrated or who has lost many gastrointestinal secretions because of vomiting,

TABLE 1-3	Normal Pulse Rates According to Age
Age	**Beats/min**
Birth	70-170
Neonate	120-140
1 year	80-140
2 years	80-130
3 years	80-120
4 years	70-115
Adult	60-100

From Eubanks DH, Bone RC: Comprehensive respiratory care, ed 2, St Louis, 1990, Mosby.

nasogastric tube drainage, or diarrhea. Hyponatremia is a low blood sodium level, which might be seen in a patient who is fluid-overloaded.

4. Bicarbonate (HCO3−)

Altered bicarbonate levels are commonly seen in patients with pulmonary conditions. The kidneys of patients with a chronically elevated arterial partial pressure of carbon dioxide ($PaCO_2$) typically retain bicarbonate to moderate the respiratory acidosis caused by the elevated carbon dioxide level. Conversely, the kidneys of patients with a chronically decreased $PaCO_2$ level excrete bicarbonate to moderate the respiratory alkalosis caused by the decreased $PaCO_2$ level.

5. Calcium (Ca++)

Hypercalcemia is an elevated calcium level, which may be associated with patients taking diuretics. Electrocardiographic changes associated with an increased calcium level include a shortened QT interval and widened, rounded T waves. Hypocalcemia is a decreased calcium level. It causes electrocardiographic changes such as lengthening of the ST segment and the QT interval.

6. Glucose

The blood glucose level is important to monitor, because it directly relates to how much glucose is available to the patient for energy for daily activities. The normal values are listed in Table 1-4. Hypoglycemia is a low blood level of glucose; it can mean that the patient is malnourished. Hyperglycemia is a high blood level of glucose; this may indicate that the patient has diabetes mellitus or Cushing's disease or is being treated with corticosteroids. More specific testing must be done to prove the diagnosis.

5. Recommend the adjustment of electrolyte therapy (code: IIIE2d) [difficulty: R, Ap]

Any abnormality should be promptly corrected so that the patient's nervous system, muscle function, and cellular processes can be optimized. Most abnormalities can be corrected by dietary adjustments or, if necessary, by oral or intravenous supplementation.

TABLE 1-4	Normal Serum Electrolyte and Glucose Levels
Normal Electrolyte Values*	
Chloride (Cl⁻)	95-106 mEq/L
Potassium (K⁺)	3.5-5.5 mEq/L
Sodium (Na⁺)	135-145 mEq/L
Calcium (Ca⁺⁺)	4.5-5.5 mEq/L
Bicarbonate (HCO₃⁻)	22-25 mEq/L
Normal Glucose Values*	
Serum or plasma	70-110 mg/100 mL (dL)
Whole blood	60-100 mg/100 mL (dL)

*These values may vary somewhat among references.

TABLE 1-5	Normal Hemoglobin, Hematocrit, and Red Blood Cell Counts for Adults and Children*		
Gender	**Adult**	**Infant**	**Child**
Hemoglobin (g/100 mL [g/dL])			
Female	12.0-16.0	12.2-20.0	11.2-13.4
Male	13.5-18.0	Same	Same
Hematocrit (mL/100 mL [mL/dL])			
Female	38%-47%		
Male	40%-54%		
Red Blood Cell Count (in millions/mL)			
Female	4.2-5.4	5.0-5.1	4.6-4.8
Male	4.6-6.2	Same	Same

*These values may vary somewhat among references.

6. Evaluate laboratory results of cardiac enzymes (code: IA4) [difficulty: R, Ap]

A panel of cardiac enzyme studies may be ordered to help differentiate between lung and heart problems in a patient with a chief complaint of dyspnea. These are the main cardiac enzymes:

a. Creatine kinase MB (CK-MB). This value will increase 4-6 hours after a myocardial infarction. See Chapter 11 for more details.

b. Troponin I (cTnI) and troponin T (cTnT). These values will increase 2-4 hours after a myocardial infarction. See Chapter 11 for more details.

c. Brain natriuretic peptide (B-type natriuretic peptide, BNP). An elevated value will be seen in a patient with congestive heart failure. A value of ≥300 pg/mL indicates mild heart failure. A value of ≥600 pg/mL indicates moderate heart failure. A value of ≥900 pg/mL indicates severe heart failure.

d. C-reactive protein (CRP). This is a nonspecific marker of inflammation that has been linked to an increased risk for myocardial infarction, stroke, and peripheral vascular disease. An increased CRP of >1 mg/dL correlates with the peak CK-MB value but occurs 1-3 days later.

High levels of the cardiac enzymes point to a cardiac problem such as a myocardial infarction or congestive heart failure. Cardiac enzyme values should be monitored to rule out a heart problem. If the cardiac enzymes are normal, look for a pulmonary cause behind the patient's dyspnea.

7. Complete blood count

a. Evaluate data in the patient record (code: IA4) [difficulty: R, Ap]

See below.

b. Recommend a complete blood count test (code: IE2) [difficulty: R, Ap, An]

A complete blood count is routinely done for all hospitalized patients, as well as for patients seen for a variety of illnesses and for routine physical examinations. The red blood cell (RBC, or erythrocyte) count, white blood cell (WBC, or leukocyte) count, and differential provide a great deal of information about the hematologic system and many other organ systems.

The key normal values for the RBC count are listed in Table 1-5. The hemoglobin and hematocrit values also are important, because they directly relate to the patient's oxygen-carrying capacity. Decreased hemoglobin and hematocrit values indicate that the patient is anemic. An anemic patient has less oxygen-carrying capacity, and as a result, more stress is placed on the heart. Hypoxemia resulting from a cardiopulmonary abnormality places this patient at great risk. A transfusion is indicated if the hematocrit is below the level the physician considers clinically safe.

An increased number of circulating erythrocytes indicates that the patient has polycythemia. When this is seen as a response to chronic hypoxemia from COPD, cyanotic congenital heart disease, or another disorder, it is labeled *secondary* polycythemia. This patient is at added risk because the thickened blood causes an increased afterload against which the heart must pump. These patients also are more prone to blood clots. With supplemental oxygen or other clinical treatment to increase the arterial partial pressure of oxygen (PaO₂) to at least 55-60 torr, the erythrocyte and hematocrit levels, over time, return to normal.

The key normal leukocyte count and differential are listed in Table 1-6. A normal leukocyte count and a normal differential reveal two things about the patient. First, no active bacterial infection is present. Second, the patient's body is able to produce the normal number and variety of WBCs to combat an infection.

A mild to moderate increase in the leukocyte count is called *leukocytosis*. It is seen as a WBC count of 11,000-17,000 per cubic millimeter (mm³). Usually, the higher the

TABLE 1-6	White Blood Cell and Differential Counts*
White Blood Cell Count (mm³)	
Adult	4500-11,000
Infant and child	9000-33,000
Differential Count	
Segmented neutrophil	40%
Lymphocytes	20%
Monocytes	2%
Eosinophils	0%
Bands	0%
Basophils	0%

*These values may vary somewhat among references.

TABLE 1-7	Normal Coagulation Study Results		
Test Name	**Normal Value**	**Critical Value**
Bleeding time	1-9 minutes	>15 minutes
Prothrombin time	11.0-12.5 seconds; 85%-100%	>20 seconds
Partial thromboplastin time	60-70 seconds	>100 seconds
Activated partial thromboplastin time	30-40 seconds	>70 seconds

count, the more severe the infection. A WBC count above 17,000/mm³ is seen in patients with severe sepsis, miliary tuberculosis, and other overwhelming infections. When a patient has an acute, severe bacterial infection, the WBC differential count shows an increased number of neutrophils. Exceptions to this are patients who are elderly, those who have acquired immunodeficiency syndrome, and those with other immunodeficiencies. These patients may have an infection but show only a mildly elevated WBC count.

Leukopenia is a low absolute WBC count of 3000-5000/mm³ or less. An acute viral infection can cause a mild to moderate decrease in the neutrophil count. A patient with a low WBC count is at great risk of bacterial or other infections.

8. Evaluate coagulation study results in the patient record (code: IA4) [difficulty: R, Ap]

Coagulation studies are routinely done for many hospitalized patients, for those who are to have surgery, and for those who have or are suspected of having a blood-clotting disorder. Also, many medications speed or slow clotting time (so-called blood thinners). It is important to review a patient's coagulation studies before drawing a blood sample or performing a procedure that may lead to bleeding. Table 1-7 lists normal coagulation study results. If the patient's clotting time is increased, the individual is at risk of bleeding. Be prepared to apply pressure to a blood sampling site (especially and arterial one) longer than expected.

9. Sputum gram stain

a. Recommend a sputum gram stain (code: IE6) [difficulty: R, Ap, An]

Whenever bronchitis or pneumonia is suspected, it is important to obtain a mucus or sputum sample for evaluation. A sample of mucus suctioned from the lungs should show only pulmonary organisms. Sputum is the mixture of mucus from the lungs and saliva from the mouth; therefore the organisms found in it may have come from either place. Recommend a Gram stain of the mucus or sputum as a quick way to initially classify any bacterial organisms.

b. Evaluate sputum gram stain results in the patient record (code: IA4) [difficulty: R, Ap]

The first step in the microbial analysis of sputum, mucus, or other body fluids or tissues is a Gram stain. Gram staining is a special process for colorizing bacteria that divides them into two groups. Gram-positive (g+) bacteria are stained violet. These are the most common types of bacteria that cause bronchitis and pneumonia. In general, penicillin or related drugs and sulfa-type antibiotics kill gram-positive bacteria. Gram-negative (g−) bacteria are stained pink. These organisms, unfortunately, are found in many of the sickest and weakest patients. Often the only way to kill gram-negative bacteria is with a specific antibiotic to which they have been proven sensitive. So-called broad-spectrum antibiotics, such as tetracycline, also may be used.

Gram staining cannot be used to identify *Mycobacterium tuberculosis* (TB) bacteria. Instead, another stain, such as the Ziehl–Neelsen stain, must be used. This is an *acid-fast* stain, and it gives the TB bacteria a red coloration. Other pathogens, such as viruses, protozoa, and fungi, cannot be identified by Gram staining. Protozoa and fungi must be identified with specialized stains. Fungi and *M tuberculosis* may take 6-8 weeks to culture.

10. Culture and sensitivity test

a. Recommend a culture and sensitivity test (code: IE6) [difficulty: R, Ap, An]

If an infection is suspected, a sample of sputum, mucus, blood, fluid, or tissue should be obtained. After Gram staining has been performed on the sample, a culture and sensitivity (C&S) study should be performed. Culturing involves actively growing any organisms to determine what they are. In a sensitivity test, the cultured organism is exposed to a variety of antimicrobial drugs.

TABLE 1-8 Normal Urinalysis Results	
Test Item	**Normal Value**
Appearance	Clear
Color	Amber yellow
pH	4.6-8.0 (average 6.0)
Specific gravity	Adult: 1.005-1.030 (usually 1.010-1.025)
	Newborn: 1.001-1.020
White blood cells	0-4
Red blood cells	0-2

b. Evaluate culture and sensitivity results in the patient record (code: IA4) [difficulty: R, Ap]

The goal of a C&S study is to determine which drug or drugs kill the pathogen most effectively. The patient then is treated with that antibiotic. It may take 1-3 days to get the C&S results back.

11. Evaluate fluid balance trends in the patient record (code: IA13a) [difficulty: R, Ap]

Fluid intake and output should be approximately equal in a normal person with a properly functioning heart and kidneys. Fluid intake includes liquids that the patient drinks or is given by nasogastric tube and intravenous fluids. Output includes urine output and fluid loss from vomiting, the nasogastric tube, or diarrhea.

To help evaluate kidney function, a urine sample routinely is taken from every patient admitted to the hospital and from pregnant women and presurgical patients. Much information about the functioning of the kidneys and other metabolic processes can be gathered from the urinalysis results. A urinalysis also is done for diagnostic purposes in patients with suspicious abdominal or back pain, hematuria, and chronic renal disease. Table 1-8 lists the normal findings for a urinalysis. Any abnormal findings should be further investigated to discover the cause.

12. Fluid balance

a. Evaluate data on trends in fluid balance (intake and output) (code: IA13a) [difficulty: R, Ap]

Intake and output usually are measured over each 8-hour shift. Insensible water loss through perspiration and breathing usually is ignored in adults, because the amount lost is relatively small and can only be estimated. Insensible water loss can be a risk in the low-birth-weight infant. Prevent this by keeping the infant's environmental temperature within 1° C of the body temperature (neutral thermal environment). Supplemental oxygen should be humidified.

Intake and output should be monitored closely in any patient who has a history of heart or kidney problems or who has a current serious cardiopulmonary disorder. Do this by adding all the patient's intake (e.g., oral, intravenous) and output (e.g., urine, blood work) for each 8-hour

BOX 1-1 Fluid Intake and Urine Output for Normal Adults
Normal, minimal daily water requirement for an adult patient is ~1500-2000 mL
Average urine output is 0.5-1.0 mL/kg/h
Polyuria is a urine output of >1500 mL/h
Oliguria is a urine output of <400 mL in 24 hours
Anuria is a urine output of <100 mL in 24 hours

shift. Box 1-1 shows the normal adult values for fluid intake and urine output; see Table 1-8 for the normal values for urine specific gravity and other urinalysis information.

b. Recommend an adjustment in patient's fluid balance (code: III2c) [difficulty: R, Ap]

The dehydrated patient will probably show some or all of the following signs and symptoms: tachycardia, hypotension, high urine specific gravity, oliguria (low urine output), low central venous pressure (CVP) and pulmonary capillary wedge pressure (PCWP), tenting of the skin when pinched, slow capillary refill, and mental confusion. This patient needs more fluid.

Often a patient with heart or kidney failure has a decreased output compared with input. This can lead to fluid overload problems, with peripheral or pulmonary edema and heart failure. The patient will probably show some or all of the following signs and symptoms: tachycardia, hypertension, low urine specific gravity, increased urine output, increased CVP and PCWP, peripheral edema in the dependent parts of the body, and pulmonary edema with breath sounds revealing crackles/rales. This patient needs to be fluid restricted and sodium restricted. If a patient is given a diuretic medication, the urine output can greatly increase to exceed the intake. Remember that the loss of 1 L of fluid results in the patient losing 1 kg (2.2 lb) of weight.

13. Evaluate intracranial pressure trends in the patient record (code: IA13a) [difficulty: R, Ap]

Intracranial pressure (ICP) is the pressure within the cranium (skull) and is normally <10 mm Hg. A person with a brain tumor or who has suffered a blow to the head resulting in cerebral edema will have an increased ICP. If a person's ICP is >20 mm Hg, the clinical outcome will significantly worsen. See Chapter 15 for more information including the use of hyperventilation.

MODULE B

Radiographic imaging

Note: It is beyond the scope of this text to cover all the features of normal radiographic images. Review standard textbooks for this as needed. This discussion is limited to items listed as testable by the NBRC.

1. Review imaging study results (code: IA9) [difficulty: R, Ap]

Look for the results of chest radiographs, computed tomography (CT), magnetic resonance imaging (MRI), positron emission tomography (PET), ventilation/perfusion ($\dot{V}/\dot{Q}$), and ultrasonography scans or studies. If possible, compare previous studies with the most recent to gain a better understanding of the patient's condition.

2. Recommend imaging studies (code: IE3) [difficulty: R, Ap, An]

A chest radiograph or other imaging study should be taken whenever a significant change in the patient's cardiopulmonary condition occurs or whenever an invasive thoracic procedure is performed. In 2006 the American College of Radiology listed the following criteria for a bedside chest radiograph: (1) daily, routine radiograph of a patient being mechanically ventilated; (2) daily, routine radiograph of a patient with an acute cardiopulmonary condition; (3) immediate radiograph after the insertion of a chest tube, endotracheal intubation, central venous catheter, pulmonary artery catheter, or nasogastric tube.

As discussed below, a given imaging method may be preferred in a specific clinical situation. See Figure 1-1 for a comparison of how a small lung tumor appears in a routine chest radiograph, a CT scan, and a PET scan.

a. Chest radiograph

A chest radiograph (chest X-ray) should be recommended in the following situations:

- After an endotracheal or tracheostomy tube has been placed or repositioned
- After the jugular/subclavian route has been used to insert a CVP or pulmonary artery (Swan–Ganz) catheter
- After a chest tube has been placed in the pleural space to remove air or fluids
- Hemoptysis (bloody sputum) is noted
- A sudden deleterious change is noted in the patient's cardiopulmonary condition
- The balloon on the pulmonary artery (Swan–Ganz) catheter has been inflated for a prolonged period, and a pulmonary infarct is suspected
- A pneumothorax is suspected
- Any invasive thoracic procedure, i.e., pleural biopsy

Exam Hint 1-3

Expect to see at least one question in which the respiratory therapist should recommend a chest radiograph to rule out or confirm a pneumothorax. Signs and symptoms that the patient may have a pneumothorax include the following: sudden chest pain with an increase in dyspnea and shortness of breath, absent breath sounds over a lung field, tracheal deviation and heart sounds shifted to the side opposite the pneumothorax, asymmetrical chest movement, hyperresonant percussion noted over the pneumothorax, a sudden increase in peak pressure or plateau pressure or both on the patient's ventilator, or air in the soft tissues, or a combination of these.

---

b. Upper-airway radiograph

An upper-airway radiograph (anterior or lateral or both) should be recommended for a patient who presents

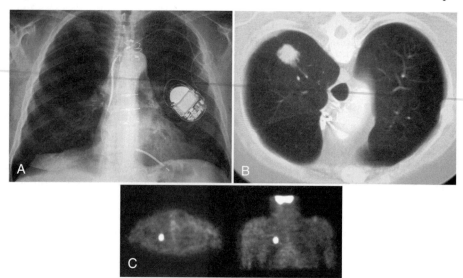

Figure 1-1 Comparison of three different radiographic imaging technologies used to view a right upper lobe coin lesion. **A,** A routine chest radiograph shows a faint shadow partially obscured by the clavicle. More obvious are the cardiac pacemaker and its wires and the sternal wires after open heart surgery. **B,** A CT scan clearly shows the white shadow caused by a dense mass. However, there is no way to tell if the mass is cancerous. **C,** A PET scan shows two views of the "hot" lesion. The lesion is proven to be cancerous because it is much more metabolically active than the surrounding tissues. Although a chest radiograph may be helpful for routine monitoring, other radiographic methods are often needed to further identify a change in the patient's condition. (From Heuer AJ, Scanlan CL: Wilkins' clinical assessment in respiratory care, ed 7, St Louis, 2014, Mosby.)

with indications of upper-airway obstruction. These can include:

- Aspirated foreign body
- Laryngeal edema
- Laryngeal tumor
- Laryngotracheal bronchitis (or croup) versus epiglottitis (see Module H for more information)

c. CT scan

A CT scan provides a more detailed image than a conventional radiograph. It is able to depict abnormalities of the lungs and mediastinum. Indications include, but are not limited to, the following:

- Tumor
- Hematoma
- Abscess and cyst
- Pleural effusion
- Aortic or other vascular abnormality (after an intravenous contrast material has been administered)
- Traumatic chest injury

d. MRI scan

An MRI scan provides images of body organs without the use of radioactive materials. The images are created when the powerful magnet of the MRI machine is turned on and off, affecting the way hydrogen atoms align within the body. A limitation of MRI is that the patient cannot have any metallic implants. In addition, most mechanical ventilators cannot be used during an MRI scan because the magnetic field will interfere with the unit. Indications for an MRI scan include, but are not limited to, the following:

- Imaging of the head, spinal cord, and surrounding structures
- Imaging of the heart and great vessels
- Imaging of the kidneys, liver, and other organs

Although not specified by the NBRC, the following should be studied, if possible: PET scans, $\dot{V}/\dot{Q}$ scans of the lungs, angiograms, and barium swallow studies.

e. PET scan

A PET scan is performed using a radioactive substance that is either inhaled or given intravenously. As the radioactive substance breaks down in the target organ, it emits a positron (a positive electron). When the positron combines with an electron, they annihilate each other with the release of two γ-rays. Detectors outside the body identify the origin of the γ-rays and can determine the functioning and metabolism of the target organ. Indications for a PET scan include, but are not limited to, the following:

- Determining the regional metabolism of the heart and brain
- Measuring the size of a myocardial infarction
- Measuring the effects of treatment on a cancerous tumor
- Determining pulmonary perfusion or ventilation

f. Ventilation/perfusion scan

A $\dot{V}/\dot{Q}$ scan is used to identify where air moves into the lungs during breathing and blood flows through the lungs. A *ventilation scan* ($\dot{V}$ scan) is performed to verify or refute the clinical suspicion that a patient has an area of the lung or lungs that is underventilated. Abnormal ventilation is seen in the case of a bronchial obstruction from a tumor or foreign body or with an alveolar problem, such as atelectasis, consolidation, or emphysema. Radioactive xenon (^{133}Xe) is mixed with oxygen and inhaled to show the lung fields. A special scanner is used to pick up the radioactivity through the chest wall. Areas of normal ventilation can be compared with underventilated areas.

A *perfusion scan* ($\dot{Q}$ scan) is performed to verify or refute the clinical suspicion that a patient has an area of pulmonary circulation that is underperfused. Abnormal perfusion is seen in the case of a pulmonary embolism, tumor, or vascular problem, such as pulmonary hypertension. Radioactive technetium (^{99m}Tc) is injected into the patient's venous system, where it is filtered out by the pulmonary circulation. As previously described, a special scanner is used to pick up the radioactivity through the chest wall. Areas of normal perfusion can be compared with underperfused areas. The ventilation scan and perfusion scan tests can be done singly or as a set.

Comparing the ventilation and perfusion results side by side enables the physician to look for areas of mismatching. Normally, ventilation and perfusion match fairly closely and result in a 1:1 mix of air and blood at the alveolar capillary membrane. A pulmonary embolism results in a $\dot{V}/\dot{Q}$ ratio of 2 (or greater):1 (or less), because normal ventilation is present and perfusion is reduced or absent. An obstructed airway with resulting atelectasis results in a $\dot{V}/\dot{Q}$ ratio of 1 (or less):2 (or greater), because ventilation is reduced or absent and perfusion is normal.

g. Angiogram

An angiogram involves the placement of a catheter into an artery or a vein. Commonly, a radiopaque dye is injected so that the flow of blood through the vessel can be observed. If a blockage is found, a balloon at the tip of the catheter may be inflated (balloon angioplasty) to flatten the blockage. Reasons to perform an angiogram include, but are not limited to, the following:

- Check blood flow through the carotid arteries and into the brain
- Check blood flow through the coronary arteries and the chambers of the heart
- Check blood flow through the pulmonary arteries when perfusion study results are inconclusive
- Perform a procedure to remove a blockage from an artery (this could include balloon angioplasty, laser atherectomy, or embolectomy)

h. Barium swallow (esophagogram)

A barium swallow (esophagogram) enables a radiographic image to be taken of the esophagus, stomach, and small intestine. Indications for a barium swallow include, but are not limited to, the following:

- Dysphagia
- Noncardiac chest pain
- Gastroesophageal reflux

3. Review the chest radiograph to determine the quality of the imaging (code: IB7a) [difficulty: R, Ap]

a. Patient identification

It is standard practice for the patient's name and identification number to be incorporated into the chest radiograph (chest radiograph film).

b. Patient positioning

The patient is positioned between the radiograph machine and the film cassette so that the high-frequency electromagnetic (X-ray) radiation penetrates the patient's body, hits the film, and provides the desired view of the internal organs. The patient is usually positioned to be viewed in one of three planes. The coronal plane image presents the person as if you were facing him or her. The transverse plane image presents the person as if you were looking down on the head to the toes (birds-eye view). The sagittal plane image presents the person in a right or left lateral view. Figure 1-2 shows the most common radiographic projections used for patients with cardiopulmonary problems. Examples of some of these positions are shown in this chapter.

If possible, the patient should be moved to the radiography department, and the chest radiograph should be taken from the *posterior to anterior* (posteroanterior, PA) position. The patient's chest is placed against the film cassette with the shoulders rolled forward. Because radiographs penetrate from back to front, the size of the heart is close to normal. The patient is instructed to take in and hold a deep breath. This reveals more clearly the lung fields, heart, and other structures. This may be contrasted with a chest radiograph taken after the patient has exhaled completely. If the patient has been correctly positioned perpendicular to the film cassette, the radiograph image will show the clavicle bones to be symmetrical and the scapulae will be rotated out.

If a portable chest radiograph must be taken because the patient is too ill to be moved from his or her bed, the *anterior to posterior* (anteroposterior, AP) position must be used. The radiographs penetrate the body from front to back. This should be noted in the chart, because this view of the organs shows the heart's size to be larger than that seen in a PA radiograph.

The standard *lateral view* is taken with the patient standing upright with both arms raised above the head and the left side against the film cassette. This is done because the heart is left of center in the chest. A lateral view is used to see behind the heart and hemidiaphragms. It can be combined with an AP or a PA view to localize lesions within the chest. This view also is used to measure the patient's anterior-to-posterior chest diameter. This is often enlarged in patients with air trapping from emphysema.

The *oblique position* provides a third angle for viewing the internal chest structures. This is especially helpful when the physician is checking the heart borders, mediastinal structures, hilar structures, and lung masses.

The *lateral decubitus position* enables fluid within the pleural space to be viewed. As little as 25-50 mL of fluid can be detected in an adult as it flows to the horizontal position. An air/fluid level in a lung cavity (cyst) also can be evaluated by the shifting of the fluid line by gravity. The *dorsal decubitus position* is used to help identify a small pneumothorax in an infant.

The *lordotic (apical lordotic) position* is used when the upper lung fields must be viewed without the clavicles and first and second ribs obscuring them. The apices, right middle lobe, and lingula can be clearly seen.

Make sure, when viewing any chest radiograph, that you are looking at the film correctly. That is, the film should be viewed as if you were looking directly at the patient's chest. For example, in a PA or AP film, if you reached out your right hand, you would touch the image of the patient's left shoulder. To help with correct viewing, the film should show the letter L over the patient's left shoulder (on your right as you look at the film). Note that sometimes the film will show the letter R over the patient's right shoulder (on your left as you look at the film).

c. Penetration/exposure

The radiologic technologist is responsible for exposing the patient to X-rays long enough to penetrate the tissues and acquire the proper exposure of the internal organs. With proper exposure time the internal structures can be differentiated. The vertebral bodies should be visible through the air column of the trachea and the shadow of the heart. Figure 1-1, A shows a properly penetrated standard chest radiograph. With underpenetration/underexposure the structures will be too white (see Fig. 1-3). With overpenetration/overexposure the structures will be too dark (see Fig. 1-4). Even if a film has been under- or overpenetrated, it may still be useful in identifying a pathological condition.

In all chest radiograph positions, the patient must take and hold a deep breath without moving as the picture is taken. If the patient is on a mechanical ventilator when an AP chest radiograph is obtained, a sigh breath should be delivered and held by the respiratory therapist to inflate the lungs fully.

It must be understood that the image seen on a chest radiograph film is the negative, or reverse, image of the densities of the structures within the chest. When viewing a radiograph film, a range of shadings will be seen progressing from white to black. *Radiopaque* items are very dense. They absorb most X-rays, preventing them

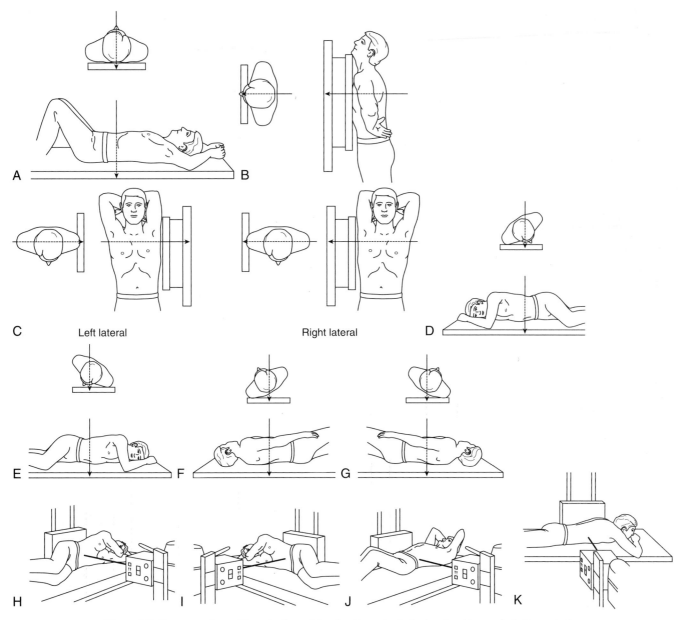

Figure 1-2 Common radiographic projections of the chest to evaluate the heart and lungs. **A,** Anteroposterior (AP) projection. **B,** Posteroanterior (PA) projection. **C,** Lateral projections. **D,** Right anterior oblique projection. **E,** PA oblique projection, left anterior projection. **F,** AP oblique projection, left posterior oblique projection. **G,** AP oblique projection, right posterior oblique projection. **H,** Left lateral decubitus. **I,** Right lateral decubitus. **J,** Dorsal decubitus. **K,** Ventral decubitus. (From Long BW, Frank ED, Ehrlich RA: Radiography essentials for limited practice, ed 4, St Louis, 2013, Saunders.)

from striking the film, and therefore appear white on the film. *Radiolucent* items have little density. They absorb few X-rays, allowing them to strike the film, and therefore appear dark on the film. Altogether, four densities are seen on a chest radiograph:

1. Air

Because air is the least dense substance, it blocks very few X-rays; most hit the film in the cassette. This causes the film to turn black. Notice that the film around the

patient's body is completely black. Because the normal lungs are air filled with little tissue, they appear almost black. Normally some lung tissue markings can be seen as wispy white shadows. Air in the stomach or intestine also appears dark compared with the surrounding tissues.

2. Tissue

The tissues of the lungs, heart, diaphragm, breasts, fat, and so on partially block the radiographs. This results in white shadows of varying opacity, depending on the density of

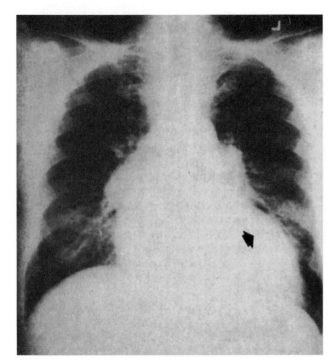

Figure 1-3 Chest radiograph of an adult showing pulmonary edema, increased pulmonary vascular markings, and an enlarged left ventricle (cardiomegaly). The cardiothoracic diameter is increased, and the arrow shows where the border of the left ventricle normally would be seen. Even though the film is underpenetrated, it can still be clinically useful. (From Des Jardins T, Burton GG: Clinical manifestations and assessment of respiratory disease, ed 6, St Louis, 2011, Mosby.)

the tissues. For example, the heart appears as a fairly solid white organ. Fluid also partially blocks radiographs. A pleural effusion is seen as a white shadow around one or both lungs.

3. Bone

The calcium in bone makes it dense enough to block most X-ray penetration; therefore the ribs, clavicles, and vertebrae are seen as fairly solid white lines. Broken ribs can be easily identified by the misalignment of their shadows.

4. Metallic

Bullets, wire sutures, metal plates, artificial heart valves, and coins completely block all radiograph penetration. This results in a sharply outlined white shadow. Medical devices, such as an endotracheal or a tracheostomy tube, nasogastric tube, or heart catheter, contain materials that completely block radiographs. Therefore these radiopaque items can be easily seen within the patient on a chest radiograph.

When the radiograph is obtained with the proper penetration and exposure, the intervertebral spaces of the spinal column are just visible. If the film is underexposed (the overall color of the film and body tissues

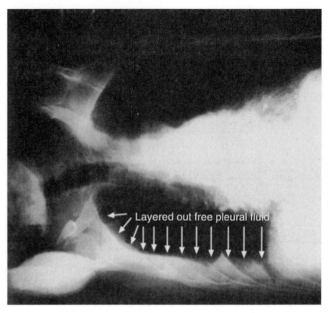

Figure 1-4 Lateral decubitus radiograph of an adult showing the shift of a small pleural effusion to the now-dependent part of the pleural space. Even though the film is overpenetrated, the layer of fluid can be seen (arrows). (From Heuer AJ, Scanlan CL: Wilkins' clinical assessment in respiratory care, ed 7, St Louis, 2014, Mosby.)

is too white), the carina or an internal catheter may not be seen. If the film is overexposed (the overall color of the film and body tissues is too black), the air-filled lung fields will be too black, and it may not be possible to detect a pneumothorax.

4. Review a chest radiograph to assess the presence of, or change in, pneumothorax or other air leaks (code: IB7e(i)) [difficulty: R, Ap]

Free air that leaks into the interstitial spaces of the lung or body cavities is abnormal in any patient. Causes of an air leak include, but are not limited to, barotrauma/volutrauma (alveolar rupture related to the use of a mechanical ventilator), a ruptured bleb (congenital or acquired blister on the visceral pleura), puncture wound through the chest wall, and needle puncture through the pleural space during the insertion of a CVP or pulmonary artery catheter via the subclavian or jugular vein. Once air under pressure is forced through a bronchial or alveolar tear into the interstitial tissues, it tends to follow the path of least resistance. This may result in air being found in any of the following areas, singly or in combination.

a. Pneumothorax

Pneumothorax is air in the pleural space. The lung tends to collapse toward the hilum. A pneumothorax is identified on the chest radiograph as an area of black, indicating air that surrounds the collapsed lung. No lung markings are visible in the air-filled space, and the edge of the lung

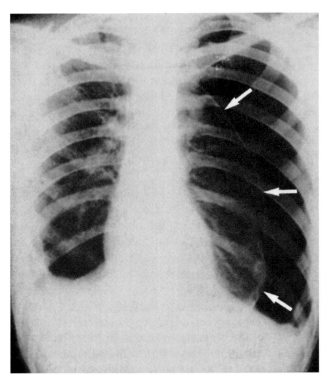

Figure 1-5 Chest radiograph of an adult male with a left-sided tension pneumothorax. The edge of the collapsed lung is shown *(arrows)*. Note how the mediastinum is shifted to the right, the right lung is compressed, and the left hemidiaphragm is depressed. (From Des Jardins T, Burton GG: Clinical manifestations and assessment of respiratory disease, ed 6, St Louis, 2011, Mosby.)

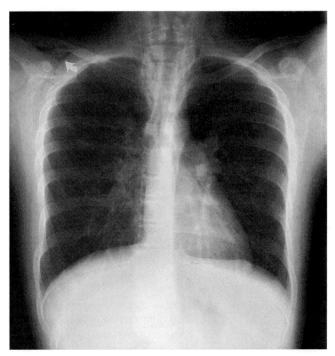

Figure 1-6 Air trapping and hyperinflation leading to air leaks. The PA chest radiograph of an 11-year-old asthmatic child shows a pneumomediastinum. The free air has further dissected into the soft tissues of the neck and right shoulder (see arrow). The horizontal ribs are caused by the hyperinflated lungs. (From Kacmarek RM, Stoller JK, Heuer AJ, editors: Egan's fundamentals of respiratory care, ed 10, St Louis, 2013, Mosby.)

can be seen (Fig. 1-5). If the air is under sufficient pressure to shift the lung and mediastinal structures to the opposite side, the condition is called a *tension pneumothorax*. This is a serious condition that can lead to the death of the patient if it is not quickly identified and treated. A pleural chest tube is always placed into the affected side to remove the air so that the lung can reexpand. (See Chapter 18 for more information on the treatment of a pneumothorax.)

b. Subcutaneous emphysema and other air leaks

Subcutaneous emphysema is air found in the soft tissues, such as the skin, axilla, shoulder, neck, or breast, of the affected side. In extreme cases, the air forces its way into skin and soft tissues throughout the body. Scattered dark areas (air pockets) appear in the various soft tissues on the chest radiograph (Fig. 1-6). *Pneumomediastinum* is air in the mediastinal space (see Fig. 1-6). *Pneumopericardium* is air in the pericardial space (Fig. 1-7). Both of these conditions can be very serious. Cardiac tamponade is created if the pressure around the heart is great enough to interfere with its function. *Pneumoperitoneum* is air in the peritoneal space. This condition can be dangerous in an infant if a large enough volume of air is below the diaphragm and its movement is limited. *Pulmonary interstitial emphysema*

(PIE) is air that has disseminated throughout the interstitial spaces of the injured lung or lungs. The lungs appear "bubbly" on the chest radiograph (see Fig. 1-7). The air may further leak into any of the previously listed locations. PIE is most commonly seen in infants with respiratory distress syndrome (RDS) who require mechanical ventilation.

5. Review a chest radiograph to assess the presence of, or change in, the mediastinum or trachea (code: IB7e(ii)) [difficulty: R, Ap]

The mediastinum is the area between the lungs that contains the heart and great vessels, trachea, hilar structures, and esophagus. In the neonate, the heart and other mediastinal structures should be approximately in the center of the chest, with the left ventricle to the left of center. In the adult, the majority of the heart and mediastinal structures should be left of center in the chest. A shift of the mediastinum (trachea and heart) is abnormal, as shown in several conditions in Figures 1-5 and 1-8. Either atelectasis or pulmonary fibrosis, if unilateral and great enough, can result in a shift *toward* the problem area. Tension pneumothorax results in a shift *away* from the problem area. Fluid in the pleural space, if great enough, results in a shift *away* from the problem area.

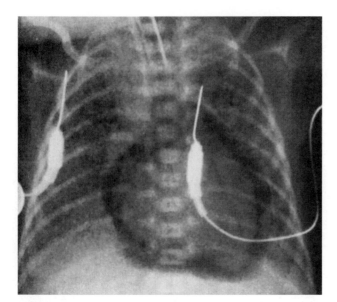

Figure 1-7 Chest radiograph of a neonate showing a pneumopericardium that resulted from pulmonary interstitial emphysema. Note the dark outline of air around the heart. Chest tubes have been placed to remove air from around the heart and the right pleural space from an earlier pneumothorax. An endotracheal tube also is seen. (From Koff PB, Eitzman DV, Neu J: Neonatal and pediatric respiratory care, St Louis, 1988, Mosby.)

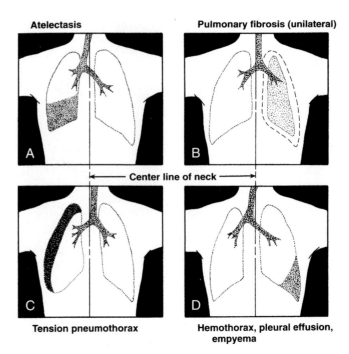

Figure 1-8 Simulated chest radiograph findings of conditions causing tracheal deviation and mediastinal shift. **A,** Unilateral atelectasis with tracheal deviation toward the affected lung. **B,** Unilateral pulmonary fibrosis with tracheal deviation toward the affected lung. **C,** Tension pneumothorax with tracheal deviation away from the affected lung. **D,** Pleural fluid with tracheal deviation away from the affected lung. The normal lung expands more than the abnormal lung during inspiration.

6. Review a chest radiograph to assess the presence of, or change in, the hemidiaphragms (code: IB7e(ii)) [difficulty: R, Ap]

The normal infant's and adult's AP or PA chest radiograph reveals a domed shape to the hemidiaphragms, with the edges turning down to acute costophrenic angles. A lateral chest radiograph reveals the same domed shape with the edges turning down to acute costophrenic angles. The edges of the hemidiaphragms should be smooth; any dips or peaks indicate an abnormality.

Both hemidiaphragms, and each separately, can be either elevated or depressed, depending on the condition of the lungs (underinflated or overinflated (hyperinflation)) and the abdominal contents. The following are commonly encountered clinical situations:

- Unilateral elevation: Atelectasis and pulmonary fibrosis (see Fig. 1-8) decrease the lung's volume; an enlarged liver pushes up on the right hemidiaphragm.
- Unilateral depression: Excessive pleural fluid, tension pneumothorax (see Fig. 1-5), check-valve bronchial obstruction from a foreign body, or an airway tumor can cause unilateral depression.
- Bilateral elevation: Free abdominal fluid, as seen with peritoneal dialysis, can push up on both hemidiaphragms.
- Bilateral depression: Asthma attack and COPD (Fig. 1-9, A and B) result in overinflation of both lungs and depression of both hemidiaphragms.

In a person with asthma, bronchitis, or emphysema (COPD), and in a newborn with meconium aspiration, both lungs are overinflated and both hemidiaphragms are depressed. Other radiographic findings include widened intercostal spaces; hyperlucent lung fields; a small, vertical heart; a small cardiothoracic diameter; and decreased vascularity of peripheral areas of the lungs, with enlarged hilar vessels. The lateral chest radiographic findings in the patient with COPD are the same, and they include anterior bowing of the sternum, increased retrosternal air space, and kyphosis. In any of the previously mentioned conditions, improvement should result in a return of the hemidiaphragm or hemidiaphragms to a position closer to normal.

7. Review a chest radiograph to assess heart position and size (code: IB7d) [difficulty: R, Ap]

The heart position and size are best evaluated from a PA chest radiograph. An AP chest radiograph will show an incorrectly large heart size. In an infant, the heart is centrally located. In an adult, the heart is more left of center. The heart size is calculated by measuring the cardiothoracic (C:T) ratio. It is the ratio of the width of the heart at the diaphragm to the widest lateral diameter inside the chest wall. The normal adult's C:T ratio is less than 0.5, or 50%, and the normal infant's C:T ratio is less than 0.6, or 60%. Figures 1-3 and 1-10 show adults with a large C:T ratio. This type of heart enlargement (cardiomegaly) is

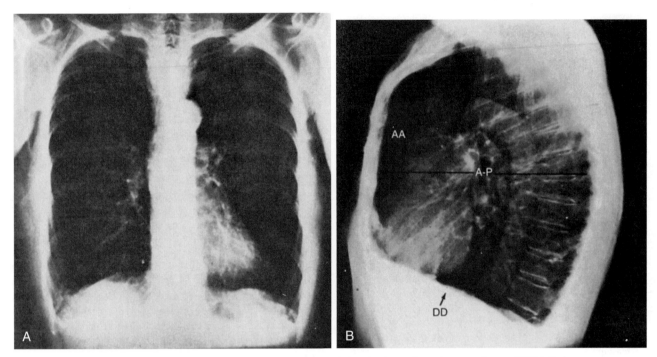

Figure 1-9 A, PA radiograph of an adult with advanced chronic obstructive pulmonary disease (COPD). Both lungs are overinflated and hyperlucent. The ribs are horizontal and spread more widely than normal. Often these patients have a cardiothoracic ratio that is smaller than normal because the heart is elongated and the lateral chest diameter is increased. **B,** Lateral radiograph of an adult with advanced COPD. Note the characteristic shape of a "barrel chest" from the overinflated lungs. The anteroposterior diameter (A-P) of the chest is increased. *AA* marks an increased anterior air space between the heart and the sternum. The angle of the manubrium and body of the sternum is more obtuse than normal. *DD* marks depressed hemidiaphragms that are flattened. (From Heuer AJ, Scanlan CL: Wilkins' clinical assessment in respiratory care, ed 7, St Louis, 2014, Mosby.)

commonly seen in patients with congestive heart failure, cor pulmonale (right-ventricular failure secondary to lung disease), and some congenital heart defects. A small C:T ratio is seen in patients who have severe COPD (emphysema and/or chronic bronchitis). The lung volumes are enlarged, which depresses the diaphragm and elongates the heart (see Fig. 1-9, A).

8. Review a chest radiograph to assess the presence of, or change in, pleural effusion (code: IB7e(i)) [difficulty: R, Ap]

Pleural fluid typically is shown on a PA or AP film as obscuring the costophrenic angle. This is because gravity tends to draw the fluid to the lowest level. Often this results in an obscuring or a blunting of the costophrenic angle of the affected side (see Fig. 1-10). In some cases, an air/fluid level is seen within the intrapleural space. The term *meniscus* is used to describe the upward curve seen in the fluid part of this intrapleural air/fluid level. Small amounts of fluid sometimes can be better visualized by taking a lateral decubitus radiograph. If the fluid is able to move freely in the pleural space, it shifts in a few minutes to the lower side (Fig. 1-4). An empyema that is loculated (fixed) by adhesions does not move when the patient lies on his or her side. If large amounts of fluid are removed by

a thoracentesis procedure, a chest radiograph should be taken to confirm the removal of fluid, the reexpansion of the lung, and that a pneumothorax did not result.

9. Review a chest radiograph to assess the presence of, or change in, pulmonary edema (code: IB7e(i)) [difficulty: R, Ap]

Pulmonary edema is watery fluid (plasma) that has leaked out of the pulmonary capillary bed into the interstitial spaces and alveoli. It is most commonly caused by left-ventricular failure (also known as *congestive heart failure*), but it can be the result of fluid overload, pulmonary capillary damage, or decreased osmotic pressure in the blood from a low level of protein.

Pulmonary edema appears on a PA or AP chest radiograph as fluffy, white infiltrates in either or both lung fields. These tend to be seen more extensively in the lower lobes as a result of gravity pulling the fluid to the basilar vessels, where it leaks out. If the root cause is left-ventricular failure, the vessels in the hila also are engorged, and the left ventricle is enlarged (see Fig. 1-3). A worsening problem results in more fluid leaking into the lungs and the appearance of more white infiltrates on succeeding chest radiographs. Once the problem has been corrected, the lungs return to normal as the fluid is reabsorbed and removed.

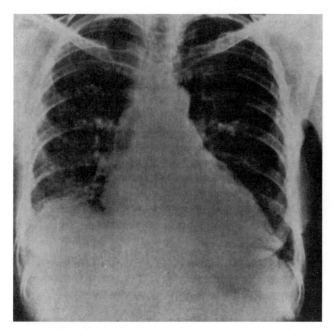

Figure 1-10 Chest radiograph of an adult showing a small pleural effusion in the right chest. Note how the costophrenic angle and hemidiaphragm are obscured by the white shadow of fluid. Also note the patient's cardiomegaly and increased cardiothoracic diameter. (From Heuer AJ, Scanlan CL: Wilkins' clinical assessment in respiratory care, ed 7, St Louis, 2014, Mosby.)

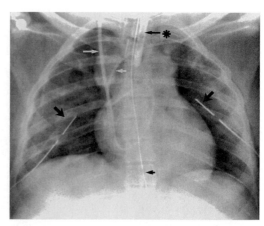

Figure 1-11 AP radiograph of an adult showing several indwelling tubes and catheters. All are radiopaque, which makes them easy to identify on the film. (1) Black arrow with asterisk shows an endotracheal tube properly located within the trachea. (2) Two large black arrows point to a pleural chest tube on each side. (3) Small black arrow shows a nasogastric tube. (4) Long white arrow shows a pulmonary artery catheter. (5) Short white arrow shows a left subclavian vein catheter. (From Heuer AJ, Scanlan CL: Wilkins' clinical assessment in respiratory care, ed 7, St Louis, 2014, Mosby.)

10. Review a chest radiograph to assess the presence and position of tubes and catheters (code: IB7b) [difficulty: R, Ap, An]

All medical devices placed into the body are made of radiopaque material. They can be seen on a chest radiograph as a white object or line.

Chest tubes are placed to remove any abnormal collection of air or fluid from the thoracic cavity so that the function of the heart and lungs returns to normal. A pleural chest tube is placed to remove air or fluid from the pleural space (see Figs. 1-7 and 1-11). The insertion site and depth of insertion of the tube depend on the patient's disorder. (See Chapter 18 for more discussion on the placement of pleural chest tubes.)

A mediastinal or pericardial chest tube is placed to remove air or fluid from either of these spaces (see Fig. 1-7). Cardiac tamponade can result from the pressure of either air or fluid compressing the heart. Most postoperative open-heart surgery patients have one or more mediastinal chest tubes in place for several days to remove any blood from around the heart. The insertion site is below the sternum, and the tube or tubes are placed posterior to the heart in the pericardial or mediastinal space or both.

On the chest radiograph, a nasogastric tube appears as a white line from the patient's nose or mouth through the esophagus and into the stomach (on the left side below the diaphragm) (see Fig. 1-11). A feeding tube may be placed as a nasogastric tube or may be surgically placed through the abdominal wall and into the stomach or small intestine. A white line on the radiograph shows its position.

A cardiac pacemaker is placed in two ways. An external pacemaker is identified on the chest radiograph by the long electrode leads that run through a vein in the right arm, through the superior vena cava, and into the right ventricle. The battery and control unit of an internal pacemaker are placed under the skin below a clavicle. The electrode leads run through the superior vena cava into the right ventricle (see Fig. 1-1).

The various venous catheters (pulmonary artery catheter, CVP catheter, umbilical artery catheter, and umbilical vein catheter) should be seen on the chest radiograph from their insertion points to their end points. See Figures 1-11 and 1-12 for the placement of several catheters.

11. Review a chest radiograph to assess the presence and position of an endotracheal or tracheostomy tube (code: IB7b) [difficulty: R, Ap, An]

The distal ends of these tubes should be seen within the lumen of the trachea and about midway between the larynx and the tracheal bifurcation to the right and left mainstem bronchi. See Figures 1-7, 1-11, and 1-12 for correct endotracheal tube placement. If an endotracheal tube is inserted too far, it will usually enter the right mainstem bronchus (Fig. 1-13). The tube should be pulled back into the trachea. See Chapter 12 for more information.

The proximal end of the tracheostomy tube (or tracheostomy button or laryngectomy tube) is seen on the film coming out of the surgical insertion site in the suprasternal notch. The distal end should be centered within

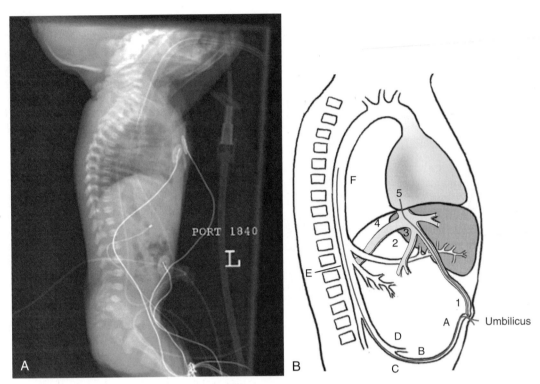

Figure 1-12 Lateral radiograph of a newborn **A,** and diagram **B,** of the course of umbilical venous and arterial catheters. The umbilical venous catheter enters through the umbilicus and passes through the umbilical vein (1), portal vein (2), ductus venosus (3), and inferior vena cava (4) and stops in the right atrium (5). The umbilical arterial catheter enters through the umbilicus and passes through the umbilical artery **A,** hypogastric artery **B,** internal iliac artery **C,** common iliac artery **D,** and abdominal aorta **E,** and stops in the thoracic aorta **F.** (From Heuer AJ, Scanlan CL: Wilkins' clinical assessment in respiratory care, ed 7, St Louis, 2014, Mosby.)

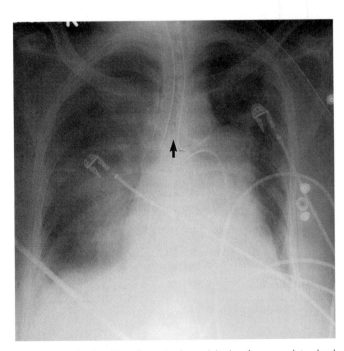

Figure 1-13 Supine AP radiograph of an adult showing an endotracheal tube with its tip in the right mainstem bronchus (arrow). The tube has been inserted too deeply and needs to be withdrawn into the trachea. (From Kacmarek RM, Stoller JK, Heuer AJ, editors: Egan's fundamentals of respiratory care, ed 10, St Louis, 2013, Mosby.)

the trachea above the carina (Fig. 1-14). All these tubes are made of a radiopaque material or have a line of radiopaque material embedded in them so that they can be easily seen on the radiograph.

Care must be taken not to push the endotracheal tube deeper into a bronchus (usually the right) or to pull it out. The tracheostomy tube and transtracheal oxygen catheter are less likely to be displaced if they receive proper care. Another radiograph should be taken to check the position of any of these tubes if clinical evidence suggests that a position may have changed.

Exam Hint 1-4

The NBRC often has a question about how to identify the location of an endotracheal tube on a chest radiograph. The distal tip of the tube should be seen in the middle of the trachea. An endotracheal tube that has been inserted too deeply will enter the right mainstem bronchus.

Note: The following items have been listed as testable on previous exams and should be reviewed, if possible:

Review a chest radiograph for an overinflated endotracheal or tracheostomy tube cuff. A properly inflated cuff fills the space between the tube and the patient's trachea so that an airtight

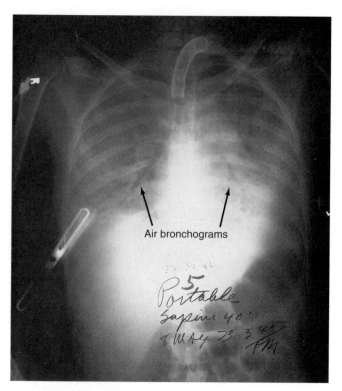

Figure 1-14 Chest radiograph of an adult showing a properly located tracheostomy tube. The overall haziness of the lung fields is typical for a patient with pulmonary fibrosis. The dark air bronchograms can be seen because the mainstem airways are patent and air filled. (From Heuer AJ, Scanlan CL, editors: Wilkins' clinical assessment in respiratory care, ed 7, St Louis, 2014, Mosby.)

seal is made. If the cuff is overinflated, it places excessive pressure on the trachea. This can cause it to dilate and be seen as a wider dark area than the rest of the tracheal air column. If this is noticed, the cuff pressure should be measured. Excessive pressure should be reduced to a safer level.

Review a chest radiograph for the size and patency of the major airways. The trachea and both the right and the left mainstem bronchi should be seen on a properly taken chest radiograph. They appear as straight, dark air columns in contrast to the white shadows of the various surrounding tissues. A white shadow within the airway may be a foreign body or a tumor. A lung tumor that presses on an airway causes the airway to narrow or be occluded.

12. Review a chest radiograph to assess the presence of foreign bodies (code: IB7c) [difficulty: R, Ap]

A foreign body is anything that is not naturally found in the chest. Metallic objects (e.g., bullets or swallowed or aspirated coins or metal buttons) are easily noticed, because they completely block any X-ray penetration through the chest and are clearly outlined on the film as solid, white shadows (Fig. 1-15). Nonmetallic foreign objects (e.g., plastic pieces from toys and foods, such as peanuts) are much more difficult to identify, because they have about the same densities as normal body tissues.

Determining the exact location of a foreign body may require taking PA, lateral, and oblique chest radiographs. Lung volumes can be compared by taking inspiratory and expiratory films. A CT scan may be the most successful method of finding a nonmetallic foreign body.

13. Review a chest radiograph to assess the presence of, or change in, consolidation (code: IB7e(i)) [difficulty: R, Ap]

A *consolidation* is a filling of the alveoli with fluid from a pulmonary infiltrate, aspirated vomitus, blood, or water. It is often segmental or lobar. A pulmonary infiltrate occurs when blood plasma (water) passes from the pulmonary vascular bed into the lung tissues. Usually this fluid moves into the lung, because the alveolar capillary membrane is damaged. On a chest radiograph, an infiltrate often appears as a faint white blurring of the lung and other associated structures. Consolidation is noticed on the chest radiograph as a dense white shadow, because fluid has completely replaced the air. The mediastinum and heart are seen in their normal locations. Figure 1-16 shows drawings of PA and lateral chest radiographs, indicating consolidation in each of the segments of both lungs. Air bronchograms also may be noticed on a radiograph that reveals consolidation. See Figure 1-14 for the dark airways within areas of white, airless lung tissue.

14. Review a chest radiograph to assess the presence of, or change in, atelectasis (code: IB7e(i)) [difficulty: R, Ap]

Atelectasis is the collapse of alveoli; no air is found in them. This problem is commonly seen postoperatively in the lower lobes of patients who have had abdominal or thoracic surgery and who do not breathe deeply because of pain. The radiograph of atelectasis shows an increase in lung markings and a decrease in the lung volumes. If it is one-sided, the mediastinum may shift toward the affected side (see Fig. 1-7, A). If it is bilateral, the mediastinum is properly located. If it is severe enough, the lungs appear uniformly white (Fig. 1-17).

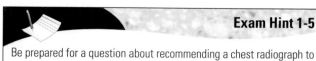

Exam Hint 1-5

Be prepared for a question about recommending a chest radiograph to check for a foreign body obstructing the upper airway or a bronchus.

MODULE C

Interview the patient.

1. Interview the patient to assess level of consciousness (code: IB1a) [difficulty: R, Ap, An]

One common way to evaluate a patient's level of consciousness is to categorize him or her as alert, stuporous, semicomatose, or comatose.

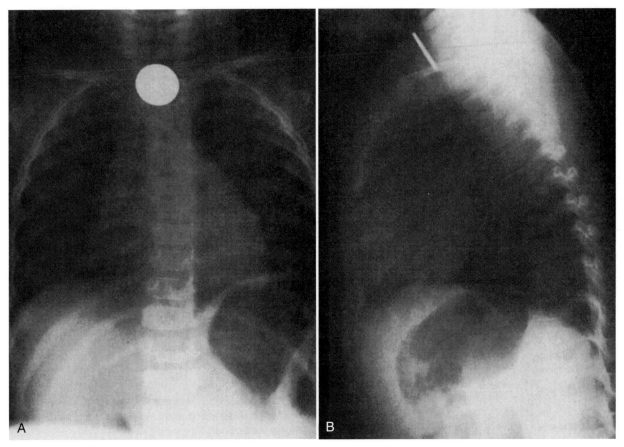

Figure 1-15 Foreign body obstruction in an 18-month-old girl. **A,** Chest radiograph with the solid white disk of a coin clearly seen in the hypopharynx. **B,** Lateral view of the chest with the edge of the coin seen as a solid white line. (From Hunter TB, Bragg DG: Radiologic guide to medical devices and foreign bodies, St Louis, 1994, Mosby.)

a. Alert

This is the normal mental state. The patient is conscious or can be fully awakened from sleep by calling his or her name. The patient can voluntarily ask logical questions and answer questions logically. The conversation is relevant to the topic under discussion. The patient's movements and actions are willful and purposeful.

b. Stuporous or lethargic

The patient is sleepy or seems to be in a trance. He or she can be aroused to respond with willful, purposeful movements and actions, but the patient may be slow. The patient may not respond to questions in a totally appropriate way.

c. Semicomatose

The patient does not perform requested movements or actions. The patient does not answer questions in an appropriate way. He or she responds defensively to pain. For example, if the right arm is pinched, it is withdrawn. Posturing of semicomatose patients includes the following:

1. Decerebrate

Legs are extended; arms are extended and rotated either inward or outward.

2. Decorticate

Legs are extended; arms are flexed, and the forearms may be rotated either inward or outward.

3. Opisthotonic

Legs, arms, and neck are extended, and the body is arched forward.

d. Comatose or coma

The patient has no spontaneous, oriented responses to the environment. Pain causes no defensive movement, but an increase in the heart and respiratory rates may occur.

Another common way to evaluate a patient's level of consciousness is to use the Glasgow Coma Scale. With this scale, a range of 3-15 points is possible; the larger the total number, the more normal the patient. A score of 15 is achieved in a patient normally awake and alert; a score of 3 is found in an unresponsive patient. Table 1-9 presents the details of the scale.

2. Interview the patient to assess orientation to time, place, and person (code: IB1a) [difficulty: R, Ap, An]

Time refers to the patient knowing the calendar date, the day of the week, and the time of day. Ask the patient,

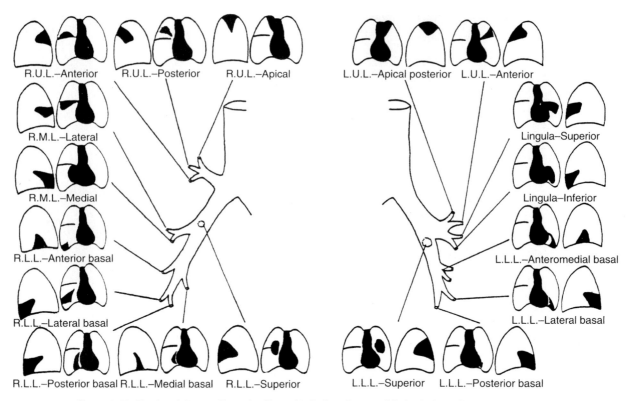

Figure 1-16 Simulated chest and lateral radiographic findings for consolidation in the various segments of both lungs. *L.L.L.,* left lower lobe; *L.U.L.,* left upper lobe; *R.L.L.,* right lower lobe; *R.M.L.,* right middle lobe; *R.U.L.,* right upper lobe. (From Cherniack RM, Cherniack L: Respiration in health and disease, ed 3, Philadelphia, 1983, Saunders.)

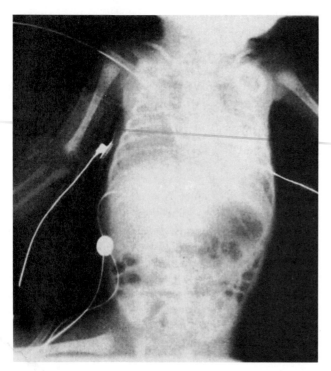

Figure 1-17 Chest radiograph of a neonate with severe atelectasis from infant respiratory distress syndrome. Also note the right apical pleural chest tube and wires to various monitoring systems. (From Des Jardins T, Burton GG: Clinical manifestations and assessment of respiratory disease, ed 6, St Louis, 2011, Mosby.)

"Do you know what day of the week it is? Do you know what the date is?" (The patient must be able to see a calendar.) "Do you know what time it is?" (The patient must be able to see a clock.) If the patient can answer these questions, he or she is oriented to time. If not, inform and show him or her. Tell the patient that you will return at a certain time. Ask the same questions when you return.

Place refers to the patient knowing where he or she is located (e.g., hospital, nursing care unit, extended care facility, home). Ask the patient, "Do you know where you are?" If the patient knows, he or she is oriented to place. If not, inform the patient of the location. Tell the patient that you will return at a certain time. Ask the same question when you return.

Person refers to the patient knowing his or her own name, address, and telephone number. The patient also should know the names of obviously important people. Ask the patient, "Do you know who the president (or the physician) is?" If not, inform the patient. Tell the patient who you are and what your job is. When you return for your next treatment, ask the patient if he remembers who you are and what you do. If the patient remembers who the president (or the physician) is and your name or job, he or she is oriented to person.

Orienting a stuporous or lethargic patient to person, place, and time may encourage the individual to cooperate more in his or her care. Pain-relieving and sedative drugs,

TABLE 1-9 Glasgow Coma Scale

Test Parameter	Response	Score*
Eyes		
Open	Spontaneously	4
	To verbal command	3
	To pain	2
	No response	1
Best Motor Response		
To verbal command	Obeys command	6
Moves arms to painful	Localizes pain	5
stimulus of knuckles	Flexion—withdrawal	4
against sternum	Flexion—abnormal movement (decorticate rigidity)	3
	Extension—abnormal movement (decerebrate rigidity)	2
	No response	1
Best Verbal Response (May Arouse by Painful Stimulus if Necessary)		
	Oriented and converses	5
	Disoriented and converses	4
	Inappropriate words used	3
	Incomprehensible sounds	2
	No response	1

*The total is obtained by adding the scores in all three areas. The range is 3-15.
From Teasdale G, Jennett B: Management of head injuries, Philadelphia, 1981, FA Davis.

stroke, injury to or edema of the brain, and other illnesses may cause disorientation to person, place, or time.

3. Interview the patient to assess emotional state (code: IB1a) [difficulty: R, Ap, An]

Acute illness or injury with great pain may result in some patients feeling fear, anxiety, or panic. Because of these feelings, the patient may be unable to concentrate closely on what you are telling him or her. This can result in directions not being understood or followed. It is important to tell the patient that you are there to help and that you need the patient to calm down so that you can help.

Chronic illness has been approached by a number of authors from varying points of view. Table 1-10 gives a presentation of a patient's reaction to chronic illness. Substitute "respiratory therapists" for "nurses" as needed.

A patient's statements and actions that indicate the *disbelief* stage of adaptation include the following:
- "I don't have (fill in the disease or condition)."
- "There is nothing really wrong with me."
- "The laboratory results are wrong."
- "The equipment is faulty."
- "The doctor/nurse/therapist is incompetent."

- Refusal to take medications.
- Refusal to take treatments or follow other physician orders.

A patient's statements and actions that indicate the *developing awareness* state of adaptation include the following:
- "The doctor/nurse/therapist doesn't know what he or she is doing."
- "It's all their fault."
- "Why is this happening to me?"
- The patient is angry about his or her illness.
- The patient may strike out verbally or physically at staff members.
- Some patients who do not get angry withdraw into a depression and wish to be left alone.

A patient's statements and actions that indicate that he or she is progressing from the *reorganization* to the *successful adaptation* stage include the following:
- "I'll never be able to do that again." (Fill in the activity.)
- "I have to get on with my life."
- "At least I'm still alive and can do this for myself."
- The patient may be sad and cry often.
- The patient may invent a nickname for his or her defect or diseased body part.
- The patient accepts the disability and focuses on his or her abilities.
- The patient works with family and others in planning for the future.

4. Interview the patient to assess ability to cooperate (code: IB1a) [difficulty: R, Ap, An]

You should be able to judge the patient's ability to cooperate. This should be based on his or her responses to your questions on level of consciousness; orientation to time, place, and person; and emotional state. An alert patient should be able to understand and follow directions. He or she should be able to take an effective treatment or cooperate in a procedure. Conversely, if the patient truly refuses the treatment or procedure, it should not be forced. Contact the patient's nurse or physician about the refusal. The physician must then decide what to do.

An alert but panicked, fearful, or anxious patient may be unable to cooperate fully until he or she is calmed by understanding who you are, what you are there to do, and why the treatment or procedure is important. Try to reassure the patient to improve cooperation.

If the patient appears alert but does not follow what you are saying, check to see whether he or she is deaf or does not speak English. An effective way to communicate must be found. Writing materials, a picture board, or a sign language interpreter is needed to communicate with a patient who is deaf. A native language translator will be needed to communicate with a patient who does not speak English.

A stuporous or very lethargic patient may be roused if you talk louder or shake the person gently. He or she

TABLE 1-10	Teaching–Learning Process in Adaptation to Chronic Illness		
Stages of Adaptation	Patient's Behavior	Nurse's Behavior	Nurse's Facilitation of the Teaching–Learning Process
Disbelief	Denies threatening condition to protect self and conserve energy; refuses to accept diagnosis; may claim to have something else; may behave so as to avoid the issue; may seem to accept diagnosis but avoids feelings about it	Allows patient to deny illness as he or she needs to; functions as noncritical listener; accepts patient's statements of how he or she feels; helps clarify patient's statements; does not point out reality	Orients all teaching to the present, not to tomorrow or next week; teaches as he or she does other nursing activities; assesses patient's level of anxiety; assures patient that he or she is safe and being observed carefully; explains all procedures and activities to the patient; gives clear, concise explanations; coordinates activities to include rest periods
Developing awareness	Uses anger as a defense against being dependent and against guilt about being sick	Listens to patient's expressions of anger and recognizes them for what they are; explores own feelings about illness and helplessness; does not argue with patient; gives dependable care with an attitude that it is necessary	Does not give anxious patient long lists of facts; continues development of trust and rapport through good physical care; orients teaching to present; explains symptoms, care, and treatment in terms of the fact that they are necessary now; does not mention long-range care needs
Reorganization	Accepts increased dependence and reorganizes relationships with significant others; members of patient's family may also use denial while they adapt to what patient's illness means to them	Establishes climate in which family and friends can express feelings about patient's illness; does not solve patient's problems but helps build communication so that patient and family can work together to solve problems	Assures family that patient is all right and safe; uses clear, concise explanations; does not argue about need for care
Resolution	Acknowledges changes seen in self; identifies with others with same problem	Encourages expression of feelings, including crying; understands own feelings of loss	Brings groups of patients with same illness together for group discussions; has a recovered person visit patient; teaches patient what he or she wants to learn (or perceives he or she needs to learn) first
Identity change	Defines self as an individual who has undergone change and is now different; "There are limits to my life because I have a disease."	Understands own feelings about patient becoming independent again	Realizes that as patient's own perceived needs are met, more mature (more progressive) needs will surface; is prepared to answer patient's questions as they arise
Successful adaptation	Can live comfortably or resignedly with himself or herself as a person who has a specific condition	Initiates closure of nurse–patient relationship	Has helped develop a relationship with the patient in which the nurse is a guide with whom the patient can consult when he or she wishes

From Kenner CV, Guzzetta CE, Dossey BM: Critical care nursing: body–mind–spirit, Boston, 1981, Little, Brown.

may or may not be able to cooperate fully. The practitioner may have to modify the treatment plan or how it is administered to compensate for the patient's lack of cooperation.

Pain relievers and sedatives may make a normally alert patient seem stuporous. If the patient has not been medicated, check with the nurse or physician to see what may have recently changed in the patient's condition.

A semicomatose patient may present the greatest problems in providing treatment or performing a procedure. These patients do not cooperate in any way but are unlikely to fight treatment either. In addition, some of their involuntary body posturings make correct positioning impossible. You must modify your equipment or procedure to accommodate the patient's inability to cooperate.

5. Interview the patient to assess level of pain (code: IB1b) [difficulty: R, Ap, An]

It has been shown that unmanaged pain can slow a patient's recovery from trauma or surgery. Because pain is a subjective feeling, only the patient can determine how severe the pain is. Some patients have a low pain threshold and report pain sooner and at a higher level than individuals with a high pain threshold. Therefore the acceptable way to determine the pain level is to have the patient rate it. Commonly, the patient is told to self-rate a pain level of 0 when no pain is felt and to assign a number up to a pain level of 10 for the most severe pain possible. Additionally, the patient should be asked to point with one finger to the area with the greatest pain. After the patient has been given a pain medication, and it has had time to take effect, the patient again is asked to rate the pain on the 0-to-10 scale. If the patient can tolerate the new pain level, it may not be necessary to

BOX 1-2 Degrees of Dyspnea

Class I	Dyspnea only on rigorous exertion ("appropriate" dyspnea)
Class II	Able to keep pace with person of same age and build on level ground without breathlessness but not on inclines
Class III	Able to walk a mile at own pace without dyspnea but cannot keep pace on level ground with normal person
Class IV	Dyspnea present after walking about 100 yards on level ground or ascending one flight of stairs
Class V	Dyspnea on low-level activity or at rest

Source: Burton GG: Practical physical diagnosis in respiratory care. In Burton GG, Hodgkin JE, editors: Respiratory care: a guide to clinical practice, ed 2, Philadelphia, 1984, JB Lippincott.

TABLE 1-11 Causes of Dyspnea Related to Preferred Body Position

Type of Dyspnea	Clinical Correlations
Orthopnea (must sit up to breathe; often occurs at night as paroxysmal nocturnal dyspnea)	Congestive heart failure
Obstructive sleep apnea (periodically stops breathing, particularly when lying on back)	Obesity; obstructive sleep apnea syndromes
Emphysematous habitus	Chronic obstructive pulmonary disease
Platypnea	Pleural effusion; dyspnea associated with various body positions
Orthodeoxia	Pulmonary fibrosis; improvement in dyspnea when patient lies flat

From Burton GG: Patient assessment procedures. In Barnes TA, editor: Respiratory care practice, Chicago, 1990, Mosby.

give more medication. However, if the pain is still too great, additional medication may be given, if allowed within the physician's orders for pain management.

6. Interview the patient to assess the presence of dyspnea (code: IB1c) [difficulty: R, Ap, An]

Dyspnea is the patient's subjective feeling of shortness of breath (SOB) or labored breathing. This is normal after vigorous exercise but abnormal in a resting patient. Orthopnea is the condition in which a patient must sit erect or stand to breathe comfortably. Lying flat causes dyspnea.

Box 1-2 classifies the degrees of dyspnea, and Table 1-11 lists various kinds of dyspnea, including orthopnea. Only class I is normal dyspnea (on severe exertion). Classes II to V are progressively severe and limiting for the patient. Any orthopnea is abnormal, and the more the patient must sit up to breathe, the more limited the patient.

The following are examples of questions to ask in evaluating dyspnea:
1. "How far can you walk before you feel short of breath?"
2. "How many flights of stairs can you climb before you experience SOB?"
3. "How far can you walk when walking as fast as your spouse?"
4. "Is there anything you do that makes the SOB worse?"
5. "Is there anything you do that makes the SOB better?"
6. "How long does the SOB last after you stop to rest?"
7. "Is the SOB worse at any particular time of the day?"
8. "Is the SOB worse at any particular time of the year?"

The following are examples of questions to ask in evaluating orthopnea:
1. "Do you wake up at night with SOB?"
2. "Does your nighttime SOB get better after you sit up on the side of your bed or in a chair?"
3. "Do you get SOB when lying down to take a nap?"
4. "Do you use extra pillows behind your head and back to help you not get SOB at night or during a nap?"
5. "How many pillows do you need to keep you from getting SOB at night or when taking a nap?"

Dyspnea, like pain, is based on the patient's level of discomfort. Some patients may complain of dyspnea, whereas others may not. The therapist can get an impression of the patient's dyspnea by how many words can be spoken continuously. A patient with severe dyspnea cannot complete even a short sentence on a single breath.

7. Interview the patient to assess exercise tolerance (code: IB1c) [difficulty: R, Ap, An]

Exercise tolerance refers to how active a person can be before feeling the need to slow down or stop. A normal person at rest should feel no difficulty breathing. During vigorous exercise, a person should be aware that he or she is working harder than normal to breathe. This is to be expected. However, after recovering from exercise, the work of breathing should again be easy.

In a person with cardiopulmonary disease, *work of breathing* (WOB) refers to the patient's subjective feeling of how difficult it is to breathe during a given activity. Patients with acute or chronic lung disease often feel that they are breathing with some difficulty with little or no activity. Because this is a subjective feeling of the patient, it is helpful to have the patient quantify it. Ask the patient to rate his or her WOB on a 1-to-10 scale, with 1 being easy breathing and 10 being extremely difficult.

If bronchospasm or secretions have increased, the patient will tell you that his or her WOB has worsened. If medications such as bronchodilators or mucolytics are effective, the patient should feel that his or her breathing is easier. Because of this, the patient can exercise more vigorously.

The patient with chronic and severe cardiopulmonary disease may describe a very restricted and limited lifestyle. Extra O_2 may have only limited benefit. The patient with chronic, but moderate, cardiopulmonary disease can live a somewhat limited but full lifestyle. Extra O_2 may help greatly at times when the patient becomes short of breath. The otherwise healthy patient with an acute cardiopulmonary disease should describe a previously full and enjoyable lifestyle. Extra O_2 may be needed now, but it is hoped that it will not be needed upon recovery.

8. Interview the patient to assess activities of daily living (code: IB1f) [difficulty: R, Ap]

The following subject areas and questions can help the therapist to further determine the patient's exercise tolerance and activities of daily living:

a. Personal grooming
- Do you get short of breath when dressing?
- What is the most difficult part of dressing?
- Are you able to wash your hair regularly?
- (For men) Are you able to shave regularly?
- Does using extra O_2 help you to do these things without getting as short of breath?

b. In-home activities
- Can you go up and down stairs without getting short of breath?
- Can you walk through your home without getting short of breath?
- Can you cook and prepare nutritious meals?
- Does using extra O_2 help you do these things without getting as short of breath?

c. Out-of-home activities
- Can you go shopping without getting short of breath?
- What clubs, church, or other organizations do you attend regularly?
- Can you do yard or garden work?
- Do you have a pet dog that you walk through the neighborhood?
- Does using extra O_2 help you do these things without getting as short of breath?

9. Interview the patient to assess smoking history (code: IB1d) [difficulty: R, Ap]

Because COPD is caused by smoking tobacco, and asthma is exacerbated by tobacco smoke and other airborne irritants, it is important to interview the patient or the patient's family about the home environment. In addition, inhaling illegal substances, such as marijuana and crack cocaine, and "huffing" from household aerosol cleaning agents can cause lung injury. If patients are assured that their responses will be kept strictly confidential within the medical record, they may be more willing to discuss these topics. If the patient is taking addictive substances, the care plan must include ways to deal with any addiction-related issues. The following questions can be asked of an adult patient and family:
- Have you ever smoked? If yes, for how long? How many packs of cigarettes a day?

- Have you ever used chewing tobacco/snuff? If yes, for how long?
- Have you used illegal drugs? What have you used? For how long?

10. Interview the patient to assess environmental exposures (code: IA1e) [difficulty: R, Ap]

Second-hand smoke in the home and work-related airborne pollutants are the main inhaled toxins that can harm the lungs. The spouse of a smoker or child of smoking parents can suffer significant lung damage along with the smoker. Smoke may also trigger bronchospasm in an asthmatic patient. Inhaled asbestos, coal, silica and other industrial dusts can lead to interstitial lung diseases. Farmers who are exposed to moldy hay, silage, bird droppings, etc., can develop allergic alveolitis problems. Ask the patient about exposure to home and environmental toxins. If there has been exposure, ask about the duration of the exposure.

11. Interview the patient to assess sputum production (code: IB1c) [difficulty: R, Ap, An]
a. Time of maximal and minimal expectoration
Interview the patient to determine the following:

1. Time of maximal expectoration
Ask the patient, "When do you cough up the most? For example, is it in the morning, after eating spicy foods, after a breathing treatment, after smoking, work, or other exposure to dusts?"

2. Time of minimal expectoration
Ask the patient, "When do you cough up the least? For example, during certain nonallergic seasons of the year or after a breathing treatment?"

b. Quantity
Some practitioners prefer to know of a specific amount such as a teaspoon, tablespoon, 10 mL, and so on. Others prefer to use subjective measures, such as "a little" or "a lot." Interview the patient to determine the following:

1. How does the quantity of sputum relate to the times of maximal and minimal expectoration and the patient's lifestyle?
Ask the patient, "Is there anything you do that increases or decreases the amount you cough out?" For example, the patient states that he coughs up 20 mL after breathing treatments but can cough up nothing after eating a bowl of ice cream.

2. Does the amount coughed up change in a cyclical way?
Ask the patient, "Do you cough up the most in the mornings or at night? Is there a work or lifestyle habit that changes how much you cough up? Is there a seasonal allergic condition that influences your asthma and sputum production?"

c. Adhesiveness of the sputum

Interview the patient to determine the following:

1. *Are there times of the day or things that you do in the day that seem to result in your secretions becoming thicker or thinner?*

2. *Do your medications (like acetylcysteine [Mucomyst]) make the secretions easier to cough out?*

3. *Do some foods make your secretions easier to cough out?*

12. Interview the patient to assess learning needs (code: IB1g) [difficulty: R, Ap]

The patient's learning needs must be assessed before an attempt is made to teach the patient. This assessment should include the patient's literacy level/education level, culture/ethnicity, and preferred learning style. Based on this information, the respiratory therapist should next determine what the patient understands of his or her condition and what the patient needs to be taught. This assessment could take place in a hospital, long-term care facility, or the patient's home. The following should improve the educational outcome.

a. Age-appropriate teaching

The patient is taught based on his or her age and ability to understand. This is most important with small children. They commonly have these fears when hospitalized:

- Fear of abandonment (separation anxiety). Small children are afraid of being abandoned in the hospital by their parents.
- Fear of the unknown. Equipment and procedures must be explained so that the child will not be left to use his or her imagination.
- Fear of punishment. Children may imagine that their illness is a punishment for doing something wrong.
- Fear of bodily harm. Explain a procedure so that the child understands what is going to happen.
- Fear of death. Children who are sick but expected to recover need to understand that they will get better. It is all right for children to feel afraid. Talking about those feelings or fear of death should be encouraged.

b. Language-appropriate teaching

Use nonmedical terms whenever possible. The patient's native language must be used so that he or she will understand the situation. A translator may be needed.

c. Education level

Patients should be taught in a manner and at a level that is matched to their education and knowledge of their medical condition.

d. Prior disease knowledge

The patient should be taught, as needed, about his or her condition.

e. Medication knowledge

The patient should be taught, as needed, about his or her medication or medications, including how the medication is to be taken (e.g., metered-dose inhaler with spacer).

The patient and family must understand the therapeutic goals and how they are to be achieved. Effective teaching methods include the following:

1. Speak at the patient's and family's level of understanding. Medical language usually reserved for peer discussions is not understandable to people without a medical background, yet using overly simple explanations can be insulting to someone who is intelligent or well educated, or both. In either case, the important information will not be perceived as intended. Give the patient written instructions as needed.

2. Describe the procedure in steps rather than as a whole process from beginning to end. Demonstrate each step for the patient.

3. Frequently ask the patient and family whether they have any questions, and then answer them.

4. Have the patient and family explain back to you in their own words how they understand what you just described.

5. Have the patient and family demonstrate back to you all procedures and techniques.

6. Reteach anything that is misunderstood.

7. Retest the patient and family as needed.

8. Document in the patient's electronic medical record what has been instructed.

> **Exam Hint 1-6**
>
> Usually one question deals with patient or family teaching. This could involve assessing a patient's or family member's learning needs, developing a teaching plan, or assessing the patient's or family member's understanding of what was taught.

MODULE D

Use *observation* (inspection) to determine the patient's cardiopulmonary condition.

1. Identify the characteristics and patency of the airway (code: IB2b) [difficulty: R, Ap, An]

Look at the patient's facial area and throat for signs of a congenital defect or traumatic injury. See Chapter 12 for more discussion on airway management.

2. Evaluate the patient's general appearance (code: IB2a) [difficulty: R, Ap, An]

Start by quickly inspecting the patient from head to toe, including how he or she is dressed and found in the room.

Ideally, this is done without the patient knowing that he or she is being observed. The patient who does not have cardiopulmonary disease should be able to lie flat in bed or on either side without any breathing difficulty. The patient with one-sided lung disease may prefer to lie with the good side down. This might be the case with lobar pneumonia, pleurisy, or broken ribs. The patient with severe airway obstruction, as seen in asthma, bronchitis, or emphysema, tends to sit up in a chair or on the edge of the bed and use locked arms and shoulders for support. This enables the patient to use accessory muscles (Fig. 1-18). The patient with orthopnea will not want to lie down flat because of the resulting SOB. This is commonly seen in patients with congestive heart failure and pulmonary edema.

a. Determine if the patient is cyanotic

Cyanosis is an abnormal blue or ashen gray coloration of the skin and mucous membranes. It is most easily seen in lightly pigmented persons by looking at the lips and nail beds. It can be seen in darker pigmented people by looking at the inner portion of the lip, the inner portion of the lower eyelid, and the nail beds. Commonly, cyanosis is said to be caused by hypoxemia and that the more bluish a patient's color, the more hypoxemic he or she is. This often is the case, but cyanosis is not an accurate measurement of a patient's oxygenation. To be safe, a patient with cyanosis should have an arterial blood gas sample drawn for PaO_2 measurement or a pulse oximetry measurement performed to evaluate oxygenation.

b. Determine if the patient has muscle wasting

Muscle wasting is an abnormal condition of decreased muscle mass. Muscle wasting can be generalized or localized, depending on the underlying cause. The term *cachectic* refers to an emaciated patient whose arms and legs are thin; the shoulder, elbow, and knee joints are prominent and the ribs are clearly outlined by deep intercostal spaces. The following are examples of conditions in which muscle wasting is seen.

1. Chronic obstructive pulmonary disease

COPD (emphysema and bronchitis) often results in muscle wasting because the patient is using an unusually large number of calories through the act of breathing. In addition, these patients often do not eat well, because a full stomach restricts the movement of the diaphragm and worsens the WOB and SOB. Because of this, they frequently are malnourished or undernourished. In addition, patients with cystic fibrosis are usually thin. This is the result of malnourishment from the gastrointestinal problems that are part of the disease and their increased work of breathing.

2. Lung cancer

Lung cancer or other cancers usually result in a loss of muscle mass. This is because the growing tumor consumes

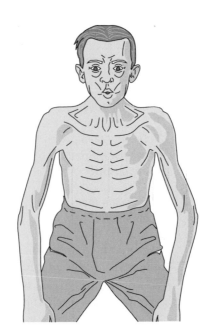

CLINICAL MANIFESTATIONS

- Use of accessory muscles to breathe
- Pursed-lip breathing
- Minimal or absent cough
- Leaning forward to breathe
- Barrel chest
- Digital clubbing
- Dyspnea on exertion (late sign)

A

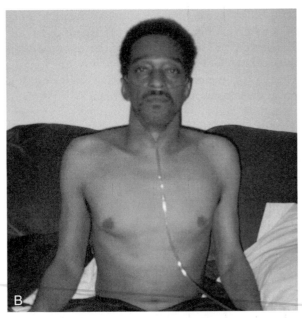

B

Figure 1-18 Typical posture seen in patients using accessory muscles of respiration. The shoulders are locked so that the accessory muscles can be used more effectively. **A,** Common clinical manifestations of a patient with COPD who is experiencing dyspnea. **B,** Patient wearing a nasal cannula and positioned to optimize the use of his accessory muscles of breathing. (Adapted from Burton GC, Hodgkin JE, editors: Respiratory care, ed 2, Philadelphia, 1984, Lippincott Williams & Wilkins.)

many calories that then are not available to the normal body tissues. These patients usually also have thin arms and legs with prominent joints in advanced disease.

3. Neurologic injuries

Neurologic injuries, such as transection of the spinal cord, result in atrophy of the affected muscles. Atrophy of the muscles is a decrease in size resulting from lack of use.

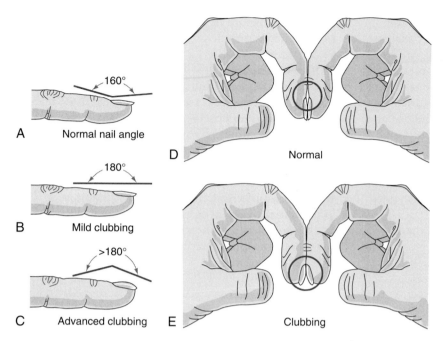

Figure 1-19 Clubbing. **A,** Normal fingernail angle is 160 degrees. **B,** Early mild clubbing appears as a flattened angle between nail and skin (180 degrees). **C,** Advanced clubbing shows a rounded (clubbed) fingertip and nail. To assess clubbing by Schamroth's diagnostic method **(D and E),** place the nails of the second digits together. Obliteration of the normal diamond-shaped space between the nails is an abnormal finding, signifying clubbing. (From Copstead LC, Banasik JL: Pathophysiology, ed 5, St Louis, 2013, Saunders.)

This is an unavoidable consequence of the permanent loss of nerve input to the affected muscles. For example, transection of the spinal cord at the first lumbar vertebra (L1) results in loss of nerve input to the legs. The patient is a paraplegic. In time, the muscles of the legs atrophy; however, if the arms are exercised, they retain normal muscle mass. If the patient has a spinal transection that results in the loss of nerve input to both the arms and the legs (quadriplegia), all of the limbs atrophy.

c. Determine if the patient is diaphoretic

Diaphoresis is profuse sweating. It normally is seen after vigorous exercise. A patient is expected to sweat after a stress test or even an oxygen-assisted walk. Diaphoresis in a patient who is resting in bed should be investigated. When the body is severely stressed, it releases adrenaline into the bloodstream. Diaphoresis is one of many bodily effects caused by the release of the hormone adrenaline. Similar sweating may be seen if a large enough dose of the drug epinephrine is given.

Diaphoresis is a nonspecific sign of serious cardiopulmonary difficulties. It may be seen any time the patient is in shock or hypoxemic. Patients with a myocardial infarct are commonly diaphoretic. The practitioner should promptly evaluate the diaphoretic patient's pulse, respiratory rate, blood pressure, and arterial blood gases.

d. Determine if the patient has digital clubbing

Clubbing of the fingers (also known as *digital clubbing*) is an abnormal thickening of the ends of the fingers. The condition can also occur in the toes. The key finding is an angle of more than 160 degrees between the top of the finger and the nail when seen from the side. Clinically, you will notice both a lateral and an AP thickening of the ends of the fingers (Fig. 1-19 shows a comparison of normal fingers and clubbed fingers). The fingernail and toenail beds may be cyanotic.

The underlying cause is not completely understood but at least in part seems to be chronic hypoxemia. This results in arteriovenous anastomosis with thickening of the tissues. The list of diseases in which clubbing is seen includes COPD, bronchogenic carcinoma, bronchiectasis, sarcoidosis, cystic fibrosis, and infective endocarditis.

e. Determine if the patient has edema

Edema is an abnormal accumulation of fluid in the interstitial spaces of the tissues and potential spaces of the body. Peripheral edema is seen when fluid leaks from the capillary bed into the tissues beneath the skin in the ankles and feet or along the back when the patient is lying supine in bed. The extent of the edema is measured by pressing a finger into the tissues. Normal skin springs back, whereas edematous skin is pitted or depressed. The pitting edema is graded as 1+ for less than ¼-in (mild), 2+ for ¼- to ½-in (moderate), and 3+ for ½- to 1-in (severe) indentation. Obviously, the deeper the pitting, the more peripheral edema the patient has.

Peripheral edema is most commonly seen in patients with congestive heart failure or cor pulmonale and those who have a fluid overload. Patients with septicemia often have peripheral edema because the blood-borne pathogen (usually *Staphylococcus*) causes abnormal capillary leakage.

Many patients with edema from heart failure also have excessive venous distention of the neck veins. The internal jugular vein and external/anterior jugular vein are observed in the normal patient by having him or her lie supine with the head elevated 30 degrees. The crest of the vein column should be seen just above the border of the midclavicle. Make a rough measure of the intravascular volume and CVP by pressing on the veins at the base of the neck. The returning blood should fill the veins and make them distend (Fig. 1-20). When the pressure is released, the veins should return to their previous level of distention just above the level of the midclavicle. Increased venous distention is noted when the veins stand out at a level above the clavicle. This is seen in patients with right-sided heart failure (cor pulmonale), cardiac tamponade, fluid overload, and COPD and when high airway pressures and positive end-expiratory pressure are needed for mechanical ventilation. The more the veins are distended, the more the patient is compromised.

It is not normal for the veins to collapse below the clavicle when the obstructing finger is removed. If this is seen, the patient should then have his or her head laid flat. Normally, when flat, the external jugular vein should be seen as partially distended. If the vein collapses on inspiration, low venous pressure is confirmed, and the patient probably is hypovolemic. This is commonly seen with dehydration, hemorrhage, or increased urine output after the use of diuretics.

A patient with heart failure also commonly has decreased capillary refill. Capillary refill is the time needed for blood to refill the capillary bed after it has been forced out. The procedure is to pinch the finger or toenail until it blanches and then release the pressure. The pink color of the nail bed should return in less than 3 seconds. Any delay in the return to pink color indicates reduced blood flow to the extremities. Cyanotic nail beds also are seen with reduced blood flow. Examples of conditions that result in decreased capillary refill include decreased cardiac output, low blood pressure from any cause, and the use of vasopressor medications.

f. Determine the patient's chest wall movement

Normal infants and adults have symmetrical chest movement when breathing at rest or during exercise. All breathing efforts are best observed when the patient is sitting up straight or standing erect and shirtless. Ideally, look at the patient from the front, back, and both sides to see the symmetry. In female patients, it may be necessary to observe only the uncovered back to judge chest movement. Any kind of asymmetrical chest movement is abnormal. The asymmetrical movement may result from an abnormality of the chest wall (kyphoscoliosis) or abdomen (enlarged liver) or from a pulmonary disorder (pneumothorax).

1. Thoracic scoliosis or kyphoscoliosis

Several variations on curvature of the spine are found. *Kyphosis* is an exaggerated AP curvature of the upper portion of the spine. *Lordosis* is an exaggerated AP curvature of the lower portion of the spine. Scoliosis is either a right or left lateral curvature of the spine. *Kyphoscoliosis* is either a right or left lateral curvature combined with an AP curvature of the spine.

Figure 1-21 shows the back view of a patient with thoracic scoliosis or kyphoscoliosis. The patient with scoliosis in Figure 1-21 tends to have more chest movement on the right side because of the right spinal curvature. The left side of the chest and left lung would inflate more than the right if the spine curved to the left. These same findings are seen in a patient with kyphoscoliosis.

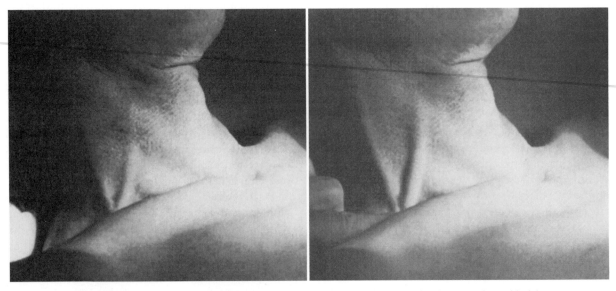

Figure 1-20 Evaluating distention of the external jugular vein. These photographs show a patient with right-sided heart failure. Note that the left photograph shows the external jugular vein distended above the level of the clavicle. The right photograph shows how pressing a finger over the external jugular vein results in its further filling with blood and distending. In a normal person, when the pressure is released, the vein collapses to just above the superior border of the midclavicle. See the text for further discussion. (From Daily EK, Schroder JS: Techniques in bedside hemodynamic monitoring, ed 5, St Louis, 1994, Mosby.)

2. Flail chest

The flail segment moves in the opposite direction from the rest of the chest (this is also known as *paradoxical movement*). That is, with inspiration, the flail segment moves inward while the rest of the chest moves outward, and during expiration, the flail segment moves outward as the rest of the chest moves inward. As the ribs heal, the segment stabilizes and moves with the rest of the chest.

3. Pneumothorax

The side with the collapsed lung does not move as much as the chest wall over the normal lung (see Fig. 1-5).

4. Atelectasis/pneumonia

The side with the atelectasis or pneumonia does not move as much as the chest wall over the normal lung (see Fig. 1-8).

Normally, an adult's diaphragm moves downward several centimeters toward the abdomen during inspiration as the chest wall moves outward. This is seen when the abdomen protrudes as its contents are forced forward.

The chest and abdomen should rise and fall together during quiet and vigorous breathing efforts. In two conditions, this normal chest and abdominal movement does not occur.

First, in patients with emphysema, severe air trapping, and a barrel chest, the diaphragm is depressed and flat rather than domed because of the air that is trapped in the lungs. On inspiration, the diaphragm still contracts, but it is unable to displace the abdominal contents downward to permit air to be drawn into the lungs. These patients do not have the expected abdominal movement during inspiration. They use the accessory muscles of inspiration to assist breathing.

Second, the normal movement does not occur in any condition in which airway resistance is increased or lung compliance is decreased. The greater negative intrathoracic pressure needed to draw the tidal volume into the lungs can cause the chest wall to collapse inward as the abdominal contents are displaced outward. The result is a kind of "seesaw" or paradoxical movement relation between the chest wall and the abdomen. On inspiration,

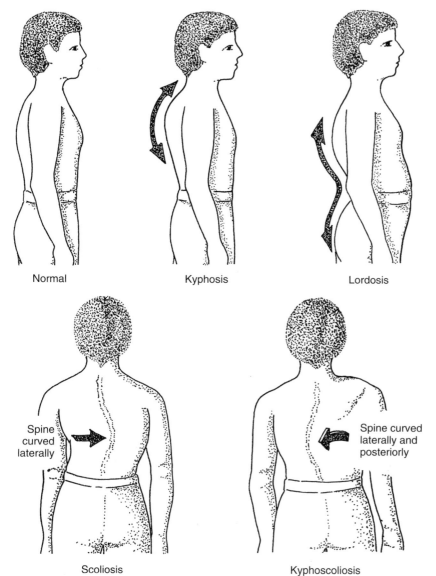

Normal   Kyphosis   Lordosis

Spine curved laterally

Spine curved laterally and posteriorly

Scoliosis   Kyphoscoliosis

Figure 1-21 Normal and abnormal spinal curves. The patient should sit or stand erect during examination.

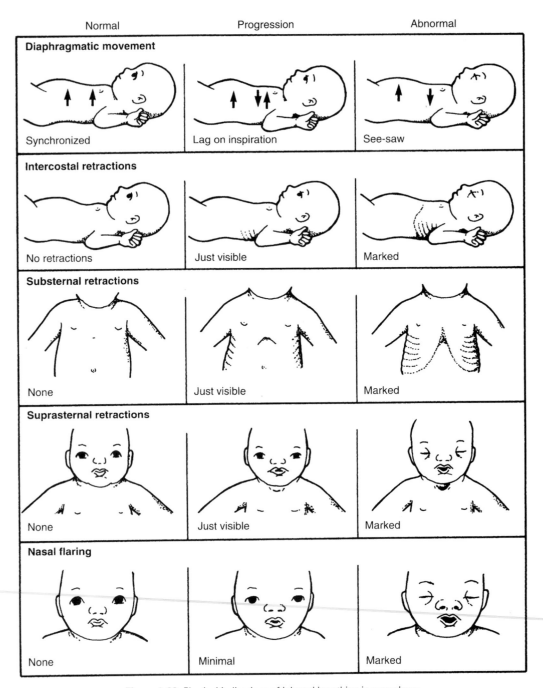

Normal	Progression	Abnormal

Diaphragmatic movement

Synchronized | Lag on inspiration | See-saw

Intercostal retractions

No retractions | Just visible | Marked

Substernal retractions

None | Just visible | Marked

Suprasternal retractions

None | Just visible | Marked

Nasal flaring

None | Minimal | Marked

Figure 1-22 Physical indications of labored breathing in a newborn.

the chest wall may move inward as the abdomen moves outward. Patients with RDS typically demonstrate this because the premature neonate's rib cage is relatively compliant compared with the stiff lungs (Fig. 1-22).

Exam Hint 1-7

Frequently a question relates to physical signs that a patient has a pneumothorax. This could include asymmetrical chest movement. The chest wall on the side with the pneumothorax will not move as much as the normal side during breathing.

g. Determine if the patient uses accessory muscles when breathing

Accessory muscles of respiration should not be needed during passive, resting breathing. They are normally used when a person is breathing vigorously during exercise. A dyspneic patient is likely to use accessory muscles even when resting. This indicates that the work of breathing is greatly increased. The primary accessory muscles of inspiration are the intercostal, scalene, sternocleidomastoid, trapezius, and rhomboid muscles. The abdominal muscles are used during active expiration. The easiest accessory muscles of inspiration to observe in action are

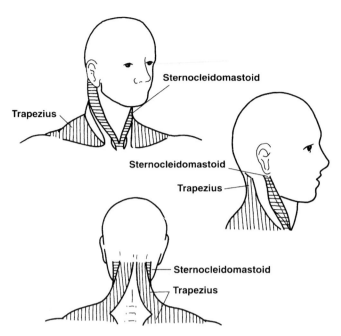

Figure 1-23 Sternocleidomastoid and trapezius accessory muscles of respiration.

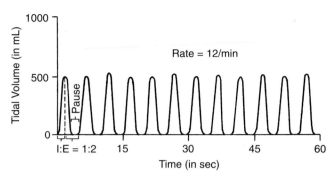

Figure 1-24 Eupnea. Pause is the time from the end of exhalation to the beginning of inspiration. *I*, Inspiratory time; *E*, expiratory time.

the sternocleidomastoids from the front and side of the patient and the trapezius from the back of the patient (Fig. 1-23). Their use is not specific for any one condition but is commonly seen in an adult patient with emphysema (see Fig. 1-18).

Contraction of the dilator nares muscles (so-called nasal flaring) during inspiration further opens the nasal passages. A person breathing comfortably should have little or no nasal flaring. A person who is exercising vigorously may show nasal flaring in an attempt to reduce airway resistance. Nasal flaring is abnormal in a patient resting in bed, and it is a sign of increased work of breathing, especially in a neonate. Examples of conditions in which nasal flaring is seen include RDS (see Fig. 1-22), acute respiratory distress syndrome (ARDS), and any condition in which pulmonary compliance is decreased or airway resistance is increased.

When a person with cardiopulmonary disease is using the inspiratory accessory muscles, intercostal or sternal retractions often are seen. A normal person breathing at rest should not have any retractions. That same person may have some minor retractions during vigorous exercise. Retractions of any kind are abnormal in any patient of any age who is resting in bed. Retractions are commonly seen in conditions in which airway resistance is increased or lung compliance is decreased. Both increase a patient's WOB. The patient must generate a more negative intrathoracic pressure to breathe, and as a result, the various soft tissues are drawn inward during inspiration.

Intercostal retractions are noticed when the soft tissues between the ribs are drawn inward during inspiration as the chest wall moves outward. Suprasternal retractions are noticed when the soft tissues *above* the sternum are drawn inward during an inspiration as the chest wall moves outward. Substernal retractions are noticed when the soft tissues *below* the sternum are drawn inward during an inspiration as the chest wall moves outward (see Fig. 1-22). Conditions in which retractions are seen include RDS, ARDS, pulmonary edema, pneumonia, asthma, bronchitis, and emphysema.

h. Determine the patient's breathing pattern (code: IB1a) [difficulty: ELE: R, Ap; WRE: An]

The various respiratory patterns can be identified by their characteristic respiratory rate, respiratory cycle, and tidal volume. Figure 1-24 shows a normal adult breathing pattern, and Figure 1-25 shows examples of normal and abnormal breathing patterns.

1. Eupnea (normal breathing)

1. Normal respiratory rate for the age of the patient (see Table 1-2)
2. Normal respiratory cycle. When timing the flow of air into and out of the lungs, the inspiratory/expiratory (I:E) ratio is about 1:2. A pause of variable time may follow exhalation of the tidal volume. This could change the true I:E ratio from 1:2 to 1:4
3. Tidal volume is normal for the size of the patient. (See Chapter 4 for calculation of a predicted tidal volume.) Inspiration is achieved without the use of accessory muscles of inspiration; exhalation is passive
4. A person usually sighs every few minutes; especially when inactive. A sigh breath typically is about 1.5 times as large as a tidal volume. It is thought to help prevent atelectasis. Frequent sighing may indicate a problem

2. Hypopnea (shallow breathing)

1. Respiratory rate usually somewhat slower than normal
2. Normal respiratory cycle
3. Tidal volume decreased for the size of the patient
4. Possible causes: deep sleep, sedation, coma, hypothermia, alkalosis, restrictive lung disease
5. May be combined with bradypnea

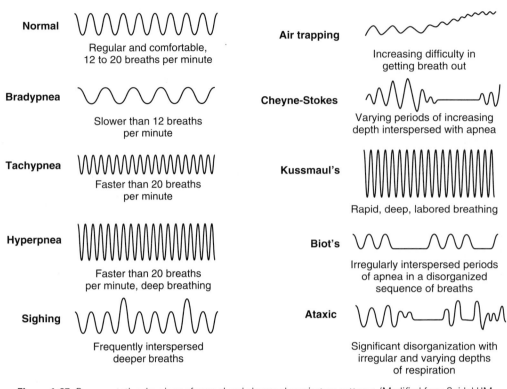

Normal
Regular and comfortable,
12 to 20 breaths per minute

Bradypnea
Slower than 12 breaths
per minute

Tachypnea
Faster than 20 breaths
per minute

Hyperpnea
Faster than 20 breaths
per minute, deep breathing

Sighing
Frequently interspersed
deeper breaths

Air trapping
Increasing difficulty in
getting breath out

Cheyne-Stokes
Varying periods of increasing
depth interspersed with apnea

Kussmaul's
Rapid, deep, labored breathing

Biot's
Irregularly interspersed periods
of apnea in a disorganized
sequence of breaths

Ataxic
Significant disorganization with
irregular and varying depths
of respiration

Figure 1-25 Representative drawings of normal and abnormal respiratory patterns. (Modified from Seidel HM, Ball JW, Dains JE, et al.: Mosby's guide to physical examination, ed 6, St Louis, 2006, Mosby.)

3. Hyperpnea (deep breathing)

1. Respiratory rate may be normal or somewhat faster
2. Normal respiratory cycle
3. Tidal volume increased for the size of the patient
4. Possible causes: acidosis, fever, pain, fear, anxiety, increased intracranial pressure
5. May be combined with tachypnea

4. Bradypnea (slow breathing)

1. Slower than normal respiratory rate
2. Expiration may be longer than normal as a result of a longer pause
3. Tidal volume may be decreased for the size of the patient
4. Possible causes: deep sleep, sedation, coma, hypothermia, alkalosis
5. May be combined with hypopnea

5. Tachypnea (rapid breathing)

1. Faster than the normal respiratory rate
2. Inspiration may be faster than normal with the help of inspiratory accessory muscles. Expiration may be shorter than normal, and expiratory accessory muscles may be used to force the air out faster. The pause seen in eupnea is absent. The I:E ratio may be 1:2 or less
3. Tidal volume may be increased for the size of the patient
4. Possible causes: acidosis, fever, pain, anxiety, increased intracranial pressure
5. May be combined with hyperpnea

6. Obstructed inspiration

1. Normal to slower respiratory rate
2. Inspiratory time is equal to or longer than expiratory time. Inspiration is aided by use of the inspiratory accessory muscles. Expiration is passive
3. Tidal volume may be normal or larger or smaller than normal, depending on how the patient adapts to the increased work of breathing. A slower rate most commonly is seen with a larger tidal volume
4. Possible causes: croup, epiglottitis, foreign body aspiration with partial airway obstruction, postextubation laryngeal edema, airway tumor, or airway trauma

7. Obstructed expiration with or without air trapping

1. Normal to slower respiratory rate
2. Expiratory time is longer than normal. Accessory muscles of inspiration and expiration may be used
3. Tidal volume may be normal or decreased for the size of the patient
4. Possible causes: asthma, emphysema, bronchitis, cystic fibrosis, bronchiectasis, airway tumor, or airway trauma. In severe cases, such as status asthmaticus, incomplete exhalation may cause air trapping

8. Kussmaul's respiration (rapid, large breaths)

1. Faster than normal rate
2. I:E ratio approaches 1:1. Both inspiratory and expiratory accessory muscles may be used

3. Tidal volume is increased for the size of the patient
4. Probable cause: acidosis (pH 7.2 to 6.95) from diabetic ketoacidosis

9. Cheyne-Stokes respiration (waxing and waning tidal volumes)

1. The respiratory rate varies from normal to faster and may include short periods of apnea
2. The respiratory cycle is normal or approximates it, except if the patient has periods of apnea
3. The tidal volumes increase and decrease over a variable time cycle. A 20-second cycle is fairly common. Periods of apnea may occur between the decreased tidal volumes
4. Possible causes: head injury, stroke, increased intracranial pressure, or congestive heart failure

10. Biot's respiration (unpredictably variable)

1. The respiratory rate may be slow with deep breaths or rapid with shallow breaths; sighing is common. Periods of apnea occur between the periods of breathing
2. The respiratory cycle varies considerably, with periods of apnea
3. Tidal volume may be larger or smaller than normal
4. Possible causes: meningitis, head (brain) injury, brain tumor, increased intracranial pressure

11. Ataxic respiration (unpredictably variable)

1. The respiratory rate varies considerably, with abrupt periods of apnea
2. The respiratory cycle varies considerably, with periods of apnea
3. Tidal volume varies unpredictably between larger and smaller than normal
4. Possible causes: lesion of the medullary respiratory centers, head (brain) injury, brain tumor, increased intracranial pressure

12. Apnea (cessation of breathing at the end of exhalation)

1. Apnea that lasts long enough to result in hypoxemia, bradycardia, and hypotension must be treated aggressively. Artificial respiration, with or without supplemental oxygen, must be started immediately
2. It is important to evaluate the patient's previous breathing pattern to determine the cause of the apnea. Normal breathing followed by apnea could result from a heart attack, stroke, or upper airway obstruction. An abnormal breathing pattern followed by apnea could be the result of worsening of the original problem
3. Evaluate the previous tidal volume variation for the reasons previously listed
4. Possible causes: airway obstruction, heart attack, stroke, or head (brain) injury

3. Determine the kind of cough the patient has (code: IB2c) [difficulty: R, Ap, An]

a. Normal cough

A normal cough has four parts:
1. The person takes a deep breath.
2. The epiglottis and vocal cords close to keep the air trapped within the lungs.
3. The abdominal and other expiratory muscles contract to increase the air pressure in the lungs.
4. The epiglottis and vocal cords open to allow the compressed air to escape explosively and remove any mucus or foreign matter.

All components must work individually and in a coordinated manner for the patient to have an effective cough. The following are possible variations used by patients who for some reason cannot cough normally.

b. Serial cough

All actions of a normal cough take place, except that the patient performs a series of smaller coughs rather than a single large one. This method of coughing may be used by postoperative patients who have too much abdominal or thoracic pain to cough normally. As the pain lessens, the patient should be able to cough normally.

c. Midinspiratory cough

All actions of a normal cough take place, except that the patient does not take as deep a breath. This midinspiratory cough can also be called a *huff cough*. Patients with emphysema and chronic bronchitis (COPD) sometimes use this to help prevent airway collapse when they cough.

A midinspiratory/huff cough also is used by patients with artificial airways. Because they cannot close the epiglottis and vocal cords, they can only take a large breath and blow out with as much force as possible. This can be an effective way to remove watery secretions.

d. Huff cough

Patients with artificial airways use this method. They cannot close the epiglottis and vocal cords; therefore they can only take a large breath and blow out with as much force as possible. This still is an effective way to remove watery secretions.

e. Assisted cough

This patient needs direct help from the therapist. The patient is given a deep breath by means of an intermittent positive-pressure breathing machine or manual ventilator. The therapist then helps the patient blow the air out quickly by pushing on the abdominal area to move the diaphragm up. This procedure is limited to conscious patients with neuromuscular defects who cannot cough effectively on their own. See Chapter 10 for a more complete discussion on normal cough and alternate coughing techniques.

4. Determine the quantity and characteristics of the patient's sputum (code: IB2c) [difficulty: R, Ap, An]

a. Quantity

Normally, a person is not aware of mucus production. The mucociliary escalator moves mucus toward the throat, where it is unconsciously swallowed. Normally mucus is uninfected and clear or white.

Typically, infections causing bronchitis or pneumonia result in the production of large amounts of mucus. The patient reports coughing and "spitting up." This mixture of mucus from the lungs and saliva from the mouth is called *sputum*. Any increase in mucus or sputum production, to the extent that the patient is aware of it, is abnormal.

As mentioned earlier, some practitioners prefer to use subjective measurements of sputum production, such as "a little," "a medium amount," or "copious." Objective measurements, such as a teaspoon, a tablespoon, or 5, 10, or 15 mL, for example, are preferred to quantify production. A marked measuring cup is needed to do this.

Note any changes in the amount of sputum the patient produces. This is best done in a timed manner, such as production per hour or per shift. It also is wise to correlate sputum production with breathing treatments or other procedures that may increase or decrease its production or clearance.

b. Characteristics

Homogeneity is best determined by letting a sputum sample stand in a test tube for several hours so that it stratifies. This is an important test to perform in a patient with a pulmonary infection or bronchiectasis. Normal sputum separates into a relatively thin surface layer of gel that floats on a lower layer of water (sol). The patient with a pulmonary infection or bronchiectasis has more viscous sputum because it contains dead bacterial cells, dead WBCs, and cellular debris from the infected lung tissues. These cells settle over time to the bottom of a sputum sample and create a third layer of sediment. Figure 1-26 shows how this layering looks in the sputum from a patient who has a pulmonary infection that eventually clears up. Table 1-12 explains other details of sputum characteristics.

Exam Hint 1-8

Usually one question requires the therapist to evaluate the patient's sputum. Examples: (1) a change from white or yellow to green indicates pneumonia; (2) a lung abscess is likely when the sputum is green and foul smelling; and (3) pink-tinged, bubbly (frothy) secretions are found with pulmonary edema.

MODULE E

Use *palpation* to determine the patient's respiratory condition.

1. Determine the patient's pulse rate, rhythm, and force (code: IB3a) [difficulty: R, Ap, An]

The HR is most commonly counted by palpating the following locations: carotid, femoral, radial, and brachial arteries and apical pulse of the heart (Fig. 1-27). The apical pulse normally is located in the area of the left midclavicular line in the fifth intercostal space. The apical pulse is

Infection

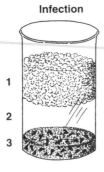

Improvement

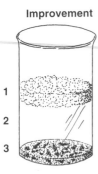

Normal

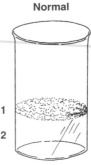

1. Gel layer: thicker than normal

2. Sol layer: thinner in ratio to gel layer than normal

3. Cellular debris: dead bacteria, WBCs, other cells

NOTE: The total volume of sputum is greatly increased

1. Gel layer: reducing toward normal

2. Sol layer: returning to normal ratio with gel layer

3. Cellular debris: thinning out as fewer dead cells are being coughed out

1. Gel layer: normal volume

2. Sol layer: normal volume and ratio with the gel layer

NOTE: The total volume of sputum is reduced to normal; also, there is no third layer of cellular debris

Figure 1-26 Evaluation of the homogeneity of sputum in the infected patient.

also known as the point of maximal impulse. The location indicates the apex of the heart (left ventricle). Other arterial sites, such as the temporal, dorsalis pedis, and posterior tibial, can be used but are more difficult to find. The pulse should be counted for a minimum of 30 seconds; counting for 1 minute provides the most accurate measure of HR.

Palpating a pulse at any of the aforementioned sites reveals the timing between the heartbeats. This rhythm is normally regular in people who are at rest or exercising at a steady level. The rhythm is felt and mentally timed as the pulse rate is counted. The period between beats should be about the same.

The respiratory effort may have some influence on the rhythm. Fairly common in children and sometimes in adults, the heart rhythm and rate increase on inspiration and decrease on expiration. This sinus arrhythmia is not really abnormal. It is caused when the negative intrathoracic pressure during inspiration draws blood more quickly into the thorax and heart. The opposite may be true during mechanical ventilation with a high peak pressure or mean airway pressure. Then the heart rhythm and rate may slow during inspiration and speed up during expiration. In any other case, an irregular rhythm indicates some sort of cardiac problem. An electrocardiogram is needed to help determine the specific cause.

TABLE 1-12	Sputum Characteristics			
Sputum Type	**Color**	**Contents**	**Illnesses**	**Odor**
Bloody (hemoptysis)	Red	Blood	Bronchogenic carcinoma; pulmonary hemorrhage; lung abscess; tuberculosis; pulmonary infarction	Typically none
Frothy or bubbly	Clear or pink	Water; plasma proteins; red blood cells	Pulmonary edema	Typically none
Mucoid	Clear or white	Water; complex sugars; glycoproteins; some cellular debris	Asthma; chronic bronchitis	Typically none
Mucopurulent	Light to medium yellow	Decreased water and complex sugars; increased cellular debris and causative organisms (if applicable); organisms are usually aerobes	Chronic and acute bronchitis	Typically none but may exist, depending on organism
Purulent	Dark yellow or green	Decreased water; greatly increased cellular debris and causative organisms (usually aerobes); complex sugars	Bronchiectasis; lung abscess; pneumonia	Depending on organism, along with clearance of mucus; also may be foul tasting to the patient; odor usually not offensive
Purulent (fetid)	Dark yellow or green	Decreased water; may contain some blood; greatly exaggerated cellular debris and causative organisms (frequently anaerobes); complex sugars	Bronchiectasis; lung abscess; cystic fibrosis	Offensive odor

From DiPietro JS: Clinical guide for respiratory care and cardiopulmonary disease, Acton, 1998, Copley Custom Publishing.

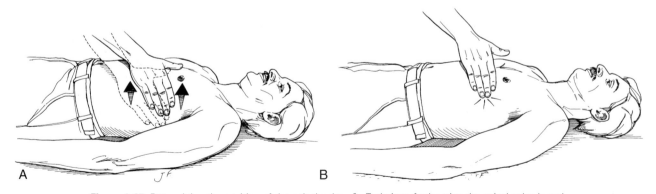

Figure 1-27 Determining the position of the apical pulse. **A,** Technique for locating the apical pulse by palpation. **B,** The apical pulse is the strongest pulse felt through the chest wall. (From Eubanks DH, Bone RC: Comprehensive respiratory care, ed 2, St Louis, 1990, Mosby.)

The force of the pulse is an indicator of the strength of the heart's contraction and BP. Normally each heartbeat should be felt with the same amount of force. A "thready" or variable force felt with each heartbeat is usually a sign of heart disease. Atrial fibrillation is an example of an irregular heart rhythm that results in an irregular force. The irregular rate and rhythm cause variable volumes of blood to be pumped with each contraction. A large volume of blood is felt as a strong pulse, whereas a small volume of blood is felt as a weak pulse.

A "bounding" or greater than normal force felt with each beat is usually a sign of hypertension. In either case, for safety's sake, the BP should be measured and compared with the patient's previous BP to see if a change has occurred.

2. Determine if there is accessory muscle activity (code: IB3b) [difficulty: R, Ap, An]

Review the above discussion on observing a patient for accessory muscle activity. See Figure 1-23 for the location of the trapezius and sternocleidomastoid muscles that can be palpated for accessory muscle use.

3. Determine if the patient has asymmetrical chest movements (code: IB3c) [difficulty: R, Ap, An]

Normally the lungs and chest move together in symmetry throughout the respiratory cycle. Asymmetrical chest wall movement during inspiration indicates a lung or chest wall problem. If the patient does not have an abnormal chest wall configuration, the problem has to be in the lungs. Less air is getting into the affected lung area or areas; therefore the chest wall does not move out as far as the chest wall over the normal lung. This is a nonspecific finding of lung disease but is also seen in pneumonia, bronchial or lung tumor, and pneumothorax.

The therapist's hands should be placed over the patient's chest to assess for asymmetrical chest movement (Fig. 1-28). The thumbs should touch at the end of expiration. The patient then is instructed to breathe in deeply as the therapist looks and feels for asymmetrical movement.

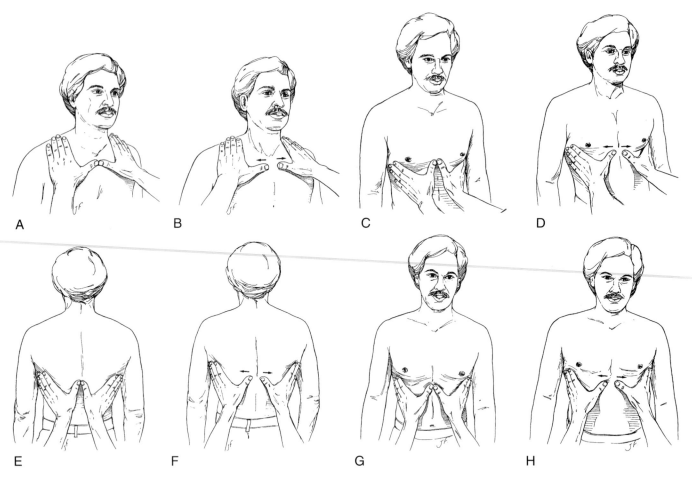

Figure 1-28 Palpation to assess symmetrical chest movement. **A,** Hand position over the apical lobes during expiration. **B,** Apical movement during inspiration. **C,** Hand position over the middle and lower lobes during expiration. **D,** Middle and lower lobe movement during inspiration. **E,** Hand position over the posterior middle lobes during expiration. **F,** Movement of the posterior middle lobes during inspiration. **G,** Hand position to check for movement of the costal margins during expiration. **H,** Costal movement during inspiration. (From Eubanks DH, Bone RC: Comprehensive respiratory care, ed 2, St Louis, 1990, Mosby.)

In Figure 1-28, A and B show the movement of the anterior apical lobes, C and D show the movement of the anterior middle and lower lobes, E and F show the movement in the posterior lower lobes, and G and H show the movement of the costal margins.

4. Determine if the patient has tactile fremitus (code: IB3c) [difficulty: R, Ap, An]

Tactile fremitus is a vibration felt through the chest wall when the patient speaks. Normally, when a sound is created in the larynx, its vibration is carried throughout the tracheobronchial tree to the lung parenchyma and to the chest wall. The intensity of the vibration or its absence gives the practitioner important information about the patient's condition.

Figure 1-29 shows various methods of detecting tactile fremitus. Some practitioners may prefer to use their fingertips, as in A and B, whereas others prefer the ulnar edge of the open or closed hand, as in C and D. The practitioner should feel all areas of the patient's chest for tactile fremitus to detect any variations and should touch the chest over both lung fields to compare their symmetry as well as anterior and posterior differences

(see Fig. 1-29, E and F). Figure 1-30 shows the posterior and anterior locations for the evaluation of tactile fremitus. Start with the supraclavicular fossae and proceed to alternate intercostal spaces. An attempt must be made to preserve the adult female patient's modesty when evaluating the anterior locations. The patient may be asked to lift the breast so that the examiner can palpate beneath it.

The procedure for evaluating tactile fremitus is to have the patient say "99" in a normal voice as the practitioner's fingers or hands are moved from location to location. This procedure is also called *palpation for bronchophony*. The "99" should be spoken at least once for each location to determine any variations. Having the patient speak more loudly or deeply should increase the intensity of the vibrations felt. The intensity of the vibrations directly relates to the density of the underlying lung and chest cavity. Conditions that increase density result in more intense vibrations. Conversely, conditions that decrease density result in less-intense vibrations. Vibrations also are reduced when they are blocked from penetrating through to the surface. Table 1-13 presents conditions that alter tactile fremitus.

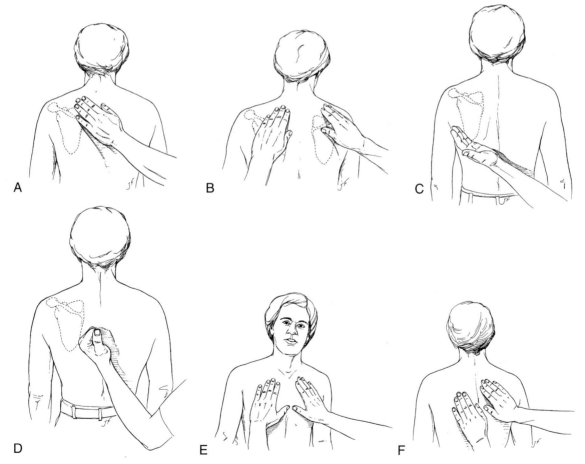

Figure 1-29 A-D, Techniques for detecting tactile fremitus. **E** and **F,** Anterior and posterior placement of the hands to detect tactile fremitus. (From Eubanks DH, Bone RC: Comprehensive respiratory care, ed 2, St Louis, 1990, Mosby.)

5. Determine if the patient has rhonchial fremitus, indicating secretions in the airway (code: IB3c) [difficulty: R, Ap, An]

Rhonchial fremitus, also known as *palpable rhonchi*, is a type of tactile fremitus noticed when vibrations from airway secretions can be felt through the chest wall as the patient breathes. They are abnormal because they indicate that the patient has a significant secretion problem. Palpable rhonchi are not detected in a patient with clear airways. Having the patient cough or suctioning the airway to remove secretions results in the reduction or complete elimination of palpable rhonchi. Remember that an airway that is completely occluded by a mucous plug or foreign body will *not* reveal palpable rhonchi, because no airflow is present. Breath sounds also are absent in this area.

Various methods are available for detecting palpable rhonchi. Some therapists may prefer to use their fingertips, whereas others prefer to use the edge of the open or closed hand. It is important to assess all areas of the patient's chest to detect the exact location or locations of the secretions.

6. Determine if the patient has crepitus (code: IB3c) [difficulty: R, Ap, An]

Crepitus (or crepitation) is the sound heard when an area with subcutaneous emphysema is gently pressed. The dry crackling-like sound resembles that of the breakfast cereal Rice Krispies in milk. A stethoscope can be used to help focus the sound to the exact location. In extreme instances, the unaided ear can detect the sound. As the fingers of one hand are sequentially pressed into the affected area, the subcutaneous air is felt to move away from the pressure points.

Subcutaneous emphysema is air under the skin that has leaked from a pneumothorax. The skin appears puffy or edematous; this is most commonly seen in the tissues on the side of the pneumothorax. The pressurized air dissects through the tissues, following the path of least resistance, and is most likely found under the skin in the axilla, neck, chest wall, and breast. In extreme cases, air is found under the skin throughout the body.

Although not dangerous, crepitus is a serious finding because it indicates that the patient has a pulmonary air leak. It may be accompanied by pneumothorax, pneumomediastinum, or pulmonary interstitial emphysema. A chest radiographic examination should be done immediately if the crepitation is a new finding.

7. Determine if the patient has any tracheal deviation (code: IB3c) [difficulty: R, Ap, An]

Normally the trachea is in a midline position within the neck and thorax. The location of the trachea is found by having the patient look straight ahead and gently inserting the index finger into the suprasternal notch of an upright or supine patient (Fig. 1-31). The trachea should be detected in the midline, with soft tissues on both sides. A trachea that is shifted off to one side is abnormal and can be caused by the following (see Fig. 1-8):

- Atelectasis, which causes the trachea to be pulled *toward* the affected side
- Pulmonary fibrosis, which causes the trachea to be pulled *toward* the most affected side
- Tension pneumothorax, which causes the trachea to be pushed *away* from the affected side
- Hemothorax, pleural effusion, and empyema, which push the trachea *away* from the affected side

Correction of the underlying pulmonary problem results in the trachea returning to its normal midline position.

TABLE 1-13	Abnormal Tactile Fremitus	
Increased		**Decreased**
Unilateral		
Pneumonia		Pneumothorax
Atelectasis		Pleural effusion
Consolidation		Bronchial obstruction
Bilateral		
Pulmonary edema		Thick chest wall (fat or muscle)
Acute respiratory distress syndrome		Chronic obstructive pulmonary disease

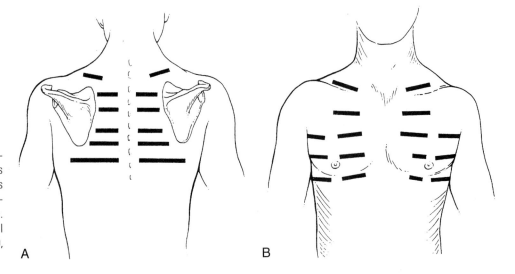

Figure 1-30 A, Locations on the posterior chest for detecting tactile fremitus and performing percussion. **B,** Locations on the anterior chest for detecting tactile fremitus and performing percussion. (From Swartz MH: Textbook of physical diagnosis, ed 6, Philadelphia, 2010, Saunders.)

A   B

8. Determine if the patient has any tenderness (code: IB3c) [difficulty: R, Ap, An]

Tenderness is an increased local sensation of pain when the chest is gently hit with the ulnar area of the fist. This tapping is done in a symmetrical pattern over the posterior and anterior lung areas and normally should not cause any pain. Intercostal tenderness is felt at the site of an inflamed pleura. Local tenderness and a history of trauma to an area of the chest lead to the conclusion of musculoskeletal pain. A chest radiograph might be indicated to determine whether any ribs have been fractured. The absence of chest wall tenderness should lead to a further investigation as to the cause of the chest pain. Consider angina pectoris (hypoxic heart pain).

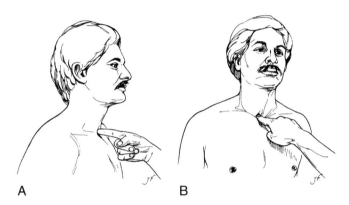

A　　　　　　　**B**

Figure 1-31 A and **B,** Detecting the position of the trachea by pressing the index finger into the suprasternal notch. From Eubanks DH, Bone RC: Comprehensive respiratory care, ed 2, St Louis, 1990, Mosby.

MODULE F

Use *auscultation* to determine the patient's respiratory condition.

1. Auscultate to assess breath sounds (code: IB5a) [difficulty: R, Ap, An]

a. Determine if the patient has bilaterally normal breath sounds

There are three types of normal breath sounds (Fig. 1-32):
1. *Normal breath sounds are also called vesicular.* These normal breath sounds are heard over all areas of normally ventilated lungs. Normal breath sounds have been variously described as "leaves rustling" or "like a gentle breeze." These faint sounds are made as air is moved through the small airways of the lungs during the breathing cycle. The inspiratory to expiratory (I:E) ratio is *heard* at about 3:1. (Do not confuse this with the *observed* I:E ratio of about 1:2.) The inspiratory sound is louder than the expiratory sound, and there is no pause between inspiration and expiration.
2. *Bronchial breath sounds are also called tracheal.* These normal breath sounds are heard over the trachea. Bronchial breath sounds have been described as being louder, harsher, and higher pitched than normal. They have a fairly uniform pitch on inspiration and expiration, with a distinct pause in the transition of flow. The I:E ratio is about 1:1.5.
3. *Bronchovesicular sounds are a cross between bronchial and vesicular.* Bronchovesicular sounds are more muffled

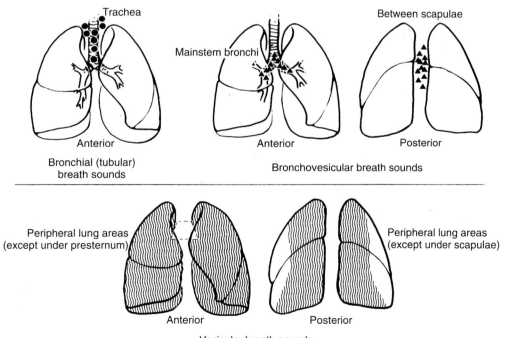

Figure 1-32 Breath sounds heard over the normal chest. (From Lehrer S: Understanding lung sounds, Philadelphia, 1984, Saunders.)

than bronchial but louder than vesicular and have the same pitch throughout inspiration and expiration. They are normally heard over the mainstem bronchi. The I:E ratio is about 1:1.

Bronchial and bronchovesicular breath sounds are abnormal if heard in any other areas except those mentioned here. When these sounds are heard over areas that should be normal vesicular, it is a sign of consolidation or atelectasis with a patent airway.

b. Determine if the patient has abnormal breath sounds

The term *adventitious* is used collectively to describe all types of abnormal breath sounds.

The following discussion is limited to variations in normal vesicular breath sounds. The abnormal presentation of bronchial and bronchovesicular breath sounds was discussed earlier.

1. Increased vesicular breath sounds

a. Found most often in children and in debilitated adults because their thinner chest walls transmit the sounds better.
b. Increased breath sounds are commonly described as harsh.

2. Decreased vesicular breath sounds

a. Most commonly caused by a pleural effusion, hemothorax, or empyema because of fluid between the lung and the stethoscope (see Fig. 1-8, D).
b. Pulmonary fibrosis resulting from decreased airflow (see Fig. 1-8, B).
c. Emphysema resulting from decreased airflow.
d. Pleural thickening resulting from dampening from the thicker pleural tissues.

Exam Hint 1-9

Remember that when an intubated patient has breath sounds from the right lung but breath sounds are absent from the left lung, the endotracheal tube has been placed into the right mainstem bronchus.

---

3. Greatly decreased or absent vesicular breath sounds

a. Pneumothorax caused by the lung being forced away from the chest wall (see Fig. 1-8, C).
b. Severe atelectasis (see Fig. 1-8, A) or severe bronchospasm that results from little or no air moving into the alveoli.
c. Endotracheal tube placement into a bronchus instead of the trachea. In this case, the right bronchus is most commonly intubated; therefore the breath sounds are absent over the left lung.
d. Large pleural effusion.
e. Obese patient.

Exam Hint 1-10

Expect to see at least one question that deals with identifying the presence of abnormal breath sounds. With proper treatment of the underlying problem, breath sounds should return to normal.

4. Unequal vesicular breath sounds

a. Pneumonia, consolidation, or atelectasis that decreases airflow into a segment or lobe.
b. Foreign body or tumor in a bronchus that decreases airflow to the distal lung.
c. Spinal or thoracic deformity that reduces airflow to the underlying lung.

5. Wheezing

Wheezing (also known as *wheeze* and *rhonchi*) has the following features or characteristics:
- They are continuous sounds.
- They are more commonly heard on expiration than inspiration.
- Low-pitched, polyphonic expiratory wheezing is commonly associated with secretions in the airways. A common term for these sounds is *rhonchi*. Common pulmonary conditions include bronchitis, pneumonia, or any other secretion-causing problem. Coughing or tracheal suctioning often causes these sounds to be modified or eliminated.
- High-pitched, *monophonic* expiratory sounds are commonly associated with closure of one large airway. This is commonly found with an airway tumor.
- High-pitched, *polyphonic* expiratory sounds are commonly associated with closure of many small airways. The term *wheeze* is commonly used to describe these sounds caused by bronchospasm in an asthmatic patient. Coughing or tracheal suctioning is unlikely to eliminate these high-pitched sounds. Effective treatment with bronchodilating medications should make the wheezing diminish and vesicular sounds return.

6. Crackles (rales)

Crackles have the following features or characteristics:
- They are more commonly heard on inspiration than on expiration.
- During inspiration, crackles are discontinuous popping sounds.
- They may be caused by the sudden opening of collapsed airways. Early inspiratory crackles are heard in patients with obstructive lung diseases such as chronic bronchitis, bronchiectasis, asthma, and emphysema. Late inspiratory crackles are heard in patients with atelectasis, pneumonia, pulmonary edema, or fibrosis.
- During expiration, crackles are caused by air passing through secretions. They are heard as gurgling or bubbling sounds during the same phase of the respiratory cycle.

7. Stridor

Stridor is heard as a harsh, monophonic, high-pitched inspiratory sound over the larynx. (It is not the normal tracheal sound.) It has these features or characteristics:

- Stridor can often be heard without a stethoscope.
- Common pediatric conditions include acute epiglottitis, laryngotracheobronchitis (croup), and laryngomalacia (congenital stridor).
- Common adult conditions include postextubation laryngeal edema and a laryngeal tumor.
- When stridor is heard on inspiration and expiration, it commonly is caused by an aspirated foreign body, tracheal stenosis, or a laryngeal tumor.

8. Friction rub

A friction rub (also known as a *pleural* friction rub) is the sound caused by the rubbing together of the inflamed and adherent visceral and parietal pleura, as seen in pleurisy. It is heard through a stethoscope and is described as loud and grating, clicking, or the creaking of old leather. The inspiratory sound frequently is reversed from the expiratory sound as the pleural tissues rub against each other in the opposite direction.

A friction rub is heard most commonly over the lower lung areas. Commonly, the sound is found at the site where the patient complains of pleural pain on breathing. Coughing and suctioning do not affect it. The causes include pulmonary infarct or any pneumonia that leads to an abscess or empyema.

Exam Hint 1-11

Expect at least one question concerning the interpretation of breath sounds or identifying a situation that might cause an abnormal breath sound. Examples include (1) absent breath sounds over an area of pneumothorax; (2) absent breath sounds over the left lung when an endotracheal tube has been misplaced into the right mainstem bronchus; (3) stridor over the larynx of a patient with epiglottitis or laryngeal edema (remember that severe stridor is a respiratory emergency, because the airway may rapidly close completely; nebulized racemic epinephrine may be given, but if there is no improvement, the patient usually is intubated to provide a secure airway); (4) wheezing in a patient with asthma. A patient with bronchospasm and good airflow will have loud wheezes. In this patient, effective medication treatment results in bronchodilation, less wheezing, and clinical improvement. However, understand that ineffective medication treatment results in less airflow. Less wheezing will be heard and the patient's condition will worsen.

---

c. Auscultate to assess heart sounds (code: IB5b) [difficulty: R, Ap, An]

The patient's heart rate and rhythm can easily be determined by listening at the point of the apical pulse (see Fig. 1-27). Heart sounds are caused by the closing of the four heart valves during a cardiac cycle. The first heart sound, S_1, is heard as a "lub" sound when the mitral (bicuspid) and tricuspid valves close after the ventricles contract during systole. The second heart sound, S_2, is heard as a "dup" or "dub" sound when the pulmonary semilunar and aortic valves close after the ventricles relax during diastole. Obviously, if a heart sound cannot be detected, the patient should be assessed for cardiac arrest. Begin CPR if needed.

d. Auscultate to assess heart rhythm (code: IB5b) [difficulty: R, Ap, An]

A steady rhythm has approximately equal amounts of time between ventricular contractions. It is considered normal to have a slight increase in the HR and faster rhythm during an inspiration than during an expiration. This is caused by the increase in blood brought into the chest during the inspiration when the intrathoracic pressure is more negative. The opposite pattern might be seen when a patient is being mechanically ventilated with high peak-airway pressures. This indicates that the venous return to the heart is decreased during a mechanically delivered inspiration.

Any sudden variations in rate and rhythm not related to the respiratory cycle are abnormal. Occasionally, a third (S_3) or fourth (S_4) heart sound is heard. A patient with these extra sounds is described as having a "gallop" rhythm. This pathologic finding is usually noted in patients with congestive heart failure.

It is difficult to determine the origin of most dysrhythmias (arrhythmias) solely on the basis of their sound patterns. A diagnostic 12-lead ECG is indicated (see Chapter 11 for details). A premature ventricular contraction (PVC) can be noted by the following rhythm characteristics: (1) the heartbeat is premature and (2) a complete compensatory pause is noted between the PVC and the following normal beat. The complete compensatory pause is the time interval of two normal heartbeats. (See the representative rhythm strip [Fig. 11-22] in Chapter 11.)

e. Auscultate to assess blood pressure (code: IB5c) [difficulty: R, Ap, An]

Measure the blood pressure on any patient to establish a baseline normal value and whenever you think a significant increase or decrease in the BP might be present. The BP should be the same on any arm or leg. However, an arm typically is used. Place the proper cuff around the arm and inflate the cuff pressure above the patient's normal value. Place the diaphragm of the stethoscope over the brachial artery, and slowly let the air out of the cuff. The first distinct sound heard as the blood flows through the artery is the systolic pressure. The last distinct sound heard is the diastolic pressure. Clinical practice is needed to determine BP accurately.

MODULE G

Perform diagnostic chest percussion (code: IB4) [difficulty: R, Ap, An].

Percussion of the chest is performed to determine normal and abnormal densities of the lungs and related structures. It must be performed properly to be a reliable

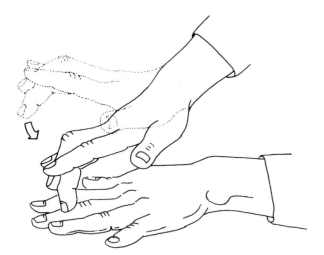

Figure 1-33 Technique for performing mediate chest percussion. (From Shapiro BA et al.: Clinical application of respiratory care, ed 4, St Louis, 1991, Mosby.)

diagnostic tool. There are two generally accepted methods of performing percussion. Both must be performed with equal force and speed, or the resulting sound will reflect the technique rather than the condition of the lungs. Do not percuss over a woman's breast tissue.

Immediate percussion involves striking the tip of the middle finger of one hand directly onto the chest wall in a symmetrical pattern. This is useful for finding large general differences in density and for finding landmarks such as the sternum and other bony structures, the liver, and the heart. Mediate percussion involves striking the tip of the middle finger of one hand onto the central section of the middle finger of the other hand (Fig. 1-33). The finger to be struck is fitted firmly between the ribs, as shown in Figure 1-30, in a symmetrical pattern. Mediate percussion is better for precisely locating an abnormal area and is used in the following discussions.

1. Determine the patient's diaphragmatic excursion

It is helpful to determine the patient's diaphragmatic excursion during both normal tidal volume breathing and maximal inspiration and expiration. Both hemidiaphragms should move the same amount during both the normal and the maximal efforts. It should be remembered that, because of the liver, the right hemidiaphragm usually is about 1 cm higher than the left.

The following procedure determines diaphragmatic excursion during tidal volume breathing:

1. The patient should sit up straight, exhale passively, and hold.
2. Percuss down the posterior chest to find the level of both hemidiaphragms. The air-filled lungs have a resonant sound, whereas the more solid tissues below the lungs have a dull sound.
3. Have the patient inhale a normal tidal volume and hold.

4. Percuss down the posterior chest to find the level of both hemidiaphragms.
5. Note the range of movement on both sides by the intercostal space when the dull sound was heard at the end of expiration and at the end of inspiration. During a quiet tidal volume breath, the adult's hemidiaphragms move down about 1.5 cm on both sides. For example, the dull sound was heard at the ninth intercostal space at the end of exhalation and the tenth intercostal space at the end of inspiration.

The following procedure determines diaphragmatic excursion during maximal expiratory and inspiratory (vital capacity) breathing:

1. The patient should sit up straight, exhale as completely as possible, and hold.
2. Percuss down the posterior chest to find the level of both hemidiaphragms. The air-filled lungs have a resonant sound, whereas the more solid tissues below the lungs have a dull sound.
3. Have the patient inhale as completely as possible and hold.
4. Percuss down the posterior chest to find the level of both hemidiaphragms.
5. Note the range of movement on both sides by the intercostal space when the dull sound was heard at the end of expiration and at the end of inspiration. During the vital capacity effort, the adult's hemidiaphragms move down about 5 cm on both sides. For example, the dull sound was heard at the seventh intercostal space at the end of exhalation and the eleventh intercostal space at the end of inspiration (Fig. 1-34).

Box 1-3 shows conditions that can affect the position of one or both hemidiaphragms.

Exam Hint 1-12

There is usually one question that relates to an abnormal percussion note. Know that a hyperresonant percussion note is heard over an area of pneumothorax.

2. Determine whether the patient has areas of altered resonance

Mediate percussion with proper technique should be performed over the posterior and anterior areas of the chest while avoiding breast tissue (see Fig. 1-30). The usual pattern is to proceed from the top down and side to side to compare for symmetrical sounds. The shoulders should be rolled forward when percussing the posterior chest to move the scapulae as much out of the way as possible. Table 1-14 shows the various types of percussion notes, their common characteristics, and example locations. Figure 1-35 shows the locations of the normal percussion sounds over the anterior chest.

A hyperresonant sound is always abnormal when found over lung areas. It indicates that more air than

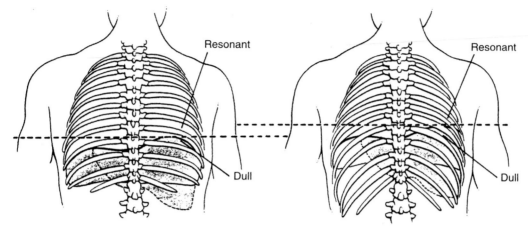

Figure 1-34 Excursion of the hemidiaphragms can be determined by percussing the patient's posterior chest. This should be done at the end of inspiration (as shown on the left) and expiration (as shown on the right). The change from a resonant (lung) sound to a dull (abdominal) sound indicates the border of the hemidiaphragm on each side. (From Swartz MH: Textbook of physical diagnosis, ed 6, Philadelphia, 2010, Saunders.)

BOX 1-3 Conditions That Affect the Position of the Hemidiaphragms

Elevated
Unilateral
Atelectasis (on the affected side)
Paralysis of the hemidiaphragm (on the affected side)
Enlarged liver (right side only)

Bilateral
Third semester of pregnancy
Obesity
Ascites
Atelectasis (if bilateral)

Depressed
Unilateral
Pneumothorax (on the affected side)
Check-valve obstruction to exhalation (on the affected side)
Pleural effusion (on the affected side)

Bilateral
COPD*
Asthma attack

---

*COPD is chronic obstructive pulmonary disease, a combination of chronic bronchitis and emphysema.

normal is present. Although emphysema can cause hyperresonance, a pneumothorax usually is the cause. Be careful not to confuse hyperresonance with the normal sound of tympany found over an air-filled stomach. An increase in the density of the underlying lung or related structures results in a dull sound at an abnormal location. This sound is associated with pneumonia, consolidation, or atelectasis when the alveoli are fluid-filled or airless; with tumor; and with pleural fluid, such as effusion, blood, pus, or chyle. Dullness over the heart and liver is normal.

MODULE H

Neonatal and pediatric assessment

1. Evaluate data in the maternal and perinatal/ neonatal patient record (code: IA10) [difficulty: R, Ap, An]

a. Evaluate the maternal and perinatal/neonatal history and data

Perinatal refers to the period toward the end of a pregnancy and for up to 4 weeks after the birth of the infant.

1. Antenatal assessment (assessment during the pregnancy)/social history

The medical and personal history of the mother is obviously important, because it directly relates to the health of the fetus she is carrying. The mother's age is important, because women younger than 16 years and older than 40 years are more likely to have a high-risk pregnancy. This is especially true if a woman older than 40 years is having her first child. *Gravida* is the term that refers to pregnancy; *primigravida* refers to a woman with her first pregnancy. *Para* is the term that refers to the woman delivering a potentially live infant; *primipara/primiparous* refers to a woman's first delivery of an infant. Box 1-4 lists a number of maternal and other factors that can result in the anticipation of a high-risk infant being born. It must be noted that about 25% of high-risk infants are born without any indication of a problem in the history.

2. Intrapartum assessment (assessment during labor)

Some of the labor and delivery/obstetric factors that can adversely affect the delivery process include premature labor (less than 38 weeks' gestation), postmature labor (greater than 42 weeks' gestation), prolapsed umbilical cord, and cesarean section. The fetal heart rate (FHR, or

TABLE 1-14	Percussion Notes and Characteristics			
Percussion Notes	**Relative Intensity**	**Relative Pitch**	**Relative Duration**	**Example Locations**
Resonant/resonance	Loud	Low	Long	Normal lung
Flat/flatness	Soft	High	Short	Sternum, spine, scapula
Dull/dullness	Medium	Medium	Medium	Liver, heart
Tympanic/tympany	Loud	High	Longer	Stomach air
Hyperresonant/hyperresonance	Very loud	Low	Long	Bilateral: emphysema, asthma Unilateral: pneumothorax, bleb

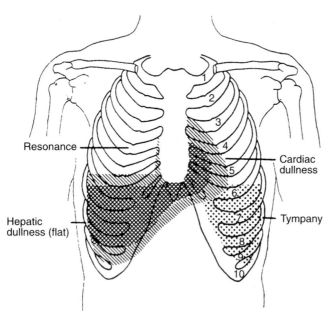

Figure 1-35 Areas over the normal anterior thorax where resonance, dullness, tympany, and flatness can be heard during percussion. (From Prior JA, Silberstein JS, Stang JM: Physical diagnosis, ed 6, St Louis, 1981, Mosby.)

fetal heart tones) usually is monitored to determine how the fetus is tolerating the stress of labor and delivery.

The FHR should range from 120 to 160 beats/min, and it is normally variable with the fetus's waking and sleeping periods. The FHR can be measured externally through the mother's abdominal wall. During a contraction of the uterus, the FHR commonly slows to near or less than 120 beats/min. This occurs because of vagus nerve stimulation during compression of the head into the birth canal (Fig. 1-36, A). The FHR returns to normal when the contraction is over. This normal decrease and increase in the FHR related to uterine contractions is called *early deceleration* or *type I dips*.

Late deceleration, or *type II dips,* are seen when the FHR slows sometime after the contraction begins and does not return to normal until sometime after the contraction is over (see Fig. 1-36, B). This is often caused by uteroplacental insufficiency from compression of the vessels in the placenta. It is frequently associated with low Apgar scores and fetal asphyxia and acidosis.

BOX 1-4   Some Factors Associated with a High-Risk Newborn Infant

Maternal Factors
Maternal age younger than 16 or older than 40 years
Low socioeconomic status
Poor nutrition
Lack of medical care during pregnancy
Smoking, drug or alcohol abuse
Underweight or overweight
Abnormal fetal growth
Hereditary anomalies
Vaginal bleeding early in pregnancy
Low maternal urinary estriol
Polyhydramnios or oligohydramnios
Toxemia of pregnancy/preeclampsia
Previous history of infant(s) with jaundice or respiratory distress or previous premature delivery
Chronic disease
Hypertension unrelated to pregnancy
Diabetes mellitus
Cardiovascular disease
Pulmonary disease
Anemia
Renal disease

Labor and Delivery/Obstetric Factors
Premature rupture of the membranes
Prolonged rupture of the membranes (>24 hours)
Premature labor (<38 weeks' gestation)
Postmature labor (>42 weeks' gestation)
Rapid or prolonged labor
Prolapsed umbilical cord
Previous or primary cesarean section
Breech or other abnormal presentation
Analgesia and anesthesia

Fetal Factors
Multiple births
Meconium in amniotic fluid
Abnormal fetal heart rate or rhythm
Fetal acidosis
Prematurity or postmaturity
Small or large for gestational age
Rh factor sensitization
Congenital malformation
Immature lecithin/sphingomyelin ratio or negative phosphatidylglycerol test
Birth trauma

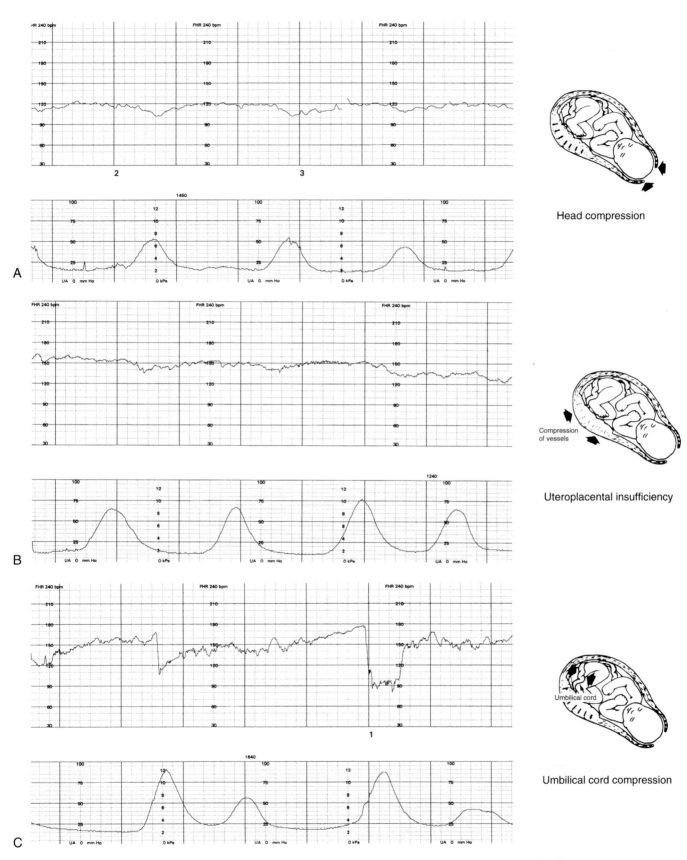

Figure 1-36 Fetal heart rate patterns showing normal early deceleration **A,** abnormal late deceleration **B,** and variable deceleration **C.**

Variable deceleration is seen when the FHR slows and increases in an unpredictable pattern in comparison with the contractions (see Fig. 1-36, C). This pattern is seen more commonly than late deceleration and is believed to be caused by compression of the umbilical cord by a body part. During the compression, little or no blood reaches the fetus. It also is often associated with low Apgar scores and fetal asphyxia and acidosis.

With late and variable deceleration, the mother's HR and BP should be monitored. Treatment includes giving the mother supplemental oxygen and placing her in a head-down, left lateral position. If the fetus is thought to be at risk of asphyxia, a cesarean section must be performed.

Other heartbeat irregularities are not related to labor and delivery. Tachycardia of greater than 160 beats/min can be associated with infection, fetal immaturity, congenital heart malformations, and the effects of maternal drugs. Bradycardia of less than 120 beats/min and decreased beat-to-beat variability (fixed heart rate) are seen with fetal asphyxia and distress.

3. Postpartum or neonatal assessment

Some of the fetal factors that can adversely affect the newborn include multiple births, meconium in the amniotic fluid, abnormal FHR or rhythm, prematurity or postmaturity, small or large size for gestational age, congenital malformation, and birth trauma.

4. Resuscitation and vital signs

All newborns require some level of resuscitation. This is usually limited to suctioning amniotic fluid out of the nose and mouth, drying the skin, providing warmth, and the tactile stimulation that comes from these procedures. Newborns with moderate Apgar scores may need to breathe in some supplemental oxygen until they are more vigorous and ventilating better. The newborn with a low Apgar score requires CPR. Table 1-15 lists the vital signs seen in a normal newborn.

5. Weight

The relationship between birth weight and gestational age is important to evaluate. In general, an infant between the 10th and the 90th percentiles of normal weight for gestational age is within normal limits. Any infant either large or small for gestational age is at increased risk of complications during and after delivery. Large postterm infants and small preterm infants are especially at risk.

b. Evaluate the lecithin/sphingomyelin ratio test

To determine the lung maturity of the fetus, a sample of amniotic fluid must be obtained by amniocentesis. The maturity of the fetus's lungs can be determined by evaluating three components of surfactant released by the developing alveolar type II cells. Recall that in a

TABLE 1-15	Normal Newborn Vital Signs
Characteristic	**Normal Range**
Heart rate	>120 beats/min
	<160 beats/min
Blood Pressure	**Systolic/Diastolic**
1000-2000 g birth weight	55 mm Hg/30 mm Hg
>3000 g birth weight	65 mm Hg/40 mm Hg
Respiratory rate	30-60 breaths/min
	Periodic breathing with apneic spells of <10 seconds common; should not be associated with bradycardia or cyanosis
Temperature	Keep abdominal skin temperature at 36.5° C
	Keep rectal (core) temperature between 35.5° C and 37.5° C

TABLE 1-16	Lecithin/Sphingomyelin (L:S) Ratio and Phosphatidylglycerol (PG) as Markers of Fetal Lung Maturity
Clinical Finding	**Interpretation**
L:S ratio ≥2:1 (2.0)	Mature lungs; <5% chance of RDS
L:S ratio 1.5:1 (1.5)	Transitional lungs; about a 50% chance of RDS
L:S ratio ≤1:1 (1.0)	Immature lungs; about a 90% chance of RDS
PG present	Mature lungs
PG absent	Immature lungs

RDS, respiratory distress syndrome.

premature neonate without sufficient surfactant in the lungs, infant respiratory distress syndrome probably will develop.

The first test of lung maturity is the lecithin/sphingomyelin (L:S) ratio. This test is a comparison of the relative amounts of these two surfactant components. In general, the more lecithin compared with sphingomyelin, the more mature the lungs. Usually a significant increase in the lecithin level occurs at about 35 weeks of gestation. A weakness of the L:S ratio test is that borderline values are difficult to interpret, and false-positive values are sometimes found.

The second test involves determining the presence of phosphatidylglycerol (PG) in the amniotic fluid. It appears at about 36 weeks of gestation and increases through the duration of the pregnancy. The laboratory reports PG as either present or absent from the sample of amniotic fluid. Its presence always indicates lung maturity. Table 1-16 provides more information about the interpretation of these two tests.

TABLE 1-17	Apgar Scoring Chart		
Sign	**0**	**1**	**2**
Heart rate	Absent	Slow (<100 beats/min)	>100
Respiratory effort	Absent	Weak cry, hypoventilation	Good strong cry
Muscle tone	Limp	Some flexion of extremities	Well flexed
Reflex response	No response	Grimace	Cough, sneeze, or cry
Response to catheter in nostril or to other cutaneous stimulation			
Color	Blue, pale	Body pink, extremities blue	Completely pink

c. Evaluate Apgar scores

The Apgar scoring system is used in the delivery room to provide a general evaluation of how a newborn infant is responding. The five parameters judged are heart rate, respiratory effort, muscle tone, reflex response, and color. Table 1-17 shows how the five parameters are scored on a scale of 0, 1, and 2. The newborn is evaluated soon after birth to calculate a 1-minute Apgar score. A 5-minute evaluation and Apgar score also are calculated. The infant is rated as good if the score is 7-10, fair if the score is 4-6, and poor if the score is 0-3. If the 5-minute score is less than 7, the newborn is rescored every 5 minutes up to 20 minutes after the delivery.

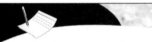

Exam Hint 1-13

Usually at least one question deals with interpretation of a newborn's given Apgar score. Also, be able to determine the Apgar score based on given information and interpret the patient's condition based on the score.

d. Evaluate gestational age (Dubowitz score)

The Dubowitz score is made up of 11 physical and 10 neurologic criteria that develop at a set rate during gestation. Ballard and co-workers modified the scoring system by simplifying it to six physical and six neurologic criteria. Figure 1-37 shows the criteria, scoring system, and scale for rating the maturity of the newborn. A score of 35-45 indicates that the infant was born between 38 and 42 weeks of gestation; this is a normal score for a term infant. A premature infant has a score of less than 35, and a postterm infant has a score of greater than 45. The maturity rating scale can be used to estimate gestational age accurately within 2 weeks.

1. Use *inspection* (observation) to determine the perinatal or neonatal patient's overall cardiopulmonary status

a. Perform inspection to assess Apgar scores (code: IB2d) [difficulty: R, Ap, An]

Review the previous information and Table 1-17 as needed. Shortly after birth, the neonate's HR, respiratory effort, muscle tone, reflex response, and color are evaluated and

each is given a score of 0, 1, or 2. The total of all five parameters is the 1-minute Apgar score. This score is a good index of how the newborn tolerated the delivery process. The 5-minute Apgar score is a good index of how the newborn's cardiopulmonary system is adjusting from fetal to postnatal conditions. A low 5-minute Apgar score is associated with increased mortality in the first month of life. Survivors have a high risk of mental impairment and cerebral palsy.

b. Perform inspection to assess gestational age (Dubowitz score) (code: IB2d) [difficulty: R, Ap, An]

The descriptions of gestational development for the criteria of physical maturity are listed in Figure 1-37. As can be seen, more points are earned for each step of gestational development. A term infant will score 3 or 4 points for each of the 12 criteria. The illustrations of gestational development for the criteria of neurologic/neuromuscular maturity can be seen in the figure; however, because the infant must be manipulated to perform the rating, the following descriptions can be helpful.

1. Posture

The infant should be supine and quiet. Simply observe how the infant positions the arms and legs. The more mature infant fully flexes the elbows, hips, and knees.

2. Square window

Flex the hand at the wrist. Exert gentle pressure to have the wrist flex as much as possible. The more mature infant has full flexibility of the hand against the forearm.

3. Arm recoil

With the infant supine, fully flex the forearms for 5 seconds. Then fully extend the forearms by pulling on the hands. When released, the more mature infant quickly returns the forearms to full flexion.

4. Popliteal angle

The infant must lie supine with the pelvis flat on the examining surface. The lower leg is flexed onto the thigh, and the thigh is fully flexed to the abdomen. One hand is used to hold the thigh in the flexed position, and the other

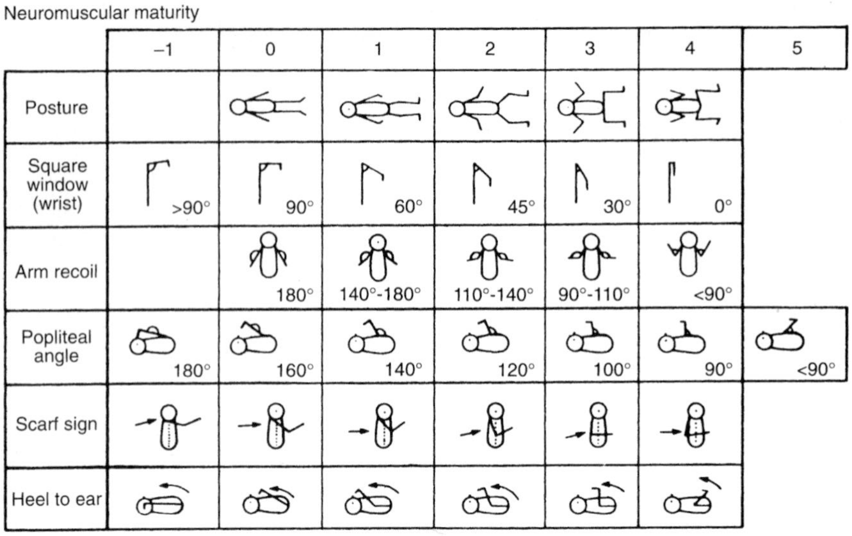

Neuromuscular maturity

	−1	0	1	2	3	4	5
Posture							
Square window (wrist)	>90°	90°	60°	45°	30°	0°	
Arm recoil		180°	140°-180°	110°-140°	90°-110°	<90°	
Popliteal angle	180°	160°	140°	120°	100°	90°	<90°
Scarf sign							
Heel to ear							

Physical maturity

Skin	Sticky, friable, transparent	Gelatinous red, translucent	Smooth, pink, visible veins	Superficial peeling and/or rash, few veins	Cracking, pale areas, rare veins	Parchment, deep cracking, no vessels	Leathery, cracked, wrinkled
Lanugo	None	Sparse	Abundant	Thinning	Bald areas	Mostly bald	
Plantar surface	Heel-toe 40-50 mm:−1 <40 mm:−2	>50 mm No crease	Faint red marks	Anterior transverse crease only	Creases ant. 2/3	Creases over entire sole	
Breast	Imperceptible	Barely perceptible	Flat areola, no bud	Stippled areola, 1–2 mm bud	Raised areola, 3–4 mm bud	Full areola, 5–10 mm bud	
Eye/Ear	Lids fused loosely: −1 tightly: −2	Lids open; pinna flat; stays folded	Slightly curved pinna; soft; slow recoil	Well-curved pinna; soft but ready recoil	Formed and firm instant recoil	Thick cartilage ear stiff	
Genitals male	Scrotum flat, smooth	Scrotum empty; faint rugae	Testes in upper canal; rare rugae	Testes descending; few rugae	Testes down; good rugae	Testes pendulous; deep rugae	
Genitals female	Clitoris prominent; labia flat	Prominent clitoris; small labia minora	Prominent clitoris; enlarging minora	Majora and minora equally prominent	Majora large; minora small	Majora cover clitoris and minora	

Maturity rating

score	weeks
−10	20
−5	22
0	24
5	26
10	28
15	30
20	32
25	34
30	36
35	38
40	40
45	42
50	44

Figure 1-37 Ballard modification of the Dubowitz Gestational Age Assessment. (From Ballard JL, Khoury JC, Wedig K: New Ballard Score, expanded to include extremely premature infants, J Pediatr 119:417, 1991.)

hand is used to extend the lower leg. The angle between the thigh and lower leg is then measured. The more mature infant has less joint flexion and a smaller angle.

5. Scarf sign

With the infant supine, take one of the infant's hands and extend it as far as possible across the neck toward the opposite shoulder. The infant is scored as follows:

0 = The elbow reaches the opposite anterior axillary line.
1 = The elbow reaches closer to the opposite anterior axillary line than the midline of the chest.
2 = The elbow reaches midway between the opposite anterior axillary line and the midline of the chest.

3 = The elbow reaches the midline of the chest.
4 = The elbow does not reach the midline of the chest.

6. Heel-to-ear maneuver

The infant should be supine on the examining table with the pelvis flat. Take the infant's foot in one hand and move it as near to the head as possible. Do not force it! The more mature infant has less joint flexibility and is unable to move the foot as near the head as a less mature infant.

c. Perform inspection to assess the results of transillumination of the chest

Transillumination of the chest is a test performed on a neonate to identify the presence of a pneumothorax. The room is darkened, and a bright light from a flashlight is

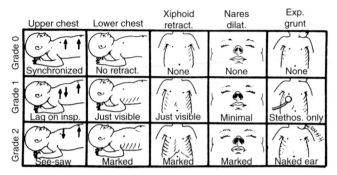

Figure 1-38 Silverman (also called Silverman–Anderson) scoring system for assessing a newborn's level of respiratory distress. A child having great difficulty breathing would have asynchrony between the chest and the abdomen, marked nasal flaring, and expiratory grunting that could be heard by the naked ear. See the text for more discussion. (Modified from Silverman WA, Anderson DH: Pediatrics 17:1, 1956.)

placed against the patient's chest. When free air is around the collapsed lung, the light creates a "halo" effect through the neonate's thin chest wall. This confirms the pneumothorax.

d. Perform inspection to determine the Silverman score (code: IB2d) [difficulty: R, Ap, An]

The Silverman score (also called the Silverman–Anderson score) is used to grade an infant's level of respiratory distress. See Figure 1-38 for the five monitored signs: upper chest movement, lower chest movement, xiphoid retractions, nasal dilation, and expiratory grunt. Each of the five signs is graded from absent (a grade of 0) to moderately present (a grade of 1) to fully present (a grade of 2). A normally breathing infant will have no signs of respiratory distress and a score of 0. An infant with great respiratory distress will have a score of 10. This child will have uncoordinated chest and abdominal movements when breathing, so-called see-saw breathing. There will be marked lower chest intercostal retractions and sub-xiphoid retractions. Inspiratory nasal dilation (flaring) will be marked. Last, an expiratory grunt can be heard with the naked ear.

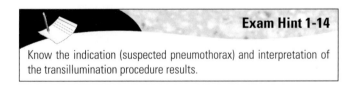

Exam Hint 1-14

Know the indication (suspected pneumothorax) and interpretation of the transillumination procedure results.

2. Review lateral neck radiographs (code: IB6) [difficulty: R, Ap]

A lateral neck or PA neck radiograph is usually taken to identify the cause of an airway obstruction or cervical spine injury. This discussion will focus on airway obstruction issues. The following usually applies to a child but can also apply to an adult.

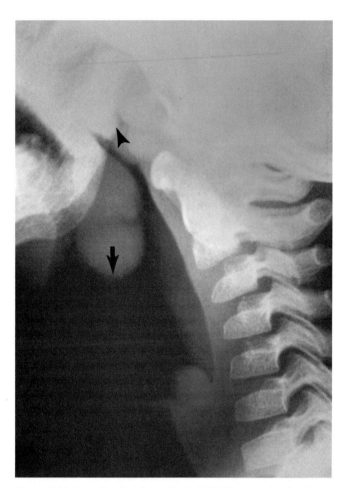

Figure 1-39 Lateral neck radiograph of a child. The arrowhead points to enlarged adenoids in the nasopharynx. The arrow points to enlarged tonsils. (From Walsh BK, Czervinske MP, DiBlasi RM: Perinatal and pediatric respiratory care, ed 3, St Louis, 2010, Saunders.)

a. Look for enlarged palatine tonsils and pharyngeal tonsils (adenoids)

The oral tonsils and adenoids in the nasopharynx are lymphoid tissues that become enlarged when infected. This is a common problem in young children and can lead to obstructive sleep apnea. Figure 1-39 shows a lateral neck radiograph showing enlarged tonsils and adenoids.

b. Look for epiglottitis

Epiglottitis is an inflammation of the epiglottis and surrounding supraglottic structures. It is a medical emergency and needs to be differentiated from nonemergency laryngotracheobronchitis. Epiglottitis is usually diagnosed on the basis of history and general physical examination and results in the child being intubated. The throat should *not* be directly observed before intubation. If a lateral neck radiograph is taken to confirm epiglottitis, it will show a white haziness in the supraglottic area. Sometimes the enlarged epiglottis seen on the film is called the "thumb sign." This is because the usually thin epiglottis is swollen and looks like the end of the thumb. Figures 1-40 and 1-41 show drawings

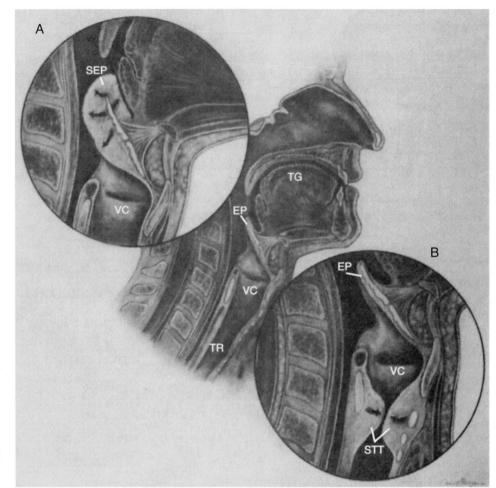

Figure 1-40 Drawing of the normal upper airway is shown in the middle. Contrast it with **A,** epiglottitis and **B,** laryngotracheobronchitis (croup). *EP,* epiglottis; *SEP,* swollen epiglottis; *STT,* swollen tracheal tissue; *TG,* tongue; *TR,* trachea; *VC,* vocal chords. (From Des Jardins T, Burton GG: Clinical manifestations and assessment of respiratory disease, ed 5, St Louis, 2006, Mosby.)

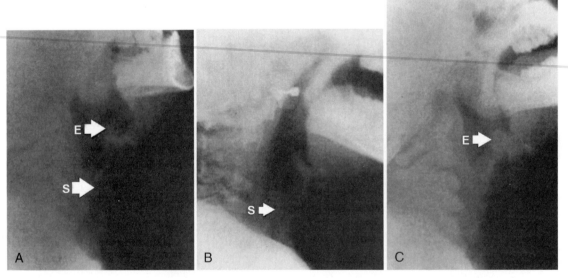

Figure 1-41 Lateral neck radiographs in children showing **A,** normal upper airway during an inspiration; **B,** laryngotracheobronchitis (croup) with haziness of the subglottic trachea from mucosal edema; and **C,** epiglottitis with a swollen, rounded epiglottis. Areas marked *E* show the epiglottis; areas marked *S* show the subglottic trachea. (From Koff PB, Eitzman DV, Neu J, editors: Neonatal and pediatric respiratory care, St Louis, 1988, Mosby.)

TABLE 1-18	General History and Physical Findings of Laryngotracheobronchitis (LTB) and Epiglottitis	
Clinical Finding	**LTB**	**Epiglottitis**
Age	3-36 months	2-4 years
Onset	Slow (24-48 hours)	Abrupt (2-4 hours)
Fever	Absent	Present
Drooling	Absent	Present
Lateral neck radiograph	Haziness in subglottic area	Haziness in supraglottic area
Inspiratory stridor	High pitched and loud	Low pitched and muffled
Hoarseness	Present	Absent
Swallowing difficulty	Absent	Present
White blood cell count	Normal (viral)	Elevated (bacterial)

From Des Jardins TR: Clinical manifestations and assessment of respiratory disease, ed 5, St Louis, 2006, Mosby.

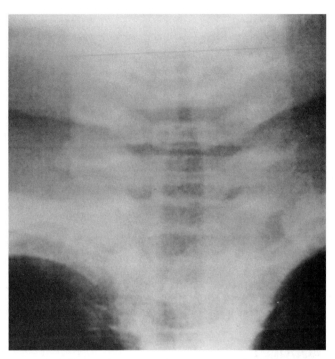

Figure 1-42 Front neck and upper chest radiograph of a child with laryngotracheobronchitis. The dark column is the trachea. Note the narrowing at the apex caused by subglottic edema below the vocal cords. This characteristic narrowing is often called the steeple sign. (From Walsh BK, Czervinske MP, DiBlasi RM: Perinatal and pediatric respiratory care, ed 3, St Louis, 2010, Saunders.)

and lateral neck radiographs of the normal upper airway and epiglottitis. Table 1-18 lists the general history and physical findings for distinguishing between the two conditions.

It must be emphasized that under no circumstances should the child be laid supine for the neck radiograph. This can result in the swollen epiglottis fatally closing over the opening to the trachea. Allow the child to sit upright in the most comfortable position.

c. Look for laryngotracheobronchitis

Laryngotracheobronchitis is subglottic edema of the mucous membranes of the larynx, trachea, and bronchi. This condition is also known as LTB, laryngotracheal bronchitis, and croup. LTB is not a medical emergency but must be differentiated from the much more serious problem of epiglottitis. Subglottic edema usually is treated with the inhalation of a cool bland aerosol or, if necessary, nebulized racemic epinephrine for mucosal vasoconstriction. A lateral neck radiograph of subglottic edema shows a white haziness in the subglottic area. This is the swollen laryngeal and tracheal tissue. The airway narrowing is sometimes obvious enough to be called the "steeple sign," "steepling," or "pencil sign." This is seen when the usually blunt end of the trachea at the vocal cords is thinned to a narrow point by the swollen mucous membrane. Figures 1-40 and 1-41 show drawings and lateral neck radiographs of the normal upper airway and laryngotracheobronchitis. Figure 1-42 is an AP neck radiograph showing the steeple sign. Table 1-18 lists the general history and physical findings for distinguishing between the two conditions.

d. Look for a foreign body (code: IB7c) [difficulty: R, Ap]

A history of sudden breathing difficulty, cough, and inspiratory stridor combined with a physical examination of the patient usually points to aspiration. Often, a lateral neck radiograph or combined chest and neck radiograph helps to confirm the presence and position of a foreign body. See Figure 1-15 for AP and lateral chest and neck radiographic images. The clearly seen solid white shape of the foreign body indicates that the object is metallic (a coin).

Plastic toy pieces and foods such as peanuts are much harder to see on a neck radiograph than are metallic objects, because their densities are closer to those found in the body. Obstructing plastic toys and food are more easily identified by looking for a narrowing or distortion of the dark air column of the upper airway and trachea.

e. Airway tumor

Airway narrowing can be caused by either a tumor within the lumen of the airway or a growth from outside the larynx, trachea, or bronchi that forces it to collapse. Mouth, throat, and lung cancers are most commonly seen in patients who use chewing tobacco (snuff) or smoke.

Exam Hint 1-15

Past exams have usually included two questions about some aspect of fetal, neonatal, or pediatric patient assessment. Be able to make a differential diagnosis between croup and epiglottitis.

TABLE 1-19   Common Physical Findings in Selected Pulmonary Conditions

Condition	Inspection	Palpation	Percussion	Auscultation
Asthma and COPD*	Hyperinflated chest	Decreased expansion	Hyperresonance	Long expiratory time
	Use of accessory muscles	Decreased fremitus	Low diaphragms	Wheezes
Atelectasis (lobar)	Inspiratory lag on affected side	Decreased fremitus	Dullness	Absent breath sounds
		Trachea and heart shifted *toward* affected side		
Consolidation (pneumonia)	Possible inspiratory lag or splinting on affected side	Rhonchial fremitus	Dullness	Bronchial breath sounds
				Bronchophony
				Pectoriloquy
Pleural effusion (large)	Inspiratory lag on affected side	Decreased fremitus	Dullness	Absent breath sounds
Tension pneumothorax	Inspiratory lag on affected side	Absent fremitus	Hyperresonance	Absent breath sounds
		Trachea and heart shifted *away* from affected side		

*COPD is chronic obstructive pulmonary disease, a combination of emphysema and chronic bronchitis.
Modified from Hinshaw HC, Murray JF: Diseases of the chest, ed 4, Philadelphia, 1980, Saunders.

MODULE I

Respiratory Care Plan

1. Determine a patient's pathophysiologic state (code: IIIF1) [difficulty: R, Ap, An]

The limitations of this text prevent an in-depth discussion of the various cardiopulmonary conditions and disorders that befall the patients to whom respiratory therapists provide care. However, some discussion of cardiopulmonary conditions is included in the following chapters as the therapeutic procedures are presented. Table 1-19 summarizes some of the key physical examination findings associated with commonly encountered clinical conditions. The NBRC's Detailed Content Outline lists the following conditions as testable:

- Apnea
- ARDS
- Asthma
- Bariatric
- Bronchiolitis
- Burn injury
- Cardiovascular
- Chronic lung disease of prematurity
- Congenital defects of newborns
- COPD
- Cystic fibrosis
- Heart failure
- Immunocompromised
- Infectious disease
- Inhalation injuries
- Lung transplantation
- Neurologic
- Neuromuscular
- Postsurgical

- Pulmonary embolism
- Pulmonary hypertension
- Shock
- Trauma

It is highly recommended that a pathology book be reviewed for guidance on how these conditions are diagnosed and managed.

Exam Hint 1-16

The NBRC is known to ask one or two questions about commonly encountered cardiopulmonary pathologies. Take the time to study at least the following: asthma, COPD (emphysema and chronic bronchitis), bacterial pneumonia, tension pneumothorax, and heart failure with pulmonary edema.

2. Recommend tuberculosis skin testing as a diagnostic procedure (code: IE1) [difficulty: R, Ap]

If a patient has a history and signs and symptoms that suggest TB, skin testing should be performed. The Mantoux test is commonly recommended. With this test, an intradermal injection of purified protein derivative of the tubercle bacillus is performed. After 48-72 hours an induration (skin wheal) is looked for. A positive reaction is confirmed by an induration of ≥10 mm. It is commonly accepted that this reaction confirms that the patient has in the past or recently been infected with tuberculosis. After this positive test, the patient should have a chest radiograph taken to look for pulmonary effects. A sputum sample should also be obtained for a culture and sensitivity test to confirm TB and the antibiotic agents that would be most effective against it.

3. Recommend allergy skin testing as a diagnostic procedure (code: IE1) [difficulty: R, Ap]

After a patient has been diagnosed with asthma, it is imperative that a treatment plan be developed. Part of this plan will include avoiding those allergens that trigger the patient's asthma attacks. In many patients it is difficult to determine which environmental allergens are causing the problem. Recommend allergy skin testing so that the triggering agents can be clearly identified. Briefly, an allergist will perform skin-prick tests or intradermal injections of suspected substances such as eggs, peanut butter, and seafood. A swelling at that site confirms the patient's allergic reaction. Minimally, the patient should avoid those allergens. The allergist may also want to begin immunotherapy (antigen desensitization) to reduce the patient's reaction to the allergen.

4. Recommend starting a treatment based on the patient's response (code: IIIE2a) [difficulty: R, Ap, An]

See below.

5. Recommend a change in the therapeutic plan if indicated (code: IIIF2) [difficulty: R, Ap, An]

For the patient to receive the best care possible, the respiratory therapist must know the indications, contraindications, complications, and hazards of the respiratory care procedures the patient will receive. The patient must be assessed before, during, and after the treatment or procedure to determine whether it was effective. The key goal of an appropriate care plan is to treat the patient's condition in the best way possible. Modifications to the care plan must be made as needed as the patient's condition changes.

The respiratory therapist should be a member of the patient care team (i.e., the physician, nurse, and others) in deciding how best to care for the patient. The following steps are necessary in developing the respiratory care plan for any patient:

1. Determine expected outcome(s) or goal(s).
2. Develop a plan to achieve success.
3. Decide how to measure whether the goal or goals have been achieved.
4. Plan a timeline to measure the patient's progress.
5. Document the patient's response to care and the final outcome.

When the patient has recovered sufficiently from illness or injury, a discharge plan will be needed to help in the transition to home or a long-term recovery facility. Typically, the discharge plan includes the following:

- Patient evaluation that determines the patient is ready for discharge. The patient needs to have recovered sufficiently to leave the hospital.
- Determination of the best place for the patient to go for further recovery and the necessary patient care resources. It must be determined whether the patient can go home or should go to an extended care facility. If the patient is to go home, it must be determined whether the family can provide the necessary care. If not, arrangements must be made for home care respiratory therapists and nurses.
- Determination that the patient's financial resources are adequate. If not, social services must be contacted to work with the patient's insurance company or other financial support agencies.

6. Recommend a treatment be terminated (code: IIIE1) [difficulty: R, Ap, An]

Patient safety should always be an important consideration during the treatment or procedure. The respiratory therapist should know the complications and hazards of any patient care activity that is performed. These are discussed in the following chapters. Be prepared to stop the treatment or procedure if the patient has an adverse reaction to it. Additionally, be prepared to recommend to the physician that the treatment or procedure be discontinued if it is likely to result in additional adverse reactions.

7. Recommend discontinuing a treatment based on the patient's response (code: IIIE2h) [difficulty: R, Ap, An]

There are typically three reasons to discontinue a patient's treatment. First, the patient has recovered and no longer needs the treatment or procedure. It is expensive and wasteful to perform unnecessary treatments. Second, the patient has had an adverse reaction and is likely to have an adverse reaction every time the treatment or procedure is repeated. For example, the patient's BP goes too high whenever he or she is placed in a head-down position for postural drainage. Third, the patient's condition is terminal, and the patient or responsible family member wants all treatment to be stopped.

BIBLIOGRAPHY

Aloan CA, Hill TV, editors: *Respiratory care of the newborn and child,* ed 2, Philadelphia, 1997, Lippincott-Raven.

American Association for Respiratory Care: Clinical practice guideline: discharge planning for the respiratory care patient, *Respir Care* 40:1308, 1995.

American Association for Respiratory Care: Clinical practice guideline: providing patient and caregiver training 2010, *Respir Care* 55(6):765–769, 2010.

Barkauskas VH, Stoltenberg-Allen K, Baumann LC, et al.: *Health physical assessment,* St Louis, 1994, Mosby.

Barnes TA, editor: *Core textbook of respiratory care practice,* ed 2, St Louis, 1994, Mosby.

Black CP: Neonatal assessment and resuscitation. In Walsh BK, Czervinske MP, DiBlasi RM, editors: *Perinatal and pediatric respiratory care,* ed 3, St Louis, 2010, Saunders.

Black CP: Examination and assessment of the neonatal patient. In Walsh BK, Czervinske MP, DiBlasi RM, editors: *Perinatal and pediatric respiratory care*, ed 3, St Louis, 2010, Saunders.

Brown MK, Mason SC: Neonatal assessment. In Hess DR, MacIntyre NR, Mishoe SC, Galvin WF, Adams AB, editors: *Respiratory care principles and practice*, ed 2, Sudbury, MA, 2012, Jones & Bartlett Learning.

Butler TJ: *Laboratory exercises for competency in respiratory care*, ed 3, Philadelphia, 2013, FA Davis.

Chipman DW, English P: Neonatal and pediatric respiratory care. In Kacmarek RM, Stoller JK, Heuer AJ, editors: *Egan's fundamentals of respiratory care*, ed 10, St Louis, 2013, Mosby.

Clochesy JM, Breu C, Cardin S, et al.: *Critical care nursing*, ed 2, Philadelphia, 1996, Saunders.

Clark WF: Comprehensive history, assessment, and documentation. In Wyka KA, Mathews PJ, Rutkowski J, editors: *Foundations of respiratory care*, ed 2, Clifton Park, NY, 2012, Delmar.

Cohen Z: Chest Imaging. In Heuer AJ, Scanlan CL, editors: *Wilkins' clinical assessment in respiratory care*, ed 7, St. Louis, 2014, Mosby.

Daily EK, Schroeder JS: *Techniques in bedside hemodynamic monitoring*, ed 5, St Louis, 1994, Mosby.

DeNunzio C, Heure AJ: Fundamentals of physical examination. In Heuer AJ, Scanlan CL, editors: *Wilkins' clinical assessment in respiratory care*, ed 7, St. Louis, 2014, Mosby.

Des Jardins T: Burton GG: *Clinical manifestations and assessment of respiratory disease*, ed 6, St Louis, 2011, Mosby.

Des Jardins T: *Cardiopulmonary anatomy & physiology*, ed 6, Clifton Park, NY, 2013, Delmar.

Eisenberg RL, Johnson NM: *Comprehensive radiographic pathology*, ed 4, St Louis, 2007, Mosby.

Eisenhuber E, Schaefer-Prokop CM, Prosch H, Schima W: Bedside chest radiography, *Respir Care* 57(3):427–443, 2012.

Erickson B: *Heart sounds and murmurs: a practical guide*, ed 3, St Louis, 1997, Mosby.

Eubanks DH, Bone RC: *Comprehensive respiratory care*, ed 2, St Louis, 1990, Mosby.

Fink JB, Hunt GE, editors: *Clinical practice in respiratory care*, Philadelphia, 1999, Lippincott-Raven.

Fischback F: *A manual of laboratory & diagnostic tests*, ed 6, Philadelphia, 2000, Lippincott Williams & Wilkins.

Formenti P, Tomicic VF, Hess DR: Imaging the thorax. In Hess DR, MacIntyre NR, Mishoe SC, Galvin WF, Adams AB, editors: *Respiratory care principles and practice*, ed 2, Sudbury, MA, 2012, Jones & Bartlett Learning.

Fydryszewski NA, Keohane EM: Clinical laboratory studies. In Heuer AJ, Scanlan CL, editors: *Wilkins' clinical assessment in respiratory care*, ed 7, St Louis, 2014, Mosby.

Galvin WF: Patient education. In Hess DR, MacIntyre NR, Mishoe SC, Galvin WF, Adams AB, editors: *Respiratory care principles and practices*, ed 2, Sudbury, MA, 2012, Jones & Bartlett Learning.

Gardner DD: Patient education and health promotion. In Kacmarek RM, Stoller JK, Heuer AJ, editors: *Egan's fundamentals of respiratory care*, ed 10, St Louis, 2013, Mosby.

Harbrecht BG, Delgado E, Tuttle RP, Cohen-Melamed MH, Saul MI, Valenta CA: Improved outcomes with routine respiratory therapist evaluation of non-intensive unit surgery patients, *Respir Care* 54(7):861–867, 2009.

Hess DR, Kacmarek RM: *Essentials of mechanical ventilation*, ed 2, New York, 2002, McGraw-Hill.

Heuer AJ: Cardiopulmonary symptoms. In Heuer AJ, Scanlan CL, editors: *Wilkins' clinical assessment in respiratory care*, ed 7, St Louis, 2014, Mosby.

Heuer AJ: The medical history and the interview. In Heuer AJ, Scanlan CL, editors: *Wilkins' clinical assessment in respiratory care*, ed 7, St Louis, 2014, Mosby.

Heuer AJ: Vital signs. In Heuer AJ, Scanlan CL, editors: *Wilkins' clinical assessment in respiratory care*, ed 7, St Louis, 2014, Mosby.

Hinski ST: *Respiratory care clinical competency lab manual*, St Louis, 2014, Mosby.

Ingram JD: Radiographic assessment. In Walsh BK, Czervinske MP, DiBlasi RM, editors: *Perinatal and pediatric respiratory care*, ed 3, St Louis, 2010, Saunders.

Johnson AL, Hampson DF, Hampson NB: Sputum color: potential implications for clinical practice, *Respir Care* 53(4):450–454, 2008.

Johnson P, Stevenson K: Pediatric advanced life support. In Walsh BK, Czervinske MP, DiBlasi RM, editors: *Perinatal and pediatric respiratory care*, ed 3, St Louis, 2010, Saunders.

Kacmarek RM, Dimas S, Mack CW, editors: *The essentials of respiratory therapy*, ed 4, St Louis, 2005, Mosby.

Kallet RH: Bedside assessment of the patient. In Kacmarek RM, Stoller JK, Heuer AJ, editors: *Egan's fundamentals of respiratory care*, ed 10, St Louis, 2013, Mosby.

Kallet RH: Interpreting clinical and laboratory data. In Kacmarek RM, Stoller JK, Heuer AJ, editors: *Egan's fundamentals of respiratory care*, ed 10, St Louis, 2013, Mosby.

Kampa IS: Clinical laboratory studies. In Wyka KA, Mathews PJ, Rutkowski J, editors: *Foundations of respiratory care*, ed 2, Clifton Park, NY, 2012, Delmar.

Kenner CV, Guzzetta CE, Dossey BM: *Critical care nursing: body–mind–spirit*, Boston, 1981, Little, Brown.

Koff PB, Eitzman DV, Neu J, editors: *Neonatal and pediatric respiratory care*, ed 2, St Louis, 1993, Mosby.

Kowalczyk N, Mace JD: *Radiographic pathology for technicians*, ed 5, St Louis, 2009, Mosby.

Lehrer S: *Understanding lung sounds*, Philadelphia, 1984, Saunders.

Mathews PJ, Cox GG: Radiology for the respiratory therapist. In Wyka KA, Mathews PJ, Rutkowski J, editors: *Foundations of respiratory care*, ed 2, Clifton Park, NY, 2012, Delmar.

Mohammed RO, Bhagat R, MacIntyre NR: Blood chemistries and hematology. In Hess DR, MacIntyre NR, Mishoe SC, Galvin WF, Adams AB, editors: *Respiratory care principles and practice*, ed 2, Sudbury, MA, 2012, Jones & Bartlett Learning.

National Asthma Education Program: *Expert Panel Report 2: guidelines for the diagnosis and management of asthma*, Publication No. 97-4051. Bethesda, MD, April 1997, National Heart, Lung, and Blood Institute, National Institutes of Health.

National Heart, Lung, and Blood Institute and World Health Organization Global Initiative for Chronic Obstructive Lung Disease (GOLD): Global strategy for the diagnosis, management and prevention of chronic obstructive pulmonary disease: executive summary, *Am J Respir Crit Care Med* 163:1256, 2001.

Oblouk Darovic G: *Hemodynamic monitoring: invasive and noninvasive clinical monitoring*, ed 3, Philadelphia, 2002, Saunders.

Pagana KD, Pagana TJ: *Manual of diagnostic and laboratory tests*, ed 3, St Louis, 2006, Mosby.

Peters RM: Chest trauma. In Moser KM, Spragg RG, editors: *Respiratory emergencies*, ed 2, St Louis, 1982, Mosby.

Restrepo RD, Cohen Z: Neurological assessment. In Heuer AJ, Scanlan CL, editors: *Wilkins' clinical assessment in respiratory care*, ed 7, St Louis, 2014, Mosby.

Rodriguez N: Neonatal and pediatric assessment. In Heuer AJ, Scanlan CL, editors: *Wilkins' clinical assessment in respiratory care*, ed 7, St Louis, 2014, Mosby.

Salyer J, DiBlasi R: Neonatal and pediatric respiratory care. In Wyka KA, Mathews PJ, Rutkowski J, editors: *Foundations of respiratory care*, ed 2, Clifton Park, NY, 2012, Delmar.

Scanlan CL: Preparing for the patient encounter. In Heuer AJ, Scanlan CL, editors: *Wilkins' clinical assessment in respiratory care*, ed 7, St Louis, 2014, Mosby.

Schellhaese DE: Examination and assessment of the pediatric patient. In Walsh BK, Czervinske MP, DiBlasi RM, editors: *Perinatal and pediatric respiratory care*, ed 3, St Louis, 2010, Saunders.

Sheard S, Rao P, Devaraj A: Imaging of acute respiratory distress syndrome, *Respir Care* 57(4):607–612, 2012.

Simmons P: History and physical examination. In Hess DR, MacIntyre NR, Mishoe SC, Galvin WF, Adams AB, editors: *Respiratory care principles and practice*, ed 2, Sudbury, MA, 2012, Jones & Bartlett Learning.

Specht NL, Stoller JK: Review of thoracic imaging. In Kacmarek RM, Stoller JK, Heuer AJ, editors: *Egan's fundamentals of respiratory care*, ed 10, St Louis, 2013, Mosby.

Spiro SG, Silvestri GA, Agusti A, editors: *Clinical respiratory medicine*, ed 4, Philadelphia, 2012, Saunders.

Tilkian AG, Boudreau CM: *Understanding heart sounds and murmur*, ed 4, Philadelphia, 2001, Saunders.

Van Leeuwen AM, Poelhuis-Leth DJ, Bladh ML: *Davis's comprehensive handbook of laboratory diagnostic tests with nursing implications*, ed 5, Philadelphia, 2013, FA Davis.

Varcelotti Watkins GA: Fundamentals of patient education. In Wyka KA, Mathews PJ, Rutkowski J, editors: *Foundations of respiratory care*, ed 2, Clifton Park, NY, 2012, Delmar.

Wang J-S, Cherng J-M, Perng D-S, Lee H-S, Wang S: High-resolution computed tomography in assessment of patients with emphysema, *Respir Care* 58(4):614–622, 2013.

Whitaker K: *Comprehensive perinatal and pediatric respiratory care*, ed 2, Albany, NY, 1997, Delmar.

Wilkins RL, Hodgkin JE, Lopez B: *Lung sounds: a practical guide*, ed 3, St Louis, 2004, Mosby.

SELF-STUDY QUESTIONS

See Appendix for answers.

1. A 67-year-old male patient with a history of COPD and heart failure has arrived in the Emergency Department with a chief complaint of dyspnea. To help with the differential diagnosis, the physician orders the patient's blood to be tested for bacteremia, CK-MB, cTnI, cTnT, and BNP. All results are negative. What is the most likely cause of the patient's dyspnea?
   A. Exacerbation of COPD
   B. Myocardial infarction
   C. Pneumonia
   D. Congestive heart failure

2. In listening to a patient's lungs, bronchial breath sounds are heard over the right lower lobe area. These would indicate which of the following?
   A. Normal lungs
   B. Pneumothorax
   C. Consolidation in the patient's right lower lobe
   D. Pleural effusion in the patient's right lower lobe

3. After feeling a sudden chest pain and shortness of breath while lifting weights, a 37-year-old man drove himself to the Emergency Department. After starting oxygen therapy on the patient, the respiratory therapist performed a physical exam. Pertinent findings included a hyperresonant percussion note on the right side and tracheal shift to the left. Based on these findings, what is the patient's most likely problem?
   A. Broken ribs on the right side
   B. Right-sided pneumothorax
   C. Broken clavicle on the right side
   D. Acute myocardial infarction

4. The respiratory therapist is called to the Emergency Department to help care for a patient who was in a car accident and has chest injuries, including broken ribs. Crepitations are felt while palpating the patient's neck. What is the most likely cause of this?
   A. The patient has a laryngeal tumor.
   B. Blood is in the back of the patient's throat.
   C. The patient has aspirated a tooth.
   D. The patient's lung has an air leak.

5. The respiratory therapist is called to help in the evaluation of a 55-year-old male patient. The following signs and symptoms are noted: oral temperature of 40° C (104.5° F), diaphoresis, respiratory rate of 22, the use of accessory muscles of respiration, and palpable rhonchi in the right lower lobe. You would suspect which of the following diagnoses?
   A. Bacterial pneumonia
   B. Heart attack
   C. Pneumothorax
   D. Viral pneumonia

6. Since being told of the diagnosis of cancer, a patient has become argumentative about the care received and threatens to hit the nurse and therapist. The patient should be evaluated for:
   A. Language barrier problems
   B. Hypercarbia
   C. Emotional state
   D. Hypoxemia

7. To help determine a patient's level of consciousness, which of the following questions should be asked?
   1. "Do you know what day this is?"
   2. "Can I see your identification wristband?"
   3. "Do you know where you are?"
   4. "How are you feeling today?"
   5. "Do you know who the president is?"

A. 3 only
B. 5 only
C. 2 and 4 only
D. 1 and 3 only

8. To help determine if a patient has orthopnea, which of the following should be asked?
    A. "How many flights of stairs can you climb?"
    B. "Do you know who the governor is?"
    C. "Do you need to use extra pillows when you sleep?"
    D. "Do any foods make it harder to cough up your secretions?"

9. In observing an infant's chest configuration, the respiratory therapist notices that it is the same size in both the AP and the lateral dimensions. This would indicate that the patient has:
    A. A normal chest
    B. Funnel chest/pectus excavatum
    C. Pulmonary emphysema with air trapping
    D. Lordosis

10. In examining a patient, the respiratory therapist notices that the patient has greatly diminished breath sounds in the right lower lobe and the trachea has shifted to the right. These signs indicate which condition?
    A. Right-sided pneumothorax
    B. Right-sided atelectasis
    C. Left-sided pneumothorax
    D. Left-sided pneumonia

11. In palpating a patient for symmetrical chest movements, it is noticed that the patient's left side does not move as much as the right side. This indicates that the patient has which condition or conditions?
    1. Emphysema
    2. Congestive heart failure
    3. Left-sided pneumonia
    4. Left-sided pneumothorax
    5. Right-sided pneumonia
    A. 2 only
    B. 3 and 4 only
    C. 4 and 5 only
    D. 1 and 2 only

12. A respiratory therapist is called to the Emergency Department to help evaluate a pediatric patient. Upon entering the room, a harsh, high-pitched sound is heard on the patient's inspiration. Which of the following is true?
    A. Sounds are tracheal.
    B. Sounds are bronchovesicular.
    C. Sounds are stridorous.
    D. Sounds are bronchial.

13. A respiratory therapist is called to evaluate a patient's breathing pattern. It is noticed that the patient's tidal volumes go from small to large to small and then stop

for 10 seconds before starting up again. The pattern repeats itself. This patient's breathing pattern would best be called:
    A. Eupnea
    B. Obstructed expiration
    C. Kussmaul's respiration
    D. Cheyne-Stokes respiration

14. A tension pneumothorax is identified by which of the following?
    1. Chest X-ray film shows a shift of the mediastinum toward the affected lung.
    2. Chest X-ray film shows elevation of the hemidiaphragm on the affected side.
    3. The patient's vital signs suddenly deteriorate.
    4. Chest X-ray film shows a depression of the hemidiaphragm on the affected side.
    5. Chest X-ray film shows a shift of the mediastinum away from the affected lung.
    6. Vital signs are essentially unchanged.
    A. 1, 2, and 6 only
    B. 3, 4, and 5 only
    C. 1, 2, and 3 only
    D. 1, 3, and 4 only

15. An adult patient is complaining of localized pain over the lower right area of the chest while breathing. When you auscultate the patient's chest, a rasping noise is heard at the point of pain on both inspiration and expiration. This is most likely:
    A. Pleural friction rub
    B. Normal breath sounds
    C. Wheeze
    D. Rhonchi

16. A 65-year-old female patient has distended external jugular veins even though her head and body are raised 45 degrees above her legs. This would indicate that she:
    A. Is hypertensive
    B. Is fluid-overloaded
    C. Has emphysema
    D. Is dehydrated

17. Tactile fremitus would be reduced in all of the following conditions EXCEPT:
    A. Pneumothorax
    B. COPD
    C. Pulmonary edema
    D. Pleural effusion

18. A frail, thin patient known to have lung cancer is admitted to the hospital. The patient's family members are also present. What should be asked of them to make sure the proper level of care is delivered?
    A. The last time the patient ate
    B. The last time the patient had a bowel movement
    C. Whether any advance directives have been documented

D. Whether the patient has brought home care medications

19. It is most important to ask a patient with a broken ankle from a recent slip on an icy sidewalk about which of the following?
    A. Level of pain
    B. Level of consciousness
    C. Work of breathing
    D. Emotional state

20. All of the following could result in a mediastinal shift on a chest X-ray film EXCEPT:
    A. Right-sided hemothorax
    B. Bilateral lower-lobe pneumonia
    C. Left-sided tension pneumothorax
    D. Right lower-lobe atelectasis

21. A patient who is suffering respiratory distress would exhibit all of the following EXCEPT:
    A. Normal respiratory rate
    B. Nasal flaring
    C. Intercostal retractions
    D. Use of accessory muscles of inspiration

22. An adult patient with a history of smoking has shown an increased anteroposterior diameter and depressed hemidiaphragms on a PA chest radiograph. It is most likely that the patient has:
    A. Pulmonary fibrosis
    B. Emphysema
    C. Taken too deep a breath
    D. Left-ventricular failure

23. After 2 days of vomiting and diarrhea caused by the flu, a 50-year-old patient is admitted. The patient's ECG shows five PVCs in 1 minute and flat T waves. What laboratory test would you recommend?
    A. Urinalysis
    B. Arterial blood gas analysis
    C. Electrolytes
    D. Complete blood count

24. A 48-year-old patient with an extensive smoking history usually coughs out about 20 mL of sputum every day. The patient developed a "chest cold" 4 days ago and has noticed increased shortness of breath and thicker secretions. What should be done at this time?
    A. Have the patient increase the flow on his home oxygen concentrator.
    B. Get a sputum sample for a culture-and-sensitivity study.
    C. Have the patient perform a 6-minute walk test.
    D. Perform percussion to determine the hemidiaphragm positions.

25. A recently home-delivered baby is brought in to the Emergency Department by the paramedics. The physician asks the respiratory therapist to help evaluate the newborn's condition. Normal vital signs for a term newborn include all of the following EXCEPT:
    A. Heart rate of 130/min
    B. Rectal temperature of 36.5° C
    C. Blood pressure of 64/40 mm Hg
    D. Respiratory rate of 20/min

26. The respiratory therapist is assisting with the delivery of a high-risk infant. After being evaluated, the infant is given a 5-minute Apgar score of 8. What should be recommended to the assisting nurse and physician?
    A. Give the infant supplemental oxygen.
    B. Give the mother supplemental oxygen.
    C. Begin bag/mask rescue breathing on the infant.
    D. Give the infant to the mother for bonding.

27. The respiratory therapist is called to the pediatrics department to help in the evaluation and care of a 4-year-old girl who has been sick with a bad cold for the past 2 days. In viewing a lateral neck radiograph of the child, the following are seen: (1) clear air column through the upper airway and (2) pointed narrowing of the tracheal air column below the larynx. What is the child's most likely condition?
    A. Laryngotracheobronchitis
    B. Aspirated a coin
    C. Epiglottitis
    D. Tonsillitis

28. A young adult who had surgery for a deviated nasal septum was accidentally given 2 L of intravenous fluid in 1 hour. Which of the following signs would point to the patient being fluid-overloaded?
    1. Tachycardia
    2. Bradycardia
    3. High urine specific gravity
    4. Peripheral edema
    5. Low urine specific gravity
    A. 3 and 4 only
    B. 1 and 3 only
    C. 2 and 5 only
    D. 1, 4, and 5 only

29. Patients with heart or lung disease commonly have shifting of mediastinal structures. In evaluating patients with cardiopulmonary disease, which of the following could result in a mediastinal shift being seen on a chest radiograph?
    1. Right-sided hemothorax
    2. Bilateral lower-lobe pneumonia
    3. Left-sided tension pneumothorax
    4. Left lower-lobe atelectasis
    5. Fibrosis of the left lung
    A. 3 only
    B. 4 and 5 only
    C. 1, 2, and 3 only
    D. 1, 3, 4, and 5 only

30. The radiologist remarks upon viewing a 65-year-old patient's PA chest radiograph that the patient has an increased cardiothoracic ratio. This indicates to you that:
    A. The patient has an athletic heart.
    B. The patient has a left pleural effusion.
    C. The patient has an abnormal heart.
    D. The patient has a left middle-lobe infiltrate.

31. A patient has acute respiratory distress syndrome and is significantly hypoxemic. It is likely that the patient will exhibit all the following EXCEPT:
    A. A normal respiratory rate
    B. Nasal flaring
    C. Intercostal retractions
    D. Use of accessory muscles of inspiration

32. An adult patient with a history of COPD and left-ventricular failure has been hospitalized. A series of diagnostic procedures is being performed. The preferred radiographic position to minimize distortion of the heart is:
    A. Anteroposterior
    B. Posteroanterior
    C. Lateral
    D. Oblique

33. An intubated patient has been moved from the operating room to the Intensive Care Unit. Upon arrival there is concern that the endotracheal tube has moved. What is the best way to determine its location?
    A. Palpate the larynx.
    B. Listen to stomach sounds.
    C. Percuss the patient's chest.
    D. Get a chest radiograph.

34. A 65-year-old patient with repeated episodes of congestive heart failure has a chest radiograph taken. The radiograph shows the left costophrenic angle to be blunted with an air/fluid level with a meniscus in the left lower-lung area. How should this be interpreted?
    A. Pleural effusion of the left lung
    B. Pulmonary edema of the left lung
    C. Pneumonia of the left lung
    D. Pulmonary embolism of the left lung

35. A 3-day-old newborn is brought into the Emergency Department with the father after they were involved in an automobile accident. The newborn is showing signs of respiratory distress with cyanosis and tachycardia. What test would you recommend to determine whether the newborn has a pneumothorax?
    A. Arterial blood gases
    B. Apgar score
    C. Transillumination
    D. Thoracentesis

36. The respiratory therapist is assisting in the delivery of a high-risk neonate. At 1 minute after birth, the following are noted:
    • Heart rate is 90 beats/min.
    • There is a weak cry.
    • Arms and legs show some flexion.
    • The baby grimaces when a nasal catheter is inserted into a nostril.
    • Extremities are blue with a pink body (acrocyanosis).
    The neonate should be given an Apgar score of:
    A. 3
    B. 5
    C. 7
    D. 9

37. An elderly patient with congestive heart failure has been treated with the diuretic furosemide (Lasix). Which serum electrolyte is the most important to monitor in this situation?
    A. Potassium
    B. Chloride
    C. Calcium
    D. Sodium

38. A newborn has been admitted to the neonatal Intensive Care Unit. The physician has determined the newborn to have a Silverman score of 5. How should this be interpreted?
    A. Within the normal range
    B. Suctioning is indicated
    C. Moderate respiratory distress
    D. Severe respiratory distress

2 Infection Control

Note: It can be anticipated that the Therapist Multiple-Choice Examination (TMC) will include an *average of 4 of 140 actual questions* (3% of the exam) on infection control. (This is based on the question mix typically found on the National Board of Respiratory Care's previous Entry Level Examinations and Written Registry Examinations.)

Remember that the TMC version you take will include 20 additional questions being evaluated for possible inclusion in other versions of the TMC. So, there will be a total of 160 questions taken. There is no way to differentiate between the 140 actual questions and the 20 questions being evaluated for future use. Please go to the Introduction for detailed information on the Therapist Multiple-Choice Examination and the Clinical Simulation Examination.

MODULE A

Adhere to infection control policies and procedures (e.g., Standard Precautions, isolation) (code: IIB5) [difficulty: R].

1. Standard precautions

Standard (formerly called Universal) Precautions are designed for the care of all patients, regardless of their diagnosis or presumed infection status. Barriers such as gloves and masks and other procedures are used to prevent contact with body fluids. This approach to patient care has been adopted because of the concern of health care workers and the public that the human immunodeficiency virus (HIV), hepatitis B, or other deadly pathogens may be spread unknowingly by contact. Box 2-1 includes specific Standard Precaution guidelines established by the Centers for Disease Control and Prevention (CDC) and the Occupational Safety and Health Administration.

2. Hand hygiene

Hand washing or sanitizing is the single most important procedure for reducing the spread of infection. An alcohol-based sanitizing foam, gel, or rinse (often with a skin softener) should be rubbed onto the hands for at least 15 s unless they are obviously contaminated or soiled with body fluids or waste. Then, the hands should be washed with plain soap and warm tap water for at least 15 s. An antimicrobial soap should be used only if called for in the infection control protocol (for example, a surgical scrub).

In any case, respiratory therapists should wash or sanitize their hands before and between each patient contact. The following times are recommended when working in a general patient care area:

- When coming on duty.
- When hands are obviously soiled or after contamination by blood or other patient body fluids. Hands should be washed, rather than using a cleansing agent, if a patient has an antibiotic-resistant infection, such as *Clostridium difficile* or methicillin-resistant *Staphylococcus aureus* (MRSA).
- Before contact with the face and mouth of a patient, especially if the patient has an artificial airway.
- Before setting up equipment or pouring medications.
- When leaving an isolation area or handling contaminated articles from an isolation area.
- After handling soiled dressings, sputum containers, urinals, bedpans, catheters, etc.
- After removing patient care gloves. When working in a restricted area, such as the operating room, burn unit, or neonatal Intensive Care Unit, policy may require hand washing before putting on gloves and entering the unit, as well as after removing the gloves.
- After personal use of the toilet.
- After using hands to cover a cough and after blowing or wiping the nose.
- Before eating or serving food.
- On completion of duty.

The most common bacterial organisms spread by personal contact are *S. aureus*, *Escherichia coli*, and *Streptococcus* species. Suspect personal contact and poor hand cleansing whenever a patient has one of these infections.

Exam Hint 2-1

Past examinations have asked about the importance of hand washing or sanitizing and the indications for it to prevent the spread of infection.

3. Respiratory hygiene/cough etiquette

To contain respiratory secretions, anyone with signs and symptoms of a respiratory infection should be told to do the following:

- Cover nose and mouth when coughing or sneezing.
- Use tissues to contain secretions.
- Throw away used tissues in the nearest waste container.

BOX 2-1   Standard Precautions to Prevent the Spread of Infection

Exclusion from Patient Contact

Any health care worker with exudative skin lesions should not work in the direct care of patients.

Personal Protective Equipment

1. Gloves should be worn under these conditions: during direct contact with blood, body fluids, secretions, mucous membranes, and wounds; when handling all items or surfaces contaminated by blood or body fluids; when performing venipuncture; or when handling intravenous catheters or monitoring devices.
2. Gloves must be changed between patients or if the gloves become torn or punctured, as with a needle-stick injury.
3. Hands should be washed immediately after the gloves are removed; the hands and any other body areas must be washed immediately if contaminated by blood or other body fluid.
4. Masks, eye goggles, or face shields, as well as gowns or aprons, should be worn when a procedure is performed that may lead to the splashing or splattering of blood, secretions, or body fluids.
5. Contaminated masks, goggles, face shields, gowns, and aprons should be removed and disposed of properly.
6. Contaminated worker uniforms should be left at the hospital for cleaning.

Needle and Instrument Precautions

1. Care should be taken when needles and sharp instruments are handled.
2. Used needles and sharp instruments should be placed into puncture-resistant containers for proper disposal; reusable needles should be placed into a puncture-resistant container for transport.
3. No attempt should be made to manually recap arterial blood gas or other needles, remove them from the syringe, or bend or cut them (needle-covering systems or methods of pushing the needle into a rubber cube are used widely; these require the use of only one hand with no touching of the needle).

Patient Specimens

1. Blood and body fluids should be placed into leak-proof, sturdy plastic bags for transportation to the laboratory.
2. The laboratory requisition form should be placed on the outside of this bag.

Cardiopulmonary Resuscitation

1. Mouth-to-mouth breathing should be avoided even though no evidence suggests that saliva transmits human immunodeficiency virus infection.
2. Mouth-to-valve mask resuscitators and manual resuscitators (bag-valve) should be readily available for use in ventilating patients.

- Cleanse the hands after contact with respiratory secretions. An alcohol-based hand rub should be used when hand washing cannot be done.
- Wear a surgical mask and sit at least 3 feet away from others.
- Droplet Precautions should be used by health care workers when working with a patient who is showing signs and symptoms of a respiratory infection.

4. Respiratory care equipment and procedures

The following guidelines are recommended to minimize the spread of infection by equipment and procedures. Follow the manufacturer's specific guidelines when applicable:

a. Each patient should have his or her own equipment.
b. Disposable equipment should be discarded after use.
c. Reusable equipment should undergo high-level disinfection or should be sterilized between patients.
d. Equipment such as O_2 masks, large-volume nebulizers, and aerosol tubing should be changed every 24 hours.
e. Ventilator breathing circuits should be changed only when they are visibly soiled with secretions or blood. If a heat–moisture exchanger is used for humidification, it may be kept with the circuit for at least 48 hours unless visibly soiled.
f. Sterile water should be used for procedures, and the unused portion should be discarded after 24 hours.
g. Add water to reservoir systems immediately before use.
h. Discard any unused water in a reservoir system before refilling.

i. Drain and discard any water collected in tubing; do *not* drain water back into the reservoir.
j. Medications should be stored under the conditions set by the manufacturer, should be discarded if they appear abnormal, and should be discarded on the expiration date.
k. Unused portions of medications should be discarded after 24 hours.
l. Sterile syringes should be used when measuring medications.
m. Sterile suction catheters should be used and sterile gloves worn whenever the patient's airway is suctioned.

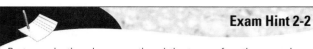

Exam Hint 2-2

Past examinations have questioned the types of routine procedures that should be performed to control the spread of infection through respiratory care equipment.

5. Isolation (transmission prevention) protocols

Transmission prevention protocols are used for patients known or suspected to be infected or colonized with epidemiologically significant pathogens that are spread through airborne or droplet transmission or by contact with dry skin or contaminated surfaces. These protocols are used in addition to Standard Precautions. The following are general guidelines and specific diseases or conditions established by the CDC for the three types of patient isolation categories. Hospitals may establish extra standards and post them at the door to the patient's room.

a. Airborne precautions

Airborne Precautions are used in addition to Standard Precautions for patients with known or suspected illnesses transmitted by airborne droplet nuclei, such as pulmonary tuberculosis (TB), varicella (chickenpox), rubeola (measles), and H1N1 avian influenza (flu), and when severe acute respiratory syndrome (SARS) is known or strongly suspected. Because droplet nuclei are small and lightweight, they can travel farther than a droplet in an air current.

1. Room placement

Patients under Airborne Precautions must be placed in an airborne infection isolation room. This negative pressure room must have 6 to 12 air changes per hour. Room air can be vented outside of the building, or it can be recirculated through a high-efficiency particulate air filter.

2. Gloves and hand washing

Use standard precautions.

3. Respiratory protection

a. If a patient is known to have or is suspected of having TB or SARS, a National Institute for Occupational Safety and Health (NIOSH)-approved respirator mask (N-95, N-99, or N-100) must be worn by all caregivers who enter the room. The respirator mask should be fit tested for the individual to ensure there are no air leaks. If the caregiver cannot wear an N-95 mask, a powered air protection respirator must be worn.
b. If a patient is known to have or is suspected of having varicella or rubeola, a NIOSH-approved respirator mask (N-95 or higher) must be worn by all *susceptible* caregivers who enter the room.

4. Eye protection

Health care workers should wear goggles or a face shield when within 3 feet of the patient.

5. Patient transport

a. Transport personnel must wear a NIOSH-approved respirator mask (N-95 or higher).
b. The patient must wear an isolation mask while out of his or her room.

6. Patient equipment

Use standard precautions.

b. Droplet precautions

Droplet Precautions are used in addition to Standard Precautions for patients known to have or suspected of having serious illness transmitted by large-particle droplets such as human influenza (flu), invasive *Haemophilus influenzae* (type b), *Neisseria meningitidis* disease including meningococcal bacteremia and meningitis, *Mycoplasma pneumoniae*, and *Bordetella pertussis*. A patient with *possible* SARS also is placed into this group until the condition is ruled out. (If SARS is confirmed, the patient is kept under Droplet, Airborne, Contact, and Standard Precautions.) Droplets can be spread by coughing, talking, or sneezing and during suctioning and bronchoscopy procedures. Droplets are larger and heavier than droplet nuclei and usually do not travel more than 3–10 feet from the patient source.

1. Room placement

A private room is preferred, but patients with the same infection may be placed in the same room. (This is known as cohorting.)

2. Gloves and hand washing

Use standard precautions.

3. Gown

Use standard precautions.

4. Respiratory protection

a. Use standard precautions.
b. Caregivers must wear an isolation mask if working within 3 feet of the patient.

5. Patient transport

a. Transport personnel must wear an isolation mask if working within 3 feet of the patient.
b. The patient must wear an isolation mask while out of his or her room.

6. Patient equipment

Use standard precautions.

c. Contact precautions

Contact Precautions are used in addition to Standard Precautions for patients known to have or suspected of having epidemiologically important organisms that can be transmitted by direct contact with environmental surfaces, such as patients with SARS, avian flu, diarrhea (for example, *C. difficile*, vancomycin-resistant enterococcus), wound infection (for example, MRSA or vancomycin-resistant *S. aureus*), respiratory syncytial virus in a young child, or localized herpes zoster (shingles).

1. Room placement

A private room is preferred, but patients with the same infection may be placed in the same room. (This is known as cohorting.)

2. Gloves and hand washing

a. Wear gloves when entering the patient's room.
b. Change gloves after contact with any contaminated item.
c. Remove gloves and wash hands before leaving the patient's room.

3. Gown

a. Wear a gown when entering the patient's room if you anticipate substantial contact with the patient, environmental surfaces, or patient items.

b. Remove the gown and wash hands before leaving the room.

4. Respiratory protection

Use standard precautions.

5. Patient transport

a. Limit transportation of the patient from the room. The patient must wear a clean gown.

b. If transportation is required, caregivers must wear a gown and gloves.

6. Patient equipment

a. Each patient should have his or her own dedicated noncritical equipment (thermometer, commode, blood pressure cuff, sphygmomanometer, stethoscope, etc.).

b. Clean and disinfect all patient care equipment after the patient has been discharged.

6. Implement infectious disease protocols

a. Avian flu (avian influenza)

Avian flu (also called "bird flu") is caused by influenza type A viruses that primarily infect poultry. Although human infections are rare, persons in contact with infected poultry or who inhale infected aerosolized droppings from infected poultry can become infected. A person who presents with a severe febrile respiratory illness and has traveled within the past 10 days from an area with an avian flu outbreak (usually China or a Southeast Asia country) should be suspected of having avian flu. Standard Precautions and Droplet Precautions are implemented for the patient. These precautions are continued for 14 days after the symptoms begin or until (1) it is proven that the patient does not have avian flu or (2) a different diagnosis is established.

See the previous discussion on Standard Precautions, respiratory hygiene/cough etiquette, and Droplet Precautions for guidance on how to prevent the spread of this infection. In addition, all health care workers should be immunized against influenza.

b. Severe acute respiratory syndrome

SARS is caused by a corona virus (CoV) (thus the common abbreviation SARS-CoV). This rare but serious pulmonary infection is spread by respiratory droplets through close person-to-person contact. If a person has a serious pneumonia or acute respiratory distress syndrome with an unknown cause and has traveled to China or a Southeast Asia country within the past 10 days, SARS infection should be considered until another cause can be found.

See the previous discussion on Standard Precautions, respiratory hygiene/cough etiquette, and Droplet Precautions for guidance on how to prevent the spread of this infection.

MODULE B

Recommend vaccinations (code: IIIE4l) [difficulty: R].

1. Pneumovax

The Pneumovax 23 (pneumococcal vaccine polyvalent) vaccine provides protection against the 23 most prevalent or invasive types of *Streptococcus pneumoniae* bacteria. Patients with serious chronic illness should be immunized to prevent them from developing this very dangerous type of pneumonia. Guidelines for immunization include the following:

Any *immunocompetent* person 2 years of age or older who has one or more of the following conditions should be immunized:

- 50 years of age or older
- Chronic cardiovascular disease (congestive heart failure and cardiomyopathies)
- Chronic pulmonary disease (chronic obstructive pulmonary disease, asthma with chronic bronchitis)
- Diabetes mellitus
- Alcoholism or chronic liver disease
- Cerebrospinal fluid leaks
- Sickle cell disease
- Splenectomy
- Lives in a special environment or social setting (Alaskan Natives and certain American Indian populations)

Any *immunoincompetent* person 2 years of age or older who has one or more of the following conditions should be immunized:

- HIV infection
- Leukemia
- Lymphoma
- Hodgkin's disease
- Multiple myeloma
- Generalized malignancy
- Renal failure or nephrotic syndrome
- Receiving immunosuppressive chemotherapy including corticosteroids
- Organ or bone marrow transplant

Revaccination is recommended in the following circumstances as long as at least 5 years have passed since the first vaccination:

1. An immunocompetent person 65 years of age or older
2. An immunoincompetent person who is at highest risk for a serious pneumococcal infection or who has a rapid drop in pneumococcal antibody levels

A third vaccination is not recommended. In general, vaccination should be performed at least 2 weeks before certain medical procedures such as elective splenectomy or immunosuppressive therapy are started. The Pneumovax

23 intramuscular or subcutaneous injection can be given at the same time as the influenza vaccination, as long as a different arm is used for each injection.

2. Influenza

Seasonal influenza (flu) vaccination begins in September or October of each year but can be given later if necessary. Two ways to be immunized are available, and each method provides protection against three strains of flu virus. The intramuscular injection vaccine contains inactivated or killed virus and is given to healthy people and those with medical conditions. The inhaled vaccine is given only to healthy individuals between 5 and 49 years of age; pregnant women are excluded.

The flu vaccine is recommended for the following groups:
- Children 6-59 months of age
- A woman who will be pregnant during the flu season
- Those who will be 50 years or older
- Anyone 6 months of age or older with a chronic heart or lung condition, including asthma
- Anyone with difficulty breathing or swallowing caused by brain injury or disease, spinal cord injury, seizure disorder, or neuromuscular disease
- Anyone who has been hospitalized or needed regular doctor visits in the past year because of chronic medical conditions such as diabetes, kidney disease, hemoglobin abnormalities, or a weakened immune system
- Those between 6 months and 18 years of age in need of regular aspirin therapy who might therefore be at risk for Reye's syndrome if they get the flu
- Residents of nursing homes or similar facilities
- Family members and caregivers of children younger than 6 months of age and anyone at risk for severe complications from influenza
- Any health care worker

The influenza vaccination injection and Pneumovax 23 intramuscular or subcutaneous injection can be given at the same time as long as a different arm is used for each injection.

MODULE C

Decontaminate respiratory care equipment.

Decontamination is the process of disassembling, washing (to remove dried secretions or other debris), rinsing, disinfecting or sterilizing, and reassembling used patient care equipment. The choice of whether to disinfect or sterilize the equipment depends on how it is used clinically, what type of pathogen is involved, and from what material the equipment is made. The process results in the equipment being free of any pathogens, so that it can be used with another patient.

Most respiratory pathogens are not spore-formers, so low-level or high-level disinfection is acceptable. Either

a glutaraldehyde solution (alkaline, acid, or buffered) or pasteurization is used in most departments for disinfecting plastic masks, hoses, etc. See Table 2-1 for details on the most commonly used methods of disinfection. (It is beyond the scope of this book to cover all methods now available.) Any department that processes its own equipment must have adequate facilities for receiving used equipment and for its disassembly, cleansing, packaging, and distribution. First, a "dirty" area must exist where contaminated equipment is brought for disassembly, scrubbing of secretions or blood, and rinsing. Equipment then is placed into the glutaraldehyde solution or a pasteurizing machine. After that, equipment is taken to a "clean" area to be rinsed, dried, reassembled, and placed into plastic bags for storage. Care must be taken not to recontaminate the equipment during this procedure. Items that must be sterilized usually are just processed through the dirty area before being sent to the central supply department, where equipment is sterilized. See Table 2-2 for details on the most commonly used methods of sterilization. (It is beyond the scope of this book to cover all methods now available.)

1. Select the appropriate agent and technique for surface disinfection (code: IIB2) [difficulty: R]

Disinfection is a procedure that significantly reduces the microbial contamination of the equipment that has been processed. All disinfection processes destroy the vegetative form (the cell) of pathogenic organisms, including the vast majority of respiratory system pathogens. However, a few *Bacillus*-type bacteria are difficult to kill because they have a particularly tough cell wall or have spores for reproduction. Spores are analogous to seeds in that they grow into bacteria under the right conditions and are resistant to drying, heat, and many chemicals that kill the bacterial cell. Therefore, a spore-forming organism may be able to reproduce itself after the cell has been killed. Obviously, disinfection can be used only on equipment that is *not* contaminated by spore-forming bacteria. Knowing what pathogen has infected the patient, if possible, can help the clinician determine the appropriate disinfection (or sterilization) method to be used on contaminated equipment. Some disinfecting agents kill different kinds of organisms, depending on the length of exposure time.

In the hospital or a long-term care facility, equipment or instruments that do not directly touch the patient (e.g., an electrocardiograph machine, ventilator, oxygen blender) are classified as *noncritical* (low risk of spreading infection) and can undergo *low-level* disinfection. Low-level disinfectants are agents capable of killing some vegetative bacteria, fungi, and lipophilic viruses. As shown in Table 2-1, alcohol and iodine solutions are widely used for the low-level disinfection of equipment surfaces.

Blood spills or splashes on equipment require special attention because of the risk of hepatitis or HIV infection.

TABLE 2-1   Commonly Used Methods of Disinfection in the Hospital Setting for Respiratory Care-Related Equipment

Method	Conditions	MICROBES EFFECTIVE AGAINST					Comments
		Bacteria	Tuberculosis (TB)	Spores	Viruses	Fungi	
Low- and Intermediate-Level Disinfection							
Pasteurization	Complete immersion in water heated to 70° C (170° F) for 30 minutes	Yes	Yes	No	Yes	Yes	Use with rubber and many plastics used in respiratory care, especially those that are sensitive to a high temperature. *Avoid use* with any item that cannot be immersed or will be damaged at this temperature.
Alcohols (70% ethyl or 90% isopropyl)	Complete immersion for several minutes or pooling of alcohol on the equipment	Yes	Yes	No	Lipophilic only	Yes	Use with metallic or plastic surfaces of large pieces of equipment that cannot be disinfected by any other means. Also may be used with most plastics. *Avoid use* with any item that cannot be immersed or will absorb or be damaged by the alcohol.
Iodines (iodine or iodophor with 70% ethyl alcohol)	Complete immersion for several minutes or pooling of the solution on the equipment	Yes	Yes	No	Yes	Yes	Use with metallic or plastic surfaces of large pieces of equipment that cannot be disinfected by any other means. Also may be used with most plastics. *Avoid use* with any item that cannot be immersed or will absorb or be damaged by the alcohol.
High-Level Disinfection: Glutaraldehyde Solutions							
Alkaline glutaraldehyde (Cidex, Cidex 7, Sporicidin)	Complete immersion for 10 minutes	Yes	Yes	No	Yes	Yes	Use with rubber and many plastics used in respiratory care, especially those that are heat sensitive. Care must be taken to thoroughly rinse items after disinfection. *Avoid use* with any item that cannot be immersed or will absorb the solution.
Acid glutaraldehyde (Sonacide)	Complete immersion for 20 minutes	Yes	Yes	No	Yes	Yes	Use with rubber and many plastics used in respiratory care, especially those that are heat sensitive. Care must be taken to thoroughly rinse items after they have been disinfected. *Avoid use* with any item that cannot be immersed or will absorb the solution.

The CDC requires that blood spills be cleaned up with a chlorine compound (bleach).

Home care patients typically will not use alcohol or iodine solutions because of the high cost. Instead, the plastics used in home care medication nebulizers, etc., usually are disinfected in a white vinegar (acetic acid) solution. A 1.25% or higher percentage solution is classified as a low-level disinfectant and will kill most vegetative bacteria (including *Pseudomonas aeruginosa*) and some fungi and viruses. However, *Mycobacterium tuberculosis*, nonlipid viruses, and spores will not be killed.

Home care equipment is often cleansed in the following way:

1. Disassemble as needed.
2. Run hot water from the tap to eliminate as many organisms as possible. Clean the sink.
3. Use hot water to wash the equipment in a detergent solution.
4. Place the equipment into a white vinegar solution for disinfection. It should soak for 60 minutes. (Grocery store-purchased white vinegar contains 5% acetic acid. However, it may be diluted with three parts of water to

TABLE 2-2	Commonly Used Methods of Sterilization in the Hospital Setting for Respiratory Care-Related Equipment	
Method	**Conditions**	**Comments**
Steam autoclave	Autoclave chamber with an internal steam pressure of 15 lb per square inch, 121° C (250° F), 15 minutes	Use with glass, cloth, bandages, unsharpened stainless steel instruments, ventilator bacteria filters. *Avoid use* with many plastics used in respiratory care, rubber, dextrose solutions, sharpened stainless steel instruments, electrical devices, or machines.
Dry heat	Autoclave chamber at 160° C to 180° C (320° F to 356° F), 2 hours	Use with glass or sharpened stainless steel instruments. *Avoid use* with many plastics used in respiratory care, rubber, dextrose solutions, electric devices, or machines.
Ethylene oxide gas	Specific guidelines vary depending on the manufacturer of the chamber and the supplies or equipment being sterilized. In general, a gas concentration of 800-1000 mg/L must be kept for 3-4 hours at 50% to 100% relative humidity and 49° C to 57° C (120° F to 135° F). Great care must be taken to predry all items before gassing and to properly aerate them after sterilization	Use with heat-sensitive and moisture-sensitive items, such as many plastics in respiratory care equipment. *Avoid use* with supply pouches or plastic films, such as aluminum foil, nylon, thermoplastic resin (Saran), Mylar, cellophane polyamide, polyester, or other films that are not penetrated by the gas, or with polyvinyl chloride (PVC) that has been sterilized previously by the manufacturer with γ-radiation.
Glutaraldehyde Solutions		
Alkaline glutaraldehyde (Cidex, Cidex 7, Sporicidin)	Complete immersion. Cidex products for 10 hours; Sporicidin for 6 hours and 45 minutes	Use with rubber and many plastics in respiratory care, especially those that are heat sensitive; care must be taken to thoroughly rinse items after they have been cleansed. *Avoid use* with any item that cannot be immersed or that will absorb the solution.
Acid glutaraldehyde (Sonacide)	Complete immersion for 1 hour at 60° C (140° F)	Use with rubber and many plastics used in respiratory care, especially those that are heat sensitive; care must be taken to thoroughly rinse items after they have been cleansed. *Avoid use* with any item that cannot be immersed or that will absorb the solution.

produce a 1.25% solution.) After use, the acetic acid must be thrown away because it will no longer be effective.

5. After soaking, the equipment should be rinsed in hot water and placed on a clean towel to air dry.

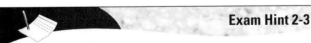

Exam Hint 2-3

Expect to see one question about using white vinegar or acetic acid to disinfect equipment in the home.

2. Implement high-level disinfection techniques (code: IIB1) [difficulty: R]

Equipment or instruments that touch surface mucous membranes and the skin but do not penetrate them are listed as *semicritical* and must undergo *high-level* disinfection (e.g., laryngoscope blades, a bronchoscope). Agents that kill all microorganisms except bacterial spores are classified as high-level disinfectants. See Table 2-1 for details on solutions used for high-level disinfection.

Bronchoscopes require special cleaning attention before being placed into a disinfecting solution. The exterior must be washed off with a gauze and low-sudsing enzymatic solution to remove all mucus. The channel cleaning brush must be used to remove any debris from the biopsy channel.

The type of equipment being cleaned will also influence which disinfection method can be used. Certain processes and agents can be used only on certain types of equipment. Table 2-1 lists the various ways to disinfect reusable patient care equipment in the hospital. Many respiratory care departments will have a pasteurization system for disinfecting reusable plastic equipment items. The equipment must be disassembled and placed onto cleaning racks so that all surfaces can be reached by the hot water (Fig. 2-1). If a toxic glutaraldehyde soak is being done, gloves must be worn when working with it or equipment that has been placed into it. In addition, the room must be well ventilated to avoid breathing in glutaraldehyde fumes.

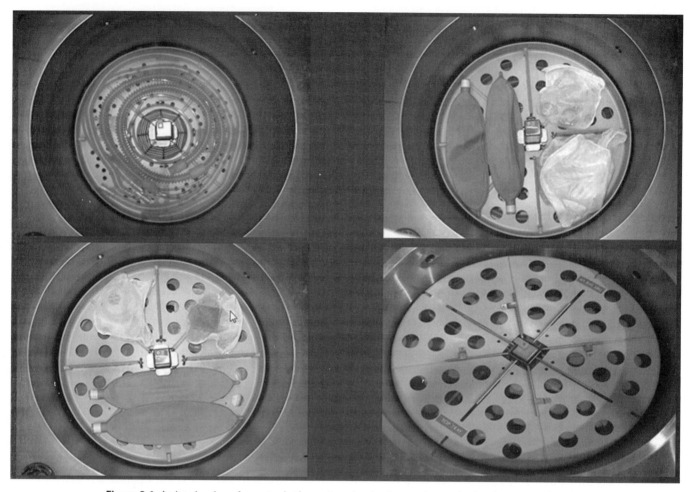

Figure 2-1 An interior view of a pasteurization system showing how equipment is placed onto one of several cleaning racks. The hot water wash will kill vegetative forms of bacteria. (Courtesy of Cenorin, Kent, Washington.)

3. Monitor the sterilization process to ensure its effectiveness (code: IIB3) [difficulty: R]

Sterilization is a procedure that destroys all living microbial organisms and renders them unable to reproduce. All sterilization procedures destroy the vegetative forms and spores of all microscopic organisms. Examples of spore-forming bacteria include *Bacillus anthracis* (anthrax), *Clostridium botulinum* (botulism), *Clostridium tetani* (tetanus), and *Clostridium perfringens* (gas gangrene). Any equipment or instruments that penetrate body tissue (e.g., a surgical scalpel, bronchoscopy forceps) are listed as *critical* (high risk of spreading infection) and must be sterilized before use on another patient. As was discussed previously, the method of sterilization depends on the type of equipment under consideration. Table 2-2 lists various methods of sterilization for reusable supplies and patient care equipment decontaminated in the hospital. Because glutaraldehyde is toxic, gloves must be worn when working with it or equipment that has been placed into it. When ethylene oxide or glutaraldehyde are being used, the room must be well ventilated to avoid breathing in any fumes.

The term *surveillance* describes the monitoring of equipment to ensure that the disinfection or sterilization process was successful and that in-use equipment is not a source of patient contamination. Processing (chemical test strip) indicators are used to ensure that the equipment was sterilized correctly. Examples include special tapes used to hold the wrapping around packages of equipment being autoclaved or placed into ethylene oxide. These tapes turn color when the autoclave has reached the proper temperature or when the correct concentration of ethylene oxide has been reached. The color change shows the user that the package was processed correctly; therefore the package contents are *probably* sterile.

To *prove* that equipment is sterile, a biologic indicator is placed into the wrapped package before sterilization. These biologic indicators are bacterial spores that are killed only if the required conditions are met. For example, the spores of *Bacillus subtilis* are placed onto strips of paper to be killed by ethylene oxide gas. An autoclave is tested for reaching its programmed temperature by placing cultures of *Geobacillus stearothermophilus* with the patient care equipment. After the equipment and biologic indicator have been sent through the sterilization process, the cultures are placed into conditions favorable for growth. If no growth occurs, they are dead; therefore no other living organisms survived.

Equipment held in storage or being used in patient care also is randomly sampled for contamination. A sample is taken for culturing of possible organisms in three ways. The first involves wiping a sterile swab onto an equipment surface and then rubbing it over a plate of growth medium or placing it into a tube of liquid broth. The second, which is used to check inside lengths of tubing, necessitates pouring a liquid broth through the tube and into a sterile container. The third involves sampling the aerosol that a nebulizer produces. A hose usually is attached to the outlet of the nebulizer. The other end of the hose is connected to a funnel, which is attached to a culture plate, where the droplets impact. In all three examples, the growth of any organism in the growth medium indicates a form of contamination. The laboratory then determines whether the organism is pathogenic. If so, measures must be taken to improve the disinfection or sterilization process.

MODULE D

Biohazardous materials

1. Make sure that biohazardous materials are handled properly (code: IIB4) [difficulty: R]

A respiratory therapist is most likely to come into contact with biohazardous materials in the form of infectious waste, body fluids, or needles and syringes. All must be handled and disposed of properly to keep the practitioner and the patient safe. Although hospital policies will vary, infectious waste and body fluids usually are placed into a red bag. The bag is removed from the patient care area and incinerated to ensure that all pathogens are killed.

Needles, syringes, or any sharp objects are placed into a sharps container, which also is red and usually is marked with a biohazard symbol. Every patient room should have a sharps container, so that used needles and syringes can be disposed of easily. If at all possible, the needle should not be recapped after use. Instead, simply drop the used needle and syringe into the slot on the container. Never force anything into the container or put a finger into it. When full, the sharps container should be sealed closed and removed for proper disposal.

BIBLIOGRAPHY

American Association for Respiratory Care (AARC): *Guidelines for the prevention of nosocomial infections*, Dallas, September 1983, *AARC Times*.

American Respiratory Care Foundation (ARCF): Guidelines for disinfection of respiratory care equipment used in the home, *Respir Care* 33:801, 1988.

Cairo JM: Principles of infection control. In Cairo JM, editor: *Mosby's respiratory care equipment*, ed 9, St Louis, 2014, Mosby.

Carroll PL: Protecting the patient and health care provider. In Wyka KA, Mathews PJ, Rutkowski JA, editors: *Foundations of respiratory care*, ed 2, Clifton Park, NY, 2012, Delmar.

Centers for Disease Control (CDC): *Interim recommendations for infection control in health-care facilities caring for patients with known or suspected avian influenza*. Retrieved August 2014, from http://www.cdc.gov/flu/avian/professional/infect-control.htm, May 21, 2004.

Chatburn RL, Kallstrom TJ, Bajaksouzian S: A comparison of acetic acid with a quaternary ammonium compound for disinfection of hand-held nebulizers, *Respir Care* 33(3):179–187, 1988.

Fink JB: Infection control and safety. In Fink JB, Hunt GE, editors: *Clinical practice in respiratory care*, Philadelphia, 1999, Lippincott Williams & Wilkins.

Fraser TG: Principles of infection prevention and control. In Kacmarek RM, Stoller JK, Heuer AJ, editors: *Egan's fundamentals of respiratory care*, ed 10, St Louis, 2013, Mosby.

Gardner DD: Infection control principles. In Hess DR, MacIntyre NR, et al.: *Respiratory care principles and practice*, ed 2, Philadelphia, 2012, Saunders.

Hoffman SW, Gildea TR: Bronchoscope cleaning and reprocessing, *AARC Times* 37(3):31–34, 2013.

Hudzicki J, Wehrman SF: Applied microbiology. In Wyka KA, Mathews PJ, Rutkowski JA, editors: *Foundations of respiratory care*, ed 2, Clifton Park, NY, 2012, Delmar.

Johnson & Johnson Medical: *Cidexplus, 28-day solution*, 1999. Arlington, TX.

Merck & Co., Inc: *Pneumovax 23 (pneumococcal vaccine polyvalent)*, July 2008. Whitehouse Station, NJ.

OSF Saint Anthony Medical Center: *Infection control precautions*, 1998. Rockford, IL.

U.S. Department of Health and Human Services: *Public health guidance for community-level preparedness and response to severe acute respiratory syndrome (SARS)*, version 2: Supplement I: Infection control in healthcare, home, and community settings. January 8, 2004.

U.S. Food and Drug Administration (FDA): *Influenza: Vaccination still the best protection*. Retrieved [date], from http://www.fda.gov/fdac/features/2006/506_influenza.html, September-October 2006.

1. A hospitalized patient who recovered from a *C. botulinum* infection received several respiratory care services. How should a nondisposable plastic pulmonary-function-testing mouthpiece be sterilized before being reused?
   A. Steam autoclave for 15 minutes.
   B. Soak in glutaraldehyde solution for 10 hours.
   C. Pasteurize for 20 minutes.
   D. Soak in an alcohol solution for 15 minutes.

2. A respiratory therapist is working with a home care patient. How should the patient be instructed to clean her small-volume nebulizer?
   1. Soak the equipment in white vinegar.
   2. Put the equipment in the oven, and turn on the broiler for 10 minutes.
   3. Rinse a nebulizer in salt water after each use.
   4. Wash the equipment in hot water with a detergent.
   A. 1 and 4 only
   B. 1 and 2 only
   C. 1, 3, and 4 only
   D. 1, 2, 3, 4

3. After a mechanical ventilator has been discontinued, what is the best method to sterilize the reusable main-flow bacteria filter?
   A. Wrapping it and soaking it in acetic acid
   B. Pasteurization
   C. Glutaraldehyde soak
   D. Steam autoclaving

4. A batch of respiratory care equipment has gone through the gas sterilization process with ethylene oxide. Routine surveillance of the equipment shows that spores of *B. subtilis* have survived the process. What should be done next?
   A. Use the equipment because this organism does not cause illness.
   B. Aerate the gas as usual, and put into use.
   C. Resterilize the equipment, and check for destruction of the spores.
   D. Wipe off the equipment with 70% alcohol to remove the spores from the equipment.

5. A retired home care patient living on a fixed income needs to be able to disinfect her respiratory therapy equipment. Which of the following would be best for her?
   A. Acetic acid
   B. Acid glutaraldehyde
   C. Ethylene oxide system
   D. Warm, soapy water

6. What is the most cost-effective way for a respiratory care department to disinfect large amounts of reusable plastic tubing and oxygen masks?

   A. 70% ethyl alcohol
   B. Steam autoclave
   C. Pasteurization
   D. Dry heat

7. A contaminated Bird Mark 7 intermittent positive-pressure breathing unit must be sterilized before use with another patient. What is the best method?
   A. Pasteurization
   B. Ethylene oxide
   C. 10-hour soak in glutaraldehyde
   D. Steam autoclave

8. A 58-year-old patient had an exacerbation of his COPD related to spring allergies. As he is being prepared for discharge from the hospital, what should the respiratory therapist recommend?
   A. Get an influenza vaccination as soon as possible.
   B. Get a tuberculosis skin test as soon as possible.
   C. Have a throat swab performed to check on a possible Streptococcus infection.
   D. Get an influenza vaccination in the fall.

9. A home care company has found that several of its tracheostomy patients have *E. coli* tracheal infections. What is the most likely cause of the infections?
   A. Poor hand-washing technique by visiting respiratory therapists
   B. Contaminated tracheostomy tubes from the manufacturer
   C. Contaminated bottles of sterile water from the manufacturer
   D. Poor hand-washing technique by patients' family members

10. A respiratory therapist notices that two people in the Emergency Department waiting room are coughing regularly. All of the following should be done EXCEPT:
   A. Have the two coughing people sit near each other.
   B. Have each person wear a face mask while waiting.
   C. Give facial tissues to the two people.
   D. Have both people sit at least 3 feet away from anyone else.

11. A patient has been confirmed to have SARS. Which of the following should be implemented to prevent the disease from spreading?
   1. The patient's health care workers must wear an N-95 face mask.
   2. The patient must wear an N-95 face mask in his or her room.
   3. Airborne precautions are used.
   4. The patient is placed in a positive air pressure room.
   5. Contact precautions are used.

A. 2 and 5 only
B. 1 and 4 only
C. 1, 3, and 5 only
D. 1, 2, 3, 4, 5

12. A home care respiratory therapist is setting up a continuous home oxygen system for a 52-year-old patient with congestive heart failure. In addition to teaching the patient about her condition and how to properly use the oxygen system, which of the following should the therapist recommend?
    A. Get the SARS vaccination.
    B. Get the Pneumovax vaccination if it has not been given already.
    C. Soak the nasal cannula in a glutaraldehyde solution for 1 hour every day.
    D. If the patient has already received the Pneumovax vaccination, she should get a booster.

13. A 47-year-old man who recently returned from a business trip to Hong Kong has a high fever and other signs and symptoms of pneumonia. SARS-CoV is among the conditions being investigated. While the patient is being evaluated, what preventative measures should be taken?
    1. Standard precautions
    2. Contact precautions
    3. Droplet precautions
    4. Airborne precautions
    A. 1 and 4 only
    B. 1 and 3 only
    C. 2 and 4 only
    D. 1, 2, 3, 4

14. An oxygen blender has just been returned from the neonatal Intensive Care Unit. What agent should be used for surface disinfection?

A. 70% ethyl alcohol
B. Acid glutaraldehyde
C. Ethylene oxide
D. Alkaline glutaraldehyde

15. An annual influenza vaccination should be given to which of the following groups?
    1. Health care workers
    2. People 50 years of age and older
    3. Children and adults with asthma
    4. Infants younger than 6 months of age
    A. 1 and 2 only   *older*
    B. 3 and 4 only
    C. 1, 2, and 3 only
    D. 1, 2, 3, 4

16. After assisting in a bronchoscopy to inspect a patient's airways, the respiratory therapist needs to clean the bronchoscope. How should the unit be disinfected?
    1. Glutaraldehyde solution
    2. Iodine solution
    3. Enzymatic detergent
    4. Hot water wash
    A. 2 only
    B. 1 and 3 only
    C. 2 and 4 only
    D. 1, 2, and 3 only

17. After working with a trauma patient in the Emergency Department, a respiratory therapist sees that there is blood on the patient's pulse oximeter. How should it be processed before being used with another patient?
    A. Wiped down with a bleach solution
    B. Low-level disinfection with an alcohol solution
    C. Sterilized by ethylene oxide
    D. High-level disinfection by glutaraldehyde

3

Blood Gas Sampling, Analysis, Monitoring, and Interpretation

Note: It can be anticipated that the Therapist Multiple-Choice Examination (TMC) will include an *average of 10 of 140 actual questions* (7% of the exam) on blood gas sampling, analysis, monitoring, and interpretation. (This is based on the question mix typically found on the National Board of Respiratory Care's (NBRC's) previous Entry Level Examinations and Written Registry Examinations.)

Remember that the TMC version you take will include 20 additional questions being evaluated for possible inclusion in other versions of the TMC. So, there will be a total of 160 questions taken. There is no way to differentiate between the 140 actual questions and the 20 questions being evaluated for future use. Please go to the Introduction for detailed information on the Therapist Multiple-Choice Examination and the Clinical Simulation Examination.

MODULE A

Recommend blood gas analysis (code: IE9) [difficulty: R, Ap, An].

Blood gas analysis and hemoximetry can be performed on a blood sample taken from a systemic artery, pulmonary artery, central vein, peripheral vein, or arterialized capillary to determine one or more of the following values: a patient's oxygen and carbon dioxide pressures, acid–base status (pH), and/or related values. However, not all values can be accurately measured from all sampling sites. See Box 3-1 for the indications for using the various blood sampling sites. An arterial blood gas (ABG) sample is the "gold" standard to which all others are compared. There are three broad, general indications to recommend an ABG sample for analysis:
- To check a patient's oxygenation status (PaO_2)
- To check a patient's acid–base status (pH)
- To check a patient's ventilation status ($PaCO_2$)

Some specific indications follow.

1. Cardiac failure
  a. Congenital defect
  b. Heart attack (myocardial infarction)
  c. Congestive heart failure with or without pulmonary edema

2. Chronic obstructive pulmonary disease (COPD)
  a. Asthma
  b. Emphysema
  c. Bronchitis
  d. Bronchiectasis

3. Any pneumonia that causes hypoxemia

4. Trauma
  a. Broken ribs
  b. Flail chest
  c. Pneumothorax
  d. Hemothorax
  e. Upper-airway trauma

5. Ventilatory failure
  a. Overdose of sedatives or pain relievers
  b. Stroke or head (brain) injury
  c. Spinal cord injury
  d. Neuromuscular diseases such as myasthenia gravis or Guillain-Barré syndrome

6. Airway obstruction
  a. Foreign-body aspiration
  b. Laryngotracheobronchitis (croup)
  c. Epiglottitis

7. Miscellaneous
  a. Smoke inhalation
  b. Carbon monoxide poisoning
  c. Near drowning
  d. Infant respiratory distress syndrome/hyaline membrane disease
  e. Acute respiratory distress syndrome (ARDS)
  f. The patient does not have an indwelling arterial line
  g. A shunt percentage calculation or alveolar–arterial O_2 pressure difference ($P[A–a]O_2$) calculation must be made
  h. Cardiopulmonary resuscitation

A limitation of any blood gas analysis is that the results reveal the condition of the patient only at the moment the sample is drawn and shortly before. Continuous patient monitoring can be done by a pulse oximeter, transcutaneous oxygen monitor, transcutaneous carbon dioxide monitor, or capnometer.

BOX 3-1   Indications for Blood Gas Analysis and Hemoximetry/CO Oximetry

Arterial Blood Gas

- Evaluate a patient's oxygenation (PaO_2, SaO_2), ventilation ($PaCO_2$), and acid–base (pH) status.
- Quantify response to a treatment such as oxygen administration or mechanical ventilation.
- Quantify diagnostic evaluations such as desaturation during an exercise test.
- Monitor the severity and progression of disease processes such as COPD.
- Calculate a patient's oxygen-carrying capability (CaO_2).
- Determine intrapulmonary shunt.

Hemoximetry/CO Oximetry

- Determine the presence and quantity of dyshemoglobins such as carboxyhemoglobin and methemoglobin.
- Determine total hemoglobin.

Central Venous Blood Gas

- Assess goal-directed therapy in a patient with sepsis, with septic shock, or after major surgery.
- Assess adequacy of perfusion in a patient with severe hemorrhagic shock, poor cardiac output, undergoing CPR, or after cardiopulmonary bypass.

Mixed Venous Oxygen Pressure ($P\bar{v}O_2$)

- Calculate a patient's oxygen-carrying capability ($C\bar{v}O_2$).
- Determine intrapulmonary shunt.

Capillary Blood Gas

- Estimate acid–base balance (capillary pH) and adequacy of ventilation ($PcCO_2$) in an infant when an ABG cannot be obtained. (A capillary blood gas sample should not be used to estimate oxygenation [PaO_2].)

Peripheral Venous Blood Gas

- Evaluate pH in patients with uremia or diabetic ketoacidosis.
- When an ABG cannot be obtained in a patient with an exacerbation of COPD, the peripheral pH and bicarbonate values will have good agreement with these arterial values. (Peripheral vein PO_2 and PCO_2 values will not correlate with arterial values.)

Monitoring is done to _continuously_ assess a patient's oxygenation and/or ventilation:

Oxygenation: pulse oximetry (SpO_2), central venous oxygen saturation ($ScvO_2$), transcutaneous oxygen ($PtCO_2$), mixed venous oxygen saturation ($S\bar{v}O_2$)

Ventilation: transcutaneous carbon dioxide ($PtcCO_2$), end-tidal carbon dioxide ($PetCO_2$)

Source: American Association for Respiratory Care: Clinical practice guideline: blood gas analysis and hemoximetry: Respir Care 58(10):1694-1703, 2013; American Association for Respiratory Care: Clinical practice guideline: capillary blood gas sampling for neonatal & pediatric patients, Respir Care 46(5):506-513, 2001; American Association for Respiratory Care: Clinical practice guideline: transcutaneous blood gas monitoring for carbon dioxide and oxygen: Respir Care 57(11):1955-1962, 2012.

MODULE B

Obtain a blood gas sample.

1. Blood gas sampling device selection and preparation

A properly prepared sampling device is essential to obtaining a blood sample that accurately reflects the patient's physiologic values.

a. Get the appropriate blood gas sampler

Obtaining an ABG sample generally involves selecting a prepackaged, sterile blood gas kit that contains the following:

- A variety of short-bevel needles: 23 or 24 gauge for radial or dorsalis pedis puncture and a 22 gauge for brachial or femoral puncture
- 3-mL syringe; many kits contain a syringe prepared with heparin as an anticoagulant
- If needed, liquid sodium or lithium heparin with an appropriate concentration
- Alcohol or iodophor (Betadine) wipes to clean the puncture site

If a blood gas kit is not available, an appropriate individual needle, 3-mL syringe, and liquid sodium or lithium heparin must be obtained. These should be available at any nursing station or from the respiratory care department.

A capillary blood gas sample requires the following:

- Several heparinized glass capillary tubes with a volume of at least 100 μL
- Metal filing (flea) to place into each capillary tube, if needed
- Plastic caps or clay to seal the tubes
- Magnet to draw the metal filing back and forth in the tube to mix the blood, if needed
- Lancet to make incision
- Moist, warm (42° C) cloth or diaper to wrap around the puncture site, or a chemical warmer
- Sterile cotton balls and bandage to place over the puncture site to aid clotting
- Isopropyl alcohol swabs (70%) to clean the puncture site
- Clean gloves to protect the practitioner's hands from any contact with spilled blood

b. Put the equipment together and make sure that it works properly

To assemble a blood gas syringe, use sterile technique to screw the selected needle onto the syringe. If the syringe does not contain heparin, it must be added. Do this by aspirating liquid heparin through the needle into the syringe. Coat the inside of the syringe with heparin by tipping the needle up, pulling the plunger back, and pushing the plunger forward to squirt the excess heparin out of the needle. This ensures that the needle and dead space of the needle are filled with heparin, and the inside of the syringe is coated. The plunger should easily slide within the barrel of the syringe. A blood clot or debris within the needle will prevent the plunger from moving and blood will not fill the syringe. Replace and safely dispose of a needle that is obstructed.

c. Make sure no air bubbles are in the syringe

Any bubbles of room air can result in errors in the patient's measured values. For example, if the patient was breathing room air, an air bubble would result in the measured oxygen level being too high. In addition, because there is virtually no carbon dioxide in room air, an air bubble would reduce the patient's measured carbon dioxide level and increase the pH. If an air bubble is found in the syringe, tilt it so that the needle is up. The bubble will rise by itself or may be raised by tapping the syringe. Remove the needle and apply a safety filter to allow air to vent from the syringe and prevent blood contamination. Push the plunger into the syringe to eject the air bubble. Cap off the hub of the syringe or needle to prevent air from entering the syringe.

d. Use the proper amount of heparin

This is a concern when liquid heparin is added to a needle and syringe. Aspirate about 1 mL of 10 mg/mL or 1000 units/mL sodium heparin through the needle into the syringe. Pull the plunger back to coat the inside of the syringe. Push the plunger forward to squirt the excess heparin out through the needle. The values of a 2- to 4-mL sample of blood should not be affected by this concentration. Remember that inadequate heparin can cause the blood sample to clot. Excessive heparin can alter the blood gas values by reducing the pH and the carbon dioxide level and increasing the oxygen level.

e. Promptly analyze the blood gas sample or cool it

Rules for cooling in an ice–water bath include:
1. Blood drawn for a shunt study needs to be cooled if not analyzed within 5 minutes.
2. Blood drawn on a patient with an elevated leukocyte or platelet count needs to be cooled if not analyzed within 5 minutes.
3. A capillary blood gas sample needs to be cooled if not analyzed within 15 minutes.
4. Blood drawn into a plastic syringe needs to be cooled if not analyzed within 30 minutes.

As a general rule, a blood gas sample should be placed into an ice–water bath to avoid any questions of accuracy. Failure to do so runs the risk of the blood's living cells consuming the available oxygen and producing carbon dioxide, which lowers the pH. Obviously, this results in incorrect measured values.

2. Arterial catheters

a. Select the appropriate catheter (code: IIA24b) [difficulty: R, Ap]

An arterial catheter (also called an arterial line) is a flexible catheter that is placed into a peripheral artery for the purposes of sampling blood or continuously monitoring the patient's blood pressure or both. The blood-sampling procedure is explained in the following discussion. Chapter 5 contains a discussion on blood pressure monitoring and illustrations of how the monitoring system is assembled.

An adult's radial artery is usually catheterized. To do so, a short needle covered with a flexible plastic catheter (an angiocatheter) is selected. Usually the needle is 23 or 24 gauge. After the angiocatheter is inserted into the artery, the needle is removed, and the catheter is left in the artery.

A newborn with a severe cardiopulmonary problem should have the catheter inserted into either of the umbilical arteries. Usually, a long, flexible umbilical artery catheter is placed into the patient and advanced into the aorta (see Fig. 1-12). If indicated, this should be done as quickly as possible after birth, before arterial spasm prevents the catheter from being advanced. If the patient weighs more than 1250 g, a 6-French (6-Fr) catheter is used; a 3.5-Fr catheter is used if the neonate weighs less than 1250 g. In addition to obtaining blood samples and monitoring the blood pressure, one can give the newborn glucose or a blood transfusion through the catheter. A neonatal patient also may have the umbilical vein catheterized.

Arterial catheters come as single units in sterile packaging. Additional stopcocks, tubing, flush solution, and an automatic solution drip device are needed. These are discussed in Chapter 5 in some detail.

b. Troubleshoot any problems with the equipment (code: IIA24b) [difficulty: R, Ap]

See the discussion in Chapter 5.

3. Perform a blood sample collection: arterial or venous catheter (code: IC6) [difficulty: R, Ap]

The general steps for obtaining an arterial, central venous, or mixed venous blood sample include:
1. Tell a conscious adult patient that you are going to take a blood sample from the arterial catheter.
2. Put gloves on both hands.
3. Remove the dead-ender cap (or syringe) from the sample (side) port on the three-way stopcock between the catheter and the intravenous (IV) tubing.
4. Screw a sterile 5- to 10-mL syringe to the sample port for removing the IV solution from the catheter. (A smaller syringe should be used for a neonate.)
5. Turn the stopcock off to the IV tubing (Fig. 3-1).
6. Pull a waste sample of IV solution and blood into the syringe. (The amount withdrawn and discarded depends on the dead-space volume from the tip of the catheter to the side port. Studies indicate that between 2.5 and 6

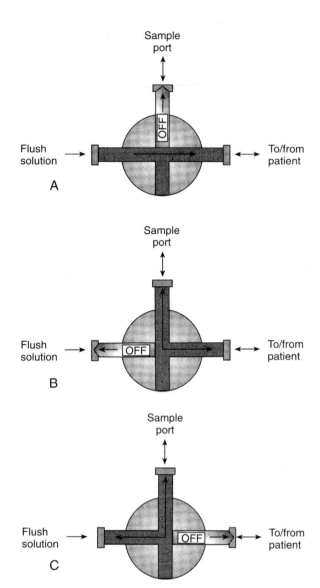

Figure 3-1 A three-way stopcock for use in an arterial line system. **A,** The normal operating position of the stopcock that allows fluid to flow to the patient (and the blood pressure to be monitored if assembled for continuous blood pressure monitoring). **B,** The stopcock position that allows blood to be withdrawn from the patient through the sample port. The flush solution port is closed. **C,** The stopcock position for flush solution to go to the sample port to clear out any blood. When the stopcock is turned to a 45-degree angle between any two ports, all of the ports are closed. (From Kacmarek RM, Stoller JK, Heuer AJ: Egan's fundamentals of respiratory care, ed 10, St Louis, 2013, Mosby.)

times this volume should be removed. Typically, this is ≤5 mL in an adult and even less in a neonate.)

7. Turn the stopcock off to all ports by turning it half-way between any two ports.

8. Attach a preheparinized sterile syringe to the sample port, turn the stopcock open to the syringe, and withdraw about 2-3 mL of arterial blood to be analyzed.

9. Turn the stopcock off to all ports by turning it half-way between any two ports.

10. Remove the blood-sample syringe, and cap off the syringe to seal it.

11. If liquid heparin is used in the syringe, roll the syringe to mix it with the blood.

12. If it will be more than 30 minutes until analysis, place the blood sample into an ice–water bath.

13. Screw the sterile waste sample syringe to the sample port for removing the blood remaining in the sample port.

14. Turn the stopcock off to the patient.

15. Pull a waste sample of IV solution into the syringe. Remove any residual blood from the hub.

16. Remove the waste sample syringe and screw the dead-ender cap (or new syringe) onto the sample port.

17. Turn the stopcock toward the sample port so that the iv solution runs into the catheter.

18. Fast flush any blood in the catheter back into the patient. Take care not to flush any air bubbles into the patient as this can cause an air embolism.

19. Remove gloves, and properly dispose of them and any other waste materials. Wash your hands.

4. Perform a blood gas sample collection: arterial puncture (code: IC6) [difficulty: R, Ap]

A number of possible variations on the technique exist. The following is a general but thorough listing of the steps and any important related information.

a. Check for a valid physician order

b. Check the patient's chart for pertinent information on supplemental oxygen being used, bleeding disorders such as hemophilia, and use of anticoagulant medications

It is important to check the patient's clotting time because a hematoma will result in a patient with a slow clotting time if extra time is not spent holding the puncture site.

c. Collect necessary equipment
   - Ice water in a cup
   - A 3-mL glass or plastic syringe
   - Appropriate needle(s)
   - Heparin, if needed
   - 70% isopropyl alcohol or iodophor swabs to clean the puncture site and a sterile 4 × 4-in gauze pad to hold over the puncture site to aid clotting
   - A seal for the needle or syringe to prevent room air contamination
   - Clean gloves to protect the practitioner's hands from any contact with spilled blood
   - Eyeglasses or goggles

d. Introduce yourself and your department to the patient

Identify the patient. Explain what you are there to do. Gain the patient's confidence so that he or she will offer full cooperation.

e. Select the puncture site

The following choices are listed in order from most to least favorable: radial, brachial, dorsalis pedis, and femoral. If the radial site is selected, try to puncture the left wrist if the patient is right-handed or vice versa.

f. If the radial or pedal site is selected, the *modified Allen test* (also known as the *Allen test*) must be performed to ensure that adequate collateral flow is present in case the artery becomes clotted because of the procedure

1. Radial artery site

See Figure 3-2 for the basic procedure. Circulation to the hand is stopped by pressing both the radial and the ulnar arteries closed. Releasing the pressure over the ulnar artery should result in the hand flushing within 5-15 seconds. This is a positive test result and proves that the ulnar artery has adequate circulation to the hand. If the hand does not flush within 15 seconds of the release of the ulnar artery, the circulation is inadequate, and the radial artery of that wrist must not be punctured. Another site must be evaluated for puncture.

2. Dorsalis pedis artery site

Press down on the dorsalis pedis artery to occlude it. Press on the nail of the great toe so that it blanches. Release the pressure on the nail, and watch for a rapid return of color. This normal test finding confirms that a good blood flow exists through the posterior tibial and lateral plantar arteries. It is safe to draw a sample from the site. A slow return of blood flow indicates poor circulation; another site must be chosen.

g. Prepare the equipment and the puncture site by using sterile technique

1. If necessary, draw up the heparin solution, flush the syringe, and discard the excess.
2. If a radial or brachial site is selected, the joint should be hyperextended with a folded towel to help stabilize it.
3. Clean the site by wiping the area with an alcohol or iodophor swab in a widening spiral motion that starts at the desired puncture site and allow time for the site to dry. Failure to allow the alcohol to dry may cause the sample to hemolyze or become contaminated.
4. Put on gloves and goggles.
5. Some prefer to anesthetize the puncture site with a 0.8- to 1.0-mL injection of 0.5%-2% lidocaine (Xylocaine) into the skin. Others think that this is unnecessary because the lidocaine injection itself will cause pain or possible vasoconstriction, making sampling more difficult. If an anesthetic is used, wait about 2 minutes for it to take effect before puncturing the skin.

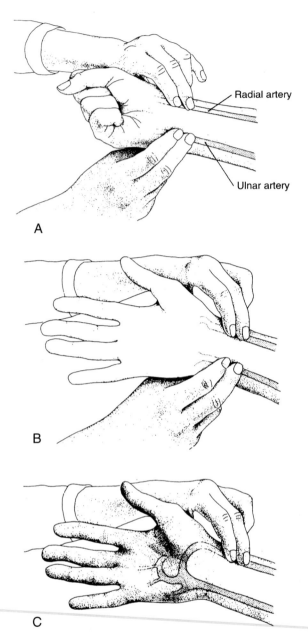

Figure 3-2 The modified Allen test. **A,** The hand is clenched into a tight fist, and pressure is applied to the radial and ulnar arteries. **B,** The hand is opened (but not fully extended); the palm and fingers are blanched. **C,** Removal of the pressure on the ulnar artery should result in flushing of the entire hand. (From Shapiro BA, Peruzzi WT, Kozlowski-Templin R: Clinical application of blood gases, ed 5, St Louis, 1994, Mosby.)

h. Draw the blood sample

1. Hold the syringe like a pencil. The radial and dorsalis pedis arteries should be entered from a 45-degree angle; the brachial and femoral arteries should be entered from a 90-degree angle (Fig. 3-3). Use the first two fingers of your free hand to palpate the pulse and hold the artery still. The bevel of the needle should be up as it enters the skin.
2. Tell the patient that he or she will "feel a stick."

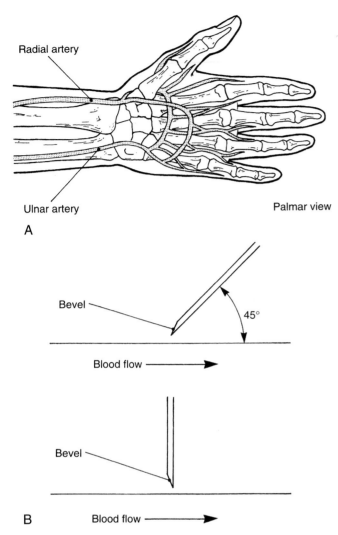

Figure 3-3 A, Radial arterial position in the lower arm and wrist. **B,** Bevel and needle positioning for radial arterial puncture and other arterial punctures, respectively. (From Lane EE, Walker JF: Clinical arterial blood gas analysis, St Louis, 1987, Mosby.)

3. The needle should enter the skin quickly to minimize pain. Carefully advance the needle into the artery. A pulsatile flow should be seen with each heartbeat. If unsuccessful, withdraw the needle to the skin, change the angle as needed, and reinsert it into the artery.
4. Withdraw about 1-2 mL of blood before removing the needle.
5. Press the sterile gauze onto the puncture site for 2-5 minutes. Check the site to ensure that clotting has occurred. Hold longer if necessary. An assistant may help with this.
6. While holding the site, seal the syringe or safely cover the needle.
7. If liquid heparin was added to the syringe, roll it to mix the heparin and blood.
8. If the blood sample will not be analyzed within 30 minutes, place the syringe into an ice–water

mix. (Failure to cool the blood sample results in a decrease in the PaO_2 value, an increase in the $PaCO_2$ value, and a decrease in the pH value.)
9. Label the syringe with the date, time, patient's name, oxygen percentage, and temperature if abnormal. Some departments may also add the patient's age and the position in which he or she was sitting or lying when the sample was drawn because of the effects they may have on oxygenation.
10. Have the sample promptly analyzed. The patient's blood gas results should be accurate if the blood sample is analyzed within 10-15 minutes if not iced and within 60 minutes if iced.
11. Properly dispose of gloves and waste materials, wash your hands, and document the procedure.
12. Return in 20 minutes to recheck the puncture site for a hematoma and good distal circulation.

Exam Hint 3-2

Commonly tested areas involve the ABG technique and possible hazards to it. Patient hazards include blood vessel trauma, hematoma, arterial clot formation, arteriospasm, and infected puncture site. In addition, the therapist may receive an accidental needle-puncture injury.

5. Perform a blood gas sample collection: arterialized capillary blood (code: IC6) [difficulty: R, Ap]

Occasionally, a sample of arterialized capillary blood from a patient must be obtained for blood gas analysis. The usual clinical situation is a neonate who has a pulmonary problem that warrants evaluation. However, because of the neonate's small arteries, a sample cannot be drawn. The steps and key points to keep in mind during the sampling procedure follow.

a. Select a highly vascularized and well-perfused site. Usually the posterolateral heel area is selected. Possible other sites include the earlobe, great toe, or finger if the heel cannot be used. No sites should be used on a neonate less than 24 hours of age because of poor peripheral circulation.
b. Warm the heel (or other site) with a warm towel, warming pad, or heat lamp for about 5-10 minutes; 42° C is ideal. Warming vasodilates the vessels and "arterializes" the capillary blood supply.
c. After warming, unwrap the site, and wipe it with an antiseptic pad.
d. Use a pediatric lance to deeply puncture the outer edge of the heel (Fig. 3-4). Blood should flow freely without squeezing the area. Wipe away the first blood drop with a sterile gauze pad. The blood will be "dearterialized" if it is squeezed out with venous blood, and the sample will be useless for blood gas analysis.
e. Insert a preheparinized capillary tube (0.075-1.0 mL) deeply into the drop of blood. The blood should easily flow through the tube and, ideally, a second sample tube is filled.

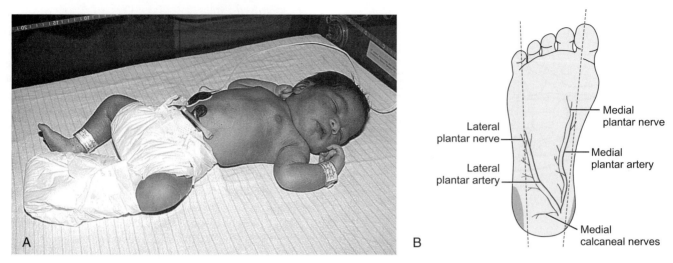

Figure 3-4 Obtaining an arterialized capillary blood sample on a newborn. **A,** The left foot is warmed to vasodilate and "arterialize" the capillary blood flow. **B,** The ideal puncture site is the outside of the heel. If necessary, the inside of the heel can also be used. Avoid puncturing the center of the heel and foot to avoid nerves and arteries. (**A,** courtesy of Marjorie Pyle, RNC, Lifecircle, Costa Mesa, CA. **A** and **B** from Perry S, Hockenberry M, Loudermilk D, Wilson D: Maternal child nursing care, ed 4, St Louis, 2010, Mosby.)

f. Place a metal filing (flea) into each tube and seal both ends of the tubes.

g. Use a magnet to draw the metal filing back and forth in the tubes to mix the blood, if needed.

h. Unless the blood samples will be analyzed within 30 minutes, place the sealed tubes into an ice–water bath.

i. Send the samples to the laboratory for analysis along with the proper paperwork unless point-of-care analysis is performed.

j. Apply pressure to stop the bleeding. Complications include infection, bone spurs, and laceration of the posterior tibial artery.

MODULE C

Analyze blood gas values.

1. Assemble a blood gas analyzer and point-of-care blood gas analyzer (code: IIA13) [difficulty: R, Ap]

Historically, a blood gas analyzer has been kept in the hospital's central laboratory. More recently analyzers have been kept in satellite labs in the Emergency Department or Intensive Care Unit. This reduces the time between a sample being drawn and analyzed and the results returned to the clinician. The need for rapid analysis has led to the development of point-of-care (POC) blood gas analyzers being used for patient transports or when data are needed quickly at the bedside. The blood gas values of PaO_2, $PaCO_2$, and pH are typically obtained from either a POC analyzer or a standard blood gas analyzer. These standard units are acceptable for all patient care situations except when carbon monoxide (CO) poisoning is known or suspected. A hemoximeter/CO oximeter is needed to measure the patient's level of carboxyhemoglobin in carbon monoxide cases. Some POC analyzers also can measure levels of serum electrolytes and other commonly needed patient values such as blood glucose, hemoglobin, and hematocrit levels.

POC analyzers can be powered through a self-contained battery or by plugging the unit into a standard alternating current electrical outlet. The units have single-use disposable cartridges that include the electrodes and calibration reagents and will hold waste samples. The following discussion covers the basic principles of operation of the electrodes in POC and standard centrally located analyzers.

a. pH electrode

The modern pH electrode has existed since the mid-1950s and is usually referred to as the *Sanz electrode* after its principal inventor. The basic principle behind the pH analyzer is its ability to measure the voltage (potential for electrical flow) between two different solutions. This is based on the different hydrogen ion (H^+) concentrations between the solutions that reflect their relative pH values. The reference electrode is immersed in a solution with a pH of 6.840 that fills a glass or plastic chamber. The blood sample, of unknown pH, is placed in a separate measuring chamber called a *cuvette*. These two chambers are separated by a special glass membrane that contains metals and sodium ions (Na^+), thus making it pH sensitive. Both chambers are kept at a stable 37° C temperature. See Figure 3-5 for a graphic representation of the pH electrode. When blood or a quality control material is introduced into the cuvette, the potential exists for hydrogen ions to replace the sodium ions in the pH-sensitive glass if the two pH's are different. The replacement is proportional to the difference in the two pH's.

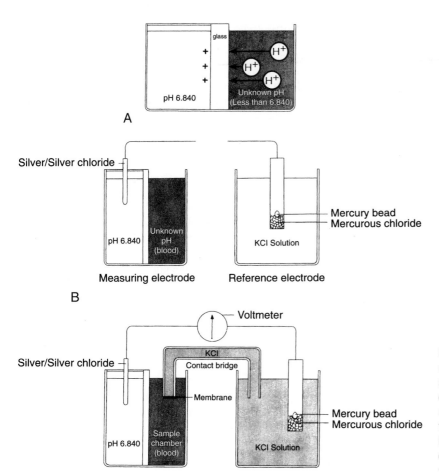

Figure 3-5 Key components of the Sanz electrode for measuring pH. **A,** A voltage develops across the pH-sensitive glass when a difference exists in the hydrogen ion concentration between the two solutions. **B,** Two separate half-cells are used for the measuring electrode and the reference electrode. **C,** The addition of a KCl contact bridge and voltmeter completes the electrical circuit and enables the pH of the patient's blood sample to be measured. (From Harrison BA, Shapiro C: Clinical application of blood gases, ed 4, St Louis, 1989, Mosby.)

b. PCO₂ electrode

The partial pressure of carbon dioxide (PCO_2) is measured in a modified pH electrode. This was first designed in the mid-1950s by Stow and further perfected by Severinghaus. Accordingly, these units are now referred to as *Severinghaus electrodes* or sometimes as *Stow-Severinghaus electrodes*. In Figure 3-6, the electrode is depicted in cross-section. It has a reference half-cell and a measuring half-cell that are enclosed within pH-sensitive glass and electrically connected by an electrolyte contact bridge. The blood sample is introduced into a cuvette heated to 37° C.

The principle of operation is based on the amount of CO_2 found in the blood sample that diffuses through the silicone elastic membrane. The CO_2 chemically combines with the bicarbonate solution to change the pH of the solution by the release of H^+. This change in H^+ concentration creates a voltage difference between the measuring and reference half-cells that is proportional to the amount of CO_2 found in the patient's blood sample.

c. PO₂ electrode

This unit is completely different from the others mentioned. It was developed in the late 1950s by Clark and thus is usually called a *Clark electrode*. It is also sometimes known as a *polarographic electrode* because of the basis of its

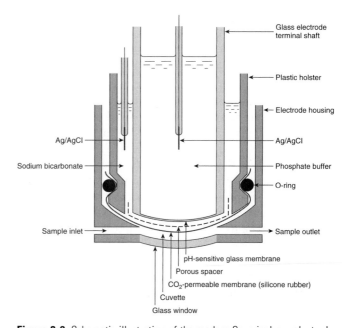

Figure 3-6 Schematic illustration of the modern Severinghaus electrode for measuring PCO_2. (From Malley WJ: Clinical blood gases: assessment and intervention, ed 2, St Louis, 2005, Saunders.)

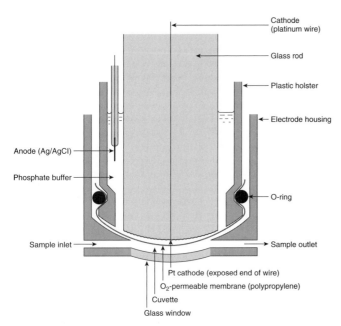

Figure 3-7 Schematic illustration of the Clark electrode for measuring PO_2. (From Malley WJ: Clinical blood gases: assessment and intervention, ed 2, St Louis, 2005, Saunders.)

operation. Figure 3-7 is a drawing of key features of the unit. A phosphate–KCl buffer solution surrounds the silver anode. A thin membrane separates the blood-filled cuvette from direct contact with the electrode but allows oxygen molecules to diffuse slowly through to contact the platinum wire cathode. The whole unit is heated to 37° C. The term polarographic comes from the addition of about 0.7 V to the cathode to make it slightly "polarized" or negative compared with the anode. This is needed to ensure that oxygen is rapidly chemically reduced (that it gains electrons) at the cathode. This creates an electric current directly proportional to the number of reduced oxygen molecules.

It must be understood that the partial pressure of oxygen (PO_2) being measured is derived from oxygen that is dissolved in the plasma. It does not come from the hemoglobin found in the erythrocytes (red blood cells). The reported value for the saturation of oxygen in the hemoglobin (SaO_2) is calculated by using a mathematical table. Under normal conditions, the calculated SaO_2 value is the same as or close to the true SaO_2 value. Carbon monoxide poisoning is the only commonly seen clinical situation during which a calculated saturation can be incorrectly high. If carbon monoxide poisoning is suspected or known, the patient's blood sample should be analyzed on a CO-oximeter unit.

2. Troubleshoot any problems with the equipment (code: IIA13) [difficulty: R, Ap]

Standard analyzers and POC analyzers are designed to self-calibrate and display information on their operation. Replace a POC testing cartridge that is not properly

functioning. Recharge a battery that is running low on reserve power. See the following discussion on quality control.

3. Perform quality control procedures for a blood gas analyzer (code: IIC2) [difficulty: R, Ap]
a. Quality control

Quality control (QC) refers to creating a measurement and documentation system to confirm the accuracy (precision) and reliability of all blood gas measurements. Accuracy or precision means that the measured physiologic values truly reflect the actual physiologic values. Reliability means that a high degree of confidence exists so that the measured values represent the patient's actual physiologic values. Both are critically important if the blood gas results are to be used to make correct clinical decisions.

b. Quality assurance

Quality assurance (QA) refers to the broader concern that the results of the blood gas measurement are not only accurate and reliable but also clinically useful. To help ensure this, the Clinical Laboratory Improvement Amendments of 1988 (CLIA 88) require that the department have written policies and procedures on items including record keeping, equipment maintenance, staff training, and the correction of errors.

c. Calibration

Calibration is the systematic standardization of the graduations of the blood gas analyzer against known values to ensure consistency. Proper calibration of the electrodes is essential to the accuracy of the blood gas values. Some general calibration steps are discussed later. The manufacturer's guidelines must be followed for the specific steps in calibration.

d. Quality control materials

A variety of QC materials are available to calibrate the electrodes for PO_2, PCO_2, and pH measurements. Their uses vary. Each of the following materials has its advantages, disadvantages, and limitations. The manufacturer of a particular brand or model of blood gas analyzer may require that a specific type of material be used in its units.

Aqueous buffers are water based and are used to check pH and PCO_2 measurements; they cannot be used to check PO_2 measurements. Commercially prepared gases are used to check PO_2 and PCO_2 measurements; they cannot be used to check pH measurements. The following CO_2 mixes may be used: 0, 5%, 10%, and 12%. The following O_2 mixes may be used: 0, 12%, 20%, 20.95% from room air, 21%, and 100%.

Tonometered liquids are exposed in the laboratory to known oxygen and carbon dioxide gas mixes until the liquids are saturated and have the same partial pressures as the gases. Three types of tonometered liquids are used. First, using human or animal serum or whole blood is

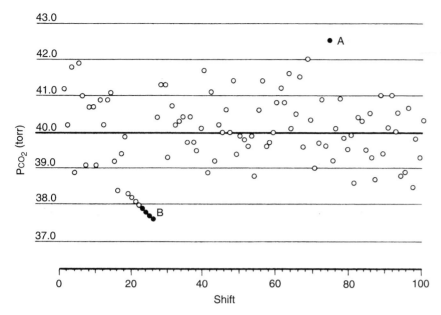

Figure 3-8 Levey-Jennings quality control chart for PaCO₂. The central horizontal line represents the mean value of 40 torr. The next lower and higher horizontal lines show 1 standard deviation (1 SD) value from the mean. The second most distant lower and higher horizontal lines are 2 SDs from the mean. The most distant horizontal lines are 3 SDs from the mean. The bottom number scale indicates 8-hour work shifts. *Open circles*, calibration values that are within 2 SDs of the mean value. They are considered to be in control. *Black circles*, calibration values that are out of control. *A* represents a random error and *B* a systematic error. (From Shapiro BA, Peruzzi WT, Kozlowski-Templin R: Clinical application of blood gases, ed 5, St Louis, 1994, Mosby.)

the most accurate method available and is used mainly to obtain PO₂ and PCO₂ levels. Although whole human blood cannot be used for pH measurements, a bovine blood product can be used to obtain all three values. Second, assayed liquids are non-water-based liquids that are pretonometered by the manufacturer and are available in sealed glass vials. They can be used to obtain PO₂, PCO₂, and pH measurements. These are very popular because of the advantages of speed and simplicity. Third, oxygenated fluorocarbon-based emulsions (perfluorinated compounds) can be used to obtain PO₂, PCO₂, and pH measurements. They are considered as accurate as whole blood without its associated risks.

e. Levey-Jennings charts

The Levey-Jennings charts (also known as *Shewhart/ Levey-Jennings* or *quality control charts*) are used to record the results of each calibration procedure. They are similarly designed, with time plotted on the horizontal scale and the analyte (PO₂, PCO₂, or pH) on the vertical scale. The vertical scale for each analyte has a central value for what is normally expected. On both sides of this normal value are standard deviation (SD) points, showing movement away from what is expected. When an analyte electrode is operating within the acceptable limits, it is said to be in control. In general, if an analyte is within 2 SDs of the normal value, it is considered to be in control.

An out-of-control situation exists whenever a single calibration value or a series of calibration values is outside established limits. A random error is an unpredictable aberration in precision that occurs when the QC material is sampled. A systematic error shows an accuracy problem and is much more serious. It must be investigated, corrected, and documented. Figure 3-8 shows examples of both random error and systematic error. Rules have been

TABLE 3-1	Westgard's Rules for Determining When an Analyzer Is Not Functioning Properly
Rule Name	**Levey-Jennings Chart**
Random Error	
1-2 SDs	The measurement is more than 2 SDs but not more than 3 SDs from the mean.
1-3 SDs	The measurement is more than 3 SDs from the mean.
R-4 SDs	Two consecutive measurements are 4 SDs or more apart.
Systematic Error	
2-2 SDs	Two consecutive measurements are either 2 SDs above or 2 SDs below the mean.
4-1 SDs	Four consecutive measurements are either 1 SD above or 1 SD below the mean.
7-trend	Seven consecutive measurements are on only one side of the mean; each measurement is progressively more out of control.
10-mean	Ten consecutive measurements are on only one side of the mean.

Modified from Lane EE, Walker JF: Clinical arterial blood gas analysis, St Louis, 1987, Mosby.
SDs, standard deviations.

established for determining whether the error is random or systematic (Table 3-1).

f. pH electrode

Note: The following guidelines are based on CLIA standards or widely reported industry standards. The various brands and models of blood gas analyzers may have different frequencies of calibration requirements, depending on their Food and Drug Administration-approved manufacturers' studies.

1. One-point calibration

1. Should be done before every sample is analyzed if one-point calibration is not automatically performed every 30 minutes
2. Performed with the near-normal QC material of 7.384 ± 0.005 pH used to set the balance potentiometer
3. Recommended every 30 minutes
4. Should be rechecked after a suspicious pH result; the blood sample should then be rerun

2. Two-point calibration

1. Should be done at least once every 8 hours when patient samples are being analyzed
2. Recommended for every 25 patient samples
3. Performed with the slope potentiometer set with a QC material of 6.840 ± 0.005 pH (this is the same pH as the reference electrode solution)
4. Performed with the balance potentiometer set with a QC material of 7.384 ± 0.005 pH

3. Three-point calibration

1. Should be done at least every 6 months on existing equipment
2. Should be done whenever a new electrode is put into use
3. Covers the physiologic range to confirm linearity; QC materials of 6.840 ± 0.005, 7.384 ± 0.005, and 7.874 ± 0.005 pH are used

g. PCO₂ electrode

1. One-point calibration

1. Should be done before every sample is analyzed if one-point calibration is not automatically performed every 30 minutes
2. Performed with 5% ± 0.03% CO_2 used to set the balance potentiometer
3. Recommended every 30 minutes
4. Should be rechecked after a suspicious PCO₂ result; the blood sample should then be rerun

The CO_2 can be directly in contact with the electrode, tonometered with an aqueous material or blood, or premixed in aqueous buffers, assayed liquids, or fluorocarbon-based emulsion.

2. Two-point calibration

1. Should be done at least once every 8 hours when patient samples are being analyzed
2. Recommended for every 25 patient samples
3. Performed with 10% ± 0.03% CO_2 to set the slope potentiometer
4. Performed with 5% ± 0.03% CO_2 to set the balance potentiometer

3. Three-point calibration

1. Should be done at least every 6 months on existing equipment
2. Should be done whenever a new electrode is put into use
3. Covers the physiologic range to confirm linearity; three PCO₂ values between 0 and 80 mm Hg should be determined
4. Room air or a gas cylinder containing up to 0.03% CO_2 can be used to set the zero point

---

Exam Hint 3-3

Past examinations have required that the following equation be solved. Remember that more than one carbon dioxide percentage can be used. *Note:* The atmospheric pressure of a gas (e.g., oxygen, carbon dioxide) may be listed by the equivalent terms of torr or mm Hg. For example, a PCO₂ of 40 torr is the same as a PCO₂ of 40 mm Hg. However, it is important to note that on the NBRC exams, the term torr is used for gas pressure.

The predicted PCO₂ value at a given CO_2 percentage is calculated with this formula:

$$P_{CO_2} = (P_B - P_{H_2O}) \times \% CO_2$$

In the above equation PCO₂ is the predicted PCO₂ in mm Hg or torr; P_B is the barometric pressure at the institution where the analysis is being performed; P_{H_2O} is the water vapor pressure based on the patient's temperature, 47 torr at 37° C/98.6° F; and %CO₂ is the percentage of CO_2 (also listed as FCO₂).

Here is an example for one-point (balance) potentiometer calibration at sea level in which PCO₂ is the predicted PCO₂ in torr, P_B is 760 torr, PH₂O is 47 torr, and %CO₂ is 5%:

1. $P_{CO_2} = (760 - 47) \times 0.05$
2. $= (713) \times 0.05$
3. $= 35.65$ or 36 torr

Therefore set the PCO₂ control at 36 torr.

---

h. PO₂ electrode
1. One-point calibration

1. Should be done before every sample is analyzed if one-point calibration is not automatically performed every 30 minutes
2. Performed with 12% ± 0.03% O_2 used to set the balance potentiometer; some analyzers are designed to use 20% ± 0.03% O_2 from a gas cylinder or draw room air (20.95% oxygen) into the unit
3. Recommended every 30 minutes
4. Should be rechecked after a suspicious PO₂ result; the blood sample should then be rerun

The O_2 can be directly in contact with the electrode, tonometered with an aqueous material or blood, or premixed in aqueous buffers, assayed liquids, or fluorocarbon-based emulsion as discussed.

2. Two-point calibration

1. Should be done at least once every 8 hours when patient samples are being analyzed
2. Should be done whenever readjustment of one-point calibration is greater than 3 torr
3. Recommended for every 25 patient samples
4. Performed with 0% ± 0.03% O_2 to set the slope potentiometer
5. Performed with 12% ± 0.03% O_2 to set the balance potentiometer; some analyzers are designed to use 20% ± 0.03% O_2 from a gas cylinder or draw room air (20.95% oxygen) into the unit

3. Three-point calibration

1. Should be done at least every 6 months on existing equipment
2. Should be done whenever a new electrode is put into use
3. Should be done to confirm linearity whenever the PO_2 value could be more than 150 torr, assuming that the balance point is set on room oxygen content; the third point should be set on 100% ± 0.03% O_2 from a gas cylinder

---

Exam Hint 3-4

Past examinations have required that the following equation be solved. Remember that more than one oxygen percentage can be used.

The predicted PO_2 value at a given O_2 percentage is calculated with this formula:

$$PO_2 = \left(P_B - P_{H_2O}\right) \times \%O_2$$

In the above equation PO_2 is the predicted PO_2 in torr; P_B is the barometric pressure at the institution where the analysis is being performed; P_{H_2O} is the water vapor pressure based on the patient's temperature, 47 torr at 37° C/98.6° F; and $\%O_2$ is the percentage of O_2 (also listed as FO_2).

Here is an example for one-point (balance) potentiometer calibration at sea level in which PO_2 is the predicted PO_2 in torr, P_B is 760 torr, P_{H_2O} is 47 torr, and $\%O_2$ is 12%:

1. $PO_2 = (760 - 47) \times 0.12$
2. $\quad = (713) \times 0.12$
3. $\quad = 85.56$ or 86 torr

Therefore set the PO_2 control at 86 torr.

Exam Hint 3-5

Often a question relates to QC. It could include reanalyzing a blood gas sample with suspicious results, rechecking out-of-control calibration results (greater than 2 SDs), or using two analyzers for cross-referencing.

BOX 3-2 Electrode Precision and Calibration Gases

Electrodes

pH ±0.01 unit.
PCO_2 ±2% (approximately ±1 mm Hg at 40 torr).
PO_2 ±3% (approximately ±2.5 mm Hg at 80 torr).
If the PO_2 is >150 torr, the precision is approximately ±10% unless three-point calibration is performed.

Calibration Gases

"Low" gas: 0% O_2 (+0.03%), 5% CO_2 (±0.03%), balance N_2.
"High" gas: 12% or 21% O_2, 10% CO_2 (both ±0.03%), balance N_2.
Suggested three-point gases: 100% O_2 (–0.03%), 0% CO_2 (+0.03%).

N_2, nitrogen; PCO_2, pressure of carbon dioxide; PO_2, pressure of oxygen.

i. Miscellaneous topics

1. Calibration gas cylinders

For economic reasons, the low-percentage oxygen and carbon dioxide gases are placed together in one cylinder, and the high-percentage oxygen and carbon dioxide gases are placed together in a second cylinder. Box 3-2 summarizes the normal precision of the electrodes discussed and the gases used in their calibration. A cylinder containing 100% oxygen and no carbon dioxide can be used for three-point calibration.

2. Temperature correction

Temperature correction is a controversial topic and refers to mathematical adjustment of a patient's PaO_2, $PaCO_2$, and pH values if his or her temperature is not 37° C. Remember that blood gas analyzers are calibrated at 37° C because it is normal body temperature. If the patient has a fever, the oxygen and carbon dioxide partial pressures in the blood will be greater than those found during the blood gas analysis. Conversely, the hypothermic patient will have lower oxygen and carbon dioxide partial pressures in the blood than those found during the blood gas analysis. The pH value will shift in the opposite direction from the PCO_2 value. Usually this small shift in values is ignored. However, because some physicians may specify that their patient's blood gases be temperature corrected, the patient's temperature should be listed on the blood gas slip. It is a simple mathematical process to temperature correct the blood gas results. Most modern analyzers perform temperature correction automatically when programmed to do so.

The 2013 American Association for Respiratory Care (AARC) Clinical Practice Guideline on blood gas analysis and hemoximetry does not recommend that temperature correction be performed. This is because the patient's values are not usually affected in a clinically significant way.

4. Perform quality control procedures for a blood gas analyzer and point-of-care blood gas analyzer (code: IIC3) [difficulty: R, Ap]

The general principles of QC and QA discussed for standard blood gas analyzers apply to POC analyzers as well. Remember to flush the electrode membrane after each use, if possible, to prevent protein buildup. If protein buildup occurs, the response time is longer than normal. Follow the manufacturer's guidelines to change an electrode membrane as needed. Make sure that no air bubbles are under the membrane or within the tubing through which the blood travels. Rerun the calibration for any of the electrodes and reanalyze the sample if you are suspicious of the result. If the electrode does not calibrate close to the reference buffer solutions or gases, it should not be used.

In a random-error situation, it is likely that the practitioner made a simple error when introducing the material or running the analyzer. Common problems include an air bubble injected into the unit or incomplete flushing of the previous sample. Usually flushing out any residual blood and then carefully injecting more of the current patient blood samples will correct the problem. Run the analyzer again to obtain new patient values or run the same patient sample through another analyzer and compare the two sets of results.

A systematic error usually indicates a problem with the analyzer, QC materials, or processes. Examples of systematic errors include misanalyzed CO_2 or O_2 standards for calibration, contaminated QC materials, or deteriorated oxygen, carbon dioxide, or pH electrode function. Each of these must be investigated until the problem is found and corrected. The unit cannot be used again until after it is proven to work properly and to give accurate results.

5. Perform blood gas analysis (code: IC7) [difficulty: R, Ap]

Modern blood gas analyzers are simple to operate. Follow the manufacturer's guidelines for insertion of the blood sample. Perform the specified steps in the analysis. Print out the results. Many current units run a self-diagnosis if any problems appear. Correct any identified problems as discussed above.

MODULE D

Perform hemoximetry.

Most hospitals have a hemoximeter in addition to a blood gas analyzer. A hemoximeter is also known as a CO oximeter or spectrophotometric oximeter. This device is the most accurate method available to measure the four different hemoglobin moieties (species or variations in the hemoglobin molecule).

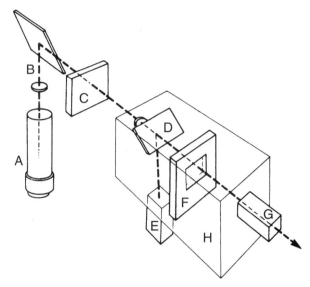

Figure 3-9 CO oximeter basic components. **A,** Thallium–neon hollow cathode light source. **B,** Lens and mirror. **C,** Monochromator with four specific wavelength filters. **D,** Light-beam splitter that diverts half of the light to the reference detector and half to the cuvette. **E,** Reference wavelength detector. **F,** Patient sample cuvette. **G,** Sample wavelength detector. **H,** Temperature-regulated block set at 37° C. (From Shapiro BA, Peruzzi WT, Kozlowski-Templin R: Clinical application of blood gases, ed 5, St Louis, 1994, Mosby.)

1. Assemble a hemoximeter (code: IIA13) [difficulty: R, Ap]

The unit is preassembled by the manufacturer. Practical experience with a unit is recommended to understand how to add a patient blood sample and perform calibration duties. (See Fig. 3-9 for a schematic drawing of a CO oximeter.) A thallium–neon hollow-cathode lamp emits light in the infrared–visible range. A device called a monochromator contains four filters and rotates through the light beam. Each filter allows only one specific wavelength to pass through it. These four monochromatic wavelengths correspond to the three isosbestic points, discussed later (shown in Fig. 3-10), and 626.6 nm. This last wavelength is poorly absorbed by all four hemoglobin moieties. It is used to find the maximal difference in absorption so that the relative amounts of the hemoglobin species can be determined.

2. Troubleshoot any problems with the equipment (code: IIA13) [difficulty: R, Ap]

The following are examples of common problems and their solutions:

- Incomplete hemolysis of the blood sample causes the light to scatter off cell fragments and lipids. Sickle cells (as in sickle cell anemia) are difficult to disrupt and may cause false oxyhemoglobin and carboxyhemoglobin readings if extra time is not taken for hemolysis. Follow the manufacturer's guidelines on the procedure for hemolyzing the red blood cells.

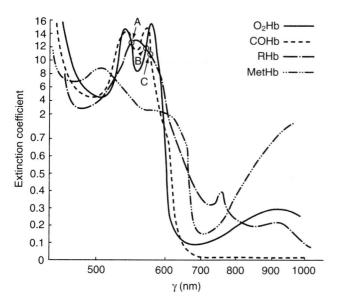

Figure 3-10 Spectral analysis of the hemoglobin moieties (species). O_2Hb is oxyhemoglobin, COHb is carboxyhemoglobin, RHb is reduced hemoglobin, and MetHb is methemoglobin. Point A shows the triple isosbestic point at 548 nm for O_2Hb, COHb, and RHb. Point B shows the double isosbestic point at 568 nm for O_2Hb and RHb. Point C shows the double isosbestic point at 578 nm for RHb and COHb. A fourth wavelength at 626.6 nm is used for comparison purposes. (From Shapiro BA, Peruzzi WT, Kozlowski-Templin R: Clinical application of blood gases, ed 5, St Louis, 1994, Mosby.)

- More than 10% methemoglobin may cause errors in the measurement of all hemoglobin moieties. Sulfhemoglobin also causes false readings. The practitioner may need to gather additional information from the chart or laboratory regarding the patient's levels of these abnormal hemoglobin moieties. CO oximetry should probably not be performed on blood samples with abnormal levels of methemoglobin or sulfhemoglobin.
- Intravenous dyes such as methylene blue, Evans blue, and indocyanine green used in various cardiac studies can absorb the same wavelengths of light used to identify the various forms of hemoglobin. The presence of these dyes results in a lower measurement of oxyhemoglobin than is actually present. Check the patient's chart for a record of dyes used. CO oximetry should probably not be used for blood gas analysis on patients who have these dyes in their systems.
- Failure to reprogram the analyzer for fetal hemoglobin instead of adult hemoglobin may produce false results. Remember to check the chart for the patient's age. Reprogram the analyzer for fetal hemoglobin for any sample taken from an infant who is only a few weeks old.
- The presence of lipid particles in the blood (hyperlipidemia) causes light scattering and results in a reading that is falsely high in total hemoglobin and percentage of methemoglobin and falsely low in percentage of oxyhemoglobin and percentage of carboxyhemoglobin. Follow the laboratory's guidelines

to determine when a patient's blood lipid value is too high for accurate use of the CO oximeter.
- The presence of air bubbles or incomplete hemolysis of blood in the cuvette causes an absorbance error. Air bubbles must be flushed out and the blood sample inserted again and reanalyzed. Make sure that all blood samples are hemolyzed according to the manufacturer's guidelines.
- Blood clots in the sample tubing prevent blood from flowing through to the cuvette. If a sample cannot be inserted into the unit, suspect and check for a blood clot. Remove any clotted tubing, replace it, and confirm that the CO oximeter is working properly.

3. Perform quality control procedures on a hemoximeter (code: IIC2) [difficulty: R, Ap]

When a blood sample is placed into the cuvette, the four monochromatic wavelengths are passed through it. The amount of absorbance at each wavelength is measured and compared with the absorbance at each wavelength by a reference sample solution. The computer integrates the data and calculates the total hemoglobin concentration and the amounts of the four hemoglobin moieties.

The total hemoglobin concentration should be calibrated when the unit is installed, at regular intervals suggested by the manufacturer, after the sample tubing is changed, after the cuvette is disassembled or changed, and whenever a suspicious reading is seen. Calibration is done by filling the cuvette with a special dye produced by the manufacturer and analyzing it by following the prescribed steps.

Routine calibration is done every 30 minutes. The unit obtains and stores absorbance readings at the four different wavelengths from a "blank" solution in the reference detector. When the same blank solution is added to the sample cuvette, the same four wavelengths are measured. Their absorption levels are normally identical. The same procedure is performed after every patient sample is analyzed.

4. Perform hemoximetry (code: IC7) [difficulty: R, Ap]

The principle of operation of a hemoximeter/CO oximeter is the comparison of the relative absorbances of four wavelengths of light by oxyhemoglobin, reduced hemoglobin, and carboxyhemoglobin. This is done by comparing the absorptions at the three isosbestic points (at which the moieties being compared have equal absorption) and a wavelength point at which the greatest difference in absorption between the two moieties is found. Each of these hemoglobin moieties has a unique spectroscopic "fingerprint" of absorbed light-wave frequencies. See Figure 3-10 for the spectral analysis of the various forms of hemoglobin. By computer integration of the data, the relative proportions of these types of hemoglobin are determined:
- Oxyhemoglobin (HbO_2 or O_2Hb), which carries oxygen to the tissues, and reduced hemoglobin (HbR or

RHb), which has given up its oxygen and picked up carbon dioxide.

- Carboxyhemoglobin (HbCO or COHb), which is nonfunctional because of the tightness with which carbon monoxide binds to the hemoglobin.
- Methemoglobin (HbMet or MetHb), which is nonfunctional because the Hb molecule is unable to combine reversibly with oxygen.
- Sulfhemoglobin (HbS or SHb), which is similar to HbMet and is also nonfunctional.
- In addition, a CO oximeter can measure the fetal hemoglobin (HbF or FHb) found in a newborn infant instead of adult oxyhemoglobin.

If the total of O_2Hb and RHb is less than 100% of the hemoglobin present, the difference has to be methemoglobin (or, rarely, sulfhemoglobin). The unit then provides data on total hemoglobin; percentages for oxyhemoglobin, reduced hemoglobin, carboxyhemoglobin, and methemoglobin; and total amounts for them in grams per deciliter of blood. Some units also calculate O_2 content.

A CO oximeter should be used to analyze a blood gas sample whenever carbon monoxide poisoning is known or suspected. In addition, a patient's MetHb should be regularly measured whenever inhaled nitric oxide is administered to reverse pulmonary hypertension.

Follow the manufacturer's guidelines on rewarming the blood sample to body temperature, hemolyzing the sample, and inserting it into the measurement cuvette. Failure to do so may result in incorrect patient values.

Exam Hint 3-6

If a patient is known to have or suspected of having carbon monoxide poisoning (e.g., removed from inside a burning building), a CO oximeter should be used for blood gas analysis. A standard or POC blood gas analyzer or standard pulse oximeter should not be used. These instruments cannot detect or measure carboxyhemoglobin.

MODULE E

Interpret blood gas analysis results.

1. Arterial blood gas results

a. Evaluate arterial blood gas results in the patient record (code: IA5) [difficulty: R, Ap]

Look in the chart for any previous ABG gas results. They should have been performed after any major change in the patient's condition or a change in treatment such as oxygen administration or mechanical ventilation.

b. Recommend blood gas analysis (code: IE9) [difficulty: R, Ap, An]

See Module A and Box 3-1 for indications for an ABG.

c. Evaluate the results of arterial blood gas analysis (code: ID6) [difficulty: R, Ap, An]

If the blood-sampling equipment preparation, the sampling procedure, and the blood gas analyzer operation were all done properly, the respiratory therapist and physician can believe that the blood gas results are accurate and reliable. However, if there was a problem with any aspect of obtaining and analyzing the blood gas sample, that sample must be discarded and a new sample obtained and analyzed.

A number of authors have written extensively on how to interpret ABGs. The system proposed by Shapiro and associates (1994) has been found to be both practical and relatively easy to understand. Most of the following discussion and tables are based on this system. This does not mean that if one has learned another system, he or she is at any disadvantage for taking the NBRC examinations.

Exam Hint 3-7

Past NBRC exams have included specific questions about ABG interpretation. The exams also incorporate blood gas results into other questions that relate to any respiratory care technique or procedure, such as oxygen therapy for a patient with COPD and adjustment of mechanical ventilation. In addition, often a question requires the interpretation of mixed venous blood gases or arterialized capillary blood gases. The examinee must be proficient in all aspects of blood gas interpretation to do well on the NBRC examination.

---

1. Assessment of oxygenation

Hypoxemia or hypoxia can rapidly become life threatening. This will often be first seen when the patient develops cardiac arrhythmias, unstable vital signs, and mental confusion or unconsciousness. Table 3-2 shows the normal PaO_2 values for the newborn, child to adult, and elderly when room air (almost 21% oxygen) is inhaled at sea level. These values decrease progressively as altitude increases. However, under most clinical conditions, this is not a factor unless working in a high-altitude setting.

A general rule is that any patient is seriously hypoxemic if the PaO_2 is less than 60 torr on room air. See Table 3-3 for guidelines on judging the seriousness of hypoxemia. Once hypoxemia is recognized, it must be corrected. The most obvious way to correct hypoxemia is to give supplemental oxygen. The clinician must realize that oxygen alone will not correct the hypoxemia if the patient is hypoventilating (increased $PaCO_2$), has heart failure, or is unable to carry or make use of the oxygen. In general, try to keep the patient's PaO_2 level between 60 and 100 torr.

Shapiro and associates (1994) suggested the following formula, in which F_IO_2 is the fraction of inspired oxygen, for determining whether the patient will be hypoxemic on room air: "If PaO_2 is less than $F_IO_2 \times 5$, the patient can be assumed to be hypoxemic on room air."

TABLE 3-2	Age-Based Acceptable Levels of Partial Pressure of Oxygen in Arterial Blood (PaO₂) When Breathing Room Air (21% Oxygen) at Sea Level

Age	PaO₂
Newborn	
Acceptable range	40-70 torr
Child to Adult	
Normal	97 torr
Acceptable range	>80 torr
Hypoxemia	<80 torr
Older Adult	
60-year-old	>80 torr
70-year-old	>70 torr
80-year-old	>60 torr
90-year-old	>50 torr

Modified from Shapiro BA, Peruzzi WT, Kozlowski-Templin R: Clinical application of blood gases, ed 5, St Louis, 1994, Mosby.

TABLE 3-3	Evaluation of Hypoxemia

CONDITIONS: ROOM AIR IS INSPIRED; THE PATIENT IS YOUNGER THAN 60 YEARS*		
Hypoxemia	**PaO₂**	**SaO₂**
Mild	60-79 torr	90-94%
Moderate	40-59 torr	75-89%
Severe	<40 torr	<75%

CONDITIONS: SUPPLEMENTAL O₂ IS INSPIRED; THE PATIENT IS YOUNGER THAN 60 YEARS	
Hypoxemia	**PaO₂**
Uncorrected	Less than room air acceptable limit (PaO₂ <80 torr)
Corrected	Within room air acceptable limit (PaO₂ >80 to <100 torr)
Excessively corrected	>100 torr

Modified from Shapiro BA, Peruzzi WT, Kozlowski-Templin R: Clinical application of blood gases, ed 5, St Louis, 1994, Mosby.
*Subtract 1 torr of O₂ from limits of mild and moderate hypoxemia for each year older than 60. A PaO₂ value of <40 torr indicates severe hypoxemia in any patient at any age.

Figure 3-11 shows a normal oxyhemoglobin dissociation curve. The saturation value is important to know because it shows how much hemoglobin is saturated with oxygen. Several important points of correlation exist between the SaO₂ and the PaO₂. (Calculated saturation values can be misleadingly high if the patient has inhaled carbon monoxide. In this situation, it is best to measure the saturation directly on a CO-oximeter–type blood gas analyzer.)

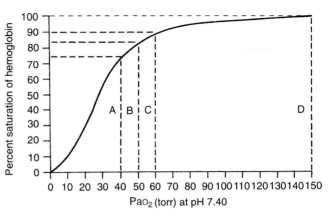

Figure 3-11 The oxygen (oxyhemoglobin) dissociation curve plots the relation between hemoglobin saturation (y axis) and plasma PaO₂ level (x axis). **A,** 75% saturation and a PaO₂ of 40 torr are normally seen in venous blood. **B,** 85% saturation and a PaO₂ of 50 torr are the minimal levels that should be allowed in a chronically hypoxemic patient. **C,** 90% saturation and a PaO₂ of 60 torr are the minimal levels that should be allowed in an acutely hypoxemic patient. **D,** Hemoglobin in the pulmonary capillaries adjacent to normal alveoli will become 100% saturated when the PaO₂ level reaches 150 torr. (Modified from Lane EE, Walker JF: Clinical arterial blood gas analysis, St Louis, 1987, Mosby.)

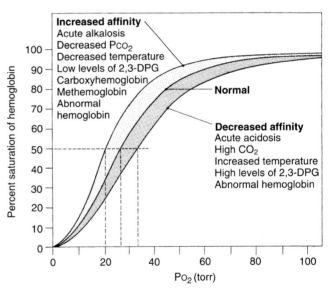

Figure 3-12 Conditions associated with altered affinity of hemoglobin for O₂. P₅₀ is the PaO₂ value at which hemoglobin is 50% saturated, normally 26.6 torr. A lower than normal P₅₀ value represents increased affinity of hemoglobin for O₂; a high P₅₀ value is seen with decreased affinity. Note that variation from the normal is associated with decreased (low P₅₀ value) or increased (high P₅₀ value) availability of O₂ to tissues (dashed lines). Shaded area, the entire oxyhemoglobin dissociation curve under the same circumstances. (From Lane EE, Walker JF: Clinical arterial blood gas analysis, St Louis, 1987, Mosby.)

Figure 3-12 shows a number of factors that can influence the oxyhemoglobin dissociation curve and how oxygen associates and dissociates from hemoglobin. In a patient with normal oxygenation, these factors are not clinically significant. However, when the PaO₂ level is less than 60 torr and the SaO₂ level is less than 90%, these factors can become an important consideration. As can be seen, a left-shifted oxyhemoglobin dissociation curve results in a lower PaO_2 value at any given saturation. This results in even less oxygen being delivered to the tissues.

Exam Hint 3-8

True shunt or venous admixture leading to ventilation/perfusion mismatching are the two most common clinical findings leading to hypoxemia.

2. Assessment of carbon dioxide and pH

The pH is the next important value to interpret because extreme acidemia/acidosis and alkalemia/alkalosis can be life threatening. The carbon dioxide value is important to interpret because it has a direct effect on the pH and indirectly affects the oxygen level. A high or low $PaCO_2$ level, by itself, is not life threatening.

Table 3-4 shows normal values for pH and $PaCO_2$ and the acceptable ranges around the mean or average. Table 3-5 shows the most widely acceptable therapeutic ranges for pH and $PaCO_2$. Values that fall outside of these ranges present a progressively greater risk to the patient.

Table 3-6 shows the definitions of Shapiro and associates for alkalosis and acidosis from a respiratory cause. An acute change in the patient's ventilation causes the following when starting from a $PaCO_2$ of 40 torr:

- If the $PaCO_2$ level increases by 20 torr, the pH decreases by 0.10 unit.
- If the $PaCO_2$ level decreases by 10 torr, the pH increases by 0.10 unit.

Thus the body can be seen as better able to compensate with metabolic buffers for a respiratory acidosis than a respiratory alkalosis.

3. Assessment of bicarbonate and base excess

Metabolic effects are evaluated by interpreting either the bicarbonate (HCO_3^-) value or the base excess/base deficit (BE/BD) value. However, remember that the bicarbonate and base excess values are *calculated*, not measured. After the measured $PaCO_2$ and pH values are determined, the bicarbonate and base excess are determined by computer algorithm or manually on the Siggaard-Andersen alignment nomogram (Fig. 3-13). Normal values are as follows:

- HCO_3^-: 24 mEq/L
- BE/BD: 0 mEq/L; ±1 mEq/L is often listed as the normal range

Values indicating metabolic alkalosis of a primary or secondary nature are:

- Bicarbonate level greater than 24 mEq/L
- BE greater than 0 or greater than ±1 mEq/L (i.e., +5 mEq/L)

Values indicating metabolic acidosis of a primary or secondary nature are:

- Bicarbonate level less than 24 mEq/L
- BE less than 0 or less than −1 mEq/L (i.e., −5 mEq/L); some laboratories report this as a BD or negative BE.

TABLE 3-4	Normal Laboratory Ranges for Partial Pressure of Carbon Dioxide in Arterial Blood ($PaCO_2$) and pH		
	Mean	**1 SD**	**2 SDs**
$PaCO_2$	40.00	8-42 torr	35-45 torr
pH	7.40	7.38-7.42	7.35-7.45

Modified from Shapiro BA, Peruzzi WT, Kozlowski-Templin R: Clinical application of blood gases, ed 5, St Louis, 1994, Mosby.
SD, standard deviation.

TABLE 3-5	Acceptable Clinical Ranges for Partial Pressure of Carbon Dioxide in Arterial Blood ($PaCO_2$) and pH
$PaCO_2$	30-50 torr*
pH	7.30-7.50

Modified from Shapiro BA, Peruzzi WT, Kozlowski-Templin R: Clinical application of blood gases, ed 5, St Louis, 1994, Mosby.
*This is the range for patients with an acute change. It does not apply to patients with long-standing disease, such as chronic obstructive pulmonary disease. These patients may have $PaCO_2$ values greater than 50 torr.

TABLE 3-6	Naming Unacceptable Values for Partial Pressure of CO_2 in Arterial Blood ($PaCO_2$) and pH
$PaCO_2$ >45 torr	Respiratory acidosis/alveolar hypoventilation/ventilatory failure
pH <7.35	Acidemia
$PaCO_2$ <35 torr	Respiratory alkalosis/alveolar hyperventilation
pH >7.45	Alkalemia

Modified from Shapiro BA, Peruzzi WT, Kozlowski-Templin R: Clinical application of blood gases, ed 5, St Louis, 1994, Mosby.

Exam Hint 3-9

The NBRC uses BE for base excess (regardless of whether it has a positive or negative value) and HCO_3^- for bicarbonate.

Exam Hint 3-10

Expect to see several arterial blood gas questions that require the interpretation of acid–base balance and oxygenation. For example, identify that a patient with COPD has an elevated carbon dioxide level and a pH in the low-normal range with a compensated respiratory acidosis. Also, expect to see ABG values included in questions about the adjustment of oxygen therapy and mechanical ventilation.

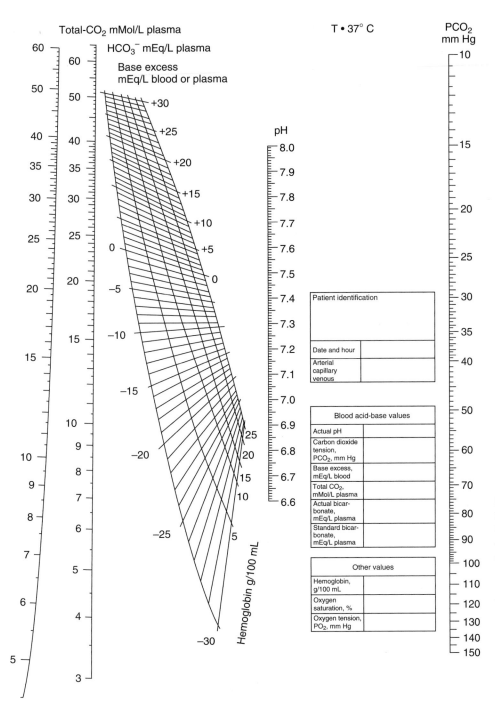

Figure 3-13 Siggaard-Andersen alignment nomogram for determining bicarbonate (HCO_3^-) and base excess (BE). To find these values, line up a straight ruler with the pH and PCO_2 values. Extend the line to find the bicarbonate HCO_3^- and BE numbers. For example, with a pH of 7.4 and PCO_2 of 40 mm Hg (torr), the base excess is seen as 0 and the HCO_3^- is seen as 24 mEq/L. (Modified from Siggaard-Andersen O: Arterial blood gas analyzers. In Burton G, Hodgkin JE, Ward JJ, eds: Respiratory care: a guide to clinical practice, ed 4, Philadelphia, 1997, JB Lippincott.)

Tables 3-7 to 3-9 show definitions of terms and classifications of the various ventilation and acid–base states. As stated earlier, there are other systems for interpreting blood gases. All are probably satisfactory for interpretation purposes and preparing for the NBRC examinations. See Figure 3-14 for a nomogram that shows the ABG relationships between $PaCO_2$, HCO_3^-, and pH. Plotting the $PaCO_2$ and pH enables the HCO_3^- to be determined as well as the extent of combined or compensated respiratory or metabolic effects.

2. Hemoximetry results

a. Evaluate hemoximetry blood gas results in the patient record (code: IA5) [difficulty: R, Ap]

Look in the chart for any previous arterial blood gas and hemoximetry results. Hemoximetry or CO oximetry is usually performed on a patient known or suspected of carbon monoxide poisoning.

TABLE 3-7   Clinical Terminology for Arterial Blood Gas Measurements

Clinical Terminology	Clinical Findings
Respiratory acidosis/alveolar hypoventilation/ventilatory failure	$PaCO_2$ >45 torr
Acute ventilatory failure	$PaCO_2$ >45 torr; pH ≤7.35
Chronic ventilatory failure	$PaCO_2$ >45 torr; pH 7.36-7.40
Respiratory alkalosis/alveolar hyperventilation	$PaCO_2$ <35 torr
Acute alveolar hyperventilation	$PaCO_2$ <35 torr; pH >7.45
Chronic alveolar hyperventilation	$PaCO_2$ <35 torr; pH 7.41-7.45
Acidemia	pH <7.35
Acidosis	Pathophysiologic condition in which the patient has a significant base deficit (plasma bicarbonate level below normal)
Alkalemia	pH >7.45
Alkalosis	Pathophysiologic condition in which the patient has a significant base excess (plasma bicarbonate level above normal)

Modified from Shapiro BA, Peruzzi WT, Kozlowski-Templin R: Clinical application of blood gases, ed 5, St Louis, 1994, Mosby.

TABLE 3-8   Evaluation of Ventilatory and Metabolic Effects on Acid–Base Status

EVALUATION OF $PaCO_2$	
$PaCO_2$ >45 torr	Respiratory acidosis/alveolar hypoventilation/ventilatory failure
$PaCO_2$ 35-45 torr	Acceptable alveolar ventilation
$PaCO_2$ <35 torr	Respiratory alkalosis/alveolar hyperventilation

EVALUATION OF $PaCO_2$ IN CONJUNCTION WITH pH*	
Acceptable Alveolar Ventilation ($PaCO_2$ from 35 to 45 torr)	
pH >7.50	Metabolic alkalosis
pH 7.30-7.50	Acceptable pH
pH <7.30	Metabolic acidosis
Alveolar Hypoventilation ($PaCO_2$ >45 torr)	
pH >7.50	Partially compensated metabolic alkalosis
pH 7.30-7.40	Chronic ventilatory failure
pH <7.30	Acute ventilatory failure
Alveolar Hyperventilation ($PaCO_2$ <35 torr)	
pH >7.50	Acute alveolar hyperventilation
pH 7.40-7.50	Chronic alveolar hyperventilation
pH 7.30-7.40	Compensated metabolic acidosis
pH <7.30	Partially compensated metabolic acidosis

Modified from Shapiro BA, Peruzzi WT, Kozlowski-Templin R: Clinical application of blood gases, ed 5, St Louis, 1994, Mosby.
$PaCO_2$, partial pressure of CO_2 in arterial blood.
*Some authors use a narrower pH range for these classifications.

TABLE 3-9   Primary Blood Gas Classification

	CO_2	pH	Bicarbonate	BE
Ventilatory Imbalance				
Acute alveolar hypoventilation	I	D	N	N
Chronic alveolar hypoventilation	I	N	I	I
Acute alveolar hyperventilation	D	I	N	N
Chronic alveolar hyperventilation	D	N	D	D
Metabolic Imbalance				
Uncompensated acidosis	N	D	D	D
Partially compensated acidosis	D	D	D	D
Uncompensated alkalosis	N	I	I	I
Partially compensated alkalosis	I	I	I	I
Compensated acidosis or alkalosis	I or D	N	I or D	I or D

Modified from Shapiro BA, Peruzzi WT, Kozlowski-Templin R: Clinical application of blood gases, ed 5, St Louis, 1994, Mosby.
D, decreased; I, increased; N, normal range; BE, base excess.

b. Recommend hemoximetry blood gas analysis (code: IE9) [difficulty: R, Ap, An]

See Module A and Box 3-1 for indications for an ABG with hemoximetry analysis.

c. Evaluate the results of a hemoximetry analysis (code: ID6) [difficulty: R, Ap, An]

If the blood-sampling equipment preparation, the sampling procedure, and blood gas analyzer operation were all done properly, the respiratory therapist and physician can believe that the blood gas results are accurate and reliable. However, if there was a problem with any aspect of obtaining and analyzing the blood gas sample, that sample must be discarded and a new sample obtained and analyzed.

The CO-oximeter-type blood gas analyzer gives values for O_2Hb, RHb, COHb, and MetHb/SHb. Each of these hemoglobin moieties can be displayed in terms of grams per deciliter, percentage of the whole and added together for a total hemoglobin value. Table 3-10 shows normal adult hemoglobin values. The amounts of carboxyhemoglobin and methemoglobin should be subtracted from the total hemoglobin amount to find the amount of functional hemoglobin. Any increase in the COHb or MetHb levels above those listed is abnormal and results in even less normal hemoglobin to carry oxygen. The patient with carbon monoxide poisoning is at greatest risk. A COHb level of 30% saturation or greater can be fatal. By subtraction, the O_2Hb (SaO_2) level can be no greater than 70% with a resulting PaO_2 of less than 40 torr.

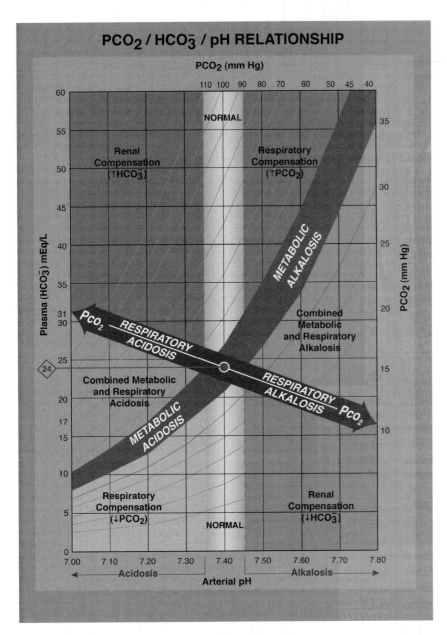

Figure 3-14 Nomogram showing the relationship between pH, PCO_2, and HCO_3^-. To use the nomogram, first find the pH. Next, follow the vertical pH line until it crosses the diagonal PCO_2 line. At the intersection, go left to find the HCO_3^- value. The nomogram can also be used to determine if there has been renal/metabolic or respiratory compensation for an acid–base imbalance. Combined metabolic and respiratory acidosis or alkalosis can also be seen. (From Des Jardins T, Burton GG: Clinical manifestations and assessment of respiratory disease, ed 6, St Louis, 2011, Mosby.)

TABLE 3-10	Normal Hemoglobin Values for Adults
Total hemoglobin (THb)	Men: 13.5-18.0 g/dL Women: 12.0-16.0 g/dL 15.0 g/dL is often listed as an average for both
Oxyhemoglobin	94-100% of THb (reported as SaO_2) of 94-100%
Carboxyhemoglobin	Nonsmokers: <1.5% (0.225 g/dL) of THb Smokers: 1.5-10% of THb
Methemoglobin	0.5-3% (0.075-0.45 g/dL) of THb
Oxygen content (arterial sample)	15-23 g/dL

g/dL, grams per deciliter (sometimes listed as g/100 mL); SaO_2, O_2 saturation in arterial blood.

EXAMPLE 1

The following example shows how to calculate the amount of functional hemoglobin and saturation for a patient with normal COHb and MetHb levels:

$$
\begin{array}{r}
15.0 \text{ g total Hb} \\
- 0.225 \text{ g COHb} \\
\hline
14.775 \text{ g} \\
- 0.15 \text{ g MetHb} \\
\hline
14.625 \text{ g functional Hb}
\end{array}
$$

$$
\begin{array}{r}
100\% \text{ potential saturation of } O_2Hb \text{ in arterial blood} \\
- 1.5\% \text{ saturation of COHb} \\
\hline
98.5\% \\
- 1.5\% \text{ saturation of MetHb} \\
\hline
97\% \text{ saturation of arterial blood } (SaO_2 \text{ of } 97\%)
\end{array}
$$

EXAMPLE 2

The following example is for a patient with an elevated COHb level and a normal MetHb level:

$$
\begin{array}{r}
15.0 \text{ g total Hb} \\
- 3.0 \text{ g COHb} \\
\hline
12.0 \text{ g} \\
- 0.15 \text{ g MetHb} \\
\hline
11.85 \text{ g functional Hb}
\end{array}
$$

$$
\begin{array}{l}
100\% \text{ potential saturation of O}_2\text{Hb in arterial blood} \\
- 20\% \text{ saturation of COHb} \\
\hline
80\% \\
- 1.5\% \text{ saturation MetHb} \\
\hline
78.5\% \text{ saturation of arterial blood (SaO}_2 \text{ of 78.5\%)}
\end{array}
$$

Exam Hint 3-11

If a significant difference is found in hemoglobin saturation values between a standard pulse oximeter, a standard or POC analyzer, and a CO oximeter, suspect that the patient has an elevated CO level. Only the CO oximeter value will be accurate if the patient has CO poisoning.

TABLE 3-11 Normal and Abnormal Mixed Venous Blood Gas Values

Normal Values

Average:	$S\bar{v}O_2$, 75%; $P\bar{v}O_2$, 40 torr; $P\bar{v}CO_2$, 46 torr; pH 7.35
Range:	$S\bar{v}O_2$, 76-70%; $P\bar{v}O_2$, 43-37 torr; $P\bar{v}CO_2$, 46-44 torr; pH 7.36-7.34

Critically Ill Patient

	$P\bar{v}O_2$ (Torr)		$S\bar{v}O_2$ (%)	
	Average	Range	Average	Range
Excellent cardiovascular reserves	>37	40-35	>70	75-68
Limited cardiovascular reserves	>32	35-30	>60	68-56
Failure of cardiovascular reserves	<30	<30	<56	<56

Modified from Shapiro BA, Peruzzi WT, Kozlowski-Templin R: Clinical application of blood gases, ed 5, St Louis, 1994, Mosby.

3. Mixed venous blood gases

a. Evaluate mixed venous blood gas results in the patient record (code: IA5) [difficulty: R, Ap]

Look in the chart for any previous mixed venous blood gas results. A mixed venous blood sample can be taken from the pulmonary artery of any patient who has a pulmonary artery (Swan-Ganz) catheter. This is a true mixed venous sample and should not be confused with a blood sample taken from an arm vein or other venous site. The symbol $P\bar{v}$ is the prefix for mixed venous blood gas values of oxygen and so forth.

Normal mixed venous blood gas values are: $S\bar{v}O_2$, 75%; $P\bar{v}O_2$, 40 mm Hg; $P\bar{v}CO_2$, 46 mm Hg; and pH 7.35. (Table 3-11 provides details on normal mixed venous blood gas values and their interpretation in patients with cardiovascular disease.)

b. Recommend mixed venous blood gas analysis (code: IE9) [difficulty: R, Ap, An]

See Module A and Box 3-1 for indications for mixed venous blood gas analysis.

c. Evaluate the results of a mixed venous blood gas analysis (code: ID6) [difficulty: R, Ap, An]

In the critically ill patient, it is just as important to measure the mixed venous blood gases as it is to measure the arterial blood gases. The venous blood gas values reveal what has happened as the arterial blood has passed through the body. Oxygen has been extracted, and carbon dioxide has been added to the hemoglobin. The difference between the arterial and the venous oxygen levels reflects oxygen consumption by the body as well as cardiac output.

Because of this, the most critical mixed venous blood gas values to measure are the $S\bar{v}O_2$ and $P\bar{v}O_2$. It is generally accepted that a $P\bar{v}O_2$ value of less than 30 torr or an $S\bar{v}O_2$ value of less than 56% indicates that the patient has tissue hypoxia. Both values can be obtained by analyzing a mixed venous blood sample taken through a pulmonary artery catheter. If the patient has a fiber-optic catheter, the $S\bar{v}O_2$ value can be monitored continuously. This is extremely helpful if the patient is unstable or having frequent changes in inspired oxygen or ventilator settings. (Pulmonary artery catheters are discussed in more detail in Chapter 5.)

4. Central venous blood gases

a. Evaluate central venous blood gas results in the patient record (code: IA5) [difficulty: R, Ap]

Look in the chart for any previous central venous blood gas results. They are most likely to be seen in a patient with sepsis or shock who has a central venous pressure (CVP) catheter.

b. Recommend central venous blood gas analysis (code: IE9) [difficulty: R, Ap, An]

See Module A and Box 3-1 for indications for central venous blood gas analysis.

c. Evaluate the results of a central venous blood gas analysis (code: ID6) [difficulty: R, Ap, An]

Although not identical measurements, the previous discussion on mixed venous blood gases and Table 3-11 would generally apply to the interpretation of central venous blood gases. If the patient's CVP catheter offers continuous oxygen saturation, the clinical goal is a central venous oxygen saturation ($ScvO_2$) value of >70% saturation.

In a patient with normal cardiovascular function, the correlation between $PcvCO_2$ and $PaCO_2$ should be about 6 torr. A large difference between a patient's $PcvCO_2$ and $PaCO_2$ can indicate inadequate circulation. This can be seen in a patient with severe hemorrhagic shock or low cardiac output, after ineffective CPR efforts, or after cardiopulmonary bypass.

5. Arterialized capillary blood gases

a. Evaluate arterialized capillary blood gas results in the patient record (code: IA5) [difficulty: R, Ap]

See Module A and Box 3-1 for indications for arterialized capillary blood gas analysis. Look in the chart for any previous arterialized capillary blood gas results in a neonatal or pediatric patient.

b. Recommend arterialized capillary blood gas analysis (code: IE9) [difficulty: R, Ap, An]

This method of obtaining a blood gas sample is limited to neonatal or pediatric patients when an arterial sample cannot be obtained.

c. Evaluate the results of arterialized capillary blood gas analysis (code: ID6) [difficulty: R, Ap, An]

Because this is not a true ABG sample, the following limitations are placed on interpreting the results.

- The capillary pH value has a good correlation with the arterial pH value.
- The capillary CO_2 ($PcCO_2$) value has a fair correlation with the $PaCO_2$ value.
- The capillary O_2 (PCO_2) value does not correlate well with the PaO_2 value.

Based on these limitations, an arterialized capillary blood pH value can be clinically useful. The capillary CO_2 value should be viewed with suspicion. It should not be the only parameter monitored to judge the infant's ability to ventilate; however, the combination of a low pH and elevated CO_2 value indicates hypoventilation. Evaluate the infant's vital signs, breathing efforts, chest radiograph, and so on to determine respiratory status.

Unfortunately, the capillary O_2 value is practically useless for judging the infant's oxygenation. Some infants may have a fairly close correlation with the PaO_2 level, whereas others do not. No way is known to

predetermine those that will match and those that will not. Many practitioners view a low capillary oxygen level as a sign of clinical hypoxemia. The AARC Clinical Practice Guideline for Oxygen Therapy in the Acute Care Hospital notes that a capillary PO_2 level of less than 40 torr documents neonatal hypoxemia. An ABG sample remains the best way to determine the patient's respiratory status.

MODULE F

Pulse oximetry

1. Evaluate pulse oximetry results in the patient record (code: IA13f) [difficulty: R, Ap]

Pulse oximetry (SpO_2) spectroscopically analyzes arterial blood to noninvasively determine the percentage of hemoglobin that is saturated with oxygen. It has become a standard of care whenever a patient's oxygenation must be continuously monitored. In general, the SpO_2 correlates with the SaO_2 and PaO_2. So, an SpO_2 value of 92% or greater indicates that the patient is adequately oxygenated (assuming normal hemoglobin concentration and cardiac function). Past values should be compared with current readings to monitor the patient's progress or response to treatment.

2. Recommend pulse oximetry for noninvasive monitoring (code: IE8) [difficulty: R, Ap, An]

Pulse oximetry is indicated in the following situations: during anesthesia and intraoperative monitoring of oxygenation, postoperatively when the patient is still sedated, when the patient is receiving sedatives or analgesics that can blunt the airway protective reflexes, during bronchoscopy, during a sleep study, during periods of respiratory distress, and for evaluating the effectiveness of oxygen therapy. An exception to the use of standard pulse oximetry is when there is known or suspected carbon monoxide poisoning.

3. Perform pulse oximetry (code: IC2) [difficulty: R, Ap]

Pulse oximetry has gained wide acceptance because it offers a way to continuously and noninvasively monitor a patient's oxygenation. The reported SpO_2% is the percentage of oxyhemoglobin. This information and the patient's heart rate are shown on a light-emitting diode (LED) display. More expensive units store the information in memory and/or print out a copy of the SpO_2 percentage and pulse rate to be placed into the patient's chart if necessary. In infants, a probe is usually placed on the hands or feet. In adults, sensors are available that can be placed on the fingers, toes, bridge of the nose, forehead, and earlobe. See examples in Figure 3-15. Choose a sensor designed to fit the site that is selected.

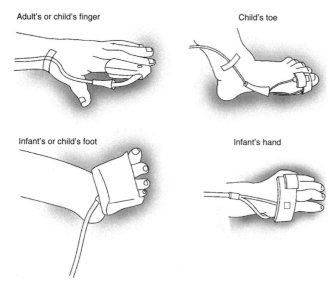

Figure 3-15 Examples of pulse oximeter sensors for the finger, hand, toe, and foot. (From Malley WJ: Clinical blood gases: assessment and intervention, ed 2, St Louis, 2005, Saunders.)

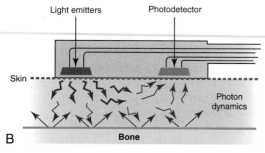

Figure 3-16 Essential functions of pulse oximeters. **A,** Basic components and features of a transmission-type pulse oximeter that is applied to a finger. The transducer sends red and infrared light waves through the finger to the photodiode. The processor compares the transmitted light to the received light and calculates the SpO₂ percentage and heart rate. **B,** Basic components of a reflectance-type pulse oximeter that would be applied to the forehead. The transducer sends red and infrared light waves through the skin where they are reflected off the skull to the photodiode. The processor compares the transmitted light to the received light and calculates the SpO₂ percentage and heart rate. (**A,** Modified from Gardner R: Pulse oximetry: is it monitoring's "silver bullet?" *J Cardiovasc Nurs* 1:79-83, 1987; **B,** From Keogh BF, Kopotic RJ: Recent findings in the use of reflectance oximetry: a critical review. *Curr Opin Anaesthesiol* 18:649-654, 2005.)

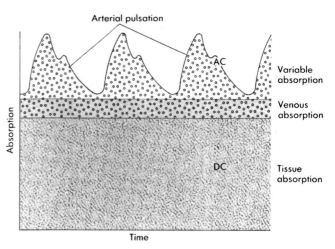

Figure 3-17 Pulse oximetry signal strength. The strong surge of blood through the artery with each heartbeat results in variable absorption of the light emitted by the pulse oximeter. Venous and tissue absorption of light is stable when the heart is at rest. This absorption difference is used to find the patient's artery and measure the heart rate. (AC, variable absorption; DC, stable absorption). (From Mottram CD: Ruppel's Manual of pulmonary function testing, ed 10, St Louis, 2013, Mosby.)

Pulse oximetry makes practical use of two physical principles. The first is spectrophotometry, which is used to analyze the transmission of wavelengths of light through the blood and body tissues. First-generation, standard pulse oximeters analyze two wavelengths of light. One wavelength is 660 nm and the other is between 920 and 940 nm, depending on the manufacturer. The 660-nm wavelength can be seen as red and is preferentially absorbed by O₂Hb. The 920- to 940-nm wavelength is not visible, because it is in the infrared range. It is preferentially absorbed by RHb (see Fig. 3-16). More advanced pulse CO oximeters analyze several more wavelengths of light and can evaluate carboxyhemoglobin and other forms of hemoglobin.

The second principle is plethysmography. It is used to find and then evaluate the amplitude of the arterial pulse waveform. Figure 3-17 shows the plethysmographic arterial waveform. When the pulse oximeter sensor is placed at a site on a patient, the fingertip for example, the two wavelengths of light shine through the blood, tissues, and bone within the finger. It is important that the sending LED and receiving (photodiode) sensors be opposite each other. Most units have a signal strength display that indicates when the photodiode is receiving a strong signal, and the patient's pulse has been detected. The microprocessor is designed to detect a baseline level of light absorption by the tissues and venous blood, containing more RHb, as well as the light absorption of arterial blood, containing more O₂Hb. It can then compare the absorptions of the two wavelengths to determine the level of saturated oxyhemoglobin. This is displayed as saturation by pulse oximetry, or SpO₂.

It must be realized that because standard pulse oximeters sample only two wavelengths of light, the technology is unable to recognize the presence or quantity of the nonfunctional hemoglobin species of COHb and MetHb. Instead, an ABG sample should be drawn and sent to the laboratory to be passed through a CO oximeter for a complete fractional hemoglobin analysis. Even healthy persons have small amounts of COHb and MetHb. For this and other technical reasons, manufacturers report the following SpO_2 values for general accuracy at 1 SD for a general population: ±2% from 100% to 70% saturation and ±3% from 70% to 50% saturation. Because of these limitations, the following clinical guidelines have been created by a number of authors.

- Do not use pulse oximetry on patients with significant levels of COHb or MetHb.
- If in doubt about abnormal types of hemoglobin, analyze an ABG through a CO oximeter and compare the true SaO_2 with the SpO_2 from pulse oximetry. Pulse oximetry can be used if the correlation of values is within 4%.
- Question the SpO_2 value when the displayed heart rate is different from the actual heart rate.
- Do not use pulse oximetry when the SpO_2 reading is less than 70%.
- Pulse oximetry does not ensure adequate oxygen delivery. Hemoglobin is necessary to deliver oxygen to the tissues. If the hemoglobin is dangerously low, but oxygenated, the SpO_2 reading will probably be in the acceptable range and the patient will still by hypoxic.
- Pulse oximetry can be used on a term neonate or a neonate who weighs 1500 g or more. Smaller neonates should have oxygenation measured by a transcutaneous oxygen monitor. This is because it is too easy to hyperoxygenate a small neonate when small changes in saturation can result in wide swings in PO_2 level. The risk of retinopathy of prematurity (formerly called retrolental fibroplasia) from hyperoxia is too great in the small neonate.

The newer pulse CO oximeters (Masimo Rad-57 or Radical-7 [Irvine, CA]) analyze 7 to 12 wavelengths of light. Because of this, they can identify and measure the various normal and abnormal types of hemoglobin, such as carboxyhemoglobin (Spco) from carbon monoxide poisoning and methemoglobin (SpMet) from inhaled nitric oxide therapy. These units provide the opportunity to continuously monitor patients with elevated levels of carboxyhemoglobin and methemoglobin as they are being treated. It may not be necessary to draw as many arterial blood gas samples for analysis through a CO oximeter. If necessary, review the discussion on CO oximeters and see Figure 3-10 because the principles apply to pulse CO oximeters.

Table 3-12 lists common clinical ranges for SpO_2 values. For the aforementioned reasons, with standard pulse oximeters the minimum safe values are 2% higher than the corresponding SaO_2 value by CO oximetry. It is important that the patient have good pulsatile blood flow to the measurement site to obtain an accurate reading.

4. Evaluate the results of pulse oximetry (code: ID2) [difficulty: R, Ap, An]

The previously healthy patient who has cardiopulmonary failure should have the SpO_2 value kept at 92% or greater

| TABLE 3-12 | Recommended Clinical Ranges for True Values in Saturation of O_2 in the Hemoglobin (SaO_2), Values in Pulse Oximetry (SpO_2),* and Their Correlation with Values in Partial Pressure of O_2 in Arterial Blood (PaO_2) |

APPROXIMATE			
	SaO_2	**SpO_2**	**PaO_2 (torr)**
Adult			
Acute hypoxemia	90-95%	92-95%†	60-95
Chronic hypoxemia	85-90%	87-92%	50-60
Neonate‡			
<1500 g or in the first week of life	About 97%	92-96%	60-70
>1500 g or after the first week of life	90-96%	90-96%	50-70
>1 month of age with chronic lung disease	85-90%	87-92%	50-60

*Based on the patient having normal carboxyhemoglobin and methemoglobin levels. Elevated levels result in an erroneously high SpO_2 reading and unsuspected hypoxemia.
†African American patients should have an SpO_2 of 95% maintained to ensure adequate oxygenation.
‡The clinical goal with most neonates is to prevent both hypoxemia, defined as a PaO_2 <45 torr, and hyperoxemia, defined as a PaO_2 >90 torr.

to ensure adequate oxygenation. The patient with COPD can probably tolerate an SpO_2 value as low as 87%. In general, a neonate should have the SpO_2 level kept between 92% and 96%. See Table 3-12 for more specific guidelines. Saturations below these values indicate hypoxemia in most patients.

Note the site at which the saturation was measured. This is especially important in neonates who may have congenital heart defects. A higher saturation in the right hand, right fingers, or right earlobe compared with the rest of the body is seen in a neonate who has patent ductus arteriosus (PDA). A higher saturation in the fingers and earlobes compared with the toes is seen in a neonate who has coarctation of the aorta.

Exam Hint 3-12

The patient with carbon monoxide poisoning should *not* be evaluated with a standard pulse oximeter because the units are unable to distinguish functional oxyhemoglobin from nonfunctional carboxyhemoglobin. These pulse oximeters show only the level of functional O_2Hb. Instead, have an ABG sample run through a hemoximeter/CO oximeter blood gas analyzer on a patient with known or suspected CO poisoning. Clinical examples include a patient removed from an enclosed house fire or a patient removed from a car with the engine running. After the patient's COHb level has been determined, a pulse CO oximeter can be used to monitor the drop in COHb level as the patient is treated with 100% oxygen.

5. Pulse oximeter equipment

a. Assemble a pulse oximeter (code: IIA21) [difficulty: R, Ap]

1. Standard pulse oximeter

In most patient care situations, a first-generation, standard pulse oximeter can be used. Follow the manufacturer's suggestions for setup. Most pulse oximetry systems visually display the strength of the pulse so that the best place for the sensor can be found (Fig. 3-17). Keep bright light away from the patient site and sensor. See Figure 3-15 for a variety of sensors for application to a finger, toe, foot, or hand. There are also sensors for an ear, the bridge of the nose, and the forehead.

2. Pulse CO oximeter

A newer-generation pulse CO oximeter (for example, a Masimo Rad-57 or Radical-7 [Irvine, CA]) will be needed if a patient is known to have carbon monoxide poisoning and continuous monitoring is required. A pulse CO oximeter can identify all types of normal and abnormal hemoglobin. It can provide information on carboxyhemoglobin (SpCO), methemoglobin (SpMet), and total hemoglobin (SpHb).

b. Troubleshoot any problems with the equipment (code: IIA21) [difficulty: R, Ap]

The pulse signal will not be strong if the patient has poor circulation at the site of the oximeter probe. This can occur if the patient is hypothermic, hypotensive, or receiving a vasoconstricting medication. If the pulse signal is weak, the pulse oximetry values may not be accurate. See Table 3-13 for common sources of error and their solutions.

Exam Hint 3-13

Usually a question is related to an inaccurately low pulse oximeter reading caused by poor local perfusion. See Table 3-13 for this and other examples of causes of inaccurate readings.

MODULE G

Transcutaneous oxygen monitoring

Note: Transcutaneous monitoring (TCM) involves the continuous monitoring of oxygen, carbon dioxide, or both as they diffuse through the skin. Each gas has its own individual electrode, and a combined electrode exists for both gases.

1. Evaluate transcutaneous oxygen results in the patient record (code: IA13f) [difficulty: R, Ap]

Transcutaneous oxygen monitoring ($PtCO_2$) enables any patient's oxygenation status to be followed on a

TABLE 3-13	Sources of Error in Pulse Oximetry
Sources of Error	**Remedy**
Light interference: Xenon lamp, fluorescent light, infrared (bilirubin) light; probe fell off of patient	Cover the probe with an opaque wrap; put the probe back in place on the patient
Low perfusion: Low blood pressure, hypothermia, vasoconstricting drugs	Use earlobe, bridge of nose, or forehead instead of finger or toe; discontinue use if still unreliable
Motion artifact	Secure the probe site; ensure that the SpO_2 reading is synchronized with the heart rate
Darkly pigmented patient	Use lightly pigmented site such as tip of finger or toe; SpO_2 value may overestimate PaO_2; discontinue use if still unreliable
Artificial or painted fingernails	Remove acrylic nails; remove black, blue, green, metallic, or frosted nail polish; use a different site
Venous pulsation being read as an arterial pulsation	Loosen a tight sensor; change the finger sensor site every 2-4 hours; loosen the cause of a tourniquet-like effect
The following vascular dyes will cause low SpO_2 readings: Methylene blue, indigo carmine, indocyanine green	Do not use SpO_2

PaO_2, partial pressure of O_2 in arterial blood; SpO_2, pulse oximeter.

continuous basis. In practice, neonates are monitored much more often than adults. Check the chart for a record of the patient's transcutaneous oxygen values. It is particularly important to compare the PaO_2 value with the $PtCO_2$ value. In addition, note what the $PtCO_2$ values are when the inspired oxygen is changed, the patient's airway is suctioned, or changes are made in continuous positive airway pressure (CPAP) or mechanical ventilation. Avoid clinical situations that have previously resulted in hypoxemia.

2. Recommend transcutaneous oxygen monitoring (code: IE8) [difficulty: R, Ap, An]

$PtCO_2$ monitoring has been used for the following purposes:

- To monitor oxygenation during transportation of an unstable neonate within the hospital or between hospitals.
- To monitor intraoperative and postoperative oxygenation.

- To monitor oxygenation during changes in the inspired oxygen and during changes in mechanical ventilation and to detect hypoxemia during an equipment failure.
- To help detect a right-to-left shunt. When a neonate has a PDA, the $PtCO_2$ level is higher in the right upper chest than in the left upper chest, abdomen, or thighs.
- To help detect a coarctation of the aorta. When this defect is present, the $PtCO_2$ value is higher in the right and left upper chest than in the abdomen or thighs.
- To determine the response to an oxygen challenge test by a patient with congenital heart disease.

3. Perform $PtCO_2$ monitoring (code: IC2) [difficulty: R, Ap, An]

a. Site selection

Care must be taken to select the best site for the electrode. A bad site will give incorrect information that can lead to mistakes in patient care. See Box 3-3 for a listing of site selection guidelines.

b. Skin and electrode preparation and application of the skin electrode

An airtight seal between the skin and the electrode is necessary for accurate readings. An air leak (21% oxygen) will falsely increase or decrease the $PtCO_2$ reading from the patient's actual value. A room air leak will always cause a decrease in the $PtcCO_2$ reading. The following steps should be taken to ensure that the skin site, adhesive ring, and electrode are prepared and an airtight seal is ensured:

1. Clean the skin. Usually, cleaning with an alcohol swab is enough to remove perspiration. Oily skin should be cleaned with soap and water.
2. Adults may need to have hair shaved from the site.
3. Adults may have dead skin cells removed by placing sticky adhesive tape against the site and pulling it off.
4. Apply the adhesive ring to the skin. Make sure there are no wrinkles that could result in a leak.
5. Prepare the electrode according to the manufacturer's guidelines. This usually includes placing a drop of the electrolyte solution on the electrode surface and placing a gas-permeable membrane with a double adhesive ring over the electrode.
6. Screw the electrode into the adhesive ring to form an airtight seal (see Fig. 3-18).
7. As the electrode warms the skin, the patient values will fluctuate. Stabilization usually requires several minutes, after which the patient values should be clinically useful.

c. Limitations and patient precautions

Because the electrode is heated, it must be rotated to a different skin site on a routine basis. The general manufacturer's guidelines for site rotation are every 4-6 hours

---

BOX 3-3 Optimal Sites and Sites to Avoid with Transcutaneous Gas Monitoring

Optimal Neonatal Sites
Upper part of the chest.
Right upper chest if a preductal $PtCO_2$ value is desired.
Abdomen.
Inner aspect of either thigh.

Optimal Child or Adult Sites
Upper part of the chest.
Inner aspect of the upper arm.

Sites to Avoid
Large fat deposit.
Bony prominence.
Pressure point.
Thick skin.
Skin edema.
Hands and feet.

Conditions in Which Transcutaneous Monitoring Should Not be Used
Locally cold skin or general, deep hypothermia.
Locally decreased peripheral perfusion or general hypotension.
Patient receiving vasoconstricting drugs such as tolazoline or dopamine.
Cardiac index less than $1.9 \, L/min/m^2$ of body surface area.
Halothane anesthesia will give erroneously high transcutaneous O_2 values unless a Teflon membrane is used.

$PtCO_2$, pressure of transcutaneous oxygen.

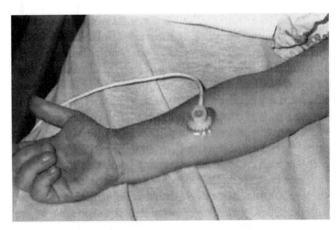

Figure 3-18 Transcutaneous oxygen (or carbon dioxide) monitor electrode properly placed onto a child's inner forearm. Note the airtight adhesive ring that holds the transducer in place. (From Jacobus C: Noninvasive monitoring in neonatal and pediatric care. In Walsh B, Czervinske MP, Diblasi RM: Perinatal and pediatric respiratory care, ed 3, St Louis, 2010, Saunders.)

for neonates weighing between 1000 and 2500 g, every 3-5 hours for neonates weighing between 2500 and 3500 g, and every 2-4 hours for neonates weighing more than 3500 g, pediatric patients, and adult patients. As a safety precaution, change the electrode on all patients at least every 4 hours, or at least every 3 hours if the patient is hypothermic. The manufacturer's range in times is based on the relative thickness of the patient's skin and the different electrode temperatures. It is important to adjust the site-rotation times on an individual patient basis. Some may tolerate longer times, and others will need more frequent rotations.

Care must be taken when removing the adhesive ring and electrode. It is possible to tear the thin, delicate skin of a premature neonate. Loosen the adhesive by running the edge of an alcohol wipe along the side that is being gently pulled up. After the electrode is removed, it is important to examine the skin; it is normal to see a red circle. This warmed, vasodilated area will stay red for some time and will gradually fade away, with no scarring or permanent injury. Rarely, the skin will have overheated and a blister is seen; this is a second-degree burn. Obviously, future site rotations must be made more frequently. Do not use this site again. Treat it as a burn, and avoid any further injury that might break the skin and lead to an infection.

4. Evaluate transcutaneous oxygen monitoring values (code: ID2) [difficulty: R, Ap, An]

It has been found that heating the electrode speeds the diffusion of oxygen through the skin. Heating also provides a closer correlation with the patient's PaO_2 value. However, it must be remembered that the $PtCO_2$ value is not the same as the PaO_2 value. Current recommendations are that any unit should give $PtCO_2$ values that are within ±15% of the PaO_2 values over the operating range of the instrument. The values should then correlate within ±15% as the patient's condition changes. This should always be confirmed.

An arterial blood gas sample should be drawn for PaO_2 every time transcutaneous oxygen monitoring is started. The PaO_2–$PtCO_2$ gradient can then be calculated as the difference between the two. For example, if the patient's PaO_2 value is 100 torr, the $PtCO_2$ value should be no less than 85 torr. If the $PtCO_2$ level decreases to 70 torr, the PaO_2 level should have decreased to no lower than 85 torr. Because of this close correlation, the patient's trend can be monitored with some assurance of accuracy. In addition, ABG samples do not need to be drawn as frequently for the PaO_2 measurement. This trending relation holds true for changes in the patient's pulmonary condition. It does not, however, hold true when the patient has cardiovascular problems such as hypotension, hypothermia, peripheral vascular disease, or cardiogenic shock with decreased tissue perfusion.

Always follow the manufacturer's recommendations for the proper electrode temperature. In general, the temperature ranges from 42.5° C for a 1000-g infant to 44° C for a 3500-g infant. A pediatric patient can tolerate a temperature of 44° C, whereas an adult can have an electrode temperature of 45° C. The higher temperatures are needed in older patients because their skin is thicker. Studies have shown that when the neonate's PaO_2 level is greater than 100 torr, the $PtCO_2$ value underestimates it. This can lead to dangerous hyperoxemia. For this reason, it is recommended that the $PtCO_2$ level be kept at less than 90 torr. In the adult, less correlation is found between the PaO_2 and the $PtCO_2$ values because of the thicker skin found in adults. The $PtCO_2$ value can still be used in the adult to follow trends in oxygenation, but the practitioner must realize that a decrease in the $PtCO_2$ value can be a result of hypoxemia, a decreased cardiac output, or cutaneous vasoconstriction. An arterial blood gas sample must be drawn to further evaluate the patient's status.

a. Correlation of $PtCO_2$ and local power consumption

As mentioned previously, the electrode is heated to above body temperature. The amount of electrical current needed to keep the electrode at a constant temperature depends on the temperature of the blood and the speed at which the blood passes beneath the electrode. This is known as local power consumption or simply local power (LP). A change in the LP value and $PtCO_2$ value can be used to indicate what is happening to the patient. For example:

- A normal LP seen with a decreased $PtCO_2$ value indicates that the patient's pulmonary problem has worsened.
- A normal LP seen with an increased $PtCO_2$ value indicates that the patient's pulmonary problem has improved.
- A decreased LP seen with a decreased $PtCO_2$ value indicates that the patient's cardiac output has worsened.
- An increased LP seen with an increased $PtCO_2$ value indicates that the patient's cardiac output has improved.

Exam Hint 3-14

If a sick neonate has normal cardiovascular status, the PaO_2 and $PtCO_2$ values should correlate with each other (but not be identical) as the patient's pulmonary condition changes; for example, the neonate has infant respiratory distress syndrome. The PaO_2 and $PtCO_2$ values probably will not correlate when the patient has cardiovascular problems; for example, the neonate is hypotensive with low cardiac output.

5. Transcutaneous oxygen monitor equipment

a. Assemble the transcutaneous oxygen monitor equipment (code: IIA21) [difficulty: R, Ap]

The electrode used for monitoring the patient's transcutaneous oxygen level is a miniaturized and modified Clark-type polarographic electrode similar to that used in the blood gas analyzer (Fig. 3-19). Some authors describe it as a Huch or Hellige electrode, named after two researchers who modified the original Clark electrode for their work with pediatric patients.

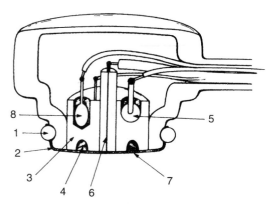

Figure 3-19 Schematic drawing of the modified Clark electrode used to monitor transcutaneous oxygen tension. 1, O-ring to hold the membrane to the electrode; 2, polypropylene membrane permeable to oxygen; 3, silver anode that surrounds the platinum cathode; 4, electrolyte chamber with solution held in place by the polypropylene membrane; 5, heating element; 6, platinum cathode; 7, electrolyte solution of sodium bicarbonate and sodium chloride held between the membrane and the electrode; and 8, negative temperature coefficient resistor that serves to regulate the temperature of the sensor. (From Shapiro BA, Peruzzi WT, Kozlowski-Templin R: Clinical application of blood gases, ed 5, St Louis, 1994, Mosby.)

Always follow the manufacturer's recommendations for the assembly and care of the equipment. Select the proper electrode for the monitor based on the physician's order for evaluating transcutaneous oxygen, carbon dioxide, or both together.

b. Troubleshoot any problems with the equipment (code: IIA21) [difficulty: R, Ap]

Problems usually associated with too much electrode drift include electrode or membrane surfaces contaminated by debris such as blood or sweat, an improperly applied membrane, a worn-out membrane, an air bubble beneath the membrane, improper gas exposed to the membrane during the calibration, exhausted electrolyte solution in the electrode, or inaccurate calibration values. After a problem is corrected, the calibration procedure should be repeated.

6. Perform quality control procedures on a transcutaneous oxygen monitor (code: IIC7) [difficulty: R, Ap]

Always follow the manufacturer's recommendations for the assembly and care of the equipment. Select the proper electrode for the monitor based on the physician's order for evaluating transcutaneous oxygen, carbon dioxide, or both together.

Two-point calibration must be performed with oxygen percentages that will cause PO_2 values beyond the clinical range that can be expected. Usually the first calibration point is a "zero" point because the electrode is exposed to no oxygen in a nitrogen-filled chamber. This point is usually quite stable. The second calibration point is found when the electrode is exposed to room air (20.95% or

0.2095 oxygen). Always follow the manufacturer's written procedures during the calibration process. Generally, when environmental conditions include a fairly stable room temperature of 25° C and 50% relative humidity, the following equation can be used to predict the room air calibration point:

$$\text{Calibration } PtCO_2 = P_B \times 0.2095$$

in which P_B is the local barometric pressure and 0.2095 is the oxygen fraction found in room air. Expose the electrode to room air to determine whether it matches the calculated calibration value. Adjust the instrument to match the calibration $PtCO_2$ if necessary. It is recommended that the room air calibration point be rechecked every 24 hours when in continuous use, after changing the membrane, or after changing the electrolyte solution. A variation of up to ±5 torr is acceptable and can be corrected by adjusting the reading on the instrument. If the variation is greater than ±5 torr, the zero point and room air calibration procedures should be repeated.

MODULE H

Transcutaneous carbon dioxide monitoring

Note: TCM involves the continuous monitoring of carbon dioxide, oxygen, or both as they diffuse through the skin. Each gas has its own individual electrode and a combined electrode exists for both gases. In addition, there are monitors that display a pulse oximeter value and transcutaneous carbon dioxide value.

1. Evaluate transcutaneous carbon dioxide results in the patient record (code: IA13f) [difficulty: R, Ap]

Transcutaneous carbon dioxide monitoring ($PtcCO_2$) enables any patient's ventilation status to be monitored on a continuous basis. In practice, neonates are monitored much more often than adults. Check the chart for a record of the patient's transcutaneous carbon dioxide values. It is particularly important to correlate these values with any ABG values, which allows comparison between the $PaCO_2$ and the $PtcCO_2$ measurements. In addition, note the $PtcCO_2$ values when changes are made in CPAP or mechanical ventilation. Avoid clinical situations that have previously resulted in hypoventilation.

2. Recommend transcutaneous carbon dioxide monitoring (code: IE8) [difficulty: R, Ap, An]

$PtcCO_2$ monitoring has been used for the following purposes:

- To monitor ventilation during transportation of an unstable infant within the hospital or between hospitals

- To monitor intraoperative and postoperative ventilation
- To monitor ventilation during changes in mechanical ventilation such as tidal volume, rate, minute ventilation, mechanical dead space, or a combination of these
- To detect hypoventilation during an accidental disconnection from the ventilator

3. Perform transcutaneous carbon dioxide monitoring (code: IC2) [difficulty: R, Ap, An]

The information on skin-site selection (see Box 3-3) and so forth presented in the preceding discussion of transcutaneous oxygen monitors applies here, as well. As with the transcutaneous oxygen electrode, it has been found that heating the $PtcCO_2$ electrode speeds the diffusion of carbon dioxide through the skin. Always follow the manufacturer's recommendations for the proper electrode temperature. Historically, the temperature of 44° C has been used with both neonates and adults. However, there may be cases in which a lower temperature, even as low as 37° C, will give good results. It must be remembered that the $PtcCO_2$ value is not the same as the $PaCO_2$ value. An arterial blood gas sample should be analyzed for $PaCO_2$ value every time transcutaneous carbon dioxide monitoring is started. Unlike transcutaneous oxygen monitoring, the correlation between $PaCO_2$ and $PtcCO_2$ values is as good in adult patients as in neonatal patients. In addition, it is not as easily influenced by changes in the patient's skin blood flow.

4. Evaluate transcutaneous carbon dioxide monitoring values (code: ID2) [difficulty: R, Ap, An]

The net effect of heating the carbon dioxide electrode and skin results in greater skin metabolism and carbon dioxide production by 4% to 5% per degree Celsius. This can result in the $PtcCO_2$ readings being 1.2 to 2 times (120%-200%) greater than the $PaCO_2$ values. Commonly, an average multiplier of 1.6 is found. The actual value varies among patients and can be found by dividing the $PtcCO_2$ value by the $PaCO_2$ value.

For example, a patient has a $PaCO_2$ level of 40 torr and a $PtcCO_2$ level of 64 torr. Calculate the gradient between the arterial and the transcutaneous values:

$$\text{Gradient} = \frac{PtcCO_2}{PaCO_2} = \frac{64}{40} = 1.6$$

As long as the patient's cardiovascular status is fairly stable, the $PaCO_2$ value can be calculated by dividing the $PtcCO_2$ value by 1.6. For example, if the patient's $PtcCO_2$ value increases to 80 torr, calculate the $PaCO_2$ value in the following manner:

$$PaCO_2 = \frac{PtcCO_2}{1.6} = \frac{80}{1.6} = 50 \text{ torr}$$

Rather than perform these calculations every time a change occurs in the patient's status, some practitioners

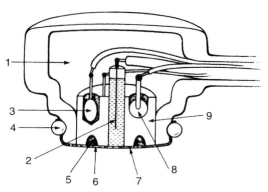

Figure 3-20 Schematic drawing of the modified Stow-Severinghaus electrode used to monitor transcutaneous carbon dioxide tension. 1, Epoxy resin; 2, glass electrode with a chlorinated silver wire, a buffer solution (the inner liquid), and a pH-sensitive glass membrane; 3, negative temperature coefficient resistor that serves to regulate the temperature of the sensor; 4, O-ring to hold the membrane to the electrode; 5, electrolyte chamber with solution held in place by the polypropylene membrane; 6, electrolyte solution of sodium bicarbonate and sodium chloride held between the membrane and the electrode; 7, polypropylene membrane permeable to carbon dioxide; 8, heating element; and 9, silver/silver chloride reference electrode. (From Shapiro BA, Peruzzi WT, Kozlowski-Templin R: Clinical application of blood gases, ed 5, St Louis, 1994, Mosby.)

divide the CO_2 values found during the calibration procedure by 1.6. This results in "real" $PaCO_2$ values being given continuously on the monitor. This change must be clearly communicated to all staff members to avoid confusion between the original $PtcCO_2$ values and values that have been reduced to arterialize them.

5. Transcutaneous carbon dioxide monitor equipment

a. Assemble the transcutaneous carbon dioxide monitor equipment (code: IIA21) [difficulty: R, Ap]

The electrode used for monitoring the patient's transcutaneous carbon dioxide level is a miniaturized and modified Stow-Severinghaus-type electrode similar to the ABG electrode (Fig. 3-20). Always follow the manufacturer's recommendations for the assembly and care of the equipment. Select the proper electrode for the monitor based on the physician's order for evaluating transcutaneous carbon dioxide.

b. Troubleshoot any problems with the equipment (code: IIA21) [difficulty: R, Ap]

Problems usually associated with too much electrode drift include electrode or membrane surfaces contaminated by debris such as blood or sweat, an improperly applied membrane, a worn-out membrane, an air bubble beneath the membrane, improper gas sample exposed to the membrane during the calibration, exhausted electrolyte solution in the electrode, or inaccurate calibration values. After a problem is corrected, the calibration procedure should be repeated.

6. Perform quality control procedures on a transcutaneous carbon dioxide monitor (code: IIC7) [difficulty: R, Ap]

Two-point calibration must be performed with carbon dioxide percentages that cause PCO_2 values beyond the expected clinical range. Usually the electrode is exposed to 5% and 10% carbon dioxide from prepared cylinders. Always follow the manufacturer's written procedures during the calibration process. Generally, when environmental conditions include a fairly stable room temperature of 25° C and 50% relative humidity, the following equation can be used to predict the two calibration points:

Calibration $PtcCO_2 = (P_B \times CO_2 \% \text{ used}) -$
$\qquad (XCO_2 \times \text{electrode temperature factor})$

in which P_B is the local barometric pressure; $CO_2\%$ is the carbon dioxide fraction exposed to the electrode, either 10% (0.10) or 5% (0.05); and XCO_2 is the correction factor used to equilibrate the $PtcCO_2$ to $PaCO_2$. (This is discussed later.)

a. Electrode temperature factor

This is a factor determined by the manufacturer based on the electrode temperature being heated to 44° C. Expose the electrode to 10% carbon dioxide in a sealed chamber to determine whether it matches the calculated calibration value. Adjust the instrument to match the calibration $PtcCO_2$ if necessary. Next, expose the electrode to 5% carbon dioxide in the sealed chamber. Again, adjust the instrument to match the calibration $PtcCO_2$ if necessary. It is recommended that the two-point calibration points be rechecked every 24 hours when in continuous use, after changing the membrane, or after changing the electrolyte solution. A variation of up to ±4 torr is acceptable and can be corrected by adjusting the reading on the instrument. If the variation is greater than ±4 torr, the two-point calibration procedures should be repeated.

MODULE I

Cardiopulmonary calculations

The purpose of the following equations is to numerically quantify the severity of a patient's lung dysfunction. If a patient's condition should deteriorate, the "number" will worsen. With successful treatment and recovery, the patient's "number" will improve.

1. Difference between the alveolar oxygen level and the arterial oxygen level

a. Calculate the difference between the alveolar oxygen level and the arterial oxygen level (code: IC10) [difficulty: R, Ap]

This gap between the alveolar oxygen level and the arterial oxygen level is called the alveolar–arterial oxygen pressure difference [$P(A-a)O_2$] Measurement of this gap or difference gives an important indication of the seriousness of the patient's condition.

Perform the following to determine the $P(A-a)O_2$:
1. Note the patient's inspired oxygen percentage.
2. Draw and analyze an ABG sample. Note the patient's PaO_2 and $PaCO_2$ values.
3. Note the patient's temperature. This is needed to determine the patient's pulmonary water vapor pressure (PH_2O). The value of 47 torr (mm Hg) is used if the patient's temperature is normal. Check published tables for the pulmonary water vapor pressure if the patient's temperature is higher or lower than normal.
4. Measure the local barometric pressure (P_B) in torr (mm Hg).
5. If possible, calculate the patient's respiratory exchange ratio. If this cannot be done, use the standard value of 0.8.
6. Calculate the patient's PAO_2 value. The formula presented here is the most commonly used of several versions:

$$PAO_2 = \left[(P_B - P_{H_2O}) F_IO_2 \right] - \frac{PaCO_2}{0.8}$$

In this equation:
- PAO_2 is the pressure of alveolar oxygen.
- P_B is the barometric pressure of air. This is 760 torr (mm Hg) at sea level; it decreases as the altitude increases.
- PH_2O is the pressure of water vapor in the lungs. This is 47 torr (mm Hg) at the normal temperature of 98.6° F/37° C. Remember that water vapor pressure increases if the patient has a fever and decreases if the patient is hypothermic.
- F_IO_2 is the fractional concentration (percentage) of inspired oxygen. Use whatever percentage of oxygen your patient is inhaling:

$\dfrac{PaCO_2}{0.8} = \text{effect of carbon dioxide and the patient's metabolism}$

The factor of 0.8 is based on how much oxygen a normal person uses in 1 minute and how much carbon dioxide is produced in 1 minute. The symbols for this metabolic value are R for respiratory exchange ratio and RQ for respiratory quotient. The following calculation is based on a normal person's metabolism:

$$R \text{ or } RQ = \frac{\dot{V}_{CO_2}}{\dot{V}_{O_2}} = \frac{200 \text{mL/min}}{250 \text{mL/min}} = 0.8$$

Because many sick patients do not react as expected, the factor has a range of 0.6-1.1, depending on oxygen consumption and carbon dioxide production. Assume that the factor is 0.8 unless you are told otherwise or measure otherwise.

7. Subtract the patient's PaO_2 value from the PAO_2 value to determine the $P(A-a)O_2$.

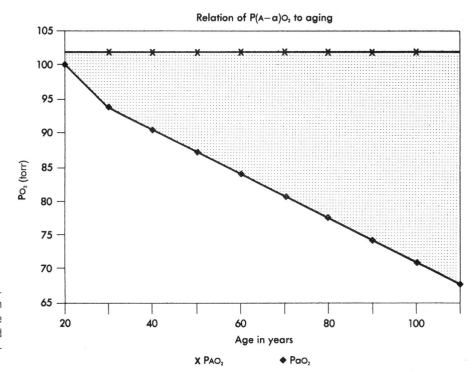

Figure 3-21 The relation of P(A–a)O₂ to aging. As the PaO₂ level naturally decreases with age, the P(A–a)O₂ level increases at the rate of approximately 3 torr per decade beyond 20 years. (From Lane EE, Walker JF: Clinical arterial blood gas analysis, St Louis, 1987, Mosby.)

b. Evaluate the results of the P(A–a)O₂ calculation (code: ID9) [difficulty: R, Ap, An]

When interpreting the patient's value, remember that the P(A–a)O₂ level in a normal young person should be no greater than 15 torr. The difference slowly increases as a normal person ages (Fig. 3-21). Lung disease causes the value to increase significantly. The following are examples of some conditions in which the measurement of the P(A–a)O₂ level aids in diagnosis or treatment:

- Patients who are hypoxemic because they are hypoventilating (increased CO₂ concentration) have a normal P(A–a)O₂ value when breathing room air. The hypoxemia can be corrected by increasing ventilation. Supplemental oxygen results in an expected increase in PaO₂ level.
- Any condition in which a low ventilation-to-perfusion ratio is found shows an elevated P(A–a)O₂ measurement when the patient is breathing room air. Supplemental oxygen results in an increase in PaO₂ level; however, the increase is not as dramatic as that seen in the hypoventilating patient. Examples include asthma, bronchitis, emphysema, or any other condition in which unequal distribution of air into and out of the lungs but relatively normal perfusion is found.
- Any shunt-producing disease or condition. Examples include ARDS and right-to-left anatomic shunt, such as could be seen in a ventricular septal defect. The P(A–a)O₂ value becomes greater as the oxygen percentage is increased. It is commonly accepted that a P(A–a)O₂ value of more than 350 torr, when 80%-100% oxygen is administered, indicates that the patient is experiencing refractory hypoxemia.

The patient probably needs to be supported by a mechanical ventilator. Commonly, positive end-expiratory pressure (PEEP) is administered so that the oxygen percentage can be reduced to a safer level.

- An indication to begin extracorporeal membrane oxygenation (ECMO) in a neonate: MacIntyre and Branson use a P(A–a)O₂ value of more than 500 torr for 4 hours. Chang uses a P(A–a)O₂ value, on 100% oxygen, of 605-620 torr for 4-12 hours.
- Any disease producing a diffusion defect. Pulmonary fibrosis from any cause results in a wider than normal P(A–a)O₂ range. Supplemental oxygen results in an increase in the PaO₂ level, but not as great an increase as desired.

The following examples are offered to aid in the calculation of P(A–a)O₂ and the interpretation of the results.

EXAMPLE 1

You are working in a major teaching hospital in Miami. The patient's physician asks you to calculate the P(A–a)O₂ on a 30-year-old patient. The following conditions exist:

- $P_B = 760$ torr
- $PH_2O = 47$ torr because your patient's temperature is 98.6° F/37° C
- $F_IO_2 = 0.21$ because the patient is breathing room air
- $PaCO_2 = 40$ torr
- $PaO_2 = 90$ torr
- $R = 0.8$

$$PAO_2 = ([P_B - PH_2O] F_IO_2) - PaCO_2/0.8$$

$$PAO_2 = ([760 - 47] 0.21) - 40/0.8$$

$PAO_2 = ([713] 0.21) - 50$

$PAO_2 = 100$ torr

$P(A-a)O_2 = 100 - 90 = 10$ torr

Interpretation: A $P(A-a)O_2$ value of 10 torr is normal for a patient of this age. It is normal to see a difference between the alveolar and the arterial oxygen levels that starts in the range of 4-12 torr and slowly increases with age (see Fig. 3-21).

EXAMPLE 2

You are working in a major teaching hospital in Denver. You are asked to calculate the alveolar–arterial difference in oxygen on a 40-year-old patient. The following conditions exist:
- $P_B = 710$ torr
- $PH_2O = 50$ torr because your patient's temperature is 100° F/38° C
- $F_IO_2 = 0.35$ because the patient is breathing 35% oxygen by mask
- $PaCO_2 = 55$ torr
- $PaO_2 = 65$ torr
- $R = 0.85$

$PAO_2 = ([P_B - PH_2O]F_IO_2) - PaCO_2/0.8$

$PAO_2 = ([710 - 50]0.35) - 55/0.85$

$PAO_2 = ([660]0.35) - 65$

$PAO_2 = 166$ torr

$P(A-a)O_2 = 166 - 65 = 101$ torr

Interpretation: The difference of 101 torr is elevated even though this patient is older than the patient in Example 1.

2. PaO$_2$/F$_I$O$_2$ (P:F) ratio

The P:F ratio is an easy bedside calculation used to assess a patient's lung function and ability to oxygenate. However, because the patient's $PaCO_2$ and airway pressures (mean airway pressure and PEEP) are not factors in the equation, an elevated carbon dioxide level and/or mean airway pressure may make the P:F ratio less useful than the $P(A-a)O_2$ value or oxygenation index.

a. Calculate the P:F ratio (ELE code: IC10) [difficulty: R, Ap]

There are two versions of the P:F ratio calculation based on how the F_IO_2 value is used. In the first version (favored by Hess and Kacmarek, Adams, Chang, and Cairo) the F_IO_2 value is used as a decimal fraction. For example, a person breathing room air would have an F_IO_2 of 0.21. So, the F value would be 0.21. Within this group, some favor the answer be given in torr, whereas others favor the answer as a simple numerical value. Both will be listed here.

In the second version (favored by Malley and Shapiro, Peruzzi, and Templin) the F_IO_2 value is the whole number for the oxygen percentage. For example, a person breathing room air would be inhaling 21% oxygen. So, the F value would be 21.

Because both versions have advocates, an example of each will be given.

Version 1

You are working in a major teaching hospital in Miami. The patient's physician asks you to calculate the P:F ratio on a 30-year-old patient. The following conditions exist:
- $P_B = 760$ torr
- $PH_2O = 47$ torr because your patient's temperature is 98.6° F/37° C
- $F_IO_2 = 0.21$ because the patient is breathing room air. So, the F value is 0.21.
- $PaO_2 = 90$ torr

$$\frac{PaO_2}{F_IO_2} = \frac{90}{0.21} = 429 \text{ or } 429 \text{ torr}$$

Version 2

You are working in a major teaching hospital in Miami. The patient's physician asks you to calculate the P:F ratio on a 30-year-old patient. The following conditions exist:
- $P_B = 760$ torr
- $PH_2O = 47$ torr because your patient's temperature is 98.6° F/37° C
- $F_IO_2 = 0.21$ because the patient is breathing room air. So, the F value is 21.
- $PaO_2 = 90$ torr

$$\frac{PaO_2}{F_IO_2} = \frac{90}{21} = 4.29$$

b. Evaluate the results of the P:F ratio (code: ID9) [difficulty: R, Ap, An]

As a result of these two calculation versions, the answers will be different by two decimal places. This leads to opposite interpretations of the answer: high is good vs low is good. Because of this, it is suggested that the basic principles of both versions be understood.

Version 1 interpretation while breathing room air

Normal: 400-500 or 400-500 torr.
Weaning trial can be attempted: ≥150 or ≥150 torr.
Acute lung injury: 200-300 or 200-300 torr.
ARDS: ≤200 or ≤200 torr.

Version 2 interpretation while breathing room air

Normal: 4.0-5.0.
Weaning trial can be attempted: ≥1.5.
Acute lung injury: 2.0-3.9.
ARDS: ≤2.0.

3. Oxygenation index

a. Calculate the oxygenation index (OI) (ELE code: IC10) [difficulty: R, Ap]

There are two versions of the OI calculation based on how the F_IO_2 value is used. In the first version (favored by the 2010 AARC Clinical Practice Guideline on inhaled nitric oxide, Hess and Kacmarek, and MacIntyre and Branson) the F_IO_2 value is used as a decimal fraction. For example, a person breathing room air would have an F_IO_2 of 0.21. So, 0.21 is used in the equation. The OI is given as a simple numerical value.

In the second version (favored by Chang and Adams) the F_IO_2 value is the whole number for the oxygen percentage. For example, a person breathing room air would be inhaling 21% oxygen. So, 21 is used in the equation. The OI is given as a simple numerical value.

Either equation results in the same answer. Because both versions have advocates, an example of each will be given.

Version 1

A critically ill neonatal patient is receiving mechanical ventilation and being considered for ECMO. The following conditions exist:

- Mean airway pressure (MAP, mPaw, Paw, or $\overline{Paw}$) is 20 cm water
- $PaO_2 = 50$ torr
- $F_IO_2 = 0.80$

$$OI = \left[\frac{F_IO_2 \times \overline{Paw}}{PaO_2} \right] \times 100$$

$$= \left[\frac{0.80 \times 20}{50} \right] \times 100$$

$$= \left[\frac{16}{50} \right] \times 100$$

$$OI = 32$$

Version 2

A critically ill neonatal patient is receiving mechanical ventilation and being considered for ECMO. The following conditions exist:

- Mean airway pressure (MAP, mPaw, Paw, or $\overline{Paw}$) is 20 cm water.
- $PaO_2 = 50$ torr
- $F_IO_2 = 80\%$ oxygen

$$OI = \frac{F_IO_2 \times \overline{Paw}}{PaO_2}$$

$$= \frac{80 \times 20}{50}$$

$$= \frac{1600}{50}$$

$$OI = 32$$

b. Evaluate the results of the OI calculation (code: ID9) [difficulty: R, Ap, An]

Although the OI calculation can be used on any patient receiving mechanical ventilation, it is most commonly used with neonatal patients. It has been shown helpful in assessing the need to initiate ECMO and to assess the effectiveness of inhaled nitric oxide. An OI of >25 is a sign of severe ventilatory failure and associated with a high mortality rate. A decreasing OI would point to improved lung function.

Exam Hint 3-15

Regardless of which calculation is performed or evaluated, the key point to remember is that the gap between inhaled oxygen and arterial oxygen widens with lung dysfunction. Diseases that cause true shunt or venous admixture result in a ventilation/perfusion mismatch. Giving supplemental oxygen will have little beneficial effect on the patient's oxygenation. PEEP is indicated and should result in a narrowed inhaled oxygen to arterial oxygen gap.

MODULE J

Respiratory care plan

1. Determine a patient's pathophysiologic state (code: IIIF1) [difficulty: R, Ap, An]

Many patients with pneumonia or other pulmonary conditions will have significant hypoxemia despite receiving supplemental oxygen. Arterial blood gas analysis is extremely important to assess the patient's condition and response to therapy. Hemoximetry/CO oximetry is essential to prove or disprove that a patient has suffered carbon monoxide poisoning.

2. Recommend starting a treatment based on the patient's response (code: IIIE2a) [difficulty: R, Ap, An]

See below.

3. Recommend a change in the therapeutic plan if indicated (code: IIIF2) [difficulty: R, Ap, An]

As part of the patient care team, you may need to evaluate the patient's blood gas values and other parameters to make a recommendation. For example, a patient with carbon monoxide poisoning is best treated by administering 100% oxygen through a nonrebreather mask. Pure oxygen reduces the half-life of COHb to 60-90 minutes. A first-generation pulse oximeter should not be used to measure this patient's saturation of oxyhemoglobin. These units are unable to identify COHb and will give misleadingly high saturation values for O_2Hb.

ABG analysis remains the "gold standard" by which all other values are judged. Typically, the arterial sample is analyzed through a standard blood gas analyzer. A CO oximeter is needed if the patient has carbon monoxide poisoning.

Mixed venous, central venous, and capillary blood-sample analysis is limited in clinical application, but very helpful in the right patient situation. However, these offer only momentary insight into the patient's condition.

Pulse oximetry and transcutaneous oxygen monitoring offer continuous information on the patient's oxygenation status. Transcutaneous carbon dioxide monitoring allows continuous monitoring of the patient's ventilation. As with all technology, these units have advantages, disadvantages, and limitations. It is up to the practitioner to make the correct choices. Some unstable patients can best be monitored through the combination of periodic evaluation of ABGs and these noninvasive continuous monitoring systems.

Exam Hint 3-16

Be prepared to make a recommendation regarding adjustment of the patient's inspired oxygen based on the PaO_2 (or related) value. Also be prepared to make a recommendation regarding adjustment of the patient's mechanical ventilation settings for tidal volume, rate, minute volume, mechanical dead space, or a combination of these based on the $PaCO_2$ (or related) value.

---

4. Recommend a treatment be terminated (code: IIIE1) [difficulty: R, Ap, An]

The hazards associated with drawing a sample of arterial blood were presented earlier. If a puncture site is not suitable, a different site must be selected. The possible burn hazard of transcutaneous monitoring was presented earlier. If blistering occurs at the probe site, move it to a different site.

5. Recommend discontinuing a treatment based on the patient's response (code: IIIE2h) [difficulty: R, Ap, An]

If blistering occurs at every transcutaneous monitoring probe site, the patient's skin is likely too sensitive to increased heat. Be prepared to recommend that transcutaneous monitoring be discontinued.

BIBLIOGRAPHY

Adams AB: Monitoring the patient in the Intensive Care Unit. In Kacmarek RM, Stoller, Heuer AJ, editors: *Egan's fundamentals of respiratory care*, ed 10, St Louis, 2013, Mosby.

American Academy of Pediatrics: Task force on transcutaneous oxygen monitors, *Pediatrics* 83(1):122, 1989.

American Association for Respiratory Care: Evidence-based clinical practice guideline: Inhaled nitric oxide for neonates with acute hypoxic respiratory failure, *Respir Care* 55(55):1717–1745, 2010.

American Association for Respiratory Care: Clinical practice guideline: blood gas analysis and hemoximetry: 2001 revision and update, *Respir Care* 46:498–505, 2001.

American Association for Respiratory Care: Clinical practice guideline: blood gas analysis and hemoximetry, *Respir Care* 58(10):1694–1703, 2013.

American Association for Respiratory Care: Clinical practice guideline: in-vitro pH and blood gas analysis and hemoximetry, *Respir Care* 38(5):505, 1993.

American Association for Respiratory Care: Clinical practice guideline: transcutaneous blood gas monitoring for carbon dioxide and oxygen, *Respir Care* 57(11):1955–1962, 2012.

American Association for Respiratory Care: Clinical practice guideline: transcutaneous blood gas monitoring for neonatal and pediatric patients: 2004 revision and update, *Respir Care* 49(9):1069–1072, 2004.

American Association for Respiratory Care: Clinical practice guideline: transcutaneous blood gas monitoring for neonatal and pediatric patients, *Respir Care* 39(12):1176, 1994.

American Association for Respiratory Care: Clinical practice guideline: capillary blood gas sampling for neonatal & pediatric patients, *Respir Care* 46(5):506–513, 2001.

American Association for Respiratory Care: Clinical practice guideline: capillary blood gas sampling for neonatal and pediatric patients, *Respir Care* 39(12):1180, 1994.

American Association for Respiratory Care: Clinical practice guideline: oxygen therapy in the acute care hospital, *Respir Care* 36(12):1410, 1991.

American Association for Respiratory Care: Clinical practice guideline: pulse oximetry, *Respir Care* 37(12):1406, 1991 (Retired).

American Association for Respiratory Care: Clinical practice guideline: sampling for arterial blood gas analysis, *Respir Care* 37(8):913, 1991 (Retired).

Beachey W: Acid–base balance. In Kacmarek RM, Stoller, Heuer AJ, editors: *Egan's fundamentals of respiratory care*, ed 10, St Louis, 2013, Mosby.

Bender JJ, Allison JR, Goehring JJ, Patel MD, Niederst SM, Douce FH: Arterial sampler filling time during arterial and venous punctures, and its relationship with mean arterial pressure in human subjects, *Respir Care* 57(11):1945–1948, 2012.

Blanchette T, Dziodzio J, Harris K: Pulse oximetry and normoximetry in neonatal intensive care, *Respir Care* 36(1):25, 1991.

Bohn DJ: Ask the expert, *Respiratory Tract* 9, February 1988.

Branson RD, Hess DR, Chatburn RL, editors: *Respiratory care equipment*, ed 2, Philadelphia, 1999, Lippincott Williams & Wilkins.

Burton GC, Hodgkin JE, Ward JJ, editors: *Respiratory care: a guide to clinical practice*, ed 4, Philadelphia, 1997, Lippincott-Raven.

Cairo JM: Blood gas monitoring. In Cairo JM, editor: *Mosby's respiratory care equipment*, ed 9, St Louis, 2014, Mosby.

Cairo JM: Establishing the need for mechanical ventilation. In Cairo JM, editor: *Pilbeam's Mechanical ventilation*, ed 5, St Louis, 2012, Mosby.

Chang DW, Hiers JH: Weaning from mechanical ventilation. In Chang DW, editor: *Clinical application of mechanical ventilation*, ed 4, Clifton Park, NY, 2014, Delmar.

Czervinske MP: Arterial blood gas analysis and other cardiopulmonary monitoring. In Koff PB, Daily KE, Schroeder JS, editors: *Techniques in bedside hemodynamic monitoring*, ed 4, St Louis, 1989, Mosby.

DiBlasi RM, Czervinske MP: Invasive blood gas analysis and cardiovascular monitoring. In Walsh B, Czervinske MP, Diblasi RM, editors: *Perinatal and pediatric respiratory care*, ed 3, St Louis, 2010, Saunders.

Elser RC: Quality control of blood gas analysis: a review, *Respir Care* 31(9):807, 1986.

Federal government releases CLIA '88 final regulations, *AARC-Times* 16(4):76, 1992.

Fell WL: Sampling and measurement of blood gases. In Lane EE, Walker JF, editors: *Clinical arterial blood gas analysis*, St Louis, 1987, Mosby.

Fink JB, Hunt GE, editors: *Clinical practice in respiratory care*, Philadelphia, 1999, Lippincott-Raven.

Garza D, Becan-McBride K: *Phlebotomy handbook*, ed 4, Stamford, 1996, Appleton & Lange.

Gentile MA, Cheifetz IM: Extracorporeal techniques for cardiopulmonary support. In MacIntyre NR, Branson RD, editors: *Mechanical ventilation*, ed 2, St Louis, 2009, Saunders.

Hess DR, Kacmarek RM: *Essentials of mechanical ventilation*, ed 2, New York, 2002, McGraw-Hill.

Huang Y-CT, Lease E, Beachey W: Gas exchange. In Hess DR, MacIntyre NR, Mishoe SC, Galvin WF, Adams AB, editors: *Respiratory care principles and practice*, ed 2, Burlington, MA, 2012, Jones & Bartlett Learning.

Jacobus C: Noninvasive monitoring in neonatal and pediatric care. In Walsh B, Czervinske MP, Diblasi RM, editors: *Perinatal and pediatric respiratory care*, ed 3, St Louis, 2010, Saunders.

Jubran A, Tobin MJ: Reliability of pulse oximetry in titrating supplemental oxygen therapy in ventilator-dependent patients, *Chest* 97:1420, 1990.

Lane EE, Walker JF: *Clinical arterial blood gas analysis*, St Louis, 1987, Mosby.

Madama VC: *Pulmonary function testing and cardiopulmonary stress testing*, ed 2, Albany, NY, 1998, Delmar.

Mahoney JJ, Hodgkin JE, Van Kessel AL: Arterial blood gas analysis. In Burton GG, Hodgkin JE, Ward JJ, editors: *Respiratory care: a guide to clinical practice*, ed 4, Philadelphia, 1997, Lippincott-Raven.

Malley WJ: *Clinical blood gases: assessment and intervention*, ed 2, St Louis, 2005, Saunders.

Malley WJ: Blood gas testing: tabletops vs handheld devices, *AARC Times* 36(6):26–29, 2013.

Marino JB: Analysis and monitoring of gas exchange. In Hinski ST, editor: *Respiratory care clinical competency lab manual*, St Louis, 2014, Mosby.

Martin RJ: Transcutaneous monitoring: instrumentation and clinical applications, *Respir Care* 35(6):577, 1990.

Mathews P, Conway L: Arterial blood gases and noninvasive monitoring of oxygen and carbon dioxide. In Wyka KA, Mathews PJ, Clark WF, editors: *Foundations of respiratory care*, Albany, NY, 2002, Delmar.

Mathews PJ, Conway L: Arterial blood gases and noninvasive monitoring of oxygen and carbon dioxide. In Wyka KA, Mathews PJ, Rutkowski J, editors: *Foundations of respiratory care*, ed 2, Clifton Park, NY, 2012, Delmar.

Mohler JG, Collier CR, Brandt W: Blood gases. In Clausen JL, editor: *Pulmonary function testing guidelines and controversies*, Orlando, 1984, Grune & Stratton.

Moran RF: Assessment of quality control of blood gas/pH analyzer performance, *Respir Care* 26(6):538, 1981.

Moran RF: CLIA regulations. I. The cure might be worse than the disease, *AARC Times* 14(11):41, 1990.

Moran RF: CLIA regulations. II. An analysis of some technical requirements, *AARC Times* 14(12):25, 1990.

Mottram CD: Blood gases and related tests. In Mottram CD, editor: *Ruppel's Manual of pulmonary function testing*, ed 10, St Louis, 2013, Mosby.

Nelson CM, Murphy EM, Bradley JK, et al.: Clinical use of pulse oximetry to determine oxygen prescriptions for patients with hypoxemia, *Respir Care* 31(8):673, 1986.

Novametrics Medical Systems: product literature on transcutaneous monitoring, Wallingford, CT.

Peters JA, Hodgkin JE, Collier CA: Blood gas analysis and acid–base physiology. In Burton GG, Hodgkin JE, Ward JJ, editors: *Respiratory care: a guide to clinical practice*, ed 3, Philadelphia, 1991, JB Lippincott.

Salyer JW: Pulse oximetry in the neonatal Intensive Care Unit, *Respir Care* 36(1):17, 1991.

Scanlan CL: Interpretation of blood gases. In Heuer AJ, Scanlan CL, editors: *Wilkins' clinical assessment in respiratory care*, ed 7, St Louis, 2014, Mosby.

Sebbane M, Claret P-G, Mercier G, Lefebvre S, et al.: Emergency Department management of suspected carbon monoxide poisoning: role of pulse CO-oximetry, *Respir Care* 58(10):1614–1620, 2013.

Shapiro BA, Kacmarek RM, Cane RD, et al.: *Clinical application of respiratory care*, ed 4, St Louis, 1991, Mosby.

Shapiro BA, Peruzzi WT, Kozlowski-Templin R: *Clinical application of blood gases*, ed 5, St Louis, 1994, Mosby.

Siobal MS: Analysis and monitoring of gas exchange. In Kacmarek RM, Stoller, Heuer AJ, editors: *Egan's fundamentals of respiratory care*, ed 10, St Louis, 2013, Mosby.

Toben B: Blood gases and associated technologies. In Wanger J, editor: *Pulmonary function testing*, ed 3, Burlington, MA, 2012, Jones & Bartlett Learning.

Walton JR, Shapiro BA: Value and application of temperature-compensated blood gas data, *Respir Care* 25(2), 1980.

Weaver LK, Churchill SK, Deru K, Cooney D: False positive rate of carbon monoxide saturation by pulse oximetry of Emergency Department patients, *Respir Care* 58(2):232–240, 2013.

Whitaker KB, Trujillo LM: Neonatal mechanical ventilation. In Chang DW, editor: *Clinical application of mechanical ventilation*, ed 4, Clifton Park, NY, 2014, Delmar.

White GC: *Equipment theory for respiratory care*, ed 3, Albany, NY, 1999, Delmar.

Wilkins RL: Analysis and monitoring of gas exchange. In Wilkins RL, Stoller JK, Kacmarek RM, editors: *Egan's fundamentals of respiratory care*, ed 9, St Louis, 2009, Mosby.

Yamamoto LG, Yamamoto JA, Yamamoto JB, Yamamoto BE, Yamamoto PP: Nail polish does not significantly affect pulse oximeter measurements in mildly hypoxic subjects, *Respir Care* 53(11):1470–1474, 2008.

1. Before drawing a blood gas sample from the radial artery, which test should be performed?
   A. Allen test
   B. Modified Allen test
   C. Blood pressure measurement
   D. Nail bed blanching

2. A patient is brought into the Emergency Department after being rescued from a house fire. She is unconscious and has facial burns. The physician believes that she is suffering from smoke inhalation. What should be recommended as the best way to evaluate her?
   A. ABGs analyzed through a CO oximeter
   B. Standard pulse oximetry
   C. ABGs analyzed through a standard blood gas analyzer
   D. Continuous $PtCO_2$ monitor

3. A respiratory therapist is ordered to draw a blood sample from your patient's radial artery. Before drawing the sample, a circulation test is performed by having the patient make a fist while pressure is applied over his ulnar and radial arteries. The patient's hand is then opened, and pressure is released from the ulnar artery. His hand color returns within 15 seconds. This would indicate that the patient's:
   A. Radial circulation is adequate
   B. Radial circulation is inadequate
   C. Ulnar circulation is adequate
   D. Ulnar circulation is inadequate

4. A respiratory therapist working in the Intensive Care Unit notices that an arterial blood sample has been sitting out for 40 minutes. It was not put in ice water. The blood gas analysis could be affected in which of the following ways?
   1. Increased PaO_2
   2. Increased $PaCO_2$
   3. Decreased PaO_2
   4. Decreased $PaCO_2$
   5. Increased pH
   6. Decreased pH
   A. 1, 2, and 6 only
   B. 3, 4, and 5 only
   C. 2, 3, and 6 only
   D. 3, 4, and 6 only

5. An arterial puncture to obtain a sample for blood gas analysis should be recommended under which of the following conditions?
   1. To measure the patient's PaO_2 level after a change in the patient's inspired O_2 concentration
   2. Suspected CO poisoning
   3. To measure the patient's $PaCO_2$ level after a change in the patient's minute volume

4. After the patient with respiratory distress has been admitted to the Emergency Department with a tension pneumothorax
   A. 1 and 2 only
   B. 1 and 3 only
   C. 2, 3, and 4 only
   D. 1, 2, 3, 4

6. Safety guidelines for the protection of the respiratory therapist who is drawing an ABG sample include which of the following?
   1. Put a glove only on the hand used to draw the sample.
   2. Put a glove only on the hand with which you feel the pulse.
   3. Put gloves on both hands.
   4. Wear goggles.
   A. 2 only
   B. 3 only
   C. 3 and 4 only
   D. 1 and 4 only

7. A 50-year-old patient has a PaO_2 value of 72 torr when breathing room air. How should this be interpreted?
   A. Normal for a person of that age
   B. Mild hypoxemia
   C. Moderate hypoxemia
   D. Severe hypoxemia

8. An acute rise in $PaCO_2$ level from 40 to 50 torr would result in the following change in pH:
   A. Rise of 0.10 unit
   B. Fall of 0.05 unit
   C. Fall of 0.10 unit
   D. Rise of 0.05 unit

9. Interpret the following arterial blood gas drawn from a patient who is breathing 40% O_2: pH, 7.37; $PaCO_2$, 62 torr; PaO_2, 54 torr; bicarbonate, 38 mEq/L; and base excess, +11 mEq/L; SaO_2, 87%.
   1. Corrected hypoxemia
   2. Uncorrected hypoxemia
   3. Metabolic alkalosis
   4. Uncompensated metabolic acidosis
   5. Compensated respiratory acidosis
   A. 1 and 4 only
   B. 1 and 3 only
   C. 2 and 4 only
   D. 2 and 5 only

10. Interpret the following arterial blood gas drawn from a patient who is breathing 35% O_2: pH, 7.29; $PaCO_2$, 37 torr; PaO_2, 86 torr; bicarbonate, 17 mEq/L; and base excess, −8 mEq/L; SaO_2, 90%.
    1. Corrected hypoxemia
    2. Uncorrected hypoxemia
    3. Compensated metabolic acidosis

4. Uncompensated metabolic acidosis
5. Compensated respiratory acidosis
   A. 2 and 4 only
   B. 1 and 4 only
   C. 2 and 5 only
   D. 1 and 3 only

11. Interpret the following arterial blood gas drawn from a patient who is breathing 21% O_2: pH, 7.57; $PaCO_2$, 20 torr; PaO_2, 117 torr; bicarbonate, 24 mEq/L; and base excess, +1 mEq/L; SaO_2, 98%.
    1. Normal oxygenation
    2. Excessively corrected hypoxemia
    3. Uncompensated respiratory alkalosis
    4. Uncompensated metabolic acidosis
    5. Compensated respiratory and metabolic alkalosis
    A. 2 and 3 only
    B. 2 and 4 only
    C. 1 and 3 only
    D. 1 and 4 only

12. Interpret the following arterial blood gas drawn from a patient who is breathing 60% O_2: pH, 7.18; $PaCO_2$, 50 torr; PaO_2, 72 torr; bicarbonate, 18 mEq/L; and base excess, −10 mEq/L; SaO_2, 94%.
    1. Uncorrected hypoxemia
    2. Corrected hypoxemia
    3. Uncorrected respiratory acidosis
    4. Uncorrected metabolic acidosis
    5. Combined metabolic and respiratory acidosis
    A. 1 and 5 only
    B. 2 and 5 only
    C. 2 and 3 only
    D. 2 and 4 only

13. Interpret the following arterial blood gas drawn from a patient who is breathing 24% O_2: pH, 7.45; $PaCO_2$, 22 torr; PaO_2, 57 torr; bicarbonate, 16 mEq/L; and base excess, −6 mEq/L; SaO_2, 91%.
    1. Corrected hypoxemia
    2. Uncorrected hypoxemia
    3. Compensated respiratory alkalosis
    4. Uncompensated respiratory alkalosis
    5. Combined metabolic and respiratory acidosis
    A. 1 and 3 only
    B. 1 and 4 only
    C. 2 and 3 only
    D. 2 and 5 only

14. Which of the following best indicates that a patient's tissues are adequately oxygenated?
    A. PaO_2, 85 torr
    B. $P\bar{v}O_2$, 30 torr
    C. $S\bar{v}O_2$, 75%
    D. SaO_2, 90%

15. Blood gas analyzer calibration values are considered to be *in control* if they are within:
    A. 1 SD of the norm
    B. 2 SDs of the norm
    C. 3 SDs of the norm
    D. 4 SDs of the norm

16. A 50-year-old patient with emphysema seems to be tiring 30 minutes into a weaning attempt on a Briggs adapter (T-piece). The best way to evaluate the patient's ventilatory status is by:
    A. Checking pH value
    B. Measuring a $PtcCO_2$ value
    C. Checking $PaCO_2$ value
    D. Measuring bedside vital capacity

17. A patient has Guillain-Barré syndrome and pneumonia. The patient has just been placed on 35% O_2 by mask. The physician asks for your suggestion on the best way to evaluate the patient's overall ability to breathe. What should be recommended?
    A. Doing a full set of pulmonary function tests
    B. Drawing an arterial blood sample for analysis
    C. Performing pulse oximetry
    D. Performing a force vital capacity measurement

18. A respiratory therapist is called to evaluate a patient who is using a pulse oximeter. Upon entering the room, it is noticed that the patient is an African-American woman with an oximeter probe on her right earlobe. The monitor shows a weak pulse signal and a fluctuating SpO_2 value. Which of the following should be done in an attempt to correct the problem?
    1. Try monitoring from a fingertip.
    2. Switch to a probe over the bridge of the nose.
    3. Cover the probe with an opaque wrap.
    4. Switch the probe to the left earlobe.
    A. 2 only
    B. 3 only
    C. 1 and 3 only
    D. 2 and 4 only

19. A respiratory therapist is working with a postanesthesia patient who is on a $PtcCO_2$ monitor. The correlation factor between the $PaCO_2$ and the $PtcCO_2$ is 1.4. The patient's previous $PtcCO_2$ level was 63 torr. The nurse has called you because it is now 75 torr. The patient's approximate $PaCO_2$ value would be calculated as:
    A. 54 torr
    B. 63 torr
    C. 75 torr
    D. 105 torr

20. A 35-year-old patient with pneumonia is receiving mechanical ventilation with PEEP. Calculate and interpret the patient's P(A–a)O$_2$ level. The following conditions exist:

    P$_B$ = 750 torr; normal is 760 torr for sea level

    P$_{H_2O}$ = 54 torr because your patient's temperature is 104° F/40° C; normal is 47 torr for a normal temperature

    F$_I$O$_2$ = 0.5 for 50% inspired oxygen; normal is 0.21 for room air

    PaCO$_2$ = 36 torr

    PaO$_2$ = 60 torr

    Respiratory exchange ratio = 0.8

    $$PACO_2 = \left[(P_B - P_{H_2O})\, F_IO_2\right] - \frac{PaCO_2}{0.8}$$

    Based on the listed conditions, what is the patient's PAO$_2$ value?
    A. 95 torr
    B. 101 torr
    C. 303 torr
    D. 312 torr

21. Based on the listed conditions, what is the patient's P(A–a)O$_2$ value?
    A. 41 torr
    B. 232 torr
    C. 243 torr
    D. 248 torr

22. How should the patient's P(A–a)O$_2$ results be interpreted?
    A. Check for a blood gas analyzer error.
    B. Normal oxygenation and ventilation.
    C. Normal for a patient of this age.
    D. Larger than normal difference.

23. A 50-year-old male patient is being treated for a pulmonary embolism. He is receiving 50% O$_2$ by mask. The results of a P(A–a)O$_2$ study indicate that his alveolar–arterial difference is 205 torr. What is the best interpretation of this study?
    A. The results are not physiologically possible.
    B. It is within the normal range.
    C. The alveolar–arterial difference is increased.
    D. The patient's condition is improving.

24. A premature neonate breathing room air has a PtcCO$_2$ electrode placed on her right thigh and a PtCO$_2$ electrode placed on her left thigh. Both have been showing stable readings over the past hour. After the patient was moved about for nursing care it is noticed that the PtCO$_2$ electrode value has increased. The PtcCO$_2$ electrode value is unchanged. What could explain this?
    A. The PtCO$_2$ electrode has pulled loose from the skin.
    B. The inspired oxygen percentage has been decreased.
    C. The patient's pulmonary condition has improved.
    D. The patient is hyperventilating.

25. After a modified Allen test is performed on a patient's right wrist, it takes 25 seconds for the patient's hand to regain its color. What should be done now?
    A. Perform an Allen test on the right wrist.
    B. Draw an arterial blood sample on the right wrist.
    C. Draw an arterial blood sample on the left wrist.
    D. Perform a modified Allen test on the patient's left wrist.

26. A 45-year-old patient has been admitted to the Emergency Department after having smoke inhalation from a house fire. The patient is wearing a nonrebreather mask set at 10 L/min of oxygen. The most appropriate way to evaluate the patient's oxygenation status is by:
    A. Pulse oximetry with a standard unit
    B. Transcutaneous oxygen monitor
    C. ABG sample run through a blood gas analyzer
    D. ABG sample run through a CO oximeter

27. Interpret the following arterial blood gas drawn when the patient was breathing 45% oxygen: pH, 7.38; PaCO$_2$, 59 torr; PaO$_2$, 64 torr; HCO$_3^-$, 39 mEq/L; and BE, +12 mEq/L; SaO$_2$, 91%.
    1. Corrected hypoxemia
    2. Uncorrected hypoxemia
    3. Metabolic alkalosis
    4. Compensated respiratory acidosis
    5. Metabolic acidosis
    A. 1 and 4 only
    B. 1 and 3 only
    C. 2 and 5 only
    D. 2 and 4 only

28. Interpret the following mixed venous blood gas drawn when the patient was breathing 40% oxygen: pH, 7.35; Pv̄CO$_2$, 46 torr; Pv̄O$_2$, 40 torr; Sv̄O$_2$, 75%.
    1. Corrected hypoxemia
    2. Uncorrected hypoxemia
    3. Metabolic acidosis
    4. Normal acid–base balance
    5. Respiratory acidosis
    A. 2 and 3 only
    B. 1 and 5 only
    C. 2 and 5 only
    D. 1 and 4 only

29. Interpret the following arterial blood gas drawn when the patient was breathing 30% oxygen: pH, 7.44; $PaCO_2$, 25 mm Hg; PaO_2, 65 mm Hg; HCO_3^-, 17 mEq/L; and BE, −7 mEq/L; SaO_2, 91%.
    1. Corrected hypoxemia
    2. Uncorrected hypoxemia
    3. Compensated respiratory alkalosis
    4. Uncompensated respiratory alkalosis
    5. Combined metabolic and respiratory acidosis
    A. 1 and 3 only
    B. 1 and 4 only
    C. 2 and 3 only
    D. 2 and 5 only

30. Which of the following clinical values indicates that a patient's tissues are hypoxemic?
    A. PaO_2 of 55 torr
    B. $P\bar{v}O_2$ of 25 torr
    C. $S\bar{v}O_2$ of 80%
    D. SaO_2 of 88%

31. A spontaneously breathing neonate is in an incubator. The patient is being monitored with a transcutaneous carbon dioxide electrode on her right upper chest. An hour ago, the patient's carbon dioxide value was 45 torr, and now it is 5 torr. The nurse tells you that no change has occurred in the neonate's condition. What is the most likely explanation for this difference?
    A. The patient has a patent ductus arteriosus.
    B. Air has leaked under the electrode.
    C. The temperature inside the incubator has been increased.
    D. The patient's cardiac output and lung condition have improved.

32. A 17-year-old patient is receiving mechanical ventilation because of apnea resulting from a drug overdose. While the patient is breathing 25% oxygen, the following ABG values are analyzed:

    PaO_2 of 155 torr

    SaO_2 of 100%

    pH of 7.42

    $PaCO_2$ of 41 torr

    BE of +2 mEQ/L

    What action should now be taken?
    A. Reduce the patient to 21% oxygen.
    B. Maintain the present settings.
    C. Recheck the blood gas analyzer.
    D. Hyperventilate the patient.

33. A neonatal patient is receiving 40% oxygen in an oxyhood. The following capillary blood gas results have just been received: pH, 7.37; PCO_2, 45 mm Hg; PO_2, 60 mm Hg; HCO_3^-, 22 mEq/L; and BE, −2 mEq/L; SO_2, 91%. Which of the blood gas values can be reliably used clinically?
    1. pH, 7.37
    2. PCO_2, 45 mm Hg
    3. PO_2, 60 mm Hg
    4. SO_2, 91%
    A. 1 and 2 only
    B. 3 and 4 only
    C. 1, 2, and 3 only
    D. 1, 2, 3, 4

34. The results of a set of arterial blood gases and central venous blood gases have been received from a patient in the Intensive Care Unit. The results show that the $PcvCO_2$ is 58 torr and the $PaCO_2$ is 43 torr. How should these results be interpreted?
    A. Disregard owing to a preanalytic error with the $PcvCO_2$.
    B. Low cardiac output.
    C. The patient is being hyperventilated.
    D. The patient is in ventilatory failure.

35. An adult patient in Denver, Colorado, is receiving 50% oxygen through an air entrainment mask. The patient's arterial blood gas values are pH, 7.41; $PaCO_2$, 38 torr; PaO_2, 85 torr; bicarbonate, 25 mEq/L; and base excess, +1 mEq/L; SaO_2, 96%. The local P_B is 745 torr. The patient's P:F ratio would be calculated as which of the following?
    A. 0.05
    B. 0.11
    C. 0.76
    D. 1.7

36. Because it is not possible to obtain an arterial blood gas sample on a newborn child, the physician orders blood gas analysis of an arterialized capillary blood sample. Which of the following should be selected as the preferred sampling site?
    A. Fingertip
    B. Earlobe
    C. Lateral area of the heel
    D. Toe tip

4 Pulmonary Function Testing

Note: It can be anticipated that the Therapist Multiple-Choice Examination (TMC) will include an *average of 6 of 140 actual questions* (4% of the exam) on pulmonary function testing. (This is based on the question mix typically found on the National Board of Respiratory Care's (NBRC's) previous Entry Level Examinations and Written Registry Examinations.)

Remember that the TMC version you take will include 20 additional questions being evaluated for possible inclusion in other versions of the TMC. So, there will be a total of 160 questions given. There is no way to differentiate between the 140 actual questions and the 20 questions being evaluated for future use. Please go to the Introduction for detailed information on the TMC and the Clinical Simulation Examination.

MODULE A

Review the patient's record for data on the following tests.

1. Pulmonary function results (code: IA6) [difficulty: R, Ap]

Be prepared to review the results of all types of pulmonary function test (PFT) results. This chapter covers the PFTs listed by the NBRC and other PFTs that have been tested by the NBRC.

2. Lung compliance (code: IA13e) [difficulty: R, Ap]

Lung compliance usually is measured in patients with stiff lungs (as found with pulmonary fibrosis) or overly compliant lungs (as found with emphysema).

3. Airway resistance (code: IA13e) [difficulty: R, Ap]

Patients with asthma or chronic bronchitis may need to have airway resistance measured as part of their bronchodilator therapy management. Airway resistance decreases if the proper type and amount of medication are taken.

4. Work of breathing (code: IA13a) [difficulty: R, Ap]

Work of breathing is the patient's subjective feeling about his or her difficulty in breathing. A normal person without cardiopulmonary disease would not feel any difficulty in breathing at rest. However, a person with cardiopulmonary disease, such as chronic obstructive pulmonary disease (COPD) or congestive heart failure, would feel an increased work of breathing, even at rest. The patient would say that he or she feels "short of breath."

MODULE B

Bedside spirometry

1. Perform bedside spirometry tests

a. Recommend lung mechanics (bedside spirometry) tests (code: IE7) [difficulty: R, Ap, An]

The bedside lung mechanics tests typically include the following:

- Lung volumes and capacities except for those requiring the residual volume (RV).
- Spirometry for nonforced or slow vital capacity (SVC).
- Forced vital capacity (FVC) and flow values derived from the FVC. These values are needed to determine the degree of impairment in patients with obstructive diseases.
- Maximum inspiratory pressure (MIP) and maximum expiratory pressure (MEP). These values indicate the patient's overall respiratory muscle strength.

Other common bedside tests are also presented in this section. Bedside spirometry tests are indicated in a patient who is showing signs of breathing difficulty and for whom the physician and respiratory therapist are considering the need for mechanical ventilation. For example, a patient with a progressive neuromuscular disease or worsening cardiopulmonary condition would show a smaller vital capacity (VC) and MIP and MEP as he or she weakens. Conversely, as a mechanically ventilated patient improves, bedside spirometry is used to evaluate the patient's spontaneous breathing for weaning. The more advanced spirometry tests, such as flow-volume loop, timed expiratory volumes, and maximum voluntary ventilation (MVV), are included later in the chapter with the pulmonary function laboratory tests.

2. Tidal volume

a. Perform the procedure (code: IC4) [difficulty: R, Ap]

The tidal volume (V_T) is the volume of gas inhaled or exhaled in each respiratory cycle. Usually the expiratory volume is measured. Realize that individual tidal

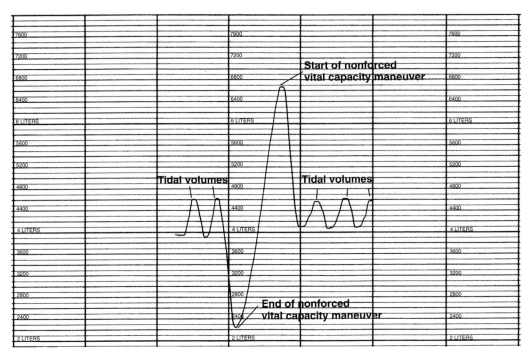

Figure 4-1 Volume–time curve tracing of tidal volumes and nonforced vital capacity.

volumes are rarely identical. Figure 4-1 shows several different tidal volumes before and after a nonforced (slow) VC. It is recommended, therefore, that the tidal volumes and respiratory rate (f) be accumulated for 1 minute (thus providing a minute volume [$\dot{V}_E$]). An average V_T is found by dividing the $\dot{V}_E$ by the f. If this cannot be done, find the average volume of at least six breaths. The average predicted tidal volume for a resting, afebrile, alert adult should be about

3 to 4 mL/lb of ideal body weight or

7 to 9 mL/kg of ideal body weight

For example, the predicted tidal volume range of a 154-lb (70-kg) patient is calculated as follows:

3 to 4 mL/lb × 154 lb = 462 to 616 mL

7 to 9 mL/kg × 70 kg = 490 to 630 mL

The patient should be allowed to relax before the test is performed so that the measured volume is accurate and not exaggerated because of any undue stress or excitement. Keeping the instructions and demonstration simple and easy to follow helps reduce the patient's anxiety. Some patients will not tolerate a full minute's tidal volume measurement. In that case, measure the accumulated tidal volumes for as long as possible and divide by the number of respirations to calculate the average.

b. Evaluate the results (code: ID4) [difficulty: R, Ap, An]

A tidal volume that is larger or smaller than expected for the patient's size requires further evaluation. A small tidal volume may be seen in patients who have a low metabolic rate, are asleep or in a coma, have a neuromuscular disease that makes them unable to breathe deeply, or are alkalotic. A large tidal volume may be seen in patients with a high metabolic rate, a fever, a dead-space-producing disease such as a pulmonary embolism, increased intracranial pressure, or an acidotic condition.

A patient with a progressive neuromuscular disease or worsening cardiopulmonary disease should have the tidal volume, respiratory rate, and other bedside spirometry values monitored closely. If the patient's condition worsens, mechanical ventilation may have to be started. The frequency of monitoring varies with the patient's condition, for example, every shift initially and hourly if the patient is critical. Conversely, as a mechanically ventilated patient improves, bedside spirometry is used to evaluate the patient's spontaneous breathing for weaning.

The patient's inspiratory-to-expiratory (I:E) ratio can also be monitored while the tidal volume is measured. The I:E ratio is the ratio of the patient's inspiratory time (T_I) to the expiratory time (T_E). It can be simply measured at the bedside with a stopwatch. Again, make sure the patient is relaxed and breathing in the normal pattern to get an accurate timing. Measure several of the patient's inspiratory times and expiratory times to figure an average for each. A spirometer that gives a printout is needed if a more complete analysis of the patient's breathing pattern is necessary.

A normal, spontaneously breathing patient has an I:E ratio of 1:2 to 1:4. A prolonged inspiratory time often is seen in patients with an upper airway obstruction. A prolonged expiratory time often is seen in patients with asthma or COPD. Any abnormal I:E ratio should be investigated. For example, patients with Kussmaul's respiration, Cheyne-Stokes respiration, or Biot's respiration will have unusual I:E ratios.

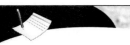

Exam Hint 4-1

The NBRC is known to test the examinee's ability to calculate (1) the T_I and T_E from a given I:E ratio and f and (2) the I:E ratio from a given T_I and T_E. These examples should help.

1. Calculate the patient's T_I and T_E when the I:E ratio is 1:2 and f is 12/min.

   a. $\dfrac{60 \text{ s/min}}{12 \text{ breaths/min}} = 5 \text{ s/respiratory cycle}$

   b. $\dfrac{5 \text{ s/respiratory cycle}}{3 \text{ parts of I and E}} = 1.66 \text{ seconds of 1 part}$

   c. $T_I = 1 \text{ part} = 1.66 \text{ seconds}$
   d. $T_E = 2 \text{ parts} = 3.32 \text{ seconds}$
2. Calculate the neonatal patient's I:E ratio when the T_I is 0.3 second and the T_E is 0.9 second.
   a. I:E = I/E = 0.3/0.9 second
   b. I/E = 1/3 (the I:E ratio is 1:3)

3. Minute volume

a. Perform the procedure (code: IC4) [difficulty: R, Ap]

The minute volume ($\dot{V}_E$) is the volume of gas exhaled in 1 minute. It usually is a more stable value than are individual tidal volumes. The minute volume is found by adding the accumulated tidal volumes for 1 minute. A simple hand-held spirometer often is used to accumulate the tidal volume breaths. If the patient cannot perform the test for 1 minute, do it for 30 seconds and double the value.

b. Evaluate the results (code: ID4) [difficulty: R, Ap, An]

The predicted range for a minute volume in a resting, afebrile, alert adult should be 5-10 L/min. The wide range is found in part because the minute volume is a product of two factors: tidal volume and respiratory rate. It is possible for either one or both of these factors to be normal, abnormally high, or abnormally low. For this reason, the minute volume must be evaluated along with the tidal volume and respiratory rate to reach any conclusion about the patient's condition. The same factors that have an impact on the tidal volume affect the patient's minute ventilation.

4. Alveolar ventilation

a. Perform the procedure (code: IC4) [difficulty: R, Ap]

Alveolar ventilation (V_A) is the amount of tidal volume that reaches the alveoli. It is calculated by subtracting the physiologic dead space (anatomic plus alveolar dead space) from the measured tidal volume. For a bedside test, it is possible to subtract only the estimated anatomic dead space. It is estimated at 1 mL/lb, or 2.2 mL/kg, of ideal body weight. The alveolar dead space measurement requires sophisticated equipment, which usually is available only in the pulmonary function testing laboratory. Clinically normal people have very little alveolar dead space.

EXAMPLE 1

A 154-lb (70-kg) person has a measured tidal volume of 500 mL and an estimated anatomic dead space of about 154 mL.

Calculated alveolar ventilation = 500 − 154 mL = 346 mL

The minute alveolar ventilation ($\dot{V}_A$) is the volume of gas that reaches the alveoli in 1 minute. It is found by multiplying the alveolar volume by the respiratory rate in 1 minute.

EXAMPLE 2

A 154-lb (70-kg) person has a measured tidal volume of 500 mL and an estimated anatomic dead space of about 154 mL. The respiratory rate is 14/min.

Calculated alveolar ventilation = 346 mL (500 − 154 mL).

Calculated minute alveolar ventilation = 14 × 346 mL = 4844 mL

b. Evaluate the results (code: ID4) [difficulty: R, Ap, An]

The following examples show how the patient's alveolar ventilation can vary considerably because of changes in the respiratory rate and tidal volume, even though the minute volume remains unchanged. These examples are included to show the importance of alveolar ventilation on the patient's arterial partial pressure of carbon dioxide ($PaCO_2$) values.

EXAMPLE 1

Normal patient: $f = 12$, tidal volume = 500 mL, anatomic dead space = 154 mL.

$$\text{Minute alveolar ventilation} \left(\dot{V}_A\right) = 12 \times (500 - 154 \text{ mL})$$
$$= 12 \times 346 \text{ mL}$$
$$= 4152 \text{ mL}$$

This patient should have a normal carbon dioxide level.

EXAMPLE 2

Tachypneic patient: $f = 24$, tidal volume = 250 mL, anatomic dead space = 154 mL.

$$\text{Minute volume} = 12 \times 250 \text{ mL} = 3000 \text{ mL}$$

$$\text{Minute alveolar ventilation} \left(\dot{V}_A\right) = 24 \times (250 - 154 \text{ mL}).$$
$$= 24 \times 96 \text{ mL}$$
$$= 2304 \text{ mL}$$

This patient should have a high carbon dioxide level.

EXAMPLE 3

Bradypneic patient: $f = 6$, tidal volume = 1000 mL, anatomic dead space = 154 mL.

$$\text{Minute volume} = 6 \times 1000 \text{ mL} = 6000 \text{ mL}$$

$$\begin{aligned}
\text{Minute alveolar ventilation } \left(\dot{V}_A \right) &= 6 \times (1000 - 154 \text{ mL}) \\
&= 6 \times 846 \text{ mL} \\
&= 5076 \text{ mL}
\end{aligned}$$

This patient should have a low carbon dioxide level.

5. Maximum inspiratory pressure

a. Perform the procedure (code: IC13) [difficulty: R, Ap]

The MIP is the greatest amount of negative pressure the patient can create when inspiring against an occluded airway. It also is known as *negative inspiratory force*. The following factors affect the test results: strength of the diaphragm and accessory muscles of inspiration, lung volume when the airway is occluded, ventilatory drive, and length of time the airway is occluded. MIP is most commonly used to determine the weanability of mechanically ventilated patients. In addition, it is used to help monitor the strength of patients with neuromuscular diseases.

A study of the literature reveals that a number of measurement devices have been assembled and that various bedside techniques have been used to determine the effort of a patient breathing naturally, an intubated patient, and a patient breathing with assistance from a mechanical ventilator. Branson et al. (1989) and Kacmarek et al. (1989) make a strong case for the use of a double one-way valve to connect the intubated patient to the manometer (Fig. 4-2). Use of the one-way valve lets the patient exhale but prevents an inhalation when the practitioner occludes the opening. This forces the patient to inhale from closer to RV with each breathing effort. Steps in the MIP procedure for a normally breathing patient include the following:

1. Obtain a pressure gauge capable of measuring at least −60 cm H_2O pressure.
2. Have the patient sit upright. Place a note in the chart if the patient is lying down.
3. Describe the procedure to the patient.
4. Simulate a demonstration of the procedure.
5. Place nose clips over the patient's nose. Have the patient seal the lips and teeth around the mouthpiece and breathe through the open port.
6. Tell the patient to exhale completely. Seal the port when RV has been reached.
7. Tell the patient to breathe in as hard as possible and hold it for 1 to 3 seconds.
8. Reteach if necessary.
9. Repeat until at least three good efforts have been performed. Record the greatest stable value seen after the first second of effort. This eliminates any artifact created by the cheeks or by chest wall movement.

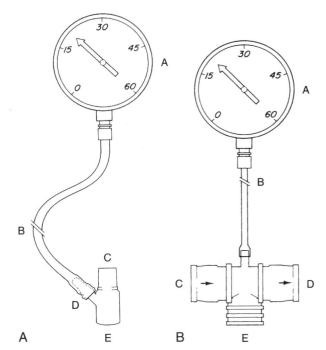

Figure 4-2 Two systems for measuring maximum inspiratory pressure (MIP) in a patient with an artificial airway. System **A,** simple occlusion. *A,* pressure manometer; *B,* connecting tubing; *C,* port to be occluded during MIP; *D,* connection of the adapter to the manometer; *E,* port to connect to the patient's airway. System **B,** one-way valve. *A,* pressure manometer; *B,* connecting tubing; *C,* inspiratory port to be occluded during the MIP effort; *D,* expiratory port; *E,* port to be connected to the patient's artificial airway. (From Kacmarek RM, Cycyk-Chapman MC, Young-Palazzo PJ, et al.: Determination of maximal inspiratory pressure: a clinical study and literature review, Respir Care, 34:868, 1989.)

b. Evaluate the results (code: ID12) [difficulty: R, Ap, An]

Patients of either gender and of any age should be able to generate at least −60 cm H_2O. This is enough to offer assurance that the patient has enough strength and coordination to protect the airway, take a deep breath, and cough effectively. Patients with neuromuscular diseases, diseases of the respiratory muscles, thoracic injury or abnormality, and chronic obstructive lung diseases tend to have decreased strength. The patient who cannot generate at least −20 cm H_2O is at risk. This patient probably does not have the strength to cough effectively. Depending on the blood gas values and other physical parameters, the patient may need to be intubated and maintained on a mechanical ventilator.

Black and Hyatt (1969) published MIP prediction formulas for spontaneous breathing in nonintubated adults 20 to 86 years of age who are breathing from residual volume; these formulas are presented in Table 4-1. The values are in centimeters of water pressure (cm H_2O). As can be seen, the older the patient, the lower the predicted negative inspiratory force.

TABLE 4–1	Age and Gender in Predicting Maximum Inspiratory Pressure	
Gender	**Lower Limit of Normal**	
Males: 143 – (0.55 × age)	–75 cm H_2O	
Females: 104 – (0.51 × age)	–50 cm H_2O	

A patient being weaned from mechanical ventilation or with a deteriorating neuromuscular condition should have the MIP measured on a regular, frequent basis. If the patient's pressure is only –20 cm H_2O, the physician should be notified. Mechanical ventilation is probably needed.

It is important to monitor any patient for signs of undue stress and hypoxemia, such as tachycardia, bradycardia, ventricular dysrhythmias, hypertension, hypotension, and decreasing saturation on pulse oximetry. If any of these are seen, the procedure should be stopped and the patient reoxygenated and ventilated. Some patients achieve their best effort on the first or second inspiration and have decreasing effort as they continue trying. This is probably because of fatigue. Stop the procedure and record the best effort.

Exam Hint 4-2

Expect to see at least one question in which the MIP value is used to help determine whether a patient is getting stronger or weaker. If the patient's MIP is at least –20 cm H_2O (e.g., –35 cm H_2O), and other conditions are acceptable, the patient can be weaned from the mechanical ventilator. Conversely, if the patient's MIP is not at least –20 cm H_2O (e.g., –15 cm H_2O), and other conditions are unacceptable, the patient should not be weaned from the mechanical ventilator.

6. Maximum expiratory pressure

a. Perform the procedure (code: IC13) [difficulty: R, Ap]

The MEP is the greatest amount of positive pressure the patient can create when expiring from total lung capacity (TLC) against an occluded airway. It also is known as a *maximum expiratory force*. The following factors affect the test results: patient cooperation and effort, strength of the expiratory muscles, lung volume when the airway is occluded, ventilatory drive, and length of time the airway is occluded. The MEP is used to determine the weanability of mechanically ventilated patients and to monitor the strength of patients with neuromuscular diseases.

As with the MIP test, a study of the literature reveals that a number of measurement devices have been assembled and that various bedside techniques have been used to determine the effort of a patient breathing naturally and the effort of one who is intubated and breathing

by way of a mechanical ventilator. A strong case can be made for the use of a double one-way valve to connect the intubated patient to the manometer (see Fig. 4-2). Use of the one-way valves lets the patient inhale but prevents an exhalation when the practitioner occludes the expiratory opening. This forces the patient to exhale from closer to TLC with each breathing effort. However, the expiratory efforts should not be held for longer than 3 seconds. This test is similar to the Valsalva maneuver and can cause a reduction in cardiac output because of the high intrathoracic pressure.

Steps in the MEP procedure for a normally breathing patient include the following:

1. Obtain a pressure gauge capable of measuring at least +60 cm H_2O pressure.
2. Have the patient sit upright. Place a note in the chart if the patient is lying down.
3. Describe the procedure to the patient.
4. Simulate a demonstration of the procedure.
5. Place nose clips over the patient's nose. Have the patient seal the lips and teeth around the mouthpiece and breathe through the open port.
6. Tell the patient to inhale completely. Seal the port when TLC has been reached.
7. Tell the patient to breathe out as hard as possible. Hold it for 1 to 3 seconds.
8. Reteach if necessary.
9. Repeat until at least three good efforts have been performed. Record the greatest stable value seen after the first second of effort. This eliminates any artifact created by the cheeks or chest wall movement.

It is important to monitor any patient for signs of undue stress and hypoxemia, such as tachycardia, bradycardia, ventricular dysrhythmias, hypotension, and decreasing saturation on pulse oximetry. If any of these is seen, the procedure should be stopped and the patient reoxygenated and ventilated.

b. Evaluate the results (code: ID12) [difficulty: R, Ap, An]

Clinically normal people of either gender and of any age should be able to generate at least 80 cm H_2O. Patients with neuromuscular diseases, thoracic injury or abnormality, and COPD tend to have decreased strength. An MEP of +40 cm H_2O is probably enough to offer assurance that the patient has enough strength and coordination to cough effectively to clear secretions. However, depending on the blood gas values and other physical parameters, the patient may need to be intubated and maintained on a mechanical ventilator.

Black and Hyatt published MEP prediction formulas for spontaneously breathing, nonintubated adults 20 to 86 years of age who are breathing from TLC; these formulas are presented in Table 4-2. The values are in centimeters of water pressure. As can be seen, the older the patient, the lower the predicted maximum expiratory force.

7. Vital capacity

a. Perform the test (code: IC4) [difficulty: R, Ap]

The nonforced (slow) vital capacity (VC or SVC) is the greatest volume of gas the patient can exhale after the lungs have been completely filled. The therapist should demonstrate the procedure to the patient. He or she must understand that there is no need to blow out fast while emptying the lungs. The measurement device can be a simple hand-held spirometer if a printout of the result is not needed. A portable, computer-based spirometer can be used, if needed, to generate a printout of the results or a graphic tracing. Normally at least three efforts are made, and the largest is recorded.

b. Evaluate the results (code: ID4) [difficulty: R, Ap, An]

See Figure 4-1 for a graphic tracing of a nonforced VC. Compare it with the tracing on Figure 4-3, which shows an FVC. In a patient with normal lung function, the same volume should be found in a nonforced VC and an FVC. A patient with asthma or COPD will usually have a smaller FVC than nonforced VC because of small airway collapse during the maximum effort. The following discussion on the FVC includes predicted values for male and female patients and guidelines on VC and FVC interpretation.

TABLE 4–2	Age and Gender in Predicting Maximum Expiratory Pressure	
Gender	**Lower Limit of Normal**	
Males: 268 – (1.03 × age)	+140 cm H$_2$O	
Females: 170 – (0.53 × age)	+95 cm H$_2$O	

The VC and other simple spirometry values are commonly measured at the bedside in patients with neuromuscular disease and those who are being weaned from mechanical ventilation. A VC that is increasing toward the normal, predicted patient value is a good sign, because it indicates that the patient is recovering. If the VC is decreasing, the patient is probably becoming weaker and will not be able to cough out secretions effectively. Mechanical ventilation may be needed. See Module C for more discussion on the vital capacity. See Chapter 15 for more discussion on how the VC is used to evaluate a patient's need for mechanical ventilation.

8. Peak flow

a. Perform the test (code: IC3) [difficulty: R, Ap]

The *peak flow* (PF), or *peak expiratory flow rate*, is the highest flow rate seen in a patient's forced expiratory effort. The PF usually is found at the start of an FVC effort. It can be measured at the bedside on some portable pulmonary function testing units, but it is most commonly done on a portable, disposable peak flowmeter. Select a unit that is appropriate for the patient. An adult peak flowmeter should be able to measure a flow of up to 850 L/min (about 14 L/s), and a pediatric unit should be able

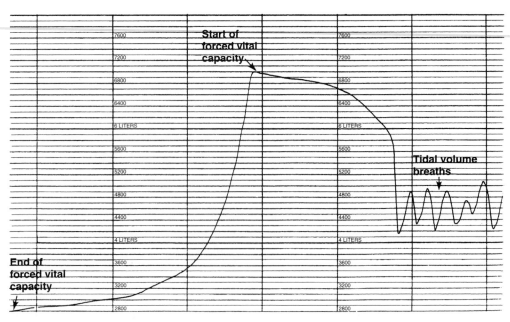

Figure 4-3 Tracing of tidal volumes and forced vital capacity.

to measure a flow of up to 400 L/min (about 7 L/s). The patient is instructed to take in as deep a breath as possible and blow it out as hard as possible. The therapist should demonstrate the procedure. It is not necessary for the patient to push out all air for several seconds until completely empty. The patient should tightly seal the lips around the mouthpiece to prevent leaks. Nose clips are recommended but not required. A good patient effort must be repeated three times. Record the highest recorded value in liters per minute (or liters per second, depending on the unit).

b. Evaluate the results (code: ID3) [difficulty: R, Ap, An]

The peak flow and forced expiratory volume in 1 second (FEV_1) are the bedside measurements most commonly used to evaluate the response of a patient with asthma or COPD to inhaled bronchodilator medications. If the medication dose is effective, the patient's peak flow will increase significantly from the premedication value. Many peak flowmeters come with adjustable markers for the National Asthma Education Program's "color zone" scheme:

- *Green zone:* Peak flow is 80% to 100% of predicted or personal best.
- *Yellow zone:* Peak flow is 50% to 79% of predicted or personal best.
- *Red zone:* Peak flow is less than 50% of predicted or personal best.

Current asthma guidelines state that if an asthma patient's peak flow is in the green zone, the medications are adequately controlling the asthma. If the peak flow is in the yellow zone, the patient's medications are not adequately controlling the asthma. Increased doses are indicated if ordered by the physician. If the peak flow is in the red zone, the patient's medications are not adequately controlling the asthma. The patient needs more bronchodilator medication. The home care patient should get medical help as soon as possible. Each patient should have his or her individually calculated color zones marked on the peak flowmeter to guide medication usage. The patient should be instructed on the meaning of the zones and the proper use of medications. See Module C for more discussion of the peak flow.

MODULE C

Pulmonary function testing laboratory studies

1. Recommend exhaled nitric oxide as a diagnostic procedure (code: IE11) [difficulty: R, Ap, An]

Exhaled nitric oxide (eNO) is measured in patients with known or suspected eosinophilic (airway) inflammation. The test has been shown to be most useful for evaluating patients with asthma but may also be of use in patients with COPD. The patient should be told not to eat, drink, or smoke for at least 1 hour before the test. If other pulmonary function tests are scheduled, the exhaled nitric oxide test should be performed first. This is because the other tests, such as spirometry, exercise testing, and methacholine challenge testing, can change the eNO results.

The patient's exhaled breath is analyzed through a chemiluminescence analyzer for the level of nitric oxide in parts per billion (ppb). The patient is instructed to exhale completely (to residual volume), insert the mouthpiece, and inhale as much as possible (to TLC) through the eNO device. The inhaled gas is scrubbed of any NO that may be found in room air. The patient then slowly exhales through the eNO device at a controlled rate of 0.05 L/s. This results in an exhaled NO plateau of several seconds that is analyzed for the patient's value. The patient must perform at least two acceptable eNO efforts that are within 10% of each other. The two acceptable values are averaged for the final reported value.

The following normal ranges have been established for exhalation of a breath at the controlled rate of 0.05 L/s:

- Adult: 15 to 25 ppb, with an upper limit of normal of 35 ppb.
- Child: 5 to 22 ppb, with an upper limit of normal of 25 ppb.

Actual patient values greater than these indicate increased eosinophilic activity. In other words, a patient with asthma is having more airway inflammation and is not under control. The physician would probably consider increasing the dose of corticosteroids or other controlling medications. In addition, the following conditions have been shown to increase exhaled nitric oxide during an exacerbation: chronic bronchitis (COPD), pneumonia, alveolitis, bronchiolitis obliterans, bronchiectasis, sarcoidosis, or a condition with a chronic cough. Conversely, reduced eNO is found in smokers and patients with cystic fibrosis.

2. Recommend exhaled carbon monoxide as a diagnostic procedure (code: IE11) [difficulty: R, Ap, An]

Exhaled carbon monoxide (variously abbreviated as eCO, ECO, COexh, COExh, and breath CO, or BCO) is currently measured to determine if a patient has been smoking. This is especially important before a patient undergoes a single-breath carbon monoxide diffusing capacity test. Because this test uses a small amount of inhaled carbon monoxide to determine the patient's lung diffusion, any additional CO from smoking will cause incorrect test results. So, the eCO should be measured before the test is performed. Do not perform the test if recent smoking has been confirmed.

When a patient is enrolled in a smoking cessation program, the eCO level can be measured to find out if he or she has smoked recently. Knowing that the eCO level will be checked can act as an additional motivator to avoid smoking.

In addition, there is current research attempting to quantify a measureable link between increased exhaled carbon monoxide and airway inflammation. An increased eCO could be used as an early indicator of an exacerbation of asthma, COPD, or cystic fibrosis.

There are currently several types of exhaled CO monitors. The Smokerlyzer ED50 and Micro+ versions (Bedfont Scientific Ltd, Kent, UK) are easy to use hand-held devices. The patient is instructed to hold his or her breath for 20 seconds and then slowly exhale through the disposable mouthpiece into the unit. (The breath hold allows the carboxyhemoglobin (COHb) level to equilibrate with the alveolar CO level.) In general, an eCO of ≥ 7 parts per million confirms that the patient has been smoking.

3. Screening spirometry

a. Perform screening spirometry (code: IC5) [difficulty: R, Ap]

Screening spirometers are portable, simple hand-held devices that can be used in a physician's office or at the bedside (see Fig. 4-4). They can be used to measure VC, FVC, and the FEV_1 through FEV_6. General indications for screening spirometry include:

1. Rule out airway obstruction in a patient with respiratory symptoms.
2. Assess the presence/absence of airflow obstruction in a patient at risk for COPD (e.g., smokers).
3. Assess the severity of airflow obstruction in a patient with dyspnea or other respiratory symptoms.

The key screening spirometry maneuver is an FVC. The patient is instructed to take in as deep a breath as possible and blow it out as hard as possible. The therapist should demonstrate the procedure. It is necessary for the patient to push out all air for at least 6 seconds or until the lungs are completely empty. The patient should be wearing nose clips and tightly seal the lips around the mouthpiece to prevent leaks. A good patient effort must be repeated three times. The highest recorded values are recorded in liters. If the patient cannot perform an FVC, a nonforced VC may be performed. Note this in the chart.

b. Evaluate the results (code: ID5) [difficulty: R, Ap, An]

The Global Initiative for Chronic Obstructive Lung Disease standards recommend that the FEV_1/FVC test be used for assessing airflow obstruction and COPD. The critical finding is an FEV_1/FVC of <70%. In other words, if a patient's forced expiratory volume in 1 second is less than 70% of the FVC (or VC), the patient has an airflow obstruction problem. The lower the exhaled percentage, the worse the airflow obstruction. Because this is only a screening test, the physician should order more comprehensive pulmonary function testing to accurately measure the level of disability and diagnose the patient's disease.

4. Recommend pulmonary function testing (code: IE7) [difficulty: R, Ap, An]

Because the pulmonary function testing laboratory has more advanced equipment and specially trained personnel,

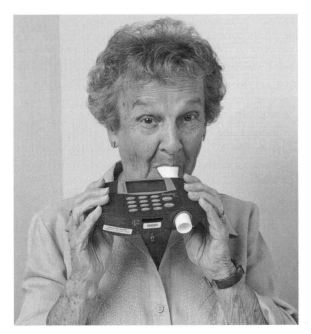

Figure 4-4 Patient using a screening spirometer. These types of simple portable devices are widely used in a physician's office to initially screen for COPD or asthma. (Courtesy of ndd Medical Technologies, Inc., Andover, MA.)

the more challenging cases requiring a pulmonary diagnosis are sent there for testing. The following tests either are specifically listed as testable by the NBRC or have been tested in recent examinations.

5. Forced vital capacity

a. Perform the test (code: IC23) [difficulty: R, Ap]

The FVC is the greatest volume of gas that the patient can exhale as rapidly as possible after the lungs have been completely filled. Normally, the FVC is the same volume as that found in a slow or nonforced VC. Careful instructions, demonstrations, and coaching are needed to ensure that the patient's efforts are the best possible. At least three proper efforts must be obtained.

If the measurement instrument does not give a printout, simply record the patient's efforts in the chart. If the measurement instrument does give a printout, include copies of the efforts. See Figure 4-3 for the tracing of a properly performed FVC. The tracing allows comparison of the volumes exhaled in a series of 1-s intervals. Because of this, the tracing often is referred to as a *volume–time curve.* Note that the start of the effort is smooth and without interruption. The initial fast flow of gas from the upper airway is seen as the nearly vertical part of the tracing. The rest of the tracing is smooth without any coughing or other interruptions in the patient's effort. The tracing becomes progressively more horizontal as the end of the effort is reached. Encourage the patient to try to push out as much air as possible as the end approaches. To provide an acceptable FVC, the patient must show

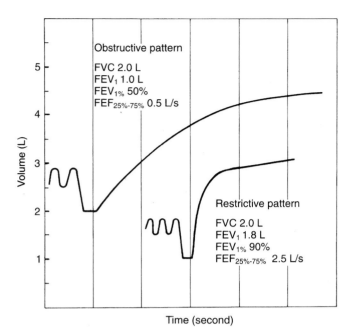

Figure 4-5 Forced vital capacity (FVC) tracings showing an obstructed flow pattern and a restrictive flow pattern. Note that the patient with the obstructed pattern has a slower than normal exhalation, whereas the patient with the restrictive pattern has a faster than normal exhalation. (From Ruppel G: Manual of pulmonary function testing, ed 6, St Louis, 1994, Mosby.)

maximum effort without coughing or closing the glottis, and the expiratory effort must last at least 6 seconds. The patient's final 2 seconds of expiratory effort should show no appreciable airflow. Each of the three recorded, accepted FVCs must show these traits and a close similarity of the patient's efforts.

b. Evaluate the results (code: ID22) [difficulty: R, Ap, An]

Figure 4-3 was made on a chain-compensated, water-seal spirometry system. Note how the tracing progresses from the right to the left. The Stead-Wells system shows the same tracing "upside down" compared with the chain-compensated system. The tracing starts on the left and moves to the right (Fig. 4-5). Other tracings may show either the chain-compensated or the Stead-Wells tracings in a mirror image or opposite shape.

Exam Hint 4-4

The NBRC can show an FVC tracing from any system and expect it to be interpreted. The start of the FVC effort can be determined by the near-vertical portion of the tracing and the relatively small expiratory reserve volume (ERV) compared with the inspiratory reserve volume (IRV). You must be able to determine the various volumes and capacities from a spirometry tracing.

Normal racial/ethnic differences in the FVC must be taken into consideration. Most modern pulmonary function systems automatically adjust the predicted values for racial differences when so programmed by the operator. If not, the predicted values should be mathematically adjusted by the therapist. The predicted normal values, in liters, for the FVC in Caucasian patients were reported by Morris et al. (1971) as:*

Men : $[(0.148 \times \text{Height in inches}) - (0.025 \times \text{Age})]$
$$- 4.24 \ [\text{SD (1 standard deviation) } 0.58]$$

Women : $[(0.115 \times \text{Height in inches}) - (0.024 \times \text{Age})] - 2.85 \ (\text{SD } 0.52)$

EXAMPLE

Calculate the predicted FVC for a 50-year-old Caucasian man who is 6 feet (72 in.) tall.

$$
\begin{aligned}
\text{FVC} &= [(0.148 \times \text{Height in inches}) - (0.025 \times \text{Age})] - 4.24 \\
&= [(0.148 \times 72) - (0.025 \times 50)] - 4.24 \\
&= (10.656 - 1.25) - 4.24 \\
&= 9.406 - 4.24 \\
&= 5.166 \, \text{L}
\end{aligned}
$$

African-Americans are known to have a smaller lung capacity than Caucasians of the same height. For this reason, a 10%-15% adjustment should be made for the predicted FVC and TLC of an African-American patient. In other words, the predicted values for this patient are 85% to 90% of those of a comparable Caucasian patient.

Adjustments for Hispanic and Asian populations are not so well documented. It has been reported that the predicted FVC values should be adjusted downward by 20%-25% for Asians.

It has been commonly accepted that a measured FVC that is at least 80% of the adjusted FVC is considered to be within normal limits for adults of all races/ethnic backgrounds. In addition, the FEV_1 and TLC measurements have been included in this 80% of predicted rule. More recent studies by Knudson et al. (1987) and Paoletti et al. (1985) suggest that normal values for most tests should be determined by finding the percentage of predicted value above which 95% of the population would be seen (the so-called normal 95th percentile). Even though this method finds 5% (1 in 20) of healthy nonsmokers to be abnormal, it offers more realistic predicted values. It is normal to see a decline in the FVC with age.

Restrictive problems, such as advanced pregnancy, obesity, ascites, neuromuscular disease, sarcoidosis, pulmonary fibrosis, and chest wall or spinal deformity, can result in a small FVC. Typically, all of these patients' lung volumes and capacities are small. Patients with chronic obstructive lung diseases, such as emphysema, bronchitis, asthma, cystic fibrosis, and bronchiectasis, commonly

---

*The atmospheric temperature, pressure, saturated (ATPS) to body temperature, pressure, saturated (BTPS) correction has been calculated into these equations.

have a large FVC. Typically, all of these patients' lung volumes and capacities are large. (Fig. 4-6 shows a comparison of the lung volumes and capacities of a normal, an obstructive, and a restrictive patient. See Fig. 4-7 for all of the normal lung volumes and capacities.)

The limitations of this text prevent a discussion of back-extrapolation to find the start of a less than perfect effort or the calculations for correcting volumes and flows from atmospheric temperature, pressure, saturated (ATPS) to body temperature, pressure, saturated (BTPS). However, most textbooks on pulmonary function testing discuss these topics. Because the BTPS correction reflects the patient's true effort, it is standard practice to report all flows and volumes in BTPS.

Exam Hint 4-5

You may need to calculate how close a patient's FVC or other breathing effort has come to his or her predicted value. This is known as the *patient's percentage of predicted*. It is found by this equation:

$$\frac{\text{Patient's actual test result}}{\text{Patient's predicted test value}} \times 100 = \text{Patient's \% of predicted}$$

For example, in the previous discussion on FVC, it was determined that a patient had a predicted FVC of 5.166 L. Calculate the percentage of predicted if the actual FVC result is 4.65 L:

$$\frac{4.65\,\text{L}}{5.116} \times 100 = \text{Patient's \% of predicted} = .90 \times 100 = 90\,\%$$

Therefore, the patient exhaled 90% of predicted FVC and is within the normal range for that test result.

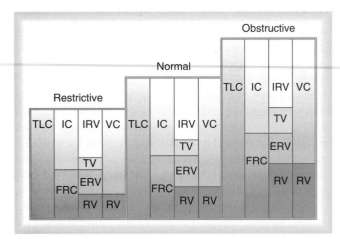

Figure 4-6 Lung volumes and capacities of normal, obstructed, and restricted patients. Note how the obstructed and restricted patients' volumes and capacities are out of proportion compared with those of the normal patient. See Figure 4-7 for more information. TLC, total lung capacity; IC, inspiratory capacity; IRV, inspiratory reserve volume; TV (or V$_T$), tidal volume; ERV, expiratory reserve volume; RV, residual volume; VC, vital capacity; FRC, functional residual capacity. (From Douce FH: Pulmonary function testing. In Kacmarek RM, Stoller JK, Heuer AJ, editors: Egan's fundamentals of respiratory care, ed 10, St Louis, 2013, Mosby.)

6. Peak flow

a. Perform the procedure (code: IC23) [difficulty: R, Ap, An]

The PF is the highest flow rate found in a patient's forced expiratory effort. Some authors refer to the PF as the *peak expiratory flow rate* (PEFR). The PF normally occurs at the beginning of the FVC effort. The instructions for the test must emphasize that the patient "blast" the air out as hard and fast as possible. It is not necessary to encourage the patient to empty his or her lungs completely to residual volume.

For bedside spirometry or home care, the patient's effort is easily measured directly with a hand-held peak flowmeter. Usually at least three efforts are required to find two that are acceptably close. PF values that are consistently low despite variable patient efforts probably indicate a malfunctioning flowmeter that should not be used. It is reasonable to record the patient's effort in liters per second, because the effort takes place in about that much time. However, do not be confused by some measurement instruments and other prediction equations giving the value in liters per minute. Simply multiply or divide by 60 to convert your patient's effort from one time frame to the other. For example, a young man's PF might be recorded as 10 L/s or 600 L/min. Cherniack and Raber (1972) published the following formulas for predicting PF in liters per second.[†]

$$\text{Men}: [(0.144 \times \text{Height in inches}) - (0.024 \times \text{Age})] + 2.225$$

$$\text{Women}: [(0.090 \times \text{Height in inches}) - (0.018 \times \text{Age})] + 1.130$$

b. Evaluate the results (code: ID22) [difficulty: R, Ap, An]

The PF is directly related to height and indirectly related to age. Therefore, the taller the patient, the greater the PF. The PF decreases with age. The PF is a rather nonspecific measurement of airway obstruction. It measures flow through the upper airways and can be reduced in patients with an upper airway problem, such as a tumor, vocal cord paralysis, or laryngeal edema.

The PF test is most often given to patients having an asthma attack as a quick and easy measurement of small airway obstruction. Current asthma guidelines state that if the peak flow of a patient with asthma is 80%-100% of predicted or personal best, he or she is in the green zone. This means that the patient's medications are adequately controlling his or her asthma. If the peak flow is 50%-79% of predicted or personal best, he or she is in the yellow zone. This means that the patient's medications are not adequately controlling the asthma. Increased doses are indicated if ordered by the physician. If the peak flow is less than 50% of predicted or personal best, the patient is in the red zone. This means that the patient's medications

---

[†]The ATPS to BTPS correction has been calculated into these equations.

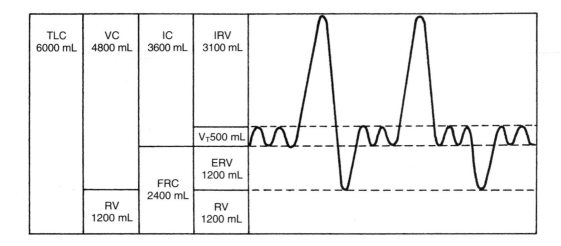

TLC 6000 mL	VC 4800 mL	IC 3600 mL	IRV 3100 mL	
			V$_T$500 mL	
		FRC 2400 mL	ERV 1200 mL	
	RV 1200 mL		RV 1200 mL	

Volumes: Four primary

A. Tidal volume (V$_T$). The volume of gas inspired *or* expired during normal respiration.
B. Inspiratory reserve volume (IRV): The maximum volume of gas that can be inspired beyond a normal inspiration.
C. Expiratory reserve volume (ERV): The maximum volume of gas that can be exhaled after a normal expiration.
D. Residual volume (RV): The volume of gas remaining in the lungs after a maximum expiration.

Capacities: Four, which include two or more primary volumes

A. Total lung capacity (TLC): The total amount of gas contained in the lungs after maximum inspiration. Includes all four primary volumes (TLC = V$_T$ + IRV + ERV + RV).
B. Vital capacity (VC): The maximum amount of gas that can be exhaled after a maximum inspiration. Includes three primary volumes (VC = V$_T$ + IRV + ERV).
C. Inspiratory capacity (IC): The maximum amount of gas that can be inspired after a normal expiration. Includes two primary volumes (IC = V$_T$ + IRV).
D. Functional residual capacity (FRC): The total amount of gas remaining in the lungs after normal expiration. Includes two primary volumes (FRC = ERV + RV).

Figure 4-7 Lung volumes and capacities for a clinically normal young man.

are not adequately controlling the asthma. The patient should seek medical help as soon as possible.

It is the respiratory therapist's responsibility to calculate the patient's color zones and mark them on the patient's personal peak flowmeter. The therapist should instruct the patient about the meanings of the color zones and the appropriate use of the prescribed medications.

Timed forced expiratory volume tests. All of the timed forced expiratory volume test results are derived from a properly performed FVC test (see Fig. 4-3). When the FVC is done correctly, the following values can be calculated and results evaluated to determine the patient's clinical condition. As discussed earlier, an FVC within 80% of predicted is interpreted as being within normal limits.

7. Forced expiratory flow 25%-75% (FEF$_{25\%-75\%}$)

a. Perform the procedure (code: IC23) [difficulty: R, Ap]

The FEF$_{25\%-75\%}$ is the mean forced expiratory flow during the middle half of an acceptable FVC (Fig. 4-8). The FVC measurement that should be used for this test is the one with the greatest combination of FVC volume and FEV$_1$. As mentioned earlier, the patient must give his or her best

effort. The measurement usually is recorded in liters per second but may be recorded in liters per minute.

b. Interpret the results (code: ID22) [difficulty: R, Ap, An]

The results are normally less than in the PF test, because the flow being measured comes from medium-sized and small airways (smaller than 2 mm in diameter). The measured results for either sex should normally gradually decline with age. A woman will have lower results than a man who is matched for age and height. A patient with a restrictive lung disease may have a normal or increased value, whereas a low value is measured in a patient with obstructive lung disease. A small FEF$_{25\%-75\%}$ value when the FVC and FEV$_1$ values are normal often is taken to indicate early small-airway disease. A normal, 68-kg (150-lb) young man should have values of 4-5 L/s or 240-300 L/min. The following formulas were developed by Morris et al. (1971) and can be used to calculate the predicted values in liters per second:

Men : [(0.047 × Height in inches) − (0.045 × Age in years)] + 2.513 (SD 1.12)

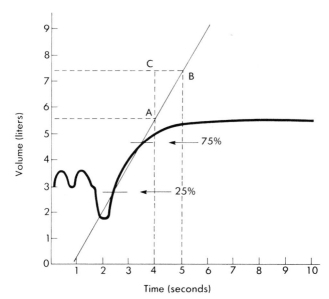

Figure 4-8 One method of determining the 25%-75% forced expiratory flow (FEF$_{25\%-75\%}$) value from an FVC tracing. First, mark the 25% and 75% points from the start of the effort. These are found by multiplying the FVC value by 0.25 and 0.75, respectively, and measuring from the start of the effort. Second, draw a line through these two points to intersect the dashed time lines at points A and B. Horizontal dashed lines are added from A and B to cross the volume scale. The FEF$_{25\%-75\%}$ value is read as the distance between A and C, or about 2 L/s. BTPS corrects this measurement. (From Mottram CD: Ruppel's Manual of pulmonary function testing, ed 10, St Louis, 2013, Mosby.)

Women: $[(0.060 \times \text{Height in inches}) - (0.030 \times \text{Age in years})]$
$+ 0.551 \ (\text{SD } 0.80)$

8. Forced expiratory volume timed (FEV$_T$)

a. Perform the procedure (code: IC23) [difficulty: R, Ap]

The FEV$_T$ is the volume of air exhaled from an acceptable FVC in the specified time. The time increments are 0.5, 1, 2, and 3 seconds or more and are listed as FEV$_{0.5}$, FEV$_1$, FEV$_2$, FEV$_3$, and so on. It is important that the FVC have a good start and a maximum effort to the end of the test.

The FEV$_1$ is the measurement most commonly used, along with the FVC, to judge the patient's response to inhaled bronchodilators, for bronchoprovocation testing to screen for asthmatic tendencies, to detect exercise-induced asthma, and for simple screening. All measured values should be corrected for BTPS.

The timed forced expiratory volumes (FEV$_{0.5}$, FEV$_1$, FEV$_2$, FEV$_3$) effectively "cut" the FVC into sections based on how much volume the patient forcibly exhales in 0.5, 1, 2, and 3 seconds. Some patients with severe obstructive lung disease require several more seconds to exhale completely. In these cases, simply keep measuring the volume exhaled in each additional second. Figure 4-9 shows an FVC tracing that is subdivided at 0.5-, 1-, 2-, and 3-s intervals. Some bedside units give a numeric value for some or all of the timed intervals; however, it is best to have a spirometer that produces a printed copy

of the patient's FVC effort. The individual volumes can be determined by marking the vertical distance on the volume scale from the baseline (TLC) to the respective arrow tips.

b. Evaluate the results (code: ID22) [difficulty: R, Ap, An]

The FEV$_T$ values often are reduced in both restrictive and obstructive lung diseases. Patients with a severe restrictive lung disease exhale almost all of their small FVC within the first second. Patients with severe obstructive lung disease show low values at all time intervals, with the volumes at FEV$_2$, FEV$_3$, and so on, becoming disproportionately smaller. The most commonly evaluated values are the FEV$_1$ and the FEV$_{1\%}$ (discussed below). The following formulas[‡] were developed by Morris et al. (1971) and can be used to calculate the predicted values for FEV$_1$ in liters:

Men: $[(0.092 \times \text{Height in inches}) - (0.032 \times \text{age in years})]$
$-1.260 \ (\text{SD } 0.55)$

Women: $[(0.089 \times \text{Height in inches}) - (0.024 \times \text{age in years})]$
$-1.93 \ (\text{SD } 0.47)$

The American Thoracic Society/European Respiratory Society (ATS/ERS) Task Force on Standardization of

---

[‡]The ATPS to BTPS correction has been calculated into these equations.

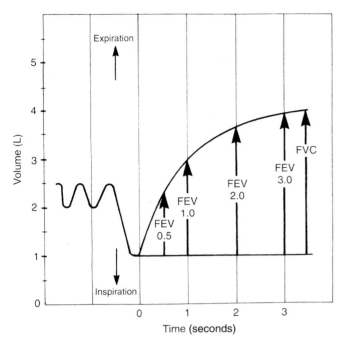

Figure 4-9 Forced vital capacity divided into $FEV_{0.5}$, $FEV_{1.0}$, $FEV_{2.0}$, and $FEV_{3.0}$. (From Ruppel G: Manual of pulmonary function testing, ed 4, St Louis, 1986, Mosby.)

Lung Function Testing has suggested the following FEV_1 severity classifications:

Mild	FEV_1 >70% predicted
Moderate	FEV_1 = 60%-69% predicted
Moderately severe	FEV_1 = 50%-59% predicted
Severe	FEV_1 = 35%-49% predicted
Very severe	FEV_1 <35%

9. Forced expiratory volume/FVC ratio [FEV_T: FVC or $FEV_{T\%}$]

a. Perform the procedure (code: IC23) [difficulty: R, Ap]

The FEV_T to FVC ratio compares, by division, the volume exhaled at 0.5, 1, 2, and 3 (or more) seconds (see Fig. 4-9) with the FVC. This results in a series of decimal fractions. These are multiplied by 100 to convert to percentages.

Because each person's FVC is unique, the FEV time interval volumes taken from the FVC also are unique. The division process described previously standardizes the FEV time interval results, regardless of the patient's FVC. Therefore, these percentage values can be standardized for all individuals despite different FVCs. The predicted values for normal patients are as follows:

$FEV_{0.5\%}$	50%-60% of the FVC
$FEV_{1\%}$	75%-85% of the FVC
$FEV_{2\%}$	90%-95% of the FVC
$FEV_{3\%}$	95%-98% of the FVC
$FEV_{6\%}$	98%-100% of the FVC

b. Interpret the results (code: ID22) [difficulty: R, Ap, An]

These values normally decrease slightly in elderly patients. Most patients with normal lungs and airways are still able to completely exhale the FVC within 4 seconds.

Patients with restrictive lung diseases often exhale the FVC more quickly than expected. This happens because these patients have a smaller than normal FVC and stiff lungs, which recoil more quickly than expected to their resting volume. See Figure 4-5 to compare the FVC curves of a patient with restrictive lung disease with the FVC curves of a patient with obstructive lung disease. A patient with restrictive lung disease exhales the FVC too quickly, and all of the derived values are higher than expected.

Patients with obstructive lung disease take longer than expected to exhale the FVC. As a result, the percentages of the FVC exhaled in the timed intervals listed are lower than normal. Of all the measured values, the $FEV_{1\%}$ is the most important. It is used as the key marker in screening spirometry. Obviously, the lower the percentage exhaled for any timed interval, the worse the obstruction to exhalation.

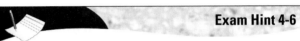

Exam Hint 4-6

Of all the timed forced expiratory volume tests, the FEV_1 is the most important to monitor. An FEV_1 of less than 70% of the FVC confirms obstructive lung disease.

10. Spirometry before and after inhalation of an aerosolized bronchodilator

a. Perform the procedure (code: IC23) [difficulty: R, Ap]

The following are common indications for the procedure:
- The patient is known to have asthma or another type of chronic obstructive lung disease.
- The patient has an $FEV_{1\%}$ of less than 70% (unless elderly).
- The effectiveness of a new bronchodilator is being evaluated.

The most commonly administered tests are the PF and $FEV_{1\%}$ from an FVC. Before starting the test, make sure that the patient has not taken a bronchodilating drug in the previous 4 to 6 hours. If no bronchodilating drugs have been administered, the test can be performed. A PF or $FEV_{1\%}$ test is performed and the value or values are measured. Then a fast-onset, beta-adrenergic type medication is given. The medication can be given by hand-held nebulizer or metered-dose inhaler. Wait about 10 to 15 minutes for the medication to take effect and the patient's blood gas values to return to normal. Then repeat the PF or

$FEV_{1\%}$ test. The percentage of improvement is calculated using this formula:

$$\text{Percentage of change} = \frac{\text{After drug airflow} - \text{Before drug airflow}}{\text{Before drug airflow}} \times 100$$

b. Evaluate the results (code: ID22) [difficulty: R, Ap, An]

To prove that the medication is effective, according to the current standard, the patient must have at least a 12% improvement in PF, $FEV_{1\%}$, or both and a 200-mL increase in exhaled volume. (The old standard required a 15%-20% improvement in flow.) It is not uncommon to see patients with asthma improve much more than this. Other patients may not have this much improvement but do show increases in airflow and FVC and say that they feel better. In these cases, the physician may decide to continue the medication.

Exam Hint 4-7

A postbronchodilator increase in PF or $FEV_{1\%}$ of at least 15% shows reversible small-airway obstruction. This indicates that a patient with asthma or COPD has responded to the inhaled bronchodilator.

11. Bronchoprovocation studies

a. Perform the procedure (code: IC23) [difficulty: R, Ap, An]

A bronchoprovocation study (also known as *bronchial provocation*) is indicated when a patient has a history indicating asthma or hyperactive airways yet has normal spirometry testing. Other indications for a bronchoprovocation study include assessing the severity of airway hyperresponsiveness; evaluating the risk of asthma developing, including occupational asthma; assessing the effectiveness of medications to control the patient's asthma; and excluding asthma during a diagnostic workup.

The most common testing regimen involves having the patient inhale increasingly higher doses of nebulized methacholine (a cholinergic (parasympathetic) drug) and measuring spirometry results. Because of this, the procedure may be referred to as a *methacholine challenge test*. Occasionally, other factors, such as exercising while breathing cold air, inhaling a histamine, or inhaling a targeted antigen, such as animal dander, are substituted for methacholine. In addition, to evaluate the effectiveness of asthma-controlling medications, the physician may order that they be withheld for a specified period. The following discussion is limited to inhaled methacholine.

Testing should not be performed on a high-risk patient, such as someone who (1) has an FEV_1 of less than 50% of predicted, (2) has had a stroke or heart attack within the past 3 months, (3) has uncontrolled hypertension, or (4) has a known aortic or cerebral aneurysm. Remember, above all, that a positive test result indicates that the patient has some level of bronchospasm.

The basic procedure is as follows:

1. Perform a baseline FVC and measure the FEV_1. These results should be within the normal range to justify continuing the testing procedure.
2. Have the patient inhale nebulized normal saline (0.9% NaCl). Repeat the FVC. A decrease in the FEV_1 of 10% or greater is a positive response. See step 6.
3. If the patient is normal, continue as follows: Have the patient inhale 0.03 mg/mL nebulized methacholine. Repeat the FVC. A decrease in the FEV_1 of 20% or greater is a positive response (for example, after the methacholine was inhaled, the patient's FEV_1 dropped from 3000 mL to 2400 mL). See step 6.
4. If the patient is normal, continue as follows: Have the patient inhale 0.06 mg/mL nebulized methacholine. Repeat the FVC. A decrease in the FEV_1 of 20% or greater is a positive response. See step 6.

If the patient is normal, continue as follows:

5. Repeat step 4 with the methacholine dose doubling each time (e.g., 0.12, 0.24, 0.48 mg/mL, and so on). Stop the testing if the patient reaches the maximum methacholine dose of 16 mg/mL.
6. Stop any further testing. Assess the patient's vital signs, breath sounds, and oxygenation. Administer a nebulized, fast-acting bronchodilator medication, such as albuterol (see Chapter 9) if needed. Report the findings to the physician in charge.
7. Repeat spirometry to demonstrate that the patient has returned to his or her baseline values. Do not discharge the patient until he or she has returned to normal.
8. Chart the findings of the testing procedure, including how much methacholine was inhaled and the patient's final FEV_1.

b. Evaluate the results (code: ID22) [difficulty: R, Ap, An]

If the patient has a 20% drop in FEV_1, the physician would interpret that to mean the patient had a positive test and has a bronchospasm-inducing condition. Inhaling a small amount of methacholine with a large drop in FEV_1 indicates a severe reaction. A negative test result is seen if the patient inhales the maximum dose of methacholine (16 mg/mL) without a significant drop in FEV_1.

12. Flow-volume loops

a. Perform the procedure (code: IC23) [difficulty: R, Ap]

The flow-volume loop is a graphic display of the flow and volume generated during a forced expiratory vital capacity (FEVC) that is immediately followed by a forced inspiratory vital capacity (FIVC). It is used to identify inspiratory or expiratory flow at any lung volume.

As with the FVC test, the patient should be coached to inhale completely and blast the air out until he or she is completely empty. When you are sure that the patient has exhaled to residual volume, coach him or her to inhale as quickly as possible until the lungs are completely full. The entire procedure needs to be done as a continuous effort. There can be no hesitation at the start, leaks, glottis closing, or coughing throughout the entire procedure.

The expiratory half of the curve is called the *maximum expiratory flow-volume* (MEFV) curve. It begins at TLC and ends at residual volume. The inspiratory half of the curve is called the *maximum inspiratory flow-volume* curve. It begins at residual volume and ends at TLC. Ideally, the two halves of the loop meet at the TLC. Flow is recorded in liters per second and graphed on the vertical (ordinate, or y) axis. Volume is recorded in liters and graphed on the horizontal (abscissa, or x) axis. Both flow and volume should be BTPS adjusted.

b. Evaluate the results (code: ID22) [difficulty: R, Ap]

Flow-volume loops have gained great popularity, because the shape of the curve is diagnostic of the patient's condition. In addition, the peak inspiratory and peak expiratory flows can be measured. If the effort is timed, all the parameters found on the previously discussed volume–time curves can be found on the flow-volume loop. The following examples show a normal flow-volume loop and representative abnormal loops.

1. Normal

A normal flow-volume loop is shown in Figures 4-10 and 4-11. First look at Figure 4-10, in which the various volumes are measured on the horizontal scale. The tidal volume (V_T) of 500 mL is the small loop within the larger VC loop. The ERV and IRV are shown on both sides of the tidal volume. The FVC is shown as the total of all three volumes. Finally, TLC and RV are marked.

Figure 4-11 shows the same normal flow-volume loop in which the various flows are measured on the vertical scale. Starting from TLC with the FEVC, the peak expiratory flow rate is seen as the greatest flow generated; it is about 9 L/s. Starting from RV with the FIVC, the peak inspiratory flow rate is seen as the greatest flow that is generated; it is about 7 L/s. It is normal for the PEFR to be greater than the peak inspiratory flow rate.

To find the instantaneous flow at any FVC lung volume, the FVC must be divided by 4 to find the 25th, 50th, and 75th percentile points. In Figure 4-11, the FVC is 4800 mL. Dividing by 4 gives 1200 mL per quarter of the FVC. These points are marked on the horizontal volume scale. If a vertical (dashed) line is drawn through these three points to the flow-volume tracing, the instantaneous flows at these volumes can be found. *Expiratory flows* are reported as follows:

- Flow at 75% of the FEVC = $\dot{V}_{max75}$ (maximum flow with 75% of the FVC remaining), or FEF$_{25\%}$

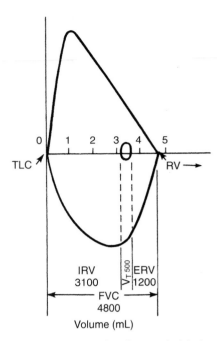

Figure 4-10 Flow-volume loop tracing of a normal adult showing the positions and values of the lung volumes. ERV, expiratory reserve volume; FVC, forced vital capacity; IRV, inspiratory reserve volume; RV, residual volume; TLC, total lung capacity.

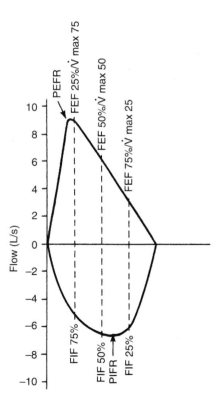

Figure 4-11 Flow-volume loop tracing of a normal adult showing the positions and values of the various inspiratory and expiratory flows. FEF, forced expiratory flow; FIF, forced inspiratory flow; PEFR, peak expiratory flow rate; PIFR, peak inspiratory flow rate.

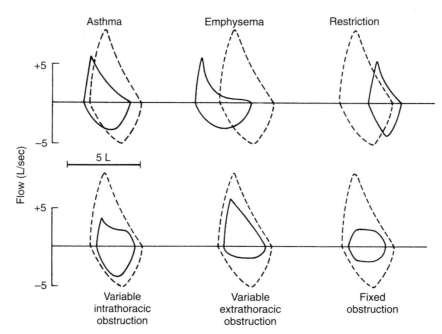

Figure 4-12 A series of abnormal flow-volume loop tracings superimposed over a dashed-line tracing of a normal loop. (From Mottram CD: Ruppel's Manual of pulmonary function testing, ed 10, St Louis, 2013, Mosby.)

- Flow at 50% of the FEVC = $\dot{V}_{max50}$ (maximum flow with 50% of the FVC remaining), or $FEF_{50\%}$
- Flow at 25% of the FEVC = $\dot{V}_{max25}$ (maximum flow with 25% of the FVC remaining), or $FEF_{75\%}$

Inspiratory *flows* are reported in this way:
- Flow at 25% of the FIVC = $FIF_{25\%}$ (forced inspiratory flow with 25% of the FVC inhaled)
- Flow at 50% of the FIVC = $FIF_{50\%}$
- Flow at 75% of the FIVC = $FIF_{75\%}$

The PEFR and $FEF_{25\%}$ or $\dot{V}_{max75\%}$ values should be about the same, because they all measure flow through the large upper airways. Either test is a good gauge of the patient's effort, because it will be low if the patient is not trying hard. The $FEF_{50\%}$ or $\dot{V}_{max50\%}$ values should approximate the $FEF_{25\%-75\%}$ values, because they both show flow through the medium to small airways in the middle half of the FVC effort. It is normal for the $FIF_{50\%}$ to be greater than the $FEF_{50\%}$. The $FEF_{75\%}$ or $\dot{V}_{max25\%}$ values are the best indicator of early small-airway disease because both show flow through the small airways as the patient approaches the residual volume. Note that the tracing from the $FEF_{25\%}$ or $\dot{V}_{max75\%}$ point to the residual volume is close to a straight line. In normal patients, the flow decreases in proportion to the decreasing lung volume, resulting in the straight-line tracing. Cherniack and Raber (1972) published formulas for predicting adult MEFV flows in liters per second; see the bibliography.

2. Small-airway disease

Examples of conditions that result in disease in the small airways (i.e., those less than 2 mm in diameter) include asthma, chronic bronchitis, bronchiectasis,

cystic fibrosis, and emphysema. The obstruction can be from bronchospasm, mucus plugging, or damage to the alveoli and small airways, leading to their collapse on expiration.

Figure 4-12 shows representative flow-volume loops for patients with asthma and emphysema superimposed over a normal flow-volume loop. Note that both loops are shifted to the left, toward the TLC, because the residual volumes are increased. The flows are also decreased more than normal as the patient exhales closer to the residual volume. This "scooped-out" appearance is very characteristic of small-airway disease. Having the patient inhale a bronchodilator and repeating the flow-volume loop shows the degree of reversibility. Some computer-based systems allow the before and after bronchodilator loops to be superimposed to better illustrate the amount of improvement.

3. Restriction

A restriction can be caused by a pulmonary condition, such as fibrosis; a thoracic condition, such as pleural effusion, pneumothorax, hemothorax, or kyphoscoliosis; or obesity, advanced pregnancy, or ascites pushing up on the diaphragm. Only fibrosis and kyphoscoliosis are permanent. Figure 4-12 shows a representative flow-volume loop for a patient with restrictive lung disease. Note that the volume is small and shifted to the right, toward the small residual volume.

4. Variable intrathoracic obstruction

A variable intrathoracic obstruction can be caused by a tumor or foreign body that partly blocks a bronchus. Figure 4-12 shows a representative flow-volume curve. Note

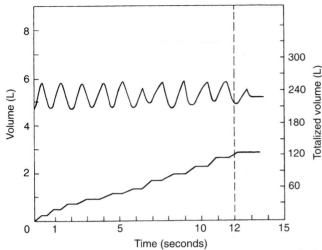

Figure 4-13 Two tracings of the same maximum voluntary ventilation effort. The saw-toothed tracing shows each individual volume effort and the respiratory rate. The stair-stepped tracing shows the cumulative volume during the 12-s effort. (From Mottram CD: Ruppel's Manual of pulmonary function testing, ed 10, St Louis, 2013, Mosby.)

that the FVC volume is almost normal, with a greatly decreased peak expiratory flow rate.

5. Variable extrathoracic obstruction

A variable extrathoracic obstruction can be caused by vocal cord paralysis, laryngeal tumor, or a foreign body that partly obstructs the upper airway. Figure 4-12 shows a representative flow-volume curve. Note that the FVC volume is almost normal, with a greatly reduced inspiratory flow. This same pattern is commonly seen in patients with obstructive sleep apnea. The $FEF_{50\%}$ will be greater than the $FIF_{50\%}$.

6. Fixed obstruction

A fixed obstruction usually is caused by a tumor in the trachea or a mainstem bronchus. Figure 4-12 shows a representative flow-volume loop. Again, the FVC volume is close to normal. Note the abnormally reduced inspiratory and expiratory flow rates. The tracing looks almost squared off, with the $FEF_{50\%}$ and $FIF_{50\%}$ values being about the same.

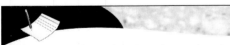

Exam Hint 4-8

Expect to see a flow-volume loop that needs to be interpreted for the patient's condition or to find a specific value, such as the vital capacity or peak flow.

13. Maximum voluntary ventilation

a. Perform the procedure (code: IC23) [difficulty: R, Ap]

The MVV is the volume of air exhaled in a specified period during a repetitive maximum respiratory effort. It is most commonly done to evaluate a patient's ability to perform a stress test. It also may be used as a preoperative screening test to help determine the patient's chance of pulmonary complications.

The patient should breathe at a volume that is greater than the tidal volume but less than the VC, at a rate of 70-120 per minute. The minimum time for the test is 12 seconds. Figure 4-13 shows two different tracings of the MVV effort. The total volume exhaled in the given period is mathematically adjusted for 1 minute so that the derived value is in liters per minute. This is done by multiplying a 5-s effort by 12 or a 12-s effort by 5. The derived value then is BTPS corrected to give the final value.

b. Interpret the results (code: ID22) [difficulty: R, Ap, An]

The results of the MVV test are among the most difficult to evaluate. This is because the patient's effort, the condition of the respiratory muscles, lung and thoracic compliance, neurologic control over the drive to breathe, and airway and tissue resistance all have an influence. Abnormalities in any of these can cause the MVV to decrease. Because more than one problem can exist, a decreased MVV does not point out the exact difficulty. A healthy young man can have an MVV of 150 to 200 L/min. Women tend to have smaller values, and the values of both genders decrease with age. Because of the many factors involved in the MVV, normal predicted values may vary by as much as ±30%. Therefore, unless the MVV is less than 70% of predicted, the patient cannot really be considered abnormal.

Cherniack and Raber (1972) published the following equations[§] for predicting the MVV in liters per minute:

$$\text{Males}: [(3.03 \times \text{Height in inches}) - (0.816 \times \text{Age in years})] - 37.9$$

$$\text{Females}: [(2.14 \times \text{Height in inches}) - (0.685 \times \text{Age in years})] - 4.87$$

The following considerations are important in the evaluation of an abnormally low MVV value:

1. Did the patient try his or her best? The respiratory therapist must make a professional judgment that the patient made his or her best effort. An objective way of judging this is to multiply the patient's FEV_1 by 35 to estimate the MVV. They should be close to the same volume. For example, if the patient's FEV_1 is 3 L, the estimated MVV is 105 L/min (3 L × 35). An MVV that is much less than this indicates that the patient did not try very hard. Conversely, an MVV value that is much greater than this indicates that the FEV_1 value is too low and should be repeated.

[§]The ATPS to BTPS correction has been calculated into these equations.

2. What is the condition of the patient's respiratory muscles? Patients with neuromuscular abnormalities probably will not be able to breathe much deeper than the normal tidal volume or keep up the effort required for the duration of the test. Because of this, their results will be low.

3. What is the patient's lung/thoracic compliance? Patients with low compliance probably will not be able to sustain the workload required by the MVV test. However, some patients are able to compensate for a small tidal volume by increasing their respiratory rate enough to generate an MVV value within normal limits. A printout of the MVV test would show a smaller than expected volume moved at a higher than expected respiratory rate.

4. What is the patient's neurologic control over the drive to breathe? Patients who have had an injury to the brain may have an abnormal drive to breathe. Because of this, they produce a low MVV.

5. What is the patient's airway and tissue resistance? Patients with increased airway resistance usually have a low MVV result. This problem may also cause air trapping and force the patient to stop the effort. Increased tissue resistance, such as is seen in pulmonary edema, obesity, and ascites, also results in a low MVV value.

Despite the difficulties in determining the cause of a decreased MVV value, the test may prove helpful in preoperative evaluation and cardiopulmonary stress testing. Any patient with a lower than normal MVV value is at an increased risk of postoperative atelectasis and pneumonia. The risks of pulmonary complications related to MVV are low when the patient reaches 75% to 50% of predicted, moderate when the patient reaches 50% to 33% of predicted, and high when the patient reaches less than 33% of predicted. Patients with known moderate to severe COPD usually have to stop exercise testing because of their inability to breathe. An MVV value of less than 50 L/min is a good predictor of this.

14. Single-breath nitrogen washout test and closing volume

a. Perform the procedure (code: IC23) [difficulty: R, Ap]

The single-breath nitrogen washout (SBN_2) is used to measure two things: (1) the evenness of the distribution of ventilation into the lungs during inspiration and (2) the emptying rate of the lungs during exhalation. It is a helpful diagnostic test in any adult patient who is known to have or suspected of having obstructive airway disease. The NBRC uses the phrase *nitrogen washout distribution test* for its examinations.

The closing volume is one part of the SBN_2 test. It marks the lung volume when small-airway closure begins and is used as an early indicator of small-airway disease.

The SBN_2 test is done by analyzing the nitrogen (N_2) percentage exhaled after an inspiratory vital capacity (IVC)

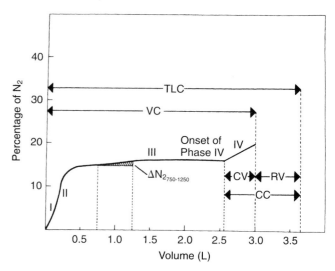

Figure 4-14 Tracing of a normal single-breath nitrogen washout test showing the four phases and other features. CC, closing capacity; CV, closing volume; ΔN_2 750-1250, nitrogen percentage found in the 500 mL of gas exhaled between 750 and 1250 mL of the vital capacity; RV, residual volume; TLC, total lung capacity; VC, vital capacity. (From Mottram CD: Ruppel's Manual of pulmonary function testing, ed 10, St Louis, 2013, Mosby.)

of 100% oxygen. It is beyond the scope of this book to go into detail on all the steps of the procedure; however, the general steps include instructing the patient to perform an IVC test while inhaling oxygen. The patient is told to exhale slowly and evenly until the lungs are empty again, without any breath holding. The exhaled gases are sent through a rapid N_2 analyzer to measure the percentage, a spirometer to measure the volume, and a graphing device.

b. Evaluate the results (code: ID22) [difficulty: R, Ap, An]

Figure 4-14 shows a normal tracing, which shows these phases:

- ***Phase I*** shows gas exhaled from the anatomic dead space of the upper airway. Because it is made up of 100% oxygen, the nitrogen percentage shows a zero reading.
- ***Phase II*** shows a mix of dead-space gas and alveolar gas. The nitrogen percentage increases rapidly as the pure oxygen is exhaled and nitrogen-rich gas from the alveoli is brought out. The first 750 mL of gas that includes these first two phases is not used in the evaluation of the distribution of ventilation.
- ***Phase III*** shows a fairly level plateau as alveolar gas from the lower lobes with a stable mix of oxygen and nitrogen is exhaled. Phase III is further evaluated in the following two ways:

1. ΔN_2 750-1250 looks at the increase in the nitrogen percentage found in the 500 mL of gas exhaled between 750 and 1250 mL of the VC. It is normally no more than 1.5% in healthy young adults. It increases to 3%-4.5% in healthy older adults. Patients with severe airway and lung disease, such as emphysema, may have a finding of 6%-10% or more.

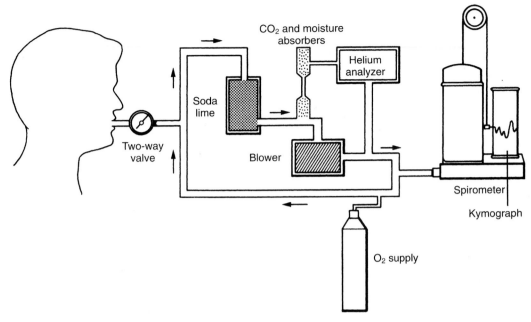

Figure 4-15 Schematic drawing of the key components of a helium dilution system for measuring functional residual capacity. (From Beauchamp RK: Pulmonary function testing procedures. In Barnes TA, editor: Respiratory care practice, St Louis, 1988, Mosby.)

2 .The slope of phase III is found by drawing a straight line from the point at which 30% of the VC is exhaled to the point at which phase IV begins. It is normally no more than 0.5%-1% N_2 per liter of exhaled volume in healthy young adults, but it may vary widely.

- *Phase IV* is seen as a sharp increase in the nitrogen percentage and continues to residual volume. This is seen when the nitrogen-rich gas from the upper airways continues to be exhaled as the basilar airways became compressed and close off near the end of the VC effort.

The start of phase IV is called the *closing volume* (CV). It marks the lung volume when small-airway closure begins and is an early indicator of small-airway disease. The CV does not occur in healthy young adults until after about 80% to 90% of the VC has been exhaled. The closing capacity (CC) is found by adding the closing volume to the residual volume (found by another test). Healthy young adults have a CC that is about 30% of their TLC.

Problems can be indicated as follows: increase in the $\Delta N_{2\ 750\text{-}1250}$ or the slope of phase III, and especially early onset of phase IV; increased closing volume; and increased closing capacity. The diseases or conditions that can cause these abnormal test results are small-airway disease, congestive heart failure with pulmonary edema, and obesity.

15. Functional residual capacity by the helium dilution method

a. Perform the procedure (code: IC23) [difficulty: R, Ap, An]

The functional residual capacity (FRC) is the volume of gas left in the lungs at the end of a normal expiration. It cannot be measured through spirometry. The FRC is needed to calculate a patient's RV and TLC. It is necessary to know a patient's RV, FRC, and TLC to diagnose and determine the severity of obstructive lung disease and restrictive lung disease.

The helium (He) dilution method basically involves diluting the resident gases in the lungs (mainly nitrogen and oxygen) with helium to mathematically determine the FRC. This also is called the *closed-circuit* method, because the patient and circuit are sealed off. Figure 4-15 shows a schematic drawing of the components that make up the circuit. These include a two-way valve to switch the patient from breathing room air to the helium mix, soda lime to absorb the patient's exhaled carbon dioxide from the circuit, a combined carbon dioxide (CO_2) and water vapor absorber to prevent these gases from entering the helium analyzer, the helium analyzer, a variable speed blower to move the gases through the circuit, a spirometer for monitoring tidal volumes, an attached kymograph to trace the patient's breathing pattern, and an oxygen supply to meet the patient's needs. The helium supply is not shown.

It is beyond the scope of this text to cover all the steps in the helium dilution test; however, the following features of the procedure are important to know. Add enough helium to the room air in the circuit to create a 10%-15% He mix. At the end of a normal exhalation, the patient is switched to breathing the mix so that the FRC can be determined. The patient breathes the gas mix until the helium is evenly distributed throughout the lungs and the helium percentage is stable. Typically, the test is performed for up to 7 minutes, if needed, to reach an equilibrium point. Extending the test longer may help to reach a stable equilibrium point in abnormal patients. The calculation of RV is rather complex and usually is done through the computer built into the pulmonary function system. Spirometry also must be performed, because the ERV is subtracted from the FRC to find the RV. Commonly the test is repeated. The patient should be allowed to breathe room air for 5 minutes between tests to clear the helium from the lungs. Patients with severe obstructive lung disease may need more time. Bates et al. (1971) published the following equations[§] for calculating the normal FRC in liters:

$$\text{Males}: (0.130 \times \text{Height in inches}) - 5.16$$

$$\text{Females}: (0.119 \times \text{Height in inches}) - 4.85$$

Goldman and Becklake (1959) published the following equations[§] for calculating the normal RV in liters:

$$\text{Males}: [(0.069 \times \text{Height in inches}) + (0.017 \times \text{Age in years}) - 3.45$$

$$\text{Females}: [(0.081 \times \text{Height in inches}) + (0.009 \times \text{Age in years}) - 3.90$$

b. Evaluate the results (code: ID22)
[difficulty: R, Ap, An]

A normal young man has an FRC volume of about 2400 mL. As shown in Figure 4-7, it is composed of the ERV and the RV. The FRC and RV values are invaluable for diagnosing obstructive and restrictive lung diseases. See Figure 4-6 for the relative volumes and capacities for a normal patient, a patient with an obstructive pattern, and a patient with a restrictive pattern. Note that the obstructive patient has a disproportionate increase in the RV, with a resulting decrease in the FVC. The TLC may be normal, as shown, or, more commonly, lung capacity may be increased. The patient with restrictive disease has a proportionate decrease in all the lung volumes and capacities. It is commonly accepted that the normal limits of TLC are about ±20% of the predicted value. This ±20% of the normal limit applies to the FRC and RV values as well. In other words, obstructive lung disease can be diagnosed by an RV, FRC, or TLC that is more than 120% of the predicted value. Common examples of obstructive diseases include asthma, bronchitis, and emphysema. Restrictive lung disease can be diagnosed by an RV, FRC, or TLC that is less than 80% of the predicted value. Examples of restrictive diseases include fibrotic lung disease, air or fluid in the pleural space, obesity, kyphoscoliosis, pectus excavatum, and neuromuscular weakness or paralysis.

The following factors are important to ensure that the measured values are accurate:

- The system must not have any leaks. A leak can result in overestimation of the FRC, because the lost helium results in a lower final helium percentage. A leak also can result in failure of the final helium percentage to stabilize as expected.
- The patient must be breathing on the system long enough for the helium to reach all the lung units and reach equilibrium. Usually this takes about 7 minutes; however, patients with severe obstructive

lung disease will need more time and may never reach an equilibrium state. This results in an underestimation of the FRC.

16. Functional residual capacity by the nitrogen washout method
a. Perform the procedure (code: IC23)
[difficulty: R, Ap]

As discussed in the helium dilution method, the nitrogen (N_2) washout method is used to find the FRC so that the RV can be derived from it and TLC calculated. It is necessary to know a patient's RV, FRC, and TLC to diagnose and determine the severity of obstructive lung disease and restrictive lung disease.

The nitrogen washout method basically involves having the patient breathe in 100% oxygen until all the resident nitrogen is removed from the lungs. It also is called the *open-circuit* method, because the patient inspires as much oxygen as needed to displace the nitrogen to a reservoir for measurement.

Figure 4-16 shows a schematic drawing of the components that make up the automated nitrogen washout system and circuit. These include a solenoid valve to switch the patient from breathing room air to breathing pure oxygen, an oxygen source with demand valve, a nitrogen analyzer with recorder, a pneumotachometer, and a microprocessor that directs all the necessary activities for the test. It is beyond the scope of this text to go into the complete procedure for the test; however, the following features should be known. The circuit is filled with pure oxygen. The patient is switched from room air to oxygen at the end of a normal exhalation so that the nitrogen in the FRC can be determined. Typically, the test is performed for up to 7 minutes or until the nitrogen percentage falls below a target level. This target percentage has been reported by various authors as 1% (best results) up to 3%. Extending the test longer may help to reach a target level in patients with increased airway resistance or an increased lung volume. As before, the calculation of RV is rather complex and is usually done through the computer built into the pulmonary function system. Spirometry also must be performed, because the ERV is subtracted from the FRC to find the RV. Commonly the test is repeated. The patient should be allowed to breathe room air for at least 15 minutes between tests to clear the oxygen from the lungs. Patients with severe obstructive lung disease may need more time.

Predicted patient values for the FRC and RV can be determined with the same equations listed in the previous discussion of the helium dilution method of determining FRC.

b. Evaluate the results (code: ID22)
[difficulty: R, Ap, An]

As discussed earlier for the helium dilution test, the FRC and RV values are invaluable for diagnosing obstructive and restrictive lung diseases. When done properly, the

---

[§]The ATPS to BTPS correction has been calculated into these equations.

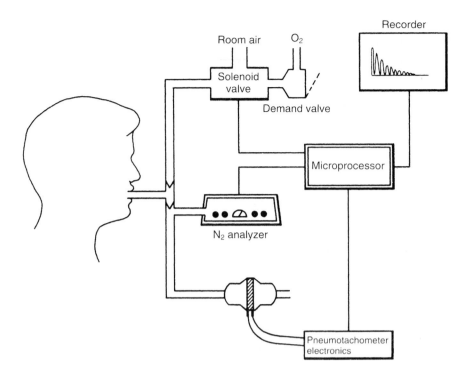

Figure 4-16 Schematic drawing of the key components of the automated nitrogen washout system for measuring functional residual capacity. (From Beauchamp RK: Pulmonary function testing procedures. In Barnes TA, editor: Respiratory care practice, St Louis, 1988, Mosby.)

helium dilution and nitrogen washout tests reveal similar patient values. If the nitrogen percentage is graphed over time, the shape of the washout curve also can be helpful for evaluating the degree of airway obstruction. Both the normal and the abnormal tracings show rapid nitrogen washout from the upper-airway dead space. However, as the test continues, a patient with obstructive lung disease shows a progressive slowing of the nitrogen washout rate.

The following considerations are important to ensure that the measured values are accurate:

- The system must not have any leaks. A leak would be noticed as a sudden increase in the nitrogen percentage after a steady decrease. This results in overestimation in the FRC value.
- The patient must be breathing on the system long enough for the nitrogen to be washed out of all the lung units. Usually this takes less than 7 minutes; however, patients with severe obstructive lung disease need more time and may never reach the targeted percentage. This results in underestimation of the FRC.

17. Total lung capacity

a. Perform the procedure (code: IC23) [difficulty: R, Ap]

The TLC is the volume of air in the lungs after inhalation of a VC. As discussed earlier, the patient's TLC must be determined to diagnose obstructive or restrictive lung disease.

See Figure 4-7 for an example of the relationships between lung volumes and capacities. As can be seen, the TLC can be found by adding several combinations of volumes and capacities. Most commonly, it is calculated by adding

the FRC to the inspiratory capacity (IC) found through spirometry. However, be prepared to add or subtract various combinations of volumes and capacities to find the TLC.

b. Evaluate the results (code: ID22) [difficulty: R, Ap, An]

The TLC results cannot be interpreted without looking at the volumes and capacities that compose it. Figure 4-6 shows representative TLC patterns for a normal patient and a patient with an obstructive pattern and one with a restrictive pattern. Note that with the abnormal patterns, the FRC and its components, the ERV and RV, are out of proportion. Patients with emphysema, bronchitis, or asthma often show the obstructive pattern with a large FRC of trapped gas. Patients with fibrotic lung disease, thoracic deformities, or obesity often show the restrictive pattern, with a decreased FRC and other lung volumes.

Some practitioners use the general rule that a TLC more than 120% of predicted indicates an obstructive pattern, and a TLC less than 80% of predicted indicates a restrictive pattern. However, this may be an oversimplification. It is more reliable to calculate the RV to TLC (RV:TLC) ratio. This takes into account the interrelation of the two. Normal healthy adults have an RV:TLC ratio of 0.20 (20%) to 0.35 (35%). An increased RV:TLC ratio is commonly seen in patients with emphysema and an increased RV. However, if the patient's TLC is increased in proportion to the RV, the ratio may be within normal limits. A decreased RV:TLC ratio is commonly seen in patients with fibrotic lung disease. The ratio will be normal, however, if the patient's TLC is decreased in proportion to the RV. Table 4-3 shows the relationships of the lung volumes and capacities, TLC, and RV:TLC ratio found in a number of conditions.

TABLE 4-3 Lung Volumes and Capacities Seen in Various Disorders

Disorder	VC	IC	ERV	FRC	RV	TLC	RV:TLC
Asthma or airway disease	D	N	D	N, I	I	N, I*	I
Emphysema	N	N	N	I	I	I	N, I
Diffuse parenchymal disease							
Early	N	N	N	D	N	N	N
Advanced (all volumes and capacities equally reduced)							
Space-occupying lesions	N	N	N	N	D	N	
Obesity	N	N	D	N, I†	N	N	I
Thoracic/skeletal disease	D	D	D	D	N	D	I

D, decreased; ERV, expiratory reserve volume; FRC, functional residual capacity; I, increased; IC, inspiratory capacity; N, normal; RV, residual volume; TLC, total lung capacity; VC, vital capacity.

*When airway resistance is greater than about 3.5 cm H_2O/L/s.

†When the weight:height (pounds:inches) ratio is greater than 5:1.

Modified from Snow MG: Determination of functional residual capacity, Respir Care 34:586, 1989.

Exam Hint 4-9

Most examinations have at least one table that must be interpreted to determine whether the patient has obstructive lung disease or restrictive lung disease. The "20% rule" can help with this determination. Obstructive lung disease is identified by lung volumes (TLC, FRC, RV) that are 20% or more *greater* than predicted (more than 120% of predicted). Restrictive lung disease is identified by lung volumes (TLC, FRC, RV) that are 20% or more *smaller* than predicted (less than 80% of predicted).

---

18. Body plethysmography

The body plethysmography unit (sometimes called the *body bubble* or *body box*) is a sealable chamber large enough for an adult to sit inside. Auxiliary equipment includes a differential-pressure pneumotachometer, a monitor/storage oscilloscope, a computer, and a recording device (Fig. 4-17). The plethysmograph can be used to measure (1) the FRC and, from that, the RV and TLC; (2) lung compliance; and (3) airway resistance. Each of these tests is discussed later.

a. Thoracic gas volume

1. Perform the procedure (code: IC23) [difficulty: R, Ap]

The volume of gas measured in the lungs at the end of exhalation by a plethysmograph is called the *thoracic gas volume* (TGV). When the unit has been accurately calibrated and the test properly performed, the plethysmograph provides a more accurate FRC volume measurement than either the helium dilution or the nitrogen washout method. Once the TGV is determined, the RV can be derived from it and the TLC calculated. It is necessary to know a patient's RV, FRC, and TLC to diagnose and determine the severity of obstructive lung disease and restrictive lung disease.

It is not possible to go into a complete discussion of the procedure; however, the following steps are important. The unit must be sealed so that it is airtight during the patient's

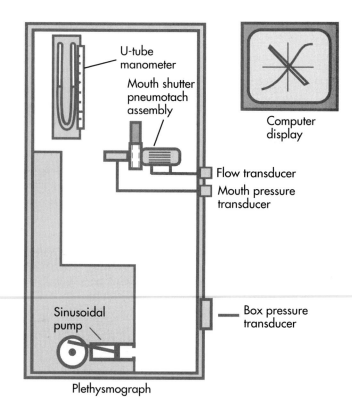

Figure 4-17 Schematic drawing of the layout of a body plethysmograph with its components. The patient sits within the sealed plethysmograph chamber for the tests. (From Mottram CD: Ruppel's Manual of pulmonary function testing, ed 10, St Louis, 2013, Mosby.)

breathing. The patient is instructed to breathe a normal tidal volume through the pneumotachometer. At the end of exhalation (FRC), a shutter is closed on the pneumotachometer so that no air leaks. The patient is instructed to continue to make tidal volume breathing efforts. The computer integrates the following two pressure changes: (1) a decrease in mouth pressure as the patient attempts to inhale and (2) an increase in plethysmograph chamber pressure as the patient's chest expands. The patient's TGV

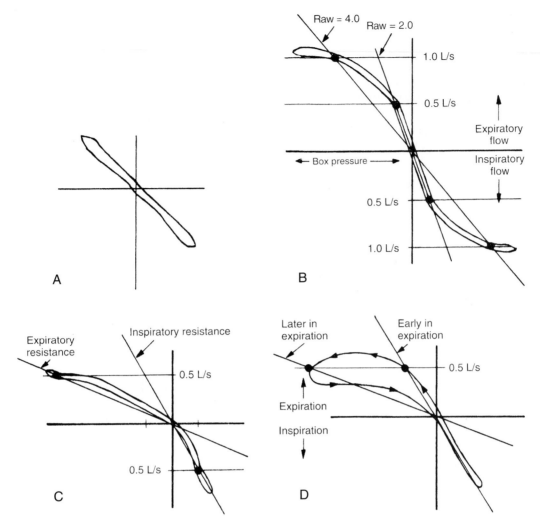

Figure 4-18 Examples of body plethysmography tracings. **A,** A normal thoracic gas volume loop. **B,** A normal inspiratory and expiratory loop for airway resistance (Raw). Note that it is symmetrical. This patient has an Raw of 2 cm H_2O/L/s at the standard flow of 0.5 L/s. As the flow increases, the Raw increases as a result of the increased turbulence. The Raw of 4 cm H_2O/L/s seen at the flow of 1 L/s should not be recorded as the patient's value. **C,** A patient whose expiratory resistance is greater than his or her inspiratory resistance. In this case, either both resistances should be recorded in the chart or just the expiratory resistance if only one can be recorded. **D,** A significant difference between early and late expiratory resistance. This is commonly seen in patients with obstructive airway disease, such as emphysema. Record the late resistance, because it better represents the patient's disease condition. (From Zarins LP, Clausen JL: Body plethysmography. In Clausen JL, editor: Pulmonary function testing guidelines and controversies, Orlando, 1984, Grune & Stratton.)

is then determined at FRC. Figure 4-18, A, shows a normal TGV loop on the oscilloscope. Through spirometry, the patient's ERV, RV, and TLC can be calculated.

2. Evaluate the results (code: ID22)
[difficulty: R, Ap, An]

The interpretation of the TGV and TLC results from a body plethysmograph is about the same as the interpretation of the FRC and TLC results from the helium dilution or nitrogen washout methods. (Review these earlier discussions if needed.) The only difference would be if the TGV were significantly larger than the FRC. This would indicate that the patient has trapped gas that was measured only in the plethysmograph. The TGV is commonly larger than the FRC

measured by the preceding two methods when the patient has COPD. This is because it includes *all* the gas found in the thorax. That gas may be found in normal alveoli connected by a patent airway to the atmosphere, but the TGV may also include gas trapped in emphysematous blebs and bullae, pneumothorax, pneumomediastinum, and so forth.

b. Lung compliance
1. Perform the procedure (code: IC12)
[difficulty: R, Ap]

Lung compliance (CL) is the volume change per unit of pressure change in the lungs. It is recorded in liters or milliliters per centimeter of water pressure (L (or mL)/cm H_2O). A lung compliance test is indicated in a patient with

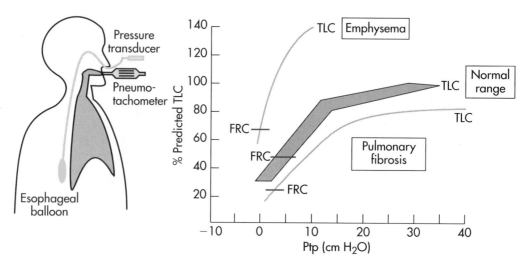

Figure 4-19 Measurement of CL with the esophageal balloon technique. A balloon is swallowed to the midthoracic level, filled with air, and connected to a pressure transducer to measure intrapleural pressure. The patient sits within a body plethysmograph and breathes through a pneumotachometer to measure mouth pressure and gas flow. The graph shows a tracing for a patient with normal compliance. In contrast, the patient with emphysema has an increased TLC and increased compliance; the patient with pulmonary fibrosis has a decreased TLC and decreased compliance. (From Ruppel G: Manual of pulmonary function testing, ed 9, St Louis, 2009, Mosby.)

a known or suspected condition that causes the lungs to be either overly compliant (as in emphysema) or noncompliant (as in pulmonary fibrosis).

The patient must swallow a balloon 10 cm long to the midthoracic level. A catheter connects the proximal end of the balloon to a pressure transducer outside the patient. Air is injected into the balloon, and the transducer is calibrated accurately to measure changes in intrathoracic pressure as the patient breathes. The patient is then placed into a body plethysmograph that is sealed. He or she is told to breathe through the differential-pressure pneumotachometer to measure lung volumes. The patient is then instructed to inhale slowly from the resting level (FRC) to TLC. As this is done, the pneumotachometer shutter is periodically closed to measure the intrathoracic pressure decrease at the increasing volumes (Fig. 4-19). As the patient slowly exhales from TLC, the shutter is again periodically closed to measure the increasing intrathoracic pressure as the patient returns to FRC volume. Lung compliance is usually calculated from the pressure and volume points of FRC and FRC plus 500 mL (for a tidal volume).

2. Evaluate the results (code: ID11)
[difficulty: R, Ap, An]

Normal CL in an adult is 0.2 L/cm H_2O. Through other methods, the normal adult's thoracic compliance has been determined also to be 0.2 L/cm H_2O. However, because the lungs tend to recoil smaller and the thorax cage tends to expand out, the two opposing forces offset each other somewhat. Because of this, the lung/thoracic compliance is calculated as 0.1 L (or 100 mL)/cm H_2O.

A number of diseases and conditions can affect lung, thoracic, and lung/thoracic compliance. Patients with emphysema are known to have a higher than normal lung compliance. Their lungs are overly distended. Decreased lung compliance is seen in pulmonary fibrosis (from sarcoidosis, silicosis, or asbestosis), lung tumor, pulmonary edema, atelectasis, pneumonia, or decreased surfactant. Decreased thoracic compliance is seen in patients with kyphoscoliosis, pectus excavatum, obesity, enlarged liver, or advanced pregnancy. All these conditions result in small, stiff lungs.

c. Airway resistance
1. Perform the procedure (code: IC23)
[difficulty: R, Ap]

Airway resistance (Raw) is the difference in pressure between the alveoli and the mouth that develops as air flows into and out of the lungs. It is recorded in centimeters of water pressure per liter of gas moved per second (cm H_2O/L/s). The test is performed on patients with a known or suspected condition of increased airway resistance. These conditions include asthma, emphysema, and chronic bronchitis (COPD). The test confirms the patient's condition. Then it is used to help determine the proper dose of bronchodilator medications to help manage the disease.

The patient is placed into a plethysmograph that is sealed. He or she is instructed to breathe through a differential-pressure pneumotachometer. With the pneumotachometer shutter open, the patient is told to pant several tidal volumes of about 500 mL at a rate of 1 breath per second. Data on flow rate, tidal volume, mouth pressure changes, and chamber pressure changes are recorded and graphed (Fig. 4-20). Then the shutter is closed at the patient's resting FRC volume. The patient is told to continue panting at the same volume and rate. Again, flow rate, tidal volume, mouth pressure changes, and chamber pressures are recorded and

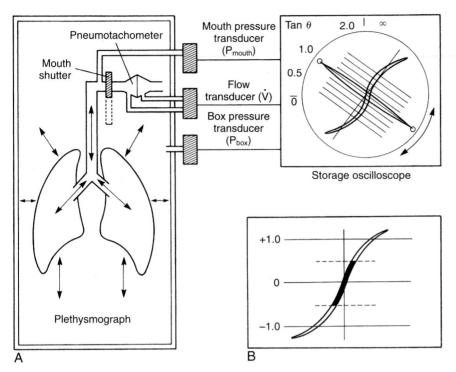

Figure 4-20 Measurement of Raw. **A,** The body plethysmograph in which the patient sits during the test. Tidal volume panting against an open and then closed pneumotachometer shutter is displayed on the storage oscilloscope. **B,** A printout of the pressure changes as the patient pants a tidal volume of 500 mL/s. (From Ruppel G: Manual of pulmonary function testing, ed 6, St Louis, 1994, Mosby.)

graphed. The computer integrates the data to calculate the patient's airway resistance during tidal volume breathing.

2. Evaluate the results (code: ID12)
[difficulty: R, Ap]

Airway resistance is the pressure difference developed per unit of flow. This pressure is required to overcome the friction of moving the tidal volume through the airways into the lungs. It can be thought of as the ratio of alveolar pressure to airflow. It is calculated by this formula:

$$Raw = \frac{\text{Atmospheric pressure} - \text{Alveolar pressure}}{\text{Flow}}$$

Ruppel (2003) reported that the normal adult's airway resistance ranges from 0.6 to 2.4 cm $H_2O/L/s$. The standard inspiratory and expiratory flow rate during the test is 0.5 L/s (500 mL/s). This is to standardize air turbulence during the test. The usual components of airway resistance found in an adult are as follows:

- Upper airway including the nose and mouth (50%)
- Trachea and bronchi larger than 2 mm in diameter (30%)
- Airways less than 2 mm in diameter (20%)

Increased airway resistance is abnormal. It is most readily noticed if the problem is in the upper airway, trachea, or major bronchi, because most resistance is normally found there. Patients with asthma, bronchitis, and emphysema have most of their resistance in the airways that are 2 mm or less in diameter. Because of this, significant disease must be present before a large enough airway resistance is noticed to alert the therapist or physician to the problem. Figure 4-18, B-D, shows normal and increased expiratory

resistance curves. Madama (1998) lists the following airway resistance values and their severity:

Raw (cm $H_2O/L/s$)	Severity
2.8 to 4.5	Mild
4.5 to 8	Moderate
Over 8	Severe

19. Diffusing capacity
a. Perform the procedure (code: IC23)
[difficulty: R, Ap]

The diffusing capacity (DL or DLCO) tests look at the capacity for carbon monoxide to diffuse through the lungs into the blood. Carbon monoxide is used, because its high affinity for hemoglobin virtually eliminates blood as a barrier to diffusion. The measured value can then be correlated to the ability of oxygen to diffuse through the lungs. This test is indicated when it is important to know the extent of lung disability causing hypoxemia. This is most common with patients having emphysema, but it also is important in patients with fibrotic lung disease.

At the time of this writing, the single-breath carbon monoxide diffusing capacity test (DLCO-SB) is the only version that has a widely adopted standard technique for administration. It is recorded in milliliters of carbon monoxide (CO) per minute per millimeter of mercury at 0° C, 760 mm Hg, and standard temperature, pressure, dry conditions (STPD).

The following are key steps in the procedure. A reservoir or spirometer is filled with a mix of 0.3% CO, 10% He, 21% O_2, and the balance of N_2 (Fig. 4-21). The patient is connected to the apparatus and breathes room air while being

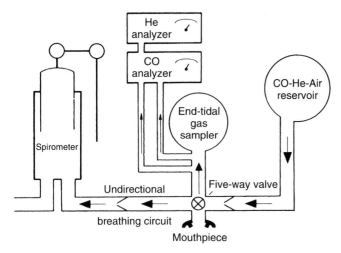

Figure 4-21 Schematic drawing of the components and breathing circuit used to perform a DLCO-SB test. Analysis of the patient's exhaled helium (He) and carbon monoxide (CO) percentages is critical to the test. (From Ruppel G: Manual of pulmonary function testing, ed 6, St Louis, 1994, Mosby.)

instructed in the test. After the patient is told to exhale completely (to RV), the practitioner switches the patient to the gas mix. The patient is instructed to rapidly inhale an IVC. A shutter automatically closes so that the patient cannot exhale for 10 s. This allows time for some of the carbon monoxide to diffuse into the patient's bloodstream.

After the breath hold, the shutter opens, and the patient is told to exhale to resting volume. The equipment is designed to automatically let 750 to 1000 mL of exhaled gas pass through to the spirometer. The next 500 mL of gas is diverted into the end-tidal gas sampler. This sample is then analyzed for He% and CO%. The remainder of the patient's exhaled volume is passed through into the spirometer. The various measured parameters are integrated into the equations in the computer to give the patient's DLCO-SB value.

This test is done only after the patient has been measured for both RV and TLC. That is because the patient's lung volume directly affects the diffusibility of carbon monoxide.

b. Evaluate the results (code: ID22) [difficulty: R, Ap, An]

Interpretation is limited to the results of the DLCO-SB test. Ruppel (2009) reported that the average resting normal adult DLCO-SB is 25 mL CO/min/mm Hg STPD. Gaensler and Wright (1966) reported the following DLCO-SB prediction equations, with values in mL/CO/min/mm Hg STPD:

Males : [(0.250 × Height in inches) − (0.177 × Age in years)] + 19.93

Females : [(0.284 × Height in inches) − (0.177 × Age in years)] + 7.72

It should be noted that a number of other authors have developed their own prediction equations. In general, patients who show DLCO-SB results within ±20% of the predicted values (80% to 120% of predicted) are considered to be within normal limits. A patient who has actual results that

are significantly below the predicted values (<80% of predicted) has a problem with lung diffusion. Figure 4-22 shows a number of common conditions that can lead to poor lung diffusion. The following factors also should be taken into consideration when interpreting the measured values:

- Increased hematocrit and hemoglobin values result in an increased DLCO, whereas decreased values result in a decreased DLCO. An actual value should be used to calculate a patient's DLCO.
- An increased carboxyhemoglobin level results in a decreased DLCO. Patients who smoke should be instructed not to smoke the night before the test so that the COHb level will decrease to normal.
- An increased alveolar carbon dioxide level results in a lowered alveolar oxygen level. This, in turn, results in an increased DLCO. A decreased alveolar carbon dioxide level results in a decreased DLCO.
- Increased altitude results in an increased DLCO. This is probably a concern only if the patient is tested in a mountainous area.
- An increased pulmonary capillary blood volume results in an increased DLCO.
- The patient should breathe room air for at least 4 minutes before the test is repeated.
- It is well known that diffusibility is directly related to lung volume. This is the reason that African Americans have lower diffusion rates than Caucasians. To eliminate this as a factor in interpreting the DL value, it is necessary to divide the diffusion value by the TLC. African Americans have the same normal values as Caucasians when this calculation is performed.

MODULE D

Pulmonary function equipment

1. Hand-held spirometers

a. Assemble the necessary equipment (code: IIA19) [difficulty: R, Ap]

Hand-held spirometers are used to perform the following tests at the patient's bedside:

1. Tidal volume (V_T)
2. Vital capacity (depending on the spirometer, either a maximum effort (forced vital capacity, FVC) or a nonforced effort (vital capacity, VC))
3. Minute volume ($\dot{V}_E$)

A variety of hand-held spirometers are available. The *Wright respirometer* is a turbine-type device that is used in this discussion because it has been widely used for many years (see Fig. 4-23). In addition, a double one-way valve assembly and mouthpiece need to be attached at the patient port. Nose clips should be worn to prevent a leak. The double one-way valve is used so that the patient inhales room air and exhales through the device. This prevents cross-contamination between patients. The unit itself is gas sterilized.

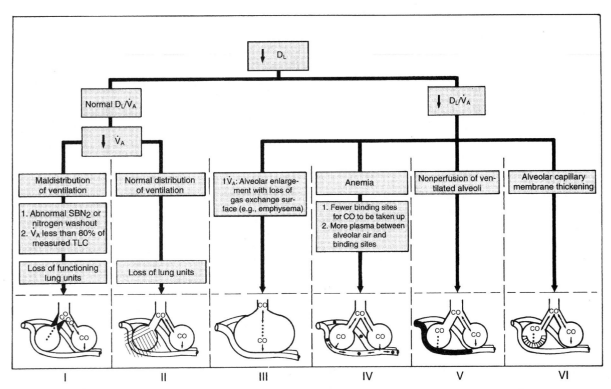

Figure 4-22 Six factors that can cause decreased lung diffusion (D_L). Factors I and II result in a decrease in D_L that is in proportion to the decrease in alveolar volume. Factors III, IV, V, and VI result in a decrease in D_L that is greater than the decrease in alveolar volume. Therefore these latter conditions are more harmful to the patient's pulmonary function and well-being. SBN_2, single-breath nitrogen washout; TLC, total lung capacity; $\dot{V}_A$, alveolar ventilation. (From Ayers LN, Whipp BJ, Ziment I: A guide to the interpretation of pulmonary function tests, ed 2, New York, 1978, Roerig.)

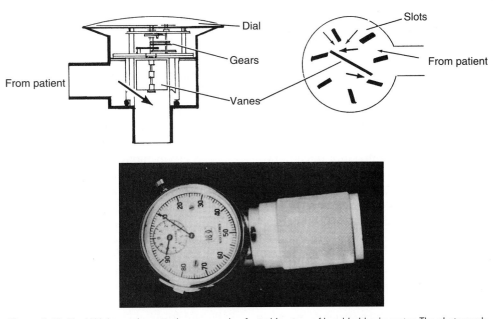

Figure 4-23 The Wright respirometer is an example of a turbine type of hand-held spirometer. The photograph shows one of several versions. All feature a scale that shows 1-L and 100-mL increments for measuring tidal volume. Another scale is used for minute volume because it accumulates up to 100 L. The cut-away drawings show the internal vanes and gears that translate flow into volume displayed on the two scales. (From Cairo JM: Mosby's respiratory care equipment, ed 9, St Louis, 2014, Mosby.)

The Wright respirometer is accurate with expiratory flows between 3 L/min and 300 L/min (0.05 L/s (50 mL/s) and 5 L/s). It should not be used with pediatric patients with small tidal volume breaths because the inertia of the spinning vane and gears will result in an inaccurately low volume reading. Patients should blow only a nonforced VC through the unit. An FVC of >5 L/s can distort and damage the vane and gears.

b. Troubleshoot any problems with the equipment (code: IIA19) [difficulty: R, Ap]

All units must work properly and have all ancillary equipment properly connected to be airtight. Any leaks will result in a loss of flow and volume. Tighten any loose connections and repeat the procedure if necessary. No volume will be measured if the patient exhales through the expiratory port rather than the patient port.

2. Screening spirometers

a. Assemble the necessary equipment (code: IIA19) [difficulty: R, Ap]

All screening spirometers convert one type of physical information or signal to another (e.g., converting an airflow or pressure signal to an electrical signal). See Figure 4-24 for schematic drawings of common principles of operation. Any type should be acceptable for performing screening spirometry. Make sure that the unit you select is capable of performing the ordered tests. Be sure that you select a unit capable of printing out a hard copy of the patient's test results and spirometry tracings if they are required for the chart. All screening spirometers are electrically powered. Many contain a micropressor and can measure all of the standard spirometry volumes and flow. All of these spirometers require additional items, such as patient nose clips and a mouthpiece. A double one-way valve system can also be added to direct gas flow properly through the equipment and to minimize cross-contamination between patients. Two widely used types of screening spirometers are discussed below.

1. Differential-pressure (flow-sensing) pneumotachometer

Some articles refer to a differential-pressure pneumotachometer as a *Fleisch-type* device. These units have a resistive element (tubes or mesh screen) in the flow tube. The faster the flow of gas through the flow tube, the greater the pressure difference before and after the resistance. Hoses connect the flow tubes before and after the resistive element to the differential-pressure transducer. The transducer converts this pressure difference into an electrical signal. A microprocessor calculates the various patient values from this information (see Fig. 4-24, A).

Assembly requires the addition of the patient's mouthpiece to the inspiratory port so that no air leak occurs. The expiratory port should be kept completely open so that the only obstruction to the patient's airflow is from the resistive element. A volume calibration check is performed by forcing a known amount of air from a super syringe (certified volume standard syringe) through the pneumotachometer. Minimally, several repetitions of a known 3-L volume should reveal identical measured volumes. As long as the measured volumes are within ±3% or 50 mL (whichever is less), the unit is acceptably accurate.

Common problems with accuracy include an air leak around the mouthpiece; cracked, disconnected, or obstructed pressure-relaying hoses; water condensation or mucus on the resistive element; or obstructed upstream or downstream port. The resistive element is usually heated to minimize any condensation.

2. Heat-transfer pneumotachometer

Some articles refer to a heat-transfer pneumotachometer as a *thermistor-type device* or *heated-wire anemometer*. These units have a heated thermistor that is cooled as the gas flows past it. The temperature transducer automatically increases and measures the flow of electricity to the thermistor to keep it at the required temperature. A microprocessor calculates the various patient values from this information. The earlier discussion on assembly, calibration, and troubleshooting applies to the heat-transfer pneumotachometers, except that no pressure-relaying hoses are present (Fig. 4-25).

b. Troubleshoot any problems with the equipment (code: IIA19) [difficulty: R, Ap]

All units must work properly and have all ancillary equipment properly connected to be airtight. Any leaks will result in a loss of volume, flow, or pressure. Tighten any loose connections and repeat the procedure if necessary. All pressure hoses must be kept free of water or mucus. Any plugging will prevent the pressure changes from being transmitted to the pressure transducer.

3. Gas analyzers

a. Assemble the necessary equipment (code: IIA22) [difficulty: R, Ap]

The CO, He, O_2, and specialty gas analyzers are needed for a variety of special tests, as described earlier and summarized here:

1. Carbon monoxide is analyzed in the single-breath carbon monoxide diffusing capacity test.
2. Helium is analyzed in the single-breath carbon monoxide diffusing capacity test and the helium dilution test to find the FRC.
3. Oxygen is analyzed in the single-breath carbon monoxide diffusing capacity test and the helium dilution test to find the FRC.
4. Nitrogen is analyzed in the single-breath nitrogen washout test and the nitrogen washout method of finding the FRC.

Check the label on the tank to be sure it is the correct gas at the correct percentage. Review Table 6-1 for color codings for tanks, if needed. Each specialty gas has its own diameter index safety system reduction valve to connect to

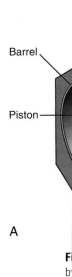

A

and Stead-Wells u
lating patient info

Gas analyzers
oxide and other
and lung diffusi
absorber should
FVC tests becaus
however, it must
last more than 1.
edly into the clos
added to the circ
to breathe repeat
ing is a checklist
lem solving:

1. Make sure
   too low).
2. Use a 7-L b
3. Make sure
   nections a
4. Check the
   correctly,]
   adjustable
5. Make sure
   circuit for
   lung diffu
6. Add oxyge
   tests.
7. Make sur
   properly.
8. Do not be
   is present
   near-verti

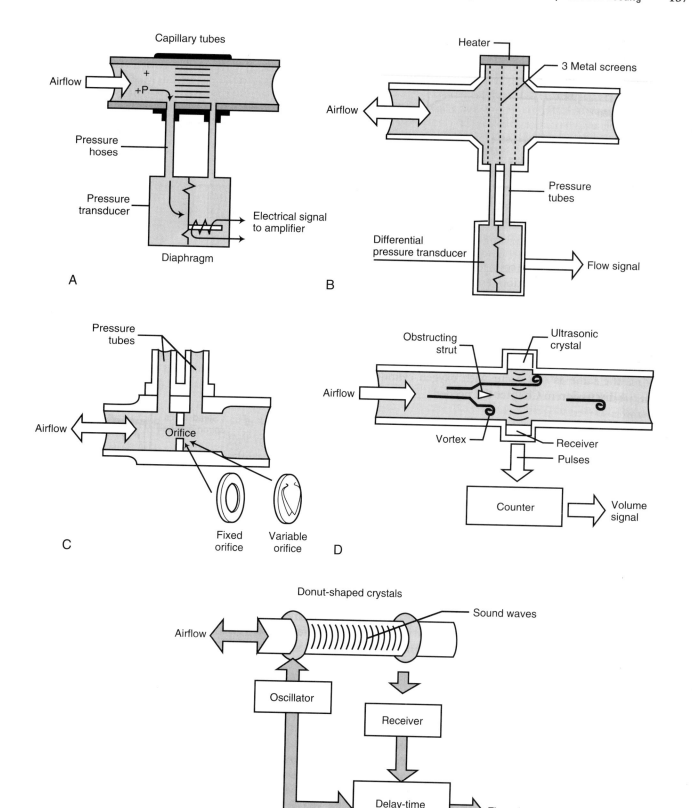

Figure 4-24 Principles of operation for pneumotachometers used for pulmonary function screening. **A,** Differential-pressure (Fleisch-type) device. **B,** Screen-type device. **C,** Fixed and variable orifice device. **D,** Vortex ultrasonic device. **E,** Nonvortex device. (Redrawn from Sullivan WJ, Peters GM, Enright PL: Pneumotachography: theory and clinical applications, Respir Care 29:736, 1984.)

Protective s

Figure 4-25
Ruppel G: Ma
Mosby.)

the tank. A
outlet to th

   b. Trou
      (cod
The probl
pressure-r
hoses are
Review the

MODUL

Quality a

1. Perfor
   functi
Every pul
a quality
maintena
formed a
the progr
dards. Al
adopted
equipmer
bration a
software
be recorc
tion mus
   See th
rometers
encounte
The foll
tory equ
modern
ware wit
   Volur
respirom
volume d
gas fills
These sy
to room

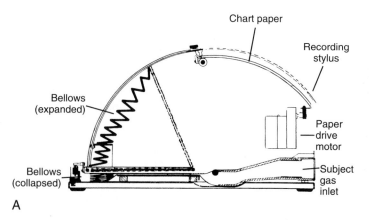
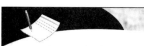
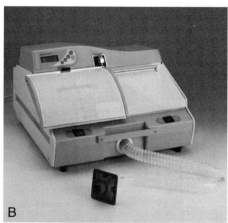

Figure 4-29 Wedge-type spirometer. **A,** The cutaway view shows the fan-like bellows that opens and closes with the patient's breathing efforts. This results in the writing stylus marking on the moving graph paper. **B,** The photograph shows a wedge-type spirometer with its patient breathing circuit, graph paper, and stylus. (**A** and **B:** Modified from Vitalograph Medical Instrumentation, Product Brochure, Lenexa, KS.)

1. Use a super syringe with at least a 3-L capacity to pump air repeatedly into and out of the unit. A reading that is accurate to within ±3%, or ±50 mL, should be measured. The flow rates should be varied to ensure that they do not affect the measured volumes. Volumes of 1 and 2 L also should be pumped into the unit to check for linearity.
2. To check for leaks in the circuit, perform the following steps:
   a. Pump a 3-L volume into the bellows.
   b. Close the mouthpiece to the atmosphere to seal the circuit.
   c. Add a weight to the bell to speed up any small leaks.
   d. Turn on the kymograph at a slow speed and put the pen on the paper to record any decrease in volume.
   e. If a leak is noted, locate and seal it.
3. Turn on the kymograph to its various speeds and check its accuracy with a stopwatch. The manufacturer's literature should tell how far the kymograph will travel at its set speeds.
4. Compare the thermometer reading with that of a laboratory-quality unit.
5. Replace or repair any component that fails to meet the manufacturer's standards or those established by the ATS/ERS.

e. Body plethysmography equipment
See Figure 4-17 for the basic components of the system. The plethysmograph chamber must be airtight when the door and all vents are closed. This can be confirmed by attaching a pressure manometer to a chamber port and applying a known volume or pressure into the sealed chamber. The pressures should be identical between the chamber pressure gauges and the outside pressure

manometer. The differential-pressure pneumotachometer must also read accurately when a known volume is pumped through it. Most manufacturers have a series of calibration check procedures listed in the equipment literature.

> **Exam Hint 4-10**
>
> Commonly, examinations have at least one question that deals with recommending tests for assessing a patient with airway obstruction or evaluating the results of PFTs on a patient with airway obstruction. This can include interpreting a table of data, a volume-time tracing, or a flow-volume loop or calculating the results of a before-and-after bronchodilator study.

2. Perform quality control procedures for gas analyzers (code: IIC1) [difficulty: R, Ap]
   a. Nitrogen washout equipment for measuring functional residual capacity
See Figure 4-16 for the basic setup and breathing circuit of a nitrogen washout system. Review the troubleshooting of volume-displacement and pneumotachometer spirometers; they are used with the nitrogen washout procedure to find the FRC. The nitrogen washout-type RV test uses an emission spectroscopy ionization chamber analyzer for nitrogen. It is more commonly called a *Geissler tube ionizer*. It uses a vacuum pump to draw a gas sample into the ionization chamber. The intensity of the light spectrum given off by the ionized nitrogen directly relates to its percentage in the sample. A two-point calibration check should be performed at least every 6 months to check for linearity. It involves the following steps:

1. Draw a room-air sample into the unit and check the nitrogen meter reading. It should read about 78% nitrogen.
2. Adjust the meter reading, if necessary, to the manufacturer's specified value.
3. Turn off the needle valve so that no air can be drawn into the unit.
4. Check to see that the nitrogen meter reading decreases to zero nitrogen as the vacuum pump removes all gas from the ionization chamber.

Linearity (three-point calibration) can be checked by introducing 5%-10% nitrogen into the unit to see whether the nitrogen meter measures that value. If all three points match, there is even greater confidence in the accuracy of the measurements. Do not use an analyzer that is inaccurate.

Exam Hint 4-11

Most examinations include one question that deals with either calibrating a piece of pulmonary function equipment or troubleshooting and fixing a problem with equipment. A common question area involves a 3-L super syringe being used to perform volume calibration. The measured volume is at least 50 mL less than the 3 L pumped into the spirometer. This indicates a leak in the system.

---

b. Helium dilution equipment for measuring functional residual capacity

See Figure 4-15 for the basic setup of the helium dilution equipment and breathing circuit. Again, review the troubleshooting of volume-displacement and pneumotachometer spirometers; they are used with the helium dilution procedure to find the FRC. Both the helium dilution FRC test and the lung diffusion tests require the analysis of helium in the gas mixture. A thermal conductivity analyzer typically is used. It operates under the principle of a Wheatstone bridge, in which differences in gas density lead to different cooling rates of heated thermistor beads. The different rates of cooling change electrical resistances and cause different electrical currents to flow. In a helium analyzer, the greater the helium concentration, the faster the thermistor bead cools, and the more electricity flows through the circuit. This is then read off a meter as the helium percentage.

The thermal conductivity helium analyzer should be linear over the clinically used range of helium to an accuracy of ±0.2% He. Minimally, a two-point calibration should be performed. A room-air sample can be drawn into the analyzer and should read zero helium. A known helium concentration may then be added and analyzed (for example, heliox, which contains 80% helium and 20% oxygen). A third point can be checked if needed by analyzing another known helium percentage.

MODULE F

Respiratory care plan

1. Determine a patient's pathophysiologic state (code: IIIF1) [difficulty: R, Ap, An]

Even though a physician must legally determine the patient's diagnosis, a therapist should be able to understand the cause, pathophysiology, diagnosis, treatment, and prognosis for patients with cardiopulmonary disorders. The interpretation of patient data that are tested by the NBRC was discussed earlier. Figure 4-30 shows an algorithm demonstrating several key pulmonary function differences between normal people and those with common pulmonary conditions. The following is a brief summary of the PFT test results that would indicate an obstructive or restrictive lung condition.

a. Obstructive airway disease

The patient with severe obstructive lung disease shows low gas flow at all time intervals. The RV will usually be increased as a result of air trapping. This will increase the FRC and often the TLC. Despite the increased lung volume, the patient's diffusing ability is usually decreased. Examples of conditions that cause obstructive lung disease include asthma, emphysema, bronchitis, and bronchiolitis. Excessive mucus, foreign bodies, and airway tumors also cause bronchospasm and air trapping.

b. Restrictive lung disease

In restrictive lung disease, all lung volumes and capacities are reduced, and lung diffusion is reduced. Expiratory flows such as FEV_1 are increased owing to the increased recoil of the lungs. Examples of conditions that cause restrictive lung disease include fibrosis, pulmonary edema, hemothorax or pneumothorax, acute or infant respiratory distress syndrome, chest wall deformities, obesity, and various neuromuscular disorders.

2. Recommend starting a treatment based on the patient's response (code: IIIE2a) [difficulty: R, Ap, An]

See below.

3. Recommend a change in the therapeutic plan if indicated (code: IIIF2) [difficulty: R, Ap, An]

The care plan depends on the patient's diagnosis and the degree of limitation. If the patient has reversible small-airway disease, he or she should be counseled to stop smoking and avoid all airborne irritants. Inhaled or systemic bronchodilators or both should be prescribed to relax the airways as much as possible. If the patient has restrictive lung disease, he or she should be counseled to avoid any airborne irritants. Whether any medications or other procedures can be performed to offer some relief depends on the specific cause of the patient's disorder.

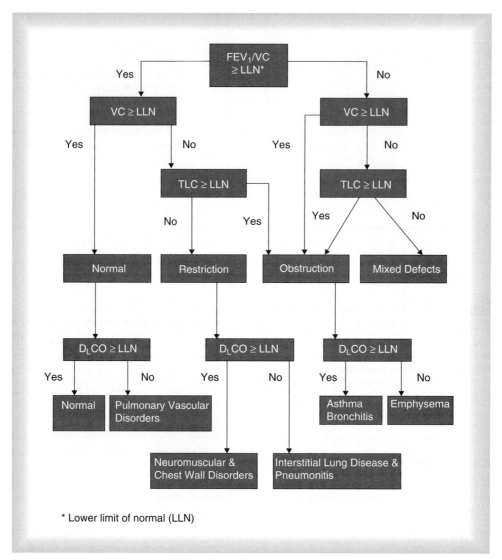

Figure 4-30 An algorithm that can be used to help guide the decision-making process to determine whether a patient is normal (within the lower limit of normal) or has one of five different pulmonary conditions. See the text for a discussion of each of the decision-making points. (From Gardner RM et al.: Computer guidelines for pulmonary laboratories, Am Rev Respir Dis 134:628, 1986.)

4. Recommend a treatment be terminated (code: IIIE1) [difficulty: R, Ap, An]

Pulmonary function testing is often performed to assess bronchodilator therapy in a patient with suspected or known asthma or COPD. If a medication is not beneficial to the patient, the physician should be informed so that it can be discontinued.

5. Recommend discontinuing a test based on the patient's response (code: IIIE2h) [difficulty: R, Ap, An]

Some pulmonary function tests, such as repeated FVC or maximum voluntary ventilation efforts, can be very strenuous for patients with COPD. They can result in severe coughing and bronchospasm. If this happens, the physician should be informed and the testing stopped.

Exam Hint 4-12

Most examinations have tested the examinee's understanding and interpretation of data to determine whether a patient has obstructive or restrictive lung disease. This usually involves the assessment of patient data on a table. A key finding in patients with obstructive lung disease is air trapping, which results in an RV, FRC, and TLC greater than 120% of predicted. A key finding in patients with restrictive lung disease is an RV, FRC, and TLC less than 80% of predicted.

BIBLIOGRAPHY

American Association for Respiratory Care: Clinical practice guideline: spirometry—1996 update, *Respir Care* 41:629, 1996 (Retired).

American Association for Respiratory Care: Clinical practice guideline: single-breath carbon monoxide diffusing capacity, *Respir Care* 44:539, 1999 (Retired).

American Association for Respiratory Care: Clinical practice guideline: static lung volumes—2001 revision and update, *Respir Care* 46:531, 2001 (Retired).

American Association for Respiratory Care: Clinical practice guideline: infant/toddler pulmonary function tests—2008 revision and update, *Respir Care* 53:929, 2008.

American Association for Respiratory Care: Clinical practice guideline: methacholine challenge testing, *Respir Care* 46:523, 2001 (Retired).

American Association for Respiratory Care: Clinical practice guideline: body plethysmography—2001 revision and update, *Respir Care* 46:506, 2001 (Retired).

American Association for Respiratory Care: Clinical practice guideline: assessing response to bronchodilator therapy at point of care, *Respir Care* 40:1300, 1995 (Retired).

American Thoracic Society: Standardization of spirometry—1987 update, *Am Rev Respir Dis* 136:1285, 1987.

Ayers LN, Whipp BJ, Ziment I: *A guide to the interpretation of pulmonary function tests*, ed 2, New York, 1978, Roerig.

Bates DV, Macklem PT, Christie RV: *Respiratory function in disease*, ed 2, Philadelphia, 1971, Saunders.

Beauchamp RK: Pulmonary function testing procedures. In Barnes TA, editor: *Respiratory care practice*, Chicago, 1988, Mosby.

Black LF, Hyatt RE: Maximal respiratory pressures: normal values and relationship to age and sex, *Am Rev Respir Dis* 99:696, 1969.

Branson RD, Hurst JM, Davis Jr K, et al.: Measurement of maximal inspiratory pressure: a comparison of three methods, *Respir Care* 34:789, 1989.

Buist SA, Ross BB: Predicted values for closing volumes using a modified single-breath nitrogen test, *Am Rev Respir Dis* 111:405, 1975.

Busse WW: What is the best pulmonary diagnostic approach for wheezing patients with normal spirometry? *Respir Care* 57:39–49, 2012.

Cairo JM: Assessment of pulmonary function. In Cairo JM, editor: *Mosby's respiratory care equipment*, ed 9, St Louis, 2014, Mosby.

Cannefax E, Enright P: Pulmonary function testing. In Hess DR, MacIntyre NR, Mishoe SC, Galvin WF, Adams AB, editors: *Respiratory care principles and practice*, ed 2, Burlington, MA, 2012, Jones & Bartlett Learning.

Chen CC, Chang CH, Tsai YC, Tseng CW, Tu ML, Wang CC, et al.: Utilizing exhaled carbon monoxide measurement with self-declared smoking cessation: enhancing abstinence effectiveness in Taiwanese outpatients, *Clin Respir J*, Online first: December 18, 2013. http://dx.doi.org/10.1111/crj.12096

Cherniack RM: *Pulmonary function testing*, ed 2, Philadelphia, 1992, Saunders.

Cherniack RM, Raber MD: Normal standards for ventilatory function using an automated wedge spirometer, *Am Rev Respir Dis* 106:38, 1972.

Clausen JL, editor: *Pulmonary function testing guidelines and controversies*, Orlando, 1984, Grune & Stratton.

Clausen JL: Clinical interpretation of pulmonary function test, *Respir Care* 34:638, 1989.

Crapo RO: Reference values for lung function tests, *Respir Care* 34:626, 1989.

Devici SE, Deveci F, Acik Y, Ozan AT: The measurement of exhaled carbon monoxide in healthy smokers and non-smokers, *Respir Med* 98(6):551–556, 2004.

de Souza LC, da Silva CT, Lugon JR: Evaluation of the inspiratory pressure using a digital vacuometer in mechanically ventilated patients: analysis of the time to achieve the inspiratory peak, *Respir Care* 57:257–262, 2012.

Douce FH: Pulmonary function testing. In Kacmarek RM, Stoller JK, Heuer AJ, editors: *Egan's fundamentals of respiratory care*, ed 10, St Louis, 2013, Mosby.

Enright PL: Should we keep pushing for a spirometer in every doctor's office? *Respir Care* 57:146–153, 2012.

Enright PL, Hodgkin JE: Pulmonary function tests. In Burton GG, Hodgkin JE, Ward JJ, editors: *Respiratory care: a guide to clinical practice*, ed 4, Philadelphia, 1997, Lippincott-Raven.

Gaensler EA, Wright GW: Evaluation of respiratory impairment, *Arch Environ Health* 12:146, 1966.

Gardner RM: Pulmonary function laboratory standards, *Respir Care* 34:651, 1989.

Gardner RM, Clausen JL, Cotton DJ, Crapo RO, Hankinson JL, Johnson Jr RL: Computer guidelines for pulmonary laboratories, *Am Rev Respir Dis* 134:628, 1986.

Global Initiative for Chronic Obstructive Lung Disease Executive Summary: *Global strategy for the diagnosis, management, and prevention of COPD*, Bethesda, MD, December 2009, National Heart, Lung, and Blood Institute. and the World Health Organization (Geneva Switzerland), 2009. Available at http://www.goldcopd.org

Goldman HI, Becklake MR: Respiratory function tests: normal values at median altitudes and the prediction of normal results, *Am Rev Tuberculosis* 79:457, 1959.

Hayes D, Kraman SS: The physiologic basis of spirometry, *Respir Care* 54:1717–1726, 2009.

Hess D: Measurement of maximal inspiratory pressure: a call for standardization, *Respir Care* 34:857, 1989.

Hunt GE: Diagnostic procedures at the bedside. In Fink JB, Hunt GE, editors: *Clinical practice in respiratory care*, Philadelphia, 1999, Lippincott Williams & Wilkins.

Kacmarek RM, Cycyk-Chapman MC, Young-Palazzo PJ, et al.: Determination of maximal inspiratory pressure: a clinical study and literature review, *Respir Care* 34:868, 1989.

Knudson RJ, Kaltenborn WT, Knudson DE, Burrows B: The single-breath carbon monoxide diffusing capacity, *Am Rev Respir Dis* 135:805, 1987.

Knudson RJ, Lebowitz MD, Holberg CJ, Burrows B: Changes in the normal maximal expiratory flow-volume curve with growth and aging, *Am Rev Respir Dis* 127:725, 1983.

Kory RC, Callahan R, Syner JC: The Veterans Administration-Army cooperative study of pulmonary function. I. Clinical spirometry in normal men, *Am J Med* 30:243, 1961.

MacIntyre NR: Diffusing capacity of the lung for carbon monoxide, *Respir Care* 34:489, 1989.

MacIntyre NR: Spirometry for the diagnosis and management of chronic obstructive pulmonary disease, *Respir Care* 54:1050–1057, 2009.

MacIntyre NR, Selecky PA: Is there a role for screening spirometry? *Respir Care* 55:35–42, 2010.

Madama VC: *Pulmonary function testing and cardiopulmonary stress testing*, ed 2, Albany, NY, 1998, Delmar.

Morris JF, Koski A, Johnson LC: Spirometric standards for healthy nonsmoking adults, *Am Rev Respir Dis* 103:57, 1971.

Mottram CD: *Ruppel's manual of pulmonary function testing*, ed 10, St Louis, 2013, Mosby.

Myers TR, Op't Holt T: Asthma. In Hess DR, MacIntyre NR, Mishoe SC, Galvin WF, Adams AB, editors: *Respiratory care principles and practice*, ed 2, Sudbury, MA, 2012, Jones & Bartlett Learning.

National Institutes of Health: *Practical guide for the diagnosis and management of asthma*, Atlanta, 1997, US Department of Health and Human Services. Pub No 97-4053.

Paoletti P, Viegi G, Pistelli G, et al.: Reference equations for the single-breath diffusing capacity, *Am Rev Respir Dis* 132:806, 1985.

Sachs MC, Enright PL, Hinkley Stukovsky KD, Jiang R, et al.: Performance of maximum inspiratory pressure tests and maximum inspiratory reference equations for 4 race/ethnic groups, *Respir Care* 54:1321–1328, 2009.

Single breath carbon monoxide diffusing capacity (transfer factor): recommendations for a standard technique, *Am Rev Respir Dis* 136:1299, 1987.

Sivagnaname Y: Utility of measuring exhaled carbon monoxide (ECO) level in addition to pulmonary function test (spirometry) in the monitoring of chronic obstructive pulmonary disease (COPD), *Int J Med Sci Public Health*, Online First: December 31, 2013. http://dx.doi.org/10.5455/ijmsph.2013.181220131

Snow MG: Determination of functional residual capacity, *Respir Care* 34:586, 1989.

Togores B, Bosch M, Agusti AG: The measurement of exhaled carbon monoxide is influenced by airflow obstruction, *Eur Respir J* 15(1):177–180, 2000.

Wallace JL, George CM, Tolley EA, Winton JC, et al.: Peak expiratory flow in bed? A comparison of 3 positions, *Respir Care* 58:494–497, 2013.

Wanger J: *Pulmonary function testing*, ed 3, Burlington, MA, 2012, Jones & Bartlett Learning.

Whitman RA, Holland SA: Pulmonary function testing. In Wyka KA, Mathews PJ, Rutkowski J, editors: *Foundations of respiratory care*, ed 2, Clifton Park, NY, 2012, Delmar.

Zamel N, Altose MD, Speir Jr WA: Statement on spirometry, *Chest* 3:547, 1983.

SELF-STUDY QUESTIONS   *See Appendix for answers.*

1. Which of the following statements is/are true of the MEP test?
   1. A pressure of −20 to −25 cm H_2O usually is adequate.
   2. A pressure of +20 to +25 cm H_2O usually is adequate.
   3. A pressure of +40 cm H_2O is usually adequate.
   4. It is a good indicator of the patient's ability to cough.
   5. The patient should hold the effort for 1 to 3 seconds.
   A. 3 only
   B. 1 and 2 only
   C. 3 and 4 only
   D. 3, 4, and 5 only

2. The predicted FVC value for African-Americans is:
   A. 10% to 15% higher than that for Caucasians
   B. The same as for Caucasians
   C. 10% to 15% less than that for Caucasians
   D. 20% to 25% less than that for Caucasians

3. Which of the following test results is/are needed to calculate TLC?
   1. FRC
   2. RV
   3. V_T
   4. ERV
   5. IC
   6. VC
   A. 1 and 3 only
   B. 5 and 6 only
   C. 1 and 4 only
   D. 2 and 6 only

4. A normal MEFV loop test would show:
   A. $FEF_{50\%}$ less than $FIF_{50\%}$
   B. Predicted lung diffusion ability
   C. $FEF_{50\%}$ greater than $FIF_{50\%}$
   D. A normal FRC

5. A patient with a neuromuscular disease has been having serial bedside spirometry performed. Over the past 4 hours, her VC and MIP values have been decreasing. How should this be interpreted?
   A. Her strength is improving.
   B. She is not giving her best effort.
   C. She has undiagnosed asthma.
   D. Her condition is worsening.

6. An order is received to perform the following bedside spirometry tests on a patient: tidal volume, FVC, and peak flow. Which device would you take with you to perform the tests?
   A. Stead-Wells water-seal spirometer
   B. Maximum inspiratory pressure manometer
   C. Differential-pressure pneumotachometer
   D. Body plethysmograph

7. Before a patient does an FVC test, the pneumotachometer should have the following done:
   A. The gas analyzer should be calibrated.
   B. A CO_2-absorbing material should be placed in line with the circuit.
   C. A 3-L volume should be pumped into and out of the circuit.
   D. The kymograph speeds should be checked.

8. To help in the diagnosis of a patient with a questionable history of wheezing and possible asthma, which of the following would be the best test?
   A. Bronchoprovocation study
   B. Flow-volume loop
   C. Before-and-after bronchodilator study
   D. Airway resistance (Raw)

9. A patient has just been tested for C_L in a body plethysmograph. The patient's compliance was determined to be $0.2\,L$ $(200\,mL)/cm\ H_2O$. Based on this, the patient most likely has:
   A. Asthma
   B. Pulmonary fibrosis
   C. Emphysema
   D. Normal lungs

10. Calculate a patient's inspiratory time and expiratory time when he has an I:E ratio of 2:1 and a respiratory rate of 15/min.
    A. 1.3 seconds for inspiration and 2.7 seconds for expiration
    B. 1.7 seconds for inspiration and 3.3 seconds for expiration
    C. 2.7 seconds for inspiration and 1.3 seconds for expiration
    D. 3.3 seconds for inspiration and 1.7 seconds for expiration

11. When a patient performs an MEP test, it is important that he or she:
    A. Blow out all air before starting the effort
    B. Breathe in a V_T and blow out hard
    C. Inhale to TLC and blow out hard
    D. Exhale a V_T breath and inhale as hard as possible

12. A patient weighs $45\,kg$ (100 lb). The patient's predicted V_T would be:
    A. $250\,mL$
    B. $350\,mL$
    C. $450\,mL$
    D. $550\,mL$

13. An order is received to calculate a patient's alveolar ventilation. The patient's respiratory rate is 16, and average V_T is $580\,mL$. The patient weighs $170\,lb$. The patient's alveolar ventilation is:
    A. $410\,mL$
    B. $510\,mL$
    C. $750\,mL$
    D. $2720\,mL$

14. A patient has an $FEV_{1\%}$ that is calculated to be 80% of his or her FVC. On the basis of this finding, the patient probably:
    A. Has COPD
    B. Has a laryngeal tumor
    C. Has a fibrotic lung disease
    D. Is clinically normal

Note: Refer to the following figure for questions 15, 16, 17, and 18.

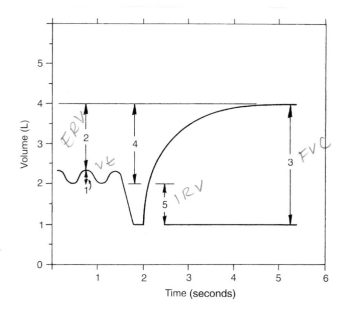

15. Which section of the spirometry tracing represents the FVC?
    A. 2
    B. 3
    C. 4
    D. 5

16. Which section of the spirometry tracing represents the V_T?
    A. 1
    B. 2
    C. 3
    D. 4

17. Which section of the spirometry tracing represents the inspiratory reserve volume?
    A. 2
    B. 3
    C. 4
    D. 5

18. Which section of the spirometry tracing represents the expiratory reserve volume?
    A. 1
    B. 2
    C. 3
    D. 4

19. The VC is made up of:
    1. RV
    2. FRC
    3. ERV
    4. V_T
    5. IRV
    A. 2 and 4 only
    B. 3 and 4 only

C. 1, 2, and 3 only
D. 3, 4, and 5 only

20. Which of the following are true of the PF measurement?
    1. It is usually seen at the end of the patient's FVC effort.
    2. It increases with height.
    3. It increases with age.
    4. It decreases with age.
    5. It is usually seen at the beginning of the patient's FVC effort.
    A. 4 and 5 only
    B. 1, 2, and 3 only
    C. 2, 4, and 5 only
    D. 1, 2, and 4 only

21. A respiratory therapist is having a patient perform the MIP test. His three attempts produce these results: $-15\,cm\,H_2O$, $-45\,cm\,H_2O$, and $-20\,cm\,H_2O$. The best explanation for these values is that:
    A. The patient is starting from the FRC.
    B. The equipment has a large leak.
    C. The patient is starting from the RV.
    D. The patient is not trying his best every time.

22. The physician wants to know whether a new bronchodilator would be helpful to the patient with asthma. The physician orders a before-and-after bronchodilator study. The patient has the following peak flow values: $7.5\,L/min$ before the medication and $9.4\,L/min$ after the medication. Calculate the patient's percentage change.
    A. −25%
    B. 1.25%
    C. 25%
    D. 80%

23. Complete spirometry is performed on a 50-year-old patient, revealing the following data:

	Predicted	Actual	% Predicted
TLC (L)	5.9	8.1	137
RV (L)	1.1	1.8	164
FVC (L)	5.0	2.6	52
FEF$_{25\%-75\%}$ (L/s)	4.2	1.5	36
FEV$_1$/FVC	75%	20%	27

How should the data be interpreted?
    A. Mild restrictive lung disease
    B. Severe restrictive lung disease
    C. Mild obstructive lung disease
    D. Severe obstructive lung disease

24. A nitrogen washout test for residual volume has been performed on a patient for 7 minutes and has not reached the desired nitrogen percentage. What could explain this situation?
    A. There is an oxygen leak into the system.
    B. The patient has an abnormally high respiratory exchange ratio.

C. The patient has severe air trapping.
D. Nitrogen has been absorbed into the patient's tissues.

25. A patient has been scheduled for a battery of pulmonary function tests. He tells you that he is so nervous about the testing that he has smoked four cigarettes in the past 2 hours. Which of the following tests is most likely to be adversely affected by this?
    A. FRC
    B. Lung diffusion
    C. Raw
    D. FVC

26. After spirometry is performed, it is important that patient flow rates be reported at
    A. ATPS
    B. BTPS
    C. STPD
    D. ATPD

27. A patient is performing a residual volume test on a water-seal spirometer in the pulmonary function laboratory. After breathing on the system for 1 minute, the patient takes out the mouthpiece and complains of being short of breath. What is the most likely problem in the pulmonary function system?
    A. The carbon dioxide absorber was accidentally left in the circuit.
    B. There is too much water around the spirometer bell.
    C. The carbon dioxide absorber has been left out of the circuit.
    D. Nose clips were left off of the patient.

28. Which of the following studies produces the most accurate determination of the TLC in a patient with severe emphysema?
    A. Single-breath nitrogen washout test
    B. Seven-minute nitrogen washout test
    C. Helium dilution test
    D. Body plethysmography test

29. The pulmonary function testing laboratory has recently acquired an exhaled nitric oxide analyzer. Which patient population should it be used with?
    A. History of COPD
    B. History of asthma attacks
    C. History of acute respiratory distress syndrome
    D. History of asbestos exposure

30. Before a patient performs a forced vital capacity test, all of the following should be done to the water-sealed spirometer EXCEPT:
    A. Make sure the circuit is airtight.
    B. Place carbon dioxide-absorbing material in line with the circuit.
    C. Pump a 3-L volume into and out of the circuit to check for leaks.
    D. Check the kymograph speeds.

31. A properly performed FVC test will not have:
    1. **Any coughing or leaks**
    2. **A weak patient effort**
    3. **An unsatisfactory start to the test**
    4. **Excessive variability among test results**
    A. 1 and 2 only
    B. 2 and 3 only
    C. 1, 2, and 4 only
    D. 1, 2, 3, 4

32. A patient has a suspected diagnosis of asthma. Which of the following tests would be the least helpful in assessing the patient for this condition?
    A. Before-and-after bronchodilator study
    B. Flow-volume loop
    C. Diffusion study
    D. Bronchoprovocation testing

33. A patient with a history of COPD has been admitted. To help clarify the patient's diagnosis as emphysema or asthma, which of the following should the respiratory therapist recommend?
    A. Flow-volume loop
    B. Maximum voluntary ventilation
    C. Spirometry before and after an inhaled beta agonist
    D. Peak flow test

Note: Refer to the following figure for questions 34, 35, and 36.

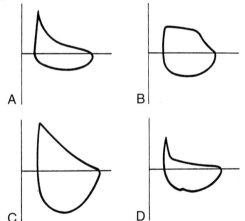

34. Which of the flow-volume loops represents the most severe small-airway obstruction?
    A. Tracing A
    B. Tracing B
    C. Tracing C
    D. Tracing D

35. Which of the flow-volume loops represents a fixed large-airway obstruction?
    A. Tracing A
    B. Tracing B
    C. Tracing C
    D. Tracing D

36. Tracing A represents a patient with asthmatic bronchitis, and tracing C represents the same patient 1 hour after receiving an inhaled bronchodilator medication. What conclusion can be reached?
    A. The patient's condition is treatable.
    B. The patient is not giving his or her best effort.
    C. The patient's condition has worsened.
    D. The patient needs another bronchodilator treatment.

37. As the PFT lab respiratory therapist, you have received an order to perform exhaled nitric oxide (eNO) analysis, spirometry testing, and residual volume testing on a 10-year-old girl with a history of wheezing and chronic cough. First, you perform the eNO analysis and find the girl's eNO value to be 35 ppb. How should this information be interpreted?
    A. The value is within normal limits, and the other testing should continue.
    B. The analyzer must be recalibrated to room air and the test repeated.
    C. The patient's value is increased from normal.
    D. The patient's other tests need to be performed first and the eNO test repeated.

38. Before performing a lung diffusion test on a patient, which of the following should be measured?
    A. Exhaled carbon monoxide
    B. Exhaled carbon dioxide
    C. Exhaled nitric oxide
    D. Exhaled oxygen

39. A Wright respirometer can be used for all of the following bedside spirometry tests EXCEPT:
    A. Tidal volume
    B. Minute volume
    C. Vital capacity
    D. Forced vital capacity

5

Advanced Cardiopulmonary Monitoring

Note: It can be anticipated that the Therapist Multiple-Choice Examination (TMC) will include an *average of 4 of 140 actual questions* (3% of the exam) on advanced cardiopulmonary monitoring. (This is based on the question mix typically found on the National Board of Respiratory Care's (NBRC's) previous Entry Level Examinations and Written Registry Examinations.)

Remember that the TMC version you take will include 20 additional questions being evaluated for possible inclusion in other versions of the TMC. So, there will be a total of 160 questions taken. There is no way to differentiate between the 140 actual questions and the 20 questions being evaluated for future use. Please go to the Introduction for detailed information on the Therapist Multiple-Choice Examination and the Clinical Simulation Examination.

MODULE A

Exhaled carbon dioxide analysis

1. Capnography (exhaled CO₂ monitoring)

a. Review capnography data in the patient record (code: IA13f) [difficulty: R, Ap]

Capnography is the analysis of graphic waveforms and numeric data from a patient showing the pattern and partial pressure of exhaled carbon dioxide ($P_{ET}CO_2$ or PetCO₂). It is wise to look for previous capnography data before measuring the patient's exhaled CO_2 level again. Look for numeric values as well as a printout of the tracing of exhaled CO_2. Be prepared to compare the previous information with the new data to help evaluate the patient's condition. It is also useful to compare the patient's CO_2 pressure in arterial blood ($PaCO_2$) with the capnography information, even though they should not be expected to be the same.

b. Recommend capnography (code: IE8) [difficulty: R, Ap, An]

There are three broad categorical reasons to recommend capnography.
1. Verify the correct placement of an artificial airway. It is a clinical standard that all endotracheal tube (ETT) and laryngeal mask airway (LMA) placements be confirmed by capnography. If the ETT is within the patient's trachea or a mainstem bronchus, or the LMA has sealed the larynx, the exhaled tidal volume

gas will contain carbon dioxide. Conversely, if the tube is in the esophagus, no carbon dioxide will be detected. Either waveform capnography or a disposable colorimetric unit may be used. Capnography should also be used during patient transportation to confirm the correct placement of the ETT. See the discussion in Chapter 12 for more information.
2. Assess pulmonary circulation and respiratory status. When a patient's cardiopulmonary condition is unstable, the exhaled carbon dioxide value changes faster than the pulse oximeter value. Capnography can be used to screen for a pulmonary embolism and to assess the effectiveness of cardiopulmonary resuscitation (CPR) efforts. If the $P_{ET}CO_2$ is <10 mm Hg, compressions should be improved. If the patient's spontaneous circulation should improve, the $P_{ET}CO_2$ will increase. See the discussion in Chapter 11 for more information.
3. Optimize mechanical ventilation. Tidal volume and mechanical dead-space changes will cause a corresponding change in exhaled carbon dioxide. As discussed below, in some patients capnography can be used as a monitoring tool to decrease the need for frequent arterial blood gas sampling for a $PaCO_2$ value. Volumetric capnography is used to calculate the V_D/V_T ratio, as discussed below.

c. Perform capnography to gather clinical information (code: IC2) [difficulty: R, Ap]

The capnometer is a device that measures the concentration of CO_2 in an exhaled gas sample from a patient. (Capnography involves graphically displaying the information provided by the capnometer.) The principle of operation of most bedside capnometer units is based upon carbon dioxide's absorption of infrared light in a narrow wavelength band (4.3 μm). Infrared light at this wavelength is passed through the gas sample to a receiving unit. The difference between what is transmitted and what is received is directly related to how much carbon dioxide is in the gas sample. In other words, the greater the difference between the sent and the received infrared light, the greater the concentration of carbon dioxide in the gas sample.

The capnometer is calibrated by comparing a gas sample without carbon dioxide (possibly room air) with a second gas sample containing a known amount of carbon dioxide. The first gas sample without CO_2 should give a "zero" reading. Adjust the calibration control to zero if needed. The second sample usually contains 5% to 10% carbon dioxide. The capnometer should display a CO_2 level that matches the amount in the known gas sample. Adjust the calibration control as necessary. The carbon dioxide level can be documented as a percentage or fraction (F_ACO_2) or as a partial pressure (P_ACO_2).

The capnograph is a strip chart recorder that provides a copy of the patient's exhaled carbon dioxide curve. There are at least two paper speeds that are useful for different purposes. The fast speed is most useful for evaluating sudden changes in the patient's condition. Each individual breath is easily seen (Fig. 5-1). The slow speed is most useful for trend monitoring (Fig. 5-2).

Two different gas sampling methods exist: mainstream and sidestream. The mainstream method involves having the infrared sensing unit at the airway; usually it is attached directly to the endotracheal/tracheostomy tube. If the patient is on a ventilator, the sampling adapter must be placed between the ETT and the ventilator circuit (with or without mechanical dead space). All inspired and expired gas passes through the sensor (Fig. 5-3).

The sidestream method employs a capillary tube placed so that a small sampling of the patient's exhaled gas can be drawn into the capnometer for analysis. It is not necessary for the patient's entire breath to pass through the sampling adapter; therefore it can be used in an unintubated

patient by placing the sampling catheter a short distance into a nostril. This can also be done with a special nasal cannula that delivers oxygen into one nostril and transports exhaled CO_2, via the other nasal prong, to the capnometer. If the patient is on a ventilator, the sampling adapter must be placed between the ETT and the ventilator circuit (with or without mechanical dead space). Remember that the patient's exhaled tidal volume (V_T) and minute volume ($\dot{V}_E$) are reduced by the amount that is drawn into the capnometer (Fig. 5-4).

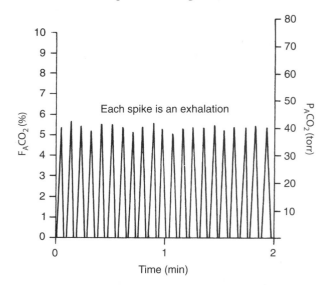

Figure 5-2 Normal capnograph tracing taken at a slow speed. The percentage of exhaled alveolar CO_2 is shown on the left vertical scale as F_ACO_2. The partial pressure of exhaled alveolar CO_2 is shown on the right vertical scale as P_ACO_2. The slow speed results in a blending of parts **A, B,** and **C** of the fast-speed tracing (Fig. 5-1). Each spike is part **C** of the curve and marks an exhalation. A slow-speed tracing is more useful in trend monitoring of a patient than a fast-speed tracing.

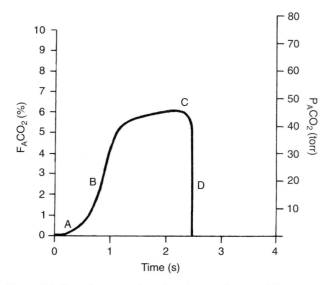

Figure 5-1 Normal capnograph tracing taken at a fast speed. The percentage of exhaled alveolar CO_2 is shown on the left vertical scale as F_ACO_2. The partial pressure of exhaled alveolar CO_2 is shown on the right vertical scale as P_ACO_2. (*Note:* Gas pressure can be listed as mm Hg or torr.) The tracing of exhaled gas can be divided into these four components: **A,** the beginning of exhalation, which shows no carbon dioxide in the upper-airway anatomic dead space; **B,** the addition of alveolar gas, rich in carbon dioxide, to the anatomic dead-space gas, which causes a rapid rise in measured CO_2 level; **C,** pure alveolar gas with a stable amount of CO_2, which causes a plateau—the end-tidal CO_2 point is shown at **C,** just before inspiration; and **D,** inspiration with a rapid drop in carbon dioxide concentration to zero. Compared to a slow-speed tracing, a fast-speed tracing is more useful for determining the cause of a patient's changing condition.

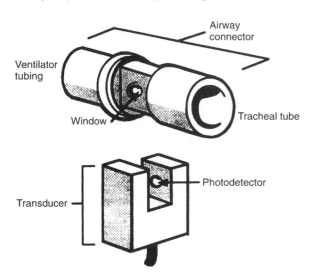

Figure 5-3 Schematic drawing of a mainstream exhaled carbon dioxide analyzer sensor. The infrared sensor is attached to the patient's airway so that all of the exhaled and inhaled gas passes through it. (From Szaflarski NL, Cohen NH: Use of capnography in critically ill patients. Heart Lung 20:363-374, 1991.)

d. Evaluate the results of the procedure (code: ID2) [difficulty: R, Ap, An]

It is known that carbon dioxide diffuses from the higher concentration in the tissues to the venous blood and is transported to the lungs to be exhaled. Figure 5-5 shows the normal physiology behind capnography. This diffusion or "flow" of CO_2 results in a measurable gradient or difference. In a healthy, upright-sitting person, a close relationship exists between carbon dioxide levels in both venous blood and arterial blood and the amount of exhaled carbon dioxide gas. The carbon dioxide level at the end of exhalation is most frequently monitored during patient care. This is called the end-tidal carbon dioxide pressure ($P_{ET}CO_2$). When ventilation and perfusion match well, as in a healthy person, the gradient between the arterial carbon dioxide level ($PaCO_2$) and the $P_{ET}CO_2$ is between 2 and 3 torr (mm Hg), with a range of 1-5 torr. The gradient will show the $P_{ET}CO_2$ level to be less than the $PaCO_2$ level. This is because the $P_{ET}CO_2$ value is an average of exhaled carbon dioxide levels from all lung areas.

Box 5-1 lists normal values of capnography. Three factors influence capnography's use and the interpretation of the results.

1. The first factor is the patient's metabolism. The average resting adult produces about 200 mL of CO_2 per minute, and fever and exercise increase this value. Hypothermia, sleep, and sedation decrease CO_2 production. Exhaled CO_2 is monitored during a CPR attempt to determine the effectiveness of circulation and ventilation attempts and to decide if the efforts should be continued or stopped. If no carbon dioxide is being exhaled despite proper CPR procedures, the physician may conclude that the patient's metabolism has stopped altogether and death has occurred.

There would then be nothing to gain by continuing CPR efforts. Conversely, a significant increase in exhaled CO_2 is strong sign of effective CPR efforts or the return of a spontaneous heart beat.

2. Although not a major factor, the patient's cardiac output (CO) is another factor that influences the use of capnography. Sepsis, which might double a patient's CO, reduces the partial pressure of CO_2 (PCO_2) by only a few torr. Cardiogenic shock, which reduces the CO, raises the PCO_2 only a few torr.

3. The third and most important factor is alveolar ventilation. A doubling of alveolar ventilation, under steady-state conditions for carbon dioxide production, results in a halving of the PCO_2 levels in

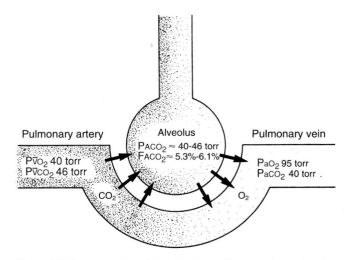

Pulmonary artery

$P\bar{v}O_2$ 40 torr
$P\bar{v}CO_2$ 46 torr

CO_2

Alveolus
$PACO_2 \approx$ 40-46 torr
$FACO_2 \approx$ 5.3%-6.1%

O_2

Pulmonary vein

PaO_2 95 torr
$PaCO_2$ 40 torr

Figure 5-5 Representation of the alveolar–capillary membrane showing the diffusion of oxygen and carbon dioxide and the arterialization of venous blood. Also shown are alveolar CO_2 values measured by capnography.

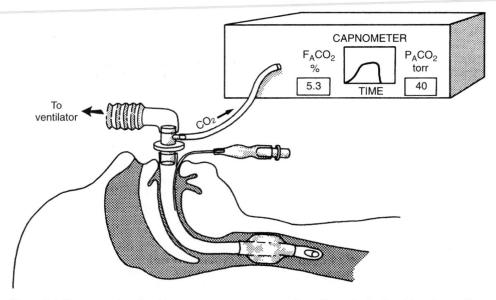

CAPNOMETER

F_ACO_2
%
5.3

TIME

P_ACO_2
torr
40

To ventilator

CO_2

Figure 5-4 Representation of a sidestream capnometry system. A capillary tube is placed into the ventilator circuit to sample the exhaled and inhaled gases.

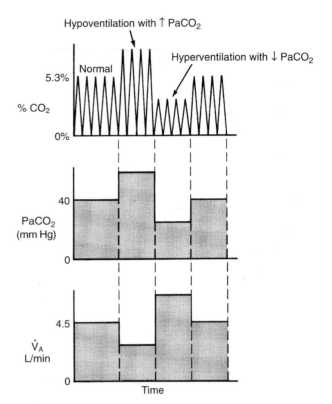

Figure 5-6 Relationship between alveolar ventilation, $PaCO_2$, and exhaled percentage CO_2. (From Pilbeam SP: Mechanical ventilation: physiological and clinical applications, ed 4, St Louis, 2006, Mosby.)

> **Box 5-1   Normal Blood Gas and Capnography Values (Based on a Sea-Level Barometric Pressure of 760 torr)**
>
> *$PaCO_2$[†] is 40 torr (range of 35-45 torr).*
> *$P\overline{v}O_2$[‡] is about 46 torr.*
>
> *The pressure of exhaled alveolar CO_2 (P_ACO_2*) ranges from 35 to 43 torr with the breathing cycle.*
>
> *The pressure of exhaled end-tidal ($PetCO_2$*) ranges from 35 to 43 torr. This shows the carbon dioxide level varying between the arterial and the mixed venous blood levels. This value normally trends with the $PaCO_2$ level.*
>
> *The normal trend between the pressures of arterial CO_2 and end-tidal CO_2 is about 2-3 torr, with a range of 1-5 torr. In other words: $P(a–et)CO_2$ is about 2-3 torr.*
>
> *The percentage of end-tidal CO_2 (F_ACO_2) is about 4%-6% and trends with the $PaCO_2$ level.*
>
> ---
>
> * The abbreviations $PetCO_2$, $P_{ET}CO_2$, P_ACO_2, and F_ACO_2 may be seen listed in the literature as end-tidal CO_2. The NBRC typically uses the abbreviation $P_{ET}CO_2$ for end-tidal CO_2.
> † $PaCO_2$ is the partial pressure of carbon dioxide in arterial blood.
> ‡ $P\overline{v}CO_2$ is the partial pressure of carbon dioxide in mixed venous blood.
> *Note:* Gas pressure can be listed as mm Hg or torr.

arterial blood and alveolar gas. However, a reduction of alveolar ventilation to half of its previous level will result in the $PaCO_2$ and P_ACO_2 levels being doubled (Fig. 5-6).

Tidal volume (V_T) and respiratory rate are directly related to alveolar ventilation. Of the two, tidal volume is more important because it relates to the patient's dead space (V_D) to V_T ratio (V_D/V_T). A decrease in the patient's V_T level results in less alveolar ventilation and a rise in PCO_2 level. Conversely, an increase in the V_T level results in more alveolar ventilation and a drop in the PCO_2 level.

Capnography is most accurate and correlates best with the $PaCO_2$ level if the patient's ventilation and perfusion match. The more ventilation and perfusion mismatching there is, or the more unstable the pulmonary perfusion is, the wider or less reliable is the gradient between the patient's arterial carbon dioxide and alveolar carbon dioxide levels. The following procedures should be performed to help understand the patient's condition and interpret the capnography results.

> **Exam Hint 5-1**
>
> Remember that mm Hg (millimeters of mercury) and torr are equivalent units of pressure. The NBRC uses these two units for different items in its questions. It uses mm Hg for blood pressure (BP) measurements and torr for blood gas values (such as $PaCO_2$ and $P\overline{v}O_2$). However, in questions referring to capnography, the NBRC has used both mm Hg and torr in its questions that relate to exhaled CO_2 (such as P_ACO_2 and $P_{ET}CO_2$).

2. Arterial–end-tidal carbon dioxide gradient

a. Review arterial–end-tidal carbon dioxide gradient data in the patient record (code: IA13f) [difficulty: R, Ap]

The arterial–end-tidal carbon dioxide gradient [$P(a–et)CO_2$] is the difference between the arterial and the end-tidal carbon dioxide values. This shows how efficiently carbon dioxide diffuses out of the arterial blood and into the alveoli for a normal exhalation. The normal gradient is 2-3 torr, with a range of 1-5 torr. However, in a patient with cardiopulmonary disease, the gradient will widen. The patient's previous $P(a–et)CO_2$ value should be checked before performing the test again. A narrowing or widening of the gradient would indicate a change in the patient's condition.

b. Recommend arterial–end-tidal carbon dioxide gradient measurement (code: IE8) [difficulty: R, Ap, An]

Recommend a $P(a–et)CO_2$ gradient measurement in a patient with cardiopulmonary disease to determine the baseline difference or to assess a change in condition. The possible gradient ranges from 6 to 20 torr in unstable patients with cardiopulmonary abnormalities. Once the gradient has been determined, it may be possible to monitor the patient's ventilatory condition by capnography alone. It may be possible to less frequently draw an arterial blood sample to measure the $PaCO_2$ level.

c. Perform the bedside procedure to gather clinical information (code: IC2) [difficulty: R, Ap]

Follow these steps to determine the $P(a-et)CO_2$ gradient:
1. Simultaneously: (1) draw an arterial blood gas (ABG) sample for $PaCO_2$ measurement and (2) have the patient exhale normally through the capnography unit to obtain an end-tidal gas sample for P_ACO_2 measurement.
2. The difference is the $P(a-et)CO_2$ gradient. The end-tidal sample commonly shows a lower CO_2 level than the arterial sample.

EXAMPLE 1

A patient is seen in the recovery room after surgery and has the following PCO_2 levels: $PaCO_2$ = 40 torr, $PetCO_2$ = 36 torr. Calculate the patient's arterial–end-tidal carbon dioxide gradient, as follows:

$$\begin{aligned} PaCO_2 &= 40 \text{ torr} \\ PetCO_2 &= \underline{-36 \text{ torr}} \\ P(a-et)CO_2 &= 4 \text{ torr} \end{aligned}$$

The usefulness of this gradient is demonstrated when monitoring a patient's spontaneous breathing during weaning or making ventilator changes in the tidal volume or minute volume. It may be possible to avoid drawing as many ABG samples.

EXAMPLE 2

The patient in Example 1 is seen later and has the following capnography reading: $PetCO_2$ = 54 torr. The patient's $PaCO_2$ level can be easily estimated by addition:

$$\begin{aligned} PetCO_2 &= 54 \text{ torr} \\ P(a-et)CO_2 \text{ gradient} &= \underline{+4 \text{ torr}} \\ \text{estimated } PaCO_2 &= 58 \text{ torr} \end{aligned}$$

It can be concluded that the patient is not breathing as deeply as before. Appropriate action should be taken to awaken the patient, further reverse the anesthesia, or begin artificial ventilation.

d. Evaluate the results of the procedure (code: ID2) [difficulty: R, Ap, An]

A wider than normal $P(a-et)CO_2$ gradient indicates abnormal ventilation and/or perfusion. As the patient's cardiopulmonary condition improves, the gradient should narrow closer to normal. It is also helpful to look at the patient's capnography tracing for any abnormalities. Review the components of a fast-speed capnography tracing in Figure 5-1 to understand a normal person's expiratory pattern. Figure 5-7 shows eight different abnormal fast-speed capnography tracings. See the figure legend for an explanation of each problem. As the

patient returns to normal, the tracing should approach that shown in Figure 5-1.

3. Arterial–residual volume carbon dioxide gradient

a. Review arterial–residual volume carbon dioxide gradient data in the patient record (code: IA13f) [difficulty: R, Ap]

The arterial–residual volume carbon dioxide gradient ($P[a-RV]CO_2$) is the difference between the arterial and the residual volume carbon dioxide values. This shows how efficiently carbon dioxide diffuses out of the arterial blood and into the alveoli during a maximum exhalation. The normal gradient is 4-6 torr and should be less than 7 torr. However, in a patient with cardiopulmonary disease, the gradient will widen. The patient's previous $P(a-RV)CO_2$ value should be checked before performing the test again. A narrowing or widening of the gradient would indicate a change in the patient's condition.

b. Recommend the arterial–residual volume alveolar carbon dioxide gradient procedure (code: IE8) [difficulty: R, Ap, An]

If a patient has an abnormal capnography tracing or an increased $P(a-et)CO_2$ gradient, it is likely that he or she has cardiopulmonary disease with significant ventilation and perfusion mismatching. A $P(RV-et)CO_2$ gradient measurement should be recommended to further evaluate the patient's condition.

c. Perform the procedure to gather clinical information (code: IC2) [difficulty: R, Ap]

Follow these steps to determine the $P(a-RV)CO_2$ gradient:
1. Simultaneously: (1) draw an ABG sample for $PaCO_2$ measurement and (2) have a cooperative patient exhale maximally through the capnography unit for the carbon dioxide level at residual volume.
2. The difference is the $P(a-RV)CO_2$ gradient. The alveolar sample commonly shows a lower CO_2 level than the arterial sample.

d. Evaluate the results of the procedure (code: ID2) [difficulty: R, Ap, An]

The graphic results will be similar to those shown in Figure 5-8. The wider the gradient, the greater the ventilation to perfusion ($\dot{V}/\dot{Q}$) mismatching. A gradient of more than 13 torr is considered to be markedly abnormal. This may be the case in patients with chronic obstructive pulmonary disease (COPD), pulmonary emboli, left-heart failure (LHF), or hypotension.

When comparing the normal (solid line) tracing in Figure 5-8 with the $\dot{V}/\dot{Q}$ mismatching (dashed line) tracing, note the increased gradient at end-tidal CO_2. With continued exhalation to residual volume, the LHF and COPD patients have a narrowing of the gradient. This can be used clinically to follow these patients' progress and

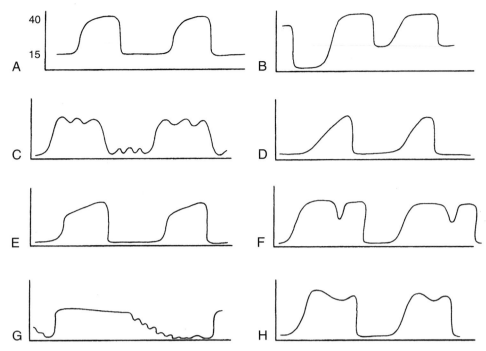

Figure 5-7 A series of abnormal fast-speed capnography tracings. **A,** A mechanically ventilated patient with a malfunctioning exhalation valve. Note that the baseline CO_2 level is elevated because the patient's exhaled breath is measured during an inspiration. Correction of the exhalation valve should result in normal inhalation and exhalation. **B,** This rapidly rising baseline gas pressure and failure to return to baseline is usually seen when moisture or secretions block the capillary tube. Clearing the obstruction enables the patient's gas to again reach the analyzer. **C,** Distortions in the tracing from incomplete exhalation. These may be caused by hiccups, chest compressions during CPR, or inconsistent tidal volume efforts during an asthma attack. **D,** An obstructive lung disease patient with ventilation and perfusion mismatching. There is no alveolar plateau with a stable CO_2 level. Inhaling a bronchodilator should result in the tracing returning closer to normal. **E,** A patient with restrictive lung disease showing no plateau of alveolar gas emptying. This is because the alveoli do not empty evenly. **F,** A sudden drop in carbon dioxide level in the middle of an exhalation indicates that the patient attempted inspiration. This "cleft" is usually seen when a patient who has been pharmacologically paralyzed begins to regain movement. **G,** Uneven carbon dioxide levels seen at the end of exhalation can be caused by the following: (1) the patient's heartbeat pumping fresh blood and CO_2 to the emptying lungs; the cardiogenic oscillations should match the heart rate; (2) the ventilator's exhalation valve is fluttering open and closed. **H,** The alveolar plateau is biphasic. This has been seen in patients with lungs that are different in compliance and ventilation/perfusion matching (e.g., single lung transplantation). (From Shapiro BA, Peruzzi WT, Kozlowski-Templin R: Clinical application of blood gases, ed 5, St Louis, 1994, Mosby.)

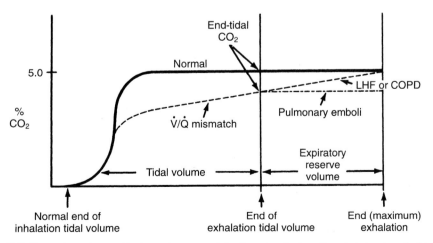

Figure 5-8 Comparison of several fast-speed capnograph tracings showing how the exhaled carbon dioxide level changes as the patient exhales to residual volume. A normal tracing is matched against abnormal tracings of pulmonary emboli, left-heart failure (LHF), and chronic obstructive pulmonary disease (COPD). The normal patient has the same end-tidal CO_2 level as the residual volume CO_2 level, showing good matching of ventilation and perfusion. LHF and COPD patients have a narrowing of the gradient as residual volume is approached. The patient with a pulmonary embolism keeps the same gradient at the residual volume as that found at the end of the tidal volume. (From Pilbeam SP: Mechanical ventilation: physiological and clinical applications, ed 4, St Louis, 2006, Mosby.)

response to treatment. The patient with a large pulmonary embolism will not have such a narrowing of the gradient as he or she exhales to residual volume. This patient's gradient will narrow to normal as the embolism is resolved and the physiologic dead space returns to normal.

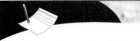

Exam Hint 5-2

Past exams have often had one question that requires the interpretation of capnography results, especially the end-tidal CO_2 value (PetCO2). Examples include a change in alveolar ventilation, shallow breathing, or a CPR attempt.

4. Capnography equipment

a. Assemble capnography equipment (code: IIA21) [difficulty: R, Ap]

As discussed earlier, capnography is used to measure a patient's exhaled carbon dioxide level and display the expiratory waveform pattern and/or numerical data. There are two different types of capnometer systems. Their main difference is in how the gas is sampled from the patient. Figure 5-3 shows the patient connection for a mainstream capnometer. Figure 5-4 shows a sidestream capnometer. Both work equally well if the patient is intubated. The capnometer connector is attached between the ETT and the ventilator circuit or T-piece (Briggs adapter). The sidestream unit may also be used with a spontaneously breathing patient because the capillary tube can be placed into a patient's nostril for gas sampling. The following are components of a capnometer system:

- *Airway attachment:* The mainstream and sidestream units must have both inhaled and exhaled gas pass through the sensor or connector, respectively. Connections must be airtight and free of obstructions.
- The *gas sampling capillary tube* of the sidestream unit must be kept clear of water or secretions.
- *Capnometer:* Periodically calibrate the unit with two gases of different CO_2 content. Room air is used for the "zero" value, and either 5% or 10% CO_2 in a pre-analyzed cylinder is used for the "high" value. Both values should calibrate within the manufacturer's specifications.
- *Capnograph:* Check that the paper speeds and marker work properly.

b. Troubleshoot any problems with the equipment [code: IIA21] [difficulty: R, Ap]

Capnometer systems have relatively few problems. The sidestream capnometer units must be kept dry. An external water trap is located between the capillary tube and the capnometer itself. Make sure that the water is drained periodically. Either capnometer system can be disconnected from the patient. This is seen as a drop in the exhaled carbon dioxide level to zero. The alarm should activate if it has been set.

c. Perform quality control procedures on capnometer equipment (code: IIC1) [difficulty: R, Ap]

Both mainstream and sidestream capnometer units are calibrated using two reference points. Room air is used to set the zero (low) point, and either 5% or 10% carbon dioxide from a cylinder is used to set the high point. Follow the manufacturer's guidelines regarding how much adjustment for the low point or the high point can be tolerated. Do not use a machine that cannot be properly calibrated.

MODULE B

Dead space to tidal volume ratio

1. Perform the dead space to tidal volume calculation (code: IC10) [difficulty: R, Ap]

Dead space is that part of the tidal volume that does not participate in gas exchange (wasted ventilation). A patient's dead space may be anatomic and/or alveolar. The dead space to tidal volume calculation (V_D/V_T) is performed to document the amount of a patient's dead space. There are several clinical situations, such as a pulmonary embolism, that can justify the procedure. Review previous data before repeating the test to understand if the patient's condition has changed or is abnormal. Be prepared to compare the previous information with the new data to help evaluate the patient's current condition.

The procedure is the mathematical comparison of a person's dead-space volume with tidal volume. Steps in the procedure are as follow (Fig. 5-9):

1. Determine the *average* exhaled CO_2 ($P_{\overline{E}}CO_2$) level by either of these methods:
   a. Collect the patient's entire exhaled gas sample over several minutes in a large airtight bag. Count the number of breaths that occurred. Calculate the average tidal volume breath by dividing the total exhaled volume by the total rate. Put all or part of this gas sample through the blood gas analyzer to determine the PCO_2 value.
   b. Have the patient's exhaled gas pass through a capnometer that can give you an average value (not end-tidal CO_2). The number of breaths should be averaged for greater PCO_2 accuracy. Measure or calculate the patient's average tidal volume over the time of the test.
2. Draw an arterial sample at the same time that you are performing either step 1a or step 1b. Have the blood sample analyzed for $PaCO_2$ level.
3. Calculate the results using either of two methods.

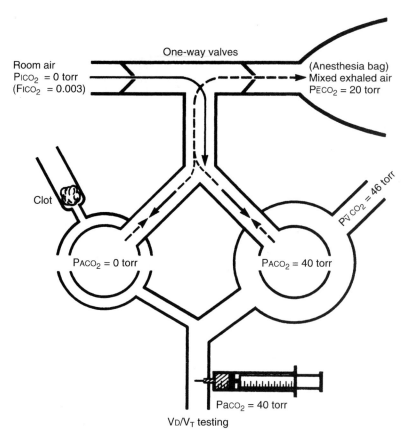

Figure 5-9 A schematic presentation of the procedure for gathering patient samples for calculating the dead space to tidal volume ratio (V_D/V_T). An anesthesia or other airtight bag is used to gather all exhaled gas to determine the average exhaled carbon dioxide pressure. An arterial sample is collected for $PaCO_2$ determination. (From Pilbeam SP: Mechanical ventilation: physiological and clinical applications, ed 4, St Louis, 2006, Mosby.)

a. Determine the decimal fraction or percentage of dead space

Place both carbon dioxide values into the following formula, which is derived from the original Bohr formula:

$$V_D/V_T \text{ (or } V_D) = \frac{(PaCO_2 - P_{\bar{E}}CO_2)}{PaCO_2}$$

In this formula:

V_D/V_T or V_D is the patient's physiologic dead space,

$PaCO_2$ is the patient's arterial carbon dioxide pressure,

$P_{\bar{E}}CO_2$ is the patient's average exhaled carbon dioxide pressure.

The following example is based on an abnormal adult:

$$PaCO_2 = 45 \text{ torr}$$
$$P_{\bar{E}}CO_2 = 18 \text{ torr}$$
$$V_D = \frac{(45 - 18)}{45}$$
$$= \frac{27}{45} = 0.6$$

The patient's V_D fraction can be recorded as 0.6 or 60%. (Note that this equation must be used when the patient's tidal volume is not known.)

b. Determine the dead-space volume

Place both carbon dioxide values into this formula, which is derived from the original Bohr formula:

$$V_D/V_T \text{(or } V_D) = \frac{(PaCO_2 - P_{\bar{E}}CO_2)}{PaCO_2} \times V_T$$

In this formula:

V_D/V_T or V_D is the patient's physiologic dead space,

V_T is the average exhaled tidal volume,

$PaCO_2$ is the patient's arterial carbon dioxide pressure,

$P_{\bar{E}}CO_2$ is the patient's average exhaled carbon dioxide pressure.

The following example is based on a normal adult:

$$V_T = 500 \text{ mL}$$
$$PaCO_2 = 40 \text{ torr}$$
$$P_{\bar{E}}CO_2 = 28 \text{ torr}$$
$$V_D = \frac{(40 - 28)}{40} = \frac{12}{40} \times 500 = 0.3 \times 500 \text{ mL} = 150 \text{ mL}$$

The patient's physiologic V_D volume = 150 mL. (Note that this equation must be used when the patient's tidal volume is known.)

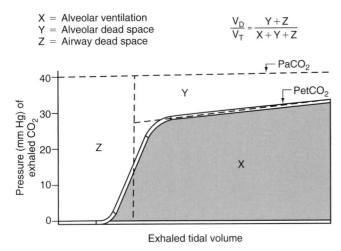

$$\frac{V_D}{V_T} = \frac{Y+Z}{X+Y+Z}$$

X = Alveolar ventilation
Y = Alveolar dead space
Z = Airway dead space

Figure 5-10 A graphic representation of the factors involved in the calculation of a patient's dead-space volume, or dead-space to tidal volume (V_D/V_T) ratio, through volumetric capnography. These units can measure exhaled carbon dioxide (by pressure or percentage) at time intervals as the patient's tidal volume is exhaled. Review Figure 5-1, as needed, for a normal capnograph tracing.

In addition, the preceding equation allows calculation of the patient's V_D/V_T ratio. In this example, it is 150/500, 0.3, or 30%, depending on how it is written.

Volumetric capnography technology allows the patient's dead space to be rapidly determined. These units can simultaneously measure the patient's exhaled tidal volume and the variable percentage of carbon dioxide found during the exhalation (Fig. 5-10). The computer that is integrated with the volumetric capnography unit then calculates the volume of dead space as a fraction of the exhaled tidal volume. Figure 5-11 shows how volumetric capnography can be set up to measure the dead space of a patient requiring mechanical ventilation. This technology permits the rapid assessment of a patient as treatment is being performed. For example, if a patient had a large pulmonary embolism resulting in significant dead space, a clot-dissolving medication such as streptokinase (Kabikinase or Streptase) or alteplase (Activase) would be given. These thrombolytic medications will rapidly dissolve the patient's pulmonary embolism. With volumetric capnography, the dead-space volume can be monitored as it normalizes when blood flow through the lungs is restored.

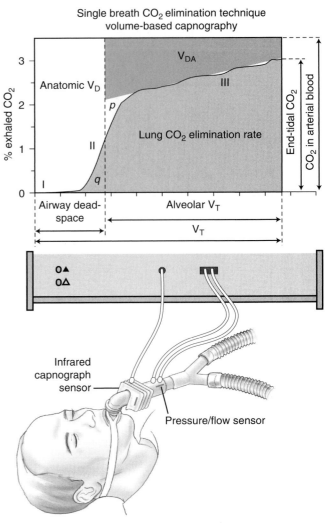

Figure 5-11 Measurement of volumetric capnography on a patient receiving mechanical ventilation. All measurements are taken between the patient's ETT and the mechanical ventilator circuit. The mainstream capnograph sensor sends data on exhaled carbon dioxide concentration to the computer within the capnograph monitor. The pressure and flow sensors send data to the computer to determine the exhaled volume. The computer integrates the information to determine anatomic dead space (white area) and alveolar dead space (dark gray area). With areas q and p being calculated as equal, the shaded area is alveolar volume where gas exchange occurs.

2. Evaluate the results of the V_D/V_T calculation (code: ID9) [difficulty: R, Ap, An]

The normal adult's V_D/V_T ratio ranges from 0.2 (20%) to 0.4 (40%). Anatomic dead space is normally greater in men than in women. The normal 3-kg neonate's dead-space to tidal volume ratio is 0.3 (30%). Physiologic dead space (also known as respiratory dead space) is gas that is breathed into the lungs but does not take part in gas exchange. This is because the alveoli are not perfused or are underperfused for the amount of gas that they receive.

Exam Hint 5-3

Past examinations have included a V_D/V_T calculation. Be prepared to calculate the value by either method. In addition, know the information needed to make the calculation, for example, average exhaled carbon dioxide value ($P_{\overline{E}}CO_2$) rather than end-tidal carbon dioxide value (PetCO$_2$).

Physiologic dead space is composed of the following:

- Anatomic dead space, or the gas in the connecting airways from the nose and mouth to the terminal bronchioles. Generally it is assumed to be about 1 mL/lb of ideal body weight, or 2.2 mL/kg of ideal body weight.
- Alveolar dead space that is composed of nonfunctioning alveoli that are ventilated but not perfused is minimal in a normal person. The previous "normal" adult example has the expected amount of dead space for his or her weight.

The following conditions or pulmonary disorders can cause the ratio to vary from the normal range:

a. Decreased V_D/V_T ratio

1. Lung resection or pneumonectomy, because the airways are removed; the patient will maintain his or her tidal volume in the other lung segments.
2. Asthma attack, because the airways are narrowed.
3. Insertion of an endotracheal or tracheostomy tube, because the upper airway is bypassed.
4. Exercise in the normal, healthy person, because the increased BP increases perfusion of the apices (Zone 1).

b. Increased V_D/V_T ratio

1. Vascular tumor in the lung, because of decreased perfusion to ventilated alveoli.
2. Pulmonary embolism, because of lack of blood flow to ventilated alveoli. Consider this if the patient is a candidate for a pulmonary embolism and suddenly deteriorates.
3. Circulatory disorders such as shock, sepsis, congestive heart failure, or CPR because of decreased blood flow to the lungs.

c. Increased dead space effect with ventilation greater than perfusion ($\dot{V} > \dot{Q}$)

1. Rapid, shallow ventilations, because the upper airway dead space is overventilated compared with the alveoli.
2. Mechanical dead space added to the ventilator circuit. This is an intentional effort to have the patient retain some of his or her exhaled carbon dioxide to correct for a respiratory alkalosis.
3. COPD (bronchitis, bronchiectasis, cystic fibrosis, emphysema), because varying degrees of bronchospasm, mucous plugging, and tissue destruction lead to increased ventilation and perfusion mismatching.

Many clinicians believe that a dead space/tidal volume ratio of 0.6 (60%) or more is an indication for mechanically ventilating the patient. A person who is wasting 60% or more of his or her ventilation will soon tire from the work of breathing and go into ventilatory failure.

Exam Hint 5-4

Remember that a pulmonary embolism is the most likely cause of a sudden increase in dead space. This concept is usually tested. In addition, there is usually a question that relates to identifying that a COPD patient will have a chronically increased V_D/V_T value.

MODULE C

Hemodynamic monitoring

The current NBRC Detailed Content Outline has been streamlined by placing all measurements related to cardiovascular function into the broad category of "hemodynamic monitoring." The following topics are included because they have been specifically listed on previous versions of the Detailed Content Outline and tested on previous versions of the NBRC's exams.

1. Blood pressure

a. Evaluate data in the patient record for a trend in BP (code: IA14) [difficulty: R, Ap]

Systemic arterial blood pressure (BP) is the force exerted against the walls of the arteries when blood is pumped through them. As one of the vital signs, the patient's BP should be found in the chart. Review it to know the patient's normal BP reading and if it has been stable or variable with the patient's changing condition.

b. Recommend blood pressure measurement (code: IE12) [difficulty: R, Ap, An]

The patient's blood pressure (BP), and other vital signs, should be monitored as often as clinically prudent. If the patient's cardiovascular or pulmonary condition is changing frequently, the BP should be measured frequently. Continuous BP monitoring is possible with the insertion of an arterial catheter and related equipment (discussed below).

c. Perform blood pressure measurement (code: IC11) [difficulty: R, Ap]

The general steps in measuring BP were described in Chapter 1. The BP is usually measured on either of the patient's arms. Necessary equipment includes the proper size of BP cuff, a sphygmomanometer to measure the pressure, and a stethoscope to hear the sounds of blood flow returning through the brachial artery. Figure 5-12 shows the basic elements of the procedure. The cuff is inflated to a pressure that is greater than the patient's systolic pressure. As the pressure in the cuff is gradually decreased, the first sound heard (Korotkoff sounds) is the systolic pressure. The pressure reading at which this sound ceases is the diastolic pressure. BP measurement can usually be performed manually by a respiratory therapist or other trained health care professional. If the BP

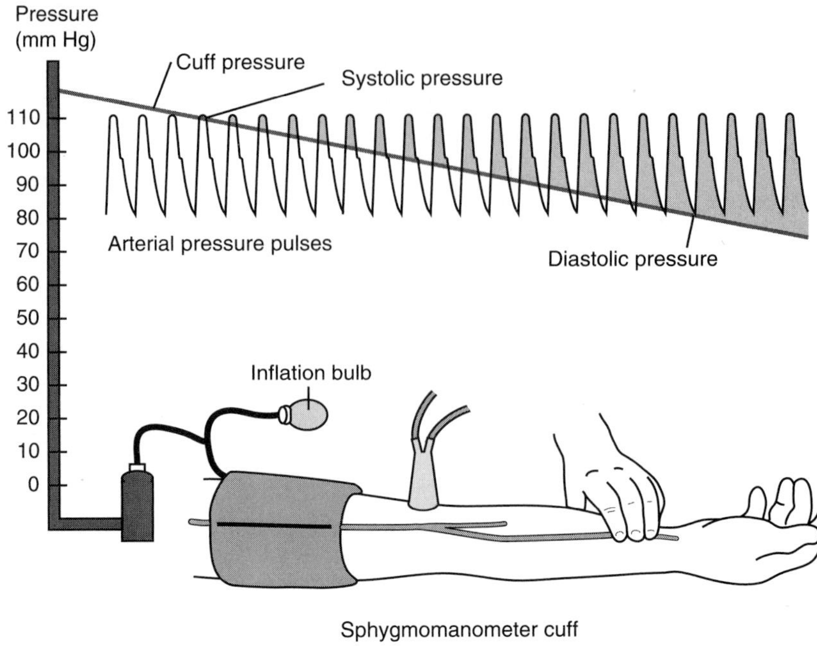

Figure 5-12 Arterial blood pressure is most commonly measured with a sphygmomanometer cuff that is inflated to a pressure greater than the patient's BP. When that happens, no palpable pulse can be felt. As the cuff pressure is gradually decreased, a respiratory therapist can listen, with a stethoscope placed over the brachial artery, for the return of blood flow. The first sound heard is systolic pressure (in this case 110 mm Hg) and the last sound heard is diastolic pressure (in this case 80 mm Hg). (Modified from Rushmer RF: Cardiovascular dynamics, ed 3, Philadelphia, 1970, Saunders. In Heuer AJ, Scanlan CL, editors: Wilkins' clinical assessment in respiratory care, ed 7, St Louis, 2014, Mosby.)

needs to be measured frequently, an automated BP measurement system can be set up on the patient's arm. This unit can be programmed to measure the BP on a schedule and can also have high and low BP alarm limits established as a safety feature.

d. Evaluate the results of the blood pressure measurement (code: ID10) [difficulty: R, Ap, An]

Review the general discussion on BP in Chapter 1. The following are normal BP values:

> Adult: less than 120/80 mm Hg

> Infants and children younger than 10 years: 60 to 100/20 to 70 mm Hg

Patients who have values that are higher or lower than these should be further evaluated. Know the following values because they represent a serious clinical problem:

Hypotension in an adult is a systolic BP of less than 90 mm Hg

Hypertension in an adult is a systolic BP of 140 mm Hg or greater, a diastolic blood pressure of 90 mm Hg or greater, or both

2. Central venous pressure monitoring

a. Evaluate data in the patient record for a trend in CVP (code: IA14) [difficulty: R, Ap]

The central venous pressure (CVP) is the pressure measured in a patient's superior vena cava, just above the right atrium (Fig. 5-13). Review previous patient data to understand whether there is an abnormality. Compare the current data with the earlier information to determine if there has been a change in the patient's condition. See Box 5-2 for normal values.

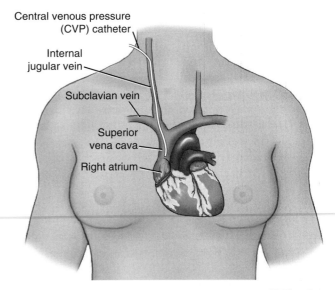

Figure 5-13 Proper position of a central venous pressure (CVP) catheter with its distal tip located in the superior vena cava, just above the right atrium. The catheter can be inserted through the internal jugular vein (as shown) or the subclavian vein. This traditional, single-lumen CVP catheter can be used to measure the pressure on the right side of the heart and to administer fluids or medications.

b. Recommend central venous pressure measurement (code: IE12) [difficulty: R, Ap, An]

The CVP is measured to know the pressure in the right atrium of the patient's heart. This information is used to help evaluate a patient's fluid status and to guide the administration or restriction of more fluids. A single-lumen CVP catheter (also called a CVP line) is inserted into patients for one or more reasons: (1) to monitor the

BOX 5-2   Normal Cardiopulmonary Values

Arterial Blood Pressure (BP)
   Adults: less than 120/80 mm Hg
   Infants and children younger than 10 years: 60-100/20-70 mm Hg
Central Venous Pressure (CVP)
   Range for a normal adult is 2-8 cm of water or 1-6 mm Hg
   Range for a normal infant is 1-5 mm Hg
   Range for a normal neonate is 3 mm Hg or less
Pulmonary Artery Pressure (PAP)
   Range for a normal adult is 15-28/5-16 mm Hg (about 25/10 mm Hg)
   Range for a normal adult mean PAP is 10-22 mm Hg
   Range for a normal child is 15-30/5-10 mm Hg
   Range for a normal neonate is 30-60/2-10 mm Hg
Pulmonary Capillary Wedge Pressure (PCWP)
   Range for a normal PCWP (mean) is 6-15 mm Hg (about 8 mm Hg)
Cardiac Output (CO)
   Range for a normal adult is 4-8 L/min
   Range for a normal neonate is 0.6-0.8 L/min
Stroke Volume (SV)
   Adults: 50-120 mL/beat
   School-age children: 35 mL/beat
   Preschoolers: 15 mL/beat
   Neonates: 5 mL/beat
Cardiac Index (CI)
   2.5-4.0 L/min/m^2 of body surface area
Arterial–Venous Oxygen Content Difference
   Range of normal is 3.0-5.5 Vol% of O_2
Shunt
   5% or less of CO
Pulmonary Vascular Resistance (PVR)
   80-240 dyn/s/cm^{-5} or
   1-3 mm Hg/L/min
Systemic Vascular Resistance (SVR)
   900-1400 dyn/s/cm^{-5}

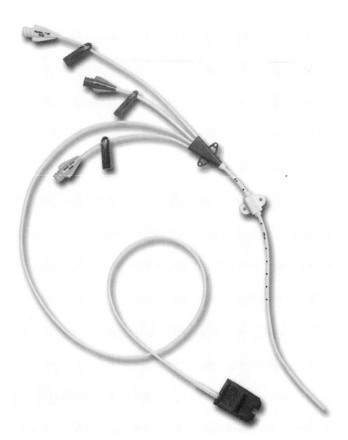

Figure 5-14 Triple-lumen CVP catheter that can be used to continuously monitor the patient's oxygen saturation of central venous blood (ScvO$_2$) in addition to measuring the right heart pressure and administering fluids and medications. (From Edwards Lifesciences LLC, Irvine, Calif.)

patient's right-sided (right atrium) heart pressure, (2) to rapidly administer a large volume of intravenous fluids, and (3) to administer cardiac medications during a CPR attempt. The development of a triple-lumen CVP catheter with integrated fiber-optic channel (Edwards Lifesciences, LLC) has enabled the continuous monitoring of central venous oxygen saturation (ScvO$_2$), in addition to the previously mentioned uses (Fig. 5-14).

c. Perform central venous pressure measurement (code: IC11) [difficulty: R, Ap]

The CVP catheter is usually inserted into the right jugular vein or right subclavian vein and advanced to just above the superior vena cava. When set up for monitoring pressure, it measures the right-atrial pressure (see Fig. 5-15 for how to perform the procedure). Note that the stopcock must be kept at the midchest (midheart) level. Usually a mark is placed at this location (on the patient's chest) for consistency. Raising the stopcock above the mark results in an incorrectly low reading. Lowering the stopcock below the mark results in an incorrectly high reading

(Fig. 5-16). Clinical practice is very important in learning how to perform this procedure. It is important that the patient breathes spontaneously if at all possible. Peak pressures during inspiration on a mechanical ventilator may artificially raise the CVP reading. Positive end-expiratory pressure (PEEP) may also raise the CVP reading. If the patient cannot be removed from the ventilator, take the reading during exhalation. Document the ventilator settings and whether the reading was taken with the patient on the ventilator. Record the data in the patient's chart or flow sheet.

Exam Hint 5-5

Past exams have asked about the proper placement of the CVP stopcock or arterial pressure transducer at the midchest (midheart) location to ensure accurate pressure measurements. Usually a mark is placed on the patient's chest for a consistent measurement point. Review Figure 5-16 for the effects of misplacement.

d. Evaluate the results of the central venous pressure measurement (code: ID10) [difficulty: R, Ap, An]

As noted earlier, the CVP is a measure of the pressure in the right atrium. The two main factors that influence the

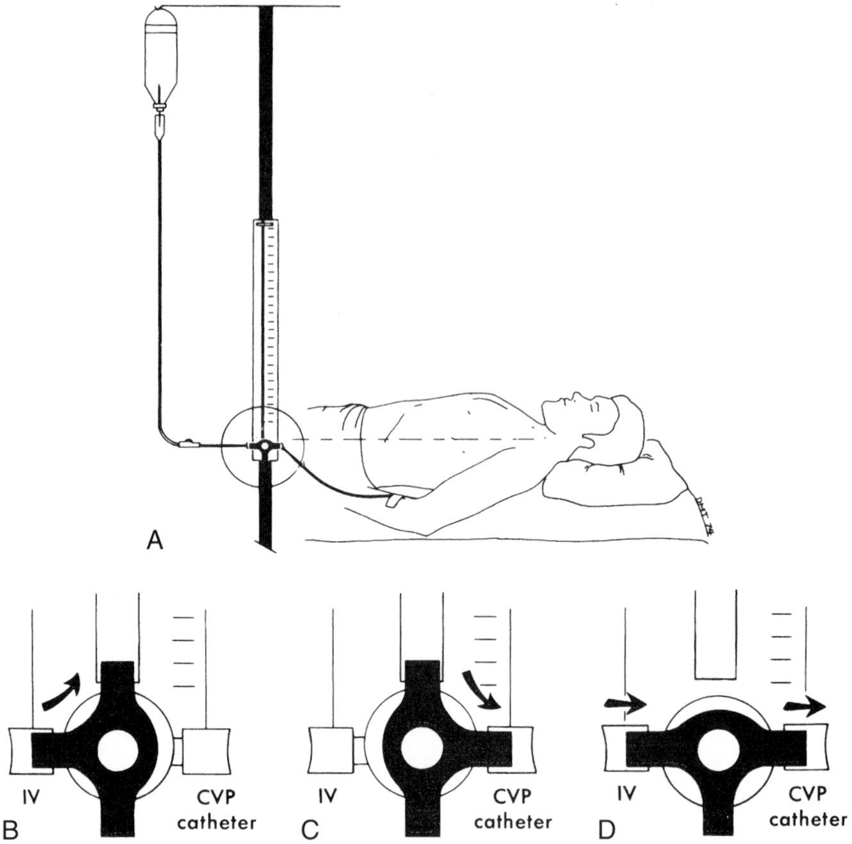

Figure 5-15 Procedure for determining the central venous pressure (CVP) with a manometer. **A,** Water-column manometer marked in centimeters, intravenous (iv) tubing, and patient in place. The patient must be placed in a horizontal position with the stopcock located at the midchest (midheart) point, as shown by the dashed line. **B,** Turn the stopcock so that the manometer fills with fluid above the expected pressure. **C,** Turn the stopcock off to the iv line so that the fluid flows from the manometer into the patient. Look at the stable fluid level for the CVP reading. **D,** Turn the stopcock so that the fluid flows from the iv line into the patient. (From Daily EK, Schroeder JS: Techniques in bedside hemodynamic monitoring, ed 5, St Louis, 1994, Mosby.)

right-atrial pressure are the blood volume returning to it and the functioning of the right ventricle (see Box 5-2 for normal CVP readings).

A decreased CVP reading usually indicates that the patient is hypovolemic. Hypotension confirms this. An increased CVP reading may suggest one of the following possibilities:

- *Fluid overload.* Check for an elevated BP and crackles in the bases of the lungs. Unfortunately, an elevated CVP reading is a late finding of this problem.
- *Tricuspid valve or pulmonic valve insufficiency or stenosis.* Abnormal electrocardiogram or echocardiogram findings or abnormal heart sounds (heart murmur) help to specify the problem.
- *Right-ventricular failure.* A right-ventricular heart attack can be identified on a diagnostic electrocardiogram. If a COPD patient with pulmonary hypertension has right-ventricular failure, the condition is called *cor pulmonale.*
- *Cardiac tamponade* (blood filling the pericardium). Watch for a drop in BP, tachycardia, and distended jugular veins. This problem can be rapidly fatal if not quickly corrected.
- *Atrial septal defect or ventricular septal defect with a left-to-right intracardiac shunt.* These congenital conditions are usually detected in a young child by an abnormal diagnostic electrocardiogram or an abnormal heart sound (heart murmur).

- *Pulmonary embolism (PE).* This condition should be suspected when a patient who has risk factors experiences a sudden onset of hypoxemia and clinical deterioration. Risk factors for a PE include immobility, atrial fibrillation, clotting abnormalities, and deep vein thrombosis. A pulmonary angiogram showing blocked blood flow through the lung(s) confirms the problem.

Exam Hint 5-6

Memorize the values listed in Box 5-2. Expect to see several questions in which these values are used as patient data or as options to answer a question. The normal values must be understood to identify any abnormal values and apply them to the patient's clinical condition.

---

3. Pulmonary artery pressure monitoring

a. Evaluate data in the patient record for a trend in PAP (code: IA14) [difficulty: R, Ap]

The pulmonary artery pressure (PAP) is the systolic and diastolic pressure found in either pulmonary artery. Review the patient's previous values before taking another pressure reading to make a comparison. Box 5-2 shows normal cardiopulmonary values.

To read the PAP, a pulmonary artery catheter (PAC) must be inserted through a vein and passed through the right atrium and right ventricle into the pulmonary artery. (The

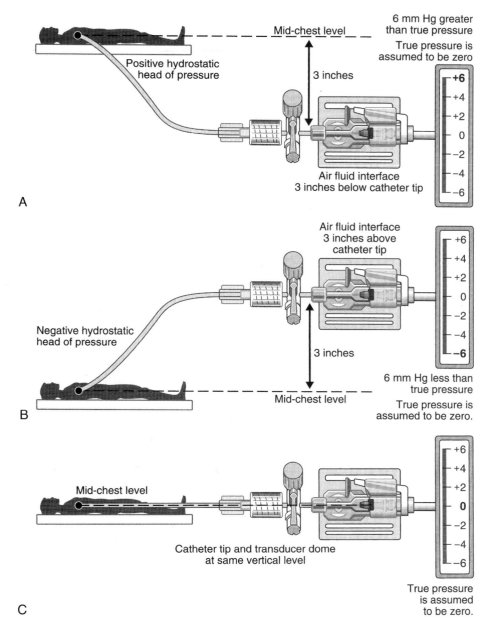

Figure 5-16 The effects of patient position compared to position of the pressure transducer. **A,** When the patient's midchest (midheart) is *above* the pressure transducer, the measured pressure will be *higher* than actual. **B,** When the patient's midchest (midheart) is *below* the pressure transducer, the measured pressure will be *lower* than actual. **C,** True pressures will be measured when the patient's midchest is the same height as the pressure manometer. All hemodynamic pressures (CVP, arterial pressure, pulmonary artery pressure, and pulmonary capillary wedge pressure) will be adversely affected if the patient and manometer heights do not match, as shown in **A** and **B**. (From Oblouk Darovic G: Hemodynamic monitoring—invasive and noninvasive clinical application, ed 3, Philadelphia, 2002, Saunders.)

NBRC often refers to this as a flow-directed pulmonary artery catheter. The PAC is also commonly called a Swan-Ganz catheter after the inventors who gave their names to a particular brand.) The common insertion sites, in descending order of preference, are the basilic vein in either the right or the left arm, the right internal jugular or subclavian vein, or the right or left femoral vein. The catheters are available in different lengths and diameters for pediatric and adult patients. Figure 5-17 shows a typical adult catheter.

b. Recommend pulmonary artery pressure measurement (code: IE12) [difficulty: R, Ap, An]

The PAP is important to measure in patients with severe pulmonary or cardiovascular instability, pulmonary hypertension, myocardial infarction, congestive heart failure, hypertension, and hypotension.

c. Perform pulmonary artery pressure measurement (code: IC11) [difficulty: R, Ap]

Figure 5-17 is an illustration of a 7-French (7-Fr) quadruple-lumen thermodilution PAC. In addition to measurement of PAP, it can be used to measure CO. Figure 5-18 illustrates how a PAC could be arranged with a pressure transducer and pressure monitor. Figure 5-19 shows a representation of the series of pressure waveforms seen as the catheter is advanced through the heart and into the wedged position in a branch of the pulmonary artery. Figure 5-20 shows a larger cutaway view of the heart with a PAC and normal heart chambers and related pressures.

To obtain an accurate PAP measurement, the equipment must be set up and calibrated properly, the distal lumen of the catheter must be patent with a continuous fluid-filled channel from the patient's bloodstream back

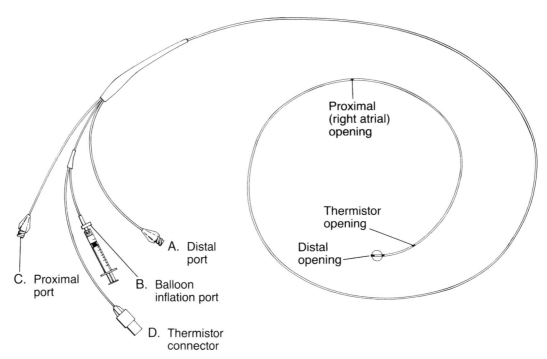

Figure 5-17 A 7-Fr quadruple-lumen thermodilution pulmonary artery catheter. **A,** Distal port goes to the tip of the catheter. It is used for measuring PAP and PCWP and for sampling blood for PvO$_2$ determination. **B,** Balloon inflation port is used to inflate the balloon for inserting the catheter and for obtaining a PCWP reading. **C,** Proximal port is used for measuring central venous pressure and for injecting iced saline for a thermodilution cardiac output (CO) study. The iced saline exits from the right atrial opening. **D,** Thermistor connector attaches to the CO computer. A bimetallic wire runs through the catheter to the thermistor opening, where it is exposed to temperature changes of the blood and cold injectate. (*Note:* Not all catheters are capable of measuring CO. Some catheters have other special features such as being able to continuously measure venous saturation or cardiac pacemaker leads.) (From Oblouk Darovic G: Hemodynamic monitoring—invasive and noninvasive clinical application, ed 3, Philadelphia, 2002, Saunders.)

to the transducer, and the catheter's balloon must be deflated. Clinical practice is important in understanding how to perform this procedure. Record the PAP data in the patient's chart or flow sheet.

d. Evaluate the results of the pulmonary artery pressure measurement (code: ID10) [difficulty: R, Ap, An]

Again, the PAP is the systolic and diastolic pressure found in the pulmonary artery (see Box 5-2 for normal values). Elevated PAP values are usually seen with the following conditions:
1. Left-ventricular failure/congestive heart failure, acute myocardial infarction, or fluid overload. To better identify the pathophysiologic problem, it is necessary to evaluate the following kinds of clinical information:
   a. The patient has a known history of heart disease or a sudden illness suggesting a heart attack.
   b. Crackles are heard in the bases of the lungs.
   c. Decreased static lung compliance is present.
   d. The patient has elevated pulmonary capillary wedge pressure.
   e. Decreased CO and/or low BP is present.

f. The normal gradient (difference) between pulmonary artery diastolic pressure (PAd) and pulmonary capillary wedge pressure (PCWP) is <5 mm Hg.

EXAMPLE

An adult male patient has the following PAC values: PAP, 35/25 mm Hg; PCWP, 22 mm Hg. Calculate the patient's pulmonary artery diastolic pressure minus pulmonary capillary wedge pressure (PAd–PCWP) gradient to help evaluate his condition.

Pulmonary artery diastolic pressure:	25 mm Hg
Minus the pulmonary capillary wedge pressure:	–22 mm Hg
The PAd–PCWP gradient is:	3 mm Hg

It can be concluded that his PAd–PCWP gradient is normal.
2. Pulmonary hypertension from COPD (usually emphysema). To better determine the pathophysiologic problem, it is necessary to evaluate the following kinds of clinical information:
   a. The patient usually has a known history of COPD.

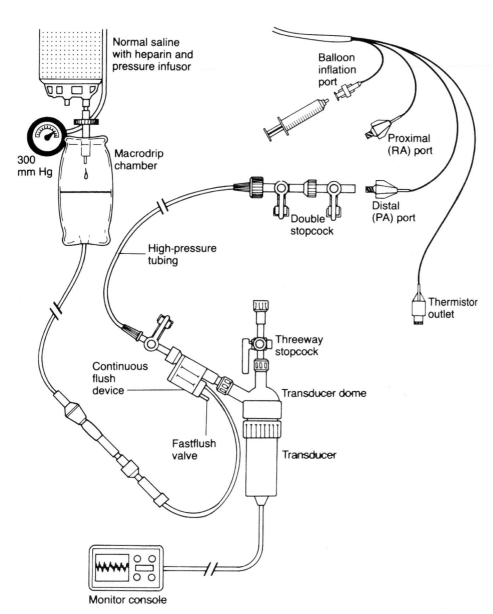

Normal saline with heparin and pressure infusor

300 mm Hg

Macrodrip chamber

High-pressure tubing

Continuous flush device

Fastflush valve

Monitor console

Balloon inflation port

Proximal (RA) port

Distal (PA) port

Double stopcock

Threeway stopcock

Transducer dome

Transducer

Thermistor outlet

Figure 5-18 The various components of the pulmonary artery monitoring system. It includes a fluid source such as normal saline that is pressurized to 300 mm Hg to maintain a flow of fluid through the tubing system. The continuous flush device (made by Sorenson) is designed to allow three drops of fluid per minute through the tubing system; pulling on the fast-flush valve gives a continuous flow of fluid to clear air or blood from the system. The transducer converts a pressure signal to an electrical signal that is sent to the monitor for display as numeric data and a pressure waveform. The high-pressure tubing transfers the patient's pressure accurately to the transducer. The double stopcocks are used to close off the tubing system or sample blood from the patient. This then connects to the distal port of the pulmonary artery catheter. This same monitoring system can be used with an arterial catheter for continuous pressure monitoring and blood sampling. (Adapted from Smith RN: Invasive pressure monitoring, Am J Nurse 9:1514, 1978. Copyright 1978 The American Journal of Nursing. Used with permission in Oblouk Darovic G: Hemodynamic monitoring—invasive and noninvasive clinical application, Philadelphia, 1987, Saunders.)

b. Systolic PAP may exceed 40 mm Hg if the problem is long-standing.

c. The PAd–PCWP gradient is greater than 5 mm Hg.

EXAMPLE

An adult female patient has the following PAC values: PAP, 35/25 mm Hg; PCWP, 8 mm Hg. Calculate the patient's PAd–PCWP gradient to help evaluate her condition.

Pulmonary artery diastolic pressure:	25 mm Hg
Minus the pulmonary capillary wedge pressure:	–8 mm Hg
The PAd–PCWP gradient is:	17 mm Hg

It can be concluded that her PAd–PCWP gradient is elevated.

3. Pulmonary hypertension from a pulmonary embolism. To better determine the pathophysiologic problem, it is necessary to evaluate the following kinds of clinical information:

a. The patient has a history of sudden vital sign instability, shortness of breath, hypoxemia, hemoptysis, and/or chest pain.

b. The systolic PAP is less than 40 mm Hg. This is because the relatively thin-walled right ventricle cannot rapidly increase its muscle mass to increase pressure.

c. The PAd–PCWP gradient is greater than 5 mm Hg if the embolism is large.

4. Pulmonary hypertension is present in a neonate with persistent pulmonary hypertension of the newborn (PPHN). This condition is often seen in the premature

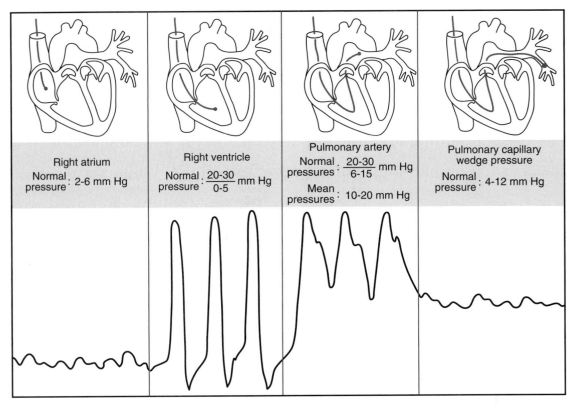

Figure 5-19 Sequence of pressures and pressure waveforms seen as the pulmonary artery catheter advances through the right atrium, right ventricle, and pulmonary artery until it wedges. Be observant of premature ventricular contractions as the catheter is advanced through the right ventricle. (From Heuer AJ, Scanlan CL: Wilkins' clinical assessment in respiratory care, ed 7, St Louis, 2014, Mosby.)

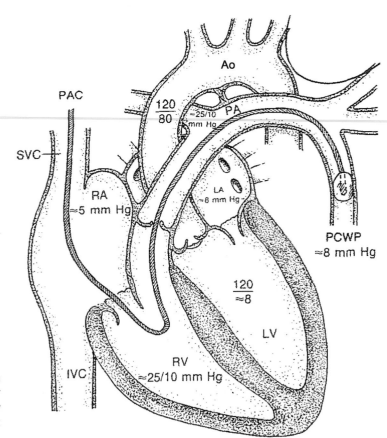

Figure 5-20 Pulmonary artery catheter (PAC) through a heart with normal chamber pressures. SVC, superior vena cava; IVC, inferior vena cava; RA, right atrium; RV, right ventricle; PA, pulmonary artery; PCWP, pulmonary capillary wedge pressure; LA, left atrium; LV, left ventricle; and Ao, aorta.

neonate with respiratory distress syndrome. When these neonates become hypoxic, the pulmonary vascular bed constricts. This causes the infant to revert back to fetal circulation. Administering 100% oxygen and hyperventilating the infant usually reverse the processes. The PAP then returns to normal.

Decreased PAP values are not frequently seen. Patients with hypovolemic shock, anaphylaxis (allergic shock), or excessive use of vasodilating drugs may have a decreased PAP. The most common clinical sign in these patients is a low systemic BP.

Exam Hint 5-7

Expect to see at least one question requiring the calculation of the PAd–PCWP gradient and at least one question requiring the result to be interpreted.

---

4. Pulmonary capillary wedge pressure monitoring

a. Evaluate data in the patient record for a trend in pulmonary capillary wedge pressure (code: IA14) [difficulty: R, Ap]

Pulmonary capillary wedge pressure (PCWP) refers to the pressure measured in the pulmonary capillary bed under no-flow conditions. It is important to review previous patient data before measuring another pressure. Normal values are listed in Box 5-2.

b. Recommend pulmonary capillary wedge pressure measurement (code: IE12) [difficulty: R, Ap, An]

Measuring the PCWP is important in patients with severe pulmonary or cardiovascular disorders, including pulmonary hypertension, myocardial infarction, congestive heart failure, fluid overload, dehydration, hypertension, and hypotension.

c. Perform pulmonary capillary wedge pressure measurement (code: IC11) [difficulty: R, Ap]

A PAC must be placed into a patient's pulmonary artery for the PCWP to be measured. The PCWP is obtained by inflating the balloon at the tip of the catheter. This temporarily obstructs that branch of the pulmonary artery so that the downstream pressure from the left ventricle is seen on the monitor (see Figs. 5-19 and 5-20). The balloon volume varies with the diameter of the catheter. The necessary volume is printed on the catheter near where the air is injected into the balloon. For example, the 5-Fr catheter balloon holds 0.8 mL of air and the 7-Fr catheter balloon holds 1.5 mL of air. It is important to inject only the required amount of air. Overinflating may burst the balloon or rupture the pulmonary artery. If the balloon wedges at less than the required volume, the catheter is probably too far down in the artery and may need to be withdrawn a short distance. The balloon is inflated only long enough to obtain the PCWP and then the balloon is deflated. Pulmonary infarction will occur if the balloon is left inflated and the blood in the pulmonary artery is stagnant and allowed to clot. Record the PCWP value in the patient's chart or flow sheet.

d. Evaluate the results of the pulmonary capillary wedge pressure measurement (code: ID10) [difficulty: R, Ap, An]

As noted earlier, the PCWP refers to the pressure measured in the pulmonary capillary bed under no-flow conditions. This pressure reflects downstream pressure from the left side of the heart. At diastole, in the patient without pulmonary hypertension or mitral valve disease, the PCWP parallels left-atrial pressure and left-ventricular end-diastolic pressure. The literature reveals that a variety of terms and initials are used to describe the same physiologic value. Do not be confused by reading about the pulmonary capillary pressure (PCP), pulmonary wedge pressure (PWP), pulmonary artery wedge pressure (PAWP), or wedge pressure.

Elevated PCWP is generally considered to be greater than 10 mm Hg and can indicate the following conditions:

1. *Intravascular fluid overload:* Review the patient's history to see if the patient is in renal failure or has recently received a large amount of oral or intravenous fluids. Perform a physical exam to determine if the patient has edema in the ankles or in the back, if the patient has been lying down. Look for jugular vein distension when the patient is lying back flat. Listen for crackles in the bases of the lungs.
2. *Left-ventricular dysfunction with congestive heart failure:* Perform the same assessment steps listed in point 1, above. In addition, look for a history of chronic heart failure or acute myocardial infarction.
3. *Mitral valve insufficiency:* Blood regurgitating back into the left atrium is shown as an elevated PCWP reading.

These conditions result in serious problems for the patient's lung function. When the PCWP reaches 20-25 mm Hg, fluid begins to leak into the pulmonary interstitium. This makes the lungs less compliant and increases the patient's work of breathing. A PCWP of 25-30 mm Hg results in frank pulmonary edema and dramatically decreases the patient's PaO_2 level.

Decreased PCWP is generally considered to be less than 4 mm Hg and can indicate the following conditions:

1. *Low intravascular volume (hypovolemia):* Review the patient's history for causes of dehydration (e.g., vomiting and diarrhea). A physical examination will show tachycardia, low BP, low urine output with a high specific gravity, tenting of the skin when pinched (showing poor turgor), and flat neck (jugular) veins when the patient is lying supine.
2. *Sepsis:* The patient's history will show infection, usually a septicemia. The physical examination will disclose tachycardia, hypotension, and oliguria, as noted in point 1. A major difference between hypoventilation and sepsis is that the patient will appear to be fluid overloaded because of the peripheral edema.

This finding is present when an infectious organism (often *Staphylococcus aureus*) causes a dilation of the peripheral vascular bed and leakage of fluids out of the vascular bed into the tissues. The patient will have weak peripheral pulses and feel warm.

5. Cardiac output

a. Evaluate data in the patient record for a trend in cardiac output (code: IA14) [difficulty: R, Ap]

Cardiac output (CO) is the volume of blood pumped in 1 minute. It is calculated as the product of heart rate (HR) for 1 minute and stroke volume (SV): CO = HR × SV. CO is a measurement of the heart's pumping ability to meet the body's needs. As always, review previous data before repeating the test. Box 5-2 lists normal values.

b. Recommend cardiac output measurement (code: IE12) [difficulty: R, Ap, An]

A CO measurement is performed on patients with serious cardiovascular disease to assess the condition of the heart. A major change in vital signs or new cardiovascular treatment justifies a measurement. Figure 5-21 shows the interplay of factors that can have an impact on a patient's CO. To measure CO, the patient must have a PAC in place that is capable of measuring CO.

c. Perform cardiac output measurement (code: IC11) [difficulty: R, Ap]

At the time of this book's publication, there are several CO methods that are commonly utilized in the cardiac catheterization laboratory. They will not be presented here.

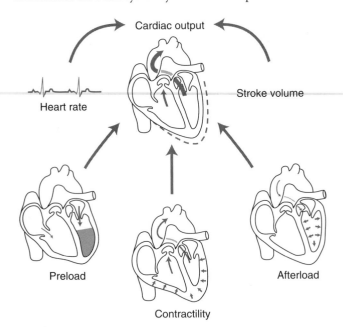

Figure 5-21 Factors that influence cardiac output (CO). CO is the product of heart rate and stroke volume (SV). SV is determined by preload (blood volume), contractility of each ventricle, and afterload (arterial resistance). (From Wilkins RL, Dexter JR, Heuer AJ: Clinical assessment in respiratory care, ed 6, St Louis, 2010, Mosby.)

This discussion is limited to Intensive Care Unit bedside procedures in which a respiratory therapist is likely to be involved. A thermodilution CO study involves using one of two special four-lumen PACs. Both catheter types require additional hardware and supplies, including a computer designed to calculate the CO.

The first type of thermodilution catheter is used to inject a cool solution into the heart. This cool solution is diluted with the patient's blood. As the blood and cool solution mix passes a thermistor at the catheter tip, the computer calculates the patient's CO based on the time required to pump the cooler blood past the thermistor (see Fig. 5-17).

This procedure requires an injectable saline solution or a 5% dextrose, ice–water bath to cool the injectate, necessary tubing and connections, thermometer, 10-mL syringes, and injector system (Fig. 5-22). It is beyond the scope of this text to describe all of the steps in the various types of adult and neonatal thermodilution CO procedures. Hands-on experience is necessary. Only the most important and common features are presented here:

- The usual injectate volume is 10 mL. The neonatal injectate volume may be reduced to 3 mL in an attempt to prevent fluid-overloading of the patient. The right atrial lumen is used for the injection.
- The usual injectate temperature is 0°C to 4°C. Some clinicians use room-air-temperature injectate because it is easier to work with. The cold injectate CO result may be more accurate because of the greater difference between its temperature and the patient's body temperature. If the patient is hypothermic, the cold injectate must be used for greater accuracy.
- Three injections are usually performed. The results are then averaged for the final CO value. Individual CO measurements that vary by more than 10% from each other probably indicate an error in the procedure. A compressed CO_2 "gun" is preferred to hand injection because the injector gun provides a smoother and more reliable injection. The injection must be completed within 4 seconds.

The "cool solution" thermodilution CO procedure has been available for more than 20 years and is widely used clinically. Its main disadvantages are that the CO value is available only intermittently, it is a time-consuming procedure, and patients with heart failure are given significant amounts of additional fluid for each CO calculation.

The second type of thermodilution CO catheter uses a thermal filament (a heated wire) that wraps around the catheter (Fig. 5-23). With this catheter, the computer periodically directs electricity to the filament. This results in periodic warming of the blood from the heated wire. The computer calculates the patient's CO by determining the time needed to pump the heated blood past the thermistor at the tip of the catheter. The advantages of the "heated wire" CO catheter are that it gives an updated CO value every 30 seconds, requires no additional time from the nurse or respiratory therapist after the initial setup, and does not add any additional fluid to the patient's intake.

d. Calculate the cardiac output value (code: IC10) [difficulty: R, Ap]

The following formula can be used to calculate a predicted CO for the adult patient. This value can then be compared with the actual patient CO.

$$CO = \frac{BSA \times 125}{0.045}$$

BSA is the body surface area and can be calculated mathematically or determined from a data table (Fig. 5-24). See the following discussion on cardiac index (CI) for information on calculating BSA.

The following two methods can be used to calculate the patient's CO:

1. A computer calculates the CO when either thermodilution method is used. As long as the procedural steps are done properly and the patient and catheter variables are programmed into the computer, the results should be reliable. This method is widely used at the bedside.

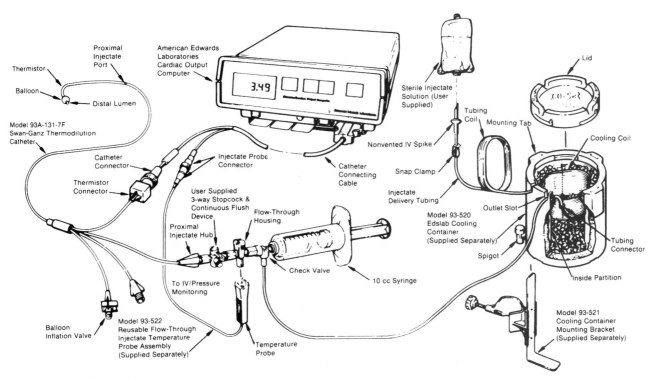

Figure 5-22 Complete system for performing thermodilution cardiac output studies. (From Edwards Lifesciences LLC, Irvine, Calif, 1985.)

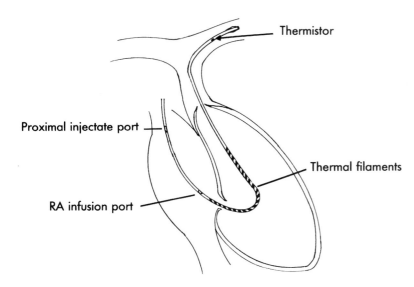

Figure 5-23 View of the right side of the heart showing a continuous cardiac output thermodilution pulmonary artery catheter in proper position. Note the thermal filaments that heat the passing blood. The resulting temperature change is detected by the thermistor in the pulmonary artery. (From Daily EK, Schroeder JS: Techniques in bedside hemodynamic monitoring, ed 5, St Louis, 1994, Mosby.)

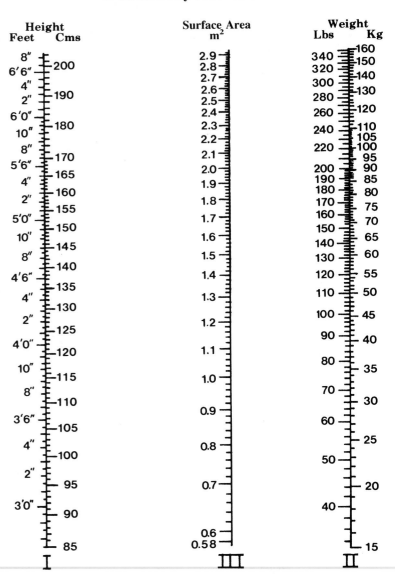

Dubois body surface chart

Figure 5-24 DuBois Body Surface Chart (as prepared by Boothby and Sandiford of the Mayo Clinic). *Directions:* To find the body surface of a patient, locate the height in inches (or centimeters) on scale I and the weight in pounds (or kilograms) on scale II. Place a straightedge (ruler) between these two points, which will intersect scale III at the patient's surface area value. (From Boothby WM, Sandiford RB: Boston Med Surg J 185:337, 1921.)

2. The Fick method of measuring CO is the "gold standard" by which all others are compared. Unfortunately, it is difficult to perform at the bedside and is primarily utilized in the cardiac catheterization laboratory. The patient's inhaled and exhaled gases must be analyzed for PO_2 level to calculate his or her oxygen consumption. In addition, arterial and mixed venous blood samples must be taken and analyzed for oxygen level to calculate the arterial–venous oxygen content difference ($C[a-v]O_2$). The following example shows fairly standard values for an adult:

$$CO\ (mL/min) = \frac{oxygen consumption\ (mL/min)}{arterial\ O_2\ content\ (Vol\,\%)-venous\ O_2\ content\ (Vol\,\%)}$$

In this equation:

Vol% is the volume percentage of milliliters of oxygen/ 100 mL of blood,

Oxygen consumption is 250 mL/min,

Arterial oxygen content is 20 Vol%,

Mixed venous content is 15 Vol%

Therefore:

$$CO = \frac{250\ mL/min}{20\ Vol\,\%-15\ Vol\,\%} = \frac{250\ mL/min}{5\ Vol\,\%} = \frac{250}{0.05}$$
$$= 5000\ mL/min = 5\ L/min$$

e. Evaluate the results of the cardiac output measurement (code: ID10) [difficulty: R, Ap, An]

As listed in Box 5-2, the healthy, resting adult has a CO in the range of 4-8 L/min, and a healthy, resting neonate has a CO in the range of 0.6-0.8 L/min.

CO can increase markedly in a person with a healthy heart who is stressed or exercising, has a fever, or has any other reason for an increased metabolism. All these conditions increase the person's demand for oxygen, which is primarily met by increasing CO. (To a lesser extent, the tissues extract more oxygen from the blood.) Sepsis is the most commonly seen condition that results in a high CO.

There are many possible causes of a decreased CO. The most common are hypovolemia, increased peripheral resistance, and heart failure. A patient with low CO often has a low BP. If the CO and BP are too low, the patient will develop metabolic acidosis from peripheral hypoxemia. Death can result if this is not quickly corrected.

6. Stroke volume

a. Evaluate data in the patient record for a trend in stroke volume (code: IA14) [difficulty: R, Ap]

Stroke volume (SV) is the volume of blood ejected with each heartbeat. It is the difference between the volume of blood in each ventricle at the end of diastole (preload) and the volume left in the ventricles at the end of systole (after ejection [*afterload*]). It is helpful to review the patient's previous CO and SV data before performing another SV measurement.

b. Recommend stroke volume measurement (code: IE12) [difficulty: R, Ap, An]

An SV (and CO) measurement is performed on patients with serious cardiovascular disease to assess the condition of the heart. A major change in vital signs or new cardiovascular treatment justifies a measurement. As shown in Figure 5-21, preload, contractility of each ventricle, and afterload can influence a patient's SV.

c. Calculate the stroke volume (code: IC10) [difficulty: R, Ap]

The normal SV is based on a person's age. See Box 5-2 for normal values. SV can be determined through a cardiac ultrasound procedure or can be calculated from the patient's HR and CO measurements.

For example, calculate an adult patient's SV when the HR is 100 beats/min and CO is 8 L (8000 mL):

$$SV = \frac{CO}{HR} = \frac{8000 \text{ mL}}{100 \text{ beats/min}} = 80 \text{ mL}$$

The stoke volume is not the entire preload volume. The SV portion of the preload that is pumped out of the ventricle is referred to as the *ejection fraction*. Under normal conditions, an adult will have an ejection fraction of 0.6-0.75. This means the ventricle ejects an SV that is usually 60% to 75% of the preload volume.

d. Evaluate the results of the stroke volume calculation (code: ID10) [difficulty: R, Ap, An]

The SV is the same for both ventricles except under pathologic conditions. Usually, however, only the left ventricle is of concern. The Frank-Starling curve shows us that as the heart muscle is stretched with greater volume, it contracts and pumps more completely, resulting in a larger SV. A left ventricle that has been damaged by a myocardial infarction

does not pump as effectively and the SV decreases. A drop in SV results in a decrease in CO unless the HR can increase to compensate for the difference. This is seen in many patients with heart disease. In addition, when a healthy right ventricle continues to pump more blood than the damaged left ventricle, the unpumped blood backs up into the pulmonary circulation and results in pulmonary edema (congestive heart failure).

7. Cardiac index

a. Evaluate data in the patient record for a trend in cardiac index (code: IA14) [difficulty: R, Ap]

The cardiac index (CI) is the cardiac output (CO) per square meter of body surface area. Review any previous information on CI before performing another calculation.

b. Recommend a cardiac index measurement (code: IE12) [difficulty: R, Ap, An]

If CO is being determined, the CI should also be calculated for additional information on heart function.

c. Calculate the cardiac index (code: IC10) [difficulty: R, Ap]

Because CI is the CO per square meter of body surface area, both CO and body surface area must be known. CO is usually measured by the thermodilution CO method via a special PAC. The BSA can be determined from the DuBois Body Surface Chart as shown in Figure 5-24. The body surface area can also be determined with the following equation:

$$BSA = \frac{1 + \text{weight in kilograms} + (\text{height in centimeters} - 160)}{100}$$

EXAMPLE

A 166-lb/75-kg, 5 feet 10 in/152-cm man has a CO of 6 L/min. According to the DuBois Body Surface Chart, he has a BSA of 1.92 m². His CI is calculated as:

$$CI = \frac{CO}{BSA} = \frac{6 \text{ L/min}}{1.92 \text{ m}^2} = 3.125 \text{ L/min/m}^2$$

d. Evaluate the results of the cardiac index calculation (code: ID10) [difficulty: R, Ap, An]

An adult's normal, resting CI is 2.5-4 L/min/m² of BSA. The CI is a much more accurate way of determining if the patient's oxygen demands are being met compared to simply looking at the CO. For example, a resting CO of 4 L/min is considered normal. This CO might be fine for a small adult but not for a large one. The CI takes into account the difference in body size. A normal CI indicates that the patient is receiving enough oxygen to meet the body's needs. A low CI should be a cause for concern; it usually indicates that the patient is not getting enough blood and oxygen to his or her tissues. Check to see if the patient's CO and BP are also low and if the patient has hypoxemia or acidosis. If these conditions exist, they must be corrected as quickly as possible to prevent dire consequences. A high CI indicates that the patient is pumping more blood than appears to be necessary. Investigate why this is occurring. See the earlier discussion on CO and the factors that affect it to understand the factors that affect CI as well.

8. Mixed venous blood sampling

a. Evaluate data in the patient record for a trend in mixed venous oxygen (code: IA14) [difficulty: R, Ap]

Mixed venous blood sampling involves taking blood from either the pulmonary artery or the superior vena cava. The gold standard for this procedure involves the analysis of true mixed venous blood taken from the pulmonary artery through a PAC. The pressure of mixed venous oxygen ($P\bar{v}O_2$) and the saturation of mixed venous oxygen ($S\bar{v}O_2$) represent tissue oxygenation. This is because the blood has returned *from* the body after having some of its oxygen extracted. (Remember that PaO_2 and SaO_2 represent the supply of oxygen *to* the tissues.) Another option involves the use of a CVP catheter equipped with fiber-optic technology for the measurement of the saturation of central venous oxygen ($ScvO_2$). As always, the $P\bar{v}O_2$ or $ScvO_2$ value(s) should be reviewed before performing another measurement.

b. Recommend a mixed venous oxygen measurement (code: IE12) [difficulty: R, Ap, An]

Recommend a mixed venous oxygen measurement if it is clinically important to know the patient's level of tissue oxygenation. Low $P\bar{v}O_2$, $S\bar{v}O_2$, and $ScvO_2$ values are often seen in patients with heart failure because the slow flow of blood through the tissues results in more oxygen being extracted. In addition, $P\bar{v}O_2$ and $S\bar{v}O_2$ values are needed to calculate a patient's arterial–venous oxygen content difference or shunt percentage.

Because of technical difficulties and increased risks associated with the placement of a PAC, the placement of a triple-lumen CVP catheter with fiber-optic channel for $ScvO_2$ monitoring may be recommended. This CVP catheter has been found useful in monitoring patients with increased intracranial pressure, heart failure, heart surgery, and severe sepsis. Information from either catheter is very helpful in managing these critically ill patients.

c. Perform mixed venous oxygen measurement (code: IC11) [difficulty: R, Ap]

A patient with a functioning PAC can have a sample of blood withdrawn through it and analyzed for the $P\bar{v}O_2$ value (and the other blood gas values as well). There are currently three methods of performing the bedside procedure.

1. Perform the procedure through the distal lumen of a PAC as it is being inserted

This method is employed when trying to determine whether there is a ventricular septal defect. The procedure is commonly done on neonates with suspected congenital heart defects, but may be used in adults as well. Using sterile technique, blood samples are withdrawn serially from the right atrium, the right ventricle, and sometimes the pulmonary artery.

Normally, the $P\bar{v}O_2$ and $S\bar{v}O_2$ values are the same in all blood samples. The patient with a ventricular septal defect shows a significant increase in $P\bar{v}O_2$ and $S\bar{v}O_2$ values when measurements are taken from the right atrium, the right ventricle, and the pulmonary artery. This is because the oxygenated blood from the left ventricle is forced though the ventricular septal defect to raise the oxygen value of the right-ventricular blood. In other words, the $P\bar{v}O_2$ and $S\bar{v}O_2$ values will be higher in the right ventricle and pulmonary artery than the right atrium.

2. Use a PAC with reflectance oximetry capability

These catheters have fiber-optic bundles built into them and use technology similar to that used in pulse oximeters (Fig. 5-25). The processing unit sends two narrow wavebands of light down the transmitting fiber-optic bundle to be illuminated on the passing blood in the pulmonary artery. Oxyhemoglobin in the red blood cells absorbs some of the light. The rest is reflected. The receiving fiber-optic bundle picks up some of this light and transmits it back to the monitoring unit.

$S\bar{v}O_2$ is determined by the monitoring unit based on the light waves that were transmitted and received. Care must be taken when using this catheter in patients with elevated carboxyhemoglobin or methemoglobin levels. As with pulse oximetry, carboxyhemoglobin and methemoglobin will be interpreted as oxyhemoglobin. Thus inaccurately high readings will be seen.

An actual mixed venous blood sample can be taken with this catheter through the distal lumen as described next. The advantage of the reflectance oximetry system is that it provides continuous monitoring of the patient's venous oxygen level. In addition, high and low saturation alarms can be set. The alarms would warn the clinician of a problem with the patient or the equipment. For example, a sudden decrease in the $S\bar{v}O_2$ value could indicate the patient is hypoxemic or the tip of the catheter has become lodged in the wall of the artery. The situation must be investigated.

3. Use the distal lumen of a "standard" PAC

A true mixed venous blood sample is obtained by withdrawing blood from the distal lumen of the catheter. This is the same lumen that is used for the PAP and PCWP readings. Using sterile technique, a 5- to 10-mL syringe is used to withdraw the heparinized solution in the lumen until about 1-2 mL of blood is removed. A second preheparinized syringe is then used to withdraw about 2 mL of mixed venous blood. It is important to withdraw the intravenous (iv) solution and blood at a rate no faster than 0.5 mL per second. Withdrawing at a faster rate can

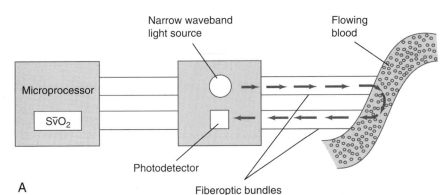

Narrow waveband light source

Flowing blood

Microprocessor

$S\bar{v}O_2$

Photodetector

Fiberoptic bundles

A

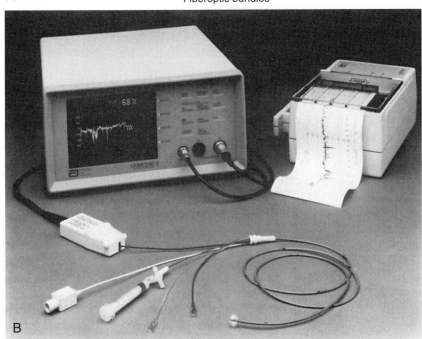

B

Figure 5-25 Mixed venous oxygen saturation ($S\bar{v}O_2$) can be monitored continuously by reflection spectrophotometry (spectroscopy) in the appropriate pulmonary artery catheter (PAC). (Note that the same technology is used in a CVP catheter that measures continuous central venous oxygen saturation.) **A,** Detail of the fiber-optic bundles in the catheter. Specific wavelengths of light are directed at passing blood. Some of the light is absorbed by the passing red blood cells and some is reflected back to the photodetector. The microprocessor calculates the percentage $S\bar{v}O_2$. **B,** Components of the system include (1) microprocessor that connects to the catheter, displays the $S\bar{v}O_2$ % values, and has high and low saturation alarms; (2) strip-chart recorder to copy the saturation values over time; and (3) fiber-optic reflective spectroscopy-type PAC. The catheter can also be used for measuring pulmonary artery pressure, pulmonary capillary wedge pressure, and cardiac output and for obtaining a mixed venous blood gas sample. **A,** from Mottram CD: Ruppel's manual of pulmonary function testing, ed 10, St Louis, 2013, Mosby. **B,** Courtesy of Abbott Critical Care Systems, Mountain View, Calif.

pull preoxygenated blood back through the capillary bed and give falsely elevated oxygen values. After sampling the blood, the lumen must be fast-flushed with the heparinized solution to prevent the blood from clotting (see Fig. 5-18). Flush for several seconds until the solution flows freely. This blood sample may be reliably analyzed for $S\bar{v}O_2$, $P\bar{v}O_2$, and $P\bar{v}CO_2$ values.

4. Use a central venous catheter with reflectance oximetry capability

As discussed earlier, this CVP catheter has gained acceptance in monitoring the status of patients with a variety of conditions. Clinical studies have shown that the $ScvO_2$ values will track patient changes in a manner similar to the $S\bar{v}O_2$ and $P\bar{v}O_2$ values from a PAC. In other words, if the patient's $S\bar{v}O_2$ and/or $P\bar{v}O_2$ values increase (or decrease), so will the $ScvO_2$ values. However, because the $ScvO_2$ values are less consistent than true mixed venous oxygen values, the patient's clinical goal for $ScvO_2$ monitoring is >70% saturation.

d. Evaluate the results of the mixed venous blood measurement (code: ID10) [difficulty: R, Ap, An]

This topic is discussed in some detail in Chapter 3. The normal values follow:

$P\bar{v}O_2$ of 40 torr (range of 37 to 43 torr)
$S\bar{v}O_2$ of 75% (range of 70% to 76%)

True mixed venous blood oxygen values are useful for monitoring the patient's oxygen consumption. The most accurate methods of calculating percentage shunt and CO (Fick method) use mixed venous blood oxygen values with arterial blood oxygen values. A $P\bar{v}O_2$ value of less than 30 torr or an $S\bar{v}O_2$ value of less than 56% is considered to show tissue hypoxemia. The situation must be quickly treated. Increase the inspired oxygen percentage as needed. Low SV and CO measurements can be increased by giving digoxin (Lanoxin) or other inotropic agents. Low BP can be increased by administering vasopressors such as dopamine hydrochloride (Intropin) or norepinephrine (Levophed).

9. Arterial–venous oxygen content difference

a. Evaluate data in the patient record for a trend in arterial–venous oxygen content difference (code: IA14) [difficulty: R, Ap]

The difference between arterial oxygen content and venous oxygen content $[C(a - \bar{v})O_2]$ is a calculation of oxygen consumption by the body. It is the difference between the oxygen content of arterial blood and the oxygen content of mixed venous blood. Box 5-2 lists normal values. As always, check previous values to compare with present values to determine if the patient's condition has changed.

b. Recommend an arterial–venous oxygen content measurement (code: IE12) [difficulty: R, Ap, An]

The $C(a - \bar{v})O_2$ measurement should be recommended when it is necessary to know a patient's oxygen consumption, such as with heart failure or sepsis management.

c. Perform an arterial–venous oxygen content difference measurement (code: IC11) [difficulty: R, Ap]

The following steps must be performed to make the arterial–venous oxygen content calculation:

1. Draw and analyze an arterial blood gas sample.
2. Simultaneously draw and analyze a mixed venous blood gas sample.
3. Determine the patient's hemoglobin value.
4. Place the data into the calculations shown in the next discussion.

d. Calculate the arterial–venous oxygen content difference (code: IC10) [difficulty: R, Ap]

As mentioned in the previous discussion, the arterial–venous oxygen content difference is found by subtracting venous blood oxygen content from arterial blood oxygen content. These two values must first be calculated separately and then subtracted as shown in these three steps:

1. CaO_2 is the content of oxygen in arterial blood, or Vol% of oxygen in arterial blood (Vol% is mL of oxygen/100 mL of blood):

$$CaO_2 = (Hb \times 1.34 \times SaO_2) + (PaO_2 \times 0.003)$$

2. $C\bar{v}O_2$ is the content of oxygen in mixed venous blood, or Vol% of oxygen in mixed venous blood:

$$C\bar{v}O_2 = (Hb \times 1.34 \times S\bar{v}O_2) + (P\bar{v}O_2 \times 0.003)$$

3. Therefore:

$$C(a - \bar{v})O_2 = CaO_2 - C\bar{v}O_2$$

EXAMPLE

Your patient has the following clinical data:

PaO_2 = 95 torr

SaO_2 = 97% or 0.97

$P\bar{v}O_2$ = 40 torr

$S\bar{v}O_2$ = 75% or 0.75

15 g/dL = the patient's hemoglobin concentration

1.34 = mL of oxygen/g of Hb in the patient (the value of 1.39 mL of oxygen/g of Hb is occasionally used)

0.003 = the oxygen-carrying capacity of blood plasma per torr PO_2

Therefore:

1. $CaO_2 = (Hb \times 1.34 \times SaO_2) + (PaO_2 \times 0.003)$
   $= (15 \times 1.34 \times 0.97) + (95 \times 0.003)$
   $= (19.5) + (0.3)$
   $= 19.8$ Vol %

2. $C\bar{v}O_2 = (Hb \times 1.34 \times S\bar{v}O_2) + (P\bar{v}O_2 \times 0.003)$
   $= (15 \times 1.34 \times 0.75) + (40 \times 0.003)$
   $= (15.1) + (0.1)$
   $= 15.2$ Vol %

3. $C(a - \bar{v})O_2$ difference $= (CaO_2$ of 19.8 Vol % $) - (C\bar{v}O_2$ of 15.2 Vol % $)$
   $= 4.6$ Vol %

e. Evaluate the results of the arterial–venous oxygen content difference (code: ID10) [difficulty: R, Ap, An]

The normal range for the $C(a - \bar{v})O_2$ difference is 3-5.5 Vol%. Measurements in this range show normal levels of oxygen consumption by the tissues, CO, and cardiopulmonary function. (See Fig. 5-26 for a graphic presentation of $C(a - \bar{v})O_2$ on the oxyhemoglobin dissociation curve.) A $C(a - \bar{v})O_2$ difference of greater than 5.5-6 Vol% is seen in patients with a low CO. As the blood flows more slowly than normal through the tissues, more oxygen is consumed per milliliter of blood. The $S\bar{v}O_2$ and $P\bar{v}O_2$ values drop and the $C(a - \bar{v})O_2$ difference widens.

A $C(a - \bar{v})O_2$ difference of less than 4 Vol% in the healthy patient commonly indicates good cardiovascular reserve with an increased CO. As the blood flows more quickly than normal through the tissues, less oxygen is consumed per milliliter of blood. The $S\bar{v}O_2$ and $P\bar{v}O_2$ values increase and the $C(a - \bar{v})O_2$ difference narrows. The septic patient may have a narrowed $C(a - \bar{v})O_2$ difference because of peripheral shunting and decreased oxygen consumption by the tissues caused by the infection. The $C(a - \bar{v})O_2$ difference is necessary to accurately calculate the percentage of pulmonary shunting as discussed next.

10. Shunt study

a. Evaluate data in the patient record for a trend in shunt (code: IA14) [difficulty: R, Ap]

Shunt ($\dot{Q}s/\dot{Q}t$) is the amount of blood pumped by the heart that passes through the lungs but does not participate in gas exchange. A PAC must be inserted into the patient for a shunt study to be performed. Review previous ($\dot{Q}s/\dot{Q}t$) study results and compare with current information to see if there has been a change in the patient's status. See Box 5-2 for normal values.

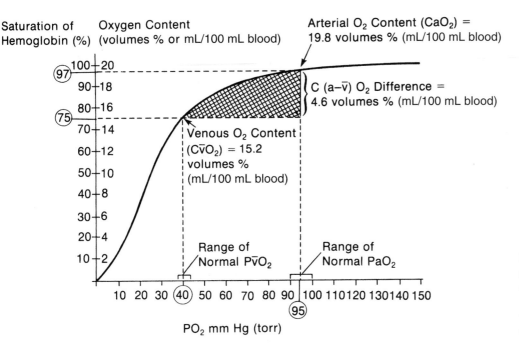

Figure 5-26 Oxyhemoglobin dissociation curve showing normal oxygen saturations and pressures in arterial and venous blood. From these, the normal $C(a-v)O_2$ difference of 4.6 Vol% can be calculated.

b. Recommend a shunt study (code: IE12) [difficulty: R, Ap, An]

A shunt study is very useful to find out how much ventilation-to-perfusion mismatch a patient has. Most patients with refractory hypoxemia and requiring mechanical ventilation have an increased amount of pulmonary shunting. When an optimal PEEP study is performed, a shunt study should be done with each change in the PEEP level.

c. Perform a shunt study (code: IC11) [difficulty: R, Ap]

Steps in the bedside shunt procedure include:
1. Measure the patient's fractional concentration of inspired oxygen (F_IO_2).
2. Simultaneously draw arterial and mixed venous blood samples.
3. Have both blood samples analyzed for SO_2 and PO_2 levels.
4. Calculate the percentage of shunt as shown next.

d. Calculate the shunt percentage (code: IC10)

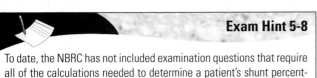

Exam Hint 5-8

To date, the NBRC has not included examination questions that require all of the calculations needed to determine a patient's shunt percentage. However, examinations have included questions that relate to calculating components of the shunt equations. These have included calculating CaO_2, $C\bar{v}O_2$, and $C(a-\bar{v})O_2$.

[difficulty: R, Ap]

There are a number of possible variations on the methods and equations for calculating shunt percentage. Only the two most commonly used equations are presented here.

1. Modified clinical shunt equation

$$\dot{Q}_s/\dot{Q}_t = \frac{P(A-a)O_2 \times 0.003}{C(a-\bar{v})O_2 + [P(A-a)O_2 \times 0.003]}$$

In this equation:

PAO_2 is the partial pressure of oxygen in the alveoli calculated from the alveolar oxygen equation

PaO_2 is the partial pressure of oxygen in the arterial blood

0.003 is the oxygen-carrying capacity of blood plasma per mm Hg PO_2

$C(a-\bar{v})O_2$ is the oxygen content of arterial blood minus the oxygen content of mixed venous blood

This formula requires that the patient's hemoglobin be 100% saturated. This does not happen until the PaO_2 level reaches 150 torr at any given F_IO_2. An obvious clinical limitation is that very ill patients never reach 100% saturation even when breathing 100% oxygen. Also, putting patients on more than 80% oxygen, even for just the duration of the test, may lead to some denitrogenation absorption atelectasis. This results in an incorrectly high shunt percentage calculation.

EXAMPLE

Modified clinical shunt equation.

The subsequent example shows the modified clinical shunt calculation with the following environmental and patient information:

P_B (local barometric pressure) = 760 torr for sea level in this example

P_{H_2O} = 47 torr; water vapor pressure in the lungs at normal body temperature

F_IO_2 = 100% or 1.0

PaO_2 = 155 torr

$PaCO_2$ = 40 torr

SaO_2 = 100% or 1.0

$P\bar{v}O_2$ = 40 torr

$S\bar{v}O_2$ = 75% or 0.75

0.8 is the normal respiratory quotient (an exact value can be determined by a metabolic study)

15 g/dL is the patient's hemoglobin concentration

0.003 is the oxygen-carrying capacity of blood plasma per torr PO_2

1.34 mL is the oxygen/g of Hb in the patient (the value of 1.39 mL of oxygen/g of Hb is occasionally used)

Preliminary calculations:
1. Oxygen content of arterial blood

$$CaO_2 = (Hb \times 1.34 \times SaO_2) + (PaO_2 \times 0.003)$$
$$= (15 \times 1.34 \times 1.0) + (155 \times 0.003)$$
$$= (20.1) + (0.5)$$
$$= 20.6 \text{ Vol } \%$$

2. Oxygen content of mixed venous blood

$$C\bar{v}O_2 = (Hb \times 1.34 \times S\bar{v}O_2) + (P\bar{v}O_2 \times 0.003)$$
$$= (15 \times 1.34 \times 0.75) + (40 \times 0.003)$$
$$= (15.1) + (0.1)$$
$$= 15.2 \text{ Vol } \%$$

3. Partial pressure of oxygen in the alveoli: the alveolar oxygen equation is used for this. (Review Chapter 3 if necessary.)

$$PAO_2 = [(P_B - PH_2O) \times F_IO_2] - \frac{PaCO_2}{0.8}$$
$$= [(760 - 47) \times 1.0] - \frac{40}{0.8}$$
$$= [713] - 50$$
$$= 663 \text{ torr}$$

Final calculation:

$$\dot{Q}_s/\dot{Q}_t = \frac{P(A-a)O_2 \times 0.003}{C(a-\bar{v})O_2 + [P(A-a)O_2 \times 0.003]}$$
$$= \frac{(663 - 155) \times 0.003}{(20.6 - 15.2) + [(663 - 155) \times 0.003]}$$
$$= \frac{(508) \times 0.003}{5.4 + [(508) \times 0.003]}$$
$$= \frac{1.5}{5.4 + 1.5}$$
$$= \frac{1.5}{6.9}$$
$$= 0.217 \text{ or } 21.7\% \text{ shunt}$$

2. Classic shunt equation

This equation is widely used because of the clinical limitations of the clinical shunt equation:

$$\dot{Q}_s/\dot{Q}_t = \frac{CO_2 - CaO_2}{CcO_2 - C\bar{v}O_2}$$

In this equation:

CcO_2 is the content of oxygen in the end pulmonary capillary blood

CaO_2 is the content of oxygen in the arterial blood

$C\bar{v}O_2$ is the content of oxygen in the mixed venous blood

The patient should be inspiring 30% oxygen or more to calculate the oxygen content of end pulmonary capillary blood. This much oxygen should cause the PAO_2 value of the ventilated alveoli to reach 150 torr or more, which results in 100% saturation of the hemoglobin of the end pulmonary capillary blood (ScO_2). Most patients who are sick enough to warrant a shunt determination will be on at least 30% oxygen. If not, the ScO_2 value must be determined by using the oxyhemoglobin dissociation curve.

A PAC is needed to sample mixed venous blood for $P\bar{v}O_2$ and $S\bar{v}O_2$ levels in both of these equations. An arterial blood gas sample is also needed. There are clinical situations in which either of these equations will work and will result in the same answer.

EXAMPLE

Classic shunt equation

The subsequent example shows the classic shunt calculation with the following environmental and patient information:

P_B = 760 torr for sea level in this example

PH_2O = 47 torr; water vapor pressure in the lungs at normal body temperature

F_IO_2 = 30% or 0.3

PaO_2 = 95 torr

$PaCO_2$ = 40 torr

SaO_2 = 97% or 0.97

$P\bar{v}O_2$ = 40 torr

$S\bar{v}O_2$ = 75% or 0.75

0.8 is the normal respiratory quotient (an exact value can be determined by a metabolic study)

15 g/dL is the patient's hemoglobin concentration

0.003 is the oxygen-carrying capacity of blood plasma per torr PO_2

1.34 mL of oxygen/g of Hb in the patient (the value of 1.39 mL of oxygen/g of Hb is occasionally used)

Preliminary calculations:
1. Oxygen content of arterial blood

$$CaO_2 = (Hb \times 1.34 \times SaO_2) + (PaO_2 \times 0.003)$$
$$= (15 \times 1.34 \times 0.97) + (95 \times 0.003)$$
$$= (19.5) + (0.3)$$
$$= 19.8 \text{ Vol } \%$$

2. Oxygen content of mixed venous blood

$$C\bar{v}O_2 = (Hb \times 1.34 \times S\bar{v}O_2) + (P\bar{v}O_2 \times 0.003)$$
$$= (15 \times 1.34 \times 0.75) + (40 \times 0.003)$$
$$= (15.1) + (0.1)$$
$$= 15.2 \text{ Vol}\%$$

3. Partial pressure of oxygen in the alveoli: the alveolar oxygen equation is used for this. (Review Chapter 3 if necessary.)

$$PAO_2 = [(P_B - PH_2O) \times F_iO_2] - \frac{PaCO_2}{0.8}$$
$$= [(760 - 47) \times 0.3] - \frac{40}{0.8}$$
$$= [214] - 50$$
$$= 164 \text{ torr}$$

4. Oxygen content of pulmonary capillary blood

$$CcO_2 = (Hb \times 1.34 \times ScO_2) + (PAO_2 \times 0.003)$$
$$= (15 \times 1.34 \times 1.0) + (164 \times 0.003)$$
$$= 20.1 + 0.492$$
$$= 20.1 + 0.5 \text{ (Rounded off to one decimal place)}$$
$$= 20.6 \text{ Vol}\%$$

Final calculation:

$$\dot{Q}_s/\dot{Q}_t = \frac{CcO_2 - CaO_2}{CaO_2 - C\bar{v}O_2}$$
$$= \frac{20.6 - 19.8}{19.8 - 15.2}$$
$$= \frac{0.8}{4.6}$$
$$= 0.174 \text{ or } 17.4\% \text{ shunt}$$

e. Evaluate the results of the shunt study calculation (code: ID10) [difficulty: R, Ap, An]

As noted earlier, shunt is the amount of blood pumped by the heart that does not participate in gas exchange through the lungs. It is wasted CO and wasted effort by the heart. The healthy person has a shunt of 5% or less of CO. This shunted blood has a low oxygen content and dilutes the oxygen content of all the blood. The larger the percentage of shunted blood, the more the heart and body are stressed. Many clinicians believe that an indication for mechanical ventilation is a shunt of 15% to 20%. Most agree that a shunt of more than 30% can be life threatening. A ventilator is used to reduce the patient's work of breathing and oxygen consumption. Also, supplemental oxygen can be carefully controlled, and PEEP may be added to increase the patient's functional residual capacity as needed.

11. Pulmonary vascular resistance

a. Evaluate data in the patient record for a trend in pulmonary vascular resistance (code: IA14) [difficulty: R, Ap]

Pulmonary vascular resistance (PVR) is the total resistance of the pulmonary vascular bed to the blood being pumped through it by the right ventricle. This resistance

is also called *afterload* and can be calculated when other cardiopulmonary studies are performed.

b. Recommend a pulmonary vascular resistance measurement (code: IE12) [difficulty: R, Ap, An]

It is valuable to know the PVR in any case in which restricted blood flow through the lungs is known or suspected. This could include a patient with COPD, a pulmonary embolism, pulmonary hypertension, or PPHN. If therapeutic procedures are effective, the patient's PVR should be decreased toward normal. For example, inhaled nitric oxide therapy has been shown to be effective in reducing the PVR of a newborn with PPHN.

c. Perform a pulmonary vascular resistance measurement (code: IC11) [difficulty: R, Ap]

CO, mean pulmonary BP, and pulmonary capillary wedge pressure must be known to determine the PVR. To gather the necessary hemodynamic information, the patient must have a thermodilution-type CO PAC. Measure the CO, PAP, and PCWP as described earlier.

d. Calculate the pulmonary vascular resistance (code: IC10) [difficulty: R, Ap]

The patient must have the mean PAP, PCWP, and CO measured and placed into this formula:

$$PVR = \frac{\text{mean pulmonary artery pressure (PAm)} - \text{pulmonary capillary wedge pressure (PCWP)}}{\text{cardiac output (CO)}} \times 80$$

The answer will be in units of $dyn/s/cm^{-5}$.

e. Evaluate the results of the pulmonary vascular resistance calculation (code: ID10) [difficulty: R, Ap, An]

The normal range for PVR in an adult is 1-3 mm Hg/L/min. Multiplying this value by 80 changes the result to units of $dyn/s/cm^{-5}$. PVR is listed this way in some cardiology studies. The normal range of PVR in an adult is between 80 and 240 $dyn/s/cm^{-5}$.

With a normal PVR, the difference between the pulmonary artery diastolic pressure and the pulmonary capillary wedge pressure is 5 mm Hg or less. Any of the following can cause an elevated PVR:

- Decreased oxygen in the lungs
- COPD
- Acute respiratory distress syndrome (ARDS)
- PPHN/persistent fetal circulation
- Primary pulmonary hypertension
- Pulmonary embolism
- Excessive PEEP
- Increased pulmonary blood flow from a left-to-right intracardiac shunt such as an atrial septal defect or ventricular septal defect

Additional clinical data must be gathered to confirm the diagnosis. An increased PVR is a serious problem because it can lead to right ventricular hypertrophy. The COPD patient is at risk for developing cor pulmonale—right-ventricular failure secondary to lung disease and increased PVR.

12. Systemic vascular resistance

a. Evaluate data in the patient record for a trend in systemic vascular resistance (code: IA14) [difficulty: R, Ap]

Systemic vascular resistance (SVR) is the total resistance of the systemic vascular bed to the blood being pumped through it by the left ventricle. This resistance is also called afterload and can be calculated when other cardiopulmonary studies are performed.

b. Recommend a systemic vascular resistance measurement (code: IE12) [difficulty: R, Ap, An]

Recommend an SVR measurement in a clinical situation in which there may be abnormally increased or decreased resistance to blood flow through the body. This may include a patient with hypertension or vasodilation from an anaphylactic reaction or sepsis.

c. Perform a systemic vascular resistance measurement (code: IC11) [difficulty: R, Ap]

CO, systemic BP, and CVP must be known to determine the SVR. To gather the necessary hemodynamic information, the patient must have a thermodilution-type CO PAC, arterial line, and CVP line (if this cannot be measured from the PAC).

d. Calculate the systemic vascular resistance (code: IC10) [difficulty: R, Ap]

The patient must have mean arterial pressure, CVP, and CO measured and placed into the following formula:

$$SVR = \frac{\text{mean arterial pressure (MAP)} - \text{central venous pressure (CVP)}}{\text{cardiac output (CO)}} \times 80$$

The answer will be in units of $dyn/s/cm^{-5}$.

e. Evaluate the results of the systemic vascular resistance calculation (code: ID10) [difficulty: R, Ap, An]

The normal range of SVR in the adult is 15-20 mm Hg/L/min. Multiplying this value by 80 changes the result to units of $dyn/s/cm^{-5}$. SVR is listed this way in some cardiology studies. When multiplied by 80, an adult's SVR ranges between 770-900 and 1400-1500 $dyn/s/cm^{-5}$.

A patient with hypertension will have an elevated SVR. It will also increase if the patient is given a vasoconstricting drug and decrease if the patient is given a vasodilating drug. Some allergic reactions result in anaphylaxis with a dramatic drop in the SVR and BP despite an increase in the CO.

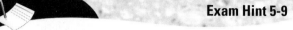

Exam Hint 5-9

Know the normal values for pulmonary and SVR. To date, the NBRC has not expected the examinee to perform all of the calculations to determine a patient's PVR or SVR. Know that a patient with COPD or PPHN will have a chronically increased PVR and a patient with a large pulmonary embolism will have a sudden increase in the PVR. With proper treatment, the PVR will decrease toward normal.

There are several ways that the cardiology version of the PVR or SVR value can be found. The preferred versions have units listed in "$dyn/s/cm^{-5}$" or "dynes sec/cm^{-5}." However, the NBRC has also listed these values in units of "dynes seconds cm^{-5}," "dynes·seconds·cm^{-5}," and "mm Hg/L/min."

13. Pressure transducers

a. Assemble the necessary equipment for the procedure (code: IIA24a) [difficulty: R, Ap]

Hemodynamic monitoring requires a transducer that converts a BP signal into an electrical signal. Select a strain-gauge-type transducer to do this. The strain-gauge transducer uses a fine wire screen that bends proportionately to the pressure put against it.

Check to see that the wire screen of the transducer is not bent, damaged, or contaminated with old blood or other debris. The transducer's wire cable and monitor-connecting prongs should not be bent or damaged. Carefully insert the prongs into the receiving jack on the monitor.

A disposable, sterile, clear plastic dome should be firmly attached to the transducer. Noncompliant pressure tubing should connect the transducer with the patient's arterial or PAC. The automatic fluid drip system (Sorenson) should be pressurized to 300 mm Hg. Heparin must be added to the fluid (usually normal saline) to prevent clotting in the patient's catheter. Because this is a continuous fluid "plumbing" system, all connections must be tightly joined to be watertight without leaks. There must be a continuous flow of fluid through the tubing system and into the patient's blood vessel. Any air bubbles must be removed or the measured pressure reading will be lower than the actual reading (see Figs. 5-18 and 5-27).

The transducer must be kept at the patient's midchest (midheart) level during calibration and measurement. Calibrate the electronics in the monitor by placing known pressures against the fluid system. The electronics should first be adjusted to zero pressure by opening the transducer to room air (atmospheric pressure). Adjust the electronic controls as needed. A sphygmomanometer is then used to pressurize the fluid system. A PAC system is pressurized to relatively low pressures such as 30 and 50 mm Hg. An arterial system is adjusted to higher pressures such as 100 and 150 mm Hg. The monitored pressure should match the sphygmomanometer pressure. If not, adjust the electronic controls on the monitor to match.

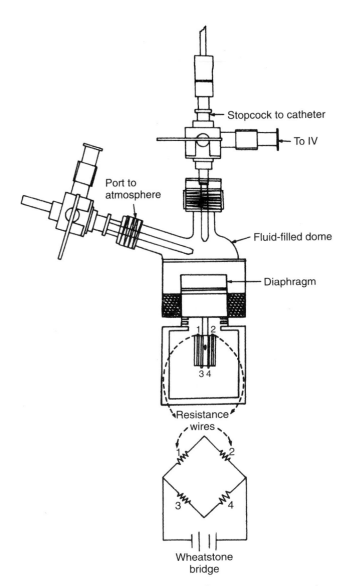

Figure 5-27 Schematic diagram of a strain-gauge pressure transducer. The wire mesh resistance wires are arranged like a Wheatstone bridge so that a pressure change results in a proportional change in the electrical resistance. (From Armstrong PW, Baigrie RS: Hemodynamic monitoring in the critically ill, Philadelphia, 1980, Harper & Row.)

b. Troubleshoot any problems with the equipment (code: IIA24a) [difficulty: R, Ap]

As mentioned previously, all connections must be watertight. If not, the IV solution will leak out when it is pressurized. This can also result in the patient's measured pressure readings being low. Stopcocks must be opened or closed properly to allow the patient's pressure to be measured by the transducer. Electronics that will not calibrate to match the known pressures should not be used.

14. Central venous catheters

a. Assemble the necessary equipment for the procedure (code: IIA24b) [difficulty: R, Ap]

Obtain the catheter type and gauge that are requested by the physician. Additional equipment includes a water-column manometer, stopcock, intravenous tubing, and IV solution system. A triple-lumen fiber-optic channel CVP catheter will be needed to measure the patient's $ScvO_2$ values.

See Figure 5-15 for the traditional assembly of the equipment and the procedure for measuring the CVP. The equipment must be properly calibrated to ensure that the data are accurate. Calibrating a CVP water-column manometer usually involves only making sure that it reads zero at atmospheric pressure.

b. Troubleshoot any problems with the equipment (code: IIA24b) [difficulty: R, Ap]

Make sure that all connections are watertight. Check the position of the stopcock if the CVP cannot be measured.

15. Arterial catheters

a. Assemble the necessary equipment for the procedure (code: IIA24b) [difficulty: R, Ap]

A neonate can have its umbilical artery catheterized. An adult usually has the radial artery catheterized. See Chapter 18 for the discussion on placing an arterial catheter. Following are the general supplies necessary for catheterizing either of these arteries for drawing blood gases and continuously monitoring BP:

- Sterile 20- or 21-gauge needle with a flexible plastic sheath. After placement into the artery, the needle is withdrawn and the sheath is left in place. A neonate needs a long catheter of the correct gauge based on his or her body weight.
- Sterile surgical drape for covering the area surrounding the insertion site.
- Disinfectant such as 70% isopropyl alcohol or Betadine solution.
- Local anesthetic such as 4% lidocaine in a syringe and needle for injection into the insertion site.
- One or two sterile 3- or 5-mL syringes for blood sampling.
- Equipment for setting up a pressurized intravenous drip system so that the catheter does not clot.

See Figures 5-18 and 5-28 for illustrations of how the pressure transducer, connecting tubing, stopcocks, infusion system, and monitoring electronics are assembled. See Figure 5-29 for a completed radial artery system. Clinical experience is needed with these types of systems.

The process of calibrating the monitor for systemic artery pressures was briefly discussed earlier. Regardless of whether the catheter is placed into a systemic artery, pulmonary artery, umbilical artery, or superior vena cava, the equipment must be properly calibrated to ensure accurate data. When performing two-point calibration, all pressures should read "zero" when exposed to atmospheric pressure. This is the low point. The high-point pressure for arterial pressure monitoring is commonly 100 mm Hg.

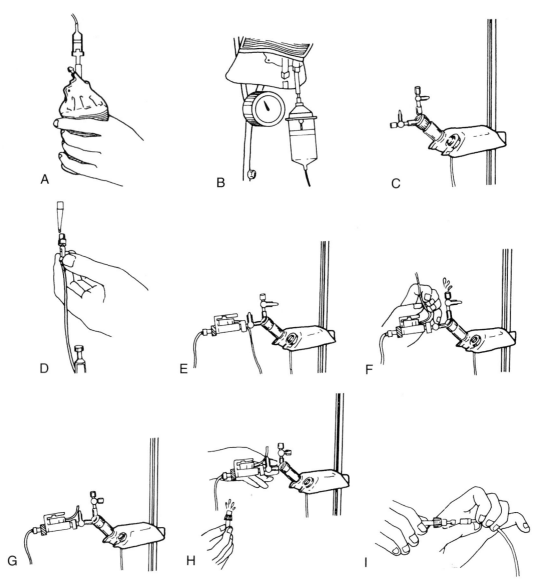

Figure 5-28 Common steps in the assembly of the tubing circuit and pressure transducer to attach to an arterial or pulmonary artery catheter (PAC). Sterile technique must be maintained at all times. (*Note:* Individual institutions will vary these steps. Clinical practice is very important in this assembly.) **A,** Obtain a 250- to 500-mL bag of sterile, normal saline. Add 1-2 units of heparin per milliliter of solution. Attach an IV line with a macrodrip chamber. **B,** Insert the solution bag into a pressure bag. Inflate the pressure to about 100 mm Hg to force the fluid through the IV tubing. The pressure bag will be inflated up to 300 mm Hg at the end of this procedure to ensure that three drops of fluid flow through the tubing per minute to keep it patent. **C,** Attach the strain-gauge pressure transducer to an IV pole. Let it and the monitor warm up. **D,** Attach the IV tubing to the continuous flush device (Sorenson Intraflow). **E,** Screw the continuous flush device into the transducer stopcock. **F,** Back-flush the continuous flush device and transducer, with open stopcocks, so that all air is removed and replaced with the saline solution. **G,** Zero and calibrate the pressure transducer and monitor. **H,** Attach high-pressure tubing to the continuous flush device. Flush the air out of it. **I,** Attach the high-pressure tubing to the patient's arterial line or PAC. Ensure that no air bubbles are present and that there is a continuous saline-to-blood connection. Accurate patient pressures should now be seen on the monitor. (From Oblouk Darovic G: Hemodynamic monitoring, Philadelphia, 1987, Saunders.)

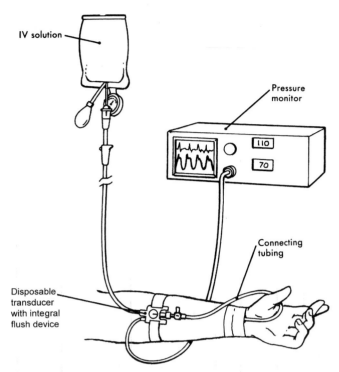

Figure 5-29 Example of a complete setup for monitoring the arterial pressure. (From Daily EK, Schroeder JS: Techniques in bedside hemodynamic monitoring, ed 5, St Louis, 1994, Mosby.)

b. Troubleshoot any problems with the equipment (code: IIA24b) [difficulty: R, Ap]

Table 5-1 lists problems, causes, prevention, and treatment for inaccurate pressure measurements with arterial or PACs. Table 5-2 specifically lists problems with arterial lines. Figure 5-30 shows common problem areas with arterial lines. PACs can have problems in the same areas. If the equipment is properly assembled, the pressure readings will be accurate. If the pressure readings are transmitted to a display monitor, the BP waveform can be seen.

16. Pulmonary artery catheter

a. Assemble the necessary equipment for the procedure (code: IIA24b) [difficulty: R, Ap]

PACs are available in several diameter sizes. The smallest can be advanced into a pediatric patient's vein. Most adults will have either a 5-Fr or a 7-Fr catheter inserted. Once the appropriate size is determined, select a catheter that provides the information that is needed. A standard 5-Fr catheter can be used to measure PAP and pulmonary capillary wedge pressure, and a mixed venous blood sample can be withdrawn from it for analysis. A 7-Fr thermodilution CO catheter can perform all the functions just mentioned and in addition provide a CVP measurement and measure CO through the computer (see Figs. 5-17 and 5-22). A 7-Fr fiber-optic catheter can measure continuous $S\bar{v}O_2$ as well as PAP, PCWP, CVP, and CO by the thermodilution method. Mixed venous blood can also be sampled for analysis.

The 5- and 7-Fr catheters are packaged self-contained as a single unit. The general assembly of the related tubing circuit and pressure transducer was discussed earlier and illustrated in Figures 5-18 and 5-28. Clinical experience is needed. Make sure that all connections are watertight, the transducer calibrates accurately, and the balloon inflates and deflates properly.

The process of calibrating the monitor for PAPs or systemic artery pressures was briefly discussed earlier. Regardless of whether the catheter is placed into a systemic artery, pulmonary artery, umbilical artery, or superior vena cava, the equipment must be properly calibrated to ensure accurate data. When performing two-point calibration, all pressures should read "zero" when exposed to atmospheric pressure. This is the low point. The high-point pressure for PAP monitoring is commonly 30 mm Hg.

b. Troubleshoot any problems with the equipment (code: IIA24b) [difficulty: R, Ap]

See Table 5-3 for a listing of the problems seen with PACs and their causes, prevention, and treatment. Figure 5-30 shows common problem areas with the related pressure tubing and equipment.

17. Cardiac output computer

a. Assemble the necessary equipment for the procedure (code: IIA24b) [difficulty: R, Ap]

The manufacturers of CO PACs (e.g., Edwards Laboratories LLC) also make thermodilution CO computers. However, the computer is usually designed for use with only their brand of catheter. Make sure that you have a compatible catheter and computer.

Figure 5-17 shows a thermodilution CO PAC. Note the thermistor connection to the CO computer and the proximal port where the cooled solution is injected. See Figure 5-22 for the assembly of the CO computer to the catheter. In addition, the computer must be programmed with the size of catheter, injectate volume, and injectate temperature.

b. Troubleshoot any problems with the equipment (code: IIA24b) [difficulty: R, Ap]

An error in the CO value can be caused by an error in programming the computer or by not injecting the cooled solution through the proximal port in the required 4 s.

18. Continuous mixed venous oxygen saturation monitor

a. Assemble the necessary equipment for the procedure (code: IIA24b) [difficulty: R, Ap]

The manufacturers of continuous mixed venous oxygen saturation PACs (e.g., Edwards Laboratories LLC) also make the required monitor. However, the monitor is usually designed for use with only their brand of catheter. Make sure that you have a compatible catheter and monitor.

TABLE 5-1	Inaccurate Pressure Measurements		
Problem	**Cause**	**Prevention**	**Treatment**
Damped waveforms and inaccurate pressures	Partial clotting at catheter tip	Use continuous drip with 1 unit of heparin/1 mL of IV fluid. Hand flush occasionally. Flush with large volume after blood sampling. Use heparin-coated catheters.	Aspirate, then flush catheter with heparinized fluid (*not* in PAW position).
	Tip moving against wall	Obtain more stable catheter position.	Reposition catheter.
	Kinking of catheter	Restrict catheter movement at insertion site.	Reposition to straighten catheter. Replace catheter.
Abnormally low or negative pressure reading	Incorrect air reference level (above midchest level)	Maintain transducer air reference port at midchest level; rezero after patient position changes.	Remeasure level of transducer air reference and reposition at midchest level; rezero.
	Incorrect zeroing and calibration of monitor	Zero and calibrate monitor properly.	Recheck zero and calibration of monitor.
	Loose connection	Use Luer-Lok stopcocks.	Check all connections.
Abnormally high pressure reading	Pressure trapped by improper sequence of stopcock operation	Turn stopcocks in proper sequence when two pressures are measured on one transducer.	Thoroughly flush transducers with IV solution; rezero and turn stopcocks in proper sequence.
	Incorrect air reference level (below midchest level)	Maintain transducer air reference port at midchest level; recheck and rezero after patient position changes.	Check air reference level; reset at midchest and rezero.
Inappropriate pressure waveform	Migration of catheter tip (e.g., in RV or PAW instead of in PA)	Establish optimal position carefully when introducing catheter initially. Suture catheter at insertion site and tape catheter to patient's skin.	Review waveform; if RV, inflate balloon; if PAW, deflate balloon and withdraw catheter slightly. Check position under fluoroscope and/or radiograph after reposition.
No pressure available	Transducer not open to catheter Amplifiers still on cal, zero, or off	Follow routine, systematic steps for pressure measurement.	Check system, stopcocks.
Noise or fling in pressure waveform	Excessive catheter movement, particularly in PA	Avoid excessive catheter length in ventricle.	Try different catheter tip position.
	Excessive tubing length	Use shortest tubing possible (<3-4 feet).	Eliminate excess tubing.
	Excessive stopcocks	Minimize number of stopcocks.	Eliminate excess stopcocks.

From Daily EK, Schroeder JS: Techniques in bedside hemodynamic monitoring, ed 5, St Louis, 1994, Mosby.
PA, pulmonary artery; PAW, pulmonary artery wedge; RV, right ventricle.

See Figure 5-25 for a photograph of a continuous mixed venous oxygen saturation PAC and its connection to the required monitor and analyzer. Make sure the monitor is properly connected to the catheter. Calibrate the equipment as directed by the manufacturer so that accurate patient values will be measured.

b. Troubleshoot any problems with the equipment (code: IIA24b) [difficulty: R, Ap]

Errors can result from the catheter and monitor not being properly connected or the analyzer not being properly calibrated.

MODULE D

Respiratory care plan

1. Determine a patient's pathophysiologic state (code: IIIF1) [difficulty: R, Ap, An]

See Figure 5-31 for examples of diagnostic pathways. These can be used to help the clinician evaluate all the patient data. The diagnosis or pathophysiologic state can be determined by following the data on a given pathway. Normal values and common conditions associated with abnormal values were discussed earlier in this chapter.

TABLE 5-2   Problems Encountered with Arterial Catheters

Problem	Cause	Prevention	Treatment
Hematoma after withdrawal of needle	Bleeding or oozing at puncture site	Maintain firm pressure on site during withdrawal of catheter and for 5-15 minutes (as necessary) after withdrawal. Apply elastic tape (Elastoplast) firmly over puncture site.	Continue to hold pressure to puncture site until oozing stops.
		For femoral arterial puncture sites, leave a sandbag on site for 1-2 hours to prevent oozing. If patient is receiving heparin, discontinue 2 hours before catheter removal.	Apply sandbag to femoral puncture site for 1-2 hours after removal of catheter.
Decreased or absent pulse distal to puncture site	Spasm of artery	Introduce arterial needle cleanly, nontraumatically.	Inject lidocaine locally at insertion site and 10 mg into arterial catheter.
	Thrombosis of artery	Use 1 unit of heparin/1 mL of IV fluid	Arteriotomy and Fogarty catheterization both distally and proximally from the puncture site result in return of pulse in more than 90% of cases if brachial or femoral artery is used.
Bleed-back into tubing, dome, or transducer	Insufficient pressure on IV bag Loose connections	Maintain 300 mm Hg pressure on IV bag. Use Luer-Lok stopcocks; tighten periodically. Keep all connecting sites visible. Observe connecting sites frequently.	Replace transducer. "Fast flush" through system. Tighten all connections.
Hemorrhage	Loose connections	Use built-in alarm system. Use Luer-Lok stopcocks.	Tighten all connections.
Emboli	Clot from catheter tip into bloodstream	Always aspirate and discard before flushing. Use continuous flush device. Use 1 unit of heparin/1 mL of IV fluid. Gently flush <2-4 mL.	Remove catheter.
Local infection	Forward movement of contaminated catheter Break in sterile technique Prolonged catheter use	Carefully suture catheter at insertion site. Always use aseptic technique. Remove catheter after 72-96 hours. Inspect and care for insertion site daily, including dressing change and antibiotic or iodophor ointment.	Remove catheter. Prescribe antibiotic.
Sepsis	Break in sterile technique Prolonged catheter use	Use percutaneous insertion. Always use aseptic technique. Remove catheter after 72-96 hours.	Remove catheter. Prescribe antibiotic.
	Bacterial growth in IV fluid	Change IV fluid bag, stopcocks, dome, and tubing every 24-48 hours. Do not use IV fluid containing glucose. Use sterile dead-ender caps on all ports of stopcocks. Carefully flush remaining blood from stopcocks after blood sampling.	

From Daily EK, Schroeder JS: Techniques in bedside hemodynamic monitoring, ed 5, St Louis, 1994, Mosby.

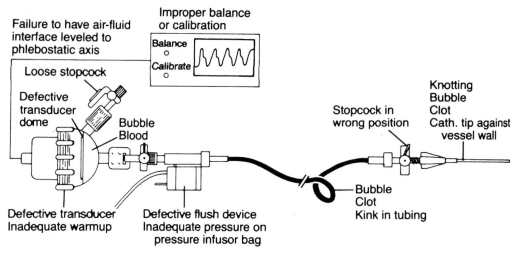

Figure 5-30 Common problem areas with arterial and pulmonary artery catheters. (From Oblouk Darovic G: Hemodynamic monitoring—invasive and noninvasive clinical application, ed 3, Philadelphia, 2002, Saunders.)

TABLE 5-3	Problems Encountered with Pulmonary Artery Catheters

Problem	Cause	Prevention	Treatment
Phlebitis or local infection at insertion site	Mechanical irritation or contamination	Prepare skin properly before insertion. Use sterile technique during insertion and dressing change. Insert smoothly and rapidly. Use Teflon-coated introducer. Attach silver-impregnated cuff to introducer. Change dressings, stopcocks, and connecting tubing every 24-48 hours. Remove catheter or change insertion site every 4 days.	Remove catheter. Apply warm compresses. Give pain medication as necessary.
Ventricular irritability	Looping of excess catheter in right ventricle	Suture catheter at insertion site; check chest film.	Reposition catheter; remove loop.
	Migration of catheter from PA to RV	Position catheter tip in main right or left PA.	Inflate balloon to encourage catheter flotation out to PA.
	Irritation of the endocardium during catheter passage	Keep balloon inflated during advancement; advance gently.	Advance rapidly out to PA.
Apparent wedging of catheter with balloon *deflated*	Forward migration of catheter tip caused by blood flow, excessive loop in RV, or inadequate suturing of catheter at insertion site	Check catheter tip by fluoroscopy; position in main right or left PA. Check catheter position on radiography film if fluoroscopy is not used. Suture catheter in place at insertion site.	Aspirate blood from catheter; if catheter is wedged, sample will be arterialized and obtained with difficulty. If wedged, slowly pull back catheter until PA waveform appears. If not wedged, gently aspirate and flush catheter with saline; catheter tip can partially clot, causing damping that resembles damped PAW waveform.

TABLE 5-3	Problems Encountered with Pulmonary Artery Catheters—cont'd		
Problem	**Cause**	**Prevention**	**Treatment**
Pulmonary hemorrhage or infarction, or both	Distal migration of catheter tip Continuous or prolonged wedging of catheter Overinflation of balloon while catheter is wedged Failure of balloon to deflate	Check chest film immediately after insertion and 12-24 hours later; remove any catheter loop in RA or RV. Leave balloon deflated. Suture catheter at skin to prevent inadvertent advancement. Position catheter in main right or left PA. Pull catheter back to pulmonary artery if it spontaneously wedges. Do not flush catheter when in wedge position. Inflate balloon slowly with only enough air to obtain a PAW waveform. Do not inflate 7-Fr catheter with more than 1-1.5 mL of air. Do not inflate if resistance is met.	Deflate balloon. Place patient on side (catheter tip down). Stop anticoagulation. Consider "wedge" angiogram. Intubate with double-lumen ETT. Surgery, if severe hemorrhage
"Overwedging" or damped PAW	Overinflation of balloon Eccentric inflation of balloon	Watch waveform during inflation; inject only enough air to obtain PAW pressure. Do not inflate 7-Fr catheter with more than 1-1.5 mL of air. Check inflated balloon shape before insertion.	Deflate balloon; reinflate slowly with only enough air to obtain PAW pressure. Deflate balloon; reposition and slowly reinflate.
PA balloon rupture	Overinflation of balloon Frequent inflations of balloon Syringe deflation damaging wall of balloon	Inflate slowly with only enough air to obtain a PAW pressure. Monitor PAd pressure as reflection of PAW and LVEDP. Allow passive deflation of balloon. Remove syringe after inflation.	Remove syringe to prevent further air injection. Monitor PAd pressure.
Infection	Nonsterile insertion techniques Contamination via skin	Use sterile techniques. Use sterile catheter sleeve. Prepare skin with effective antiseptic (chlorhexidine). Apply iodophor ointment and sterile gauze dressing daily. Do not use clear semipermeable dressing. Inspect site daily. Reassess need for catheter after 3 days. Avoid internal jugular approach.	Remove catheter. Use antibiotics.
	Contamination through stopcock ports or catheter hub	Use sterile dead-ender caps on all stopcock ports. Change iv solution, stopcock, and tubing every 24-48 hours. Do not use IV solution that contains glucose.	
	Fluid contamination from transducer through cracked membrane of disposable dome	Check transducer domes for cracks. Change transducers every 48 hours. Change disposable dome after countershock. Do not use IV solution that contains glucose.	
	Prolonged catheter placement	Change catheter insertion site every 4 days.	
Heart block during insertion of catheter	Mechanical irritation of bundle of His in patients with preexisting left bundle branch block	Insert catheter expeditiously with balloon inflated. Insert transvenous pacing catheter before PA catheter insertion.	Use temporary pacemaker or flotation catheter with pacing wire.

From Daily EK, Schroeder JS: Techniques in bedside hemodynamic monitoring, ed 5, St Louis, 1994, Mosby.
ETT, endotracheal tube; LVEDP, left-ventricular end-diastolic pressure; PA, pulmonary artery; PAd, pulmonary artery diastolic; PAW, pulmonary artery wedge; RV, right ventricle.

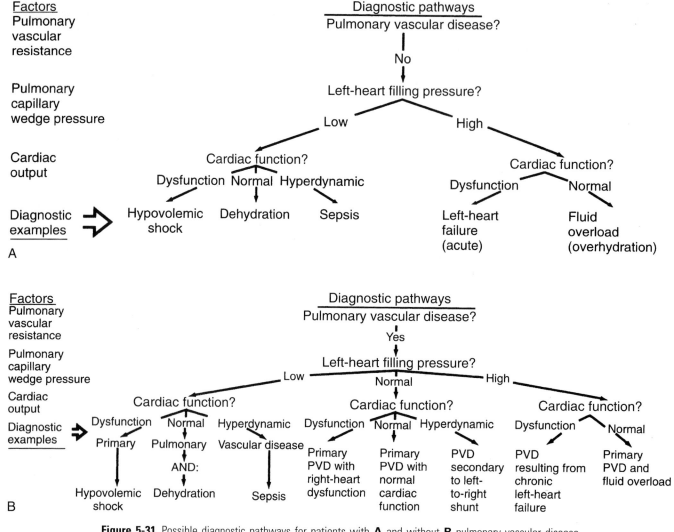

Figure 5-31 Possible diagnostic pathways for patients with **A** and without **B** pulmonary vascular disease (PVD). In both cases, the pulmonary vascular resistance, pulmonary capillary wedge pressure, and cardiac output are measured. High, normal, or low values lead down different pathways. Previous discussions and clinical experience are needed to determine the final diagnosis. Sepsis may be associated with normal left-heart filling pressures. Primary PVD may be caused by pulmonary emboli, pulmonary artery disease (vasculitis, "primary" pulmonary hypertension), respiratory distress syndromes, hypoxic vasoconstriction, or drugs. (From Osgood CF, Watson MH, Slaughter MS et al.: Respir Care 29(1):25–34, 1984.)

2. Recommend adjustment of the patient's fluid balance (code: IIIE2c) [difficulty: R, Ap]

The PCWP is often used to guide the administration or limitation of fluids to the patient. It is generally believed that a PCWP of greater than 10 mm Hg indicates fluid overload. If the PCWP is greater than 20 mm Hg, the patient will often develop pulmonary edema. Fluids should be restricted and diuretic medications (furosemide [Lasix]) given to increase urine output.

It is generally believed that a PCWP of less than 4 mm Hg indicates hypovolemia/dehydration. The usual treatment is to increase intravenous fluids.

3. Recommend starting a treatment based on the patient's response (code: IIIE2a) [difficulty: R, Ap, An]

See below.

4. Recommend a change in the therapeutic plan if indicated (code: IIIF2) [difficulty: R, Ap, An]

Each clinical problem presented in this section requires its own individualized treatment. Be prepared to make recommendations to change the inspired oxygen percentage, give fluids if the patient is dehydrated, give diuretic medications to increase urine output if the patient is fluid overloaded, give vasodilator medications if the patient is hypertensive, or give vasopressor medications if the patient is hypotensive.

5. Recommend a treatment be terminated (code: IIIE1) [difficulty: R, Ap, An]

See below.

6. Recommend discontinuing a treatment based on the patient's response (code: IIIE2h) [difficulty: R, Ap, An]

A catheter should be withdrawn if the patient develops signs or symptoms of infection at the insertion site. There is a risk of puncturing the right lung during the insertion of a central venous catheter by way of the subclavian vein (see Fig. 5-13). Assess the patient for equal, bilateral breath sounds after this procedure has been attempted. Know the signs and symptoms of a pneumothorax. Review them in Chapter 1, if needed.

Exam Hint 5-10

Closely review the following concepts because they have been tested on previous examinations.
1. Interpretation of PAP: An increased PAP is usually associated with one of the following: fluid overload, heart failure or pulmonary hypertension (increased PVR) from COPD (emphysema), pulmonary embolism, or PPHN.

2. Interpretation of pulmonary capillary wedge pressure: An increased PCWP is usually associated with one of the following: fluid overload, heart failure, mitral valve insufficiency, cardiac tamponade, or constrictive pericarditis. Treatment for fluid overload and/or heart failure usually includes restriction of fluids and administration of diuretics (Lasix) and digitalis-type drugs (Lanoxin). A decreased PCWP is usually associated with dehydration or vasodilation. Dehydration is treated with increased fluids. Vasodilation is treated with vasoconstricting drugs. When interpreting the PAP and PCWP together, it is very important to calculate the difference between the PAP diastolic pressure and the PCWP. Normally, the difference (or gradient) is 5 mm Hg or less. In other words, if the PAP diastolic pressure minus the PCWP is 5 mm Hg or less, the patient does not have pulmonary hypertension. A gradient of more than 5 mm Hg indicates pulmonary hypertension.
3. Interpretation of CO: Decreased CO is usually caused by hypovolemia or heart failure. Hypovolemia is treated with increased fluids. Heart failure is treated with digitalis-type drugs (Lanoxin). CO may also be decreased on a ventilator-dependent patient with high peak pressures or a high PEEP level because of the increased intrathoracic pressure. When this is presented in an NBRC question and a request for care is made, the best response is to decrease the PEEP.

BIBLIOGRAPHY

AARC clinical practice guideline: capnography/capnometry during mechanical ventilation, *Respir Care* 56(4):503–509, 2011.

Adams AB: Monitoring the patient in the Intensive Care Unit. In Kacmarek RM, Stoller JK, Heuer AJ, editors: *Egan's fundamentals of respiratory care*, ed 10, St Louis, 2013, Mosby.

Aggarwal NK, Kiran U, Kapoor PM, Chowdhury UK: Intraoperative central venous oxygen saturation as a surrogate for mixed venous oxygen saturation in patients undergoing cardiac surgery, *J Anesth Clin Pharmacology* 23(1):29–33, 2007.

Anton WR, Raghu G: Measuring end-tidal carbon dioxide tension at maximal exhalation to improve its utility during T-piece weaning trials, *Respir Care* 35(11):1082–1083, 1990.

Brewer LM, Orr JA, Pace NL: Anatomic dead space cannot be predicted by body weight, *Respir Care* 53(7):885–891, 2008.

Cairo JM: Assessment of cardiovascular function. In Cairo JM, editor: *Mosby's respiratory care equipment*, ed 9, St Louis, 2014, Mosby.

Cairo JM: Assessment of pulmonary function. In Cairo JM, editor: *Mosby's respiratory care equipment*, ed 9, St Louis, 2014, Mosby.

Cairo JM: Hemodynamic monitoring. In Cairo JM, editor: *Pilbeam's mechanical ventilation—physiologic and clinical applications*, ed 5, St Louis, 2012, Mosby.

Cairo JM: Assessment of respiratory function. In Cairo JM, editor: *Pilbeam's mechanical ventilation—physiologic and clinical applications*, ed 5, St Louis, 2012, Mosby.

Carlon GC, Ray Jr C, Miodownik S, Kopec I, Groeger JS: Capnography in mechanically ventilated patients, *Crit Care Med* 16(5):550–556, 1988.

Chatburn RL, Daoud EG: Ventilation. In Kacmarek RM, Stoller JK, Heuer AJ, editors: *Egan's fundamentals of respiratory care*, ed 10, St Louis, 2013, Mosby.

Chop WC, Chang DW: Monitoring in mechanical ventilation. In Chang DW, editor: *Clinical application of mechanical ventilation*, ed 4, Clifton Park, NY, 2014, Delmar.

Clark DB, Marshall SG: Mixed venous oxygen saturation measurement. II. General and specific clinical applications, *Respir Ther* 81–86, Nov/Dec 1986.

Daily EK, Schroeder JS: *Techniques in bedside hemodynamic monitoring*, ed 5, St Louis, 1994, Mosby.

Deshpande VM, Pilbeam SP, Dixon RJ: *A comprehensive review in respiratory care*, Norwalk, CT, 1988, Appleton & Lange.

DiBlasi RM, Czervinske MP: Invasive blood gas analysis and cardiovascular monitoring. In Walsh BK, Czervinske MP, DiBlasi RM, editors: *Perinatal and pediatric respiratory care*, ed 3, St Louis, 2010, Saunders.

Divertie MB, McMichan JC: Continuous monitoring of mixed venous oxygen saturation, *Chest* 85(3):423–428, 1984.

Drumheller OJ: Cardiopulmonary anatomy and physiology. In Wyka KA, Mathews PJ, Rutkowski JA, editors: *Foundations of respiratory care*, ed 2, Clifton Park, NY, 2012, Delmar.

Fahey PJ, Harris K, Vanderwarf C: Clinical experience with continuous monitoring of mixed venous oxygen saturation in respiratory failure, *Chest* 86(5):748–752, 1984.

Fink JB, Hunt GE, editors: *Clinical practice in respiratory care*, Philadelphia, 1999, Lippincott-Raven.

Galia F, Brimioulle S, Bonnier F, Vandenbergen N, Dojat M, Vincent JL, et al.: Use of maximum end-tidal CO_2 values to improve end-tidal CO_2 monitoring accuracy, *Respir Care* 56(3):278–283, 2011.

Govert JA, Hess DR: Hemodynamic monitoring. In Hess DR, MacIntyre NR, Mishoe SC, Galvin WF, Adams AB, editors: *Respiratory care principles and practice*, ed 2, Burlington, MA, 2012, Jones & Bartlett Learning.

Gravenstein JS, Jaffe MB, Paulus DA, editors: *Capnography—clinical aspects*, Cambridge, UK, 2004, Cambridge University Press.

Graybeal JM, Russell GB: Capnometry in the surgical ICU: an analysis of the arterial-to-end-tidal carbon dioxide difference, *Respir Care* 38(8):923–928, 1993.

Guo F, Chen J, Liu S, Yang C, Yang Y: Dead space fraction changes during PEEP titration following lung recruitment in patients with ARDS, *Respir Care* 57(10):1578–1585, 2012.

Harris K: Noninvasive monitoring of gas exchange, *Respir Care* 32(7):544–557, 1987.

Hess DR: Capnometry and capnography: technical aspects, physiologic aspects, and clinical applications, *Respir Care* 35(6):557–576, 1990.

Hess DR: Respiratory monitoring. In Hess DR, MacIntyre NR, Mishoe SC, Galvin WF, Adams AB, editors: *Respiratory care principles and practice*, ed 2, Burlington, MA, 2012, Jones & Bartlett Learning.

Hess DR, Branson RD: Noninvasive respiratory monitoring equipment. In Branson RD, Hess DR, Chatburn RL, editors: *Respiratory care equipment*, ed 2, Philadelphia, 1990, Lippincott Williams & Wilkins.

Heuer AJ: Vital signs. In Heuer AJ, Scanlan CL, editors: *Wilkins' clinical assessment in respiratory care*, ed 7, St Louis, 2014, Mosby.

Hirsch CA: Gas exchange and transport. In Kacmarek RM, Stoller JK, Heuer AJ, editors: *Egan's fundamentals of respiratory care*, ed 10, St Louis, 2013, Mosby.

Huang Y-CH, Lease E, Beachey W: Gas exchange. In Hess DR, MacIntyre NR, Mishoe SC, Galvin WF, Adams AB, editors: *Respiratory care principles and practice*, ed 2, Burlington, MA, 2012, Jones & Bartlett Learning.

Hunt GE: Diagnostic procedures at the bedside. In Fink JB, Hunt GE, editors: *Clinical practice in respiratory care*, Philadelphia, 1999, Lippincott-Raven.

Jacobus C: Noninvasive monitoring in neonatal and pediatric care. In Walsh BK, Czervinske MP, DiBlasi RM, editors: *Perinatal and pediatric respiratory care*, ed 3, St Louis, 2010, Saunders.

Jaquith SM: The oximetric opticath: what is it and how can it facilitate nursing management of the critically ill patient? *Crit Care Nurse* 55–58, May/June 1984.

Kallet RH: Bedside assessment of the patient. In Kacmarek RM, Stoller JK, Heuer AJ, editors: *Egan's fundamentals of respiratory care*, ed 10, St Louis, 2013, Mosby.

Kandel G, Aberman A: Mixed venous oxygen saturation: its role in the assessment of the critically ill patient, *Arch Intern Med* 143:1400–1402, 1983.

Kinasewitz GT: Use of end-tidal capnography during mechanical ventilation, *Respir Care* 25(2):169–171, 1982.

Ludwig B, Mathews LM: Cardiac and hemodynamic monitoring. In Wyka KA, Mathews PJ, Rutkowski JA, editors: *Foundations of respiratory care*, ed 2, Clifton Park, NY, 2012, Delmar.

Malinowski T: Respiratory monitoring in the Intensive Care Unit. In Wilkins RL, Krider SJ, Sheldon RL, editors: *Clinical assessment in respiratory care*, ed 3, St Louis, 1990, Mosby.

Malley WJ: *Clinical blood gases*, ed 2, St Louis, 2005, Saunders.

Marini JJ: Obtaining meaningful data from the Swan-Ganz catheter, *Respir Care* 30(7):572–585, 1985.

Marino JR: Hemodynamic monitoring. In Hinski ST, editor: *Respiratory care clinical lab manual*, St Louis, 2014, Mosby.

McSwain SD, Hamel DS, Smith PB, Gentile MA, Srinivasan S, Meliones JN, et al.: End-tidal and arterial carbon dioxide measurements correlate across all levels of physiologic dead space, *Respir Care* 55(3):288–293, 2010.

Miller K, Scanlan CL: Vascular pressure monitoring. In Heuer AJ, Scanlan CL, editors: *Wilkins' clinical assessment in respiratory care*, ed 7, St Louis, 2014, Mosby.

Mottram CD: *Ruppel's manual of pulmonary function testing*, ed 10, St Louis, 2013, Mosby.

Nuzzo PF, Anton WR: Practical applications of capnography, *Respir Ther* 12–17, Nov/Dec 1986.

Oblouk Darovic G: *Hemodynamic monitoring—invasive and noninvasive clinical application*, ed 3, Philadelphia, 2002, Saunders.

Osgood CF, Watson MH, Slaughter MS, MacIntyre NR: Hemodynamic monitoring in respiratory care, *Respir Care* 29(1):25–34, 1984.

Paulus DA: Invasive monitoring of respiratory gas exchange: continuous measurement of mixed venous oxygen saturation, *Respir Care* 32(7):535–543, 1987.

Pekdemir M, Cinar O, Yilmaz S, Yaka E, Yuksel M: Disparity between mainstream and sidestream end-tidal carbon dioxide values and arterial carbon dioxide levels, *Respir Care* 58(7):1152–1156, 2013.

Ragosta M: *Textbook of clinical hemodynamics*, Philadelphia, 2008, Saunders.

Raurich JM, Vilar M, Colomar A, Ibañez J, Avestarán I, Pérez-Bárcena J, et al.: Prognostic value of the pulmonary dead-space fraction during the early and intermediate phases of acute respiratory distress syndrome, *Respir Care* 55(3):282–287, 2010.

Reinhart K, Kuhn H, Hartog C, Bredle DL: Continuous central venous and pulmonary artery oxygen saturation in the critically ill, *Intensive Care Med* 30:1572–1578, 2004.

Restrepo RD: Cardiac output measurement. In Heuer AJ, Scanlan CL, editors: *Wilkins' clinical assessment in respiratory care*, ed 7, St Louis, 2014, Mosby.

Scanlan CL: Interpretation of blood gases. In Heuer AJ, Scanlan CL, editors: *Wilkins' clinical assessment in respiratory care*, ed 7, St Louis, 2014, Mosby.

Shapiro BA, Peruzzi WT, Kozlowski-Templin R: *Clinical application of blood gases*, ed 5, St Louis, 1994, Mosby.

Siobal MS: Analysis and monitoring of gas exchange. In Kacmarek RM, Stoller JK, Heuer AJ, editors: *Egan's fundamentals of respiratory care*, ed 10, St Louis, 2013, Mosby.

Vines DL: Respiratory monitoring in critical care. In Heuer AJ, Scanlan CL, editors: *Wilkins' clinical assessment in respiratory care*, ed 7, St Louis, 2014, Mosby.

Wemple M, Luks AM: Challenges associated with central venous catheter placement and central venous oxygen saturation monitoring, *Respir Care* 57(12):2119–2123, 2012.

White GC: *Equipment theory for respiratory care*, ed 4, Albany, NY, 2005, Delmar.

1. The waveform sequence seen during the insertion of a PAC is:
   A. RA, RV, PAP, PCWP
   B. RV, RA, PAP, PCWP
   C. RA, RV, PCWP, PAP
   D. Ao, RA, RV, PAP

2. When evaluating a patient's SV, which of the following is true?
   A. It is an indicator of the adequacy of perfusion of the body tissues.
   B. It is the output of blood for 1 minute.
   C. It has a range of 50-120 mL in the adult.
   D. It is the resistance to flow.

3. A patient with chronic bronchitis is being monitored with regular measurements of arterial blood gas values and capnometry. The following data are available:

$PaCO_2$	53 torr
PaO_2	67 torr
$P_{ET}CO_2$	33 torr
$P_{\bar{E}}CO_2$	20 torr

   Calculate the patient's V_D/V_T.
   A. 0.30
   B. 0.38
   C. 0.62
   D. 0.71

4. A 40-year-old patient recovering from ARDS is receiving mechanical ventilation with a tidal volume of 650 mL. The patient has an arterial line, a PAC, and capnometry for monitoring. The following information is gathered after a change in PEEP level:

$PaCO_2$	43 torr
PaO_2	79 torr
$P\bar{v}O_2$	32 torr
$P_{ET}CO_2$	38 torr
$P_{\bar{E}}CO_2$	22 torr

   Calculate the patient's V_D.
   A. 273 mL
   B. 319 mL
   C. 338 mL
   D. 384 mL

5. A 35-year-old patient in the Intensive Care Unit has the following hemodynamic data. Which of these data indicates a problem with the patient?
   A. SVR of 600 dyn/s/cm−5
   B. CI of 3 L/min/m² of body surface area
   C. $P\bar{v}O_2$ of 38 torr
   D. Shunt of 4%

6. A patient with a history of congestive heart failure is inadvertently given intravenous fluids of 2000 mL instead of the ordered amount of 200 mL. Which of the following is most likely to be seen?
   A. Decreased lung markings on chest radiograph
   B. Increased pulmonary capillary wedge pressure
   C. Increased PaO_2
   D. Decreased PAP

7. A patient hospitalized with leg vein thrombosis experiences sudden shortness of breath. Which of the following should be recommended to evaluate the patient's situation?
   A. Lung compliance
   B. Electrocardiogram
   C. Chest radiograph
   D. V_D/V_T

8. Capnography will be used to monitor a patient's recovery from anesthesia. What gas should be used for the zero calibration?
   A. Room air for 0% carbon dioxide
   B. Room air for 21% oxygen
   C. 5% carbon dioxide
   D. The same concentration of anesthetic gas as used with the patient

9. Hypovolemia in an adult patient would be indicated by a PCWP of:
   A. 2 mm Hg
   B. 8 mm Hg
   C. 12 mm Hg
   D. 24 mm Hg

10. An adult patient has had a PAC inserted. A normal PAP pressure in this patient would be:
    A. 8 mm Hg
    B. 25/10 mm Hg
    C. 35/15 mm Hg
    D. 120/80 mm Hg

11. Which of the following would describe the principle of operation of a capnometer?
    A. The same as that of the Clark electrode
    B. The proportionality between carbon dioxide and hydrogen ions
    C. Absorption of infrared light by carbon dioxide
    D. The same as that of the CO oximeter

12. Calculate a patient's pulmonary artery diastolic-pulmonary capillary wedge pressure (PAd–PCWP) gradient if the PAP is 30/12 mm Hg and the PCWP is 8 mm Hg.
    A. 38 mm Hg
    B. 12 mm Hg
    C. 8 mm Hg
    D. 4 mm Hg

13. A patient has an end-tidal CO_2 pressure of 30 torr and a $P(a-et)CO_2$ gradient of 4 torr. The alveolar to end-tidal gradient is in the usual direction. Based on this, the patient's $PaCO_2$ would be estimated as:
    A. 4 torr
    B. 26 torr
    C. 30 torr
    D. 34 torr

14. A patient is known to have advanced COPD. When checking the patient's V_D/V_T ratio, what would be expected?
    A. Unaffected by patient's condition
    B. Increased
    C. Normal
    D. Decreased

15. A patient is being mechanically ventilated and has a reflectance oximetry PAC in place. What $S\bar{v}O_2$ value would indicate the patient is oxygenating adequately?
    A. 40%
    B. 50%
    C. 75%
    D. 90%

16. The normal range for the $P(a-et)CO_2$ gradient is:
    A. <1 torr
    B. 1-5 torr
    C. More than 15 torr
    D. About 40 torr

17. An adult patient has been admitted for observation after suffering a concussion in a fall. The patient's arterial BP is found to be 115/78 mm Hg. How should these results be interpreted?
    A. Within normal limits
    B. Hypertension
    C. Hypotension
    D. Intracranial bleed

18. A patient with advanced emphysema is admitted to the respiratory Intensive Care Unit. The patient is placed on a 24% Venturi-type mask and has a PAC inserted. The patient's initial PVR is 9 mm Hg/L/min and his PaO_2 is 57 torr. The physician orders an increase to 28% oxygen. The resulting PVR is 5 mm Hg/L/min and PaO_2 is 63 torr. Based on this information, what would you recommend?
    A. Decrease the oxygen to 24%.
    B. Place the patient on a ventilator.
    C. Administer a bronchodilating agent such as albuterol.
    D. Keep the patient on 28% oxygen.

19. An adult patient is in the Intensive Care Unit and is being monitored with a PAC. The patient has the following parameters: PAP of 35/20 mm Hg, PCWP of 9 mm Hg, CVP of 9 cm of water. The data show that the patient:
    A. Has right-ventricular failure/cor pulmonale
    B. Has left-ventricular failure

C. Has increased PVR
D. Is hypovolemic

20. A 40-year-old patient receiving mechanical ventilation has an arterial line in place. It is noticed that there is a significant difference between the BP taken by cuff on the left arm and the BP taken by arterial line on the right arm. What could explain this difference?
    1. **A clot is at the tip of the catheter.**
    2. **There is an air bubble in the arterial line.**
    3. **The ventilator's peak pressure is too high.**
    4. **The patient has a ventricular septal defect.**
    A. 1 and 2 only
    B. 2 and 3 only
    C. 1, 3, and 4 only
    D. 1, 2, 3, 4

21. An adult patient is receiving mechanical ventilation when the following data are gathered:

	9:00 AM	11:00 AM
PaO_2	75 torr	53 torr
Pulmonary vascular resistance	120 dyn/s/cm^{-5}	340 dyn/s/cm^{-5}
Pulmonary capillary wedge pressure	8 mm Hg	10 mm Hg
Pulmonary artery pressure	25/10 mm Hg	42/21 mm Hg

How should the results be interpreted?
    A. Pulmonary edema
    B. Pulmonary embolism
    C. Pneumonia
    D. Cardiac tamponade

22. A patient is receiving mechanical ventilation with a mandatory rate of 10/min. End-tidal carbon dioxide monitoring is being done and the following data are recorded:

	4:00 PM	6:00 PM
Set tidal volume	700 mL	700 mL
Set rate	10	10
$P_{ET}CO_2$	33 torr	41 torr
$PaCO_2$	42 torr	43 torr

How can these data be explained?
    A. Alveolar ventilation has decreased.
    B. Pulmonary edema has developed.
    C. The patient is hyperventilating.
    D. The patient's CO has increased.

23. A patient has had an arterial line inserted. What should be done to ensure that accurate BP readings are obtained?
    1. **Open the stopcock to room air to zero the transducer.**
    2. **Make sure that air fills the transducer dome.**

3. Have the patient lie flat to measure the BP.
4. Fill the pressure tubing with a saline solution.
   A. 1 and 2 only
   B. 2 and 4 only
   C. 1, 2, and 3 only
   D. 1, 3, and 4 only

24. An unconscious 25-year-old patient is admitted with viral pneumonia, vomiting, and diarrhea. Mechanical ventilation is initiated and a flow-directed PAC is inserted. The following data are gathered:

Pulmonary artery pressure	22/8 mm Hg
Pulmonary capillary wedge pressure	3 mm Hg
Central venous pressure	0 mm Hg
Blood pressure	90/60 mm Hg
Pulse	142 beats/min

What is the most likely cause of these findings?
   A. Hypovolemia
   B. High ventilating pressures
   C. Bronchospasm
   D. Rupture of the balloon on the catheter

25. A 3-day postoperative open-heart surgery patient has an arterial catheter in the right radial artery for continuous BP measurements. Because of retained secretions, the respiratory therapist places the patient into a head-down position for postural drainage therapy. The nurse notices that the patient's BP is less than before being placed into this new position. After the patient is returned to the original position, the BP is the same as it was originally. How can the therapist explain the BP changes?
   A. There was an air bubble in the arterial catheter.
   B. There was a clot in the arterial catheter.
   C. The patient's body was below the level of the pressure transducer.
   D. Postural drainage positions always cause the BP to decrease.

26. A 65-year-old patient has been sick with vomiting and diarrhea for several days. Arterial and PACs are placed for monitoring blood gases and hemodynamic parameters. ABG values on 30% O_2 show the following: PaO_2, 80 torr; $PaCO_2$, 41 torr; pH, 7.44; bicarbonate, 27 mEq/L. PAC parameters show the following: PAP, 22/8 torr; PCWP, 3 torr. In addition, serum electrolytes show the following: sodium, 156 mEq/L; potassium, 4.5 mEq/L; chlorine, 120 mEq/L. Based on these data, what should be recommended?
   A. Administer a diuretic.
   B. Increase the O_2 percentage.
   C. Administer fluids intravenously.
   D. Give a chronotropic agent.

27. A patient with heart failure and pulmonary edema has an initial $P\bar{v}O_2$ value of 35 torr. After the patient is mechanically ventilated and given digitalis, the $P\bar{v}O_2$ value is 41 torr. How should this be interpreted?
   A. Improved tissue oxygenation
   B. No clinical change
   C. Decreased tissue oxygenation
   D. Worsening heart failure

28. A neonatal patient is suspected of having a ventricular septal defect. What could be done to confirm or rule out this condition?
   A. Perform capnography to monitor the $PetCO_2$ level.
   B. Perform a V_D/V_T calculation.
   C. Check the $P\bar{v}O_2$ value from the pulmonary artery.
   D. Check the $P\bar{v}O_2$ value from the right atrium and right ventricle.

29. An adult patient with congestive heart failure needs to have his fluid management and oxygen consumption monitored. What type of catheter should be used for these measurements?
   A. Radial arterial catheter
   B. Umbilical artery catheter
   C. Single-lumen CVP catheter
   D. Triple-lumen $ScvO_2$ CVP catheter

30. As the respiratory therapist assigned to the Intensive Care Unit, you are helping in the care of the following four patients: Mr. Boone is a 28-year-old male being observed after an appendectomy. Mrs. Decker is a 74-year-old female with sepsis. Mrs. Dylan is a 48-year-old female with gastritis who is receiving intravenous fluids for dehydration. Mr. Zawinal is a 42-year-old male with diabetes. The following series of BP measurements (in mm Hg) were taken on these patients:

	10:00 AM	12:00 PM	2:00 AM
Mr. Boone	125/80	122/82	120/78
Mrs. Decker	90/60	105/40	85/45
Mrs. Dylan	88/70	94/75	105/78
Mr. Zawinal	135/98	129/94	125/89

Which of these patients should have an arterial line placed?
   A. Mr. Boone
   B. Mrs. Decker
   C. Mrs. Dylan
   D. Mr. Zawinal

31. A patient with heart failure had an $ScvO_2$ value of 65% an hour ago. The patient is now showing an $ScvO_2$ value of 60%. How should these results be interpreted?
   A. Tissue hypoxia
   B. Normal oxygenation
   C. Increased CO
   D. Decreased PVR

6 Oxygen and Medical Gas Therapy

Note: It can be anticipated that the Therapist Multiple-Choice Examination (TMC) will include an *average of 10 of 140 actual questions* (7% of the exam) on oxygen and medical gas therapy. (This is based on the question mix typically found on the National Board of Respiratory Care's (NBRC's) previous Entry Level Examinations and Written Registry Examinations.)

Remember that the TMC version you take will include 20 additional questions being evaluated for possible inclusion in other versions of the TMC. So, there will be a total of 160 questions taken. There is no way to differentiate between the 140 actual questions and the 20 questions being evaluated for future use. Please go to the Introduction for detailed information on the Therapist Multiple-Choice Examination and the Clinical Simulation Examination.

MODULE A

Ensure that the patient is adequately oxygenated.

1. Minimize hypoxemia by changing the patient's position (code: IIIC2) [difficulty: R, Ap, An]

Usually a patient who is short of breath when lying supine should be repositioned to sit more upright in a Fowler's or semi-Fowler's position. This seems to work best in patients with bilateral pulmonary problems such as congestive heart failure or pneumonia. If the patient cannot sit up and the lung problem is one-sided, roll the patient so that the more functional lung is down. The good lung should be positioned up in the following exceptions:

- Undrained pulmonary abscess that should not be drained into the good lung
- Neonatal congenital diaphragmatic hernia in which the good lung should not be compressed by the bowel in the chest cavity
- Pulmonary interstitial emphysema in which, by lying on the bad lung, the air leak and functional residual capacity can be reduced

In either case, always ask the patient whether the new position helps to make breathing easier. If not, reposition the patient until breathing is more comfortable with less shortness of breath. In general, Trendelenburg is not well tolerated. A patient with a closed head injury and brain edema should not be put into the Trendelenburg position.

2. Recommend oxygen therapy (code: III3b) [difficulty: R, Ap, An]

Oxygen (O_2) must be administered in concentrations (up to 100%) that are adequate to treat hypoxemia, decrease the patient's work of breathing, or decrease the work of the heart. Because the U.S. Food and Drug Administration (FDA) has declared supplemental oxygen to be a drug, a physician's order is required to give it to a patient or to make a change in the percentage. The only exceptions are when recognized protocols exist in your institution to give oxygen under certain limited conditions. For example, all patients with a diagnosed heart attack are given a nasal cannula at 2 L/min, or all patients undergoing cardiopulmonary resuscitation (CPR) receive 100% oxygen.

See Chapter 3 (Module A) for a listing of indications for drawing blood for an arterial blood gas (ABG) measurement or checking the pulse oximeter value. This list should be fairly complete for conditions that justify the need for supplemental oxygen. In general, the goal of giving supplemental oxygen is to keep the patient's PaO_2 level between 60 and 100 torr. Exceptions include carbon monoxide poisoning, severe anemia, and CPR, when the hope is to fully saturate the hemoglobin and increase the plasma oxygen content as much as possible. Oxygen should not be given without proof of hypoxemia or another clinical justification. When those conditions have been corrected, the oxygen percentage should be adjusted accordingly.

Giving supplemental oxygen is not done without risk. The following are oxygen-related problems that may be seen clinically.

a. O₂-induced hypoventilation

This is something to watch for in patients who have an elevated carbon dioxide level and compensated respiratory acidosis caused by severe emphysema, chronic bronchitis, or both (known as chronic obstructive pulmonary disease [COPD]). A common clinical goal is to keep the PaO_2 level between 50 and 60 torr. This correlates with an SpO_2 of 88% to 92%. Check the blood gases frequently for the oxygen and carbon dioxide levels.

b. Retinopathy of prematurity *(formerly called retrolental fibroplasia)*

This type of visual impairment is found in some premature neonates who were given high levels of supplemental oxygen. The exact cause is not completely understood but is related primarily to the degree of prematurity. There is evidence that a high oxygen saturation and fluctuating retinal blood vessel oxygen levels are key contributing factors. Keeping the PaO_2 in the range of 50-60 torr for the first week and at 50-70 torr after that should help to prevent the problem.

c. Denitrogenation absorption atelectasis

Giving more than 80% oxygen can result in atelectasis of underventilated alveoli after the oxygen has been taken up by the blood.

d. Central nervous system abnormalities

A patient who is breathing 100% oxygen in a hyperbaric chamber can have muscle tremors and seizures.

e. Pulmonary O_2 toxicity

Hyperoxic acute lung injury (HALI) is a lung injury caused by inhaling a high oxygen percentage for a prolonged time. Because of variable factors, there is no exact oxygen percentage or time period that predicts when a given patient will develop HALI. In general, it appears that there is little risk if a patient breathes in ≤60% oxygen. The risk becomes progressively greater as 70% or more oxygen is inhaled. If a person were to breathe ≥90% for a prolonged time, severe, even fatal, HALI would occur.

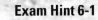

Exam Hint 6-1

The NBRC is known to ask questions that relate to the proper use of oxygen and the hazards associated with its use. Expect to see at least one question that deals with the need to decrease the oxygen percentage for a patient with COPD who has shown an increased $PaCO_2$ when given too much supplemental oxygen.

3. Minimize hypoxemia by using proper technique (code: IIIC2) [difficulty: R, Ap, An]

Use caution and plan ahead to minimize any time that the oxygen supply to the patient is disconnected or reduced. When changing equipment of any kind, have the replacement set up and tested for proper function before replacing the current setup.

It is well known that suctioning the airway reduces the patient's oxygen level. This can result in dangerous dysrhythmias. Remember to increase the patient's inspired oxygen percentage about 1 minute before, during, and for at least 1 minute after suctioning. It is acceptable and safe to give 100% oxygen to an adult for short periods like this. Remember to reduce the oxygen percentage or liter flow to the previous level once the patient is stable after the procedure. Reanalyze the percentage if possible. See Chapter 13 for the complete discussion on safety issues related to suctioning.

MODULE B

Oxygen analyzers

1. Assemble oxygen and specialty gas analyzers (code: IIA22) [difficulty: R, Ap]

Always measure the patient's inspired O_2 percentage (F_IO_2) if possible. The gas sample should be taken as close as possible to the patient to minimize the chance of dilution from room air. Record the oxygen percentage on the ABG order slip, in the department records, and in the patient's electronic medical record, if needed. As discussed in Chapter 3, the oxygen percentage must be known before the patient's PaO_2 level can be interpreted.

The oxygen liter flow is all that can be recorded with the following devices: nasal cannula, nasal catheter, simple mask, partial-rebreather mask, nonrebreather mask, and transtracheal oxygen catheter. A direct relation is found between the liter flow and the oxygen percentage, but it is not predictably accurate.

2. Troubleshoot any problems with the equipment (code: IIA22) [difficulty: R, Ap]

Because so many different models are available, consult an equipment book or the manufacturer's literature for details of the various analyzers. All portable, hand-held oxygen analyzers fall into one of the following categories: electric, physical/paramagnetic, and electrochemical.

a. Electric analyzers

These older analyzers basically operate by comparing the cooling effects of an oxygen-enriched gas sample on a heated wire versus the cooling effects of a room air gas sample on a heated wire. The oxygen-enriched gas cools faster than the room air gas. This is known as the principle of thermal conductivity. Each sample must be drawn into the analyzer through a capillary line. These analyzers are designed to work only in oxygen and nitrogen gas mixes. Do not use them around flammable gases such as those found in anesthesia. Failure to calibrate can be caused by a weak battery, a plugged capillary line, or a defect in an electrical component.

b. Physical/paramagnetic analyzers

These older analyzers make use of the fact that oxygen is attracted toward a magnetic field (paramagnetic property). The more oxygen is in a sample gas, the more the magnetic field is altered. These units can be used with all types of gases and are safe in the operating room with flammable and explosive anesthetics. A silica gel-filled container is in line with the capillary tube to dry out the sample gas before it gets to the analyzing chamber. Failure to calibrate can be caused by water or by a defect in the analyzing chamber, a weak battery, or a plugged capillary line.

c. Electrochemical analyzers: polarographic and galvanic fuel cell

Modern polarographic and galvanic analyzers employ a fuel cell that utilizes the chemical reaction in which each oxygen molecule accepts up to two electrons and becomes chemically reduced. The more oxygen there is in the gas sample, the more electrons are released from an oxidizing electrolyte solution. This is measured as an electrical current that is proportional to the oxygen percentage. These analyzers can monitor continuously and display the oxygen percentage. Both types are safe by themselves in the presence of flammable gases, but the added alarm systems are powered electrically and may make the units unsafe. Polarographic analyzers use a battery to polarize the gas-sampling probe. Because of this, they have a faster response time than do the galvanic fuel cell types. Galvanic fuel cell analyzers do not need a battery for power. However, they usually include alarms that are battery powered.

Failure to calibrate either type can be caused by a weak battery, an exhausted supply of chemical reactant in the gas-sampling probe, an electronic failure, or a damaged membrane over the probe. A damaged or torn probe will allow water, mucus, or blood onto the probe. The galvanic units must have their probes kept dry to be read accurately. Both types are pressure sensitive. High altitude causes them to display a lower-than-true oxygen percentage, and high pressure as seen in a ventilator circuit with positive end-expiratory pressure (PEEP) causes the units to display a higher-than-true oxygen percentage.

d. Specialty gas analyzers

Specialty gas analyzers (helium, nitrogen, and carbon monoxide) are used mainly with pulmonary function testing procedures and are discussed in Chapter 4. It may be necessary to use a helium analyzer if a helium and oxygen mix is given to a patient.

Nitric oxide (NO) is delivered through the INOvent delivery system (Datex-Ohmeda, Inc., Madison, WI). It is able to deliver set amounts of therapeutic NO and to continuously monitor the amount of NO given to the patient along with nitrogen dioxide (NO_2) and oxygen.

3. Perform quality control procedures for oxygen analyzers (code: IIC1) [difficulty: R, Ap]

A two-point calibration procedure is done on all oxygen analyzers by sampling room air, adjusting a calibration control if necessary to have the unit show 21% oxygen (first point or low-oxygen check), sampling 100% oxygen, and adjusting a calibration control if necessary to have the unit show 100% oxygen (second point or high-oxygen check). When room air is sampled again, the analyzer should read 21% oxygen. In general, always follow the manufacturer's guidelines for setup and calibration. If an analyzer does not pass the two-point calibration check, it should not be used.

MODULE C

Medical gas equipment

1. Oxygen and other gas cylinders, bulk storage systems, and manifolds (code: IIA12) [difficulty: R, Ap]

a. Assemble the necessary equipment

See below.

b. Troubleshoot any problems with the equipment

1. Oxygen and other gas cylinders

The various types of gases in cylinders are identified by the color code of the cylinder and the cylinder label. Note that only E cylinders have mandatory color coding. Color codings on the other cylinders are voluntary but usually are followed by the manufacturers. However, always read the label to be sure of the contents of the cylinder. The most important cylinder colors to remember are those of oxygen and air, but all are included in Table 6-1 for the sake of completeness.

Exam Hint 6-2

The NBRC is known to ask the examinee to calculate how long a certain cylinder lasts at a given gas flow. To date, only the durations of E-, H-, and K-sized oxygen cylinders have had to be calculated.

To review how to calculate the duration of flow for a particular type of cylinder, see Table 6-2 for the cylinder duration factors, the following equation, and the following examples.

Minutes of flow (divide by 60 to calculate hours)

$$= \frac{\text{Gauge pressure in psig} \times \text{Cylinder factor}}{\text{Liter flow}}$$

1. Calculate the duration of flow of an E cylinder with 1500 pounds per square inch gauge (psig) that is running at 6 L/min.

$$\text{Minutes of flow (divide by 60 to calculate hours)} = \frac{1500 \text{ psig} \times 0.28}{6 \text{ L}}$$
$$= \frac{420}{6}$$

Minutes of flow = 70 (1.16 hours, or 1 hour and 10 minutes)

2. Calculate the duration of flow of an H cylinder with 1950 psig that is running at 9 L/min.

$$\text{Minutes of flow (divide by 60 to calculate hours)} = \frac{1950 \text{ psig} \times 3.14}{9 \text{ L}}$$
$$= \frac{6123}{9}$$

Minutes of flow = 680.33 (11.34 hours, or 11 hours and 20 minutes).

---

2. Bulk storage systems

The bulk liquid oxygen (LOX) storage system is the main source of a hospital's oxygen. A reducing valve is used to decrease the gas pressure to 50 psig before it is piped throughout the hospital for easy access. Alarms will sound if the pressure is low or too high. Pressure relief valves will open if the pressure is greater than 75 psig. Zone valves are located throughout the hospital so the gas can be turned off if a leak develops or if a fire occurs.

3. Manifolds

A manifold is a piping system that connects the bulk storage system and the hospital gas piping system with a bank of H- or K-sized cylinders. These free-standing cylinders are a backup source of oxygen in case the bulk system fails. A 24-hour supply of gas must be available.

The manifold system includes a reducing valve to decrease the gas pressure to 50 psig. Check-valves are built into the manifold so that a leak in one cylinder connection cannot result in all of the gas cylinders leaking out.

2. Adjunct hardware, such as reducing valves, flowmeters, regulators, and high-pressure hose connectors (code: IIA12) [difficulty: R, Ap]

a. Assemble the necessary equipment

See below.

TABLE 6-1	Color Codes for Gas Cylinders
Gas	**Color**
Oxygen	Green (international: white)
Air	Yellow (international: black and white)
Helium	Brown
Helium and oxygen	Brown and green (check the label for the percentage of each gas) (international: brown and white)
Carbon dioxide	Gray
Carbon dioxide and oxygen	Gray and green (check the label for oxygen and the percentage of each gas) (international: gray and white)
Nitrous oxide	Blue
Cyclopropane	Orange
Ethylene	Red

TABLE 6-2	Oxygen Cylinder Duration of Flow Factors
Cylinder Size	**Factor, L/psig**
E	0.28
H	3.14
K	3.14
D	0.16
M	1.36
G	2.41

psig, pounds per square inch gauge.

b. Troubleshoot any problems with the equipment

1. Reducing valves

Reducing valves are used to reduce the high pressure seen in a bulk oxygen storage system, manifold, or gas cylinder. One or more stages (pressure-reducing steps) can be used to reach the working pressure of 50 psig. Single-stage reducing valves reach the pressure in a single step. Multiple-stage reducing valves give finer control over pressure and flow by decreasing pressure in the first stage to about 200 psig and to 50 psig in the second stage. Occasionally, three stages are seen. All reducing valves (and regulators [combined reducing valve and flowmeter]) have the following built-in safety features:

- A frangible disk that breaks to release gas pressure in the event of mechanical failure or breakage
- A fusible plug that melts to release gas pressure in the event of a fire
- American Standard Compressed Gas Cylinder Valve Outlet and Index Connections (usually called the American Standard Safety System), which prevent the accidental connection of the wrong reducing valve (or regulator) to a large gas cylinder
- The Pin Index Safety System is a special section of the American Standard System that applies to gas cylinders that are E-sized and smaller. It is designed to prevent an accidental connection of the wrong gas to a reducing valve or regulator. These reducing valves and regulators are designed with a specifically pinned yoke to wrap around the valve stem of a gas cylinder. A soft plastic O-ring washer is included to help ensure a tight seal. Figure 6-1 shows the location of the pinholes in the cylinder valve face. Table 6-3 shows the gases and pinhole positions. It is important to know the positions for oxygen and air; the others are included for the sake of completeness.

It is necessary to "crack" or blow some gas out of a cylinder before putting any reducing valve or regulator

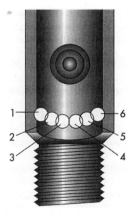

Figure 6-1 Locations of the Pin Index Safety System holes in the cylinder valve face. From Vines DL: Storage and delivery of medical gases. In Kacmarek RM, Stoller JK, Heuer AJ, editors: Egan's fundamentals of respiratory care, ed 10, St Louis, 2013, Mosby.

onto the cylinder. Do this by attaching the tank wrench to the valve stem and slowly turning the valve stem in a counterclockwise (so-called "lefty-loosy") direction to release some gas. This cracking is done to prevent any dust or debris from being forced into the reducing valve or regulator, which might cause a fire. See Figure 6-2 for a schematic drawing of an E tank of oxygen and how its yoke is connected. If the O-ring is missing or the yoke is misaligned on the post, a high-pressure gas leak will occur when the tank is opened with the tank wrench. Close off the tank to stop the leak by turning the tank wrench on

the valve stem in a clockwise direction (so-called "righty-tighty"). Investigate the yoke-to-post connection to identify causes of the leak.

2. Flowmeters

Flowmeters are designed to regulate and indicate flow. They come with the following safety features so that they cannot be attached to the wrong reducing valve, regulator, high-pressure hose, or appliance:

- Diameter Index Safety System (DISS) inlets and outlets that are specific to the various gases, so a mix-up with the wrong appliance or connector cannot occur. The DISS system applies to flowmeters that attach to all American Standard and DISS reduction valves.
- Flowmeters with quick-connect inlet adapters instead of DISS inlets. These quick-connects are designed specifically for the hospital's piped-in oxygen and air outlets. They are not interchangeable between gases or between manufacturers. Occasionally a piped oxygen outlet will jam open and will let gas rapidly escape. Insert the proper flowmeter into the outlet, and turn the flowmeter off. This stops the leak until the defective wall outlet can be repaired.

Flowmeters usually are categorized by how they react to backpressure. To complicate matters further, we must remember that the three different manufactured types of flowmeters may or may not be backpressure compensated:

TABLE 6-3	Pin Index Safety System Gases and Pinhole Locations
Gas	**Pinhole Locations**
Oxygen	2-5
Air	1-5
Oxygen/carbon dioxide (≤7%)	2-6
Oxygen/carbon dioxide (>7%)	1-6
Oxygen/helium (≤80% helium)	2-4
Oxygen/helium (>80% helium)	4-6
Nitrous oxide	3-5
Ethylene	1-3
Cyclopropane	3-6

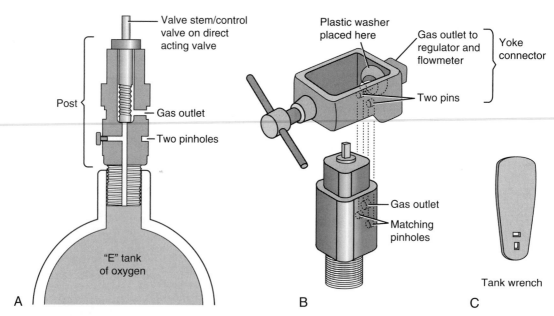

Figure 6-2 Details of an E-size tank of oxygen and its yoke connector. **A,** A cross-section through the stem (also called the control valve) of the tank shows its key features. **B,** A three-dimensional view shows how the yoke with its two pins aligns with the corresponding pinholes (locations 2 and 5) on the yoke. The plastic washer ensures a seal between the gas outlet on the stem and the yoke. (Not shown is the regulator that attaches to the yoke. See Fig. 6-6.) **C,** A tank wrench that is attached to the valve stem (also called a control valve). Turn the wrench in a counterclockwise direction to open the tank and allow gas flow; close the tank to stop gas flow by turning the wrench in a clockwise direction. Redrawn from Sills JR: Respiratory care for the health care provider, Albany, 1998, Delmar.

1. Non-backpressure-compensated (pressure-uncompensated) kinetic or Thorpe flowmeters will inaccurately indicate the flow through them in the face of backpressure. Figure 6-3, A shows an example. Note that a pressure-uncompensated flowmeter has the flow-control valve upstream of the meter. These flowmeters read accurately if they are kept upright and do not have to "push" against any backpressure. However, if laid on their sides, the "float" (a plunger or ball bearing) does not indicate the set flow. These flowmeters read a *lower* flow than that actually delivered when faced with a backpressure.

2. Backpressure-compensated (pressure-compensated) flowmeters accurately indicate the flow through them in the face of backpressure. For this reason, they should be used whenever possible. Figure 6-3, B shows an example. Note that a pressure-compensated flowmeter has the flow-control valve downstream of the meter. Because of this, these flowmeters read *accurately* in the face of backpressure as long as they are kept upright. However, if laid on their side, the float does not indicate the set flow.

In addition to reading the label, this simple test enables the practitioner to tell whether a flowmeter is backpressure-compensated:

1. Make sure the flowmeter is turned off.
2. Plug the flowmeter into a gas outlet.
3. If the float or ball bearing bounces, the flowmeter is backpressure-compensated.

3. The Bourdon flowmeter is designed similar to the Bourdon gauge in the reducing valve (Fig. 6-4). The face piece is marked in liters of flow rather than pressure. It is the flowmeter of choice in a transport situation because it may be laid flat with no effect on its flow if no backpressure is present. However, these flowmeters will display a *higher* flow than that actually delivered when faced with a backpressure.

3. Regulators

Regulators combine a reducing valve and a flowmeter (Fig. 6-5). Everything that has been discussed so far relates to regulators. Bourdon gauge reducing valves are commonly seen and can have a second Bourdon gauge added as a flowmeter (Fig. 6-6) or a Thorpe or kinetic flowmeter (see Fig. 6-5). As mentioned earlier, use a backpressure-compensated flowmeter in all situations except for patient transport.

4. High-pressure hose connectors

These connectors and other adapters connect high-pressure hoses, flowmeters, and oxygen appliances. They have DISS inlets and outlets so that the gases cannot be cross-fitted to the wrong equipment. (Note the hoses connected to the oxygen blender in Fig. 6-7.)

3. Perform quality control procedures for flowmeters (code: IIC6) [difficulty: R, Ap]

When a quality control procedure for a flowmeter is performed, it is critical that a known flow be sent through it so that the flowmeter can be checked for accuracy. This should be done without any backpressure against the flowmeter. Review the previous discussion on troubleshooting flowmeters for the effects of backpressure on non-backpressure-compensated flowmeters and Bourdon flowmeters. Do not use any flowmeter that does not give an accurate reading.

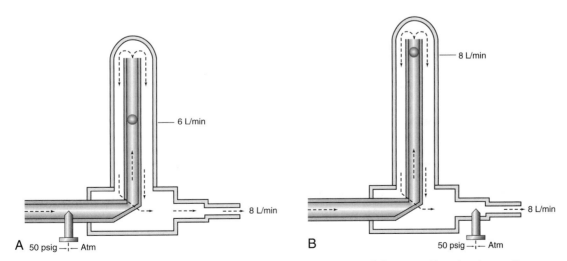

Figure 6-3 A, Non-backpressure-compensated (pressure-uncompensated) flowmeter. Note that the needle valve is upstream of the meter. In the face of backpressure, the meter will show *less* flow than is actually going to the patient. **B,** Backpressure-compensated (pressure-compensated) flowmeter. Note that the needle valve is downstream of the meter. In the face of backpressure, the meter will show the actual flow that is going to the patient. From Vines DL: Storage and delivery of medical gases. In Kacmarek RM, Stoller JK, Heuer AJ, editors: Egan's fundamentals of respiratory care, ed 10, St Louis, 2013, Mosby.

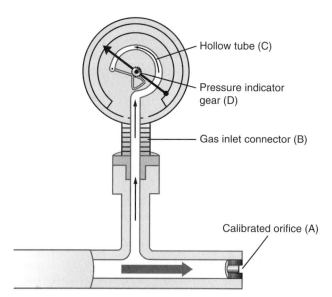

Figure 6-4 Bourdon-type non-backpressure-compensated (pressure-un-compensated) flowmeter. In the face of backpressure, the meter will show *more* flow than is actually going to the patient. From Vines DL: Storage and delivery of medical gases. In Kacmarek RM, Stoller JK, Heuer AJ, editors: Egan's fundamentals of respiratory care, ed 10, St Louis, 2013, Mosby.

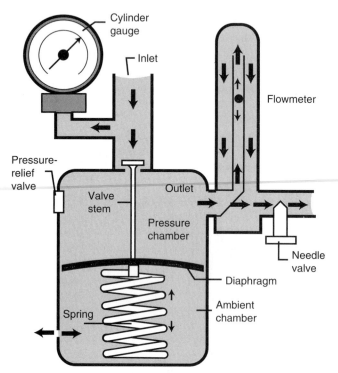

Figure 6-5 Drawing of a single-stage regulator with its components and features. The regulator has two key components: a reducing valve and a flowmeter. The reducing valve is typically a Bourdon gauge. It reduces the high pressure in the tank down to the working pressure of 50 psi for the flowmeter. The gas pressure within the tank is shown on the cylinder gauge. A Thorpe-type backpressure-compensated flowmeter is added to adjust the gas flow. From Cairo JM: Mosby's respiratory care equipment, ed 9, St Louis, 2014, Mosby.

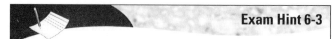

4. Pulse-dose oxygen-conserving devices (code: IIA12) [difficulty: R, Ap]

a. Assemble the necessary equipment

Three types of intermittent-flow oxygen-conserving devices are available: pulse-dose oxygen delivery devices, demand oxygen delivery systems, and hybrid units. All are used in the home care setting and save money by delivering oxygen to the patient only during inspiration. These units take the place of a regulator and flowmeter that deliver a steady flow of oxygen to the patient.

The characteristics of each unit will vary depending on the manufacturer. However, the following main operational features are found:

- A pulse-dose system delivers a bolus of oxygen at the start of the inspiratory cycle and shuts off before the end of inspiration.
- A demand system provides a continuous flow of oxygen throughout inspiration.
- A hybrid system combines features of the pulse-dose and demand systems. Cycling mechanisms vary but fall into two main categories. First, the unit may be set to time-cycle the oxygen flow on and off. Second, the patient's negative inspiratory pressure will trigger the delivery of oxygen. See Figure 6-8.

Depending on the manufacturer, the unit can be used with oxygen tanks, a low-pressure LOX system, or an oxygen concentrator. Be careful not to place a low-pressure unit on a high-pressure gas source because it will be damaged.

With a pulse-dose system, the proximal end of a special nasal cannula is attached to a pressure sensor on the pulse-dose system. It senses a decrease in pressure as the patient inspires. The sensor then opens a demand valve that delivers a burst of oxygen to the cannula. (See Fig. 6-8.) Because the nasal cannula is directly attached to the pressure sensor, a bubble-type humidifier cannot be added into the system.

Most of the units allow the respiratory therapist to work with the patient to adjust the sensor or timer to change how long the oxygen is delivered, how much is delivered, and whether the patient receives oxygen every breath or every second or third breath.

Make sure that the patient can feel a flow of gas from the cannula after he or she starts to inhale. The gas should stop during exhalation. Check the patient's pulse oximetry value at rest and during exercise to ensure that desaturation does not occur. Adjust the pressure sensor or timer to meet the patient's oxygen needs.

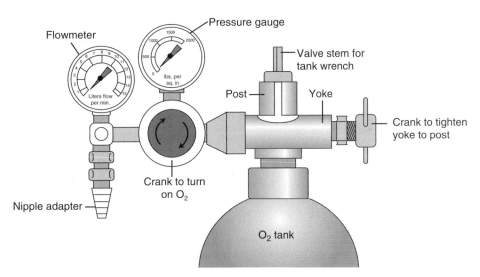

Figure 6-6 Drawing of an E tank of oxygen showing how the yoke and regulator are connected to it and their features. A Bourdon-type pressure gauge is shown. Turn the crank to let gas flow through the Bourdon-type non-backpressure-compensated (pressure-uncompensated) flowmeter. A nipple adapter is screwed on so that small-bore oxygen tubing can be connected. If the nipple adapter is unscrewed, a bubble-type humidifier or other oxygen delivery system can be attached. *Note:* This type of regulator is recommended for patient transportation if the E tank must be placed horizontally. Redrawn from Sills JR: Respiratory care for the health care provider, Albany, 1998, Delmar.

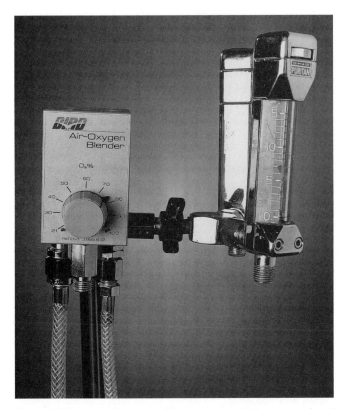

Figure 6-7 Example of an oxygen blender. Note the high-pressure air and oxygen hoses entering the bottom of the unit, the dial used to set the oxygen percentage (75%), and the blended oxygen outlet to the right. In this case, a Wye connector has been attached with two oxygen flowmeters. Courtesy VIASYS Healthcare, Palm Springs, California.

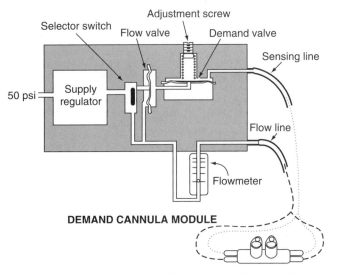

Figure 6-8 A pulse-dose oxygen delivery system with its key features shown. A specific type of nasal cannula is needed with this system. One channel transmits the negative pressure from the patient's inspiration back to the demand valve. This negative pressure opens the demand valve to allow a bolus of oxygen to travel down the second channel to the patient to inhale. From Cairo JM: Mosby's respiratory care equipment, ed 9, St Louis, 2014, Mosby.

b. Troubleshoot any problems with the equipment

If the patient cannot feel any oxygen flowing, the following should be considered: (1) the source of oxygen might be empty, (2) the tubing might be disconnected or kinked, or (3) the sensor may not be detecting the patient's effort. The patient or therapist can switch to a second oxygen source and look for disconnections or kinks in the tubing. The therapist must adjust the nasal cannula or sensor to correct for a sensitivity problem. Do not use a system that is malfunctioning and cannot be adjusted.

5. Air compressors (code: IIA12) [difficulty: R, Ap]

a. Assemble the necessary equipment

See below.

b. Troubleshoot any problems with the equipment

Air compressors are used whenever a high-pressure gas source other than oxygen is needed. All three systems are alike in that they use an electrically powered motor, filter the room air as it enters and exits the compressor, and have a condenser to remove water vapor as it leaves the compressor. See Figure 6-9.

1. Rotary-type compressors

Rotary-type compressors generate pressure with a rotating fan. They are used commonly in volume ventilators and in the home to power hand-held medication nebulizers (Fig. 6-10).

2. Diaphragm-type compressors

Diaphragm-type compressors generate pressure with a diaphragm that moves up and down within a cylinder-like piston. They also are used commonly in the home to power hand-held medication nebulizers.

3. Piston-type compressors

Piston-type compressors generate pressure through piston action within a cylinder (see Fig. 6-9). They are much more powerful than the previous two types of compressors. Because they are designed to generate pressures of 50 psig or greater, they are used in the hospital with its piped air system. They also are used in the home setting in oxygen concentrators.

Make sure that all of these units are operational by checking that the inlet and outlet filters are cleaned. Dirty filters prevent proper airflow. Check the unit's pressure gauge to make sure that it is able to meet its manufacturer's specified pressure. Empty the water trap on the condensing unit as needed.

6. Blenders (air/oxygen proportioners) (code: IIA12) [difficulty: R, Ap]

a. Assemble the necessary equipment

Oxygen blenders are designed to change the ratio of oxygen and air to blend the specific percentage of oxygen from 21% to 100% (Fig. 6-7). They are used whenever high-pressure gas is needed and the oxygen percentage may need frequent adjustment. A flowmeter may be attached to control the flow of the blended oxygen mix. There are also blenders for the specialty gases of nitric oxide and heliox (helium/oxygen). These are discussed later in the chapter. The general principles of operation of oxygen blenders discussed below also apply to the specialty gas blenders.

The oxygen and air gas sources must be pressurized to 50 psig. This can be done by taking both gases from the hospital's gas piping system or from gas cylinders with regulators. High-pressure hoses connect the gas sources

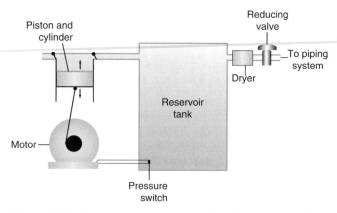

Figure 6-9 A piston-type large-volume medical air compressor. These units are used in hospitals or medical facilities. On the downstroke, the piston draws in room air that is then compressed into the reservoir tank on the upstroke. A pressure switch automatically turns the motor on and off to keep the pressure constant. As the compressed air leaves the reservoir tank, any water vapor is removed before it goes to the pressure-reducing valve. The piping system carries the air at 50 psig to any respiratory care equipment that is in use. From Vines DL: Storage and delivery of medical gases. In Kacmarek RM, Stoller JK, Heuer AJ, editors: Egan's fundamentals of respiratory care, ed 10, St Louis, 2013, Mosby.

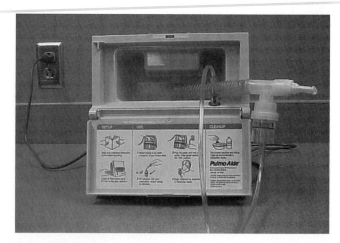

Figure 6-10 Photograph of a portable air compressor for home use. It is powered electrically with an on/off switch. Note the small-bore tubing that takes the compressed air to the small-volume nebulizer to aerosolize a medication. From Vines DL: Storage and delivery of medical gases. In Kacmarek RM, Stoller JK, Heuer AJ, editors: Egan's fundamentals of respiratory care, ed 10, St Louis, 2013, Mosby.

with the blender. The desired oxygen percentage is set simply by adjusting the knob to the desired amount. Because the blended gases are under pressure, they must be sent directly to a mechanical ventilator or other device that uses 50 psig or through an added flowmeter.

With a blender, the oxygen percentage will remain close to the desired amount even if a small decrease in one or both line pressures occurs. Always analyze the oxygen percentage to confirm that it is correct.

b. Troubleshoot any problems with the equipment

Keep the gas inlets and outlets clear of any debris. All current units give an audible whistle if one or both of the line pressures decrease to an unsafe level (often about 30 psig). If the unit has a water trap at the compressed air inlet, keep it emptied of any condensate.

7. Oxygen concentrators (code: IIA12) [difficulty: R, Ap]

a. Assemble the necessary equipment

Two different types of oxygen concentrators (also known as oxygen enrichers) are available for the delivery of continuous low-flow oxygen in the home: molecular sieve and semipermeable plastic membrane.

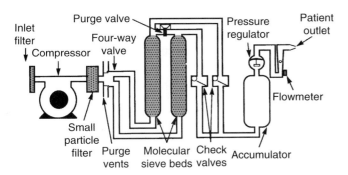

Figure 6-11 Drawing of the components of a molecular sieve oxygen concentrator. The molecular sieve beds remove nitrogen and pass oxygen through to the patient. Courtesy of Sunrise Medical, Inc., Somerset, PA.

1. Molecular sieve

Molecular sieve-type oxygen concentrators use an air compressor to push room air through two canisters of zeolite pellets (inorganic sodium–aluminum silicate) to remove nitrogen and water vapor. The remaining oxygen is delivered to the patient through a flowmeter (Fig. 6-11). With molecular sieve units, one canister of zeolite is in use while the other is purged of its water vapor and nitrogen. This alternate purge and use of the zeolite canisters is called the pressure swing absorption method. Be aware that with these units, the oxygen percentage varies inversely with the flow that is delivered (Table 6-4).

2. Semipermeable plastic membrane

Semipermeable plastic membrane oxygen concentrators make use of a very thin plastic membrane as a filter. Room air is pulled through it by a vacuum pump. Molecular oxygen and water vapor can pass through the membrane faster than nitrogen. Any excess water vapor is removed by a simple condenser system. Because some water vapor passes through with the oxygen, there is no need to add an external humidification system to the flowmeter (Fig. 6-12). The oxygen percentage is fixed at 40% in these units; however, the flow can be varied from 1 to 10 L/min, as shown in Table 6-4.

When one is deciding which type of concentrator to use, it is important to know the patient's required oxygen percentage and flow. As can be seen from Table 6-4, the molecular sieve units can deliver a higher oxygen percentage at any liter flow compared with the semipermeable plastic membrane units.

3. Portable oxygen concentrators

Some oxygen concentrators are now small enough to be carried by the patient or can be used to fill a portable oxygen tank. The Venture HomeFill II (Invacare, North Rocks, Australia) is a home-use oxygen concentrator combined with a compressor. This allows a small portable oxygen tank to be filled in the home from the

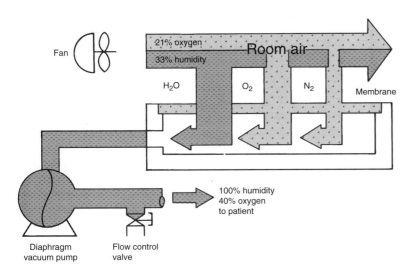

Figure 6-12 Functional schematic of a semipermeable membrane oxygen concentrator. The membrane permits more oxygen and water vapor than nitrogen to pass through. Courtesy of Oxygen Enrichment, Schenectady, NY.

TABLE 6-4	Comparison of Flow Rates and Oxygen Percentages in Oxygen Concentrators
Flow, L/min	**Approximate Oxygen Percentage**
Molecular sieve concentrator	
1-2	95-92%
3-5	92-85%
>6	<85%
Semipermeable membrane concentrator	
1-10	40%

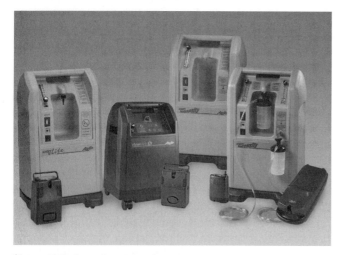

Figure 6-13 Several stationary home and portable oxygen concentrators. Note how a bubble-type humidifier can be added to the stationary concentrator to provide humidified oxygen to the patient's nasal cannula. Courtesy of AirSep, Buffalo, NY.

oxygen concentrator. The Inogen One System (Inogen, Inc., Goleta, CA) is battery powered and includes a pulse-dose nasal cannula oxygen delivery system. This unit allows the home care patient great flexibility in the home and in travel with portable oxygen delivery. Several manufacturers offer a large concentrator for the home and a smaller companion concentrator for portable use. Figure 6-13 shows examples of stationary and portable concentrators.

b. Troubleshoot any problems with the equipment

The molecular sieve-type units deliver dry gas; therefore a humidification system is frequently added to the flowmeter. With the permeable plastic membrane-type units, the condensed water vapor must be emptied from the collection jar. In both types of oxygen concentrators, it is important to check the air-inlet filter on a monthly basis to keep it clean of dust and debris. Follow the manufacturer's requirements regarding when filters should be replaced. The delivered oxygen concentration also should be checked each month. Follow the manufacturer's guidelines for its preventative maintenance needs. The molecular sieve-type units must have the zeolite pellet canisters replaced on a scheduled basis.

Some units have a visual or audio alarm that warns when a problem occurs, such as power failure, low or high pressure, or low oxygen percentage. If the unit does not have a low-oxygen percentage alarm, some home care practitioners have added an external analyzer with an alarm system. This alerts the patient to call the home care company to repair the equipment. If a patient says that he or she cannot feel any gas coming out of the cannula, have the patient place the prongs into a glass of water. If no bubbling is seen, have the patient check the tubing for a disconnection, kink, or obstruction. If the concentrator is malfunctioning, have the patient turn it off and switch to oxygen from the backup oxygen cylinder until repairs can be made.

Exam Hint 6-4

Most past examinations have included a question related to a malfunctioning oxygen concentrator used in the home. A patient may be expected to check for oxygen flowing through a cannula by placing the prongs under water to look for bubbling or by switching from the concentrator to a backup source of oxygen such as an oxygen cylinder (tank). The patient should not be expected to troubleshoot problems with the concentrator or perform maintenance work on it. That is the home care respiratory therapist's job.

8. Liquid oxygen systems (code: IIA12) [difficulty: R, Ap]

a. Assemble the necessary equipment for the procedure

A liquid oxygen (LOX) system is used in the home when it is found to be more cost-effective than an oxygen concentrator or a battery of oxygen cylinders. An additional advantage is that the patient can carry a smaller portable unit in a shoulder bag for added mobility. Carrying the unit is less conspicuous than wheeling an E cylinder about. Figure 6-14 shows the key features of a large LOX reservoir that is kept in the patient's home. Figure 6-15 shows its smaller portable companion, which can be filled from the large reservoir.

Current portable LOX systems weigh only a few pounds and can be carried over the shoulder by a strap. They can be refilled from the larger reservoir tank kept in the home. The flow rate can be adjusted to meet most patients' needs. Humidification is provided by the patient's own airway. As with any pressurized system, all fittings must be kept tight to prevent leakage.

The National Fire Protection Association has established several regulations to ensure that home LOX systems are installed safely. Key safety regulations include the following:
- Stabilize the unit to prevent it from being tipped over.
- The reservoir unit should not be set up near any radiators, steam pipes, or heat ducts to reduce the rate of oxygen loss.

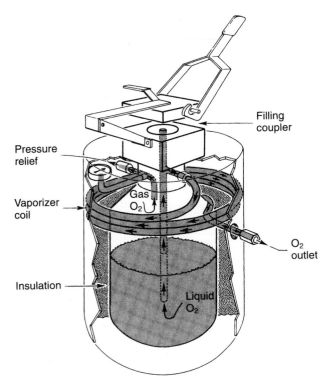

Figure 6-14 Drawing of the components of a home liquid oxygen supply unit. From Lampton LM: Home and outpatient oxygen therapy. In Brashear RE, Rhodes ML, editors: Chronic obstructive lung disease, St Louis, 1978, Mosby.

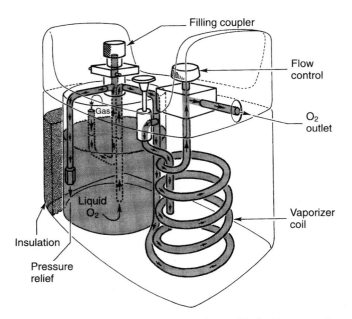

Figure 6-15 Drawing of the components of a portable liquid oxygen unit. From Lampton LM: Home and outpatient oxygen therapy. In Brashear RE, Rhodes ML, editors: Chronic obstructive lung disease, St Louis, 1978, Mosby.

- No open flames or sources of ignition can be within 5 feet of the unit.
- "No smoking" signs must be posted.
- The patient and the family must be instructed on how to use the equipment. This includes how to fill the portable unit from the large reservoir tank. That person should wear safety goggles with side shields, loose-fitting insulated gloves, and high-top boots.
- If LOX spills and contacts skin, it can cause frostbite. Medical attention should be sought immediately.
- For at least 15 minutes, avoid contact with any equipment or the floor where LOX has spilled.

b. Troubleshoot any problems with the equipment

Check that all connections are airtight to avoid spills and minimize the loss of oxygen. Make sure that the unit is functioning at its designed working pressure. Check that the pressure relief valve operates properly and that proper oxygen flow is delivered.

Exam Hint 6-5

Most past examinations have questioned the need to set up a LOX supply unit and portable unit for a home care patient or troubleshooting problems with the system. A patient may be expected to check for oxygen flowing through a cannula by placing the prongs under water to look for bubbling or by switching from the LOX system to a backup source of oxygen such as an oxygen cylinder (tank). The patient should not be expected to troubleshoot problems with the LOX system or perform maintenance work on it. That is the home care respiratory therapist's responsibility.

---

9. Heliox equipment (code: IIA17) [difficulty: R, Ap, An]

a. Assemble the necessary equipment

Heliox (helium/oxygen, He/O_2) has been used historically in the management of patients with an upper-airway obstruction. Causes include tracheal tumor, postextubation laryngeal edema, and croup. More recently, heliox has been used with success in patients with status asthmaticus. Although heliox has been used with patients experiencing an exacerbation of COPD, the clinical benefits are unproven. In any clinical situation, the key benefit of heliox is the patient's reduced work of breathing. This is the result of the decreased density of a helium/oxygen mix compared with a nitrogen/oxygen mix.

Various heliox gas mixtures come in high-pressure cylinders and require the use of an American Standard System reducing valve (or regulator) designed specifically for the gas or gas mix. As is shown in Table 6-3 and Figure 6-1, a reducing valve or regulator for an E cylinder must match the appropriate pinholes on the cylinder valve face. Corresponding high-pressure hoses also may be needed. Table 6-1 shows the color codes for the various gas cylinders. Pure helium comes in a brown cylinder, whereas helium and oxygen mixes come in brown and green cylinders. Always check the cylinder label for the exact percentage of the gases within it. Heliox comes in standard mixes of 80% He/20% O_2, 70% He/30% O_2, and 60% He/40% O_2.

The additional equipment needed depends on how the ordered heliox mixture is to be delivered to the patient.

1. Nonrebreathing mask

In most clinical situations, a respiratory therapist makes use of readily available equipment and modifies it as needed. Usually a nonrebreathing mask with a reservoir bag is used to deliver heliox to a spontaneously breathing patient. A snugly fitting mask with one-way valves and a full reservoir bag will minimize breathing of any room air. (The next module includes additional discussion on nonrebreathing masks.) A helium flowmeter can be used to set the flow of heliox to the face mask. However, if a helium flowmeter is not available, an oxygen flowmeter can be added to the reducing valve on a heliox mix cylinder. Typically, an 80/20 heliox mix is used unless the patient needs supplemental oxygen. Always set the gas flow high enough that the reservoir bag does not collapse on inspiration. The gas is humidified by attaching a bubble humidifier with sterile water to the flowmeter. Connect small-bore tubing between the humidifier nipple and the nonrebreathing mask nipple.

If the patient is being treated for asthma, the nonrebreathing mask can be modified to accept a small-volume nebulizer for bronchodilator medication delivery. (See Fig. 6-16.) Care must be taken if the nebulizer is powered by the heliox mix, as shown. Some nebulizers will not operate normally. It may be necessary to increase the heliox flow by 50% to 100% from the usual rate of oxygen flow to get the unit to operate properly. Or, simply power the nebulizer with oxygen for the treatment.

There is a risk to modifying available equipment for an unintended purposed. The inconsistency of application between therapists can put the patient at risk. The NBRC is known to ask questions about troubleshooting a nonrebreathing mask delivering heliox. Remember to keep a tight system without leaks and to set the flow high enough to prevent the reservoir bag from collapsing.

In the common situation in which an oxygen flowmeter is being used with heliox, a calculation must be done to convert the observed flow on the oxygen flowmeter to the actual flow of heliox. This is necessary because helium is less dense than oxygen. See Exam Hint 6-6 for details.

Exam Hint 6-6

Often one question requires calculation of the actual flow of a heliox mixture. The heliox factor must be known to do the calculation. One possible calculation involves figuring out the heliox flow from an observed flow through an oxygen flowmeter. The other possible calculation involves setting the observed flow through an oxygen flowmeter to achieve the desired heliox flow. See the following sample calculations.

The heliox factor must be used to determine the actual flow of heliox through an oxygen flowmeter, as follows:

Helium/Oxygen Ratio	Heliox Factor
1. 80% helium/20% oxygen	1.8
2. 70% helium/30% oxygen	1.6
3. 60% helium/40% oxygen	1.4

The following examples show how the actual heliox flow can be calculated from the observed oxygen flow seen on the flowmeter:

1. When using an 80% helium and 20% oxygen mix, multiply the observed flow by the heliox factor of 1.8.
   Example: Observed oxygen flow of 10 L/min × 1.8 = 18 L/min actual heliox flow.
2. When using a 70% helium and 30% oxygen mix, multiply the observed flow by the heliox factor of 1.6.
   Example: Observed oxygen flow of 10 L/min × 1.6 = 16 L/min actual heliox flow.
3. When using a 60% helium and 40% oxygen mix, multiply the observed flow by the heliox factor of 1.4.
   Example: Observed oxygen flow of 10 L/min × 1.4 = 14 L/min actual heliox flow.

The following examples show how to set an oxygen flowmeter to deliver a needed heliox flow by dividing the desired flow by the heliox factor:

1. When using an 80% helium and 20% oxygen mix, determine the observed flowmeter setting to deliver an actual heliox flow of 10 L/min.

   Example: $\dfrac{10\ L/min\ heliox\ desired}{1.8} = 5.6\ L/min$ set on the oxygen flowmeter.

2. When using a 70% helium and 30% oxygen mix, determine the observed flowmeter setting to deliver an actual heliox flow of 10 L/min.

   Example: $\dfrac{10\ L/min\ heliox\ desired}{1.6} = 6.3\ L/min$ set on the oxygen flowmeter.

3. When using a 60% helium and 40% oxygen mix, determine the observed flowmeter setting to deliver an actual heliox flow of 10 L/min.

   Example: $\dfrac{10\ L/min\ heliox\ desired}{1.4} = 7.1\ L/min$ set on the oxygen flowmeter.

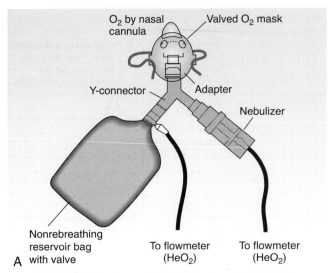

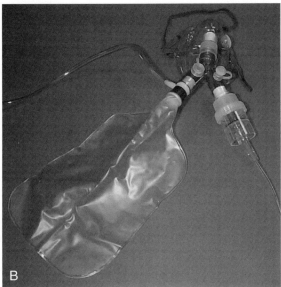

Figure 6-16 Drawing and photograph showing a modified nonrebreathing mask and reservoir bag for delivering helium/oxygen. The Y-connector allows the heliox to be breathed from the reservoir bag while the nebulizer is aerosolizing a bronchodilator medication. A separate flowmeter is used for each component. Use enough heliox flow to keep the reservoir bag from collapsing. The nebulizer can be powered by heliox, as shown, or by oxygen. From Hess DR: Nonconventional respiratory therapeutics. In Hess DR, MacIntyre NR, Mishoe SC et al., editors: Respiratory care principles & practices, Philadelphia, 2002, Saunders.

2. High-flow nasal cannula

The Precision Flow Heliox (Vapotherm, Stevensville, MD) system is able to provide a variable heliox mix through a high-flow nasal cannula (HFNC). An 80/20 heliox tank, high-pressure oxygen source, and high-pressure compressed air source are connected into a heliox blender. The oxygen percentage can be adjusted from 21% to 100% with the balance being helium. The heliox gas is humidified with the same technology that is used with other

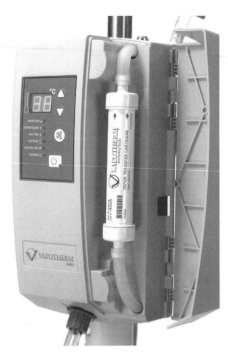

Figure 6-17 The Vapotherm 2000i high-flow nasal cannula control panel. The vapor transfer cartridge is shown inside. It can be switched out as needed and is available in adult and pediatric sizes. Courtesy of Vapotherm 2000i, Exeter, New Hampshire.

Vapotherm HFNC systems. (See Figs. 6-17 and 6-18.) A flow of 1-40 L/min is directed through the dedicated Vapotherm triple-lumen patient circuit and correctly sized nasal cannula.

3. Mechanical ventilator

Delivering a helium/oxygen mix through a ventilator presents several technical challenges. First, select a ventilator that has been approved by the U.S. FDA to deliver a heliox mix. In many ventilators, the decreased density of helium causes flow and volume sensors (usually a flow-type pneumotachometer) to read inaccurately. The CareFusion AVEA (CareFusion, Viasys Corp., San Diego, CA) is an example of a full-service ventilator that has been approved for heliox. The Aptaér Heliox Delivery System (GE Healthcare, Madison, WI) is a limited-service ventilator that is designed specifically to be used with heliox. An 80/20, 70/30, or 60/40 heliox mix can be delivered to the patient through the Pressure Support mode. Other controls include trigger (sensitivity), rise (peak flow), and end flow (to terminate inspiration).

If a ventilator is used in a non-FDA-approved manner to deliver heliox, it is recommended that pressure ventilation be used rather than volume ventilation. The risk with volume ventilation is the potential delivery of a larger tidal volume than that set on the ventilator. In addition, measure the patient's exhaled tidal volume with a bellows-type spirometer rather than a pneumotachometer.

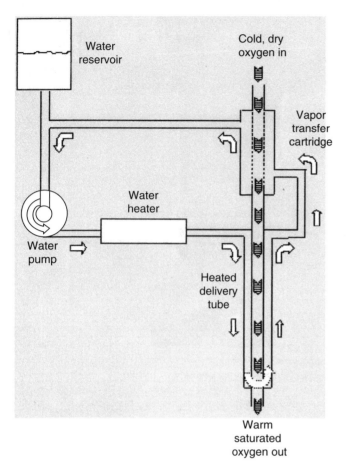

Figure 6-18 Schematic drawing of the humidification and oxygen delivery system of the Vapotherm 2000i. The vapor transfer cartridge humidifies the patient's oxygen. The patient circuit maintains the temperature of the oxygen. Modified from Kacmarek RM, Dimas S, Mack CW: The essentials of respiratory care, ed 4, St Louis, 2005, Mosby.

With any ventilator, connect the pure helium or heliox mix to the unit's internal air/oxygen proportioner (blender) through the high-pressure air inlet. High-pressure oxygen will go through on its side of the unit, as usual. If pure helium is mixed with pure oxygen, dial the oxygen percentage, as needed, to adjust the mix of the two gases. For example, giving the patient 35% oxygen results in the patient also receiving 65% helium. However, if the patient is receiving a heliox mix (e.g., 70/30), more oxygen than is set on the blender will be delivered.

In any situation in which a heliox mix is being used, *the oxygen percentage must be continuously measured.* This is done to be certain how much oxygen is being delivered and to ensure that the patient never receives less than 20% oxygen. Remember that if 100% helium is delivered through the air inlet, and the blender is set to 21% oxygen, the patient will receive pure helium and no oxygen! This would be a *fatal error.* Use a polarographic or galvanic fuel cell oxygen analyzer to monitor the patient's oxygen percentage.

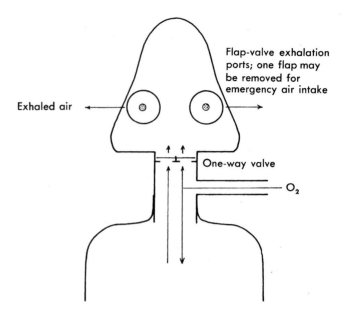

Figure 6-19 Cutaway view of a nonrebreathing mask showing gas flow. From Thalken FR: Medical gas therapy. In Scanlan CL, Spearman CB, Sheldon RL, editors: Egan's fundamentals of respiratory care, ed 5, St Louis, 1990, Mosby.

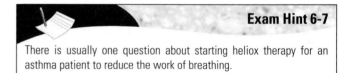

Exam Hint 6-7

There is usually one question about starting heliox therapy for an asthma patient to reduce the work of breathing.

b. Troubleshoot any problems with the equipment

When using a nonrebreathing mask, make sure that it is adjusted to give as tight a fit to the face as is practical and comfortable. All one-way valve flaps on the mask should open out for exhalation and close down on the mask during inspiration. (See Fig. 6-19.) Set the gas flow high enough that the reservoir bag does not collapse by more than one-third during inspiration.

With a mechanical ventilator, make sure that the exhaled volume is measured accurately and that alarms are adjusted to actual patient values. With either system, it is extremely important that all connections be tight because helium easily leaks out of any openings. If the oxygen percentage is too low, be prepared to make the necessary adjustments. Clinical experience is recommended with the administration of helium/oxygen mixes.

MODULE D

Initiate and adjust oxygen therapy (code: IIIC1) [difficulty: R, Ap, An].

1. Low-flow oxygen systems

Low-flow oxygen delivery systems have these characteristics:
  1. 100% oxygen is initially delivered through the appliance.

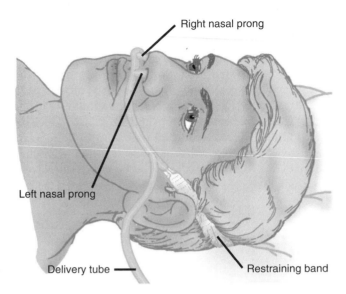

Figure 6-20 Adult wearing a low-flow nasal cannula. From Heuer AJ: Medical gas therapy. In Kacmarek RM, Stoller JK, Heuer AJ, editors: Egan's fundamentals of respiratory care, ed 10, St Louis, 2013, Mosby.

TABLE 6-5	Estimated Delivered Oxygen Percentage in Adults Based on the Oxygen Liter Flow Through a Nasal Cannula

Oxygen, L/min	Estimated Delivered Oxygen, %
1	24
2	28
3	32
4	36
5	40
6	44

2. Because the oxygen flow through the appliance may be higher, the same, or less than the patient's peak inspiratory flow, and room air (21% oxygen) may be inhaled, the final inhaled oxygen percentage can only be estimated.

3. These appliances are classified as *variable performance* because of the unknown delivered oxygen percentage.

The decision on which low-flow or high-flow oxygen delivery system to use depends on a variety of clinical factors. Be prepared to select the best system for the patient at that time. However, also be prepared to recommend or make a change in the oxygen percentage or delivery system as the patient's condition warrants.

Note: Nasal catheters will not be discussed in this text. This is because they are rarely used and not tested by the NBRC. However, the following discussion on the low-flow nasal cannula would generally apply to the nasal catheter. *Note:* Oxygen tents and aerosol tents will not be discussed in this text. This is because the NBRC will not be asking questions about them starting in 2015.

a. Low-flow nasal cannula

1. Assemble the necessary equipment

The traditional nasal cannula is a low-flow oxygen delivery tube that has been modified with two short prongs to deliver oxygen to the nostrils (Fig. 6-20). Nasal cannulas come in neonatal, pediatric, and adult sizes based on the diameter of the prongs. Care must be taken to make sure that the patient's nares are patent and are not plugged by a common cold, a deviated septum, or another unseen problem. This simple oxygen delivery device is widely used because it is more comfortable for many patients than an air entrainment mask or other types of face masks. Current clinical practice guidelines indicate that, in an adult, an oxygen flow of 4 L/min or less does not require additional humidification if the patient has a normal upper airway.

If an adult is getting from 1 to 4 L/min of oxygen and complains of nasal dryness, or if a higher flow is given, humidification will have to be provided. Often this is a bubble-type humidifier, as discussed in Chapter 8. Make sure that it is properly filled with sterile water and that the oxygen bubbles through it. Check the high-pressure pop-off valve for pressure release and a whistling sound. Before placing the cannula on the patient, check to see that the oxygen is flowing through the tubing. If available, use a cannula with curved prongs. They direct the gas flow toward the back of the nasal passages for better natural humidification and are better for patient comfort. Take care to avoid pulling the elastic restraining band too tightly around the head. Some brands loop the oxygen tubing over the ears to be drawn up snugly under the chin. Often this type is more comfortable than the types that have an elastic band.

The problem with a nasal cannula is that the delivered oxygen percentage is unreliable. Variations in the patient's respiratory rate, I:E ratio, tidal volume, and minute volume result in different inhaled oxygen percentages. This is clearly unacceptable in an unstable patient in whom PaO_2 values are being used to help judge the changing cardiopulmonary status. Because of this clinical limitation, this device and the other low-flow oxygen delivery systems in the discussions that follow should be used only with stable patients. In the adult, the delivered oxygen percentage can be estimated at approximately 4% for each liter of oxygen per minute (Table 6-5). Flows usually are limited to 6 L/min to avoid excessive irritation to the nasal passages. Flows usually are limited to no more than 1-2 L/min in infants and 4 L/min in older children. The pulse oximetry value or PaO_2 level should be checked in patients of any age whenever a flow change is made or when the patient's condition changes significantly.

2. Troubleshoot any problems with the equipment

Replace a cannula that is obviously soiled or permanently obstructed. If a bubble-type humidifier is used, refill the water as needed and replace the humidifier according to protocol.

b. Oxygen-conserving nasal cannula

1. Assemble the necessary equipment

Oxygen-conserving nasal cannulas are used for patients who need long-term, low-flow oxygen therapy and wish to reduce their costs. At least two different types of oxygen-conserving cannulas are found. Figure 6-21 shows a reservoir nasal cannula and how it operates. It has an 18-mL reservoir that fills when the patient exhales and gives up its oxygen bolus during the next inspiration. Figure 6-22 shows a pendant nasal cannula with its reservoir that hangs on the chest.

2. Troubleshoot any problems with the equipment

Both types of cannulas can have problems with tubing disconnections or kinks that can happen with any type of cannula. The only problem that is unique to both of these units is failure of the diaphragm, which moves back and forth as the reservoir fills and empties. This membrane may wear out after about a week and prevent the reservoir from filling or emptying properly. Watch as the patient breathes to make sure that the diaphragm is moving properly. If not, replace the cannula.

c. Oxygen masks: simple oxygen mask, partial-rebreathing mask, nonrebreathing mask

1. Assemble the necessary equipment

See below.

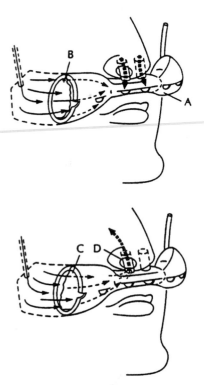

Figure 6-21 Drawing of the Oximizer reservoir nasal cannula. **A,** During exhalation, some oxygen from the patient's nasal dead space enters the reservoir. **B,** Oxygen flows into the reservoir. **C,** With inspiration, oxygen in the reservoir is inhaled. **D,** Inspired oxygen. Courtesy of CHAD Therapeutics, Lehigh Acres, Florida.

2. Troubleshoot any problems with the equipment

a. Simple oxygen mask

This mask, like all others, is designed to fit over the patient's nose and mouth and act as an oxygen reservoir for the next breath (Figs. 6-23 and 6-24). Various adult and pediatric sizes are available, and the patient should wear one that best fits the facial contours and size of the face. This is recommended for comfort, as well as to try to increase the inspired oxygen percentage by decreasing the amount of room air that is inspired. However, because a simple oxygen mask does not provide all of the patient's tidal volume

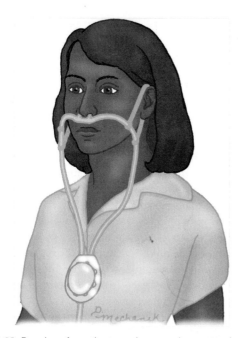

Figure 6-22 Drawing of a patient wearing a pendant reservoir nasal cannula. Courtesy of CHAD Therapeutics, LeHigh Acres, Florida; from Heuer AJ: Medical gas therapy. In Kacmarek RM, Stoller JK, Heuer AJ, editors: Egan's fundamentals of respiratory care, ed 10, St Louis, 2013, Mosby.

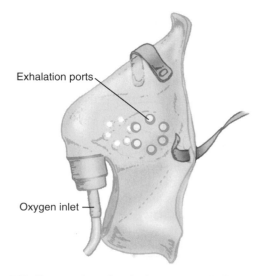

Exhalation ports

Oxygen inlet

Figure 6-23 Close-up view of a simple oxygen mask. From Heuer AJ: Medical gas therapy. In Kacmarek RM, Stoller JK, Heuer AJ, editors: Egan's fundamentals of respiratory care, ed 10, St Louis, 2013, Mosby.

gas, it is classified as a low-flow device. Exhaled breath escapes through the exhalation ports. The patient's breathing pattern affects the amount of room air that is breathed in through the same exhalation ports. These ports also are important in case the oxygen flow to the mask is cut off.

Because the oxygen reservoir in the mask is not large enough to meet the patient's tidal volume, the inspired oxygen percentage is unpredictable. Oxygen flows between 5 and 10 L/min should provide *approximately* 35% to 50% inspired oxygen. The pulse oximetry value or PaO$_2$ level should be checked whenever a flow change is made or when the patient's condition changes significantly.

A bubble humidifier is often added so that the gas is not dry. Make sure that it works properly and that oxygen is flowing through the tubing before putting it on the patient. This and all other masks use an adjustable elastic strap that goes behind the head to hold it in place.

Make sure that the mask fits snugly but not so tight as to cut off circulation.

b. Partial-rebreathing mask

The partial-rebreathing mask has a 500- to 1000-mL plastic bag added to the mask to act as an oxygen reservoir for the next breath (Figs. 6-25, 6-26, and 6-27). Child- and adult-size masks are commonly available. When properly applied, the first third of the patient's exhaled gas from the anatomic dead space is exhaled back into this bag. This gas is close to pure oxygen and has no carbon dioxide.

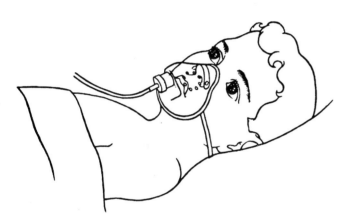

Figure 6-24 Child wearing a simple oxygen mask. From Gaebler G, Blodgett D: Gas administration. In Blodgett D, editor: Manual of pediatric respiratory care procedures, Philadelphia, 1982, Lippincott.

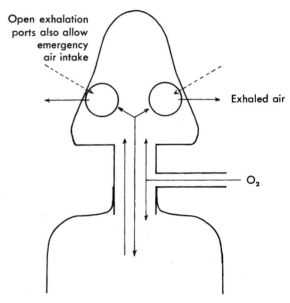

Figure 6-26 Cutaway view of a partial-rebreathing mask showing gas flow. From Thalken FR: Medical gas therapy. In Scanlan CL, Spearman CB, Sheldon RL, editors: Egan's fundamentals of respiratory care, ed 5, St Louis, 1990, Mosby.

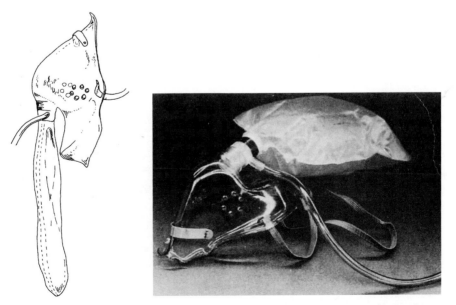

Figure 6-25 Drawing and photograph of a partial-rebreathing mask. From McPherson SP: Respiratory care equipment, ed 4, St Louis, 1990, Mosby.

Exhaled breath escapes through the exhalation ports. The patient's breathing pattern affects the amount of room air that is breathed in through the same exhalation ports. Because of this room air entrainment, a partial-rebreathing mask is classified as a low-flow device. These ports also are important in case the oxygen flow to the mask is cut off; the patient will breathe in room air. The added reservoir of oxygen results in a higher percentage being given to the patient than with a simple oxygen mask. In all cases, set an oxygen flow high enough that the reservoir bag does not collapse by more than one-third on inspiration. For example, set an initial oxygen flow of 10 L/min for an adult. When set up properly, a partial-rebreathing mask should provide *approximately* 40% to 70% inspired oxygen.

A bubble humidifier often is added so that the gas is not dry. Make sure that the high-pressure pop-off valve works properly, that the oxygen is flowing through the tubing, and that the reservoir bag has been filled before putting it on the patient. Adjust the flow as needed to ensure that the reservoir does not collapse by more than one-third on

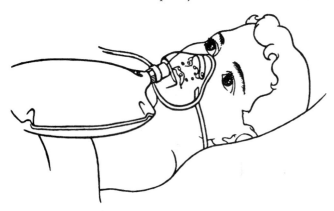

Figure 6-27 Child wearing a partial-rebreathing mask. From Gaebler G, Blodgett D: Gas administration. In Blodgett D, editor: Manual of pediatric respiratory care procedures, Philadelphia, 1982, Lippincott.

inspiration. This ensures that the mask and the reservoir are filled with as much oxygen as possible. The pulse oximetry value or PaO$_2$ level should be checked whenever the patient's condition changes significantly.

c. Nonrebreathing mask

The nonrebreathing mask initially looks like the partial-rebreathing mask with its plastic bag added as an oxygen reservoir for the next breath (Figs. 6-28 and 6-19). However, it should be noted that a one-way valve has been added between the mask and the reservoir bag. This allows the bag to be filled with pure oxygen that is available for the next breath. No exhaled gas can enter the reservoir. Two (sometimes one) one-way valves are added to the exhalation ports on the mask. In theory, with a tight-fitting mask and a high enough oxygen flow, the patient breathes in only oxygen from the mask and reservoir and no room air. However, because of leaks between the mask and the patient's face, the nonrebreathing mask is classified as a low-flow device. Exhaled breath escapes through the exhalation ports as with the partial-rebreathing mask. Not shown is an emergency pop-in valve that allows room air to be drawn into the mask if the oxygen supply is cut off. Adult and pediatric sizes are available. The mask should be conformed to fit the patient's facial contours and size as much as possible. As mentioned earlier, this is for comfort and to try to increase the inspired oxygen percentage by decreasing the amount of room air that is inspired. In theory, it is possible to deliver 100% oxygen with this mask if the oxygen flow is high enough and the mask is airtight over the face. However, experience has shown that the disposable masks that are usually available in the hospital do not prevent room air from being drawn in. In all cases, set an oxygen flow high enough that the reservoir bag does not collapse by more than one-third on inspiration. An initial oxygen flow ≥10 L/min should provide *approximately* 60% to 80% oxygen.

Valves

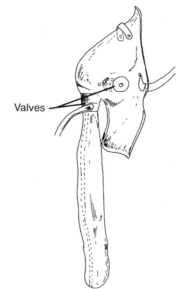
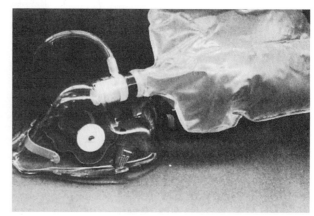

Figure 6-28 Drawing and photograph of a nonrebreathing mask. From McPherson SP: Respiratory care equipment, ed 4, St Louis, 1990, Mosby.

A bubble humidifier often is added so that the gas is not dry. Make sure that the high-pressure pop-off valve works properly, that the oxygen is flowing through the tubing, and that the reservoir bag has been filled before putting it on the patient. Adjust the flow as needed to ensure that the reservoir does not collapse by more than one-third on inspiration. This ensures that the mask and the reservoir are filled with oxygen, and that the patient's tidal volume comes completely from the reservoir bag. Try to make the mask fit as closely as possible to minimize room air entrainment. The patient's pulse oximetry value or PaO$_2$ level should be checked whenever the patient's condition changes significantly.

Exam Hint 6-8

Expect to see one question dealing with the reservoir bag collapsing on inspiration. Solve the problem by increasing the flow of therapeutic gas to the mask and bag.

Exam Hint 6-9

Expect to see one question that deals with the need to switch from a low-oxygen-percentage mask to a nonrebreathing mask to give the seriously hypoxemic patient as much oxygen as possible.

d. Transtracheal oxygen catheter

1. Assemble the necessary equipment

The transtracheal oxygen catheter is a 20-cm-long flexible, hollow plastic tube (Fig. 6-29). This low-flow oxygen delivery device is inserted into the trachea via a puncture procedure at the suprasternal notch. To date, only adults with COPD have had the procedure performed. Oxygen is delivered directly into the trachea. The patient's oxygenation can be maintained at lower oxygen flows than are needed by a regular face mask or nasal cannula. The following equipment is needed:

- Transtracheal catheter of proper size (9-Fr is the usual adult size)
- Guidewire/stylet
- Chain-link necklace to hold the catheter in place
- Regular small-bore oxygen tubing to connect to the distal end of the catheter
- Flowmeter and oxygen source
- Optional bubble humidifier with sterile water for patient comfort

Under normal working conditions, regular oxygen tubing is used to connect the oxygen source to the catheter. Oxygen flow to the catheter is set high enough to keep a satisfactory PaO$_2$ or SpO$_2$ level. Usually, this is less than previously needed by nasal cannula. When oxygen tubing is combined with a portable LOX system or a pulse-dose oxygen delivery system, the patient has a real opportunity for increased mobility and decreased cost.

2. Troubleshoot any problems with the equipment

The patient needs to be instructed to disconnect the oxygen tubing and flush the catheter with 3 mL of sterile saline twice a day. A cleaning rod also can be pushed through the catheter to make sure that no mucus accumulates. As with any tubing system, the components can become disconnected. Make sure that all connections are tight. If the saline or cleaning rod cannot be pushed through the catheter, an obstruction is likely. The patient should come into the hospital to have the catheter removed and replaced if necessary. It is possible that the proximal catheter tip has twisted into the tracheal mucosa. This can lead to subcutaneous emphysema. The patient should be instructed to turn off the oxygen to the catheter if there is sudden puffiness in the skin of the neck area. He or she should go back to using a nasal cannula for oxygen and should call the physician for guidance.

2. High-flow oxygen systems

High-flow oxygen delivery systems have these characteristics:

- A fixed, prescribed oxygen percentage is delivered through the appliance.
- The total prescribed oxygen flow through the appliance is the same as or higher than the patient's peak

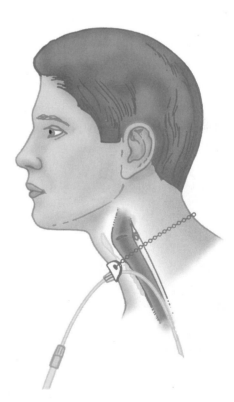

Figure 6-29 Transtracheal oxygen catheter. An adjustable chain-link necklace holds the external part of the catheter and flange secure. Standard oxygen tubing is connected to the external part of the catheter. From Heuer AJ: Medical gas therapy. In Kacmarek RM, Stoller JK, Heuer AJ, editors: Egan's fundamentals of respiratory care, ed 10, St Louis, 2013, Mosby.

inspiratory flow. Because of the high oxygen flow, no room air is inhaled.

- These appliances are classified as *fixed performance* because of the known delivered oxygen percentage.

The decision on which low-flow or high-flow oxygen delivery system to use depends on a variety of clinical factors. Be prepared to select the best system for the patient at that time. However, also be prepared to recommend or make a change in the oxygen percentage or delivery system as the patient's condition warrants.

a. Oxygen hoods

1. Assemble the necessary equipment

An oxygen hood (oxyhood) is used to provide a warmed aerosol or humidity and controlled oxygen percentage to pediatric patients who weigh no more than 18 lb (8.2 kg). (See Fig. 6-30.) Although the patient using an oxygen hood can be warmed with a radiant warmer (not tested by the NBRC) and can have oxygen delivered through a warmed or cool large-volume nebulizer (discussed in Chapter 8), this discussion will focus on an oxygen hood and patient placed inside of an incubator. This system provides better control of the environment and maintenance of body temperature. When this system is used, the following procedures should be observed:

- Use an air/oxygen blender with a flowmeter to control the oxygen percentage and flow into the hood. The flow should be at least 7 L/min to prevent the buildup of exhaled carbon dioxide. A flow of 10-15 L/min is needed to keep a stable oxygen percentage. Keeping the hood sealed as much as possible and

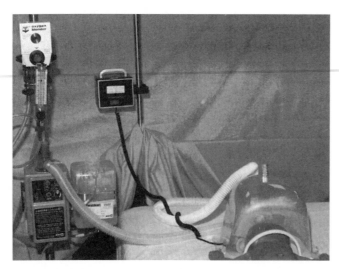

Figure 6-30 Infant in an oxygen hood. Other essential equipment includes the oxygen blender and flowmeter, humidification system, and large-bore tubing to carry the warm humidified oxygen to the hood. Supporting equipment includes the thermometer inserted through the top of the hood and an oxygen analyzer. The oxygen sensor is inside the hood next to the infant's head to measure the inspired oxygen percentage. From Barnhart SL: Oxygen administration. In Walsh BK, Czervinske MP, DiBlasi RM: Perinatal and pediatric respiratory care, ed 3, St Louis, 2010, Saunders.

minimizing the gap between the infant's neck and the opening to the hood will also help to stabilize the oxygen percentage.

- A warmed humidifier is needed to provide a high humidity level and to warm the oxygen to the infant's body temperature. Care must be taken with infants to ensure that they are neither heated nor cooled by the gas blowing over their head. A thermometer should be kept in the hood to note the temperature. Add a water drainage bag into the aerosol tubing so that condensate does not block the tubing.

- An oxygen analyzer should continuously monitor how much oxygen is inside the hood. The analyzer probe should be placed at the same level as the infant's nose. This is because oxygen is heavier than air and tends to settle toward the bottom of the hood. The advantages of the hood over the oxygen tent are that the patient's body is accessible, and the head can be reached by lifting the top off of the hood.

2. Troubleshoot any problems with the equipment

Make sure that the oxygen and aerosol delivery systems are working properly and that the oxygen percentage can be maintained. Periodically drain any water that has accumulated in the reservoir tubing. Be aware of the noise level inside the hood to minimize damage to the infant's hearing. The sound level should be monitored and kept well below 65 dB.

b. High-flow nasal cannula

1. Assemble the necessary equipment

An HFNC is designed to provide warmed and humidified oxygen at a high enough flow rate to fully meet the patient's peak inspiratory flow needs. This type of nasal cannula is better tolerated by many severely hypoxemic patients than a nonrebreathing mask because it provides 100% relative humidity at BTPS (body temperature, pressure, saturated gas) conditions, and there is no drying of the nasal mucosa. For these reasons, the HFNC has found a growing clinical application in adult, pediatric, and neonatal populations. Adults with congestive heart failure and pulmonary edema may be kept off of continuous positive airway pressure (CPAP) or mechanical ventilation through the use of an HFNC.

An HFNC may be used with some premature neonates as an alternative to CPAP or mechanical ventilation. Evidence suggests that neonatal patients receiving HFNC have a positive mouth pressure of about 3-4 cm water, which corresponds to a similar CPAP level. However, this pressure is maintained only when the mouth is closed. There is also the risk that an HFNC will create a higher CPAP level than desired. So, the smallest possible nasal cannula should be used to allow for a leak.

There are currently three classes of HFNC based upon the gas mix they deliver: 100% oxygen, 21% to 100% blended oxygen, or a heliox blended mix. Some are simple in design and inexpensive, whereas others are quite complex.

Systems that deliver 100% oxygen include the Salter Labs (Arvin, CA) high-flow cannula and humidifier and Aquinox (Smiths Medical, ASD, Inc., Kent, UK) high-flow humidification system. They feature a high efficiency bubble humidifier. (See Chapter 8 for the principles of operation of a bubble humidifier.) Systems that combine a separate oxygen blender and flowmeter with a high-flow humidification system include the Vapotherm 2000i system (Vapotherm, Exeter, NH) and Fisher & Paykel 850 and Optiflow systems (Fisher & Paykel Healthcare, Irvine, CA) with the MaxVenturi (Maxtec, Salt Lake City, UT) blender. The Vapotherm Precision Flow features its own built-in blender and flowmeter. The Vapotherm Precision Flow Heliox was discussed in Module C. All systems require a high-pressure oxygen source. All but the MaxVenturi also require a high-pressure air source.

Each HFNC has its own unique humidification system. The Vapotherm 2000i is the original HFNC and its humidification system will be briefly presented here. The Fisher & Paykel 850 and Optiflow systems are similar. Figure 6-17 shows a Vapotherm 2000i that is opened to show the vapor transfer cartridge. Water is continuously supplied into the unit and is warmed before entering the cartridge to be vaporized to humidify the patient's oxygen. The temperature can be adjusted but usually is kept at body temperature. A pediatric cartridge will be used for a flow of 1-8 L/min. An adult cartridge will be used for flows of 5-40 L/min. A triple-lumen patient circuit is attached at the bottom of the unit. (See Fig. 6-18.) The innermost lumen carries the humidified patient gas. The outer lumens transfer warmed water to maintain the desired temperature of the patient gas. The patient's nasal cannula is connected to the distal end of the circuit. There are a range of cannula sizes for neonatal, pediatric, and adult patients. The flow should be set high enough to meet the patient's inspiratory flow needs and deliver up to 100% oxygen.

2. Troubleshoot any problems with the equipment

See Chapter 8 for the discussion on troubleshooting bubble humidifiers. See the previous discussion in this chapter covering blenders and flowmeters. A backpressure-compensated (pressure-compensated) flowmeter should be used with all of these HFNC humidification systems. With the three Vapotherm systems, make sure that the proper vapor transfer cartridge is selected for the oxygen flow needed. Set the appropriate temperature. Make sure that the water supply system does not run out.

c. Air entrainment devices and masks

1. Assemble the necessary equipment

Air entrainment masks are called high-flow devices because they are designed to provide the patient with a controlled oxygen percentage at a high enough flow rate to ensure that all of the patient's inspiratory flow needs

are met (Fig. 6-31). To ensure that this happens, the total flow through the mask must be equal to or greater than the patient's peak inspiratory flow. These masks are sometimes called Venturi masks, Venti masks, jet-mixing systems, and high airflow with oxygen enrichment systems. See Table 6-6 for specific information on available air entrainment masks.

These masks are recommended in any clinical situation in which a known, precise oxygen percentage must be given to the patient who has a variable respiratory rate, inspiratory/expiratory (I:E) ratio, tidal volume, or minute volume. Common situations include a patient with COPD or a patient in respiratory failure who needs increasing oxygen percentages.

Depending on the manufacturer, the mask may come as a completed unit, may have air entrainment adapters to add to the mask, or may have an air entrainment adapter to adjust to set the desired oxygen percentage. See Table 6-6 for the recommended starting oxygen flow rate for the various oxygen percentage masks. Because it is difficult to ensure that the patient's peak inspiratory flow is matched by the gas flow through the mask, the following guidelines are recommended:

- Make sure that the total flow through the mask is at least 40 L/min in a resting patient. More may be needed if the patient is breathing rapidly.
- Provide the patient with a total flow that is four to six times his or her measured minute volume.
- The total flow through the mask can be raised by increasing the oxygen flow. This should not significantly change the oxygen percentage because more room air is entrained to keep the same ratio. However, to be certain, analyze the oxygen percentage inside

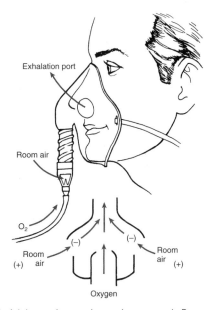

Figure 6-31 Adult wearing an air entrainment mask. Pure oxygen rapidly flows through the narrow jet. Room air is drawn in to dilute the oxygen to the desired final percentage. Modified from Malley WJ: *Clinical blood gases,* ed 2, St Louis, 2005, Saunders.

the mask to ensure that it is as prescribed. The total flow through the mask can be calculated by adding the total of the ratio parts and multiplying by the oxygen flow rate.

An air entrainment nebulizer operates essentially as discussed above and can provide 28% to 100% oxygen with humidity. This would be a better choice for giving a known oxygen percentage to a patient who would benefit from the added aerosol, for example, a patient with thick secretions. A patient with an endotracheal or tracheostomy tube is given a heated aerosol to eliminate the humidity deficit. See Chapter 8 for the principles of operation of large-volume nebulizers. See Figure 8-13 for a patient wearing an aerosol mask and air entrainment nebulizer for supplemental oxygen.

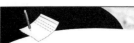

Exam Hint 6-10

It has been necessary on past exams to calculate the needed change in the oxygen flow to increase the total gas flow to meet or exceed a patient's peak inspiratory flow. This ensures that the proper oxygen percentage is delivered.

Air Entrainment Mask Calculations
Example 1
A patient is on a 28% air entrainment mask with an oxygen flow of 4 L/min. His condition worsens, and he increases his minute volume to 15 L/min. To ensure that the patient still receives his prescribed oxygen percentage, the oxygen liter flow is increased to 6 L/min. The new total flow through the mask can be calculated as follows:
   a. 28% air entrainment mask has an air/oxygen ratio of 10:1.
   b. The sum of the ratio parts is 10 + 1 = 11.
   c. Total flow = 11 × 6 L/min oxygen flow = 66 L/min.
   d. This flow is more than four times the patient's current minute volume. He should have all of his flow needs met.
   e. Reanalyze the delivered oxygen percentage to make certain that it is as prescribed.

Example 2
A patient is wearing a 40% air entrainment mask that has the manufacturer's suggested 8 L/min of oxygen running into it. Her peak inspiratory flow is about 48 L/min (0.75 L/s). To what should her oxygen flow be changed to ensure that the total gas flow is greater than her peak inspiratory flow? The new oxygen flow to the mask can be calculated as follows:
   a. 40% air entrainment mask has an air/oxygen ratio of 3:1.
   b. The sum of the ratio parts is 3 + 1 = 4.
   c. Divide the sum of the ratio parts into the peak inspiratory flow: 48/4 = 12.
   d. Increase the oxygen flow from 8 to 12 L/min.

Some patients may complain that the gas coming through the mask is dry. To resolve this problem, some manufacturers have designed an aerosol adapter to add at the jet. A separate bland aerosol then is added to the room air (21% oxygen that enters the jet stream). Make sure that the adapter fits properly and does not interfere with or block

TABLE 6-6	Specifications for Air Entrainment Devices and Masks			
Oxygen (%)	Approximate Air/Oxygen Ratio	Total Ratio Parts	Oxygen Flow Rate L/min*	Total Flow L/min
24	25:1	26	4	104
28	10:1	11	4	44
30	8:1	9	6	54
35	5:1	6	8	48
40	3:1	4	10	40
45	2:1	3	15	45
50	1.7:1	2.7	15	40.5

*These flow rates were selected to ensure that the minimum total flow through the system would be ≥40 L/min. The manufacturers may recommend other minimal O_2 flow rates.

the jet or room air entrainment ports. Do not add a bubble-type humidifier to the jet on the mask because the high backpressure through the jet will cause the pressure-relief (pop-off) valve to open, and the oxygen will leak out.

3. Troubleshoot any problems with the equipment

There are two different ways for room air to be entrained into an air entrainment mask or nebulizer. Depending on the air entrainment mask manufacturer, the jet diameter can be changed, the air entrainment ports can be changed, or both can be changed. With an air entrainment nebulizer, only the air entrainment ports can be changed to adjust the oxygen percentage. It is important to understand the two different adjustments to know what can go wrong with them and how they can be fixed. Make sure that the correct liter flow of oxygen, jet size, and air entrainment port setting are selected to get the desired total flow and oxygen percentage.

a. Variable jet diameter

Notice that the jets have different diameters but the room air entrainment ports are the same size. You will see that the smaller the jet diameter is, the lower the oxygen percentage is. This is because as the jet becomes smaller, the lateral pressure is lower. This results in more room air being brought into the entrainment ports to dilute the oxygen and increase the total flow.

Make sure that the jets are not obstructed by mucus or anything else, or the oxygen percentage will be decreased. An obstruction downstream of the jet prevents the appropriate amount of room air from being brought into the mask. This results in the oxygen percentage increasing and the total flow decreasing.

b. Variable air entrainment ports

Notice that the jet size is fixed but the room air entrainment ports have different sizes. The smaller the entrainment

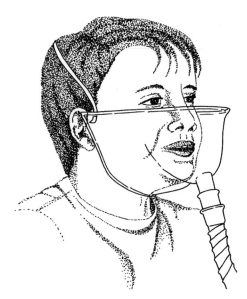

Figure 6-32 Young adult wearing a face tent.

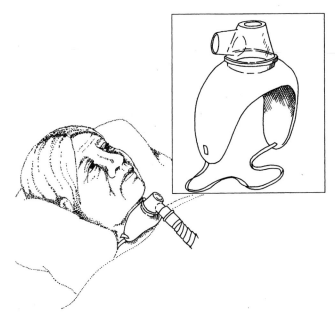

Figure 6-33 Adult wearing a tracheostomy mask/collar.

ports, the higher the oxygen percentage. This is because less room air can be entrained to dilute the oxygen. The total flow is also reduced when the entrainment ports are smaller.

Make sure that the entrainment ports are not obstructed by the patient's sheet or anything else, or the oxygen percentage will increase. An obstruction downstream of the jet prevents the appropriate amount of air from being brought into the mask. This results in the oxygen percentage increasing and the total flow decreasing.

c. Face tent

1. Assemble the necessary equipment

These masks are designed to fit around the patient's neck, under the jaw, and around the cheeks in front of the ears. The front edge should be higher than the level of the patient's nostrils (Fig. 6-32). Face tents sometimes are used to provide oxygen to a patient who cannot wear a mask or cannula because of oral or nasal trauma, burns, or surgery. The patient using a face tent should be sitting as upright as possible. A face tent usually is ordered with the oxygen run through a heated or cool large-volume nebulizer so that the gas is not dry. Make sure that the nebulizer is filled with sterile water, that the high-pressure pop-off works, and that gas is flowing through the tubing before the face tent is put on the patient. If the aerosol is heated, add a drainage bag at the low point of the tubing to collect any condensate. Flows of 5-10 L of oxygen per minute are commonly used with adults. Try to analyze the oxygen percentage close to the patient's nose and mouth to be as accurate as possible. The pulse oximeter value or PaO_2 should be checked whenever a change in the oxygen percentage is made or the patient's condition changes significantly.

2. Troubleshoot any problems with the equipment

Because oxygen is heavier than air, it tends to settle in the mask around the patient's nose and mouth if the fit is tight. However, if the mask is loose at the neck or the patient is lying flat, the oxygen will simply "pour" down out of it. This makes it difficult to know with any certainty what inspired oxygen percentage is available to the patient.

d. Tracheostomy mask/collar

1. Assemble the necessary equipment

The adult or pediatric tracheostomy mask or collar is shaped to fit over a tracheostomy tube or stoma to provide oxygen and aerosol (Fig. 6-33). Because the patient's upper airway is bypassed, a heated high-volume nebulizer is used for humidity. It is usually an air entrainment type of device so the oxygen percentage can be adjusted. Because the aerosol is heated, add a drainage bag at the low point of the tubing to collect any condensate. Make sure that the nebulizer is filled with sterile water, the high-pressure pop-off valve is working, and adequate mist is flowing through to the mask before putting it on the patient.

2. Troubleshoot any problems with the equipment

Because the tracheostomy mask is an open system without a reservoir, it is very important to set the gas flow high enough to make a "cloud" of aerosol around the tracheostomy. If an excess of aerosol can be seen around the tracheostomy during inspiration, it is likely that the desired oxygen percentage is being delivered. Analyze the oxygen percentage from inside the mask to try for as much accuracy as possible. The pulse oximeter value or PaO_2 should be checked whenever there is a flow change or an oxygen percentage change or when the patient's condition changes significantly.

e. T-piece/Briggs adapter

1. Assemble the necessary equipment

The T-piece or Briggs adapter is designed to provide air or supplemental oxygen and aerosol to an endotracheal or tracheostomy tube. It has one 15-mm inner diameter opening that fits over any endotracheal or tracheostomy tube adapter. The other two openings are 22-mm outer diameter so that aerosol tubing can be added (Fig. 6-34). A heated high-volume nebulizer is commonly used for humidity because the patient's upper airway is bypassed. The nebulizer is usually an air entrainment type of device so the oxygen percentage can be adjusted. Because the aerosol is heated, add a drainage bag at the low point of the tubing to collect any condensate. Make sure that the nebulizer is filled with sterile water, the high-pressure pop-off valve is working, and adequate mist is flowing through to the adapter before putting it on the patient.

A length of aerosol tubing must be added downstream of the T-piece to act as a reservoir so that the inspired oxygen percentage is ensured. A reservoir of 50-100 mL of aerosol tubing is commonly needed for the adult.

2. Troubleshoot any problems with the equipment

Care must be taken to adjust the gas flow so that it is high enough to meet the patient's peak inspiratory flow rate. This can be determined by watching the aerosol flow past the adapter and reservoir. Make sure that during inspiration the aerosol is still flowing past the tracheostomy or endotracheal tube and into the reservoir. Inadequate flow could cause two problems. First, room air will be inhaled and the patient's oxygen percentage will be lower than ordered. Second, the patient will rebreathe gas from the

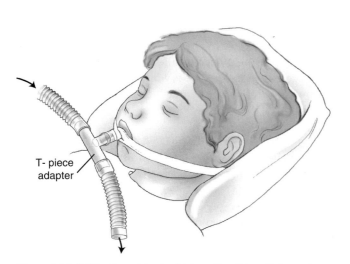

Figure 6-34 Child with endotracheal tube with a Briggs/T-piece adapter and added aerosol tubing.

Exam Hint 6-11

Know to increase the aerosol flow to a tracheostomy mask or T-piece/Briggs adapter if the aerosol cannot be seen during a patient's inspiration. The NBRC usually calls the latter device a T-piece rather than a Briggs adapter in its questions.

reservoir. This gas has just been exhaled and is high in carbon dioxide and low in oxygen.

MODULE E

Administer specialty gases (code: IIID4) [difficulty: R, Ap].

The indications for all of the specialty gases are listed in Box 6-1. Although none of these gases is used widely in respiratory care, all can be very beneficial when indicated.

1. Administer heliox therapy

Patients who benefit from He/O_2 therapy can have an upper-airway obstruction problem (tumor) or a lower-airway obstruction problem (asthma). Because helium atoms are so much smaller than nitrogen molecules, patients find that their work of breathing is greatly reduced. Normoxic patients usually are given a mix of 80% helium and 20% oxygen, whereas hypoxemic patients

---

BOX 6-1   Indications for the Special Therapeutic Gases: He/O_2 (Heliox), NO (Nitric Oxide), and O_2/CO_2 (Carbogen)

Heliox Uses
Upper-airway obstruction.
   Tracheal tumor
   Laryngotracheobronchitis (croup)
   Postextubation stridor
   Small endotracheal tube
Lower-airway obstruction.
   Status asthmaticus
   May reduce work of breathing in other conditions such as chronic obstructive pulmonary disease (COPD) or bronchiolitis.

Nitric Oxide Uses
Treatment of term and near-term (>34 weeks) neonates with hypoxic respiratory failure associated with clinical or echocardiographic evidence of pulmonary hypertension.
Possible use in acute respiratory distress syndrome (ARDS).

Carbogen Uses
Hypoplastic left-heart syndrome (HLHS).
Carbon dioxide response curve test.
Singultus (hiccup).

are given 70% helium and 30% oxygen or 60% helium and 40% oxygen. Although a patient should be given oxygen as needed, a higher oxygen percentage must result in a lower helium percentage. This will make the heliox less effective at reducing the patient's work of breathing. If even more oxygen is needed, small-bore oxygen tubing can be used to add it into the mask or reservoir bag, or a special closed system will have to be assembled from components.

Ideally any helium/oxygen delivery system should have a reservoir bag. Usually the nonrebreathing mask and the reservoir are used. The reservoir should be filled with the He/O$_2$ mix before the mask is placed on the patient's face. Again, the fit should be as tight as possible to minimize leaks. Adjust the flow so that the reservoir bag does not collapse by more than one-third during an inspiration. If it does, increase the flow. The flow should be increased if the patient complains of shortness of breath. Signs of increased work of breathing include agitation, increased use of accessory muscles of respiration, sweating, and increased respiratory rate, heart rate, and blood pressure. See the previous discussion in Module C.

2. Nitric oxide therapy

a. Recommend inhaled nitric oxide (INO) (code: IIIE4a) [difficulty: R, Ap]

See Chapter 9 for the full discussion of the various pulmonary vasodilators. This will be limited to briefly presenting INO gas. The FDA has approved INO for use as a pulmonary artery vasodilator in neonates with persistent pulmonary hypertension of the neonate (PPHN) and increased pulmonary vascular resistance (PVR). Clinical improvement is often seen when a neonate with PPHN inhales about 20 parts per million (ppm) of nitric oxide. Based on the patient's response, more or less may be needed. (See Chapter 5 for the discussion on PVR.) Under any circumstances, it is important to keep the concentration of INO as low as possible because nitric oxide combines with oxygen to form toxic NO$_2$. A level of nitrogen dioxide greater than 10 ppm can cause cell damage, hemorrhage, and pulmonary edema leading to death. In addition, as the NO$_2$ level increases, it causes an increase in the patient's methemoglobin level. Therefore, the serum level of this nonfunctional form of hemoglobin must also be monitored. Patients who receive INO are usually also receiving mechanical ventilation. To do this, special INO measurement and delivery systems are needed and levels of inspired oxygen, nitric oxide, and nitrogen dioxide must be measured. As the patient's PPHN improves, the level of INO can be reduced. This is commonly done by reducing the INO concentration in steps of 50%. For example, if 20 ppm was the original dose on nitric oxide, it would be reduced in steps of 10 ppm, then 5 ppm, and so on until there is 1 ppm or less. The neonate is assessed at each decreasing step to be sure that the pulmonary artery pressure does not increase.

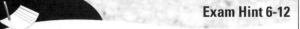

b. Administer inhaled nitric oxide (code: IIID4) [difficulty: R, Ap]

See Chapter 16 for the full discussion on the equipment needed to administer INO.

3. Administer O$_2$/CO$_2$ (carbogen) therapy (code: IIID4) [difficulty: R, Ap]

Carbon dioxide is available in tanks of pure CO$_2$ or a mix of 5%:95% or 7%:93% (carbon dioxide:oxygen ratio). Carbogen is used during cardiopulmonary bypass procedures to maintain the patient's PaCO$_2$. Common clinical uses are listed in Box 6-1. Because inhaling carbon dioxide runs counter to a person's normal exhalation of CO$_2$, the patient's PaCO$_2$ can increase with resulting respiratory acidosis. So, the patient's ABG values, vital signs, cardiac rhythm, and mental status must be monitored closely. Be prepared to decrease the carbogen percentage or stop the breathing of carbogen if the patient shows any adverse signs or symptoms.

A child with hypoplastic left-heart syndrome (HLHS) usually is being mechanically ventilated. The infant with this congenital heart defect must maintain an open foramen ovale and patent ductus arteriosus (PDA) for adequate systemic circulation (a right-to-left intracardiac shunt). Carbogen is added by small-bore tubing connecting the gas cylinder with a T-piece connected into the ventilator circuit. Usually enough carbogen flow is added to result in measurement of 1% to 4% carbon dioxide on a capnometer. Because increased carbon dioxide is a pulmonary vasoconstrictor, the PDA can be maintained. The infant's vital signs and ABG values must be closely monitored to guide the adjustment in carbogen.

The carbon dioxide response curve test is a measurement of the increase in minute volume caused by breathing different concentrations of carbon dioxide when the patient's oxygen level is normal. This pulmonary function test is performed on patients with COPD to determine whether their breathing will increase when their carbon dioxide level is increased. Depending on the method of test performed, the patient inhales between 1% and 7% carbon dioxide. The flow and concentration must be adjusted to maintain the desired carbon dioxide level as measured on a capnometer. An oxygen analyzer also should be included in the system to make sure that the patient does not inhale less than 21% oxygen.

The treatment of hiccups (singultus) usually requires only that the patient rebreathe from a paper bag. If necessary, a small amount of carbon dioxide can be added to stop the hiccups.

MODULE F

Respiratory care plan

1. Determine a patient's pathophysiologic state (code: IIIF1) [difficulty: R, Ap, An]

The goal of oxygen therapy is to correct the patient's hypoxemia. Obtain an ABG sample or perform pulse oximetry, as needed, to determine the patient's oxygenation. Review the complete discussion of these subjects in Chapter 3. The specialty gases (heliox, nitric oxide, and carbogen) are needed to help manage the specific clinical problems listed in Box 6-1.

2. Recommend starting a treatment based on the patient's response (code: IIIE2a) [difficulty: R, Ap, An]

Look for signs of hypoxemia and be prepared to recommend a change in the patient's oxygen delivery system or oxygen percentage to correct the problem. Tachycardia and tachypnea are common findings in hypoxemic patients. Proper oxygen therapy should relieve the problem so that the patient's vital signs return toward normal. An abnormal heart rhythm caused by hypoxemia should return to normal with relief of the problem. Check the patient's pulse oximeter or PaO_2 value whenever a change in the inspired oxygen percentage or a significant change in the patient's clinical condition occurs.

3. Recommend a change in the therapeutic plan if indicated (code: IIIF2) [difficulty: R, Ap, An]

Be prepared to recommend a change in the care plan depending on the patient's problem and clinical progress. Review the indications and uses of supplemental oxygen and the specialty gases.

Every patient's oxygen percentage or flow must be tailored to meet the patient's clinical goals. Usually this means keeping patients who are acutely hypoxemic at a PaO_2 level between 60 and 100 torr and an SpO_2 value between 90% and 97%. Exceptions, when the blood oxygen level is kept as high as possible, include CPR and treatment for carbon monoxide poisoning. See Chapter 3 for a complete discussion of the interpretation of ABG values.

Another exception is the patient with COPD who is hypoxemic and hypercarbic. Usually these patients'

conditions are maintained with a moderate hypoxemia. The PaO_2 level should be between 50 and 60 torr or the SpO_2 value between 88% and 92%. It is imperative to keep the oxygen in this relatively narrow range. Further hypoxemia will result in pulmonary hypertension and cor pulmonale. Cardiac dysrhythmias or arrest and death can occur if the hypoxemia is severe (<40 torr). Oxygen levels in the normal range (>60 torr) may result in blunting of the hypoxic drive. This can result in bradypnea and even greater carbon dioxide retention with corresponding acidemia. When the carbon dioxide pressure ($PaCO_2$) level exceeds 80-90 torr, some COPD patients become drowsy or somnolent. The goal of treatment is to decrease the F_IO_2 to reduce the PaO_2 level to 50-60 torr. This, in turn, stimulates the hypoxic drive so that the patient increases his or her ventilation.

4. Recommend a treatment be terminated (code: IIIE1) [difficulty: R, Ap, An]

It may be necessary to stop the use of carbogen or nitric oxide if the patient has an adverse reaction to their use.

5. Recommend discontinuing a treatment based on the patient's response (code: IIIE2h) [difficulty: R, Ap, An]

As was discussed at the beginning of the chapter, there are several possible hazards with the use of oxygen therapy. The NBRC is most likely to ask questions related to the use of or increase or decrease in oxygen in a patient with COPD. The specialty gases can be discontinued when the clinical problem (see Box 6-1) has been corrected. Discontinue supplemental oxygen when the patient is not hypoxemic while breathing room air.

Exam Hint 6-13

Know the advantages, disadvantages, and possible oxygen ranges for the various oxygen appliances discussed earlier. Be prepared to make recommendations to change from one appliance to another or to change the oxygen percentage or flow. Expect to see one question that deals with the need to reduce the inspired oxygen percentage to a patient with COPD with hypercarbia. In addition, usually one question deals with needing to increase the inspired oxygen percentage to a patient with COPD who is too hypoxemic.

BIBLIOGRAPHY

AARC clinical practice guideline: oxygen therapy in the acute care hospital, *Respir Care* 36:1410–1413, 1991.

AARC clinical practice guideline: oxygen therapy in the home or extended care facility—2007 revision & update, *Respir Care* 52:1063–1068, 2007.

American Association for Respiratory Care: clinical practice guideline: oxygen therapy for adults in the acute care facility: 2002 revision and update, *Respir Care* 47:717, 2002.

American Association for Respiratory Care: clinical practice guideline: selection of an oxygen delivery device for neonatal and pediatric patients: 2002 revision and update, *Respir Care* 47:707, 2002 (Retired).

AARC clinical practice guideline: evidence-based clinical practice guideline: inhaled nitric oxide for neonates with acute hypoxic respiratory failure, *Respir Care* 58(12):1717–1745, 2010.

Bageant RA: Oxygen analyzers, *Respir Care* 21:410–416, 1976.

Barnhart SL: Oxygen administration. In Walsh BK, Czervinske MP, DiBlasi RM, editors: *Perinatal and pediatric respiratory care*, ed 3, St Louis, 2010, Saunders.

Boatright J, Ward JJ: Therapeutic gases: manufacture, storage, and delivery. In Hess DR, MacIntyre NR, Mishoe SC, Galvin WF, Adams AB, editors: *Respiratory care principles & practices*, ed 2, Burlington, MA, 2012, Jones & Bartlett Learning.

Boatright J, Ward JJ: Therapeutic gases: management and administration. In Hess DR, MacIntyre NR, Mishoe SC, Galvin WF, Adams AB, editors: *Respiratory care principles & practices*, ed 2, Burlington, MA, 2012, Jones & Bartlett Learning.

Branson RD, Johannigman JA: Pre-hospital oxygen therapy, *Respir Care* 58(1):86-97, 2013.

Cairo JM: Administering medical gases: regulators, flowmeters, and controlling devices. In Cairo JM, editor: *Mosby's respiratory care equipment*, ed 9, St Louis, 2014, Mosby.

Cairo JM: Manufacture, storage, and transport of medical gases. In Cairo JM, editor: *Mosby's respiratory care equipment*, ed 9, St Louis, 2014, Mosby.

Dunne PJ: The clinical impact of new long-term oxygen therapy technology, *Respir Care* 54(8):1100-1111, 2009.

Elias S, Sviri S, Orenbuch-Harroch E, Fellig Y, Ben-Yehuda A, Fridlender ZG, et al.: Sildenafil to facilitate weaning from inhaled nitric oxide and mechanical ventilation in a patient with severe secondary pulmonary hypertension and a patent forament ovale, *Respir Care* 56(10):1611-1613, 2011.

Fink JB: Opportunities and risks of using heliox in your clinical practice, *Respir Care* 51(6):651-660, 2006.

Fink JB, Hunt GE, editors: *Clinical practice in respiratory care*, Philadelphia, 1999, Lippincott-Raven.

Gentile MA: Inhaled medical gases: more to breathe than oxygen, *Respir Care* 56(9):1341-1359, 2011.

Gluck EH, Onorato DJ, Castriotta R: Helium-oxygen mixtures in intubated patients with status asthmaticus and respiratory acidosis, *Chest* 98:693-698, 1990.

Green J, Frain V: Oxygen and medical gas therapy. In Wyka KA, Mathews PJ, Rutkowski, editors: *Foundations of respiratory care*, ed 2, Clifton Park, NY, 2012, Delmar.

Hess DR: Nonconventional respiratory therapeutics. In Hess DR, MacIntyre NR, Mishoe SC, et al.: *Respiratory care principles & practices*, Philadelphia, 2002, Saunders.

Hess DR: Heliox and noninvasive positive-pressure ventilation: a role for heliox in exacerbations of chronic obstructive pulmonary disease? *Respir Care* 51(6):640-650, 2006.

Heuer AJ: Medical gas therapy. In Kacmarek RM, Stoller JK, Heuer AJ, editors: *Egan's fundamentals of respiratory care*, ed 10, St Louis, 2013, Mosby.

Hollman GA, Shen G, Zeng L, Yngsdal-Krenz R, Perloff W, Zimmerman J, et al.: Helium-oxygen improves clinical asthma scores in children with acute bronchiolitis, *Crit Care Med* 26:1731-1736, 1998.

Hunt GE: Gas therapy. In Fink JB, Hunt GE, editors: *Clinical practice in respiratory care*, Philadelphia, 1999, Lippincott-Raven.

Kacmarek RM, Dimas S, Mack CW: *The essentials of respiratory care*, ed 4, St Louis, 2005, Mosby.

Kallet RH, Matthay MA: Hyperoxic acute lung injury, *Respir Care* 58(1):123-141, 2013.

Kass JE, Castriotta RJ: Heliox therapy in acute severe asthma, *Chest* 107:757-760, 1995.

Kemper KJ, Ritz RH, Benson MS, Bishop MS: Helium-oxygen mixture in the treatment of postextubation stridor in pediatric trauma patients, *Crit Care Med* 19:356-359, 1991.

Kim IK, Saville AL, Sikes KL, Corcoran TE: Heliox-driven albuterol nebulization for asthma exacerbations: an overview, *Respir Care* 51(6):613-618, 2006.

Kudukis TM, Manthous CA, Schmidt GA, Hall JB, Wylam ME: Inhaled helium-oxygen revisited: Effect of inhaled helium-oxygen during the treatment of status asthmaticus in children, *J Pediatr* 131:333-334, 1997.

Lenglet H, Szstrymf B, Leroy C, Brun P, Dreyfuss D, Ricard J: Humidified high flow nasal oxygen during respiratory failure in the Emergency Department: feasibility and efficacy, *Respir Care* 57(11):1873-1879, 2012.

Malley WJ: *Clinical blood gases*, ed 2, St Louis, 2005, Saunders.

McCoy RW: Oxygen-conserving techniques and devices, *Respir Care* 45:95-103, 2000.

McCoy RW: Options for home oxygen therapy equipment: storage and metering of oxygen in the home, *Respir Care* 58(1):65-85, 2013.

Myers TP: Use of heliox in children, *Respir Care* 51(6):619-631, 2006.

Parke RL, McGuinness SP, Eccleston ML: A preliminary randomized controlled trial to assess effectiveness of nasal high-flow oxygen in intensive care patients, *Respir Care* 56(3):265-270, 2011.

Pilbeam SP, Cairo JM, Barraza P: Special techniques in ventilatory support. In Cairo JM, editor: *Pilbeam's mechanical ventilation*, ed 5, St Louis, 2012, Mosby.

Roca O, Riera J, Torres F, Masclans JR: High-flow oxygen therapy in acute respiratory failure, *Respir Care* 55(4):408-413, 2010.

Rogers M: Administration of gas mixtures. In Walsh BK, Czervinske MP, DiBlasi RM, editors: *Perinatal and pediatric respiratory care*, ed 3, St Louis, 2010, Saunders.

Saposnick AB: Medical gases—manufacture, storage, and delivery. In Hess DR, MacIntyre NR, Mishoe SC, et al.: *Respiratory care principles & practices*, Philadelphia, 2002, Saunders.

Saposnick AB, Hess DR: Oxygen therapy: Administration and management. In Hess DR, MacIntyre NR, Mishoe SC, et al.: *Respiratory care principles & practices*, Philadelphia, 2002, Saunders.

Schaeffer EM, Pohlman A, Morgan S, Hall JB: Oxygenation in status asthmaticus improves during ventilation with helium-oxygen, *Crit Care Med* 27:2666-2670, 1999.

Shapiro BA, Harrison RA, Cane RD, et al.: *Clinical application of blood gases*, ed 4, St Louis, 1989, Mosby.

Siobal MS: Pulmonary vasodilators, *Respir Care* 52(7):885-899, 2007.

Siobal MS, Hess DR: Are inhaled vasodilators useful in acute lung injury and acute respiratory distress syndrome? *Respir Care* 55(2):144-161, 2010.

Tassaux D, Jolliet P, Thouret JM, Roeseler J, Dorne R, Chevrolet JC: Calibration of seven ICU ventilators for mechanical ventilation with helium-oxygen mixtures, *Am J Respir Crit Care Med* 160:22-32, 1999.

Venkataraman ST: Heliox during mechanical ventilation, *Respir Care* 51(6):632-639, 2006.

Vines DL: Storage and delivery of medical gases. In Kacmarek RM, Stoller JK, Heuer AJ, editors: *Egan's fundamentals of respiratory care*, ed 10, St Louis, 2013, Mosby.

Walsh BK, Brooks TM, Grenier BM: Oxygen therapy in the neonatal care environment, *Respir Care* 54(9):1193-1202, 2009.

Ward JJ: High-flow oxygen administration by nasal cannula for adult and pediatric patients, *Respir Care* 58(1):98-122, 2013.

Waugh JB, Granger WM: An evaluation of 2 new devices for nasal high-flow gas therapy, *Respir Care* 49:902-906, 2004.

White GC: *Equipment theory for respiratory care*, ed 4, Albany, NY, 2005, Delmar.

Wojciechowski WV: *Respiratory care sciences: an integrated approach*, ed 3, Albany, NY, 2000, Delmar.

1. A home care patient has a problem with his O_2 concentrator and needs to change to the H tank of O_2. If the patient's nasal cannula is receiving a flow of 3 L/min and the tank pressure is 1300 psig, how long can the patient receive O_2?
   - A. About 2 hours
   - B. About 22 hours
   - C. About 120 hours
   - D. About 1300 hours

2. What is the most likely problem to watch for in a patient with severe COPD who is receiving supplemental O_2?
   - A. Pulmonary edema from O_2 toxicity
   - B. Hypoventilation
   - C. Retinopathy of prematurity
   - D. Hyperventilation

3. An order is received to set up a HFNC on a patient. What will be needed?
   1. Humidifier
   2. High-pressure oxygen source
   3. Sterile saline
   4. Blender
   5. High-pressure air source
   - A. 2, 4, and 5 only
   - B. 2, 3, and 4 only
   - C. 1, 2, 4, and 5 only
   - D. 1, 2, 3, 4, 5

4. A respiratory therapist is making general rounds in the hospital and finds a patient whose reservoir tubing has fallen off his 40% T-piece. This would result in which of the following?
   - A. Increased inspired O_2
   - B. Increased inspired CO_2
   - C. Decreased inspired CO_2
   - D. Decreased inspired O_2

5. The risks of O_2 therapy include all of the following EXCEPT:
   - A. Pulmonary O_2 toxicity
   - B. Denitrogen absorption atelectasis
   - C. O_2-induced hyperventilation
   - D. Retinopathy of prematurity

6. A patient is wearing a face tent because of recent facial surgery. It is set at 35% O_2. The nurse moves the patient from an upright to a supine position in bed. What effect will this have on the patient's respiratory status?
   - A. Increased V_T
   - B. Increased inspired O_2
   - C. Increased inspired CO_2
   - D. Decreased inspired O_2

7. To minimize the risk of hypoxemia during a treatment or procedure, which of the following should be done?

1. Increase the O_2 percentage by 20% above the normal setting before suctioning or changing equipment.
2. Keep the O_2 percentage the same as if the patient were not hypoxemic at this time.
3. Minimize the time that the patient would be breathing room air.
4. Increase the O_2 percentage to 100% before suctioning.
5. Make sure the replacement equipment is working properly before you place it on the patient.
   - A. 1 and 3 only
   - B. 2 and 5 only
   - C. 3 and 4 only
   - D. 3, 4, and 5 only

8. An anxious 68-year-old patient with congestive heart failure will not keep the nonrebreathing mask on. What should be recommended to treat the patient's hypoxemia?
   - A. HFNC
   - B. Partial rebreathing mask
   - C. 50% air entrainment mask
   - D. 40/60 heliox mix by nonrebreathing mask

9. A patient is wearing a partial-rebreathing mask. The reservoir bag almost totally collapses during inspiration. Which of the following should be done?
   - A. Tell the patient to breathe more slowly.
   - B. Put a standard nasal cannula on the patient.
   - C. Tell the patient to breathe more rapidly.
   - D. Increase the O_2 flow.

10. When checking a home care patient's reservoir-type nasal cannula, the therapist notices that the reservoir does not fill and empty in synchrony with the patient's breathing pattern. Based on this, what should be done?
    - A. Increase the O_2 flow.
    - B. Replace the cannula.
    - C. Decrease the O_2 flow.
    - D. Switch the patient to an air entrainment mask.

11. What O_2 delivery device should be recommended for a patient who has a variable respiratory rate, I:E ratio, and V_T?
    - A. Nasal cannula
    - B. Air entrainment mask
    - C. Simple O_2 mask
    - D. Transtracheal catheter

12. The physician asks the respiratory therapist which O_2 delivery device would be best for a patient who needs about 75% O_2. What should be recommended?
    - A. Nonrebreathing mask
    - B. 6 L/min nasal cannula
    - C. Air entrainment mask
    - D. Simple O_2 mask

13. A patient has a nasal cannula and needs to be transported on a stretcher. The E-sized O_2 cylinder will have to be laid flat under the stretcher. Which flowmeter should be recommended?
    A. Backpressure-compensated Thorpe
    B. Non-backpressure-compensated Thorpe
    C. Bourdon
    D. Backpressure-compensated kinetic

14. An E cylinder of O_2 needs to be prepared for transport of a patient. A regulator with which pinhole locations should be used?
    A. 1 and 5
    B. 2 and 6
    C. 3 and 5
    D. 2 and 5

15. What is the duration of flow of an E cylinder with 1700 psig that is running at 5 L/min?
    A. 0.9 hour
    B. 1.6 hours
    C. 7.7 hours
    D. 13.7 hours

16. The respiratory therapist is called to draw an arterial blood sample from a patient who is wearing a 35% air entrainment mask. Upon entering the room, the therapist notices that the patient's covers are drawn up over the air entrainment ports of the mask. How would this affect the function of the mask?
    A. The total flow will be increased.
    B. There will be no effect.
    C. The O_2 percentage will be increased.
    D. The O_2 percentage will be decreased.

17. A phone call is received from a home care patient. The patient reports that the high-pressure pop-off valve on the bubble humidifier to the transtracheal oxygen catheter is venting. In addition, the patient cannot flush out the catheter with saline or push the cleaning rod through it. What should the patient be told to do?
    A. Remove the humidifier and double the oxygen flow rate to the catheter.
    B. Force the saline through the catheter until the obstruction is cleared.
    C. Force the cleaning rod through the catheter until the obstruction is cleared.
    D. Switch oxygen from the transtracheal catheter to a nasal cannula.

18. A 58-year-old patient with advanced emphysema is admitted with an acute exacerbation of the condition. While breathing 2 L/min of oxygen through a transtracheal oxygen catheter, the patient has the following ABG results:
    pH, 7.38
    $PaCO_2$, 57 torr
    HCO_3^-, 31 mEq/L
    PaO_2, 47 torr
    SaO_2, 80%
    Based on these findings, what should be done?
    A. Change the patient to 24% oxygen by an air entrainment mask.
    B. Initiate bilevel mask ventilation.
    C. Change the patient to a nonrebreathing mask with 10 L/min of oxygen.
    D. Increase the oxygen flow to the current system to 3 L/min.

19. A comatose patient is intubated and is receiving 35% O_2 with aerosol through a T-piece. While watching the patient breathe, the therapist notices that during each inspiration, the mist disappears from the downstream end of the T-piece. What should be recommended?
    A. Add aerosol tubing to the end of the T-piece.
    B. Change the O_2 to 30% and increase the flow.
    C. Change the O_2 to 40% and decrease the flow.
    D. Tell the patient not to breathe so deeply.

20. A 65-year-old female patient with pulmonary edema is very short of breath and hypoxemic. She is ordered to have a nonrebreathing mask with 10 L/min of oxygen going to it. However, she keeps taking off her mask because of anxiety and claustrophobia. When she removes the mask, her pulse oximeter reading drops from 90% to 82%. What should be recommended to help manage the patient?
    A. Give her a nasal cannula at 10 L/min oxygen.
    B. Sedate the patient so that she will keep her nonrebreathing mask on.
    C. Initiate CPAP by mask at 8 cm water and 40% oxygen.
    D. Begin an HFNC at ≥10 L/min oxygen.

21. An uncooperative 13-year-old patient with status asthmaticus is being treated in the Emergency Department. The physician has ordered the patient to receive a 70% helium/30% oxygen mix and continuous nebulized albuterol. What should be recommended as the best way to deliver this?
    A. Partial-rebreathing mask with reservoir bag
    B. HFNC
    C. Nonrebreathing mask with reservoir bag
    D. Through a mechanical ventilator

22. A patient with COPD is going home. After a hospital exercise test is conducted, it has been determined that the patient will require 1 L/min of supplemental oxygen only when exercising on a stationary bicycle or when the patient feels short of breath. Which of the following oxygen delivery systems should the respiratory therapist recommend?
    A. Molecular sieve oxygen concentrator
    B. Portable LOX system
    C. Semipermeable membrane oxygen concentrator
    D. Piston compressor

23. The respiratory therapist is attempting to calibrate a polarographic oxygen analyzer but finds that it cannot be done. Possible reasons for this include:
    1. The membrane is torn on the probe.
    2. The gas-sampling capillary tube is plugged with debris.
    3. The electrode solution has evaporated.
    4. The battery needs to be replaced.
    5. Water has condensed on the membrane.
    A. 1 and 3 only
    B. 2 and 3 only
    C. 3, 4, and 5 only
    D. 1, 3, 4, and 5 only

24. A patient has just been admitted through the Emergency Department with suspected CO poisoning. The physician wants the patient to receive the highest possible O_2 percentage. What should be recommended?
    A. CPAP mask at 5 cm H_2O and 40% O_2
    B. Simple mask at 6 L/min flow
    C. 50% air entrainment nebulizer to aerosol mask
    D. Nonrebreathing mask

25. A newborn infant with HLHS has just been transferred to the hospital. Mechanical ventilation is being instituted. What else can be done to help improve the neonate's heart function?
    A. Nitric oxide therapy
    B. Carbogen therapy
    C. Close the PDA
    D. Heliox therapy

26. The respiratory therapist is doing quality assurance on the department's flowmeters. After a backpressure-compensated Thorpe flowmeter is plugged in, the flow is set at 10 L/min. The flowmeter outlet is partially and then completely obstructed. Which of the following should be expected?
    A. The float will stay at the 10-L/min mark.
    B. The float will move upward in the flowmeter.
    C. The float will move upward and then downward in the flowmeter.
    D. The float will move downward and then to the bottom of the flowmeter.

27. The respiratory therapist is called to evaluate a female patient known to have advanced emphysema. She is wearing a nasal cannula at 6 L/min. The nurse says that she has become drowsy and less responsive since the oxygen was given to her an hour ago. Her ABG results on the oxygen show the following:
    PaO2, 84 torr
    PaCO2, 65 torr
    pH, 7.32

    Which of the following should be recommended?
    1. Leave her on the cannula.
    2. Change her to 24% O_2 on an air entrainment mask and repeat the ABG in 20 minutes.
    3. Change her to a simple oxygen mask and repeat the ABG in 20 minutes.
    4. Let her rest undisturbed.
    5. Monitor her closely for becoming more alert.
    A. 1 and 4 only
    B. 3 and 4 only
    C. 2 and 5 only
    D. 3 and 5 only

28. The respiratory therapist is assisting with a bronchoscopy to obtain a biopsy of a suspicious laryngeal node on a patient. Afterward, the patient complains of shortness of breath and a "tight" throat. Which of the following recommendations should be given to the physician?
    A. Give the patient an 80/20 heliox mix to breathe.
    B. Put the head of the bed down 30 degrees.
    C. Give the patient a carbogen mix to breathe.
    D. Do a 7-minute helium dilution test.

29. An adult patient who was rescued from a house fire is being received in the Emergency Department. The patient is wearing a simple oxygen mask at 5 L/min. The SpO2 value by pulse oximeter is 100%, and his SaO2 value from an ABG sample analyzed on a CO oximeter is 73%. What should be recommended at this time?
    A. Maintain the simple oxygen mask at the present flow.
    B. Change the patient to a nonrebreathing mask.
    C. Decrease the oxygen flow to the simple oxygen mask to 4 L/min.
    D. Maintain present therapy and recalibrate the CO oximeter.

30. The respiratory therapist is working with a patient who has a tracheal tumor. The patient is wearing a nonrebreathing mask with 70% helium and 30% oxygen mix. Pulse oximeter saturation is 96%. The patient says that it is getting harder to breathe and it is noticed that the reservoir bag has collapsed. The most appropriate action is to
    A. Decrease the flow of gas.
    B. Switch to a 28% air entrainment mask.
    C. Increase the flow of gas.
    D. Switch to a 60% helium and 40% oxygen mix.

31. An 8-year-old patient with asthma is going to be given a 30% oxygen and 70% helium mix of heliox through a nonrebreathing mask and reservoir bag. The physician has ordered the child to receive 7 L/min of the gas mix. Because it will be delivered through an oxygen flowmeter, what flow should be set?
    A. 3.9 L/min
    B. 4.4 L/min
    C. 9.8 L/min
    D. 11.2 L/min

32. A 36-week gestational age neonate is hypoxemic despite mechanical ventilation and has clinical

evidence of persistent pulmonary hypertension of the newborn. What can be done to correct the hypoxemia?
   A. Instill intratracheal surfactant.
   B. Begin nitric oxide therapy.
   C. Begin 10 cm water PEEP.
   D. Begin carbogen therapy.

33. A respiratory therapist is assigned to the Emergency Department of a major medical center when a 24-year-old patient with status asthmaticus is transferred by ambulance from a small, rural hospital. The patient has been given continuous bronchodilator therapy and intravenous corticosteroids and aminophylline. The patient is becoming exhausted but refuses to allow intubation and mechanical ventilation. What should be recommended?
   A. Begin heliox therapy.
   B. Begin nitric oxide therapy.
   C. Intubate and ventilate the patient despite protests.
   D. Follow the patient's wishes.

34. A neonatal patient has primary pulmonary hypertension and is receiving mechanical ventilation. After the neonate receives 20 ppm of nitric oxide therapy, PVR returns to the normal range. What should be recommended at this time?

   A. Discontinue the nitric oxide therapy.
   B. Decrease the nitric oxide to 10 ppm.
   C. Add 1% carbogen to the nitric oxide mix.
   D. Increase the nitric oxide therapy to 30 ppm.

35. A 16-year-old patient with status asthmaticus is started on a 70% helium/30% oxygen (heliox) mix through a nonrebreather mask. It is noticed that the oxygen flowmeter shows the delivery of 8 L/min of gas. What is the actual heliox gas flow?
   A. 5 L/min
   B. 8 L/min
   C. 12.8 (13) L/min
   D. 14.4 (14) L/min

36. A socially active female patient with COPD requires 2 L/min of continuous oxygen. She wishes to go with her Better Breathers Club on a bus trip to shop in Chicago. What should be recommended for her in this situation?
   A. Use a portable LOX system at 2 L/min.
   B. Take a portable E tank of oxygen with her and run it at 2 L/min.
   C. Pre-position E tanks of oxygen for her use in the various stores.
   D. Take a portable E tank of oxygen with her and run it at 1 L/min.

7 Hyperinflation Therapy

Note: It can be anticipated that the Therapist Multiple-Choice Examination (TMC) will include an *average of 2 of 140 actual questions* (1% of the exam) on hyperinflation therapy. (This is based on the question mix typically found on the National Board of Respiratory Care's previous Entry Level Examinations and Written Registry Examinations.)

Remember that the TMC version you take will include 20 additional questions being evaluated for possible inclusion in other versions of the TMC. So, there will be a total of 160 questions taken. There is no way to differentiate between the 140 actual questions and the 20 questions being evaluated for future use. Please go to the Introduction for detailed information on the TMC Examination and the Clinical Simulation Examination.

MODULE A

> Perform assisted cough for improved airway clearance (code: IIIB4) [difficulty: R, Ap].

Indications for deep breathing and coughing include retained secretions, atelectasis, the likely development of postoperative atelectasis, and the need for a sputum specimen, or they may be required as part of a bronchial hygiene therapy program. This program will usually include postural drainage therapy, positive expiratory pressure (PEP) therapy, and/or incentive spirometry (IS).

The overall phrase "directed cough" is applied to any clinical situation in which the respiratory therapist instructs a patient to cough effectively. The instructions and techniques used to generate an effective cough will vary with the clinical situation as described below. In every instance, the patient must be conscious and cooperative for the procedure to be effective. Be sure to follow standard infection control precautions and droplet nuclei precautions to control the possible transmission of a pulmonary infection from the patient.

1. Spontaneous effective cough

A spontaneous effective cough is the normal cough triggered by reflex when there are secretions or an irritation of the airway. Instruct the patient to perform these steps for a normal cough:
1. Take a deep breath.
2. Close your throat.
3. Tighten your chest muscles to build up pressure.
4. Open your throat and cough out hard. (It helps to demonstrate a strong normal cough effort.)
5. Tell the patient to cough out any secretions into a tissue or sputum specimen container.

2. Postoperative patient

A patient who has recently had an abdominal or thoracic surgery procedure may not be able to perform a spontaneous effective cough because of pain. Because of this, these patients are at an increased risk for atelectasis and pneumonia. This is especially a concern for a patient who has just had upper abdominal surgery such as cholecystectomy or splenectomy. In any situation, the patient must be properly medicated for pain control before coughing is attempted. Ideally, the patient is taught the following techniques before surgery is performed. If not, teach them postoperatively:
1. Have the patient sit up and hold his/her hands on both sides of the incision. This is to minimize traction or tension on the incision and decrease the pain. Alternatively, the therapist or the patient can hold a pillow against the incision.
2. Take in as deep a breath as possible.
3. Apply gentle hand or pillow pressure over the surgical area to "splint" the wound.
4. Perform a normal cough.
5. If the patient cannot cough normally because of pain, a series of two or three less forceful coughs can be performed.

3. Obstructive airways disease patient

A patient with chronic obstructive pulmonary disease (COPD), asthma, cystic fibrosis, or bronchiectasis is likely to experience small-airway closure if a normal cough is performed. A midinspiratory cough or huff cough may be used in this situation. Before starting, position the patient in a sitting position, bent slightly forward, with feet on the floor or supported. The patient who must lie in bed can be positioned on the preferred side with the legs flexed at the knees and hips.

a. Midinspiratory cough
1. Take in a moderately deep breath (larger than normal but not as deep as possible).
2. Briefly hold the breath.
3. Cough normally.

4. If this is not effective, perform a series of two or three coughs at relatively low flows. (It helps to demonstrate a series of reduced-effort coughs.)
5. Squeezing the knees and thighs together when coughing may help to increase the airflow and exhaled volume.

b. Forced expiratory technique cough (also known as a huff cough)

1. Take in a moderately deep breath (larger than normal but not as deep as possible).
2. Briefly hold the breath.
3. Open your throat and "huff" out two or three times. (It helps to demonstrate this "huh-huh-huh" effort.)
4. If helpful, coach the patient to perform a "chicken breath" to make a huff breath more effective (Fig. 7-1).

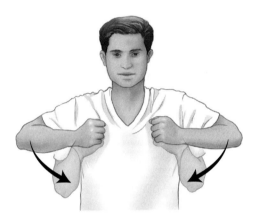

Figure 7-1 A patient performing a "chicken breath" during a huff cough effort. The elbows are raised and a quick downward movement (adduction) brings them against the sides of the chest. This helps to increase expiratory flow and volume.

Demonstrate raising the folded arms with a quick adduction movement of them against the sides of the chest.
5. After a huff cough, the patient should perform controlled, relaxed diaphragmatic breathing to regain breath control.

4. Neuromuscular/neurological disease patient

A patient with a neuromuscular disease (myasthenia gravis, Guillain-Barré syndrome, amyotrophic lateral sclerosis) or high spinal cord injury (usually a patient with quadriplegia) has decreased muscle function. Because of this, the patient is unable to take in a large breath, cough out forcefully to expel secretions, or both. The manually assisted cough and assisted inspiration techniques described below can be used singly or together to help this type of patient.

a. Manually assisted cough

There are two ways to deliver a manually assisted cough: quad cough and lateral chest compression. Both are described below.

1. Quad cough

A quad cough involves the respiratory therapist applying gentle pressure over the patient's epigastric area when he/she coughs. The therapist's hands can be placed side by side or the fingers can be interlocked for a smaller focus area (Fig. 7-2). This procedure is contraindicated in a patient who has recently eaten or is at risk for regurgitation and aspiration. Additional contraindications include pregnancy, upper abdominal surgery, or abdominal pathologies such as a hiatal hernia or abdominal aortic aneurysm.
1. Therapist places his or her hands over the patient's epigastric area below the xyphoid process.

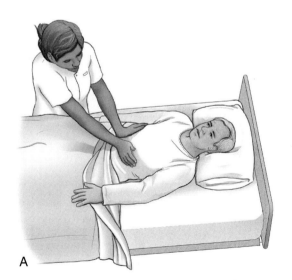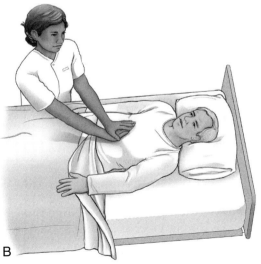

A   B

Figure 7-2 A manually assisted or "quad" cough may be applied to help a neuromuscular or neurological patient cough out secretions. There are two ways the hands can be placed over the epigastric area and below the xyphoid process. **A,** Hands are next to each other. **B,** Fingers are interlocked.

2. Have the patient take in a deep breath and hold it.
3. Tell the patient to cough hard.
4. As the patient coughs, apply gentle pressure over the epigastric area.

2. Lateral chest compression

The lateral chest compression procedure involves the respiratory therapist applying pressure over the lateral rib areas when the patient coughs. This procedure can be used when a patient cannot have pressure applied over the epigastric area. Contraindications to lateral chest compression include broken ribs, flail chest, and osteoporosis.
1. Therapist places his or her hands over the patient's lateral rib areas.
2. Have the patient take in a deep breath and hold it.
3. Tell the patient to cough hard.
4. As the patient coughs, apply gentle inward pressure over the rib areas.

b. Assisted inspiration

An assisted inspiration (also called manual hyperventilation) involves the respiratory therapist using a manual resuscitation bag to deliver a large tidal volume breath to the patient. When the patient has a normal upper airway, a properly sized face mask is attached to the bag. When the patient has an endotracheal or tracheostomy tube, the bag is connected to the artificial airway. This procedure requires careful coordination between the therapist delivering the large breath, the patient making an inspiratory effort, and possibly a second therapist delivering the manually assisted cough effort.
1. Therapist places the face mask over the patient's nose and mouth or attaches the manual resuscitation bag adapter to the endotracheal tube or tracheostomy tube.
2. Have the patient take in a deep breath.
3. At the same time, squeeze the bag to deliver a large tidal volume.
4. Remove the bag and tell the patient to cough hard.
5. If needed, a quad cough or lateral chest compression can be done to increase the cough volume and flow. Because of the quick timing of this procedure, it is more effective if a second therapist does this.

MODULE B

Perform inspiratory muscle training techniques (code: IIIB6) [difficulty: R, Ap].

Inspiratory muscle training is typically performed on a patient with COPD (chronic bronchitis and emphysema). The training is often part of a pulmonary rehabilitation program (see Chapter 17). Initially, teach the following steps to patients with obstructive airways diseases:
1. Have the patient lie in a comfortable supine position; knees can be flexed.

2. Instruct the patient to relax physically as much as possible, especially the shoulders.
3. Use soothing music, meditation, or other techniques for mental relaxation.
4. Instruct the patient to concentrate on breathing more slowly.
5. Emphasize *pursed-lip breathing*, wherein the patient, with relaxed abdominal muscles, breathes in slowly through the nose and out slowly through pursed (slightly opened) lips. Breathing with pursed lips keeps some backpressure on the airways so they stay open longer. The technique helps to improve gas exchange so the patient experiences less dyspnea.

After these first steps have been mastered, teach the following steps to patients with obstructive airways diseases:
1. The therapist places his or her hands and the patient's hands gently over the area(s) where the patient is to concentrate the breathing effort. Usually, this is the abdominal area just below the sternum. This encourages the patient to use the diaphragm more effectively and to strengthen it. With diaphragmatic breathing, the hands move out during an inspiration.
2. The same hands-on technique can be used to aid in segmental breathing over an area that is underventilated or that has atelectasis.
3. Breathing *in* against an obstruction can also increase the strength and endurance of inspiratory muscles. A variety of devices are available. One type of device is a mouthpiece with selectable openings at the other end (Fig. 7-3). The patient breathes in through the largest opening and progresses to smaller openings as tolerated.

Increasing the strength and endurance of inspiratory muscles usually requires a training schedule similar to the following:
1. Plug the nose with nose clips.
2. Inspire a normal tidal volume (V_T) at a rate of 12-15 breaths/min through the largest opening.

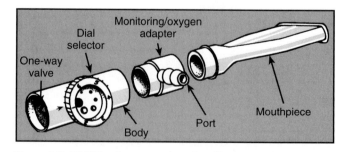

Figure 7-3 PFLEX inspiratory muscle trainer. The body of the device features a dial selector with inspiratory holes. The holes range from setting 1 (largest opening) to setting 6 (smallest opening). A one-way valve allows the patient to expire. The mouthpiece can be attached directly to the body, or a monitoring/oxygen adapter can be added between them. This adapter allows oxygen to be added to meet the patient's needs. An inspiratory force meter also can be added to determine the amount of negative pressure the patient is generating at each of the inspiratory hole settings. (Courtesy of Philips Respironics, Murrysville, PA.)

3. Continue for 10-15 minutes per day for a total of three to five times per week in the first week. If the patient notices shortness of breath, a noticeably increased pulse rate, or increased fatigue, the exercise should be stopped until the symptoms are gone. Resume the exercise when the patient is comfortable again.

4. Gradually increase the duration to about 30 minutes per session or two 15-minute sessions per day.

5. When this schedule can be tolerated easily three times per week, switch to the next smallest hole.

6. Repeat steps *1* to *5* as tolerated. The most beneficial exercise is tiring but not exhausting. The device may be adjusted to the next larger hole setting if the patient becomes too tired. The whole process usually takes 4-6 weeks before positive results are seen.

7. A maintenance program necessitates that exercise be done every other day.

MODULE C

Incentive spirometry

1. Perform hyperinflation by incentive spirometry (code: IIIB5) [difficulty: R, Ap]

Incentive spirometry (IS) is a technique whereby a patient is encouraged to breathe deeply by seeing his or her inhaled volume on the spirometry device. When the patient is coached to inhale maximally and hold the breath for 5 seconds (if possible), it is called a sustained maximal inspiration (SMI). With IS and SMI, the patient receives positive feedback by seeing that the inspired volume gradually increases as his or her condition improves. IS is indicated in any cooperative patient who has developed or is likely to develop atelectasis and can perform the procedure. Clinical situations and individuals in which atelectasis is likely to be seen include postoperative thoracic or abdominal surgery, the aged, the obese, inadequate sigh, cardiopulmonary disease, and quadriplegia and/or dysfunctional hemidiaphragm(s). It is not recommended that IS, *by itself*, be routinely used in postoperative upper-abdominal or coronary artery bypass patients to prevent atelectasis. Rather, IS may be used in conjunction with pain control, early mobilization, deep breathing, and directed cough to help prevent postoperative pulmonary complications.

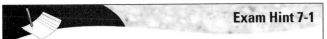

Exam Hint 7-1

IS is preferred over intermittent positive-pressure breathing (IPPB) for the prevention or treatment of atelectasis in patients who can perform IS properly.

Because the goal of IS is to prevent or treat atelectasis, the patient should inhale a near-normal inspiratory capacity (IC). The patient can benefit more by holding the IC for a 5-second SMI effort.

Before the operation, the cooperative surgical patient should have the IC measured at the bedside or calculated from a pulmonary function test in which vital capacity (VC) is measured (review Chapter 4 for IC information). The IC is measured again postoperatively.

Before you start to provide instruction, make sure that the patient is alert and cooperative enough to follow instructions. The patient's respiratory rate should be less than 25 breaths/min if the procedure is to be performed properly. Use the following steps in teaching IS:

1. Have the patient sit in semi-Fowler's position, on the edge of the bed, or up in a chair.

2. Set an initial goal of twice the patient's measured bedside V_T.

3. Tell the patient the purpose of the treatment and how to perform it properly.

4. Simulate the procedure for the patient.

5. Put the unit within easy reach, and keep it upright.

6. Have the patient exhale normally (to functional residual capacity), seal the lips around the mouthpiece, and inspire maximally through the unit in a slow, controlled effort.

7. Have the patient hold the IC for 5 seconds (if possible) before exhaling.

8. Proceed to extend the patient's goal as tolerated and indicated earlier.

9. The patient should repeat the deep breath through the IS device at regular intervals while awake. There is no standard frequency for IS breaths. Clinical trials have included: (1) at least 10 times every 1 to 2 hours, (2) 10 breaths, five times per day, (3) 15 breaths every 4 hours.

10. After each IS breath the patient should have a brief rest period with normal breathing. This will help to prevent tiring the patient and hyperventilation.

Monitor your patient's progress in the following ways:

1. If the patient cannot meet the initial goal, reconsider whether this is the best form of treatment. IPPB might be a better choice for providing a deep breath.

2. Stop the treatment temporarily if the patient has signs of hyperventilation, such as dizziness or tingling of the fingertips. A few minutes of normal breathing should result in a normal feeling again. Have the patient take longer rest periods between maximal breaths.

3. Stop the treatment if the patient complains of acute chest pain. It is possible to cause pulmonary barotrauma by breathing in as deeply as possible. Evaluate the patient's pulmonary condition and call the physician if indicated.

2. Recommend changes in incentive spirometry (code: IIIE3e) [difficulty: R, Ap, An]

See Table 7-1 for IS guidelines. The following guidelines are also suggested:

1. Set the initial IC goal at twice the V_T.

2. Increase the goal in 200-mL increments as the patient tolerates.

TABLE 7-1	Guidelines for the Use of Incentive Spirometry
Bedside Spirometry Value	**Treatment Modality**
IC >80% of the preoperative value	No treatment needed unless radiographic or clinical evidence of atelectasis exists.
IC (of an adult) <2.5 L, or VC >10 mL/kg	Incentive spirometry is indicated.
FVC <70% of predicted or VC <10 mL/kg	Intermittent positive-pressure breathing is indicated.

IC, inspiratory capacity; VC, vital capacity; FVC, forced vital capacity. See Figure 4-7 for the lung volumes and capacities. In normal people the VC and FVC should be the same.

3. Set a final IC goal of greater than 12 mL/kg of ideal body weight, or set a VC goal of greater than 15 mL/kg of ideal body weight.
4. A normal person should have an IC of about 75% of his or her VC. For example, a predicted VC of 5.166 L was calculated for a male patient in Chapter 4. His predicted IC would be calculated as 5.166 L × 0.75 = 3.875 L. However, because of natural variations in people, he might inhale only 80% of this (3.1 L) and still be considered within normal limits. Use this as a guideline for anticipating a patient's maximum IC, and do not expect your patient to inhale a greater IC than is physically possible.

Consider increasing the IS goal if the patient is easily able to reach the set goal or if the patient's breath sounds are diminished in the bases. Consider decreasing the IS goal if the patient cannot reach the set goal because it is too large, if the patient is frustrated and discouraged at his or her inability to reach the set goal, or if excessive surgical site pain prevents the patient from reaching the set goal.

MODULE D

Incentive spirometry equipment

1. Assemble incentive spirometry equipment (code: IIA15) [difficulty: R, Ap]

Two basic types of IS equipment exist: flow-oriented and volume-oriented units.

a. Flow-oriented incentive spirometers

With a flow-oriented unit, the patient breathes in a flow great enough to raise one or more plastic balls in calibrated cylinders (Fig. 7-4). The patient is encouraged to try to keep the ball (or balls) suspended by breathing in more deeply. Encourage the patient to breathe in *slowly* to suspend the balls for as long as possible. Have the patient watch as the balls are held up by the inspired

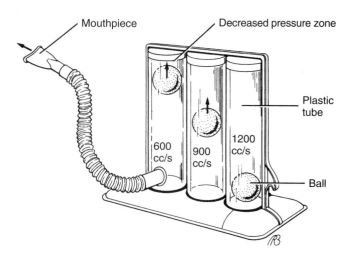

Figure 7-4 Triflo II incentive deep-breathing exerciser. This is an example of a flow-oriented incentive spirometer. (From Eubanks DH, Bone RC: Comprehensive respiratory care, ed 2, St Louis, 1990, Mosby.)

breath to provide positive reinforcement for doing a good job. The patient is not helped by breathing in a fast, short breath and having the balls pop up and down. Patients who cannot generate enough inspiratory flow to use a flow-oriented unit should use a volume-oriented unit instead.

Volume is calculated in a flow-oriented unit by multiplying the flow per second needed to suspend the ball(s) by the number of seconds that the ball(s) is suspended. For example:

$$600 \text{ mL/s} \times 2 \text{ s} = 1200 \text{ mL IC}$$

Assemble the device by attaching the flow tube to the unit and the mouthpiece to the flow tube.

b. Volume-oriented incentive spirometers

With a volume-oriented unit, the patient breathes in a set volume goal from the reservoir bellows (Fig. 7-5). In general, volume-oriented units are preferred over flow-oriented units. This is because volume-oriented units have less imposed work of breathing on the patient. In addition, patients who use a volume-oriented unit will tend to inhale a larger volume than when using a flow-oriented unit.

Some volume-oriented units have a whistle or other signal built into them to warn if the breath is too fast. Some units also have a small built-in leak so the patient must continue inspiring to keep the bellows suspended. Have the patient watch as the bellows is suspended for positive reinforcement for doing a good job. Volume is marked on the bellows container. If the unit has a built-in leak, multiply the volume inspired by the time the bellows is suspended. For example:

$$800 \text{ mL} \times 3 \text{ s} = 2400 \text{ mL IC}$$

Assemble the device by attaching the flow tube to the unit and the mouthpiece to the flow tube.

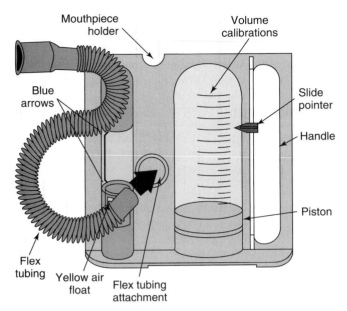

Figure 7-5 Voldyne 5000 volumetric exerciser. This is an example of a volume-oriented incentive spirometer. (Courtesy of Teleflex/Hudson RCI, Research Triangle Park, North Carolina.)

2. Troubleshoot any problems with incentive spirometry equipment (code: IIA15) [difficulty: R, Ap]

In either type of incentive spirometer, an obstruction to the flow tube or mouthpiece or a built-in leak in the calibrated cylinders stops airflow. With a flow-oriented unit, no balls will rise despite the patient's inspiratory effort. With a volume-oriented unit, the bellows will not rise despite the patient's inspiratory effort. Clearing the obstruction or sealing the leak allows either unit to work properly.

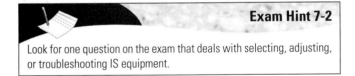

Exam Hint 7-2

Look for one question on the exam that deals with selecting, adjusting, or troubleshooting IS equipment.

MODULE E

Respiratory care plan

1. Determine a patient's pathophysiologic state (code: IIIF1) [difficulty: R, Ap, An]

Review the information in Chapter 1 that deals with the interpretation of breath sounds and chest radiograph findings that would indicate atelectasis or pneumonia. If areas with atelectasis are opened, the patient's breath sounds should improve. Areas that previously had diminished breath sounds should now have normal (vesicular) breath sounds.

2. Recommend starting a treatment based on the patient's response (code: IIIE2a) [difficulty: R, Ap, An]

Atelectasis can usually be managed by a combination of postoperative pain management, ambulation, deep-breathing exercises, directed cough, and IS. The right combination will depend on the patient's circumstances. IS is easier and less expensive than IPPB to treat atelectasis if the patient can properly perform the procedure. See Table 7-1 for guidelines on the indications for IS or IPPB.

3. Recommend a change in the therapeutic plan if indicated (code: IIIF2) [difficulty: R, Ap, An]

The following should be considered when the patient's response is evaluated:
- The opening of atelectatic areas would be signaled by the return of normal rather than diminished or absent breath sounds.
- Be prepared to measure V_T, VC, and IC to determine the patient's goals and evaluate his or her progress.
- The patient may have an increase in sputum production if the deep-breathing exercises and IS open up atelectatic areas. The patient may have a more productive cough because of a greater VC.
- If IS is not correcting the patient's atelectasis, another form of therapy such as IPPB or PEP should be tried.

4. Recommend a treatment be terminated (code: IIIE1) [difficulty: R, Ap, An]

Usually, IS is a safe procedure. Rarely, a patient will take a deep breath and cause a spontaneous pneumothorax. Acute chest pain and shortness of breath could be symptoms of a pneumothorax from barotrauma. A chest radiograph would be needed to confirm or deny the presence of a pneumothorax. Stop the treatment if a pneumothorax is suspected.

Be prepared to pause the current treatment if the patient is having a minor adverse reaction to it. Some patients will hyperventilate during the procedure and will feel dizzy or light-headed. If this happens, the patient should be told not to take any deep IS breaths for a few minutes. The dizziness should go away, and the patient should be able to resume the IS procedure. Direct the patient to continue to inhale deeply but at a slower rate.

5. Recommend discontinuing a treatment based on the patient's response (code: IIIE2h) [difficulty: R, Ap, An]

A treatment can be discontinued for one of three reasons. First, an adverse reaction to or complication of the treatment can lead to the treatment being discontinued. For example, IS, like IPPB, should not be performed on a patient with an untreated pneumothorax. Other reasons to discontinue the treatment include inadequate pain control, exacerbation of bronchospasm, hypoxemia from removal of the patient's oxygen mask, and fatigue.

If these problems are corrected, it may be possible to begin IS treatment again.

Second, ineffective treatment may lead to treatment discontinuation. If the patient cannot perform a proper IS treatment (unconscious, physically unable to perform, inadequate inspiratory volume), another way to treat atelectasis should be found. This could include IPPB. (see Chapter 14 for the discussion.) The physician would order this change in therapy.

Third, if the patient has recovered and no longer needs a hyperinflation therapy treatment, it should be discontinued. As the postsurgical patient recovers, walks about, and performs proper coughing and deep-breathing exercises, any atelectasis will be corrected. In many cases, IS can be stopped within a week after surgery. The physician should order that IS be discontinued.

Exam Hint 7-3

Understand the indications for IS versus those for IPPB. Be prepared to recommend a change in IS volume or to change from IS to IPPB.

BIBLIOGRAPHY

American Association for Respiratory Care: clinical practice guideline: directed cough, *Respir Care* 38(5):495–499, 1993 (Retired).

American Association for Respiratory Care: clinical practice guideline: incentive spirometry: 2011, *Respir Care* 56(10): 1600–1604, 2011.

American Association for Respiratory Care: clinical practice guideline: intermittent positive pressure breathing: 2003 revision & update, *Respir Care* 48(5):540–546, 2003.

American Association for Respiratory Care: clinical practice guideline: incentive spirometry, *Respir Care* 36(12):1402, 1991.

Butler TJ: *Laboratory exercises for competency in respiratory care*, ed 3, Philadelphia, 2013, FA Davis.

Cairo JM: Lung expansion devices. In Cairo JM, Pilbeam SP, editors: *Mosby's respiratory care equipment*, ed 8, St Louis, 2010, Mosby.

Cairo JM: Lung expansion therapy devices. In Cairo JM, editor: *Mosby's respiratory care equipment*, ed 9, St Louis, 2014, Mosby.

Douce FH: Incentive spirometry and other aids to lung inflation. In Barnes TA, editor: *Core textbook of respiratory care practice*, ed 2, St Louis, 1994, Mosby.

Eubanks DH, Bone RC: *Comprehensive respiratory care, a learning system*, ed 2, St Louis, 1990, Mosby.

Fink JB: Bronchial hygiene and lung expansion. In Fink JB, Hunt GE, editors: *Clinical practice in respiratory care*, Philadelphia, 1999, Lippincott Williams & Wilkins.

Fink JB: Volume expansion therapy. In Burton GG, Hodgkin JE, Ward JJ, editors: *Respiratory care: A guide to clinical practice*, Philadelphia, 1997, Lippincott-Raven.

Fink JB, Hess DR: Secretion clearance techniques. In Hess DR, MacIntyre NR, Mishoe SC, editors: *Respiratory care principles & practice*, Philadelphia, 2002, Saunders.

Fisher DF: Lung expansion therapy. In Kacmarek RM, Stoller JK, Heuer JK, editors: *Egan's fundamentals of respiratory care*, ed 10, St Louis, 2013, Mosby.

Hess DR: Sputum collection, airway clearance, and lung expansion therapy. In Hess DR, MacIntyre NR, Mishoe SC, Galvin WF, Adams AB, editors: *Respiratory care: principles and practice*, ed 2, Burlington, MA, 2012, Jones & Bartlett Learning.

Hirsh CA: Airway clearance therapy. In Kacmarek RM, Stoller JK, Heuer AF, editors: *Egan's fundamentals of respiratory care*, ed 10, St Louis, 2013, Mosby.

Johnson NT, Pierson DJ: The spectrum of pulmonary atelectasis: pathophysiology, diagnosis, and therapy, *Respir Care* 31:1107, 1986.

Mang H, Obermayer A: Imposed work of breathing during sustained maximal inspiration: comparison of six incentive spirometers, *Respir Care* 34:1122, 1989.

Paisani Dde M, Lunardi AC, da Silva CC, Porras DC, Tanaka C, Carvalho CR: Volume rather than flow incentive spirometry is effective in improving chest wall expansion and abdominal displacement using optoelectronic plethysmography, *Respir Care* 58(8):1360–1366, 2013.

Rutkowski JA: Hyperinflation therapy. In Wyka KA, Mathews PJ, Clark WF, editors: *Foundations of respiratory care*, Albany, 2002, Delmar.

Rutkowski JA: Pulmonary hygiene and chest physical therapy. In Wyka KA, Mathews PJ, Rutkowski J, editors: *Foundations of respiratory care*, ed 2, Clifton Park NY, 2012, Delmar.

Scuderi J, Olsen GN: Respiratory therapy in the management of postoperative complications, *Respir Care* 34:281, 1989.

Shapiro BA, Kacmarek RM, Cane RD, et al.: *Clinical application of respiratory care*, ed 4, St Louis, 1991, Mosby.

Walsh BK: Airway clearance techniques and lung volume expansion. In Walsh BK, Czervinski MP, DiBlasi RM, editors: *Perinatal and pediatric respiratory care*, ed 3, St Louis, 2012, Saunders.

Wilkins RL: Lung expansion therapy. In Wilkins RL, Stoller JK, Kacmarek RM, editors: *Egan's fundamentals of respiratory care*, ed 9, St Louis, 2009, Mosby.

Wojciechowski WV: Incentive spirometers, secretion evacuation devices, and inspiratory muscle training devices. In Barnes TA, editor: *Core textbook of respiratory care practice*, ed 2, St Louis, 1994, Mosby.

1. A patient is quite weak and is unable to raise the ball marker on a flow-oriented incentive spirometer to meet the set goal. The patient is becoming discouraged. What should be recommended?
   A. Have the patient continue trying.
   B. Recommend that the patient be switched to IPPB.
   C. Change the patient to a volume-oriented unit.
   D. Discontinue the treatment because it is not effective.

2. A 16-year-old postoperative appendectomy patient has clear breath sounds and normal vital signs. What should be recommended to prevent atelectasis?
   A. CPAP at 5 cm H_2O
   B. PEP therapy
   C. IPPB
   D. IS

3. If pulmonary function results are not available, what initial IS goal should be set?
   A. The IC measured at the bedside
   B. The VC measured at the bedside
   C. Three times the V_T measured at the bedside
   D. Twice the V_T measured at the bedside

4. A 12-year-old patient with cystic fibrosis will be discharged to go home. What type of directed cough should be recommended to improve secretion removal without causing airway collapse?
   A. Chicken breath
   B. Quad
   C. Splinted
   D. Lateral chest compression

5. A patient has just performed several excellent IS efforts. The patient complains of tingling fingers and dizziness. What should be done?
   A. Have the patient continue with additional IS maneuvers.
   B. Check the patient's fingers and forehead for cyanosis.
   C. Call the patient's physician to cancel the treatment order.
   D. Tell the patient to relax and breathe quietly.

6. A patient has a flow-oriented type of IS device. The patient is attempting but is unable to inhale forcibly through it. What is the most likely problem?
   A. The inspiratory tube is obstructed.
   B. The patient is not really trying.
   C. The flow resistance is set too high.
   D. The bellows is in the locked-down position.

7. A patient is using a flow-oriented IS device. With good coaching, the patient can raise a ball with 900 cc/s of flow and can keep it elevated for 1.5 seconds. What is the patient's IC?
   A. 450 mL
   B. 900 mL
   C. 1350 mL
   D. 1800 mL

8. A patient has been using an inspiratory muscle-training device. The patient is currently on the third largest of six settings and has been breathing comfortably through it 4 days/week over the past 2 weeks. What should now be recommended?
   A. Keep breathing through the same inspiratory hole.
   B. Breathe through the smallest hole.
   C. Breathe through the largest hole.
   D. Breathe through the next smallest hole.

9. A 17-year-old male patient is a quadriplegic after breaking his neck in an automobile accident. He has a tracheostomy tube, atelectasis, and retained secretions. What should be recommended to treat any atelectasis and to improve his cough?
   1. **Quad cough**
   2. **IS**
   3. **IPPB**
   4. **Assisted inspiration**
   A. 4 only
   B. 2 and 3 only
   C. 1 and 4 only
   D. 1, 2, and 3 only

10. A 40-year-old cooperative female patient had her gallbladder removed 2 days ago. She now has a low-grade fever and her chest X-ray shows signs of atelectasis in the right lower lobe. What should be done first to treat the problem?
    A. IS
    B. PEP therapy
    C. Nasotracheal suctioning
    D. IPPB therapy

11. A 75-year-old patient with a recent stroke causing right-sided weakness and dysphasia has a complication of atelectasis. The patient's IC is measured at 1.0 L. What therapy would be most appropriate to treat the patient's atelectasis?
    A. IS
    B. IPPB therapy
    C. PEP therapy
    D. Postural drainage therapy

12. A patient with advanced COPD is anxious and is feeling short of breath after returning from a medical procedure. What should the respiratory therapist recommend?
    A. Turn up the oxygen flow rate to the patient's nasal cannula.
    B. Inhale through the PFLEX inspiratory muscle trainer.
    C. Use pursed-lip breathing.
    D. Exhale through the Flutter valve unit.

13. A female patient is using a flow-oriented type of incentive spirometer at a rate of 20 times per minute. She is able to suspend the ball marker for 1 second at her targeted IC. How could the treatment be improved?
    A. Increase her target volume by 500 mL.
    B. Have her breathe at a slower rate and hold the volume longer.
    C. Have her exhale more rapidly.
    D. Lower her target volume by 100 mL and raise her respiratory rate to 25 times per minute.

14. A respiratory therapist is called to evaluate a female patient who has been using a volume-oriented incentive spirometer for 2 days since her cholecystectomy procedure. She has been following a patient-directed protocol and is easily able to inspire the 1.5-L goal set on the unit. What should be recommended?
    A. Increase her goal to 3 L.
    B. Switch her to a flow-oriented-type unit with a 1.5-L goal.
    C. Increase her volume goal to 2 L.
    D. Stop the protocol and begin IPPB treatments.

15. A patient with obstructive airways disease should be taught all of the following cough techniques EXCEPT:
    A. Sit up and lean forward slightly.
    B. Breathe in a volume larger than the V_T but less than the VC.
    C. Perform a normal cough.
    D. Perform a midinspiratory cough.

16. If IS has been successful, which breath sounds should be heard in the areas where atelectasis was noted before the treatment was started?
    A. Bronchial
    B. Bronchovesicular
    C. Vesicular
    D. Tracheal

17. A patient is recovering from a neuromuscular disease and the physician wishes to speed up the process of strengthening the patient's inspiratory muscles. What technique should the respiratory therapist recommend?
    A. PFLEX inspiratory muscle trainer
    B. Maximal inspiratory pressure
    C. Maximal expiratory pressure
    D. Trendelenburg positioning

8 Humidity and Aerosol Therapy

Note: It can be anticipated that the Therapist Multiple-Choice Examination (TMC) will include an *average of 8 of 140 actual questions* (6% of the exam) on humidity and aerosol therapy. (This is based on the question mix typically found on the National Board of Respiratory Care's (NBRC's) previous Entry Level Examinations and Written Registry Examinations.)

Remember that the TMC version you take will include 20 additional questions being evaluated for possible inclusion in other versions of the TMC. So, there will be a total of 160 questions taken. There is no way to differentiate between the 140 actual questions and the 20 questions being evaluated for future use. Please go to the Introduction for detailed information on the TMC Examination and the Clinical Simulation Examination.

MODULE A

Humidity and aerosol therapy

1. Maintain adequate humidification (code: IIIA6) [difficulty: R, Ap]

Most patients receive supplemental humidity or aerosol delivered to their airways and lungs for one of three reasons. First, patients with excessive pulmonary secretions benefit from the inhalation of extra humidity or an aerosol to reduce the viscosity (thickness) of their secretions. This makes it easier for the secretions to be coughed or suctioned out. Second, supplemental oxygen (O_2) or another medical gas from the central delivery system or cylinders is absolutely dry. Adding humidity or aerosol to the O_2 or medical gas prevents drying of the mucous membrane. Third, supplemental humidity can be used to deliver aerosolized medications. On occasion, a patient will require humidity or aerosol therapy because of hypothermia or cold air reactive airways. See Figure 8-1 for an algorithm to help guide the decision-making process when a patient is receiving a dry medical gas or has thick secretions. The AARC Clinical Practice Guideline from 2012 on humidification during invasive and noninvasive mechanical ventilation has these recommendations:

1. Every patient receiving invasive mechanical ventilation should receive humidification.
2. Passive humidification (a heat–moisture exchanger (HME)) is not recommended during noninvasive mechanical ventilation.
3. Active humidification (such as a wick-type humidifier) is suggested for noninvasive mechanical ventilation.
4. When a small tidal volume is being delivered, an HME should not be used because it will increase the patient's dead space and can increase the $PaCO_2$.
5. An HME should not be used as part of the prevention strategy for ventilator-associated pneumonia.
6. If an HME is used during invasive mechanical ventilation, it should provide a minimum of 30 mg H_2O/L.
7. When active humidification is being provided during invasive mechanical ventilation, the following criteria should be met at the Y-piece of the circuit: (1) the humidity level should be between 33 and 40 mg H_2O/L, (2) the gas temperature should be between 34° C (93.2° F) and 41° C (105.8° F), and (3) 100% relative humidity (RH) should be provided.

a. Indications for humidity therapy

1. *Humidification of dry therapeutic medical gases in patients with a normal upper airway*

Body humidity is the water saturation condition of the gas in the lungs. Under normal conditions with air, it is 43.9 (44) mg/L absolute humidity (AH) and 46.90 (47) mm Hg at 37° C (98.6° F). In other words, air is always warmed to body temperature and saturated with water by the time it reaches the lungs. As can be seen in Table 8-1, both water content and vapor pressure in the lungs vary with the patient's temperature.

Humidity deficit is the difference between the body humidity conditions and the room air (or other gas) conditions. Some humidity deficit is normal because the air must be warmed to body temperature and saturated by the time it reaches the lungs, and room conditions are rarely similar to those in the lung. The humidity deficit is eliminated through warming and humidifying of inhaled air by the respiratory passages.

The clinical practice guidelines of the American Association for Respiratory Care state that supplemental humidity is not needed for O_2 at flows of 4 L/min or less. This includes nasal cannulas and some air entrainment mask settings. As long as the patient has a normal upper airway and the hospital has an RH of about 40%, the patient should be able to fully saturate the gas with no adverse effects. Some clinicians believe that *any* O_2 flow through a nasal cannula should be humidified to prevent the local mucosa from drying out. Usually, an unheated bubble-type humidifier is used to deliver

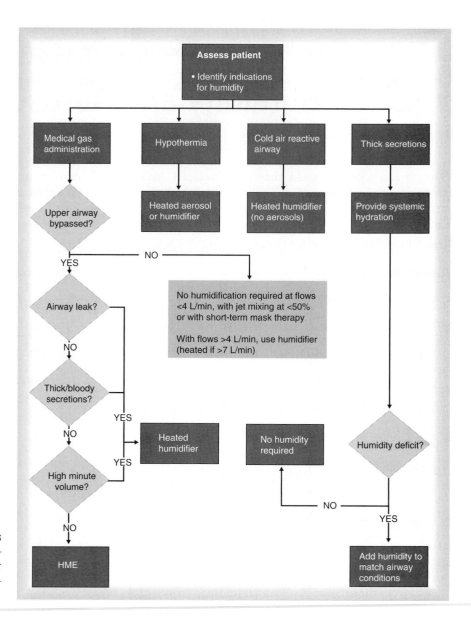

Figure 8-1 An algorithm for determining a patient's need for humidity or aerosol therapy. *HME,* heat–moisture exchanger. (From Kacmarek RM, Stoller JK, Heuer AJ, editors: Egan's fundamentals of respiratory care, ed 10, St Louis, 2013, Mosby.)

about 40% RH at room temperature. The patient then is able to fully saturate the gas. All agree that dry O_2 at flows of greater than 4 L/min by any device must be humidified.

2. Elimination of the humidity deficit in a patient with a bypassed upper airway

A patient with an endotracheal tube or tracheostomy tube is not able to humidify his or her inhaled gas. This creates a large humidity deficit that must be eliminated by providing a therapeutic humidity source. Failure to do so will result in drying of the mucous membrane and plugging of mucus. A heated humidifier is recommended and should be set to deliver gas at 34° C (93.2° F) to 41° C (105.8° F) to provide close to 100% RH to the patient. In any patient situation, the humidity deficit will be eliminated if saturated air is delivered at body temperature.

3. Reduction of airway resistance

Strong evidence suggests that patients with exercise-induced and cold air-induced asthma are less likely to experience bronchospasm if they inhale warmed, humidified gas while exercising. The clinical goal in this case is to prevent an increase in airway resistance. For most people who live in a cold winter climate, this is as simple as covering their nose and mouth with a scarf.

b. Indications for aerosol therapy

1. Humidification of dry therapeutic medical gases

Aerosol particles heated to body temperature can fully saturate inhaled carrier gas through evaporation of some of the particles. This is indicated in patients who need the humidity *and* a medicinal aerosol. This way is not preferred for delivering just humidity to a patient, and it is possible to overhydrate the airway, especially in neonates, through long-term aerosol therapy. Aerosol particles can

| TABLE 8-1 | Saturated Air Values for Absolute Humidity and Vapor Pressure under Room and Body Temperature Ranges* |

°C	°F	Absolute Humidity, mg/L	Vapor Pressure, mm Hg
1	70	18.35 (18)	18.62 (19)
22	71.6	19.42 (19)	19.79 (20)
23	73	20.58 (21)	21.02 (21)
33	92	35.61 (36)	37.59 (38)
34	93	37.57 (38)	39.75 (40)
35	95	39.60 (40)	42.02 (42)
36	97	41.70 (42)	44.40 (44)
37†	98.6	43.90 (44)	46.90 (47)
38	100	46.19 (46)	49.51 (50)
39	102	48.59 (49)	52.26 (52)
40	104	51.10 (51)	55.13 (55)
41	106	53.70 (54)	58.14 (58)

*The warmer the air is, the more water it can hold.
†So-called normal body temperature; it normally varies under different conditions.

carry bacteria and other pathogens, whereas humidity (water vapor) alone cannot.

2. Soothing of an irritated upper airway

Two generally accepted indications exist for delivery of a bland aerosol (sterile water or normal saline solution) to soothe an irritated upper airway: (1) after extubation and (2) laryngotracheobronchitis (or pediatric croup). Generally, a cool (room temperature) aerosol is delivered to reduce airway edema.

3. Delivery of medications to the airways and lungs

Respiratory therapists give many medications to patients, and these medications obviously must reach the target area. Table 8-2 gives the particle size of each medicinal aerosol and its most likely deposition area.

4. Increased clearance of secretions

Traditionally, many patients with a mild case of bronchitis were given breathing treatments with a bland aerosol to help them mobilize secretions. The aerosol was thought to add enough liquid to the secretions to enable the patient to cough them out. The patient, as is now understood, can cough more effectively because the aerosol irritates the airway, and the patient's own bronchial/submucosal glands pour out additional mucus. This reflex is mediated by the vagus nerve. This form of therapy probably is not indicated in most situations. It is clinically more effective to increase the patient's oral or intravenous fluids so that the bronchial/submucosal glands can produce secretions that are not thick.

5. Induced sputum production for a sputum specimen

See Module B for the discussion.

| TABLE 8-2 | Aerosol Particle Sizes and Their Likely Deposition Points in the Airways and Lungs |

Location	MMAD* Particle Size, μm
Nose or mouth to larynx	10 and Larger
Trachea to terminal bronchioles	9-5
Respiratory bronchioles to alveoli	5-2
Lung parenchyma (alveoli)	1-3

Note: Some controversy exists over the size of the particles that deposit in the airways and lungs. This table lists what seems to be a majority opinion. Aerosol particle diameter sizes are listed in units of micrometers, which are one-thousandth of a millimeter. As a point of clarification, most references list the symbol for a micrometer as a *u*; others use the international system unit of micrometer, which is symbolized as μm.
*Mass median aerodynamic diameter (MMAD) is defined as the aerosol diameter around which the mass is equally divided, that is, 50% of the aerosol mass is found in particles smaller than the MMAD, and 50% of the aerosol mass is found in particles larger than the MMAD.

2. Interview the patient to determine sputum production (code: IB1c) [difficulty: R, Ap, An]

Find out from the patient approximately how much sputum is produced in a day. Also, find out if certain times of the day are more productive or less productive than others. Try to relate this to breathing treatments, medications, activities, meals, and allergies.

3. Use inspection to assess the patient's cough, sputum amount, and sputum characteristics (code: IB2c) [difficulty: R, Ap, An]

The patient's sputum characteristics (e.g., consistency, color, smell) and amount must be known if the effectiveness of humidity or aerosol therapy is to be assessed. Review the related discussion in Chapter 1, and see Table 1-12. Try to relate this information to breathing treatments, medications, activities, meals, and allergies.

4. Auscultation to assess breath sounds (code: IB5a) [difficulty: R, Ap, An]

Review the discussion in Chapter 1, if necessary. The presence of expiratory crackles (also called rhonchi) would indicate airway secretions. If the patient is able to cough out the secretions, abnormal breath sounds, such as crackles, should improve. If the patient's secretions are thick (high viscosity), then aerosol therapy, as well as increased fluid intake, is indicated.

Exam Hint 8-1

Be prepared to recommend starting or changing humidity or aerosol therapy to help reduce humidity deficit or to help in the management of increased secretions.

MODULE B

Sputum induction

1. Perform a sputum induction (code: IC21) [difficulty: R, Ap]

Patients who have few, if any, secretions but from whom a sputum specimen is needed can have sputum production induced. Typically, the patient inhales an aerosol of hypertonic saline solution for about 5–10 min. Often a 7% solution is given; but, a range of 1.8% to 10% has been reported. Any nebulizer is acceptable. However, an ultrasonic nebulizer (USN) is often used because it produces a dense mist of small particles. A sputum induction is usually performed on a patient known or suspected of having a fungal infection, tuberculosis infection, or lung cancer. It is important to obtain the proper sputum container for the patient's condition. If the patient is thought to have tuberculosis, the procedure should be done in the early morning before breakfast. Hypertonic saline should not be used to obtain a sputum specimen for a general bacterial culture. This is because the high salt content will inhibit the growth of most bacteria.

2. Evaluate the results of the sputum induction procedure (code: ID20) [difficulty: R, Ap, An]

Because the purpose of the procedure is to obtain a sputum sample, it can be considered successful when the patient has a strong cough that produces a sputum sample. Saliva is not acceptable. Often the procedure is repeated over several days to improve the odds of getting a good sputum sample.

Because hypertonic saline is irritating to the airways, a patient with asthma may develop bronchospasm. Always monitor the patient's breath sounds during and after the procedure. If hypertonic saline causes bronchospasm, the treatment should be stopped. It may be necessary to administer a beta-agonist (sympathomimetic) bronchodilator to reverse the bronchospasm. Any future sputum induction procedures should be done with normal saline (0.9%) or hypotonic saline (0.45%). See Box 9-2 for details on these solutions.

MODULE C

Humidity generators (humidifiers) and administrative devices

1. Humidity delivered through small-bore tubing

a. Assemble bubble-type humidifiers (code: IIA3) [difficulty: R, Ap]

Bubble-type humidifiers are used on patients with a normal upper airway who need some supplemental humidity

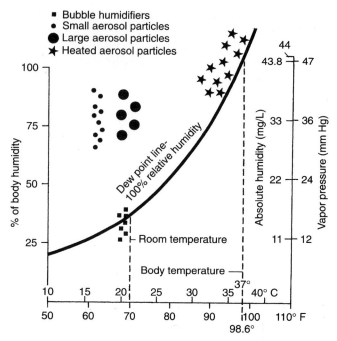

Figure 8-2 Comparison of humidity content by bubble-type humidifiers and various nebulizers.

because of the dryness of medical O_2. These devices usually are not heated and, in fact, deliver gas cooled to below room temperature. They provide around 40% RH at the delivered gas temperature. The rest of the humidity has to be made up by the patient (Figs. 8-2 and 8-3). If clinically indicated, a wraparound type of heater can be added to raise the temperature of the delivered gas and reduce the patient's humidity deficit.

Three different types of these humidifiers are designed to add some humidity to dry O_2 delivered through small-bore tubing: traditional bubble humidifiers, jet humidifiers, and underwater jet humidifiers.

a. Bubble humidifiers. Bubble humidifiers use a perforated capillary tube or a porous diffusion head to break the O_2 into small bubbles (see Fig. 8-3). This allows for greater surface area contact of the O_2 with the water and raises the RH by evaporation. The water level in the reservoir must be kept within the manufacturer's specifications and, if possible, as full as possible. The lower the water level is, the lower the RH is, because less time exists for evaporation. The faster the O_2 flow is, the lower the RH is.

b. Jet humidifiers. Jet humidifiers create an aerosol baffled out of the delivered gas flow. The RH is increased through evaporation of some of the aerosol droplets. These units deliver a higher RH than is delivered by bubble humidifiers. They have the additional advantage of delivering the same RH at higher flow levels and as the water level drops.

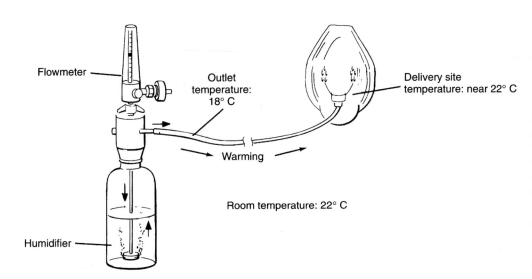

Figure 8-3 Oxygen leaving the outlet of a bubble-type humidifier is cooler than room temperature because of evaporation. Some warming toward room temperature occurs as the oxygen travels through the tubing to the patient. (From Scanlan CL: Humidity and aerosol therapy. In Scanlan CL, Spearman CB, Sheldon RL, editors: Egan's fundamentals of respiratory care, ed 5, St Louis, 1990, Mosby.)

c. Underwater jet humidifiers. Underwater jet humidifiers create water vapor and an aerosol. The aerosol is not baffled out as it is in jet humidifiers; therefore, these units deliver the highest RH. They can deliver the same humidity level at high gas flows and as the water level drops. Aerosol particles can carry pathogens, so strict infection control standards must be met to protect the patient. The water and the humidifier must be changed at least every 24 hr. If the patient needs the highest-possible-delivered RH, a jet humidifier or an underwater jet humidifier would be a better choice than a bubble type.

b. Troubleshoot any problems with the equipment (code: IIA3) [difficulty: R, Ap]

Many simple bubble humidifiers come prepackaged with sterile water and can be used for many short-term patients (e.g., those in the recovery room) or for a single long-term patient. When the water runs low, they are discarded. Bubble and other types of humidifiers consist of a reservoir jar for the water and a Diameter Index Safety System (DISS) O_2 connector lid that screws on. Turn on the flowmeter and make sure that O_2 flows through the delivery tube and bubbles into the water. Failure to bubble usually indicates that the lid and the jar are not screwed together tightly or that the delivery tube is plugged. If the tube cannot be cleared, it must be replaced.

Most of the newer bubble-type units have a pop-off type of high-pressure relief valve that is released if the pressure builds up to 40 mm Hg or 2 psi. Pinch closed the small-bore tubing to build up pressure and test the pop-off valve. Feel for the gas to escape from the valve. Many valves whistle to signal a gas leak. Do not use a unit with a pop-off valve that does not open under pressure.

1. Nasal cannula

As has been discussed earlier, current guidelines state that humidity does not need to be added to these devices if the

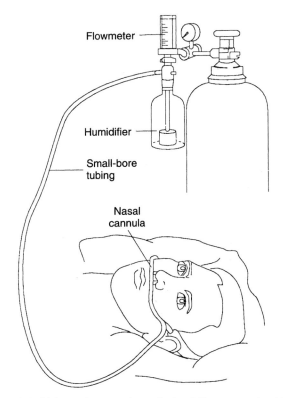

Figure 8-4 Adult wearing a nasal cannula that delivers oxygen humidified by a bubble-type humidifier. (From Guidelines for disinfection of respiratory care equipment used in the home, Respir Care 33:801, 1988.)

flow is 4 L/min or less. However, some patients complain of nasal dryness and discomfort if the cannula's O_2 is not humidified. The physician and the practitioner may believe that the patient's discomfort warrants the addition of a bubble-type humidifier. Agreement has been reached on the addition of humidity to flows greater than 4 L/min. See Figure 8-4 for a humidified nasal cannula setup. See Chapter 6 for the discussion on a high-flow nasal cannula.

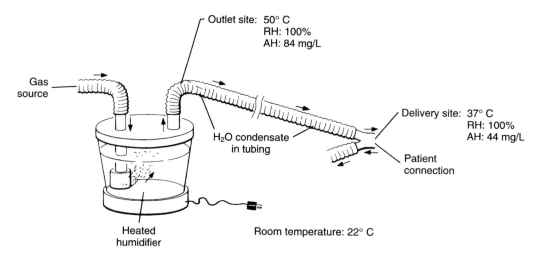

Figure 8-5 Gases leaving the outlet of a heated humidifier are hot and saturated with water vapor. As cooling occurs in the tubing, vapor condenses and absolute humidity (AH) decreases, whereas relative humidity (RH) remains at 100% (saturated). Note that almost half of the original vapor is "lost" to condensate in this example. (From Wilkins RL, Stoller JK, Kacmarek RM: Egan's fundamentals of respiratory care, ed 9, St Louis, 2009, Mosby.)

2. Oxygen masks

According to the AARC Clinical Practice Guidelines on oxygen therapy, it is unnecessary to add humidity to any adult's oxygen mask with an O_2 flow of 4 L/min or less. Humidity should be added to any mask with more than 4 L/min of O_2 added. This would include simple O_2 masks at higher flows, higher O_2 percentage air entrainment masks, partial-rebreathing masks, and nonrebreathing masks.

2. Humidity delivered through large-bore tubing

Most patients who need delivery of humidity through large-bore tubing have had the upper airway bypassed by an endotracheal or tracheostomy tube; therefore, they cannot humidify inspired gas in the normal manner. In other cases, humidity is added because the patient is receiving dry medical O_2. In both situations, a heated humidifier is recommended. It should be set to deliver gas warmed close to body temperature to provide 80% to 100% RH. The following humidity-generating devices deliver conditioned gas to the patient through large-bore (22-mm inner diameter (ID)) tubing.

a. Assemble large-volume humidifiers (code: IIA3) [difficulty: R, Ap]

There are two basic types of large-volume humidifiers: bubble humidifiers and pass-over humidifiers. All have an adjustable heater so the water in the reservoir is at or greater than body temperature. This enables them to provide up to 100% of the patient's body humidity. With all of these units, the temperature of the inspired gas must be measured near the patient. Ideally, the gas temperature is kept the same as the patient's to provide 100% RH. As discussed above, these units are used to provide humidity when the patient's upper airway is bypassed by an endotracheal or tracheostomy tube (Fig. 8-5).

Bubble humidifiers have been widely used in the past with a mechanical ventilator. They are also used with other types of systems, such as a tracheostomy mask, for delivering humidity with or without oxygen. These devices operate the same way as an efficient bubble-type humidifier, as described above. The inspiratory gas must flow through the heated water for evaporation to occur. *Note:* The Bennett Cascade is a classic example of these types of humidifiers (Fig. 8-6). Even though these units are no longer available, the NBRC refers to this type of device as a cascade-type humidifier.

Pass-over humidifiers are now commonly used with a mechanical ventilator, continuous positive airway pressure system, or high-flow nasal cannula. They are also used to provide humidity to a tracheostomy mask. There are three subtypes of pass-over humidifiers: reservoir, wick, and membrane.

With a reservoir-type humidifier, the patient's gas supply is directed over the surface of a reservoir of hot water. Evaporation occurs as the gas passes over the surface of the water. The Fisher & Paykel MR 850 heated humidifier is an example (Fisher & Paykel Healthcare, Irvine, CA).

The wick-type heated humidifier employs a wick, often made of sponge or paper, to soak up water for evaporation (Fig. 8-7). The water, wick, or both are heated so that 100% RH can be delivered. The Hudson RCI Conchatherm IV is an example (Hudson Respiratory Care, Temecula, CA).

The membrane-type humidifier makes use of a hydrophobic membrane to separate the patient's gas from the water source. Water vapor will pass through the membrane, but not aerosolized water droplets or pathogens. The Vapotherm 2000i is an example (Vapotherm, Annapolis, MD). This unit is designed to provide humidity to a high-flow nasal cannula (see Figs. 6-17 and 6-18 in Chapter 6).

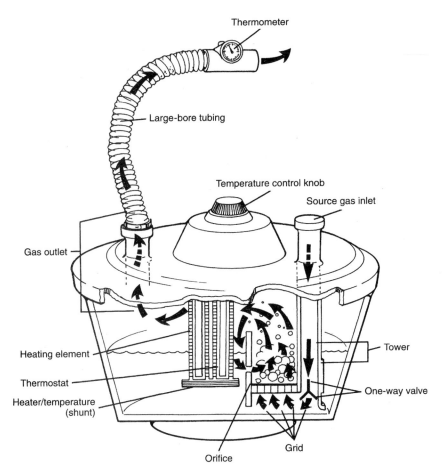

Figure 8-6 Cascade-type humidifier. (From Scanlan CL: Humidity and aerosol therapy. In Scanlan CL, Spearman CB, Sheldon RL, editors: Egan's fundamentals of respiratory care, ed 5, St Louis, 1990, Mosby.)

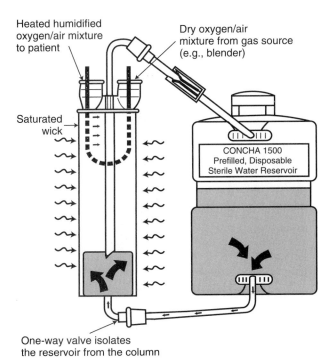

Figure 8-7 Functional diagram of a wick-type humidifier with an automatic water feed system. Water automatically enters a warmed reservoir, where it is drawn up the wick. Dry gas flows past the wick, where evaporation takes place before the gas is directed to the patient. (Redrawn from Hudson Respiratory Care, Temecula, CA. In Cairo J, Pilbeam S: Mosby's respiratory therapy equipment, ed 8, St Louis, 2010, Mosby.)

All of these units also are used with mechanical ventilators or other systems because they have very little resistance to the gas flowing through them as evaporation occurs. Some units are designed for use with a heated wire ventilator circuit and feature an automatic water feed system and a servo-controlled thermostat to keep the water and the circuit at the same temperature. This minimizes condensation.

b. Troubleshoot any problems with the equipment (code: IIA3) [difficulty: R, Ap]

Humidifiers must be assembled properly, especially when they are used to humidify a mechanical ventilator. Any loose connections may result in an air leak and loss of tidal volume (V_T). Make sure the water level is maintained properly.

Some cooling occurs as heated gas passes through unheated large-bore tubing, which results in condensation (so-called "rain out") that must be drained away. Placing a water trap into the lowest point of the tubing drains the water and helps keep the tubing clear. Remember to continue to look periodically for water puffing or sloshing back and forth in the tubing. Make sure that any condensate is drained out of the tubing and thrown away. Do not drain the condensate toward the patient or back into the water reservoir because any microorganisms in the tubing or condensate could reproduce in the reservoir. To avoid condensation, heated wire tubing is used with many ventilator circuits.

3. Heat–moisture exchangers

a. Assemble a heat–moisture exchanger (code: IIA3) [difficulty: R, Ap]

An HME is a passive humidifier that recycles the patient's own exhaled water vapor. The HME contains a highly absorbent material that is warmed and moistened when a patient's exhaled breath passes through it. The patient's next inspiration is warmed and humidified by the water absorbed within the HME. These units are not as efficient

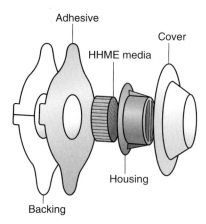

Figure 8-8 A humidity–heat–moisture exchanger (HHME) that can be placed over a patient's open tracheostomy stoma. The HHME will store humidity and heat from the patient's exhaled breath. Upon inspiration, the cool room air is warmed and moistened. (From Cairo JM: Mosby's respiratory care equipment, ed 9, St Louis, 2014, Mosby.)

as the humidifiers described earlier and are not able to provide 100% of body humidity to a patient. If possible, select an HME that has these characteristics: (1) is at least 70% efficient (provides at least 30 mg/L water vapor), (2) has a low compliance if used with a ventilator circuit, (3) is lightweight, (4) has little dead space, and (5) has little flow resistance.

Many brands of HME are available for either of two clinical applications. The first clinical use involves a patient with a tracheostomy tube. A 15-mm-ID opening allows the HME to be attached to the tube; the other end of the HME is open to room air. This type is small and convenient to use for many patients with a permanent tracheostomy. In addition, it improves a patient's mobility. If the patient has a tracheal stoma, a humidity–heat–moisture exchanger can cover the neck opening (Fig. 8-8). This device is able to capture humidity and heat from the patient's exhaled gas. With the next inhalation, the humidity and heat are breathed back in. The second clinical use involves patients who require mechanical ventilation (Fig. 8-9). The patient end of the HME is a 15-mm-ID opening that can attach to the endotracheal or tracheostomy tube; the other end of the HME has a 22-mm-ID opening so the ventilator circuit or supplemental oxygen can be attached.

b. Troubleshoot any problems with the equipment (code: IIA3) [difficulty: R, Ap]

HMEs typically come preassembled by the manufacturer. The 15-mm-ID opening must be placed over the patient's endotracheal or tracheostomy tube. The other opening of the HME can be connected to the ventilator circuit or

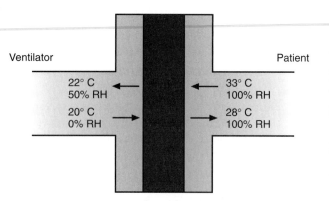 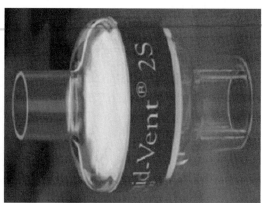

Figure 8-9 Heat–moisture exchanger (HME) for use with a mechanical ventilator. **Left,** Cut-away functional drawing shows the *(left)* ventilator side and *(right)* patient side of an HME. During exhalation, the warmed and saturated air (33 °C and 100% relative humidity (RH)) from the patient passes through the HME in the water-absorbing material. During inhalation, the cooler and drier room air is warmed and becomes more saturated with water vapor as it passes through the HME to the patient. **Right,** Photograph of an HME. The opening on the left side has a 15-mm ID and connects to the patient's endotracheal tube. The opening on the right side has a 22-mm ID and can have a ventilator circuit or T-piece attached for supplemental oxygen and aerosol. (Courtesy of Teleflex Medical Hudson RCI, Research Triangle Park, North Carolina and Cairo J, Pilbeam S: Mosby's respiratory therapy equipment, ed 8, St Louis, 2010, Mosby.)

oxygen source, if needed. Follow the manufacturer's recommendation regarding how frequently the HME should be replaced—often every 24 hr. However, current guidelines indicate that they can be used safely for at least 48 hr, possibly up to a week.

Secretions or blood coughed into the HME can obstruct the flow of gas and thus make it difficult or impossible for the patient to breathe. The HME must be removed and discarded if it becomes obstructed. Replace it with a new one. An HME should *not* be used with a patient who is known to cough out large quantities of secretions or blood.

MODULE D

Aerosol generators (nebulizers) and administrative devices

1. Ultrasonic nebulizers

a. Assemble a USN (code: IIA4) [difficulty: R, Ap]

Large-volume ultrasonic units often are chosen for delivery of bland solutions to the lower airways because of the small particle size and high output. (So-called "bland aerosols" are composed of particles of water or saline rather than medicated aerosols.) USNs work by converting electrical energy into high-frequency sound energy, which creates aerosol particles. The frequency is vital because it results in a stable aerosol with a mean particle size of about 3 mm in diameter. This is an ideal size for penetrating deeply into the lungs to the smallest airways. The only control on these units is used for amplitude (power), and it controls the aerosol output. The range is usually up to 3-6 mL/min, depending on the model. This output is greater than that possible with most pneumatic nebulizers. The aerosol can be carried to the patient via a built-in fan or by an outside O_2 source (Fig. 8-10). The warm aerosol that is created minimizes the patient's humidity deficit.

Historically, USNs have not been chosen for upper airway aerosol deposition or for administration of pharmacologically active medications such as bronchodilators, mucolytics, and antibiotics. These medications may not nebulize at the same rate as the saline diluent, which creates the risk that a very concentrated dose may be delivered at the end of treatment. Some medications may be mechanically broken down by the high-frequency vibration and rendered useless.

Recently, small-volume USN units have been designed to specifically nebulize medications into the circuit of a mechanical ventilator (Fig. 8-11). Depending on the manufacturer, the USN can be powered electrically by the ventilator, by any electrical outlet, or by batteries. These units are designed to rapidly nebulize the small volume of medication (with or without diluent). The tidal volume breath carries the medication into the patient's airways. Be aware that even though drugs have been given this way,

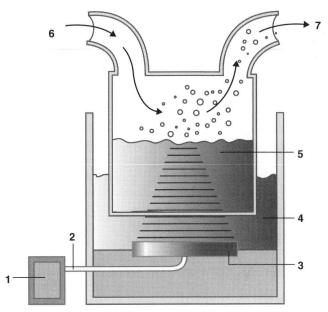

Figure 8-10 Functional diagram of a large-volume ultrasonic nebulizer. 1, electrically powered radio-frequency generator; 2, shielded electrical cable; 3, piezoelectric crystal transducer; 4, couplant chamber filled with water; 5, solution cup with saline or medication; 6, gas enters the solution cup; 7, aerosol particles are carried out to the patient. (Modified from Barnes TA, editor: Core textbook of respiratory care practice, ed 2, St Louis, 1994, Mosby.)

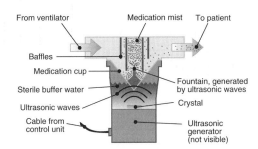

Figure 8-11 Small-volume ultrasonic nebulizer. The functional components are the same as described for Figure 8-10. This small USN is designed to be added into a mechanical ventilator circuit to provide aerosolized medications. (Courtesy Siemens, Tarrytown, NY.)

pharmaceutical companies have not included the delivery of undiluted medications in their dosing information.

b. Troubleshoot any problems with the equipment (code: IIA4) [difficulty: R, Ap]

Always follow the manufacturer's instructions when you are setting up the delivery system. Figure 8-10 shows the common features, and Table 8-3 describes how to troubleshoot many common problems. Many clinical difficulties seem to involve keeping the proper fluid levels in the couplant chamber and the solution cup. If the sterile water in the couplant chamber is too low, the vibration cannot reach the solution cup and no aerosol will be produced. If the saline level in the solution cup is too low or too

TABLE 8-3	Ultrasonic Nebulizer Troubleshooting	
Symptom	**Possible Problem**	**Suggested Check**
Unit installed and connected as specified, but pilot light does not turn on when switch is turned to the "on" position	Electrical outlet defective Circuit breaker tripped Fuse blown	Check outlet with lamp or other appliance Reset the circuit breaker, or change fuse on the power switch; if the circuit breaker continues to trip or the fuse blows again, service is needed
Unit installed and connected as specified; power pilot light turns on, normal ultrasonic activity visible in nebulizer chamber, but no aerosol output occurs	Nebulizer chamber contaminated	Wash nebulizer chamber; decontaminate
Unit installed and connected as specified; power pilot light turns on, but little ultrasonic activity is visible in the nebulizer chamber, and aerosol output is low (even when on the No. 10 power setting)	Couplant water excessively aerated Nebulizer module and couplant water too cold Diaphragm distorted, permitting air bubbles to interfere with proper transmission of vibrational energy into the nebulizer chamber	Wait for deaeration Use warmer couplant water Check to see that diaphragm is properly shaped and installed; be sure that the concave (recessed) side faces the interior of the chamber Clean couplant compartment and replace couplant water
Same as symptom described previously but at a lower power setting	Power setting too low to start and establish nebulization	Turn output control knob to maximum power setting, then reduce to desired setting
Unit installed and connected as specified, and power pilot light turns on. "Add couplant" light is on, and no ultrasonic activity is visible in the nebulizer chamber	Insufficient couplant water	Add water to the couplant compartment
Unit installed and connected as specified, and power pilot light turns on. "Add couplant" light is off, but no ultrasonic activity is visible in the nebulizer chamber	Power supply overheated and its thermostatic control opened	The cooling air has been restricted, or cooling fins need cleaning. The switch will reset when the equipment returns to room temperature
Liquid reservoir filled and properly connected to nebulizer chamber, but chamber does not fill *(for continuous-feed system only)*	Foreign material or air bubbles in feed tubes Liquid level control in nebulizer chamber plugged with foreign material Air leaks at tube connection or reservoir cap	Flush the system Clean or flush the system Tighten all connections by pushing tubes into fittings

From Op't Holt T: Aerosol generators and humidifiers. In Barnes TA, editor: Respiratory care practice, Chicago, 1988, Mosby.

high, the vibrational energy will not focus properly on the surface of the saline solution, and no aerosol will be produced. Water should not be allowed to condense and fill low points in the large-bore tubing; if it does, ultrasonic particles will liquefy as the carrier gas is forced to pass through the condensate. The exiting gas would be humidified through evaporation but would carry no aerosol particles. If the carrier gas is O_2 blended with air through an air-entrainment system, any backpressure could result in an increase in the O_2 percentage and a decrease in the total flow. Remember to always measure the O_2 percentage near the patient.

2. Large-volume pneumatic nebulizers

a. Assemble the necessary equipment (Code: IIA4) [Difficulty: R, Ap]

Large-volume nebulizers (LVNs) that are pneumatically powered share the common feature of having a liquid reservoir of at least 250 mL. Usually an LVN is used to produce a bland aerosol for a period of several hours. (So-called "bland aerosols" are composed of particles of water or saline rather than medicated aerosols.) These nebulizers also typically entrain room air to increase the total gas flow. They share the following common features:

- All are powered by compressed air or O_2 that is delivered through a flowmeter. As the gas flow drops, the aerosol output decreases.
- All make use of Bernoulli's principle with a compressed gas jet that is used to entrain liquid, room air, or both into the main gas flow. Because of this jet action, these devices are also called jet nebulizers.
- All have a capillary tube that allows the liquid to flow *up* to the jet for nebulization. (Remember that with bubble-type humidifiers, O_2 flows *down* the capillary tube.)
- All have a baffle against which the aerosol is sprayed to create a more uniform particle size.

Many, but not all, pneumatic nebulizers allow for a changeable inspired O_2 percentage. Provided that the jet is powered by O_2, the air-entrainment ports can be opened up to increase air entrainment and increase total flow (lowering the inspired O_2 percentage) or closed down to decrease air entrainment and decrease total flow (raising the inspired O_2 percentage). The O_2 percentage usually can vary from 35% to 100%. Remember to always analyze the inspired O_2 percentage near the patient because both water in the aerosol tubing and backpressure decrease the entrained air and raise the O_2 percentage.

In the clinical setting in which a patient must receive an aerosolized medication on a continuous basis, an LVN is more convenient to use than a small-volume nebulizer (SVN). This is because the SVN must have more medication added every few minutes. The continuous administration of an aerosolized bronchodilator to a severely asthmatic patient would warrant the use of an LVN. Because the medication concentration will change over time, the LVN must be emptied and refilled every 5 hr. See Module E for the discussion on medication delivery systems.

b. Troubleshoot any problems with the equipment (code: IIA4) [difficulty: R, Ap]

Most pneumatic nebulizers have an appearance that is similar to that of bubble-type humidifiers. Key components include a large reservoir jar and a top with a DISS O_2 connector and a capillary tube to the jet. Make sure the nebulizer is screwed firmly onto the oxygen flowmeter and that the component parts are attached and work properly. Keep the capillary tube and jet clear of debris to keep the aerosol output from dropping. These units allow for variable O_2 percentages. Keep the air entrainment ports open so that proper gas mixing occurs and the desired O_2 percentage is provided (Fig. 8-12). If water is present in the large-bore tubing or if the tubing is pinched, less room air will be entrained, and the delivered oxygen percentage will be higher than ordered. Keep the reservoir's water level at the proper level. If the water level drops to below the refill line, no water will be drawn up the capillary tube to the jet. If the water is filled to above the maximum line, the jet may not operate properly. Heating of the water, aerosol, or both is accomplished in one of the following ways:

- A heated metal rod is immersed into the reservoir water through a port in the top of the nebulizer. A dial is used to control how hot the rod gets. Water temperature varies depending on how deep it is, so as the water level drops, the remaining water gets hotter. It is very important that the gas temperature near the patient be measured and that the water level be kept stable to prevent burning of the airway. The heated rod presents the risk of burns to a practitioner who accidentally touches it. It must be disinfected between patients and changed as often as the nebulizer is changed. Because of these issues, these units are unlikely to be seen in clinical practice.
- Two other systems use variations on this idea of directly heating the water in the reservoir jar. The first heats the water as it passes through the capillary tube. The second type directly heats only a small amount of the reservoir water just before it

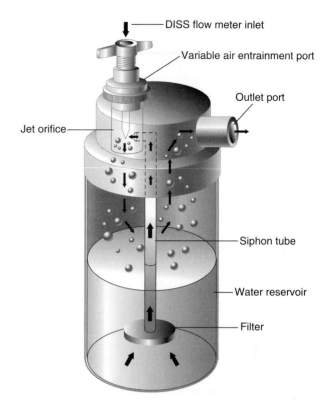

Figure 8-12 Large-volume air entrainment nebulizer. Negative pressure created at the jet draws water up the siphon tube to be aerosolized. The negative pressure also entrains room air so that a variable oxygen percentage can be delivered to the patient. (From Kacmarek RM, Stoller JK, Heuer AJ, editors: Egan's fundamentals of respiratory care, ed 10, St Louis, 2013, Mosby.)

is aerosolized. Each has the advantage of a short warm-up time compared with the heated metal rod systems. Some units have an external temperature probe for placement in the aerosol tubing. The probe acts as a servo-controller of the heating unit for better temperature regulation.
- A flexible heater is wrapped around the outside of the reservoir. A dial is used to control how hot the heater gets. The water temperature increases as the water level drops. Monitor the gas temperature near the patient for safety purposes.
- A clip-on heating base plate can be added to special reservoir jars with a metal plate. These are preferable to the previously mentioned types because they ensure a constant temperature to the aerosol as the water level drops.

Heating the water or aerosol reduces the patient's humidity deficit and usually is done if the secretions are thick. See Figure 8-2 for the location of the aerosol particles and their relationship with the dew point and with the patient's body humidity.

3. Aerosol delivery systems

Large-bore tubing (also known as *aerosol tubing* or *corrugated tubing*) is needed to connect the aerosol generator with the patient. This tubing has a 22-mm ID so it can be connected to a face mask, T-piece, etc.

a. Aerosol masks

The aerosol mask looks similar to the simple O_2 mask, except that it has larger side ports for exhalation and a 22-mm outer diameter adapter for attachment of the large-bore tubing (Fig. 8-13). This often is considered to be a low-flow O_2 mask because the ports are open to room air; therefore, it is difficult to ensure that the patient receives the set O_2 percentage. If the flow is high enough that aerosol mist can be seen flowing out of the side ports during an inspiration, little or no room air is being inspired and the aerosol mask is now a high-flow device. Some clinicians have increased the total flow through an aerosol mask by using a Y adapter to combine the large-bore tubing coming from two LVNs. In any case, it is best to analyze the O_2 percentage inside the mask to be sure of what the patient is inhaling. Any of the previously mentioned humidity or aerosol devices can be used and powered by compressed air or O_2.

b. Face tents, tracheostomy masks, tracheostomy collars, and Briggs adapter/T-piece

A face tent, a tracheostomy mask and collar, and Briggs adapter (T-piece) are discussed in Chapter 6. All have a 22-mm-ID adapter so that large-bore tubing can be added to them. Any of the previously mentioned humidity or aerosol devices can be used with these and are powered by compressed air or O_2.

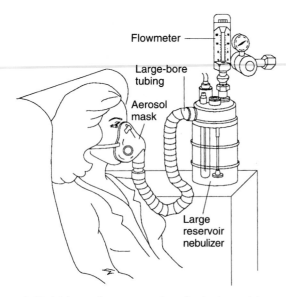

Figure 8-13 Adult wearing an aerosol mask who is receiving supplemental oxygen and aerosol from a heated large-volume nebulizer. As the warmed, humidified gas cools on its way to the patient, condensation will result in water draining to the lowest part of the large-bore tubing. (From Guidelines for disinfection of respiratory care equipment used in the home, Respir Care 33:801, 1988.)

Labels on figure: Flowmeter; Large-bore tubing; Aerosol mask; Large reservoir nebulizer

---

MODULE E

Medication delivery systems

1. Small-volume nebulizers

a. Administer medications by nebulizer (Code: IIID1) [Difficulty: R, Ap]

The 2012 AARC Clinical Practice Guideline on selecting an aerosol delivery device has stated that any medication delivery system will be effective provided it is suited to the patient's ability to use the device. These suitability factors include the patient's age, physical ability, and cognitive ability; the medication availability for the device; and the patient–device interface. In any clinical situation, when the patient is not able to use the delivery system, another one must be used. See Table 8-4 for age-related guidelines for selecting a medicated aerosol delivery device. Figure 8-14 shows an algorithm for determining which device might be best suited to the patient.

TABLE 8-4	Age-Related Guidelines for Selecting a Medicated Aerosol Delivery Device
Aerosol Delivery Device and Patient Interface	**Age**
SVN with face mask or hood	Infant
SVN with face mask	≤3 years
SVN with mouthpiece	≥3 years
LVN with face mask	≥3 years
MDI with valved holding chamber/spacer and mask	<4 years
MDI with valved holding chamber/spacer	≥4 years
DPI	≥4 years
MDI	≥5 years
Breath-actuated MDI	≥5 years
Breath-actuated SVN	≥5 years

SVN, small-volume nebulizer; *LVN,* large-volume nebulizer; *MDI,* metered-dose inhaler; *DPI,* dry powder inhaler.

b. Assemble the necessary equipment (code: IIA4) [difficulty: R, Ap]

For the purposes of this discussion, an SVN is powered by compressed air or oxygen unless specified otherwise. (See the vibrating-mesh nebulizer discussion that follows.) An SVN is designed to hold a relatively small volume of fluid (typically 3–5 mL) and to nebulize liquid medications such as bronchodilators, mucolytics, or antibiotics for inhalation. Compressed air or O_2 can be used to generate the aerosol. These units employ a jet and operate under the same physical principles as the LVNs described earlier. Because of this jet action, an SVN is also called a jet nebulizer.

Two different types of SVNs exist: mainstream and sidestream. *Mainstream nebulizers* are designed so the main flow of gas to the patient comes through the aerosol as it is produced. A second high-pressure gas flow is used to power the jet to create the aerosol. *Sidestream nebulizers* are

designed so the aerosol is produced from the main flow of gas and is supplemented by the jet's gas flow. Many manufacturers produce disposable medication SVNs, typically sidestream (Fig. 8-15), for intermittent positive-pressure breathing circuits or hand-held circuits. Select the nebulizer that produces a particle size that matches the therapeutic target.

Figure 8-16 shows a typical SVN circuit. The nebulizer consists of a medication reservoir and a manifold (top piece) that contains a capillary tube and a baffle. The two pieces must be unscrewed so the liquid medication can be added and then must be reassembled. Small-bore oxygen tubing is attached to the reservoir or manifold, depending on the manufacturer, and to the flowmeter. A mouthpiece completes the assembly. When the compressed air or O_2 flowmeter is turned to the manufacturer's suggested flow (typically 4–8 L/min), an aerosol should be continuously produced. Typically, 3–5 mL of

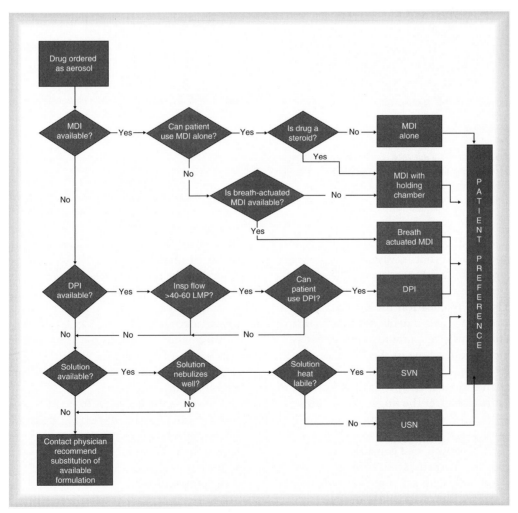

Figure 8-14 An algorithm for determining the best medication delivery device. Provided that the ordered medication is available in a metered-dose inhaler, that would be the first choice. Other variables would lead to the selection of a dry powder inhaler, small-volume nebulizer, or ultrasonic nebulizer. *MDI,* metered-dose inhaler; *DPI,* dry powder inhaler; *SVN,* small-volume nebulizer; *USN,* ultrasonic nebulizer. (From Kacmarek RM, Stoller JK, Heuer AJ, editors: Egan's fundamentals of respiratory care, ed 10, St Louis, 2013, Mosby.)

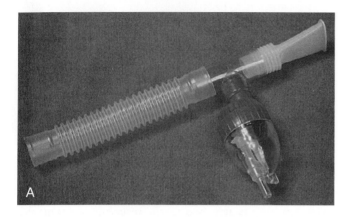

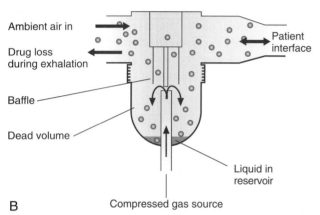

B   Compressed gas source

Figure 8-15 Example of a jet type of small-volume nebulizer for medications. A, Photograph of a standard jet nebulizer showing the medication reservoir, mouthpiece, and reservoir tube. B, Schematic drawing of standard jet nebulizer showing the internal features of jet and baffle. (From Cairo JM: Mosby's respiratory care equipment, ed 9, St Louis, 2014, Mosby.)

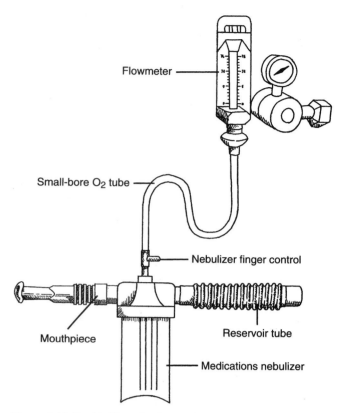

Figure 8-16 Hand-held small-volume nebulizer with mouthpiece, reservoir tube for medication, and finger control to limit wasted medication. (Adapted from Guidelines for disinfection of respiratory care equipment used in the home, Respir Care 33:801, 1988.)

medication will be nebulized in about 10 min. To reduce the amount of medication that is wasted into room air, a length of aerosol tubing (shown) or a collection bag can be added to the manifold. The reservoir tube or bag serves to hold O_2 and medication for the next inspiration. To further reduce waste, a nebulizer finger control can be added. This allows the patient to power the nebulizer by covering the open hole in the "T." Uncovering the hole permits the gas to exit; thus, the medication is not nebulized and wasted. Only a limited number of patients will be able to master the finger and inspiration coordination needed for this technique. If successful, the inspired medication will be maximized. However, the treatment time will be lengthened considerably. Despite these efforts to maximize medication delivery, all SVNs will have some residual drug volume that will not be nebulized. Some medication will be left in the reservoir and wasted.

Practitioners face two possible risks when they use SVNs. First, any aerosolized medications that escape into the room air may be inhaled. It is possible that the practitioner, or anyone else nearby, may have an allergic

or other adverse reaction. Second, nebulized secretions from the patient's airway and lungs may be inhaled; this may place the practitioner or others at risk for acquiring a pulmonary infection from the patient. Although actual problems such as these rarely occur, they are possible. If either of these situations is a concern, an SVN with one-way valves and a downstream particle filter should be used. This filter will trap any exhaled aerosol droplets (Fig. 8-17). A filtered SVN is recommended when pentamidine isethionate (NebuPent) is nebulized. A filtered SVN should be used for any other antibiotic or medication that should not contaminate the room air.

A breath-enhanced nebulizer (BEN) is an advancement over a standard jet nebulizer (Fig. 8-18). When the patient inhales, additional room air is entrained through the jet and baffle. This results in an increase in the inhaled particle mass and significantly reduces the medication wasted to the atmosphere.

A breath-actuated nebulizer (BAN) is a further advancement over a standard jet nebulizer (Fig. 8-19). With this device, the medication is nebulized only when the patient inhales. Because of this, no aerosolized medication is wasted into the atmosphere. If the patient (usually a child) cannot inhale deeply enough to

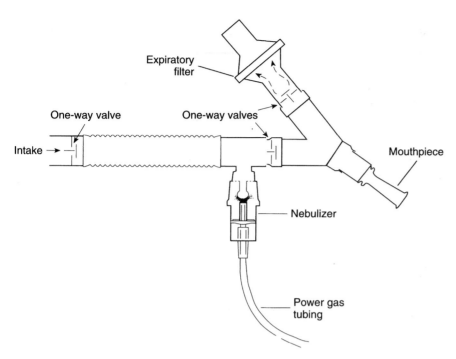

Figure 8-17 Diagram of the Respirgard II small-volume nebulizer system showing one-way valves and an expiratory filter to scavenge exhaust aerosol. (From Rau JL Jr: Respiratory care pharmacology, ed 5, St Louis, 1998, Mosby.)

automatically trigger the nebulizer, the unit can be operated manually to match inspiration with nebulization.

A vibrating-mesh nebulizer (VMN) does not use a compressed gas source to operate. Instead, it needs a battery or AC/DC electrical source to rapidly vibrate a plate with many very small holes in it (the mesh). The medication solution is pushed or pulled through the mesh holes, which results in aerosol droplets that are 2–6 μm in mass median aerodynamic diameter. Unlike the other types of gas-powered jet nebulizers, the particle size is uniform whether the patient is inhaling room air, oxygen, or a helium/oxide mix. Unlike a USN, a VMN can be used with all liquid medications without any risk of breaking down the drug. There are hand-held VMN units for home use as well as units that can be added into a mechanical ventilator circuit. All VMN units are more efficient than any type of jet nebulizer and aerosolize virtually all of the medication.

c. Troubleshoot any problems with the equipment (code: IIA4) [difficulty: R, Ap]

If a jet nebulizer fails to generate aerosol, make sure that the pieces are properly assembled, the liquid medication is at the proper depth (typically 3–5 mL), and the capillary tube is not plugged with debris. If the capillary tube is plugged, liquid will not be drawn up to the jet. Sometimes, the capillary tube can be cleared by running it under sterile water or pushing a needle through the channel. Do not use a nebulizer that does not generate an aerosol. The therapist must be sure that the patient can properly assemble, disassemble, and operate the SVN. If the patient cannot, another medication delivery system, such as a dry powder inhaler (DPI) or a metered-dose inhaler (MDI), should be recommended.

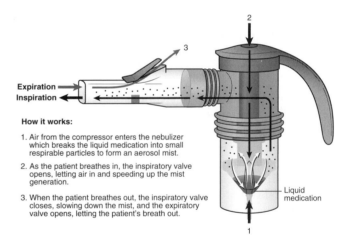

How it works:
1. Air from the compressor enters the nebulizer which breaks the liquid medication into small respirable particles to form an aerosol mist.
2. As the patient breathes in, the inspiratory valve opens, letting air in and speeding up the mist generation.
3. When the patient breathes out, the inspiratory valve closes, slowing down the mist, and the expiratory valve opens, letting the patient's breath out.

Figure 8-18 Schematic drawing of the Sprint breath-enhanced nebulizer (BEN) showing its internal functioning and gas flow. A BEN unit is more efficient at creating a dense aerosol than a standard jet nebulizer. (From PARI Respiratory Equipment, Midlothian VA.)

2. Metered-dose inhalers (code: IIA23) [difficulty: ELE: R, Ap, An]

a. Administer medications by MDI (code: IIID1) [difficulty: R, Ap]

The 2012 AARC Clinical Practice Guideline on selecting an aerosol delivery device has stated that any medication delivery system will be effective provided it is suited to the patient's ability to use the device. These suitability factors include the patient's age, physical ability, and cognitive ability; the medication availability for the device; and the patient–device interface. In any clinical situation, when the patient is not able to use the delivery system, another

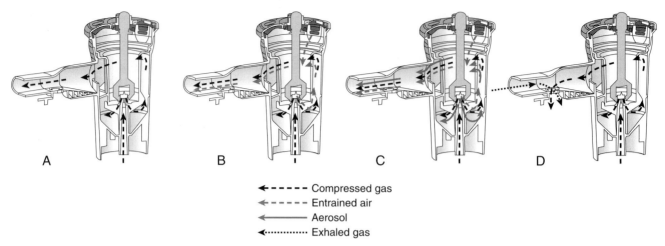

← - - - - - Compressed gas
← - - - - - Entrained air
←————— Aerosol
←············· Exhaled gas

Figure 8-19 Series of schematic drawings of the AeroEclipse BAN II. A breath-actuated nebulizer (BAN) is the most efficient type of jet nebulizer because the medication is aerosolized only when the patient inhales through it. **A,** Compressed gas passes through the unit without nebulizing and wasting medication. **B,** When the patient begins to inhale through the unit, the actuator moves down. **C,** The negative pressure resulting from inhalation pulls the diaphragm and actuator down. This seals the nozzle cover and nebulizes the medication. **D,** When the patient exhales, the diaphragm and actuator move up. This stops the nebulizer. The patient exhales through a one-way valve in the mouthpiece. (From Trudell Medical International, London, Ontario, Canada.)

one must be used. See Table 8-4 for age-related guidelines for selecting a medicated aerosol delivery device. See Figure 8-14 for an algorithm for determining which device might be best suited to the patient.

b. Assemble the necessary equipment (code: IIA5) [difficulty: R, Ap]

The following discussion focuses on gas-powered MDIs that are used with the great majority of inhaled medications. All MDIs are designed to dispense a premeasured amount of medication into the airway. Each activation of the MDI delivers a set dose of medication to the patient. Available medications include beta-agonist (sympathomimetic) and anticholinergic (parasympatholytic) bronchodilators, corticosteroid drugs, and antibiotics (see Chapter 9 for details on the medications). All gas-powered MDIs operate in the same way. They contain several milliliters of medication and compressed hydrofluoroalkane (HFA) gas inside of a metal container with a built-in jet nozzle. Because of the compressed gas used to disperse the medication, these units are also called a pressurized metered-dose inhaler. (The older MDI units that contained the environmentally hazardous propellant chlorofluorocarbon have been replaced by HFA gas units.) An exception to the above discussion is the Respimat Soft Mist Inhaler. This MDI unit creates a medication mist by spring compression rather than the release of compressed HFA gas.

With most MDIs, tipping the metering chamber over and back upright results in its filling with medication. A plastic actuator opens the jet when it is pressed into the container (Fig. 8-20). A new medication canister must be "primed" so that medication is ready to be inhaled. Tip

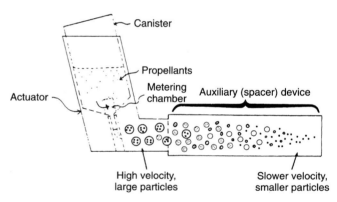

Figure 8-20 The effect of a spacer on aerosol particle size and velocity coming from a metered-dose inhaler. (From Gardenhire D: Rau's Respiratory care pharmacology, ed 7, St. Louis, 2008, Mosby.)

the metering chamber and press the actuator two or three times until the mist can be seen to come out. The patient then can inhale the medication through the built-in mouthpiece or added spacer or valved holding chamber (VHC). After inhaling the medication, the patient must disassemble the MDI unit and VHC, and cap the MDI to keep out any debris. Many of the newer MDIs will include a counter to record each activation. This helps the patient know when to get a new medication canister. Otherwise, the patient must keep a record of each activation.

c. Troubleshoot any problems with the equipment (code: IIA5) [difficulty: R, Ap]

When assembling the MDI, make sure that the medication canister nozzle fits into the jet of the actuator. If they are misaligned, no medication can be released. If needed, a spacer or VHC can be added to the actuator.

See the following discussion. To keep the jet channel open, patients should be instructed to use warm, soapy water daily to wash out the actuator. It can air dry overnight.

Some patients (e.g., those with arthritis of the fingers) may have difficulty squeezing the canister into the actuator to dispense the medication. In these cases, it may be possible to substitute a breath-activated MDI or add an MDI holder that can be squeezed easily to push the canister into the actuator. If a patient cannot properly manipulate an MDI with or without a spacer/valved holding chamber, the therapist should recommend a DPI or SVN medication delivery system.

3. Spacers and valved holding chambers for an MDI

a. Assemble the necessary equipment (code: IIA5) [difficulty: R, Ap]

The addition of a spacer or a valved holding chamber (VHC) between the actuator and the patient's mouth has been shown to increase the amount of inhaled medication. These devices slow down the aerosol so that less of it impacts on the back of the throat. This should result in fewer systemic adverse effects such as the risk of oral thrush (candidiasis fungal infection) with an MDI-powered corticosteroid. Also, the patient with poor hand and breathing coordination wastes less medication.

b. Troubleshoot any problems with the equipment (code: IIA5) [difficulty: R, Ap]

A spacer is a simple, open extension tube that is placed between the actuator and the patient. Its main advantage over direct inhalation from the MDI mouthpiece is that the aerosol plume expands and slows down so that more medication is inhaled (see Fig. 8-20). The patient should be told to refrain from exhaling through the spacer because any remaining medication will be blown out and wasted. Some spacers are designed for use with a ventilator circuit when an MDI-based medication is to be given. The spacer should be placed into the inspiratory limb of the ventilator circuit, about 18 in. from the patient. Typically, the MDI is activated during the expiratory phase so the medication can fill the spacer and inspiratory tubing before the next inspiration.

A VHC holds more medication than a spacer. The valves prevent the medicine from being exhaled out through the unit. The valves also allow the patient to inhale several times from the unit and get more medication than through a simple spacer. This is especially helpful with children or small adults with small tidal volume breaths. If available, a nonelectrostatic (antistatic) VHC should be used. The lack of electrical charge allows all of the medication in the chamber to be inhaled rather than having some particles attracted to the chamber walls. Some VHC units have a built-in whistle that sounds if the patient is inhaling too quickly. Several types of hand-held spacers or VHCs are available (Fig. 8-21). Some spacers are designed to fit with only one actuator, whereas others adapt to fit with any actuator. A face mask comes attached to some VHC units so that pediatric patients or uncooperative adults can be given the medication. When a mechanically ventilated patient requires an MDI medication, an adapter or VHC must be added into the ventilator circuit (Fig. 8-22). As discussed above, a VHC is preferred because more of the medication will be delivered into the patient.

Patients should be instructed that there is no need to wash out the spacer or VHC on a regular basis. The gradual buildup of powder inside the unit does not affect its function. If the spacer or the holding chamber becomes visibly soiled, it can be washed out with warm, soapy water. After rinsing, it can be left out to air dry.

4. Dry powder inhalers

a. Administer medications by DPI (code: IIID2) [difficulty: R, Ap]

The 2012 AARC Clinical Practice Guideline on selecting an aerosol delivery device has stated that any medication delivery system will be effective provided it is suited to the patient's ability to use the device. These suitability factors include the patient's age, physical ability, and cognitive ability; the medication availability for the device; and the patient–device interface. In any clinical situation, when the patient is not able to use the delivery system, another one must be used. See Table 8-4 for age-related guidelines for selecting a medicated aerosol delivery device. See Figure 8-14 for an algorithm for determining which device might be best suited to the patient.

b. Assemble the necessary equipment (code: IIA6) [difficulty: R, Ap]

DPIs dispense a dry medicinal powder into the patient's airways and lungs when inhaled (Fig. 8-23). The drug manufacturer sells both the medication and the dispenser to the patient. DPIs that can provide the following classes of medications are now available: maintenance and fast-acting beta-agonist (sympathomimetic) bronchodilators, anticholinergic (parasympatholytic) bronchodilators, inhaled corticosteroids, an antiviral agent, and human insulin.

Some DPI units are designed to deliver a single dose of medication. A new gelatin capsule that contains the medication must be loaded with each treatment. Examples include the Rotahaler (albuterol (Ventolin)), the Spiriva inhaler (tiotropium), and the Aerolizer (formoterol (Foradil)). (The Spinhaler for the delivery of cromolyn sodium (Intal) is no longer available.) (See Chapter 9 for details on all medications.)

Other DPI units are multidose delivery systems that contain many doses of medication within a reservoir. Examples include the Turbuhaler for formoterol (Foradil), the Turbuhaler for terbutaline (Bricanyl), and the Pulmicort Turbuhaler (for budesonide), all of which contain 200 doses; the Diskus (for salmeterol

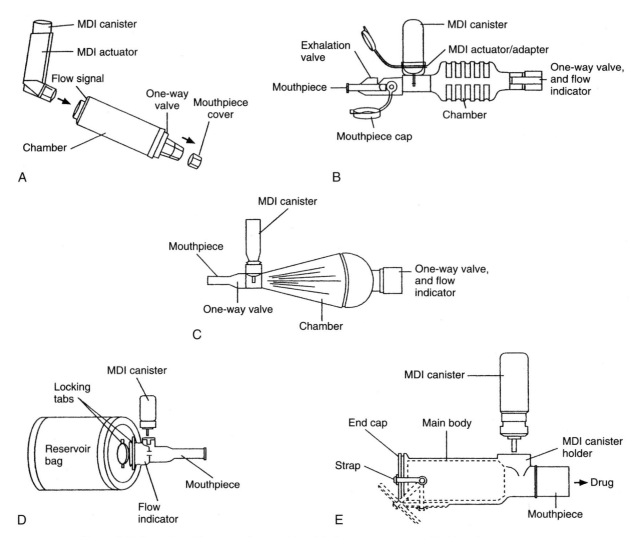

Figure 8-21 Examples of five types of metered-dose inhaler spacers and valved holding chambers. **A,** Aero-Chamber (Monaghan Medical Corp.); **B,** MediSpacer (Allegiance Healthcare, Inc.); **C,** Aerosol Cloud Enhancer (DHD, Inc.); **D,** InspirEase (Schering, Inc.); and **E,** OptiHaler (Healthscan, Inc.). (From Gardenhire D: Rau's respiratory care pharmacology, ed 7, St Louis, 2008, Mosby.)

(Serevent)), the Advair Diskus (combination of salmeterol and fluticasone propionate), and the Flovent Diskus (fluticasone propionate)), all of which contain 60 doses; and the Diskhaler (for zanamivir (Relenza)), which contains four or eight doses. (See Chapter 9 for details on all medications.)

Note that the Turbuhaler device and the Diskus device both are being used to deliver three different types of medications. Make sure the patient knows to check the label on the unit if the same type of DPI device is being used for more than one medication.

Single-use DPI units require several steps to prepare the medication before inhalation. Steps typically include the following: (1) disassemble the device, (2) properly place the first medication capsule into the device, and (3) adjust the device to pierce the capsule. With all subsequent doses, the empty capsule from the previous treatment must be

removed before the new capsule can be placed. The therapist must oversee that the patient is properly performing these steps. Patients who are too young to follow directions, who cannot physically perform the steps, or who do not have the mental capacity to understand the steps should not be using one of these DPI devices.

Multiuse DPI devices are simpler to use. However, steps must be followed to properly fill the medication from the reservoir and to prepare the unit for inhalation. Both Turbuhaler and Diskus units include a counter to keep track of how many doses have been taken. When the reservoir of medication is empty, a new DPI device must be purchased. As was discussed earlier, the patient must be able to demonstrate the ability to prepare the unit before it should be used. The therapist must be ready to recommend another medication delivery system, if needed.

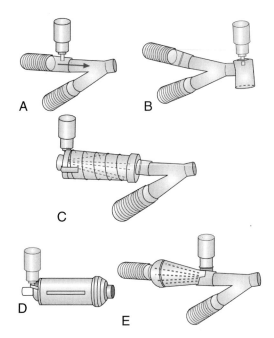

Figure 8-22 Examples of MDI adapters and valved holding chambers (VHCs) for insertion into a mechanical ventilator circuit. Examples A and B are simple adapters for the MDI. Examples C, D, and E are VHCs. Whenever possible, a VHC should be used to increase the amount of medication delivered to the patient. (Modified from Dhand R, Tobin MJ: Bronchodilator delivery with metered-dose inhalers in mechanically ventilated patients, Eur Respir J 9:585, 1996.)

c. Troubleshoot any problems with the equipment (code: IIA6) [difficulty: R, Ap]

See the manufacturer's literature for proper steps to follow in using the DPI unit. Patient practice is essential to make sure that the unit is used properly. If it does not operate properly, it must be replaced. DPI units as a group have the following limits: (1) If the unit becomes wet or is used in a high-humidity environment, the powder can congeal and clog up the unit. Less medication powder will be inhaled. (2) The user must be able to rapidly inhale the powder. If the patient's peak inspiratory flow is not at least 40–60 L/min, less medication will be inhaled. It will not leave the dispenser, or it will impact in the back of the throat rather than being inhaled into the airways and lungs. Patients who are younger than 5 years of age and patients with severe airway obstruction probably will not be able to use a DPI properly. An MDI or an SVN should be used instead to deliver the needed medications.

MODULE F

Respiratory care plan

1. Determine a patient's pathophysiologic state (code: IIIF1) [difficulty: R, Ap, An]

Hearing expiratory crackles (also called rhonchi) in the more central airways would indicate that the patient has retained secretions. The patient with many secretions should be helped by the addition of a bland aerosol or mucolytic medication and should be better able to clear these medications effectively. This should cause the patient to feel better and to have improved vital signs, oxygenation, breath sounds, and spirometry values. The use of a bland aerosol therapy can cause bronchospasm in some asthmatic patients. The development of wheezing after aerosol therapy could indicate that the patient has bronchospastic tendencies. An aerosolized bronchodilator medication may be needed. Patients with thick, dry (inspissated) secretions can have their airways occluded if aerosol therapy causes the secretions to absorb water and swell. If the patient is not able to cough out the thinned secretions, suctioning equipment must be available to remove them. Hearing normal breath sounds after humidity or aerosol therapy and a productive cough would indicate that all central airway secretions have been removed. Note whether the patient is able to more easily cough out any secretions after humidity or aerosol therapy. It is also important to evaluate the consistency of the secretions. Improved hydration should make the secretions more watery (less viscous).

2. Recommend starting a treatment based on the patient's response (code: IIIE2a) [difficulty: R, Ap, An]

Changes in the patient's secretion volume and consistency may result in a change in the type of humidity and/or aerosol therapy needed. Be prepared to decrease humidity and/or aerosol therapy if the patient's secretions are decreased in volume and easy for the patient to cough out. In contrast, be prepared to increase humidity and/or aerosol therapy if the patient's secretions are thick and difficult to cough out.

3. Recommend a change in the therapeutic plan if indicated (code: IIIF2) [difficulty: R, Ap, An]

As discussed above, be prepared to recommend a change in humidity or aerosol therapy as well as a change in the type of device used to deliver the humidity or aerosol. Often a patient

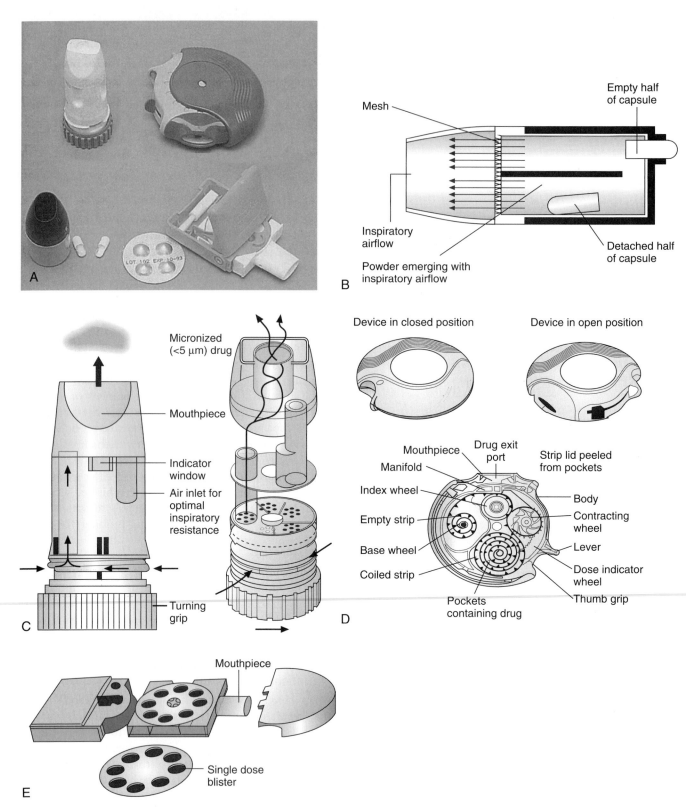

Figure 8-23 Examples of four types of dry powder inhaler. **A,** Photograph of the single-dose Rotahaler *(lower left)*, the multidose Turbuhaler *(top left)*, the multidose Diskus *(top right)*, and the multidose Diskhaler *(lower right)*. **B,** Cross-section of the Rotahaler showing how it must be held horizontally when used. **C,** Internal views of the Turbuhaler showing how it dispenses a single dose from its 200-dose reservoir of medication. **D,** Operation and cross-section through the Diskus. It has a strip with 60 doses of medication, which are individually opened and inhaled. **E,** Disassembled Diskhaler showing the medication wheel, which can contain four or eight doses of medication. (From Cairo J, Pilbeam S: Mosby's respiratory therapy equipment, ed 8, St Louis, 2010, Mosby.)

must be coached in the ideal breathing pattern to maximize the deposition of medications into the upper or lower airway. Following are recommended breathing patterns.

a. Upper airway deposition

Particles 10 μm or larger are more likely to impact the upper airway (oropharynx, larynx, trachea, and mainstem bronchi) when the patient is coached to do the following:
1. Inhale at a normal or faster speed (the flow should be greater than 30 L/min).
2. Inhale a normal V_T.
3. Breathe in a normal pattern.

b. Lower airway and alveolar deposition

Particles measuring 2–5 μm are more likely to deposit on the smaller airways (respiratory bronchioles) and in the alveoli when the patient is coached to do the following:
1. Inhale at a slow speed (the flow should be less than 30 L/min).
2. Inhale an inspiratory capacity (IC).
3. If possible, hold the full breath for 10 s before exhaling.
   Obviously, not all patients can perform these techniques perfectly, but to the extent that they can, the medication is deposited where needed and the treatment is more effective.

4. Recommend a change in humidification (code: IIIE3c) [difficulty: R, Ap]

Be prepared to change the type of humidity and aerosol delivery system used from among those discussed in this chapter based on the patient's condition. Review the indications, contraindications, uses, and limitations of the various systems.

a. Adjust the temperature of the aerosol

In general, a cool humidity or aerosol system is used with patients with the following conditions:
- Laryngotracheobronchitis (or pediatric croup)
- Upper airway irritation, such as after extubation or a bronchoscopy procedure

In general, a body-temperature humidity or aerosol system is used with patients with the following conditions:
- Bypassed upper airway (endotracheal or tracheostomy tube)
- Thick secretions
- Hypothermia
- Maintenance of a neutral thermal environment for the neonate

b. Change the output of aerosol by the equipment

Neonates are sensitive to overhydration, so long-term aerosol therapy for them should be avoided or minimized. Adult patients with heart failure or pulmonary edema also should not be given long-term aerosol therapy. Instead, a pass-over-type humidifier can be used.

The adult patient with thick secretions may be aided by long-term aerosol therapy of a dense mist, usually by a USN run at body temperature. Secretions often are liquefied and made easier to cough or suction out. The child with croup usually is given a dense mist of a cool bland aerosol in a mist tent. This therapy usually is needed for only a few days. Be wary of fluid overload if the mist is needed for a longer period. A significant gain in daily weight would indicate fluid overload.

5. Recommend a treatment be terminated (code: IIIE1) [difficulty: R, Ap, An]

The most common reason to stop a treatment is an adverse reaction to an inhaled medication. Check the patient's heart rate for tachycardia in response to inhaling a beta-agonist medication. Many consider a 20% increase in heart rate to be clinically significant. If this should happen, assess the patient and notify the physician, if necessary. The treatment may need to be paused until the heart rate returns to normal. If tachycardia returns, the treatment should be stopped.

6. Recommend discontinuing a treatment based on the patient's response (code: IIIE2h) [difficulty: R, Ap, An]

Based on the previous discussion, be prepared to stop a treatment or procedure if necessary. After further evaluation, it may be possible to continue again. However, if the patient has a serious adverse reaction, the treatment or procedure should be discontinued. Usually, this would be done after consultation with the patient's physician.

Exam Hint 8-5

Past exams have had a question that deals with recognizing that the patient is having an adverse reaction. Be prepared to stop therapy if the patient has bronchospasm or becomes short of breath when swollen secretions obstruct airways.

BIBLIOGRAPHY

Adams DA: Humidity and aerosol therapy. In Wyka KA, Mathews PJ, Rutkowski J, editors: *Foundations of respiratory care*, ed 2, Clifton Park, NY, 2012, Delmar.

Altobelli N: Aerosol and humidity therapy. In Kacmarek RM, Dimas S, Mack CW, editors: *The essentials of respiratory care*, ed 4, St Louis, 2005, Mosby.

American Association for Respiratory Care: Aerosol consensus statement, *Respir Care* 36:916, 1991.

American Association for Respiratory Care: Clinical practice guideline: humidification during invasive and noninvasive mechanical ventilation, *Respir Care* 57:782, 2012.

American Association for Respiratory Care: Clinical practice guideline: aerosol delivery device selection for spontaneously breathing patients, *Respir Care* 57:613, 2012.

American Association for Respiratory Care: Clinical practice guideline: selection of device for delivery of aerosol to the lung parenchyma, *Respir Care* 41:647, 1993.

American Association for Respiratory Care: Clinical practice guideline: bland aerosol administration, *Respir Care* 38:1196, 1993.

American Association for Respiratory Care: Clinical practice guideline: bland aerosol administration—2003 revision & update, *Respir Care* 48:529, 2003 (Retired).

American Association for Respiratory Care: Clinical practice guideline: care of the ventilator circuit and its relation to ventilator associated pneumonia, *Respir Care* 48:869, 2003.

American Association for Respiratory Care: Clinical practice guideline: delivery of aerosols to the upper airway, *Respir Care* 39:803, 1994.

American Association for Respiratory Care: Clinical practice guideline: humidification during mechanical ventilation, *Respir Care* 37:877, 1992.

American Association for Respiratory Care: Clinical practice guideline: selection of aerosol delivery device, *Respir Care* 37:891, 1992.

American Association for Respiratory Care: Clinical practice guideline: selection of aerosol delivery device for neonatal and pediatric patients, *Respir Care* 40:1325, 1995 (Retired).

Ari A, Areabi H, Fink JB: Evaluation of aerosol generator devices at 3 locations in humidified and non-humidified circuits during adult mechanical ventilation, *Respir Care* 55:837, 2010.

Arunthari V, Bruinsma RS, Lee AS, Johnson MM: A prospective, comparative trial of standard and breath-acutated nebulizer: efficacy, safety, and satisfaction, *Respir Care* 57:1242, 2012.

Barnes TA, editor: *Core textbook of respiratory care practice*, ed 2, St Louis, 1994, Mosby.

Branson RD, Gentile MA: Is humidification always necessary during noninvasive ventilation in the hospital? *Respir Care* 55:209, 2010.

Dolovich MB, Hess DR, Dhand R, Smaldone GC: Device selection and outcomes of aerosol therapy: evidence-based guidelines, *Chest* 127:335, 2005.

Fink J: Aerosol drug therapy. In Kacmarek RM, Stoller JK, Heuer AJ, editors: *Egan's fundamentals of respiratory care*, ed 10, St Louis, 2013, Mosby.

Fink J, Ari A: Humidity and aerosol therapy. In Cairo JM, editor: *Mosby's respiratory care equipment*, ed 9, St Louis, 2014, Mosby.

Fink J, Ari A: Humidity and bland aerosol therapy. In Kacmarek RM, Stoller JK, Heuer AJ, editors: *Egan's fundamentals of respiratory care*, ed 10, St Louis, 2013, Mosby.

Fink JB: Humidity. In Fink JB, Hunt GE, editors: *Clinical practice in respiratory care*, Philadelphia, 1999, Lippincott-Raven.

Fink JB, Dhand R: Aerosol drug therapy. In Fink JB, Hunt GE, editors: *Clinical practice in respiratory care*, Philadelphia, 1999, Lippincott-Raven.

Fink JB, Rubin BK: Aerosols and administration of medication. In Walsh BK, Czervinske MP, DiBlasi RM, editors: *Perinatal and pediatric respiratory care*, ed 3, St. Louis, 2010, Saunders.

Gardenhire DS: *Rau's respiratory care pharmacology*, ed 8, St Louis, 2012, Mosby.

Hess DR: Humidity and aerosol therapy. In Hess DR, MacIntyre NR, Mishoe SC, et al.: *Respiratory care principles & practices*, ed 2, Burlington, MA, 2012, Jones & Bartlett Learning.

Hess DR: Aerosol delivery devices in the treatment of asthma, *Respir Care* 53:699, 2008.

Hess DR: Aerosol therapy. In Dantzker DR, MacIntyre NR, Bakow ED, editors: *Comprehensive respiratory care*, Philadelphia, 1995, Saunders.

Hess DR: The delivery of aerosolized bronchodilator to mechanically ventilated intubated adult patients, *Respir Care* 35:399, 1990.

Prabhakaran S, Shuster J, Chesrown S, Hendeles L: Response to albuterol MDI delivered through an anti-static chamber during nocturnal bronchospasm, *Respir Care* 57:1291, 2012.

Rubin BK: Pediatric aerosol therapy: new devices and new drugs, *Respir Care* 56(9):1411–1423, 2011.

White GC: *Equipment theory for respiratory care*, ed 3, Albany, NY, 1999, Delmar.

SELF-STUDY QUESTIONS

See Appendix for answers.

1. Ten minutes into a hand-held nebulizer treatment given to deliver albuterol (Proventil), the patient complains of dizziness and tingling fingers. What should be done?
   A. Advise the patient to breathe in the same pattern.
   B. Change the medication.
   C. Tell the patient to breathe more slowly.
   D. Advise the patient to breathe deeper and faster.

2. A patient is being given a bronchodilator medication by SVN powered by 5 L/min of O_2. While watching the patient breathe, the respiratory therapist notices that during each inspiration, the mist disappears from the downstream end of the SVN. What should be recommended?
   A. Add 100 mL of aerosol tubing as a reservoir.
   B. Increase the oxygen flow.
   C. Decrease the oxygen flow.
   D. Tell the patient not to breathe so deeply.

3. A 3-year-old patient with asthma is about to be discharged and needs to take an inhaled bronchodilator medication at home. What device should be recommended?
   A. MDI
   B. SVN with mouthpiece
   C. DPI with VHC
   D. MDI with VHC

4. An order has arrived to perform an induced sputum procedure on a patient suspected of having tuberculosis. What should be the first choice to nebulize for the patient?
   A. 7% saline
   B. 0.9% saline
   C. 0.45% saline
   D. Distilled water

5. What breathing pattern should be recommended for an aerosolized medication to be deposited primarily in the larger airways?
   1. Inhale a V_T.
   2. Inhale an IC.
   3. Inhale slowly.
   4. Inhale at a normal speed.
   5. Breathe in a normal pattern.
   A. 2 and 3 only
   B. 1, 4, and 5 only
   C. 4 and 5 only
   D. 2 and 4 only

6. A physician calls a respiratory therapist to evaluate a 40-year-old patient with bronchitis and to make a recommendation for an aerosol delivery system. The patient's breath sounds indicate the presence of large-airway secretions. Despite a good cough effort, the patient has difficulty in raising them. What should be recommended?
   A. Use a hand-held nebulizer with 3 cc of normal saline every 4 hr.
   B. Place the patient into a mist tent.
   C. Start a continuous USN to an aerosol mask.
   D. Start a cascade-type humidifier to an aerosol mask.

7. A patient's humidity deficit is going to be the *smallest* under which of the following conditions?
   A. Breathing in regular hospital room air at 72° F and 40% RH
   B. Breathing in outside air at 80° F and 50% RH
   C. Breathing in 6 L/min of O_2 through a nasal cannula running through an unheated bubble humidifier
   D. Breathing in 40% O_2 at 95° F through a pass-over-type humidifier to an aerosol mask

8. A USN would be recommended for aerosol therapy for the following reason:
   A. It delivers a wide variety of aerosol droplets.
   B. Its aerosol droplets are between 10 and 20 μm in diameter.
   C. It delivers a uniform aerosol droplet of about 3 μm in diameter.
   D. It can be used to nebulize bland aerosols and liquid medications into an aerosol.

9. A patient has an endotracheal tube. Which of the following devices would be the *least* effective in reducing this patient's humidity deficit?
   A. Wick-type humidifier set at 35° C
   B. Membrane-type humidifier set at 35° C
   C. Unheated bubble-type humidifier
   D. Ultrasonic nebulizer

10. An adult patient with chronic bronchitis has a normal temperature. To fully saturate the inhaled air, how much AH must be provided by the humidifier?
    A. 35° C
    B. 47 mm Hg

C. 760 mm Hg
D. 44 mg/L

11. A patient's heated humidifier unit has a water reservoir temperature of 40° C. The humidified gas is traveling through large-bore tubing to the patient. Which of the following statements are true?
    1. Condensation will occur.
    2. The gas will warm and expand as it travels to the patient.
    3. The gas will remain saturated.
    4. The RH will decrease.
    5. The RH will increase.
    A. 1 and 3 only
    B. 3 and 4 only
    C. 2, 3, and 5 only
    D. 1, 2, and 4 only

12. The pop-off valve is whistling on a patient's bubble humidifier to a 35% O_2 air entrainment mask. What could be the problem?
    A. The reservoir jar is not screwed tightly into the top of the humidifier.
    B. The air entrainment mask should be set at 28% O_2.
    C. The small-bore tubing is pinched.
    D. The air entrainment mask should be set at 40% O_2.

13. A humidity or aerosol system delivering body-temperature gas is used in all the following situations EXCEPT:
    A. Patient with a tracheostomy
    B. Twenty-month-old infant with laryngotracheobronchitis
    C. Patient with chronic obstructive pulmonary disease with thick secretions
    D. Hypothermic near-drowning victim

14. A patient's small-volume medication nebulizer is not putting out as much aerosol as it was a short time ago. To correct the problem, which of the following should be checked?
    1. Make sure the fluid level is correct.
    2. Make sure the one-way valve is patent.
    3. Make sure the jet is patent.
    4. Make sure the O_2 can flow down the capillary tube.
    5. Make sure the fluid can flow up the capillary tube.
    A. 1 and 2 only
    B. 3 and 4 only
    C. 2 and 4 only
    D. 1, 3, and 5 only

15. A patient has pneumonia and needs an inhaled antibiotic. What size particle generator should be recommended to treat the problem?
    A. 20–50 μm
    B. 10–20 μm

C. 2–5 μm

D. 1–3 μm

16. A USN has a flashing couplant indicator light. The respiratory therapist notices that the output has decreased from what it was earlier. The most likely problem is:

A. Too much water in the solution cup

B. Too much water in the couplant chamber

C. Not enough water in the couplant chamber

D. A loose electrical cable

17. A respiratory therapist notices that water has collected at the low point of the large-bore tubing of your patient's heated aerosol system. The aerosol is "puffing" out of the end of the tubing. What should be done?

A. Add water to the reservoir jar.

B. Empty water from the reservoir jar.

C. Empty the water from the large-bore tubing into a wastewater jar.

D. Empty the water from the large-bore tubing into the reservoir jar so it is not wasted.

18. The physician wants a patient with a tracheostomy to inhale room air that is fully saturated at body temperature. The selected device must be able to meet the following criteria:

1. Deliver 40% RH

2. Deliver 100% RH

3. Provide 47 mm Hg vapor pressure

4. Provide 44 mm Hg vapor pressure

5. Deliver 44 mg/L AH

A. 2 and 4 only

B. 1, 3, and 5 only

C. 1 and 4 only

D. 2, 3, and 5 only

19. It is best to coach a patient to breathe in the following pattern for particle deposition in smaller airways and alveoli:

1. Inhale a V_T.

2. Inhale rapidly.

3. Inhale an IC.

4. Hold the breath for up to 10 s before exhaling.

5. Inhale at a slow speed.

A. 1 and 2 only

B. 3, 4, and 5 only

C. 1 and 5 only

D. 1, 2, and 4 only

20. When doing patient rounds, a respiratory therapist notices that very little aerosol is going from an LVN to a patient's tracheostomy mask. Which of the following could be the problem?

1. The water level is above the refill line on the nebulizer's reservoir jar.

2. The nebulizer is not screwed tightly into the DISS connector on the flowmeter.

3. The nebulizer jet is obstructed.

4. The water level is below the refill line on the nebulizer's reservoir jar.

5. The capillary tube is obstructed.

A. 1 and 2 only

B. 3 and 4 only

C. 1, 4, and 5 only

D. 2, 3, 4, and 5 only

21. A 64-year-old patient with a long smoking history and a diagnosis of chronic bronchitis has been admitted again with complaints of shortness of breath and productive cough. Which of the following questions should be asked to gain an understanding of the patient's problem to better guide aerosol therapy?

1. Has the volume of your secretions changed over the past week?

2. How many hours do you sleep a night?

3. Are there any medications that make your breathing easier?

4. How many flights of stairs can you climb without stopping?

A. 1 and 3 only

B. 2 and 4 only

C. 1, 2, and 3 only

D. 1, 2, 3, 4

22. A 30-year-old patient with asthma has frequent business trips by airplane. What type of nebulizer should be recommended for her liquid medications?

A. Breath-enhanced nebulizer

B. Standard nebulizer

C. Vibrating-mesh nebulizer

D. Breath-activated nebulizer

23. A 40-year-old female patient has been sick with the flu for 8 days and was admitted to the hospital with dehydration and pneumonia. Intravenous fluids and antibiotics were started. She was given an aerosol mask with 35% oxygen and continuous aerosol of normal saline nebulized through a USN system. An hour later, she reported worsening shortness of breath. Her breath sounds revealed crackles that were not there before this therapy was started. What is the most likely cause of these changes?

A. The dehydration is worse.

B. Her influenza is worse.

C. Her secretions have swollen.

D. She is allergic to the normal saline.

24. A 40-year-old patient has just been intubated and started on mechanical ventilation. It is anticipated that this will be needed for at least several days. What should be the first choice for humidification?

A. Heated cascade-type humidifier

B. SVN every 4 hr

C. Heated heat–moisture exchanger

D. VMN every 2 hr

25. A 14-year-old patient with severe asthma has just been given a new medication of inhaled corticosteroid by a DPI. After rapidly inhaling the medication, the patient begins to cough vigorously. Breath sounds reveal increased wheezing in all lung fields. What should be recommended?
    A. Have the patient inhale rapidly through the DPI to make sure all of the medication has been received.
    B. Have the patient inhale slowly through the DPI to make sure all of the medication has been received.
    C. Stop taking the DPI medication.
    D. Increase the dose of DPI medication until the patient's wheezing goes away.

26. A patient with congestive heart failure is having an exacerbation of the condition. The physician is going to support the patient's breathing with noninvasive ventilation while being aggressively treated. What should be recommended for humidification?
    A. Heat–moisture exchanger
    B. Wick-type of humidifier
    C. Large-volume nebulizer
    D. No need for added humidity

27. Complications of bland aerosol therapy include all of the following EXCEPT:
    A. Increased humidity deficit
    B. Aerosol-induced bronchospasm
    C. Fluid overload in an infant
    D. Swollen secretions that may block airways

28. An alcoholic patient has been admitted with a high fever and a productive cough. A pulmonary abscess is suspected. What sputum characteristics should be evaluated to help assess the effectiveness of aerosol and other therapy?
    1. Specific gravity
    2. Smell
    3. Consistency
    4. Platelet count
    5. Color
    A. 2 and 3 only
    B. 4 and 5 only
    C. 1, 2, and 3 only
    D. 2, 3, and 5 only

9 Pharmacology

MODULE A

Therapist-administered medications

1. Administer medications

See below. This chapter covers the classes of medications listed by the NBRC that are given to patients with cardiopulmonary conditions. Many of the medications described in this module are given as an aerosol and administered by respiratory therapists. See Chapter 8 for specific information on the MDI, SVN, and DPI devices.

   a. Administer aerosolized preparations by metered-dose inhaler (MDI) (code: IIID1) [difficulty: R, Ap]

See below. (*Note:* As of January 1, 2014, all chlorofluorocarbon-powered MDI have been banned. All MDIs must now be powered by hydrofluoroalkane (HFA) propellants.)

   b. Administer aerosolized preparations by small-volume nebulizer (SVN) (code: IIID1) [difficulty: R, Ap]

See below.

   c. Administer aerosolized preparations by dry powder inhaler (DPI) (code: IIID2) [difficulty: R, Ap]

   d. Administer medications by endotracheal instillation (code: IIID3) [difficulty: R, Ap]

See Chapter 11 for the discussion on giving medications via the endotracheal tube during a cardiopulmonary resuscitation effort.

2. Increased duration and combination medications

Since the last edition of this text, there have been two significant advances in the three classes of inhaled bronchodilator medications commonly given by respiratory therapists. The adrenergic, anticholinergic, and corticosteroid medications open the airways, resulting in reduced airway resistance and easier breathing. The first major advance is the approval of ultralong-acting beta-agonist and ultralong-acting anticholinergic medications. These new drugs last 24 hours and are taken only once a day (Anoro, Breo).

The second major development involves combining a drug from two classes into one preparation. Currently there are combinations of adrenergic and corticosteroid drugs (Advair, Dulera, Symbicort, Breo) and adrenergic and anticholinergic drugs (Combivent Respimat, Anoro).

These two advances simplify the patient's efforts and increase prescription compliance. As of this writing, there are no Food and Drug Administration (FDA)-approved combinations of anticholinergic and corticosteroid drugs or adrenergic, anticholinergic, and corticosteroid drugs. However, be watchful for the approval of new drug combinations.

3. Guidelines for duration of action

Tables 9-1 and 9-2 list the onset, peak, and duration times of the adrenergic and anticholinergic drugs, respectively. Knowing the duration of a drug enables the physician to select the best medication for the patient's situation. The general guidelines for drug duration include:
1. Ultrashort acting: 1-3 hours. Ultrashort-acting drugs, such as epinephrine, are typically used during brief medical procedures or treatments.
2. Short acting: 4 to <12 hours. Short-acting drugs, such as albuterol, are used as "rescue" drugs for a patient with an asthma or chronic obstructive pulmonary disease (COPD) exacerbation.
3. Long acting: 12 hours. Long-acting drugs, such as arformoterol, are used as "controller" drugs with stable asthma or COPD patients and need be taken only twice a day.

TABLE 9-1	Inhaled Beta-Agonist Bronchodilator Agents*

Drug	Brand Name(s)**	Receptor Preference	Adult Dosage	Time Course (Onset, Peak, Duration)
Ultrashort Acting				
Epinephrine	Adrenaline, Adrenalin chloride	α, β	SVN: 0.1% solution (1:100), 0.25-0.5 mL	Onset: 3-5 minutes Peak: 5-20 minutes Duration: 1-3 hours
Isoetharine	Isoetharine HCl, Dey-Lute Isoetharine	β_2	SVN: 1% solution, 0.25-0.5 mL (2.5-5.0 mg) qid	Onset: 1-6 minutes Peak: 15-60 minutes Duration: 1-3 hours
Racemic epinephrine	MicroNefrin, S2, AsthmaNefrin, Nephron	α, β	SVN: 2.25% solution, 0.25-0.5 mL qid (5.63-11.25 mg) qid	Onset: 3-5 minutes epinephrine Peak: 5-20 minutes Duration: 0.5-2 hours
Short Acting				
Metaproterenol	Alupent	β_2	SVN: 0.4%, 0.6%, tid, qid Tab: 10 or 20 mg, tid, qid Syrup: 10 mg/5 mL, 2 tsp tid, qid	Onset: 1-5 minutes Peak: 60 minutes Duration: 2-6 hours
Albuterol	AccuNeb	β_2	SVN: 0.5% solution, 0.5 mL (2.5 mg); 0.63 mg, Proventil hydrofluoroalkane 1.25 mg, and 2.5 mg unit dose, tid, qid	Onset: 15 minutes Peak: 30-60 minutes Duration: 5-8 hours
	Proventil HFA, Ventolin HFA, ProAir HFA		MDI: 90 mcg/puff, 2 puffs tid, qid	
	VoSpire ER		Tab: 2, 4, and 8 mg, bid, tid, qid Syrup: 2 mg/5 mL, 1-2 tsp tid, qid	Duration: Up to 12 hours
Levalbuterol	Xopenex	β_2	SVN: 0.31 mg/3 mL tid; 0.63 mg/3 mL tid; or 1.25 mg/3 mL tid; concentrate 1.25 mg/0.5 ml tid	Onset: 15 minutes Peak: 30-60 minutes Duration: 5-8 hours
	Xopenex HFA, Xopenex Pediatric		MDI: 45 mcg/puff, 2 puffs q4-6 hours, ≥4 years of age	
Long Acting				
Arformoterol	Brovana	β_2	SVN: 15 mcg/2 mL unit dose, bid	Onset: 15 minutes Peak: 30-60 minutes Duration: 12 hours
Formoterol	Perforomist	β_2	SVN: 20 mcg unit-dose vial bid	Onset: 15 minutes
	Foradil		DPI: 12 mcg/inhalation bid	Peak: 30-60 minutes
	Foradil Certihaler		DPI: 8.5 mcg/inhalation bid	Duration: 12 hours
Salmeterol	Serevent Evohaler HFA†	β_2	MDI: 25 mcg/puff, 2 puffs bid	Onset: 20 minutes
	Serevent Diskus	β_2	DPI: 50 mcg/blister bid	Peak: 3-5 hours Duration: 12 hours
Ultralong Acting				
Indacaterol	Arcapta	β_2	DPI: 75 mcg/puff, 1 inhalation per day	Onset: <15 minutes Peak: 15 minutes Duration: 24 hours
Ultralong Acting (Combined with an Anticholinergic Agent)				
Vilanterol (β_2) and umeclidinium (anticholinergic)	Anoro	β_2	DPI: 25 mcg vilanterol and 62.5 mcg umeclidinium, 1 inhalation daily	Onset: <5 minutes Peak: 5-15 minutes Duration: 24 hours

bid, twice daily; tid, three times daily; qid, four times daily; SVN, small-volume nebulizer; MDI, metered-dose inhaler; DPI, dry powder inhaler; mg, milligram (1/1000 g); mcg, microgram (1/1000 mg—*Note:* The abbreviation μg may be used instead of mcg).
A valved holding chamber is recommended with MDI administration to prevent accidental eye exposure.
*Detailed prescribing information should be obtained from the manufacturer's package insert.
**Lists of brand names may not be current owing to frequent additions and deletions by manufacturers.
Modified from Gardenhire DS: Rau's respiratory care pharmacology, ed 8, St Louis, 2012, Mosby.

TABLE 9-2   Inhaled Anticholinergic Bronchodilator Agents*

Drug	Brand Name(s)**	Adult Dosage	Time Course (Onset, Peak, Duration)
Short Acting			
Ipratropium bromide	Atrovent hydrofluoroalkane	MDI: 17 mcg/puff, 2 puffs qid SVN: 0.02% solution (0.2 mg/mL), 500 mcg tid, qid	Onset: 15 minutes Peak: 1-2 hours Duration: 4-6 hours
	Atrovent solution	Nasal spray: 21 mcg/spray; 2 sprays per nostril 2-4 times daily (dosage varies)	
Ipratropium bromide and albuterol	Combivent Respimat	Mechanical MDI: ipratropium 20 mcg/puff and albuterol 100 mcg/puff, 1 inhalation 4-6 times per day	Onset: 15 minutes Peak: 1-2 hours Duration: 4-6 hours
	DuoNeb	SVN: 3 mL: ipratropium 0.5 mg and albuterol 2.5 mg, qid	
Long Acting			
Aclidinium bromide	Tudorza	DPI: 400 mcg/inhalation, 1 inhalation bid	Onset: 15 minutes Peak: 1-6 hours Duration: 12 hours
Ultralong Acting			
Tiotropium bromide	Spiriva HandiHaler	DPI: 18 mcg/inhalation, 1 inhalation daily (one capsule)	Onset: 30 minutes Peak: 1-3 hours Duration: 24 hours
Ultralong Acting (Combined with a Beta-Adrenergic Agent)			
Umeclidinium (anticholinergic) and vilanterol (β_2)	Anoro	DPI: 62.5 mcg umeclidinium and 25 mcg vilanterol, 1 inhalation daily	Onset: <5 minutes Peak: 5-15 minutes Duration: 24 hours

bid, twice daily; tid, three times daily; qid, four times daily; SVN, small-volume nebulizer; MDI, metered-dose inhaler; DPI, dry powder inhaler; mg, milligram (1/1000 g); mcg, microgram (1/1000 mg—*Note:* The abbreviation µg may be used instead of mcg).
A valved holding chamber is recommended with MDI administration to prevent accidental eye exposure.
*Detailed prescribing information should be obtained from the manufacturer's package insert.
**Lists of brand names may not be current owing to frequent additions and deletions by manufacturers.
Modified from Gardenhire DS: Rau's respiratory care pharmacology, ed 8, St Louis, 2012, Mosby.

4. Ultralong acting: 24 hours. Ultralong-acting drugs, such as tiotropium, are used as "controller" drugs with stable asthma or COPD patients and need be taken only once a day.

4. Adrenergic (sympathomimetic) agents

a. Recommend their use (code: III4b)
[difficulty: R, Ap, An]

A variety of names have been used to describe this class of medications derived from adrenaline, including beta agonists, beta-adrenergic agonists, catecholamines, sympathomimetic amines, sympathomimetic bronchodilators, and β-adrenergic bronchodilators. The preferred term is *beta agonist* because these medications stimulate the β_2 receptors in the airway smooth muscle. This stimulation causes the airway muscles to relax, resulting in bronchodilation. Be prepared to recommend the use of these types of medications in patients with asthma and COPD (e.g., emphysema, chronic bronchitis).

A brief review of the autonomic nervous system helps in understanding how the beta-agonist medications (and anticholinergic medications) work and some side effects of their use. The autonomic nervous system is not under voluntary control. It is an automatic system designed to regulate metabolism and the vital signs. This system is made up of two branches: the sympathetic nervous system and the cholinergic (parasympathetic) nervous system. The lungs, heart, and most other organs are innervated by both branches. The blood vessels in the mucous membranes are innervated only by the sympathetic branch. The cholinergic nervous system is usually dominant and keeps the body functioning normally. The sympathetic nervous system is an "emergency" system that is dominant only during great stress (sometimes called the "fight or flight" system). Adrenaline (or epinephrine) is released by the adrenal glands in these emergencies. Adrenaline causes a number of effects, including one that many respiratory patients need—bronchodilation. The sympathetic nervous system has the following three types of receptors that are located in different organs and are affected by adrenaline and related medications.

1. α_1-Receptors are located in the blood vessels of the mucous membranes (other tissues are not included in this discussion). Vasoconstriction results when α_1-receptors are stimulated.
2. β_1-Receptors are located in the heart. Tachycardia, increased stroke volume, and possibly arrhythmias result when β_1-receptors are stimulated.
3. β_2-Receptors are located in the airways. Bronchodilation results when β_2-receptors are stimulated.

BOX 9-1   Clinically Observed Side Effects of Beta-Agonist Aerosolized Bronchodilators (from the Most Commonly Seen to the Least Commonly Seen)

Tremor: gentle, uncontrollable, involuntary muscle shaking.
Palpitations and tachycardia: irregular heartbeats and fast heart rate.
Headache.
Increased blood pressure: possibly from both the α_1-adrenergic effect on blood vessels and tachycardia.
Nervousness and irritability.
Dizziness.
Nausea.
Decreased PaO_2 level from a worsening of the ventilation/perfusion ratio.

PaO_2, partial pressure of O_2 in arterial blood.

Although the medications listed in this section are chemically derived from adrenaline, they are somewhat different in their structures. Therefore, the desired effects and unwanted side effects vary. Box 9-1 lists the side effects of the sympathomimetic bronchodilators. Clinically, the most dangerous of these side effects are palpitations, tachycardia, and hypertension. If possible, avoid drugs with unnecessary α_1 and β_1 effects.

b. Administer the prescribed medication (code: IIID1, 2) [difficulty: R, Ap]

Table 9-1 lists the onset, peak, and duration times for the various medications and the administration method, strength, and dosages. Depending on the patient's ability to manage an SVN, MDI, or DPI, select the best medication and delivery device that meets his or her needs. The respiratory therapist must make sure that the patient knows the features of the device and can use it properly. Be prepared to recommend a change if needed. Aerosolized beta-agonist bronchodilators are usually recommended and given under one of the three following situations:

1. Acute bronchospasm with severe shortness of breath. This patient needs rapid relief. Recommend a fast-acting medication such as albuterol. The current asthma-management and COPD-management guidelines list albuterol and similar medications as "rescue" agents. Because these drugs tend to have a shorter duration of action, they can be referred to as short-acting beta-agonist (SABA) medications.

2. Chronic but stable bronchospasm with moderate shortness of breath. These patients need a dependable medication of longer duration such as salmeterol or formoterol. They are considered to be "controller" agents with a duration of 12-24 hours. Because of their longer duration, they can be called long-acting beta-agonist (LABA) medications. Several medications also come in oral preparations. The oral forms are especially helpful when taken in the evening to help the patient get a good night's sleep. It is very important that the patient also have a prescription for a fast-acting rescue drug in case of sudden bronchospasm.

3. Laryngeal edema or bleeding from a bronchoscopy biopsy site. The laryngeal edema problem requires the administration of a medication that reduces the swelling of the mucous membrane of the larynx and epiglottis. Laryngeal edema can result from a direct injury or irritation of the upper airway, such as postextubation edema or laryngotracheobronchitis (croup). In addition, if the patient has anaphylaxis from an allergic reaction, laryngeal edema and hypotension are often present. If bleeding results from a biopsy during a bronchoscopy, the cut blood vessels must be made to constrict and to form clots. In cases of laryngeal edema or biopsy bleeding, nebulized racemic epinephrine (MicroNefrin) is given because it stimulates α_1-receptors. This results in vasoconstriction of the mucosal and deeper blood vessels. Therefore the laryngeal edema swelling is reduced, and biopsy bleeding stops. In the case of anaphylaxis with hypotension and laryngeal edema, intravenous epinephrine is needed to treat both life-threatening problems.

Exam Hint 9-1

A fast-onset medication (albuterol [Proventil, Ventolin], levalbuterol [Xopenex]) is used to treat a patient with acute bronchospasm. A long-duration medication (salmeterol [Serevent] or formoterol [Foradil]) is used to treat a patient with chronic, stable bronchospasm. A vasoconstricting medication (racemic epinephrine [MicroNefrin, Nephron]) is used to treat airway edema or bleeding.

Exam Hint 9-2

The NBRC rarely asks questions about a specific drug dose. However, the following drug doses should be known. The standard adult dose of albuterol (AccuNeb) for an SVN is 0.5 mL (2.5 mg), three or four times a day. The standard adult dose of levalbuterol (Xopenex) for an SVN is 1.25 mg, three times a day.

5. Anticholinergic (parasympatholytic) agents

a. Recommend their use (code: IIIE4b) [difficulty: R, Ap, An]

As briefly described above, the cholinergic (parasympathetic) half of the autonomic nervous system regulates the cardiopulmonary system under normal circumstances. It maintains normal airway diameter, heart rate, and blood pressure. The anticholinergic (also called antimuscarinic) medications promote bronchodilation by suppressing the action of the cholinergic nervous system. This results in the sympathetic nervous system dominating and causing bronchial smooth muscle relaxation and bronchodilation. The anticholinergic medications have been found to be more effective in helping patients with COPD (emphysema and/or chronic bronchitis) than in helping patients with asthma. Be prepared to recommend an anticholinergic (or antimuscarinic) medication in COPD patients.

b. Administer the prescribed medication (code: IIID1, 2) [difficulty: R, Ap]

See Table 9-2 for information on the anticholinergic medications. The first generation of short-acting anticholinergic medications (featuring ipratropium bromide) last about 4-6 hours. The continued development of anticholinergic medications has resulted in long-acting anticholinergic (LAAC) drugs (featuring aclidinium bromide) that last 12 hours. Tiotropium bromide, a super LAAC drug, lasts 24 hours.

Many patients with COPD and asthma will be treated with a combination drug that includes a medication from both the sympathomimetic and the anticholinergic groups. Depending on the patient's ability to manage an SVN, MDI, or DPI, select the best medication and delivery device that meets his or her needs. The respiratory therapist must make sure that the patient knows the features of the device and can use it properly. Be prepared to recommend a change if needed.

6. Anti-inflammatory agents

a. Inhaled corticosteroids

1. Recommend their use (code: IIIE4c) [difficulty: R, Ap, An]

An inhaled corticosteroid (ICS) affects the respiratory system in two ways: it potentiates the effects of the beta-agonist agents and it stops the inflammatory response seen in the airways of asthmatic patients after exposure to an allergen. This prevents mucosal edema from developing. The patient with chronic airway edema, as seen with asthma or COPD, should be given an ICS. When an ICS is used as directed, relatively little systemic (bodily) absorption occurs. However, it is best to monitor the patient, especially small children taking ICS for an extended period, for any side effects. Current guidelines for asthma and COPD management classify ICS as controller medications. A patient taking an ICS should also be prescribed a SABA as a rescue medication.

The patient who is diagnosed with status asthmaticus should have systemic corticosteroids promptly administered by the intravenous (iv) route. Examples of commonly used systemic corticosteroids include methylprednisolone (Medrol and Solu-Medrol), prednisone (Hydeltrasol), prednisolone (Meticortelone and Delta-Cortef), cortisone (Cortone), and hydrocortisone (Cortef and Solu-Cortef). These drugs can be lifesavers if used properly. However, prolonged use of large oral or IV doses can lead to serious systemic complications including, but not limited to, immunosuppression, adrenal gland insufficiency, hyperglycemia, and osteoporosis. If a patient has been taking systemic corticosteroids for an extended time, he or she should be gradually weaned from them after an ICS has been started. It is dangerous to suddenly stop an oral or intravenous corticosteroid that has been used for a prolonged time.

2. Administer the prescribed medication (code: IIID1, 2) [difficulty: R, Ap]

Table 9-3 shows specific strength and dosage information for the ICS. In general, an ICS is taken twice a day at 12-hour intervals. Note that there are now four inhaled medications (Advair, Symbicort, Dulera, and Breo) that combine a corticosteroid and a LABA. The patient who is using any ICS medication must gargle and rinse out his or her mouth after each use. If not, the patient runs the risk of developing a fungal infection of the mouth and throat.

Note: Although past Written Registry Examinations have included a question concerning nonsteroidal anti-inflammatory drugs, they are not included in the current detailed content outline. They are included here for the sake of completeness. There are several different types of over-the-counter medications. None is as powerful an anti-inflammatory as the corticosteroid drugs. Note the other clinical uses of acetylsalicylic acid and ibuprofen:

- Acetylsalicylic acid (e.g., Bayer aspirin): anti-inflammatory, mild analgesia, antipyretic, blocks platelet aggregation (clot formation)
- Ibuprofen (Advil, Motrin): anti-inflammatory, mild analgesia, antipyretic
- Antihistamine (Claritin): anti-inflammatory

b. Cromolyn sodium

1. Recommend its use (code: IIIE4c) [difficulty: R, Ap, An]

Cromolyn sodium (Intal) is indicated to prevent an asthma attack. This is accomplished by coating the mast cells found in the airways so that they do not degranulate and rupture. Without pretreatment, the mast cells of asthmatic patients would rupture when exposed to immunoglobulin E (IgE) from their allergen(s). This mast cell rupture would result in the spilling of leukotriene agents, histamine, and other chemical mediators that cause the bronchospasm, airway edema, and increased airway secretions of an asthma attack.

2. Administer the prescribed medication (code: IIID1, 2) [difficulty: R, Ap]

When cromolyn sodium is taken at least 1 week before exposure to the allergen, the allergic reaction is prevented or reduced. The drug was first approved for the prevention of asthma. An SVN is used to aerosolize the liquid form. It is now also available as a nasal spray for allergic rhinitis and an oral solution to help control the gastrointestinal problems found with mastocytosis. See Table 9-4 for detailed information.

TABLE 9-3	Inhaled Corticosteroid Agents*	
Drug	**Brand Name(s)****	**Formulation and Dosage**
Long Acting		
Beclomethasone dipropionate hydrofluoroalkane	QVAR	MDI: 40 mcg/puff and 80 mcg/puff Adults ≥12 years: 40-80 mcg twice daily[†], or 40-160 mcg bid[‡] Children ≥5 years: 40-80 mcg twice daily
Budesonide	Pulmicort Turbuhaler	DPI: 200 mcg/actuation Adults: 200-400 mcg bid[†], 200-400 mcg bid[‡], 400-800 mcg bid[§] Children ≥6 years: 200 mcg bid, 400 mcg maximum dose
	Pulmicort Flexhaler	DPI: 90 mcg/actuation, 180 mcg/actuation Adults: 180-360 mcg bid usual dose range, 720 mcg bid maximum Children ≥6 years: 180 mcg bid usual dose, 360 mcg bid maximum
	Pulmicort Respules	SVN: 0.25 mg/2 mL, 0.5 mg/2 mL, 1 mg/ml Children 1-8 years: 0.5 mg total dose given once daily or twice daily in divided doses[†,‡]; 1 mg given as 0.5 mg bid or once daily[§]
Budesonide and formoterol fumarate HFA	Symbicort	MDI: 80 mcg budesonide with 4.5 mcg formoterol/actuation, 2 puffs bid; 160 mcg budesonide with 4.5 mcg formoterol/actuation Adults and children ≥12 years: 160 mcg budesonide and 9 mcg formoterol bid, 320 mcg budesonide and 9 mcg formoterol; maximum daily dose: 640 mcg budesonide and 18 mcg formoterol
Flunisolide hemihydrate HFA	Aerospan	MDI: 80 mcg/puff Adults ≥12 years: 2 puffs bid, adults no more than 4 puffs daily Children 6-11 years: 1 puff daily, no more than 2 puffs daily
Fluticasone propionate	Flovent HFA	MDI: 44 mcg/puff, 110 mcg/puff, 220 mcg/puff Adults ≥12 years: 88 mcg bid[†], 88-220 mcg bid[‡], or 880 mcg bid[§] Children 4-11 years: 88 mcg bid
	Flovent Diskus	DPI: 50, 100, 250 mcg Adults: 100 mcg bid[†], 100-250 mcg bid[‡], 1000 mcg bid[§] Children 4-11 years; 50 mcg twice daily
Fluticasone propionate and salmeterol	Advair Diskus	DPI: 100 mcg fluticasone/50 mcg salmeterol, 250 mcg fluticasone/50 mcg propionate/salmeterol, or 500 mcg fluticasone/50 mcg salmeterol Adults and children ≥12 years: 100 mcg fluticasone/50 mcg salmeterol, 1 inhalation twice daily, about 12 hours apart (starting dose if not currently on inhaled corticosteroids (ICS)) Maximum recommended dose 500 mcg fluticasone/50 mcg salmeterol bid Children ≥4 years: 100 mcg fluticasone/50 mcg salmeterol, 1 inhalation bid, about 12 hours apart (for those who are symptomatic while taking an ICS)
	Advair HFA	MDI: 45 mcg fluticasone/21 mcg salmeterol, 115 mcg fluticasone/21 mcg salmeterol, or 230 mcg fluticasone/21 mcg salmeterol Adults and children ≥12 years: 2 inhalations bid, about 12 hours apart
Ciclesonide	Alvesco	MDI: 40 mcg/puff, 80 mcg/puff Adults and children ≥12 years: 80-160 mcg bid[†], 80-320 mcg bid[‡]
Ultralong Acting		
Mometasone furoate and formoterol fumarate HFA	Dulera	MDI: 100 mcg mometasone and 5 mcg formoterol, 200 mcg mometasone and 5 mcg formoterol Adults and children 12 years: ≤400 mcg mometasone and 20 mcg formoterol daily if previously on a medium dose of corticosteroids; ≤800 mcg mometasone and 20 mcg formoterol daily if previously on a high dose of corticosteroids
Mometasone furoate	Asmanex Twisthaler	DPI: 110 mcg/actuation, 220 mcg/actuation Adults and children ≥12 years: 220-880 mcg daily Children 4-11 years: 110 mcg daily
Ultralong Acting with a Beta Agonist		
Fluticasone and vilanterol	Breo	DPI: 100 mcg fluticasone and 25 mcg vilanterol per actuation, 1 puff daily

bid, twice daily; tid, three times daily; qid, four times daily; SVN, small-volume nebulizer; MDI, metered-dose inhaler; DPI, dry powder inhaler; mg, milligram (1/1000 g); mcg, microgram (1/1000 mg—*Note:* The abbreviation µg may be used instead of mcg).

A valved holding chamber is recommended with MDI administration to prevent accidental eye exposure.

*Detailed prescribing information should be obtained from the manufacturer's package insert.

**Lists of brand names may not be current owing to frequent additions and deletions by manufacturers.

[†]Recommended starting dose if on bronchodilators alone.

[‡]Recommended starting dose if on ICS previously.

[§]Recommended starting dose if on oral corticosteroids previously.

Modified from Gardenhire DS: Rau's respiratory care pharmacology, ed 8, St Louis, 2012, Mosby.

It is very important to understand that the drug is taken *only* for prophylactic purposes to prevent an asthma attack. It is contraindicated during an asthma attack. A patient experiencing acute bronchospasm should be treated with a fast-onset beta-adrenergic bronchodilator, as previously discussed.

c. Recommend the use of leukotriene modifiers (code: IIIE4c) [difficulty: R, Ap, An]

Leukotrienes are chemicals found in airway mast cells that are released during an asthma attack. These released leukotriene chemicals stimulate bronchospasm, airway edema, and increased airway secretions. The leukotriene-modifier medications (also called leukotriene antagonists) work to reduce the number of leukotriene chemicals that are released or to block the effects of leukotrienes on the airways. By accomplishing this, the patient's asthma symptoms are reduced or eliminated. See Table 9-4 for detailed information on the medications in this group.

As with cromolyn sodium, it is very important to understand that all of these drugs are taken *only* for prophylactic purposes to prevent an asthma attack. They are contraindicated during an asthma attack. A patient experiencing acute bronchospasm should be treated with a fast-onset beta-adrenergic bronchodilator, as previously discussed.

d. Recommend the use of a monoclonal antibody (code: IIIE4c) [difficulty: R, Ap, An]

As presented above, the leukotriene chemicals that are released from mast cells during an asthma attack will cause bronchospasm, airway edema, and secretions. This leukotriene release is caused when sensitized IgE binds to mast cells and causes their rupture. The monoclonal antibody medication omalizumab (Xolair) binds to the IgE so that it cannot adhere to the mast cells. Therefore, the mast cells are stable and do not rupture. Xolair has been approved for older children and adults with uncontrolled moderate to severe asthma. It is given by subcutaneous injection every 4 weeks. In some patients, the use of Xolair may allow for a reduction in high-dose corticosteroids and rescue-type medications. It is very important to understand that this drug is taken *only* for prophylactic purposes to prevent an asthma attack. It is contraindicated during an asthma attack. A patient experiencing acute bronchospasm should be treated with a fast-onset beta-adrenergic bronchodilator, as previously discussed.

TABLE 9-4	Inhaled Nonsteroidal Antiasthma Agents*	
Drug	**Brand Name(s)****	**Formulation and Dosage**
Cromolyn-Like (Mast Cell Stabilizers)		
Cromolyn sodium	Intal inhalation solution	SVN: 20 mg/amp or 20 mg/vial Adults and children ≥2 years: 20 mg inhaled 4 times daily
	Nasalcrom	Spray: 40 mg/mL (4%), gives 5.2 mg of drug Adults and children ≥2 years: 1 spray each nostril, 3-6 times daily every 4-6 hours
	Gastrocrom	Oral concentrate: 100 mg/5 mL Adults and children ≥13 years: 2 ampules qid, 30 minutes before a meal and at bedtime Children 2-12 years: 1 ampule qid, 30 minutes before a meal and at bedtime
Antileukotrienes		
Montelukast	Singulair	Tablets: 10, 4, and 5 mg cherry-flavored chewable; 4-mg packet of granules Adults and children ≥15 years: one 10-mg tablet daily in evening Children 6-14 years: one 5-mg chewable tablet daily Children 2-5 years: one 4-mg chewable tablet or one 4-mg packet of granules daily Children 6-23 months: one 4-mg packet of granules daily
Zafirlukast	Accolate	Tablets: 10 and 20 mg Adults and children ≥12 years: 20 mg (1 tablet) bid, without food Children 5-11 years: 10 mg bid
Zileuton	Zyflo, Zyflo CR	Tablets: 600 mg Adults and children ≥12 years: one 600-mg tablet qid. CR: 2 tablets bid, within 1 hour of morning and evening meals
Monoclonal Antibody		
Omalizumab	Xolair	Adults and children ≥12 years: subcutaneous injection every 4 weeks; dose dependent on patient's weight and serum IgE level

bid, twice daily; qid, four times daily; SVN, small-volume nebulizer; mg, milligram (1/1000 g).
*Detailed prescribing information should be obtained from the manufacturer's package insert.
**Lists of brand names may not be current owing to frequent additions and deletions by manufacturers.
Modified from Gardenhire DS: Rau's respiratory care pharmacology, ed 8, St Louis, 2012, Mosby.

7. Mucolytic or proteolytic agents

a. Acetylcysteine

1. Recommend its use (code: IIIE4d) [difficulty: R, Ap, An]

N-acetylcysteine/acetylcysteine/NAC (Mucomyst, Mucosil) is a mucolytic drug that has been widely used for many years with patients who have thick (viscous) mucus or mucus plugs. However, its use for the mucolytic effect is now controversial and some authors have advocated for the discontinuation of its clinical use. In the past, the NBRC has included questions about when acetylcysteine (Mucomyst) would be indicated as a mucolytic.

Know that there are two clinical concerns with this medication. Acetylcysteine has a bad odor (rotten eggs) that may lead to nausea and vomiting in some patients. Of greater concern is the stimulation of bronchospasm in some asthmatic patients. Therefore it is wise to pretreat these patients with a fast-onset aerosolized beta-adrenergic bronchodilator before acetylcysteine is nebulized. Because of the lack of proven clinical effectiveness and the noted hazards, acetylcysteine is no longer recommended in patients with cystic fibrosis. It may still be used with chronic bronchitis patients as long as the noted precautions are taken.

2. Administer the prescribed medication (code: IIID1, 2) [difficulty: R, Ap]

Mucomyst is usually administered with an SVN or with intermittent positive-pressure breathing (IPPB). Most adult patients are given up to 3-5 mL of the 10% or 20% solution. The 20% solution is often diluted with an equal volume of normal saline solution. Direct instillation of 1-2 mL of the drug into the trachea has been used to liquefy secretions. The manufacturer recommends that all medication in a vial be used within 96 hours or discarded. It should be stored in the refrigerator. A slightly purple color is commonly seen after the vial has been opened, but it can still be used safely. See Table 9-5 for specific information.

b. Deoxyribonuclease

1. Recommend its use (code: IIIE4d) [difficulty: R, Ap, An]

Dornase alfa (Pulmozyme) is a proteolytic drug that has been approved for use in the treatment of patients with cystic fibrosis. It works by breaking up strands of DNA found in the secretions of these patients with a pulmonary infection. (*Note:* The NBRC refers to this drug as recombinant human deoxyribonuclease.)

2. Administer the prescribed medication (code: IIID1, 2) [difficulty: R, Ap]

Usually a single daily dose of 2.5 mL of solution (containing 2.5 mg of dornase alfa) is inhaled by SVN. Store the drug in a refrigerator, and protect it from strong light. It has no serious side effects. See Table 9-5 for detailed information.

c. Hypertonic saline

1. Recommend its use (code: IIIG4c) [difficulty: R, Ap, An]

The various saline solutions (and sterile water) are known collectively as "bland" aerosols, because they have no direct pharmacologic effect on the lungs and airways. When they are inhaled as aerosols, however, a vagal nerve-mediated reflex causes the bronchial/submucosal glands to release more watery secretions. Therefore a saline aerosol is commonly used to help liquefy secretions and induce a patient to expel sputum. See Chapter 8 for the discussion on the use of hypertonic saline for an induced sputum procedure. Recent clinical experience has shown hypertonic saline to be an effective mucolytic in cystic fibrosis patients.

2. Administer the prescribed medication (code: IIID1, 2) [difficulty: R, Ap]

The various saline solutions are given through an SVN or IPPB treatment or, more commonly, mixed with a bronchodilator medication. See Table 9-5 and Box 9-2 for information on the various saline solutions.

d. Observe the patient to assess cough, sputum amount, and characteristics (code: IB2c) [difficulty: R, Ap, An]

The respiratory therapist should objectively evaluate the patient's cough and sputum production before and after a mucolytic has been administered. This will provide evidence of the medication's effectiveness. See Chapter 1 for further discussion and Table 1-12 for sputum characteristics.

TABLE 9-5	Inhaled Mucoactive Agents*		
Drug	**Brand Name(s)****	**Adult Dosage**	**Use**
N-acetylcysteine	10%, 20% Mucomyst	SVN: 3-5 mL	Bronchitis; efficacy not proven
Saline solutions: 0.45%, 0.9%, 5%-10%	Hyper-Sal (7% solution)	SVN: 3-5 mL, as ordered. USN: 3-5 mL, as ordered.	Sputum induction, secretion mobilization
Dornase alfa	Pulmozyme	SVN: 2.5 mg/ampule, one ampule daily	Cystic fibrosis

SVN, small-volume nebulizer; USN, ultrasonic nebulizer; mg, milligram (1/1000 g).
*Detailed prescribing information should be obtained from the manufacturer's package insert.
**Lists of brand names may not be current owing to frequent additions and deletions by manufacturers.
Modified from Gardenhire DS: Rau's respiratory care pharmacology, ed 8, St Louis, 2012, Mosby.

BOX 9-2 Saline Solutions Used as Mucolytics

Normal Saline Solution, 0.9% Saline
Direct instillation into the airway:
- Infants may be given about 1 mL before airway suctioning.*
- Adults may be given several milliliters before airway suctioning.*

Aerosol: Most medication nebulizers hold 3-5 mL that are nebulized several times daily.

Miscellaneous:
- Usually is well tolerated because it is isotonic to the body.
- Particle size is fairly stable as nebulized.

Hypotonic Saline Solution, 0.45% Saline
Direct instillation into the airway: Same as with normal saline solution.

Aerosol: Same as with normal saline solution; many practitioners use this concentration in ultrasonic nebulizers.

Miscellaneous: Particles tend to shrink because of evaporation, which results in smaller particles than nebulized that are closer to isotonic; impaction is more likely in the smaller airways.

Hypertonic Saline Solution, 1.8%-10% Saline
Aerosol: Some practitioners use a large-reservoir nebulizer with a heater to generate the aerosol. Hypertonic saline solution is most commonly used to induce a cough and sputum sample for cytologic studies (e.g., lung cancer) or for fungal or mycobacterial (e.g., tuberculosis) culture. It should not be used for a general bacterial culture because the high salt concentration inhibits the growth of most bacteria. Hypertonic saline has also been found useful as a mucolytic in cystic fibrosis patients.

Miscellaneous: Particles tend to enlarge because of the absorption of water vapor, which results in larger particles than nebulized that are closer to isotonic; impaction is more likely in the upper airway. This concentration is the most likely to cause bronchospasm in asthma patients because it is the furthest from isotonic and, therefore, the most irritating. It may be necessary to pretreat the patient with a SABA bronchodilator.

*Saline should *not* be routinely instilled into the patient's tracheal tube. See Chapter 13 for the suctioning procedure.

8. Antimicrobials

a. Recommend the use of antimicrobials (code: IIIE4f) [difficulty: R, Ap]

The terms antimicrobial, anti-infective, and antibiotic refer to natural or synthetic chemicals that are toxic to bacteria and other microorganisms. Table 9-6 lists the most commonly found respiratory tract pathogens. See Table 9-7 for a summary of the antimicrobial agents used against them. Table 9-8 lists specific information on the five currently approved aerosolized antimicrobial agents given by respiratory therapists and likely to be tested by the NBRC. They are discussed below. Be aware that other systemic antimicrobial medications have been given by aerosol despite not having FDA approval.

b. Administer the prescribed medication (code: IIID1, 2) [difficulty: R, Ap]

1. Antibacterial agents: tobramycin, aztreonam

Tobramycin (TOBI) and aztreonam (Cayston) are used to control chronic pulmonary infection with the gram-negative bacteria *Pseudomonas aeruginosa*. The currently approved treatment course involves either drug being taken for 28 days. The patient then discontinues the medication for 28 days. This treatment cycle has been shown to control the infection without antibiotic resistance developing.

TOBI has been approved for use in children 6 years and older with cystic fibrosis. It is taken through the PARI LC Plus SVN. No other medications are to be mixed with the TOBI in the nebulizer.

Cayston has been approved for use in children ≥7 years with cystic fibrosis. Because of the risk of an allergic reaction to the drug and bronchospasm, all patients should have a pulmonary function screen done before its start. The patient should be given a fast-onset beta-adrenergic

TABLE 9-6 Common Respiratory Pathogens in Approximate Order of Frequency

	Gram Positive	Gram Negative	Cell Wall Deficient
Bacteria	Streptococcus pneumoniae	Haemophilus influenzae	Mycoplasma
	Staphylococcus aureus*	Klebsiella pneumoniae	ACID-FAST
	Streptococcus faecalis (Enterococcus)	Pseudomonas aeruginosa*	Mycobacterium tuberculosis*
		Serratia species*	
Viruses	Rhinovirus	Varicella virus*	
	Adenovirus	Herpes simplex virus*	
	Respiratory syncytial virus	Cytomegalovirus*	
Fungi	Candida albicans*	Histoplasma capsulatum	
	Aspergillus species*	(Ohio Valley)	
	Pneumocystis carinii	Coccidioides immitis (Southwest U.S.)	
Protozoa	Toxoplasma gondii*		
	Cryptosporidium*		

*Seen most frequently in debilitated or immunosuppressed hosts.

TABLE 9-7 Classification of Antibiotic Agents Commonly Used against Pulmonary Infections

Class or Group	Agents	Spectrum	Major Toxicity
Aminoglycosides	Streptomycin	Primarily tuberculostatic	Vestibular, renal
	Tobramycin, TOBI aztreonam, Cayston	*Pseudomonas aeruginosa* lung	Auditory, renal infection in cystic fibrosis patients
	Gentamicin, Garamycin	Gram-negative rods, including *Pseudomonas* and *Proteus*	Vestibular, renal
Antifungal agents	Ketoconazole, Nizoral	Major agent for systemic fungal disease	Gastrointestinal upset
	Amphotericin B	Major agent for systemic fungal disease	Renal, gastrointestinal
Antituberculosis agents	Isonicotinic acid hydrazide, Isoniazid	Used for both prophylaxis and treatment	Hepatic
	Ethambutol, rifampin	Used for tuberculostatic therapy	Retinal (maculopathy), hepatic
Antiviral agents	AZT, Retrovir	Stops reproduction in retroviruses; used against HIV	Anemia
	ribavirin, Virazole	Same spectrum, used against respiratory syncytial virus; experimental against HIV	
Cephalosporin	Cephalothin, Keflin, Cephalexin	Like penicillin, with antistaphylococcal effects	Renal (usually not severe)
Chloramphenicol	Chloromycetin	Broad spectrum; used for *Haemophilus* if it is ampicillin resistant or if patient is allergic	Bone marrow
Macrolide	Erythromycin, Erythrocin	Like penicillin (used in penicillin allergy); drug of choice for *Mycoplasma*	Gastrointestinal
Penicillin	Penicillin G	Gram-positive organisms; *Staphylococcus aureus* often resistant	Allergy
Semisynthetic penicillins	Ampicillin, Omnipen, Amoxicillin	Gram-positive organisms, gram-negative *Haemophilus influenzae*; variable against gram-negative rods	Diarrhea and rash, especially with viral disease (mononucleosis)
	Oxacillin, Prostaphlin	Like penicillin, with antistaphylococcal effects	Allergy
	Geopen	Like penicillin, with antipseudomonas effects	Sodium overload-congestive failure
Sulfonamides	Pentamidine isethionate	Prophylaxis against *Pneumocystis*	Impaired renal and liver function
	NebuPent, Pentam 300; trimethoprim and sulfamethoxazole, Bactrim	Used against *Pneumocystis carinii*	Impaired renal and liver function
Tetracyclines	Tetracycline, Achromycin	Broad spectrum; useful against Haemophilus and Mycoplasma infections	Fungal overgrowth in bowel or vagina; hepatic with large IV doses

TABLE 9-8 Inhaled Antimicrobial Agents*

Drug	Brand Name	Adult Dosage	Use
Pentamidine isethionate	NebuPent	SVN†: 300 mg of powder in 6 mL of sterile water; once every 4 weeks	Prophylaxis against *Pneumocystis carinii* pneumonia
Ribavirin	Virazole	SPAG‡: 6 mg of powder in 300 mL of sterile water (20 mg/mL solution); given for 12-18 h/day for 3-7 days	Respiratory syncytial virus
Tobramycin	TOBI	SVN§: 300 mg/5 mL ampule, bid, 28 days on and 28 days off drug DPI¶: Four 28 mg capsules inhaled bid, 28 days on and 28 days off drug	*Pseudomonas aeruginosa* in cystic fibrosis patients
Aztreonam	Cayston	SVN§§: 75 mg/vial, tid, 28 days on and 28 days off drug	*P. aeruginosa* in cystic fibrosis patients
Zanamivir	Relenza	DPI: 5 mg/inhalation Adults and children ≥5 years for prophylaxis; ≥7 years for treatment: 2 inhalations (one 5-mg blister per inhalation) bid about 12 hours apart for 5 days	Influenza

bid, twice daily; DPI, dry powder inhaler; SVN, small-volume nebulizer.
*Detailed prescribing information should be obtained from the manufacturer's package insert.
†NebuPent is used only with the Respirgard II SVN.
‡Virazole is used only with the SPAG (small-particle aerosol generator) nebulizer.
§TOBI is used with an approved nebulizer system, including PARI LC Jet Plus, Hudson T Updraft II, and Marquest II.
¶TOBI Podhaler is used to deliver the dry powder medication.
§§Cayston is used with an approved Altera nebulizer system.
Modified from Gardenhire DS: Rau's respiratory care pharmacology, ed 7, St Louis, 2008, Mosby.

bronchodilator before taking Cayston. The drug is then aerosolized in the Altera Nebulizer System. Carefully monitor the patient's breath sounds and vital signs for signs of an allergic reaction during the first treatment. If the patient has difficulty breathing, stop the treatment and notify the physician.

2. Antiviral agents: zanamivir and ribavirin

Zanamivir (Relenza) is approved for the treatment of influenza in adults and children older than 5 years of age. To be effective, Relenza must be started within the first 2 days of symptoms and continued for 5 days. If taken early enough in the course of the infection, the patient's symptoms should be reduced and the course of the infection shortened. Relenza is available in a multidose DPI packet. The medication packet is loaded into the Diskhaler delivery device for inhalation (see Fig. 8-23 in Chapter 8).

Ribavirin (Virazole) is most commonly used in the treatment of infants and young children who have bronchiolitis or pneumonia from the respiratory syncytial virus (RSV). Patients requiring treatment for their condition usually are very sick and have complicating factors such as prematurity or cardiopulmonary disease. They require the treatment course of 3-7 days of nebulization of the drug for 12-18 hours per day. Only the small-particle aerosol generator can be used for the procedure. This is because it is specifically designed to nebulize the 1- to 2-mm-size particles necessary for alveoli penetration so that it can kill the virus. Virazole is also known to be effective against influenza types A and B and the herpes simplex virus. Because of the risk of side effects to health care providers, a scavenging system must be used with Vibrazole to ensure that none of the particles escape into room air.

3. Antiprotozoal agent: pentamidine isethionate

Pentamidine isethionate (NebuPent) has been approved for the prophylactic treatment of the protozoal organism *Pneumocystis carinii*. Patients with an impaired immune system, such as those with acquired immunodeficiency syndrome (AIDS) or organ transplant recipients, are most likely to suffer from *P. carinii* pneumonia. (*Note:* This may also be called *Pneumocystis jiroveci* pneumonia.) Currently, these patients are given a single 300-mg dose of NebuPent mixed with 6 mL of sterile water once every 4 weeks through the Respirgard II SVN. This unit also features an expiratory scavenging filter to prevent any droplets from entering the room air (see Fig. 8-17 in Chapter 8).

Some patients must be pretreated with an inhaled bronchodilator to prevent bronchospasm before the NebuPent is inhaled. Do not mix the two medications in the Respirgard II or use the Respirgard II for any medication other than NebuPent. Mixing NebuPent with normal saline or a bronchodilator can result in a precipitation of the medications. When given by the inhalation route, there are few systemic side effects. There is also an intramuscular or intravenous form of pentamidine called Pentam 300. Bactrim (trimethoprim and sulfamethoxazole) is preferred over systemic pentamidine because there are fewer and less serious side effects.

Exam Hint 9-3

There is usually one question that considers the need for an antimicrobial medication to treat a pulmonary infection. Know these antimicrobial agents and what they are used to treat:

- Penicillin (e.g., penicillin G, ampicillin) to treat gram-positive bacteria
- Gentamicin (Garamycin) to treat gram-negative bacteria
- Isoniazid (INH) to treat *Mycobacterium tuberculosis*
- Aerosolized TOBI or aztreonam (Cayston) to treat *Pseudomonas* pneumonia in children with cystic fibrosis
- Aerosolized pentamidine isethionate (NebuPent) for prophylactic treatment of *P. carinii*
- Aerosolized ribavirin (Vibrazole) to treat RSV in young children

---

9. Pulmonary vasodilators

a. Recommend pulmonary vasodilators (code: IIIE4a) [difficulty: R, Ap]

Pulmonary vasodilators are often indicated in the treatment of pulmonary artery hypertension (PAH). The pathologic effects of PAH include vasoconstriction, proliferation of blood vessels, narrowing and remodeling of small pulmonary arteries, and thrombosis of small pulmonary arteries. These vascular changes result in increased pulmonary artery pressure and increased pulmonary vascular resistance (PVR), which results in right-ventricular failure (see Chapter 5 for more discussion.) A diagnosis of persistent pulmonary hypertension of the newborn (PPHN) is often given to a newborn with PAH. Causes of PPHN include respiratory distress syndrome (RDS) in a premature neonate, meconium aspiration syndrome, pneumonia, sepsis, pulmonary hypoplasia, congenital diaphragmatic hernia, and some congenital heart defects. If PVR is high enough, pulmonary blood flow will be diverted through the ductus arteriosus and foramen ovale. This will result in the return to fetal circulation and systemic hypoxemia.

Common causes of PAH in an adult are sleep-disordered breathing and COPD. It is critically important to prevent the chronic hypoxemia caused by those conditions to reduce the patient's pulmonary artery pressure. Some adult patients have idiopathic PAH, meaning that the cause is unknown. Failure to control an adult's PAH will necessitate lung transplantation to avoid an early death.

A wide variety of medical therapies are available to treat the complex causes of PAH. It is beyond the scope of this text to present the wide variety of biochemical pathways of these medications. The following are current FDA-approved medications and routes of administration:

1. Supplemental oxygen

Supplemental oxygen (up to 100%) is indicated to keep the PaO_2 >60 torr and SaO_2 or SpO_2 >90%. A patient with COPD or obstructive sleep apnea should be using supplemental oxygen to prevent hypoxemia.

2. Oral medications

1. Sildenafil (Viagra, Revatio) has been shown to be effective in adults with PAH and infants with PPHN. In addition, sildenafil has been shown to prevent rebound PAH in infants with PPHN when inhaled nitric oxide (INOmax) has been stopped.
2. Calcium channel blockers such as oral diltiazem (Verapamil) are first-line medications in patients with mild PAH.
3. The endothelin receptor antagonist tracleer (Bosentan) has also been approved for PAH. Because of the risk of hepatic toxicity, liver function tests must be performed monthly.

3. Intravenous or subcutaneous medications

1. Calcium channel blockers such as diltiazem (Cardizem, Cartia, Diltia) and nifedipine (Nifedical, Procardia) can be given as an intravenous bolus, if needed. Once the hypertensive crisis has been controlled, the patient is converted to an oral medication.
2. Epoprostenol (Veletri) is taken once a week by way of a permanent intravenous catheter.
3. Treprostinil (Remodulin) or epoprostenol (Flolan) must be given by continuous intravenous drip to patients with the most serious cases of PAH.
4. Treprostinil (Remodulin) has been approved for continuous subcutaneous infusion with a pump. This option gives the patient full mobility.
5. Iloprost (Ilomedine) is taken every 8-12 weeks by intravenous catheter.

4. Inhaled medications

1. INOmax has been approved for the treatment of term and near-term (>34 weeks gestational age) neonates with hypoxic respiratory failure associated with PAH. The INOmax can be given continuously through a nasal cannula, a continuous positive airway pressure system, or a mechanical ventilator.
2. Iloprost (Ventavis) has been approved for inhalation six to nine times per day at intervals of no less than two hours. The inhaled solution is aerosolized through either the I-Neb AAD or the Prodose AAD system.
3. Treprostinil (Tyvaso) has been approved for inhalation four times per day at approximately four-hour intervals while awake. The aerosolized solution is taken by way of the Tyvaso Inhalation System.

b. Administer INOmax (code: IIID4) [difficulty: R, Ap]

See Chapter 16 for the discussion on administering INOmax.

Exam Hint 9-4

The NBRC specifically lists sildenafil (Viagra, Revatio), prostacyclin agents (treprostinil [Remodulin, Tyvaso], iloprost [Ventavis], epoprostenol [Flolan, Veletri]), and INOmax as pulmonary vasodilators.

MODULE B

Therapist-recommended medications

1. Recommend the use of theophylline (code: IIIE4b) [difficulty: R, Ap, An]

The family of drugs called xanthines includes theophylline and caffeine. Historically, theophylline was used as a bronchodilator agent in patients with asthma and COPD. Current asthma and COPD guidelines recommend that theophylline *not* be used during an exacerbation of either disease. Instead, beta-agonist, anticholinergic, and corticosteroid medications should be used. Rarely, a xanthine agent (intravenous Aminophylline, oral Elixophyllin) is used to aid the breathing of an asthma or COPD patient when the other bronchodilator medications have not been able to manage the patient's problem. Xanthine agents should be used with great caution because it is very difficult to regulate the proper serum level. Serious side effects of a high xanthine level include central nervous system stimulation, nausea and vomiting, tachycardia, tachypnea, and diuresis.

Caffeine citrate (Cafcit) has been approved for oral or intravenous administration to a neonate with apnea of prematurity. The physician may also choose to give Aminophylline for the same purpose. Both have been shown to stimulate the breathing of neonates with apnea. In most cases, as the child's central nervous system matures, breathing is properly regulated and caffeine administration can be discontinued.

2. Recommend a surfactant agent (code: IIIE4k) [difficulty: R, Ap]

Exogenous surfactant has been approved by the FDA for the prevention or treatment of infant RDS in premature neonates. These neonates have immature lungs that lack natural surfactant. As a result, atelectasis develops. Surfactant has also been successfully used to treat infants with meconium aspiration syndrome, pulmonary hemorrhage, and pneumonia. These four surfactant agents have been approved for instillation into the airways:

1. Beractant (Survanta) is a bovine lung extract.
2. Poractant alfa (Curosurf) is a pig lung extract.
3. Calfactant (Infasurf) is a bovine lung extract.

4. Lucinactant (Surfaxin) is a synthetic form of surfactant.

The 2013 American Association for Respiratory Care clinical practice guideline on surfactant replacement therapy updated its 1994 guideline. See the 2013 document for additional information to support these recommendations:

1. Surfactant replacement therapy should be performed by qualified personnel with the proper intubation and resuscitation equipment.
2. Prophylactic surfactant is recommended when a neonate with RDS is suspected of having a surfactant deficiency.
3. Therapeutic or rescue surfactant is highly recommended after a neonate with RDS has been intubated and placed onto a mechanical ventilator.
4. Multiple doses of surfactant should be given rather than a single dosage.
5. At this time, naturally derived forms of surfactant are recommended over the synthetic form.
6. Surfactant should not be delivered by aerosol.

Dosages for all of the medications are based on the infant's weight. Once one of them is instilled into the neonate's airways, be prepared to make rapid changes in the mechanical ventilator settings. This is because the lungs will rapidly become more compliant. The set pressure will need to be reduced so that the neonate is not overventilated, resulting in barotrauma. In addition, the oxygen percentage can usually be rapidly reduced.

3. Diuretics

a. Recommend the adjustment of fluid balance (code: IIIE2c) [difficulty: R, Ap]

A patient who is fluid overloaded or has congestive heart failure and pulmonary edema will often exhibit the following signs: peripheral edema, jugular vein distension, crackles for breath sounds, cyanosis, tachycardia, and hypotension. Arterial blood gas results will show hypoxemia. A chest radiograph will show an enlarged heart and pulmonary infiltrates. Shortness of breath is the most common symptom.

Treatment of the patient will include fluid restriction and diuresis to rapidly decrease the patient's fluid volume. Review Box 1-1 in Chapter 1 for normal fluid intake and output values.

b. Recommend a diuretic (code: IIIG4j) [difficulty: R, Ap]

Diuretics are most commonly indicated in patients who are fluid overloaded or have hypertension. The following are examples of diuretics commonly used to treat these problems:

- Furosemide (Lasix)
- Bumetanide (Bumex)
- Torsemide (Demadex)
- Chlorothiazide (Diuril)

These are some of the most powerful diuretics in use. They produce a rapid increase in urine output. They basically prevent the kidneys from retaining sodium so that water is excreted. A side effect of their use is a loss of potassium through the kidneys.

Another category of diuretic is used in patients who have an increased intracranial pressure (ICP). The increased ICP is usually attributable to cerebral edema from a head injury. Examples of medications used to treat an increased ICP include the following:

- Mannitol (Osmitrol)
- Sterile urea (Ureaphil, Urevert)

These medications have a high molecular weight and, through osmosis, "pull" fluid from the brain into the bloodstream. Therefore they are sometimes called osmotic diuretics. The medication, after crossing into the kidney, prevents the reabsorption of water and increases urine output.

c. Evaluate data in the patient record for electrolytes (code: IA4) [difficulty: R, Ap]

If a patient with fluid overload has been given a diuretic such as Lasix, all electrolytes, especially the serum potassium level, should be checked regularly. Lasix and related diuretic medications cause the kidneys to excrete potassium in addition to sodium and water. The so-called potassium-sparing diuretics (e.g., spironolactone [Aldactone], amiloride [Midamor], triamterene [Dyrenium]) can lead to an increased potassium level. (Review Table 1-4 in Chapter 1 for the normal electrolyte values.)

d. Recommend a blood test for electrolytes (code: IE2) [difficulty: R, Ap]

If a patient has been given a diuretic, such as Lasix, his or her serum electrolyte values should be regularly measured. The normal value for serum potassium (K+) is 3.5-5.5 mEq/L. A potassium level of less than 3.5 mEq/L is dangerous because it increases the risk of cardiac arrhythmias such as premature ventricular contractions. Replacement potassium is needed. It is usually given by the intravenous route because that is faster than when taken orally.

Be prepared to recommend the administration of any electrolyte that is less than the low end of the range. Conversely, be prepared to recommend withholding an electrolyte supplement if the serum level is greater than the upper end of the range.

Exam Hint 9-5

There will usually be at least one question about (1) recommending the use of a diuretic in a patient who is fluid overloaded or (2) the side effects of using a diuretic. A diuretic drug such as furosemide (Lasix) tends to cause the loss of potassium through the kidneys. Know to check the serum potassium level. Remember that the normal potassium level is 3.5-5.5 mEq/L. If the patient has the signs of dangerous hypokalemia (see Chapter 1), know to recommend that replacement potassium be given.

4. Recommend a sedative or hypnotic (code: IIIE4g) [difficulty: R, Ap]

Sedatives and hypnotics are medications that affect the brain to induce calming in a patient who can be either simply anxious or very agitated and uncooperative. A patient would be given a sedative in the following situations: (1) when he or she is struggling against a necessary intubation or the mechanical ventilator, thus worsening his or her condition; (2) when he or she is displaying self-destructive behavior because of a drug reaction; and (3) before a medical procedure, like bronchoscopy, for so-called conscious sedation. The effects on the patient are dose related. Low to moderate doses sedate (calm) the patient, and higher doses induce sleep (hypnosis). Three different groupings of these types of medications exist. The most widely used are the benzodiazepines, because they have fewer side effects and fewer drug interactions and are less likely to cause addiction than are the barbiturate drugs. The benzodiazepine agents can be pharmacologically reversed. The barbiturates are widely used during general anesthesia to induce sleep rapidly. Commonly used examples of the sedative/hypnotic agents include the following:

- Benzodiazepine minor tranquilizers: midazolam (Versed), diazepam (Valium), lorazepam (Ativan), chlordiazepoxide (Librium), alprazolam (Xanax), triazolam (Halcion), flurazepam (Dalmane)
- Nonbarbiturate sedative–hypnotics: meprobamate (Miltown), glutethimide (Doriden), chloral hydrate (Noctec)
- Barbiturate sedative–hypnotics: pentobarbital sodium (Nembutal), secobarbital sodium (Seconal), phenobarbital (Luminol), thiopental sodium (Pentothal)
- The intravenous anesthetic agents propofol (Diprivan) and dexmedetomidine HCl (Precedex) are also used for procedural sedation and to sedate a patient receiving mechanical ventilation

The benzodiazepine antagonist drug flumazenil (Romazicon) is indicated in the reversal of benzodiazepine agents such as Valium and Librium. Unconscious patients usually awaken quickly once the proper dose of flumazenil is given. Monitor the patient for signs of seizure activity related to the rapid reversal of the benzodiazepine medication. The patient should be observed for 2 hours in case resedation occurs. In this case, flumazenil can be readministered.

5. Recommend an analgesic (code: IIIE4h) [difficulty: R, Ap]

Analgesics are medications that control or block pain after an injury or a surgical procedure. Morphine or similar narcotic-type analgesic drugs are indicated to control moderate to severe pain. Morphine also is indicated to treat the pain of a myocardial infarction and to produce vasodilation in the patient with pulmonary edema. Additionally, pain-relieving agents, when given in large enough doses, will sedate or induce sleep. The patient who is both in pain and agitated may be treated with a combination of an analgesic and a sedative (e.g., moderate doses of morphine and diazepam). The two drugs potentiate each other. The physician may instead decide to give the patient a larger dose of morphine rather than both drug types. Examples of commonly used analgesics include the following:

- Morphine sulfate (MS, Duramorph) injection; Oramorph SR, tablets
- Tylenol with codeine tablets
- Oxycodone (Percocet, OxyContin)
- Hydrocodone (Vicodin)
- Hydromorphone (Dilaudid)
- Meperidine (Demerol)
- Propoxyphene (Darvon)

Patients receiving sedatives or analgesics, or both, must be closely monitored. Each type of medication can cause respiratory center depression if given in great enough doses. The patient may hypoventilate and even experience apnea and death. It is especially important to monitor a patient with COPD who is given morphine for the off-label management of dyspnea. Narcotic analgesic agents (e.g., morphine) and some other analgesic medications can become habit-forming or addictive if used for a prolonged period.

The narcotic antagonist drug naloxone (Narcan) counteracts the effects of narcotic agents such as morphine, heroin, and codeine. It can be given intravenously or intranasally for absorption by the mucous membranes. Narcan does not reverse benzodiazepine or barbiturate drugs. (Give flumazenil (Romazicon) to reverse the benzodiazepine drugs.) Remember that the patient who was given an accidental overdose of morphine to control pain will feel pain again when Narcan is administered.

Exam Hint 9-6

There is usually a question about recommending a drug for pain control. If the patient has severe pain from trauma or surgery, recommend morphine sulfate or a similar narcotic analgesic agent. Remember that too much narcotic can cause apnea. Narcan is the reversing agent for a narcotic overdose.

6. Recommend neuromuscular blocking agents (code: IIIE4i) [difficulty: R, Ap]

The NBRC may use the terms "paralytic agents" and "muscle relaxants" when describing medications that cause a medically induced paralysis. It would be more correct to call these medications neuromuscular blocking agents. They work by blocking nerve transmission from reaching skeletal (voluntary) muscles, and complete paralysis follows. They are most commonly used as part of balanced anesthesia before major thoracic or abdominal surgery. These drugs also are used in the Intensive Care Unit to stop a patient from fighting against an intubation or to prevent the patient from struggling against the mechanical ventilator. All of these agents are given intravenously and act rapidly. Obviously, in all these cases, the patient stops breathing and must receive mechanical ventilation. Examples of the commonly used neuromuscular blocking agents include the following:

- Depolarizing blocker: succinylcholine chloride (Anectine)
- Nondepolarizing blockers: pancuronium bromide (Pavulon, long duration), vecuronium bromide (Norcuron, intermediate duration), atracurium besylate (Tracrium, short duration), mivicurium (Mivacron, very short duration)

The nondepolarizing blockers (e.g., Pavulon) are preferred for their longer duration of action. Although all these agents induce complete paralysis of all voluntary muscles, they have little or no effect on the involuntary muscles or autonomic nervous system. Some patients may have a minor, passing change in heart rate and blood pressure. Remember that these patients are able to hear, are able to feel pain, and are completely awake and alert to their surroundings. Care must be taken to sedate the patient for anxiety and give analgesics for pain. Talk to the patient normally, and move the patient periodically to prevent pressure sores.

The nondepolarizing neuromuscular blocking agents can be reversed so that the patient can breathe and move again. These intravenous medications include neostigmine bromide (Prostigmin; preferred) and edrophonium (Tensilon). It should be noted that these reversing agents cause an outpouring of oral and bronchial secretions. Atropine is given to prevent this. The reversing agents have no effect on the depolarizing neuromuscular blocker succinylcholine chloride. Patients given this drug usually regain movement within 15 minutes after the medication is stopped.

7. Recommend vaccines (code: IIIE4I) [difficulty: R]

See Chapter 2 for the discussion on vaccination to prevent influenza, severe acute respiratory syndrome from the coronavirus, and *Streptococcus pneumoniae*.

8. Recommend cardiovascular drugs (code: IIIE4e) [difficulty: R, Ap]

See Chapter 11 for the discussion on drugs that may be used during CPR efforts.

Exam Hint 9-7

Expect several questions that require the respiratory therapist to recommend the use of medications in the classes discussed previously. Know the indications for these groups of medications and the main medications in each group.

MODULE C

Drug dosage calculations (math review)

Exam Hint 9-8

The NBRC examination content outline does not specifically list drug dosage calculations. However, some previous examinations have included one calculation.

The problems are easier to solve by remembering the following:
1. One milliliter (1 mL) or 1 cubic centimeter (1 cc) of water = 1 gram (g) of mass.
2. Most drug doses are listed in milligrams instead of grams. Convert grams to milligrams by moving the decimal point three places to the right (the same as multiplying by 1000). For example, 0.5 g = 500 mg.
3. Know how to interconvert fractions, decimal fractions, and percentages. For example: 1:100 = 1/100 = 0.01 = 1%.

One common way to solve any drug dosage calculation is by creating a proportional problem. The drug concentration must be converted into a fractional form. The proportional problem can then be set up to solve for the unknown *amount of active ingredient*. For example:

1. How much active ingredient would be in 0.5 mL of 1% strength adrenaline?

A 1% (1:100) drug concentration means that there is 1 part of active ingredient in 100 parts of the solution, or 1 mL or 1 g of active ingredient in 100 mL or 100 g of the solution. This can be set up in the following proportion:

$$\frac{1 \text{ mL active ingredient}}{100 \text{ mL total solution}} = \frac{\text{unknown active ingredient or } x}{0.5 \text{ mL solution}} \text{ (cross multiply)}$$

$$100x = 0.5 \text{ mL (divide both sides of the equation by 100)}$$

$$x = 0.005 \text{ mL} = 0.005 \text{ g} = 5 \text{ mg of active ingredient}$$

2. How much active ingredient would be in 0.25 mL of a medication solution with 5.0% active ingredient?

A 5% drug concentration means that there are 5 parts of active ingredient in 100 parts of the solution, or 5 mL or 5 g of ingredient in 100 mL or 100 g of the solution. This can be set up in the following proportion:

$$\frac{5 \text{ mL active ingredient}}{100 \text{ mL total solution}} = \frac{\text{unknown active ingredient or } x}{0.25 \text{ mL solution}} \text{ (cross multiply)}$$

$$100x = 1.25 \text{ mL (divide both sides of the equation by 100)}$$

$$x = 0.0125 \text{ mL} = 0.0125 \text{ g} = 12.5 \text{ mg of active ingredient}$$

Thus the *amount of active ingredient* can be calculated if the drug concentration is given in either fraction or percentage form.

The next two examples deal with calculating the *volume of medication solution* needed to deliver a desired amount of active ingredient. With these types of questions, it is necessary to convert to consistent units, usually converting grams to milligrams.

3. How much 0.5% Proventil would be needed to give a patient 2.5 mg of active ingredient by SVN?

A 0.5% (1:200) drug concentration means that there is 1 part of active ingredient in 200 parts of the solution, or 1 mL or 1 g of

Continued

active ingredient in 200 mL or 200 g of the solution. This converts to 1000 mg/200 mL. Set up the following proportion:

$$\frac{1000 \text{ mg active ingredient}}{200 \text{ mL total solution}} = \frac{2.5 \text{ mg}}{x \text{ mL solution}} \text{ (cross multiply)}$$

$$x = 0.5 \text{ mL of active ingredient}$$

4. How much 4% Xylocaine would be needed to give a patient 100 mg of active ingredient by hand-held nebulizer before a bronchoscopy?

A 4% drug concentration means that 4 parts of active ingredient are in 100 parts of the solution, or 4 mL or 4 g of active ingredient in 100 mL or 100 g of the solution. This converts to 4000 mg/100 mL. Set up the following proportion:

$$\frac{4000 \text{ mg active ingredient}}{100 \text{ mL total solution}} = \frac{100 \text{ mg}}{x \text{ mL solution}} \text{ (cross multiply)}$$

$$4000x = 10,000 \text{ mL (divide both sides of the equation by 4000)}$$

$$x = 2.5 \text{ mL of Xylocaine should be given.}$$

Thus the *volume of medication* solution needed to deliver a given amount of active ingredient can be calculated if the drug concentration is given in either fraction or percentage form.

MODULE D

Respiratory care plan

1. Determine a patient's pathophysiologic state (code: IIIF1) [difficulty: R, Ap, An]

The respiratory therapist should be able to determine when the patient is having cardiopulmonary problems that could require an inhaled medication. Review, if needed, information presented in Chapters 1, 3, 4, and 5 that deals with bedside assessment, blood gases, pulmonary function tests, and advanced cardiopulmonary monitoring.

2. Recommend starting a treatment based on the patient's response (code: IIIE2a) [difficulty: R, Ap, An]

Patients with stable asthma or COPD will often require several inhaled medications including bronchodilators and corticosteroids. The patient with life-threatening status asthmaticus will require multiple treatment procedures. These are likely to include many of the following: admission into the Intensive Care Unit, supplemental oxygen, monitoring of vital signs, electrocardiogram monitoring, serial arterial blood gases, continuous pulse oximetry, periodic bedside spirometry, heliox, intubation, and/or mechanical ventilation. Inhaled medications for this patient can include SABAs given hourly or continuously and anticholinergic medications. Systemic medications will probably include a corticosteroid and an antileukotriene agent. Last, a theophylline agent may be added. The goal is to resolve the asthmatic crisis.

After the patient has been stabilized, long-term care can be planned. This is likely to include LABAs, an ICS, and other preventative agents. If the patient has a pulmonary infection, the correct antimicrobial drug should be used to treat the problem.

3. Recommend a change in the therapeutic plan if indicated (code: IIIF2) [difficulty: R, Ap, An]

This chapter discusses medications that can be used to help treat many commonly seen cardiopulmonary conditions. When these medications are used properly for the appropriate patient condition, there is a good chance of recovery. The patient's vital signs and other clinical indicators will improve. The patient will report feeling better.

However, if the patient's signs and symptoms do not indicate improvement, be prepared to recommend a change in the medication. This may involve changing a dose or switching to another medication. Stop any medication to which the patient is having an allergic reaction. Tell the patient's physician about the problem, and ask for further orders.

4. Recommend a treatment be terminated (code: IIIE1) [difficulty: R, Ap, An]

As mentioned earlier, Box 9-1 lists the side effects most often seen with beta-adrenergic bronchodilators. The most serious problem is tachycardia. In some cases, patients may have cardiac arrhythmias. A common clinical guideline requests the treatment be discontinued if the patient's heart rate increases by more than 20% during the treatment. The patient should be monitored to confirm that the heart rate slows. Chart the information, and notify the nurse.

5. Recommend discontinuing a treatment based on the patient's response (code: IIIE2h) [difficulty: R, Ap, An]

The physician discontinues treatment for one of two reasons. First, the patient has recovered and no longer needs a medication. Some asthma patients may fully recover and not need any medications. However, it is more common to determine the right medications to control the condition so that the patient does not need to use rescue medications. Patients with emphysema or chronic bronchitis (COPD), or both, are likely to always need medications.

Second, the patient has a serious adverse reaction to the medication. As discussed earlier, Box 9-1 lists the adverse reactions to the beta-adrenergic bronchodilators. Repeated episodes of tachycardia or cardiac arrhythmias, or both, could lead to the physician discontinuing their use.

6. Recommend a change of drug (code: IIIE4m) [difficulty: R, Ap, An]

Be prepared to recommend changing an ineffective medication to another one. Also be prepared to recommend a second medication be taken in addition to one that is currently prescribed. Usually these recommendations relate to revising the pharmacologic care of an asthma or COPD patient. See the previous discussions of the bronchodilator and corticosteroid medications.

Exam Hint 9-9

Expect to see a question in which the decision has to be made to stop the bronchodilator treatment because the patient's heart rate increases by *more than 20%* from the baseline. For example, stop the treatment in the following situation: The pretreatment heart rate is 100 beats/min and the heart rate during the treatment increases to greater than 120 beats/min.

---

7. Make a recommendation to change the drug dosage (code: IIIE4m) [difficulty: R, Ap, An]

a. Bronchodilators

Make a recommendation to increase the amount of medication if the patient's bronchospasm is not reversed and no adverse side effects are present. Bedside spirometry should be performed regularly to evaluate the patient's peak flow. The two most important bedside spirometry values to monitor are the peak flow and forced expiratory volume in 1 second. Often, a 15%-20% improvement in either one or both of these parameters after the inhalation of an aerosolized bronchodilator is used as a clinical indication that the medication works and the patient has reversible bronchospasm. (See Chapter 4 for more specific guidelines.)

Make a recommendation to decrease the amount of medication if the patient is having serious side effects such as tachycardia or palpitations. The current guidelines on the pharmacologic management of asthma list the medications that should be used according to the categorization of the patient's asthmatic condition. All asthmatic patients should have a rescue inhaler that is a short-acting, rapid-onset beta-adrenergic bronchodilator. The medications albuterol (Proventil, Ventolin) and levalbuterol (Xopenex) are widely used for quick relief. For chronic persistent asthma, several additional medications are taken for long-term control. These include an ICS (beclomethasone, triamcinolone), an inhaled long-acting beta-adrenergic bronchodilator (salmeterol), and a preventive agent (cromolyn sodium or zafirlukast). Patients with the most severe persistent asthma also require a corticosteroid medication in syrup or pill form and sustained-release theophylline. It is recommended that the National Institutes of Health guidelines and others, as listed in the bibliography, be reviewed for complete information.

Exam Hint 9-10

A bedside peak flow improvement of about 15% after a bronchodilator treatment shows that the medication is effective. See Chapter 4 to review how to perform the calculation and other peak flow guidelines.

---

b. Mucomyst or saline solutions

Make a recommendation to increase the amount of medication if the patient's secretions are still too thick to cough or suction and if no adverse side effects to the medication exist. Make a recommendation to decrease the amount of medication if the patient's secretions are watery enough for expectoration or suctioning or if side effects to the drug (e.g., bronchospasm) exist.

8. Make a recommendation to change the concentration of a medication (code: IIIE4m) [difficulty: R, Ap, An]

The various saline solutions and sterile water are known collectively as bland aerosols, because they have no direct pharmacologic effect on the lungs and airways. They are used to increase the volume of liquid in an SVN after the medication has been added. Most of these nebulizers work most efficiently when they hold about 3-5 mL of liquid. Usually a normal saline solution (0.9% sodium chloride) is added.

Adding little or no saline to the medication results in the patient inhaling a very concentrated solution or the nebulizer not functioning properly. The nebulizer will aerosolize the medication within a few minutes, and the patient should quickly feel the beneficial effects of the treatment. However, depending on the nature of the medication, the patient might find it to be quite irritating to the airway. Coughing or bronchospasm could result. Side effects (e.g., tachycardia) should be monitored when sympathomimetic agents are administered, because the medication enters the bloodstream so quickly.

If more saline is added, the solution will be less concentrated. The nebulizer will take longer to aerosolize the medication because of the added volume, and relief of symptoms will take longer. However, it will be less likely to irritate the airway. Side effects with sympathomimetic agents could be less severe, because the drug is given over a longer period. However, remember that increasing the amount of saline makes no difference in the total amount of medication in the nebulizer for the patient. Tachycardia or other side effects may still be seen if the total amount of medication is given.

Saline-only aerosol treatments, as for induced sputum, are more effective at higher concentrations of saline. See Box 9-2 for complete information on the saline solutions.

BIBLIOGRAPHY

AARC Clinical Practice Guideline: Surfactant replacement therapy, *Respir Care* 58(2):367–375, 2013.

AARC Clinical Practice Guideline: Evidence-based clinical practice guideline: inhaled nitric oxide for neonates with acute hypoxic respiratory failure, *Respir Care* 58(12):1717–1745, 2010.

Arnold HM, Sawyer AM, Kollef MH: Use of adjunctive aerosolized antimicrobial therapy in the treatment of *Pseudomonas aeruginosa* and *Acinetobacter baumannii* ventilator-associated pneumonia, *Respir Care* 57(8):1226–1233, 2012.

Au JP, Ziment I: Drug therapy and dosage adjustment in asthma, *Respir Care* 31:415, 1986.

Aucoin RG: Pharmacology. In Walsh BK, Czervinske MP, DiBlasi RM, editors: *Perinatal and pediatric respiratory care*, ed 3, St Louis, 2010, Saunders.

Bills GW, Soderberg RC: *Principles of pharmacology for respiratory care*, ed 2, Albany, NY, 1998, Delmar.

Cairo JM: Sedatives, analgesics, and paralytics. In Cairo JM, editor: *Pilbeam's mechanical ventilation*, ed 5, St Louis, 2012, Mosby.

Canadian Asthma Consensus Guidelines, 2003: Canadian Pediatric Asthma Consensus Guidelines, *CMAJ* 173(6 Suppl): S1–S56, 2003.

Carter C, Solberg C: Respiratory pharmacology. In Hess DR, MacIntyre NR, Mishoe SC, et al.: *Respiratory care: principles and practices*, Philadelphia, 2002, Saunders.

Colbert BJ, Kennedy BJ: *Integrated cardiopulmonary pharmacology*, ed 2, Upper Saddle River, NJ, 2008, Prentice Hall.

Colbert BJ, Mason BJ: *Cardiopulmonary drug guide*, Upper Saddle River, NJ, 2003, Prentice Hall.

Colice GL: New drugs for asthma, *Respir Care* 53(6):688, 2008.

Cottrell GP, Surkin HB: *Pharmacology for respiratory care practitioners*, Philadelphia, 1995, FA Davis.

DesJardins T, Burton GG: *Clinical manifestations and assessment of respiratory disease*, ed 6, St Louis, 2011, Mosby.

Dhand R: The role of aerosolized antimicrobials in the treatment of ventilator-associated pneumonia, *Respir Care* 52(7):866–884, 2007.

Donohue JF: Safety and efficacy of β agonists, *Respir Care* 53(5):618, 2008.

Elias S, Sviri S, Orenbuch-Harroch E, Fellig Y, Ben-Yehuda A, Fridlender ZG, et al.: Sildenafil to facilitate weaning from inhaled nitric oxide and mechanical ventilation in a patient with severe secondary pulmonary hypertension and a patent foramen ovale, *Respir Care* 56(10):1611–1613, 2011.

Fink JB, Rubin BK: Aerosols and administration of medication. In Walsh BK, Czervinske MP, DiBlasi RM, editors: *Perinatal and pediatric respiratory care*, ed 3, St Louis, 2010, Saunders.

Gardenhire DS: *Rau's respiratory care pharmacology*, ed 8, St Louis, 2012, Mosby.

Gardenhire DS: Airway pharmacology. In Kacmarek RM, Stoller JK, Heuer AJ, editors: *Egan's fundamentals of respiratory care*, ed 10, St Louis, 2013, Mosby.

Geller DE: Aerosol antibiotics in cystic fibrosis, *Respir Care* 54(5):658, 2009.

Global Initiative for Chronic Obstructive Lung Disease Executive Summary: *Global strategy for the diagnosis, management, and prevention of COPD, National Heart, Lung, and Blood Institute*, Bethesda, MD, December 2009, World Health Organization (Geneva, Switzerland), 2009. Available at: http://www.gold-copd.org

Global Initiative for Asthma (GINA), National Heart, Lung, and Blood Institute, National Institutes of Health: *GINA Report, Global Strategy for Asthma Management and Prevention*, December 2009. Retrieved from www.ginasthma.org

Hill F: *Delmar's respiratory care drug reference*, Albany, NY, 1999, Delmar.

Howder CL: *Cardiopulmonary pharmacology: a handbook for respiratory practitioners and other allied health personnel*, ed 2, Baltimore, 1996, Williams & Wilkins.

Kondili E, Alexopoulou C, Prinianakis G, Xirouchaki N, Vaporidi K, Georgopoulos D: Effect of albuterol on expiratory resistance in mechanically ventilated patients, *Respir Care* 56(5):626–632, 2011.

Levine SR, McLaughlin AJ: *Pharmacology in respiratory care*, New York, 2001, McGraw-Hill.

Malmeister M: Pharmacology associated with respiratory care. In Fink JB, Hunt GE, editors: *Clinical practice in respiratory care*, Philadelphia, 1999, Lippincott-Raven.

McLaughlin AJ, Levine SR: *Respiratory care drug reference*, Gaithersburg, MD, 1997, Aspen.

Melani AS: Nebulized corticosteroids in asthma and COPD, an Italian appraisal, *Respir Care* 57(7):1161–1174, 2012.

Moini J: *Cardiopulmonary pharmacology for respiratory care*, Burlington, MA, 2012, Jones & Bartlett Learning.

Myers TR: Guidelines for asthma management: a review and comparison of 5 current guidelines, *Respir Care* 53(6):751, 2008.

National Asthma Education and Prevention Program, National Heart, Lung, and Blood Institute, National Institutes of Health: Expert Panel Report III: *Guidelines for the diagnosis and management of asthma*, NIH Publication No. 08-4051. Bethesda, MD, 2007, National Institutes of Health. Retrieved from http://www.nhlbi.nih.gov/guidelines/asthma/asthgdln.htm

Op't Hold TB: Inhaled beta-agonists, *Respir Care* 52(7):820–832, 2007.

Phua G-C, MacIntyre NR: Inhaled corticosteroids in obstructive airway disease, *Respir Care* 52(7):852–858, 2007.

Restropo RD: A stepwise approach to management of stable COPD with inhaled pharmacotherapy: a review, *Respir Care* 54(8):1058–1081, 2009.

Restropo RD: Use of inhaled anticholinergic agents in obstructive lung disease, *Respir Care* 52(7):833, 2007.

Rogers M: Administration of gas mixtures. In Walsh BK, Czervinske MP, DiBlasi RM, editors: *Perinatal and pediatric respiratory care*, ed 3, St Louis, 2010, Saunders.

Rowe BH, Edmonds ML, Spooner CH, Camargo CA: Evidence-based treatments for acute asthma, *Respir Care* 46(12):1380–1391, 2001.

Rubin BK: Mucolytics, expectorants, and mucokinetic medications, *Respir Care* 52(7):859, 2007.

Sessler CN, Gay PC: Are corticosteroids useful in late-stage acute respiratory distress syndrome? *Respir Care* 55(1):43–55, 2010.

Siegel RE: Emerging gram-negative antibiotic resistance: daunting challenges, declining sensitivities, and dire consequences, *Respir Care* 53(4):471–479, 2008.

Siobal MS: Pulmonary vasodilators, *Respir Care* 52(7):885–899, 2007.

Siobal MS, Hess DR: Are inhaled vasodilators useful in acute lung injury and acute respiratory distress syndrome? *Respir Care* 55(2):144–161, 2010.

Sioris K, Engebretsen K: Respiratory pharmacology. In Hess DR, MacIntyre NR, Mishoe SC, Galvin WF, Adams AB, editors: *Respiratory care principles and practice*, ed 2, Burlington, MA, 2012, Jones & Bartlett Learning.

Sobande PO, Kercsmar CM: Inhaled corticosteroids in asthma management, *Respir Care* 53(5):625, 2008.

Witek TJ, Schachter EN: *Pharmacology and therapeutics in respiratory care*, Philadelphia, 1994, Saunders.

Wyka KA: Cardiopulmonary pharmacology. In Wyka KA, Mathews PJ, Rutkowski, editors: *Foundations of respiratory care*, ed 2, Clifton Park, NY, 2012, Delmar.

Zanelli SA, Kaufman D: Surfactant replacement therapy. In Walsh BK, Czervinske MP, DiBlasi RM, editors: *Perinatal and pediatric respiratory care*, ed 3, St Louis, 2010, Saunders.

SELF-STUDY QUESTIONS

See Appendix for answers.

1. A patient with a fluid overload problem has been given a dose of furosemide (Lasix) intravenously. Following rapid diuresis in the patient, an arrhythmia is noticed that did not exist before the medication was given. What should be recommended?
   A. Check the patient's potassium level.
   B. Give more furosemide.
   C. Defibrillate the patient's heart.
   D. Give the patient epinephrine.

2. A 2-month-old infant has periods of apnea that result in bradycardia and cyanosis. What medication should be recommended to treat the apnea periods?
   A. Lidocaine (Xylocaine)
   B. Neostigmine (Prostigmin)
   C. Caffeine citrate (Cafcit)
   D. Albuterol (Proventil)

3. A respiratory therapist is working in the Emergency Department when an automobile crash victim arrives by ambulance. The patient is conscious, screaming, and hysterical from the extreme pain of a broken lower leg. What should be recommended for sedation?
   A. Morphine sulfate (Duramorph)
   B. Ibuprofen (Advil)
   C. Succinylcholine chloride (Anectine)
   D. Ipratropium bromide (Atrovent)

4. An asthma patient is discontinuing systemic corticosteroid. The patient will continue taking aerosolized bronchodilator. The physician wants to know what should be recommended for an inhaled corticosteroid (ICS).
   A. Naloxone (Narcan)
   B. Neostigmine bromide (Prostigmin)
   C. Beclomethasone dipropionate (QVAR)
   D. Methylprednisolone (Solu-Medrol)

5. The results of a patient's pulmonary function tests show that the peak expiratory flow rate increased the most when an aerosolized sympathomimetic drug and an aerosolized anticholinergic drug were inhaled. The physician wants to know what should be recommended for this patient.
   A. Beclomethasone dipropionate (Vanceril) and montelukast (Singulair)
   B. Ipratropium and albuterol (Combivent Respimat)
   C. Ipratropium bromide (Atrovent) and cromolyn sodium (Intal)
   D. Salmeterol (Serevent) and fluticasone (Advair Diskus)

6. A patient was extubated 30 minutes ago. The patient is hoarse and complains of "tightness in my throat"; inspiratory stridor can be heard. The drug of choice for treating this problem is:
   A. Racemic epinephrine (MicroNefrin)
   B. Acetylcysteine (Mucomyst)
   C. Levalbuterol (Xopenex)
   D. Isoetharine (Isoetharine HCl)

7. A patient has COPD with a bronchospasm component. Which of the following classes of medications would be helpful?
   1. SABA
   2. ICS
   3. LAAC
   4. LABA
   A. 2 and 4 only
   B. 1 and 3 only
   C. 2, 3, and 4 only
   D. 1, 2, 3, 4

8. An order is received to administer 5 mL of albuterol (Proventil) by hand-held nebulizer. What should be done?
   A. Confirm that the order was written and give the treatment.
   B. Have the shift supervisor give the treatment.
   C. Call the physician to check on the medication dose.
   D. Give 0.5 mL of medication because the physician probably intended that dosage.

9. A 10-year-old cystic fibrosis patient has a pulmonary infection and thick secretions. What should be recommended to help the patient cough out the secretions?
   A. Nebulized 0.9% (normal) saline solution
   B. Instillation of acetylcysteine (Mucomyst) into the patient's lungs
   C. Nebulized dornase alfa (Pulmozyme)
   D. Nebulized acetylcysteine (Mucomyst)

10. How much active ingredient would be found in 0.6 mL of 2.25% racemic epinephrine (Micronefrin)?
    A. 0.0267 mg
    B. 13.5 mg
    C. 26,700 mg
    D. 13.5 g

11. A respiratory therapist is about to administer an aerosolized bronchodilator to an adult patient. The patient's pretreatment pulse rate before starting is 85 beats/min. The treatment should be stopped if the patient's pulse rate reaches:
    A. 90 beats/min
    B. 100 beats/min
    C. 110 beats/min
    D. 120 beats/min

12. A patient is being given an aerosolized beta-agonist (sympathomimetic) drug for the first time. Monitoring should be done for what possible adverse effects?
    1. **Bradycardia**
    2. **Tremor**
    3. **Headache**
    4. **Nervousness and irritability**
    5. **Tachycardia**
    A. 1 and 2 only
    B. 2 and 4 only
    C. 3, 4, and 5 only
    D. 2, 3, 4, and 5 only

13. A patient is being discharged and will receive an aerosolized controller-type bronchodilator therapy at home. The best medication for this chronically sick but stable patient is:
    A. Arformoterol (Brovana)
    B. Metaproterenol (Alupent)
    C. Levalbuterol (Xopenex)
    D. Albuterol (Ventolin)

14. A patient has an order for an induced sputum sample to be analyzed for tuberculosis. The best medication for this is:
    A. Dornase alfa (Pulmozyme)
    B. 10% saline solution
    C. Acetylcysteine (Mucomyst)
    D. Isonicotinic acid hydrazide INH

15. After finishing an aerosolized dose of acetylcysteine (Mucomyst), a patient has breath sounds that reveal wheezing. These were not present at the start of treatment. What medication should be given before the next Mucomyst treatment?
    A. Levalbuterol (Xopenex)
    B. Sterile water
    C. Salmeterol (Serevent)
    D. 0.9% saline solution

16. A respiratory therapist is working the night shift when a 17-year-old patient with status asthmaticus is admitted through the Emergency Department. The patient has already been given Combivent Respimat and an ICS medication. The intern on-call asks for your recommendation on what additional medication to give the patient. What should be recommended?
    A. Formoterol (Foradil)
    B. Terbutaline (Brethaire)
    C. Albuterol (Proventil)
    D. Theophylline (Aminophylline)

17. A 16-year-old female patient has severe and chronic asthma. Her physician wishes to change her medications to prevent her from having asthma attacks. All of the following medications would be helpful EXCEPT:
    A. Zileuton (Zyflo)
    B. Epinephrine (Adrenaline)
    C. Cromolyn sodium (Intal)
    D. Zafirlukast (Accolate)

18. A patient with COPD is being given a new inhaled adrenergic bronchodilator medication by SVN. Within 3 minutes, the patient complains of palpitations. The patient's pulse rate was 85 beats/min before the treatment and is now 125 beats/min. What should be done?
    A. Change to a different medication.
    B. Discontinue the order.
    C. Stop the treatment.
    D. Add more saline to dilute the medication.

19. A respiratory therapist has finished giving an 8-year-old female patient with asthma an IPPB treatment with 0.5 mL of albuterol (Proventil). It is noticed that the patient's heart rate has increased 15% from before the treatment. Her breath sounds are now clear. What should be recommended to the physician for the patient's next treatment?
    A. Give her 0.5 mL of metaproterenol (Alupent).
    B. Discontinue her treatments altogether.
    C. Add more normal saline to the Proventil.
    D. Decrease the Proventil to 0.3 mL.

20. The respiratory therapist is called to the recovery room to assist in the care of a patient who returned 2 hours ago from having a bowel resection. The patient is apneic and on a mechanical ventilator. Which medication(s) could be used to wean the patient from the machine?
    1. **Flumazenil (Romazicon)**
    2. **Naloxone (Narcan)**
    3. **Dopamine (Intropin)**
    4. **Succinylcholine chloride (Anectine)**
    5. **Diazepam (Valium)**
    A. 5 only
    B. 1 and 4 only
    C. 2 and 3 only
    D. 1 and 2 only

21. How much medication solution is needed to give the patient 20 mg of the active ingredient? The solution contains 5% active ingredient.
    A. 0.1 mL
    B. 0.4 mL
    C. 1 mL
    D. 40 mL

22. An anxious 10-year-old asthma patient is being given a breathing treatment with levalbuterol (Xopenex). The patient's initial heart rate of 110 breaths/min has now increased to 120 breaths/min. What should be done?
    A. Continue the treatment as ordered.
    B. Stop the treatment and inform the physician.
    C. Change to albuterol and continue the treatment.
    D. Cut the medication dose in half and continue.

23. The laboratory results of a patient's sputum sample indicate that the patient has a gram-positive pulmonary infection. Which of the following medications should be recommended?
    A. Ribavirin (Virazole)
    B. Penicillin (Ampicillin)
    C. TOBI
    D. Gentamycin (Garamycin)

24. An 18-month-old infant is diagnosed with bronchiolitis from RSV. Which medication should be recommended?
    A. Ribavirin (Virazole)
    B. Pentamidine isethionate (NebuPent)
    C. Gentamycin (Garamycin)
    D. Trimethoprim and sulfamethoxazole (Bactrim)

25. The respiratory therapist is called to help assess a premature neonate. The patient is having difficulty breathing, and RDS is suspected. All of the following could be recommended EXCEPT:
    A. Flumazenil (Romazicon)
    B. Beractant (Survanta)
    C. Calfactant (Infasurf)
    D. Poractant alfa (Curosurf)

26. A 20-year-old asthmatic patient has received a standard dose of levalbuterol (Xopenex). Breath sounds reveal loud, bilateral wheezes. Over the course of the treatment, the patient's heart rate changed from 98 to 105 beats/min. What would you recommend?
    A. Stop the treatment and notify the physician.
    B. Repeat the treatment and monitor the patient.
    C. Switch the medication to albuterol (Ventolin).
    D. Add theophylline (aminophylline) to the intravenous line.

27. A 10-year-old female patient with status asthmaticus has been admitted to the hospital. The physician plans to start her on continuous nebulization of a fast-onset rescue inhaled bronchodilator medication. Which of the following should be recommended as part of her care plan?
    1. Admit her to the Intensive Care Unit.
    2. She should be given salmeterol (Serevent).
    3. She should be given levalbuterol (Xopenex).
    4. ECG and pulse oximeter monitoring should be done.
    5. She should be given an intravenous corticosteroid.
    A. 2 and 4 only
    B. 2, 4, and 5 only
    C. 1, 3, 4, and 5 only
    D. 1, 2, 3, 4, 5

28. A mechanically ventilated patient who has been paralyzed with a neuromuscular blocking agent should be given a sedative agent for what reason?
    A. Sustain the paralysis.
    B. Control pain.
    C. Improve patient–ventilator synchrony.
    D. Relieve anxiety.

29. A patient had a bronchoscopy procedure and biopsy taken of a suspected lung tumor. After the biopsy, uncontrolled bleeding occurs. What should be given to control the bleeding?
    A. Instill epinephrine through the bronchoscope at the site of the bleeding.
    B. Administer heparin by intravenous line.
    C. Administer nebulized albuterol (Proventil) by SVN.
    D. Administer lidocaine (Xylocaine) by an intravenous line.

30. A 15-year-old patient with cystic fibrosis has large amounts of thick secretions. There is no sign of infection. What should be administered to help manage the secretion problem?
    A. Salmeterol (Serevent)
    B. 5% saline
    C. Normal (0.9%) saline
    D. Acetylcysteine (Mucomyst)

31. A home care patient with asthma has finished a standard dose of 0.25 mL of albuterol (Ventolin). After waiting 15 minutes, the patient performs a peak flow measurement, which shows 65% of personal best. What should be done to improve the patient's condition?
    A. Decrease the dose of albuterol.
    B. Add an intravenous corticosteroid.
    C. Maintain the present therapy.
    D. Increase the dose of albuterol.

32. A premature neonate is being mechanically ventilated in the neonatal Intensive Care Unit. The neonatologist believes that the patient has pulmonary hypertension. What should be recommended?
    A. Instill lucinactant (Surfaxin) into the lungs.
    B. Administer INOmax.
    C. Give aerosolized umeclidinium and vilanterol (Anoro).
    D. Give aerosolized aclidinium (Tudorza).

33. An adult patient is panicking and fighting against the mechanical ventilator. All of the following may be used to control the patient on the ventilator EXCEPT:
    A. Flumazenil (Romazicon)
    B. Pancuronium bromide (Pavulon)
    C. Succinylcholine (Anectine)
    D. Morphine sulfate (Duramorph)

34. A patient is in shock from an allergic reaction to a bee sting. In addition, the patient has inspiratory stridor from laryngeal edema. What is the best medication to use to help raise the patient's blood pressure and help her breathing?
    A. Intravenous epinephrine (Adrenalin)
    B. Oral ibuprofen (Advil)
    C. Nebulized racemic epinephrine (Nephron)
    D. Intravenous naloxone (Narcan)

35. A 10-year-old boy with cystic fibrosis has been having recurrent episodes of *P. aeruginosa* pneumonia. What should be recommended to prevent further episodes?
    A. Instill pentamidine (Pentam) into the trachea by way of a suction catheter.
    B. Administer pentamidine (NebuPent) once a month by SVN.
    C. Isonicotinic acid hydrazide (INH) should be taken twice a week for 6 months.
    D. TOBI should be taken by SVN every other month.

36. A 4-month-old pediatric patient has chronic lung disease secondary to recovering from RDS. The patient now has pneumonia caused by RSV and is on a mechanical ventilator. What can be given to improve the patient's condition?
    A. Intravenous racemic epinephrine (MicroNefrin)
    B. Ribavirin (Virazole) by SPAG II nebulizer
    C. Intratracheal beractant (Survanta)
    D. Cromolyn sodium (Intal) by SVN

37. A 35-year-old patient has AIDS and was previously treated for *P. carinii* pneumonia. What can be used to prevent the infection from reoccurring?
    A. Trimethoprim and sulfamethoxazole (Bactrim) by pill
    B. Pentamidine (NebuPent) by SVN
    C. TOBI by small-volume inhaler
    D. Zanamivir (Relenza) by MDI

38. A 58-year-old female patient with congestive heart failure is being treated with 40% oxygen and diuretics. Within 3 hours she has lost 1500 mL of urine and her pulse oximeter reading has improved from 84% to 93% saturation. Her electrocardiogram shows a heart rate of 110 beats/min with the new observation of premature ventricular contractions. Her recent serum electrolyte values show a potassium level of 3.1 mEq/L. What recommendation could be made in her care?
    A. Give her intravenous potassium.
    B. Decrease her oxygen to 35%.
    C. Continue her diuretic medications.
    D. Restrict her intake of potassium.

39. A patient has been diagnosed with severe COPD. The physician has asked for your recommendations on medications to optimize the patient's breathing. The patient says, "I don't want…to take medicine…all day long." What should be recommended to maximize bronchodilation and convenience?
    1. Fluticasone and vilanterol (Breo)
    2. Mometasone and formoterol (Dulera)
    3. Ipratropium and albuterol (Combivent Respimat)
    4. Umeclidinium and vilanterol (Anoro)
    5. Tiotropium (Spiriva)
    A. 4 only
    B. 1 and 5 only
    C. 3 and 4 only
    D. 1, 3, and 5 only

10 Airway Clearance Therapy

Note: It can be anticipated that the Therapist Multiple-Choice Examination (TMC) will include an *average of 3 of 140 actual questions* (2% of the exam) on airway clearance therapy (ACT). (This is based on the question mix typically found on the National Board of Respiratory Care's (NBRC's) previous Entry Level Examinations and Written Registry Examinations.)

Remember that the TMC version you take will include 20 additional questions being evaluated for possible inclusion in other versions of the TMC. So, there will be a total of 160 questions taken. There is no way to differentiate between the 140 actual questions and the 20 questions being evaluated for future use. Please go to the Introduction for detailed information on the TMC Examination and the Clinical Simulation Examination.

MODULE A

Airway clearance therapy

Airway clearance therapy (ACT) is the overall phrase for any physical or mechanical method used to change airflow to improve the removal of airway secretions by coughing. (The phrase bronchopulmonary hygiene is also used to encompass the airway clearance therapies.) A patient with cystic fibrosis, bronchiectasis, pneumonia, chronic obstructive pulmonary disease, or asthma might require some form of ACT if he or she is unable to cough out accumulated secretions. ACT encompasses everything from simple, direct patient contact methods (directed cough and deep breathing, chest physiotherapy (CPT)) to intermediately complex devices (positive expiratory pressure (PEP), oscillatory PEP) and technologically complex, expensive equipment (high-frequency chest wall oscillation (HFCWO), intrapulmonary percussive ventilation (IPV), mechanical insufflation–exsufflation (MIE)). This chapter presents all of these options and how they may be best used for optimal secretion clearance. (If ACT methods are unsuccessful, nasotracheal suctioning [Chapter 13] or bronchoscopy [Chapter 18] can be done to remove the secretions.)

Many researchers, the American Association for Respiratory Care (AARC), and other agencies have investigated the various ACT methods and their applications in various patient populations. These findings have been published in several clinical practice guidelines (listed in the bibliography) and summarized here based on the pathological condition of the patient population.

Cystic fibrosis

1. All cystic fibrosis patients need some form of ACT.
2. No single ACT method has been proven to be better than another.
3. Children with cystic fibrosis must be taught age-appropriate forms of ACT (see Fig. 10-1).
4. Choose the type of ACT that the patient (or adult caregiver) likes and will faithfully perform on a long-term basis.

Uncomplicated pneumonia

1. CPT is not recommended for uncomplicated pneumonia.

Chronic obstructive pulmonary disease

1. ACT is not recommended if the patient can cough out his/her secretions.
2. If needed, the patient can be taught effective coughing techniques. (See Chapter 7.)
3. An ACT method may be used if the patient is unable to cough out his or her secretions.

Postoperative child or adult

1. ACT is not routinely needed.
2. Incentive spirometry is not routinely needed to prevent atelectasis.
3. The patient should be mobilized and ambulated as soon as possible to prevent atelectasis or pneumonia.

Neuromuscular disease

1. An assisted cough technique (huff cough, quad cough) should be used if an adult patient's peak cough flow (peak flow) is <270 L/min (4.5 L/s). (See Chapter 7.)
2. No other form of ACT can be recommended because of the lack of clinical evidence showing effectiveness.
3. If an ACT method is to be used, none has been proven to be better than another.

The overall conclusions of these clinical practice guidelines are:

1. No ACT method is demonstrably better than another.
2. When dealing with a child, the ACT method must match the child's ability to do it.
3. The patient (or caregiver) must like the ACT method or he or she will not continue to do it.

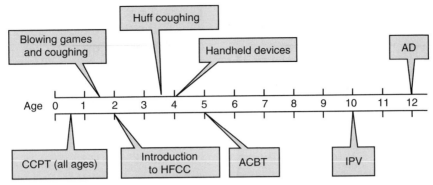

Figure 10-1 Approximate age at which a child is first able to perform an airway clearance therapy procedure. CCPT, conventional chest physiotherapy; HFCC, high-frequency chest compression (also known as high-frequency chest wall oscillation); ACBT, active cycle breathing technique; IPV, intrapulmonary percussive ventilation; AD, autogenic drainage. Hand-held devices refers to positive expiratory pressure therapy devices. (From Lester MK, Flume PA: Airway-clearance therapy guidelines and implementation, Respir Care 54(6): 733, 2009.)

4. If an ACT method has become ineffective, try others until the best method is found.

Because of the relative lack of specific guidelines, it is up to the respiratory therapist to assess the patient's physical, mental, and emotional condition to determine which ACT method(s) to try. Because the available methods range from the simple to the complex, the patient's age and ability must be considered. Figure 10-1 shows the various therapies that can be applied based on a child's age. For example, it would be useless to try to train a 2-year-old to perform IPV. In addition, look at Figure 10-2 for two algorithms that can be used to help choose between CPT, oscillatory therapy, or suctioning to remove secretions.

Often, more than one form of ACT is used during a given therapy session. Regardless of what mechanical device may be used to help mobilize secretions, the patient must still be able to cough them out. So, an effective cough is critical for any ACT method to be effective. See Chapter 7 for the discussion on directed cough or another forced expiratory technique (FET) such as the huff cough and quad cough. Two additional secretion clearance techniques will be presented here.

Active cycle breathing technique

Active cycle breathing technique (ACBT) involves the patient going through phases of breathing control (gentle diaphragmatic breathing), thoracic expansion exercises (large breaths with relaxed exhalation), and a FET (huff cough) (Fig. 10-3). The ACBT can be repeated until the patient's secretions have been cleared out. Children of about 5 years of age can be taught these techniques. ACBT can be performed by itself or combined with another ACT procedure. Most often, ACBT is combined with postural drainage. The usual steps in an ACBT cycle include:

1. The patient sits upright or in a postural drainage position.
2. Controlled, relaxed diaphragmatic breathing is performed.
3. Three or four cycles of a deep inhalation with a relaxed exhalation are performed.
4. Steps 2 and 3 are repeated as peripheral secretions enter the central airways.
5. One or two forced exhalations (huffs) are performed to clear secretions.
6. Steps 2 through 5 are repeated until all secretions have been cleared.

Autogenic drainage

Autogenic drainage (AD) involves the patient breathing at three progressively larger lung volumes to move secretions from the peripheral airways to the central airways where a huff cough can clear them (Fig. 10-4). The smallest breaths are in the tidal volume (V_T) and expiratory reserve volume (ERV) range and designed to "unstick" any secretions. Middle-sized breaths follow and expand into the inspiratory reserve volume. These larger breaths are designed to collect secretions into the larger airways. Last, large breaths approaching the vital capacity (VC) range are done to evacuate the secretions by huff breaths. Often the child will need to be about 12 years of age to master these complex steps. AD can be performed by itself in the sitting position or combined with postural drainage. The usual steps in AD include:

1. The patient sits upright or in a postural drainage position.
2. Several low-volume breaths are done to unstick any secretions. The patient should breathe slowly in through the nose, hold the breath for 2-3 seconds, and exhale slowly through the mouth.
3. About 10 medium-volume breaths are done to collect secretions into the larger airways.
4. The patient should resist the urge to cough as the secretions gather.
5. About 10 large-volume breaths are performed.

6. Several huff coughs are done to evacuate the secretions.
7. Steps 2 through 6 can be repeated until all secretions have been cleared.

Exam Hint 10-1

Be prepared to recommend starting any ACT procedure or changing from one ACT procedure to another based on the patient's response.

MODULE B

Chest physiotherapy

Chest physiotherapy (CPT) is the preferred phrase for the procedures of postural drainage, percussion, and vibration that can be done to help mobilize a patient's secretions toward the central airways for coughing and removal. Other terms and abbreviations for these activities include

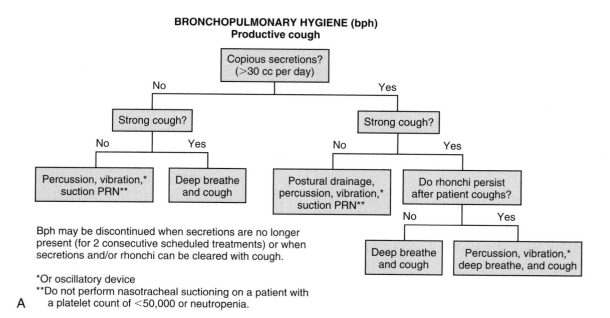

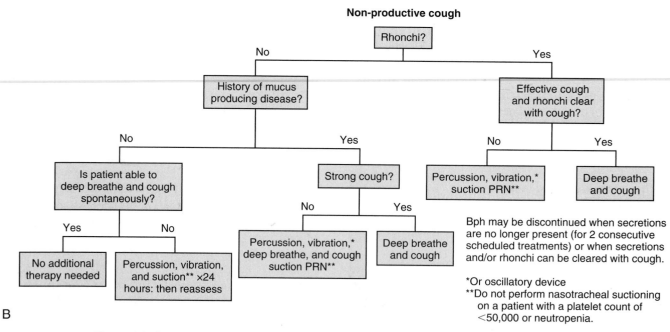

Figure 10-2 A, Algorithm for determining bronchopulmonary hygiene (bph) options for a patient with a productive cough. **B,** Algorithm for determining bph options for a patient with a nonproductive cough. (*Note:* Rhonchi are also known as expiratory crackles.) (Bronchial Hygiene Algorithm from the Cleveland Clinic Respiratory Therapy Consult Service Handbook. Courtesy of the Cleveland Clinic.)

chest physical therapy, conventional chest physiotherapy, postural drainage therapy (PDT), bronchopulmonary drainage, bronchial hygiene therapy, and postural drainage, percussion, and vibration.

1. Perform postural drainage (code: IIIB1) [difficulty: R, Ap, An]

Postural drainage therapy (PD or PDT) and turning involve moving the patient so that all lung segments are ventilated and gravity can be used to help mobilize any accumulated secretions. The AARC *Clinical Practice Guideline* on PDT (1991) was used to help develop the following information. See Box 10-1 for indications for turning, postural drainage, percussion, and vibration. Contraindications are listed in Box 10-2, and recommended actions for problems are listed in Box 10-3. Beyond the patient assessment issues listed in Box 10-4, the following should be evaluated to determine whether PDT is needed:

- PDT is not indicated if an optimally hydrated patient is producing less than 25 mL of secretions per day with the procedure.
- A dehydrated patient should have apparently ineffective PDT continued for at least 24 hours after the patient is

rehydrated. The combination of rehydration and PDT may help to mobilize previously thick secretions.

- PDT is not indicated in a patient producing more than 30 mL of secretions daily (if the PDT treatments do not increase the sputum production) because the patient is already able to expectorate the sputum effectively.

Turning involves rotating the patient's body in the longitudinal (head-to-toe) axis to promote unilateral or bilateral lung expansion. Patients can be turned from the back to one side, side to side, or one side to back to other side, depending on their needs. The bed may be moved to any head-up or head-down position, as the patient needs and tolerates. Patients should be turned every 1-2 hours as tolerated. The patient can turn himself or herself, be turned by a caregiver, or be placed in a bed that is motorized and programmed to change positions in a set pattern.

Postural drainage (bronchopulmonary drainage) involves positioning the patient to clear secretions or prevent the accumulation of secretions. The patient's body is angled so that the bronchus of a particular segment is as vertical as possible. Gravity pulls the secretions toward a major bronchus or the trachea; the secretions are then either expectorated or suctioned. The anatomy of the pulmonary lobes with their segments and respective bronchi should be reviewed (Fig. 10-5).

Note that each segment and its bronchus adjoin the right or left mainstem bronchus at a particular angle. This critical angle determines the positioning that must be used to drain the various segments. Obviously, positioning the patient incorrectly does nothing to drain the desired segment. Auscultation, palpation, and percussion of the chest should lead the practitioner to know where the secretions are located.

Individual segments should be drained when the physician's order specifies them or when the practitioner determines that secretions are present. Individual segments are generally drained for 3-15 minutes. Drainage may be provided for a longer period in special situations. Postural drainage and the external manipulation of the patient's thorax (percussion and vibration) can be very strenuous or contraindicated in some patients. Watch for hypoxemia

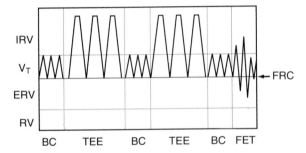

Figure 10-3 Breathing volumes and secretion clearance efforts during the active cycle breathing technique. See the text for discussion. Breathing efforts: BC, breathing control; TEE, thoracic expansion exercise; FET, forced expiratory technique. Lung volumes: IRV, inspiratory reserve volume; V$_T$, tidal volume; ERV, expiratory reserve volume; RV, residual volume. ERV and RV make up the functional residual capacity, FRC. (From Fink JB: Forced expiratory technique, directed cough, and autogenic drainage, Respir Care 52(9), 1210, 2007.)

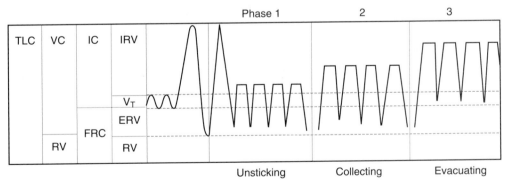

Figure 10-4 Breathing volumes used during autogenic drainage. See the text for discussion. Lung volumes: IRV, inspiratory reserve volume; V$_T$, tidal volume; ERV, expiratory reserve volume; RV, residual volume. ERV and RV make up the functional residual capacity, FRC. Vital capacity (VC) is made up of the IRV, V$_T$, and ERV. TLC is total lung capacity.

BOX 10-1   Indications for Turning, Postural Drainage, and Percussion and Vibration

Turning
- Patient unable to change his or her body position (e.g., the patient has a cerebral injury or neuromuscular disease, is being mechanically ventilated, or has been medicated to cause sedation or paralysis)
- Atelectasis or the potential for its development
- Hypoxemia associated with a particular position; if one-sided lung disease is present, the patient is typically turned so that the affected lung is superior
- Patient with an artificial airway

Postural Drainage
- Mobilize retained secretions so that they can be coughed or suctioned; patient has difficulty expectorating secretions but produces more than 25-30 mL/day; evidence or indications that a patient with an artificial airway has retained secretions

- Atelectasis that is known or is believed to be caused by a mucous plug
- Patient diagnosed with cystic fibrosis, bronchiectasis, or cavitating lung disease
- Foreign body in an airway
- Removal of aspirated foreign body or stomach contents

Percussion and Vibration
- Patient receiving postural drainage who has a large volume of thick sputum; this suggests that external manipulation of the thorax would assist gravity in its movement toward a more central airway

Based on information found in American Association for Respiratory Care: Clinical practice guideline: postural drainage therapy, Respir Care 36:1418, 1991.

BOX 10-2   Contraindications for Turning/Postural Drainage and Percussion and Vibration

Turning/Postural Drainage*
All positions are contraindicated for patients with the following:
1. Unstabilized head or neck injury, or both (absolute)
2. Active hemorrhage and hemodynamic instability (absolute)
3. ICP[†] greater than 20 mm Hg
4. Recent spinal surgery, such as a laminectomy, or acute spinal injury
5. Active hemoptysis
6. Empyema
7. Bronchopleural fistula
8. Pulmonary edema as a result of congestive heart failure
9. Large pleural effusions
10. Advanced age, anxiety, or confusion and intolerance of position changes
11. Fractured rib(s) with or without flail chest
12. Healing tissue or surgical wound

Trendelenburg position is contraindicated in patients with the following:
1. ICP greater than 20 mm Hg
2. Sensitivity to increased ICP (e.g., neurosurgery, cerebral aneurysms, eye surgery)
3. Uncontrolled hypertension
4. Distended abdomen
5. Esophageal surgery
6. Recent gross hemoptysis (especially if associated with lung cancer that was recently treated surgically or by radiation therapy)
7. Uncontrolled airway if at risk for aspiration (recent meal or tube feeding); many authors consider <1 hour after eating as a contraindication

Reverse Trendelenburg position is contraindicated in patients who are:
1. Hypotensive
2. Receiving a vasoactive medication

Percussion and Vibration
1. All of the previously listed contraindications
2. Subcutaneous emphysema (several authors list an untreated pneumothorax as an absolute contraindication)
3. Spinal anesthesia or recent epidural spinal infusion for pain control
4. Recent thoracic skin grafts or skin flaps
5. Thoracic burns, open wounds, or skin infections
6. Recently placed transvenous or subcutaneous pacemaker (especially true if a mechanical percussor/vibrator is to be used)
7. Suspicion of pulmonary tuberculosis
8. Lung contusion
9. Bronchospasm
10. Osteomyelitis of the ribs
11. Osteoporosis
12. Clotting disorder (coagulopathy)
13. Complaints of chest wall pain

In addition, a number of authors have listed the following as contraindications to percussion and vibration:
1. Not over bare skin
2. Not over buttons, zippers, folded clothes, or seams of clothing
3. Not over female breast tissue
4. Not over the spine, sternum, or kidneys
5. Not over an area with a known lung tumor

*These are relative contraindications except those marked as absolute.
[†]ICP, intracranial pressure.
Based on information found in American Association for Respiratory Care: Clinical practice guideline: postural drainage therapy, Respir Care 36:1418, 1991.

---

or an increase in dyspnea. If the patient normally is being administered supplemental O_2, it should be continued while the patient is in the drainage positions. Some patients need supplemental O_2 only when in certain positions, and it must be made available to them.

Coughing should be encouraged after each segment is drained. The patient should not cough in a head-down position, however, because of the risk of increased intracranial pressure. Have the patient sit up to cough vigorously.

BOX 10-3 Hazards/Complications, with Recommended Actions, and Limitations of Postural Drainage and Percussion and Vibration

Hazards/Complications

- *Hypoxemia.* The patient known to be hypoxic or prone to hypoxemia during the procedure should be given a higher inspired O_2 percentage. Administer 100% O_2 to any patient who becomes hypoxic during the procedure. Stop the treatment, return the patient to the original resting position, make sure ventilation is adequate, and consult with the physician before continuing.
- *Increased intracranial pressure or acute hypotension during the procedure.* If either of these complications occurs, stop the treatment, return the patient to the original resting position, and consult with the physician before continuing.
- *Pulmonary hemorrhage.* If this occurs, stop the treatment, return the patient to the original resting position, and call the physician immediately. Give the patient supplemental O_2 and keep an open airway until the physician responds.
- *Pain or injury to the patient's muscles, ribs, or spine.* Stop the therapy that appears to be causing the problem. Carefully move the patient to a more comfortable position, and call the physician before continuing.
- *Vomiting and aspiration.* Stop the treatment, apply suction as needed to clear the airway, give supplemental O_2, maintain a patent airway, return the patient to the original resting position, and call the physician immediately.
- *Bronchospasm.* If this develops, stop the treatment, return the patient to the original resting position, and give or increase the supplemental O_2 while calling the physician. Give the patient any aerosolized bronchodilators that the physician orders.
- *Arrhythmia.* If this occurs, stop the treatment, return the patient to the original resting position, and give or increase supplemental O_2 while calling the physician.

Limitations

- Be careful to give PDT only to those patients who would benefit from it. Do not rely on past experiences with other patients when you judge current situations.
- Patients with ineffective coughs may be unable to clear their airways as well as desired.
- Critically ill patients are difficult to position optimally.

Based on information found in American Association for Respiratory Care: Clinical practice guideline: postural drainage therapy, Respir Care 36:1418, 1991.

BOX 10-4 Assessment of the Patient's Needs for Postural Drainage Therapy (PDT)*

Excessive production of sputum
Ineffectiveness of cough
Patient history of PDT that was helpful in treating past problem (e.g., bronchiectasis, cystic fibrosis, lung abscess)
Abnormal breath sounds (e.g., decreased breath sounds, crackles, or rhonchi, suggesting airway secretions)
Change in the patient's vital signs
Abnormal chest radiograph finding consistent with infiltrates, atelectasis, or mucous plug

*These problems should be assessed together to evaluate the patient's need for PDT. Not all patients experience all of these problems. The seriousness of these problems should be assessed by the clinician in determining which patients will benefit from PDT.
Based on information found in American Association for Respiratory Care: Clinical practice guideline: postural drainage therapy, Respir Care 36:1418, 1991.

a. Pulmonary drainage positions

1. *Lower lobes*

a. Posterior basal segment (Fig. 10-6)

1. The patient lies face down on the bed. A pillow is placed beneath the hips.
2. The foot of the bed is elevated 18 inches or 30 degrees.
3. If ordered, perform percussion or vibration over the lower ribs near the spine on either or both sides, depending on whether one or both segments are to be drained. Note the shaded areas in Figure 10-6.

b. Lateral basal segment (Fig. 10-7)

1. The patient is shown in a position to drain the right lateral basal segment. The left lateral basal segment would be drained by placing the patient in the same position on the opposite side.
2. The patient lies one-fourth turn up from the face-down position. A pillow may be placed in front of the patient for support or between the knees for comfort.
3. The foot of the bed is elevated 18 inches or 30 degrees.
4. If ordered, percussion or vibration would be performed over the posterolateral areas of the lower ribs. See the shaded areas in Figure 10-7.

c. Anterior basal segment (Fig. 10-8)

1. The patient is shown in a position to drain the left anterior basal segment. (*Note:* This combined segment is the anatomic equivalent of the medial basal segment and anterior basal segment of the right lung.) The right anterior basal and medial basal segments would be drained by placing the patient in the same position on the opposite side.
2. The patient lies straight up on his or her side. Pillows may be used in front or behind the patient (or both) for positioning or between the knees for comfort.
3. The foot of the bed is elevated 18 inches or 30 degrees.
4. If ordered, percussion or vibration would be performed over the lower ribs below the axilla. See the shaded areas in Figure 10-8.

d. Superior segment (Fig. 10-9)

1. The patient lies face down on the bed. A pillow is placed beneath the hips.
2. The bed is flat.
3. If ordered, percussion or vibration would be performed over the middle of the back below the scapula on either or both sides of the spine, depending on whether one or both segments are to be drained. See the shaded areas in Figure 10-9.

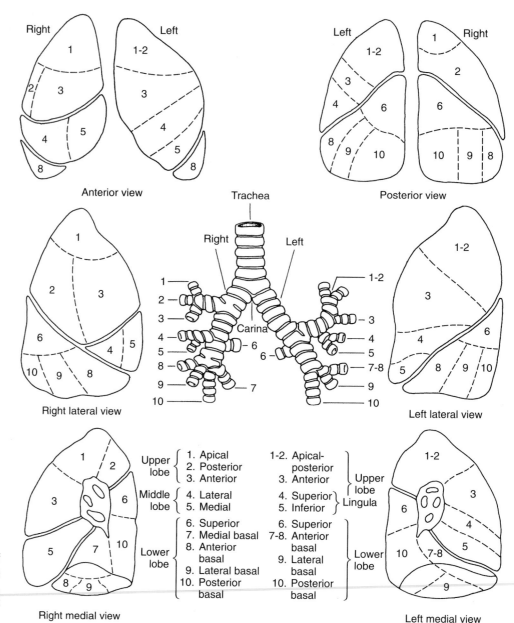

Figure 10-5 Names and locations of the lung segments and their respective bronchi. (From Shibel EM, Moser KM, editors: Respiratory emergencies, St Louis, 1977, Mosby.)

	Right	Left
Upper lobe	1. Apical 2. Posterior 3. Anterior	1-2. Apical-posterior 3. Anterior
Middle lobe	4. Lateral 5. Medial	} Upper lobe Lingula
		4. Superior 5. Inferior
Lower lobe	6. Superior 7. Medial basal 8. Anterior basal 9. Lateral basal 10. Posterior basal	6. Superior 7-8. Anterior basal 9. Lateral basal 10. Posterior basal } Lower lobe

2. Right middle lobe and left lingula

a. Right lateral and medial segments (Fig. 10-10)

1. The same position is used to drain both segments.
2. The patient lies one-fourth turn up from the back-down position. A pillow may be placed in back of the patient for support or between the flexed knees for comfort.
3. The foot of the bed is elevated 14 inches or 15 degrees.
4. If ordered, percussion or vibration would be performed below the right nipple area in a male patient. See the shaded area in Figure 10-10. Percussion and vibration may not be possible on a female patient.

b. Left superior and inferior lingula segments (Fig. 10-11)

1. The same position is used to drain both segments.
2. The patient lies one-fourth turn up from the back-down position. A pillow may be placed in back of the patient for support or between the flexed knees for comfort.
3. The foot of the bed is elevated 14 inches or 15 degrees.
4. If ordered, percussion or vibration would be performed below the left nipple area in a male patient. See the shaded area in Figure 10-11. Percussion and vibration may not be possible on a female patient.

3. Upper lobes

a. Posterior segment (Fig. 10-12)

1. The patient leans forward 30 degrees. This can be over the back of a chair (as shown in Fig. 10-12) or in bed. A pillow can be used to lean against or support the chest.
2. If ordered, percussion or vibration would be performed over the upper portion of the back on either or both sides of the spine, depending on whether one or both segments are being drained. See the shaded areas in Figure 10-12.

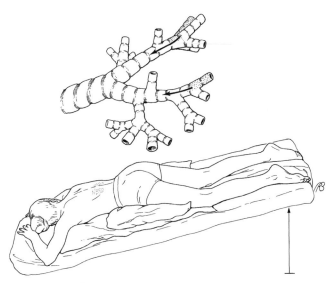

Figure 10-6 Drainage position for the posterior basal segments of both lower lobes. (From Eubanks DH, Bone RC: Comprehensive respiratory care, ed 2, St Louis, 1990, Mosby.)

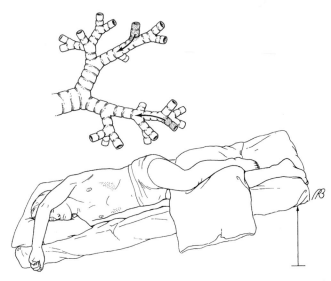

Figure 10-8 Drainage position for the anterior basal segment of the left lower lobe. The same segment in the right lung would be drained by positioning the patient similarly on the left side. (From Eubanks DH, Bone RC: Comprehensive respiratory care, ed 2, St Louis, 1990, Mosby.)

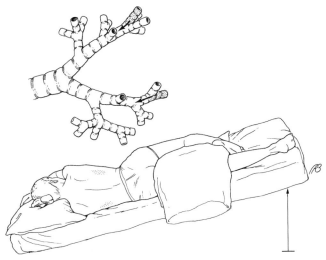

Figure 10-7 Drainage position for the lateral basal segment of the right lower lobe. The same segment in the left lung would be drained by positioning the patient similarly on the right side. (From Eubanks DH, Bone RC: Comprehensive respiratory care, ed 2, St Louis, 1990, Mosby.)

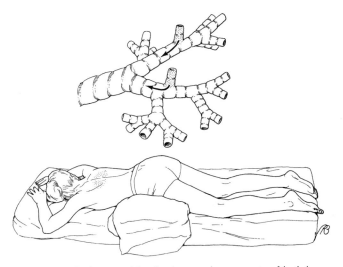

Figure 10-9 Drainage position for the superior segments of both lower lobes. (From Eubanks DH, Bone RC: Comprehensive respiratory care, ed 2, St Louis, 1990, Mosby.)

b. Apical segment (Fig. 10-13)

1. The patient leans backward 30 degrees. This can be done in bed (as shown in Fig. 10-13) or in a chair. A pillow can be leaned against to support the lower portion of the back.
2. If ordered, percussion or vibration would be performed between the clavicle and the top of the scapula on either or both sides, depending on whether one or both segments are being drained. See the shaded areas in Figure 10-13.

c. Anterior segment (Fig. 10-14)

1. The patient lies supine in bed with a pillow placed under the knees. This enables the abdominal muscles to relax so that the patient can breathe more easily.

2. If ordered, percussion or vibration would be performed between the clavicle and the nipple of a male patient on either or both sides, depending on whether one or both segments are being drained. See the shaded areas in Figure 10-14. Percussion and vibration may not be possible on a female patient.

Some authors may list slightly different positions or several additional positions. The most commonly accepted postural drainage positions have been presented. The postural drainage positions in the infant are basically the same as those in the adult. Positioning can be accomplished more easily by using pillows. Figure 10-15 shows the various segmental drainage positions.

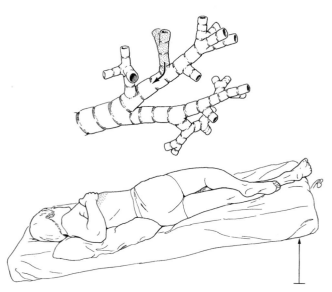

Figure 10-10 Drainage position for the lateral and medial segments of the right middle lobe. (From Eubanks DH, Bone RC: Comprehensive respiratory care, ed 2, St Louis, 1990, Mosby.)

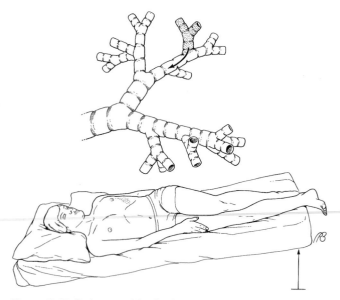

Figure 10-11 Drainage position for the superior and inferior segments of the lingula. (From Eubanks DH, Bone RC: Comprehensive respiratory care, ed 2, St Louis, 1990, Mosby.)

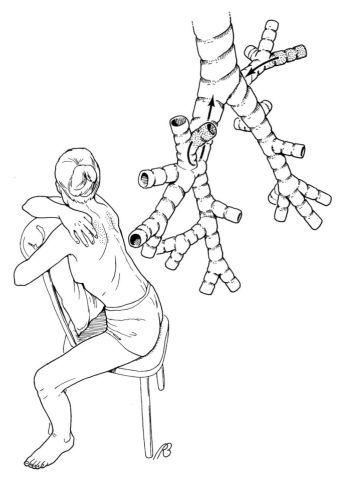

Figure 10-12 Drainage position for the posterior segments of both upper lobes. (From Eubanks DH, Bone RC: Comprehensive respiratory care, ed 2, St Louis, 1990, Mosby.)

2. Perform percussion (code: IIIB1) [difficulty: R, Ap, An]

Percussion (also known as clapping, cupping, and tapotement) is the act of rhythmically striking the adult patient's chest with cupped hands over an area with secretions. A properly cupped hand traps air against the chest and causes a popping sound. The wrists, elbows, and shoulders should be kept as loose as possible to enable the practitioner to keep the proper loose waving motion of the hand and minimize fatigue (Fig. 10-16). Infants can be percussed by putting the index, middle, and ring fingers together into a kind of three-sided tent, or by using specially designed palm cups. This enables the practitioner to percuss a small area of the chest wall. Percussion is performed throughout the breathing cycle and can be done with one or both hands. Percussion should not be painful to the patient. As an added precaution, most authors recommend that the chest be covered lightly with the patient's gown or towel. Percussion should not be done over buttons or zippers or female breast tissue.

Percussion will not help to move secretions if the patient is not in the proper postural drainage position.

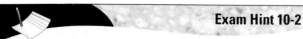

Exam Hint 10-2

The examination usually contains at least one question that deals with knowing the correct position to drain a particular lobe. The lower lobes are usually tested. The question may give information on an opaque area seen on the chest radiograph. The therapist is expected to know what segment or lobe needs to be drained. Review Figure 1-16 for a drawing showing areas of consolidation.

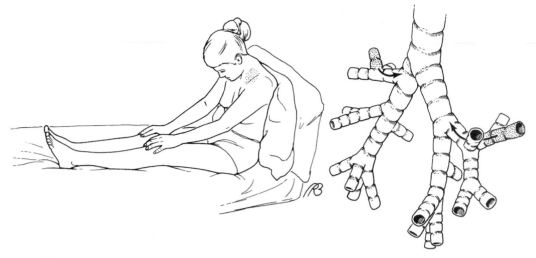

Figure 10-13 Drainage position for the apical segments of both upper lobes. (From Eubanks DH, Bone RC: Comprehensive respiratory care, ed 2, St Louis, 1990, Mosby.)

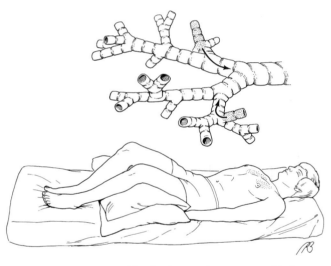

Figure 10-14 Drainage position for the anterior segments of both upper lobes. (From Eubanks DH, Bone RC: Comprehensive respiratory care, ed 2, St Louis, 1990, Mosby.)

(See the previous discussion on the drainage positions.) When the patient is properly positioned, percussion should help to vibrate the secretions more quickly down a vertical bronchus. Percussion is recommended for 5 minutes or longer in each position. Some patients, however, may not tolerate this length of treatment; 1 minute seems to be the shortest time for some therapeutic benefit. No agreement exists on the ideal manual rate of percussion. The practitioner must vary the rate, depending on how the patient feels and what seems to produce the best clearance of secretions. Recent research indicates that the ideal percussion rate is about 13-15 Hz (Hertz or cycles per second). Because this is faster than humanly possible, a mechanical percussor (discussed below) can be used to percuss the patient's chest.

3. Perform vibration (code: IIIB1) [difficulty: R, Ap, An]

Vibration is the gentle, rapid shaking of the chest wall directly over the lung segment that is being drained. It may be performed alone or with percussion. The practitioner places his or her hands side by side if the chest area is large enough or one on the other for a smaller chest area. The elbows are locked with the arms straight (Fig. 10-17). When performing vibration on a small area, such as a child's chest, a mechanical percussor/vibrator may be more effective than manual vibration (Fig. 10-18). During manual or mechanical vibration, the patient's chest is gently but effectively shaken during exhalation. The patient should exhale at least the complete tidal volume (V_T) as the chest wall is vibrated. Blowing out the ERV should help to clear out more secretions. A vibration rate of 200/min (about 3/s) has been recommended as ideal to help move secretions. The literature differs as to how the patient should exhale during the procedure. Both breathing out slowly through pursed lips and breathing out forcefully through an open mouth have been recommended. A pursed-lip exhalation pattern seems reasonable if the patient has a problem with bronchospasm and air trapping. A patient without this problem should exhale forcefully because this helps to clear more secretions. Vibration should be performed for several expiratory efforts or until it is no longer effective in helping to mobilize secretions.

4. Recommend changing the postural drainage position (code: IIIE3a) [difficulty: R, Ap]

During the treatment, the patient's secretions may be found to be more effectively drained if he or she is repositioned from what would seem to be the ideal angle. The patient's airway anatomy may be different from what is expected. Patients with chronic lung disease, such as cystic fibrosis or bronchiectasis, often know what positions

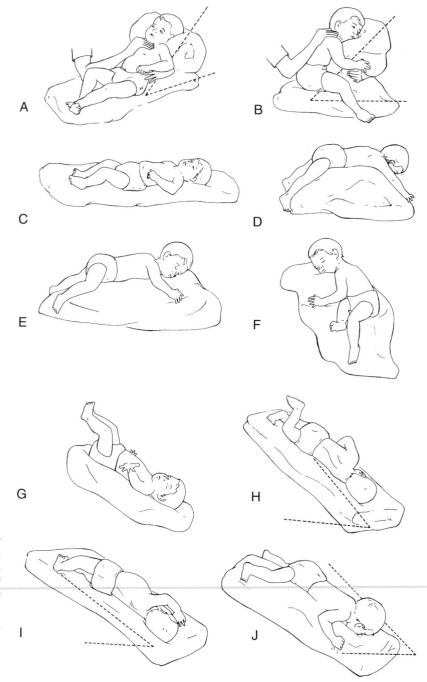

Figure 10-15 Drainage positions in infants. **A,** Apical segment of upper lobes. **B,** Posterior segments of upper lobes. **C,** Anterior segments of upper lobes. **D-F,** Superior segments of lower lobes. **G** and **H,** Anterior basal segments of both lower lobes (H on right and left sides). **I,** Segments of the right middle lobe and lingula (shown). **J,** Posterior basal segments of the lower lobes. (From Crane LD: Physical therapy for the neonate with respiratory disease. In Irwin S, Tecklin JS, editors: Cardiopulmonary physical therapy, ed 3, St Louis, 1995, Mosby.)

and angles are best for draining their lungs. Follow their advice if it produces good results.

Some patients cannot tolerate being properly positioned because their underlying lung or heart disease is aggravated by the unnatural body position. This is most commonly seen in the head-down positions to drain the lower lobes. Watch for signs of hypoxemia and shortness of breath (SOB). The patient may have to be placed in a better-tolerated but less-desirable position. As long as some downward angle to the bronchus exists, mucus will drain. Each patient must be evaluated on an individual basis.

The following treatment revisions may also be beneficial:

a. Change the length of treatment time

Lung segments should generally be drained for 3-15 minutes. If the patient is tolerating the position, and secretions are still being cleared, the position can be held longer. Stop the treatment if the patient is showing any signs of intolerance.

The total time of the procedure is recommended to be no longer than 30-40 minutes if all segments are treated because the patient may become exhausted by the various position changes. If so, the practitioner

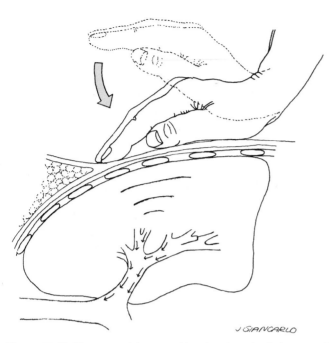

Figure 10-16 Movement of the cupped hand at the wrist during manual chest percussion. (From Shapiro BA, Kacmarek RM, Cane RD, et al.: Clinical application of respiratory care, ed 4, St Louis, 1991, Mosby.)

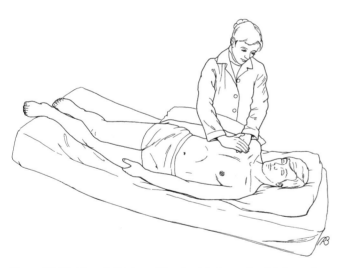

Figure 10-17 Manual vibration of the chest during postural drainage therapy. (From Eubanks DH, Bone RC: Comprehensive respiratory care, ed 2, St Louis, 1990, Mosby.)

must select the worst segments to be drained first. Several drainage sessions may be needed to drain all of the involved segments.

b. Change the treatment techniques used

Be prepared to modify the postural drainage, percussion, and vibration procedures, depending on how the patient tolerates them. For example

- Some patients cannot tolerate certain positions, especially head down, because of pain, SOB, hypoxemia, or elevated blood pressure.

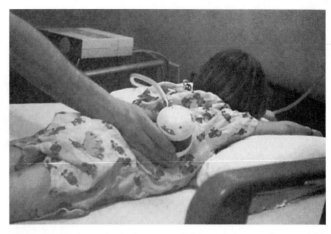

Figure 10-18 A mechanical percussor/vibrator being used on a child. (From Walsh BK, Czervinske MP, DiBlasi RM, editors: Perinatal and pediatric respiratory care, ed 3, St Louis, 2010, Saunders.)

- Percussion rate, pressure, and hand position may need to be modified, depending on the patient's tolerance, chest size, and secretion clearance.
- It may not be possible to percuss or vibrate female patients in the right middle lobe and left lingular positions because of breast tissue.
- Hypoxemia should be prevented with supplemental O_2 as needed. Pulse oximetry could be performed before and during the procedure to monitor the patient's O_2 saturation.
- Patients with cardiac disease should have their heart rate, heart rhythm, and blood pressure monitored. Check the heart rate before the procedure and with each position change.
- Postoperative or trauma patients may not tolerate certain positions, percussion, or vibration because of pain.
- Patients with copious secretions that cannot be expectorated (e.g., those who are not alert or have a tracheostomy) should not be positioned in a compromising situation. Suctioning equipment must be available.
- Patients with asthma, COPD, or obesity may not tolerate any head-down positions because of increased SOB.

c. Organize the sequence of drainage positions and treatment techniques

Differences of opinion exist as to the sequence in which the segments should be drained. Some authors state that an apices-to-bases approach is better, whereas others state that a bases-to-apices pattern is preferred. It makes sense to take an apices-to-bases approach for a first treatment when all lobes are to be drained. This pattern gives the patient time to adapt to the whole procedure. It also may be safer because the practitioner can evaluate the patient through a sequence of positions that progresses from the least to the most stressful.

If the patient can tolerate all positions without any difficulties, and the lower lobes are the worst in terms

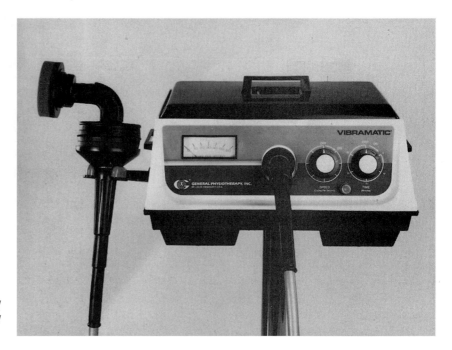

Figure 10-19 The Vibramatic/Multimatic electrically powered mechanical percussor/vibrator. (Courtesy General Physiotherapy, Inc., St Louis, MO.)

of secretions, drain the lower lobes first. If time permits, work up through the middle lobe and lingula to the upper lobes.

All of the various therapeutic options should be individualized to best meet the patient's needs. Be prepared to modify the options to use on different lung segments as the patient's condition either worsens or improves. In addition, be prepared to deliver bland and therapeutic aerosols to the patient before CPT is performed.

5. Recommend a treatment be terminated (code: IIIE1) [difficulty: R, Ap, An]

Be prepared to stop the treatment if the patient has an adverse reaction. Often this results when a patient is placed into a head-down position. Review Box 10-3 for hazards and complications of postural drainage, percussion, and vibration.

Exam Hint 10-3

Be prepared to stop the treatment if the patient becomes short of breath, becomes hypoxic, develops a headache or dizziness, or needs to cough.

6. Postural drainage therapy equipment

a. Assemble the necessary equipment for the procedure (code: IIA16) [difficulty: R, Ap]

The terms *percussor* and *vibrator* are sometimes used interchangeably. Several manufacturers produce either electrically or pneumatically powered percussors/vibrators. Some are large enough to be wheeled into the patient's

room (Fig. 10-19). Obviously, electrically powered units need a standard electrical outlet for power, and the pneumatically powered units must be plugged into a 50-psi O_2 or air source.

Hand-held battery-powered pediatric units are smaller to focus accurately on the much smaller target area of the infant's chest. Some practitioners find that an electric toothbrush with padded bristles works very well. Manual percussion of infants can be aided by using soft rubber palm cups that are available in several pediatric sizes.

Because various devices are powered by wall electrical output, 50-psi source gas, or batteries, check the power source if the device fails to work. Some units have different patient applicators and connectors. These must be fastened properly so that the vibrating action does not cause them to loosen or fall off. For example, the Vibramatic/Multimatic has several patient applicators that must be screwed into the percussion adapter, which is then screwed into the ring adapter (Fig. 10-20).

Some electrically powered units use a rubber belt and different-sized wheels to change gears and produce several vibration rates. Others electrically vary the motor speed to change the vibration rate. Some pneumatically driven units can have their percussion force and rate varied.

b. Troubleshoot any problems with the equipment (code: IIA16) [difficulty: R, Ap]

Pneumatically powered units would suddenly fail if the high-pressure hose to the wall gas outlet or the O_2 tank became disconnected. Electrically powered units would fail if the electrical cord was unplugged or the batteries were depleted.

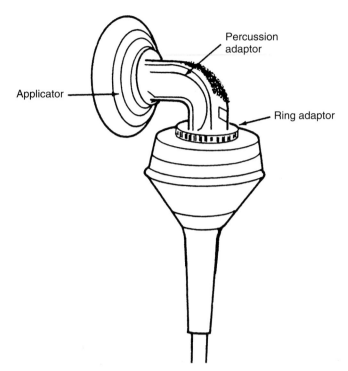

Figure 10-20 Right-angle adapter for Vibramatic chest percussor. The percussion adapter must be tightly screwed into the ring adapter, and the various patient applicators must be tightly screwed into the percussion adapter. (Courtesy of General Physiotherapy, Inc., St Louis, MO.)

MODULE C

Positive expiratory pressure therapy

Positive expiratory pressure (PEP) therapy involves having a cooperative, spontaneously breathing patient exhale against a flow-limiting orifice to create expiratory pressures between 10 and 20 cm H_2O. Because the patient's expiratory flow is limited, the faster the patient tries to exhale, the higher the airway pressure. This therapy also is called *PEP mask therapy* because many pediatric patients find it easier to exhale against a face mask rather than through a mouthpiece.

Box 10-5 lists indications for PEP therapy. In patients with air trapping because of small-airways disease (asthma or COPD), PEP therapy acts like pursed-lips breathing to keep the small airways from collapsing. This allows the trapped alveolar gas to be more completely exhaled. Patients with atelectasis, or at risk for developing atelectasis, respond well to PEP therapy if incentive spirometry is not effective. PEP seems to push air through the pores of Kohn of open alveoli into adjacent areas of atelectasis to force the alveoli open. There is evidence that PEP therapy is better than incentive spirometry or intermittent positive pressure breathing (IPPB) in the treatment of patients with postoperative atelectasis.

PEP therapy has proven effective in helping patients with chronic, copious amounts of secretions, primarily children age 4 years or older with cystic fibrosis. It also helps patients with chronic bronchitis, bronchiectasis, or

---

BOX 10-5 Indications for Positive Expiratory Pressure Therapy

To reduce air trapping in patients with emphysema, bronchitis, and asthma
To prevent or reverse atelectasis
To help mobilize retained secretions in patients older than 4 years who have cystic fibrosis, chronic bronchitis, bronchiectasis, or bronchiolitis obliterans
To maximize the delivery of aerosolized medications, such as bronchodilators, to patients receiving bronchial hygiene therapy

---

BOX 10-6 Relative Contraindications to Positive Expiratory Pressure Therapy

Untreated pneumothorax
Intracranial pressure >20 mm Hg
Active hemoptysis
Recent trauma or surgery to the skull, face, mouth, or esophagus
Patient with asthma attack or acute worsening of chronic obstructive pulmonary disease who cannot tolerate increased work of breathing
Acute sinusitis or epistaxis
Tympanic membrane rupture or other known or suspected middle ear pathology
Nausea

BOX 10-7 Hazards or Complications of Positive Expiratory Pressure Therapy

Pulmonary barotrauma
Increased intracranial pressure
Myocardial ischemia or decreased venous return to the heart
Increased work of breathing
Air swallowing that can lead to vomiting
Discomfort from mask or skin breakdown from mask pressure
Claustrophobia

---

bronchiolitis obliterans more effectively clear their secretions. Clinical evidence indicates that the PEP dilates the small airways so that air is able to pass obstructing secretions. This fills the alveoli and, on expiration, tends to force the secretions into the larger airways for coughing or suctioning. PEP therapy also seems to increase the effectiveness of inhaled aerosolized bronchodilators.

Box 10-6 lists relative contraindications to PEP therapy. No absolute contraindications exist. Box 10-7 lists hazards or complications of PEP therapy. These should be weighed against the benefits to the patient when making the recommendation to start PEP therapy. Other considerations include the patient's history of pulmonary disease and the response to CPT, ineffective cough to clear retained secretions, and breath sounds and chest radiograph findings of secretions.

PEP therapy is currently provided via two different equipment modalities, described here. The original PEP therapy devices use a fixed-orifice resistor and are presented in Part 1. The newer oscillatory PEP devices are presented in Part 2.

1. Part 1: Adjustable fixed-orifice type PEP device

a. Perform positive expiratory pressure therapy (code: IIIB3) [difficulty: R, Ap, An]

The patient must be old enough to understand instructions and be able to perform the procedure. Box 10-8 lists the steps in performing a proper PEP therapy treatment. Be prepared to adjust the expiratory resistance to meet the clinical goal of PEP therapy. Initially the resistance to exhalation should be kept low. As the training continues, the resistance the patient breathes against can be increased. The goal is to maintain a PEP of 10-20 cm H_2O with an inspiratory/expiratory (I:E) ratio of about 1:3. If the expiratory orifice is too small, the expiratory airway

---

BOX 10-8   Steps in Performing Positive Expiratory Pressure (PEP) Therapy

1. Assemble the equipment as shown in Figure 10-21. Set the expiratory resistance to the desired setting.
2. Have the conscious patient sit up straight, rest elbows on a table, and hold the PEP mask comfortably but tightly over the nose and mouth. The patient may use a mouthpiece and nose clips if preferred.
3. The patient should inhale a deeper than normal breath, but not to TLC, by using the diaphragm. The unconscious patient will inhale only a tidal volume breath.
4. The conscious patient should exhale to functional residual capacity (FRC) fast enough to generate 10-20 cm H_2O in the manometer. Have the patient look at the pressure manometer to judge how fast to exhale. The unconscious patient will exhale passively but will still benefit from the increased baseline pressure.
5. The patient should have an expiratory time that is about three times longer than the inspiratory time (an inspiratory/expiratory ratio of 1:2 to 1:4 is acceptable). The clinician can accomplish this by changing the expiratory resistor and/or having the patient change the force of exhalation.
6. Between 10 and 20 proper PEP breaths should be performed.
7. The patient should now perform a directed cough or two or three huff-type coughing efforts to raise secretions.
8. Repeat steps 2 to 7 between four and eight times (for approximately 10-20 minutes) for a full PEP treatment.

Patients in the Intensive Care Unit can perform PEP therapy as often as every hour or as rarely as every 6 hours. They should be reevaluated for treatment effectiveness every 24 hours. Patients in the acute care or home care setting can perform PEP therapy between two and four times each day. The acute care patient should be reevaluated every 72 hours; the home care patient can be evaluated at longer intervals or when a change in pulmonary status occurs.

---

pressure will be too high or the expiratory time too long. The patient will probably become fatigued. If the expiratory orifice is too large, the pressure will not be high enough to be of any benefit. In any situation, the patient will probably become tired if the total treatment time lasts longer than 20 minutes.

All of the various therapeutic options should be individualized to best meet the patient's needs. Be prepared to modify PEP therapy and CPT as the patient's condition either worsens or improves. In addition, be prepared to deliver bland and therapeutic aerosols to the patient before or during PEP therapy.

Coordinate PEP therapy with effective directed coughing, huff cough techniques, CPT, or aerosolized medication delivery. As listed in Box 10-8, PEP breaths can be alternated with huff coughs to clear secretions. Huff coughs are not full, deep coughs; rather, they are performed as follows:

1. Have the patient inhale a slow, deep breath but not to total lung capacity (TLC).
2. Hold the breath for 1-3 seconds.
3. Perform several quick, forced exhalations with an open epiglottis.
4. Small children may be taught to say "huff" with each quick exhalation. It also may help to have the young patient perform a "chicken breath" by flapping his or her arms against the sides of the chest during the exhalation.

CPT may be used before or after PEP therapy, or it may be alternated with PEP therapy, to help in the removal of secretions. Likewise, aerosolized medications may be inhaled before or simultaneously with PEP therapy. Bronchodilators and mucolytic agents should be very helpful with PEP therapy to mobilize secretions. Evaluate sputum for quantity, color, odor, and thickness.

b. Recommend a treatment be terminated (code: IIIE1) [difficulty: R, Ap, An]

During the treatment, ask the patient if he or she feels dyspnea, pain, or chest discomfort. Also monitor the patient's breath sounds, blood pressure, heart rate, and breathing pattern and rate. Monitor oxygenation by pulse oximetry, mental clarity, and skin color. Be prepared to stop the treatment if necessary. Review the contraindications listed in Box 10-6 and hazards listed in Box 10-7. If a bronchodilator or mucolytic medication is being delivered with the PEP treatment, monitor the patient for any adverse reactions to the medication.

c. Fixed-orifice PEP therapy equipment

1. Assemble the necessary equipment for the procedure (code: IIA16) [difficulty: R, Ap]

Currently, there are two hand-held fixed-orifice PEP systems that can be chosen from. Figure 10-21, A shows the Resistex unit. Basic components include the following:

- Patient mouthpiece. Nose clips can be added, if needed.

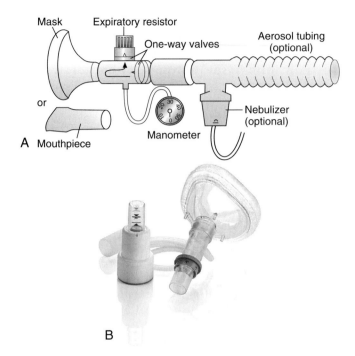

A Mouthpiece

B

Figure 10-21 Examples of fixed-orifice positive expiratory pressure (PEP) devices. **A,** The Resistex (Mercury Medical, Clearwater, FL) expiratory resistor and added components. The basic PEP assembly utilizes a transparent mask or mouthpiece, expiratory resistor, and pressure manometer with connecting oxygen tubing. If a nebulized medication is added, the following also are needed: small-volume nebulizer with T-piece, oxygen tubing to flowmeter, and large-bore tubing for an aerosol reservoir. (From Malmeister MJ, Fink JB, Hoffman GL: Positive-expiratory-pressure mask therapy: theoretical and practical considerations and a review of the literature, Respir Care 36[11]:1218, 1991.) **B,** Photograph of the DHD TheraPEP device. *(Courtesy of Smiths Medical, Dublin, OH.)* Components include a one-way valve and adapter for inspiration (a face mask is attached) and pressure generator.

- Expiratory resistor with four fixed-orifice settings.
- Pressure manometer calibrated in centimeters of water.
- Small-bore oxygen tubing to connect the expiratory resistor to the pressure manometer.
  Optional components include:
- Substitute a pediatric, small adult, or regular adult face mask for the mouthpiece. If the patient has an endotracheal or tracheostomy tube, substitute a universal airway (elbow) adapter for the mouthpiece.
- Small-volume nebulizer (SVN)—note that a metered-dose inhaler (MDI) and holding chamber can be substituted for an SVN and aerosol tubing.
- T-piece and female adapter to connect the SVN to the expiratory resistor.
- Large-bore aerosol tubing to act as a medication reservoir.
  Figure 10-21, B shows the TheraPEP device. The following basic components are included:
- Patient mouthpiece. Nose clips can be added, if needed.
- Mouthpiece adapter with hose to pressure generator.

- Inspiratory one-way valve. (Fit this into the mouthpiece if medications are not being delivered.)
- Pressure generator. Insert one of the six available fixed-orifice resistance diaphragms to suit the patient's expiratory flow goal. The pressure gauge displays the airway pressure generated during exhalation.
  The following optional components are included:
- Substitute a pediatric, small adult, or regular adult face mask for the mouthpiece.
- An SVN or MDI T-piece adapter can be inserted between the mouthpiece adapter and the one-way valve for medication delivery.
- Necessary adapters for the SVN or MDI are included.
  Procedural accessories include a basin and tissues to collect and dispose of sputum. For infection control purposes, the respiratory therapist should have gloves, mask, goggles, and gown if indicated. With either unit, if a PEP mask is used, it should be transparent, flexible, and fitted to the patient's facial contours so that no air will leak out as the pressure is increased.

As described previously and shown in Figure 10-21, the component pieces must be gathered and properly assembled. Make sure that all connections are airtight. If a leak is present, the desired PEP goal will not be reached or maintained. In addition, an air leak may be felt or a high-pitched sound may be heard. If an SVN or MDI is added, it must be tested to ensure that it works properly. Connect the SVN (or MDI) into the system, as shown in Figure 10-21, A. Add the medication and run a flow of O_2 or compressed air at 4-6 L/min through the nebulizer (as is customary). The slowed exhalation during PEP breathing should promote better deposition of medication into the small airways.

Be prepared to adjust the expiratory resistance to meet the clinical goal of PEP therapy. One of six small-exit diaphragms can be added to the pressure generator part of the TheraPEP device. Select the one that best meets the patient's clinical goal. The Resistex unit has four fixed-orifice settings from which to choose. The orifice interior diameters are 4, 3.5, 3, and 2.5 mm. Adjust the dial for the desired size to meet the patient's clinical goal. With either unit, the patient's treatment should begin with the largest opening for exhalation. If appropriate, smaller expiratory openings may be used to meet the patient's clinical goal.

2. Troubleshoot any problems with the equipment (code: IIA16) [difficulty: R, Ap]

Any leaks in the system will prevent the PEP goal from being reached. Tighten any loose connections. If the one-way valves in the Resistex or TheraPEP unit are assembled backward, the patient will inspire against a resistance instead of exhaling against it. Observe the one-way valves in use, and ask the patient if he or she finds it easy to inhale but more difficult to exhale. Move the valves to their proper positions if incorrectly placed. If an SVN is used, check that aerosol is coming from the nebulizer. If not, check the capillary tube or baffle for an obstruction; clear it by running tap water or a sterile needle through it. See Chapter 8, if necessary, for more information on fixing problems with SVNs.

2. Part 2: Adjustable vibratory-type PEP device

a. Perform vibratory positive expiratory pressure therapy (code: IIIB3) [difficulty: R, Ap, An]

The NBRC refers to this type of PEP therapy as vibratory PEP. However, because the professional literature refers to it as *oscillatory PEP* or OPEP, that terminology will be used here. OPEP has the same indications (Box 10-5), contraindications (Box 10-6), hazards (Box 10-7), and clinical benefits as PEP delivered through a fixed-orifice resistor. In theory, the airway oscillations produced with OPEP improve airway clearance better than PEP. Two widely known OPEP devices are presented here. Box 10-9 presents the basic steps in performing an OPEP treatment. Other general considerations for OPEP and related therapies are the same as those for PEP and were presented previously.

BOX 10-9 Steps in Performing Oscillatory Positive Expiratory Pressure (OPEP) Therapy

1. Assemble the equipment shown in Figure 10-22 or 10-23.
2. Ideally, have the conscious patient sit up straight with head erect. (Although not ideal, the patient may lie on either side as long as the Flutter can be held upright. The Acapella, Quake, and Aerobika may be held in any position and will work properly.)
3. The patient should inhale a deeper than normal breath, but not to TLC. Hold the breath.
4. Place the OPEP unit into the mouth, seal lips, and exhale actively. (Coach the patient to exhale about twice as fast as normal but not as fast as possible.)
5. Continue to actively exhale until the patient has reached FRC.
6. During the exhalation adjust the device so that the patient has the greatest sense of vibration felt within the lungs. With the Flutter, adjust the vertical tilt of the bowl. With the Acapella, adjust the dial at the distal end. With the Aerobika, adjust the resistance setting. With the Quake, turn the handle from slow to fast to find the ideal vibration rate. The Quake user should continue to turn the handle while breathing in through the device.
7. Repeat steps 3 to 6 while adjusting the expiratory flow rate and oscillation rate to "fine-tune" the lung maximal vibrations to mobilize secretions. Perform about 6 to 10 breaths through the OPEP device.
8. Remove the OPEP device and finish with one or two maximal efforts: Inhale to TLC, hold the breath for 2-3 seconds, and exhale as fast as possible to FRC.
9. Perform either a maximal coughing effort or midinspiratory/huff-type cough to clear out any secretions.
10. Repeat steps 3 to 9 for four to eight cycles. Total treatment time should not exceed 20 minutes.

Currently, six hand-held OPEP systems can be chosen from, based on the patient's needs. The Flutter (Fig. 10-22) is the original and has been used the most, primarily with cystic fibrosis patients. Because of its simplicity, both small children and adults can be instructed in its use. The Flutter is a pipe-shaped device with a steel ball nesting loosely inside the covered bowl. A perforated cap over the bowl keeps the ball from falling out but allows exhaled air to escape. The exhaled breath pushes the ball up in the bowl, air briefly escapes, and the ball falls back down again. When the ball falls back, backpressure is exerted against the patient's airway. The airway pressure generated during the exhalation varies from 5 to 35 cm H_2O, depending on how fast the patient exhales. The rate at which the ball flutters up and down ranges between 2 and 32 Hz (Hertz or cycles/s) and varies with the angle of the bowl. The high-frequency oscillations of backpressure on the airway caused by the fluttering steel ball are believed to help dislodge viscous secretions. The patient must sit

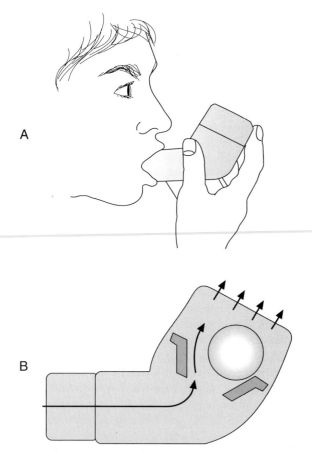

Figure 10-22 A, Patient correctly holding the Flutter for an exhalation. **B,** Cross-section drawing of the Flutter showing how the steel ball is lifted by the patient's exhaled tidal volume. When the ball drops back down into the cup, the backpressure is transmitted to the airways. (From Fink JB, Hess DR: Secretion clearance techniques. In Hess DR, MacIntyre NR, Mishoe SC, et al., editors: Respiratory care principles and practice, Philadelphia, 2002, Saunders.)

up and hold the Flutter as if it were a pipe. Through trial and error the patient varies the expiratory flow rate and angle of the bowl to find the best oscillation rate to mobilize secretions.

The RC-Cornet and the Lung Flute are two additional simple devices that, like the Flutter, reflect low-frequency sound waves down the patient's airways to thin and dislodge mucus. The RC-Cornet is a curved tube with a mouthpiece. The mouthpiece can be adjusted through five different positions to change the pressure and flow characteristics as the patient exhales through the unit. It is suggested that positions 1, 2, and 3 are best suited to a patient with COPD. Positions 4 and 5 are best suited to a patient with tenacious secretions such as found with cystic fibrosis and bronchiectasis. The device may be used at any angle, such as the patient lying down in bed. The RC-Cornet can also be combined with an SVN for a combined aerosol therapy and OPEP treatment. When used this way, the patient must sit upright. The Lung Flute is a straight tube with a mouthpiece and a long flexible reed that runs from the mouthpiece through the tube. The patient must sit upright and hold the Lung Flute down at a 45-degree angle. When blown through, the reed vibrates within the tube and sends sound waves back into the patient. In addition, the Lung Flute has been approved for a sputum induction procedure. (See the sputum induction discussion in Chapter 8 and the traditional use of hypertonic saline to stimulate a productive cough.)

In addition, there are currently three more complexly designed OPEP devices. The Acapella (Fig. 10-23, A) is available in four different models. There are two expiratory flow models that allow the practitioner to better match the patient's needs with the equipment. A third model, the Choice, can be disassembled for easy cleaning in the home or hospital. A fourth model, the Duet, is designed so that an SVN can be added without a T-piece. All models allow the user to adjust the frequency and amplitude of the oscillations. The Quake (Fig. 10-23, B) has a handle that the user turns to find the best pressure and vibration rate. With a slower rotation there is increased pressure at a lower rate. With a faster rotation there is decreased pressure with a higher rate. The Aerobika has five resistance settings, from low to high, to choose from. With any OPEP device, when the best expiratory flow, pressure, and frequency are found, the patient's secretions will be optimally mobilized. See Box 10-9 for the steps in the procedure.

If inhaled bronchodilator or mucolytic medications are ordered for the patient using the Flutter, Quake, or Lung Flute, they should be taken before the OPEP treatment. This is because these devices are not designed to be used with an SVN or MDI. The Acapella models, RC-Cornet, and Aerobika can have an SVN added to them for aerosol therapy while performing an OPEP treatment. All of the various therapeutic options should be individualized to best meet the patient's needs. Be prepared to modify OPEP therapy and CPT as the patient's condition either worsens or improves.

Coordinate OPEP therapy with effective maximal cough or huff cough techniques, CPT, or aerosolized medication delivery. As listed in Box 10-9, OPEP breaths should be alternated with directed coughing to clear secretions. Huff coughs are not full, deep coughs; rather, they are performed as follows:

1. Have the patient inhale a slow, deep breath but not to TLC.
2. Hold the breath for 1-3 seconds.
3. Perform several quick, forced exhalations with an open epiglottis.
4. Small children may be taught to say "huff" with each quick exhalation. It also may help to have the young patient perform a "chicken breath" by flapping his or her arms against the sides of the chest during the exhalation.

CPT may be used before or after OPEP therapy, or it may be alternated with OPEP therapy, to help in the removal of secretions. Aerosolized bronchodilators and mucolytic agents should be very helpful with OPEP therapy to mobilize secretions. Evaluate sputum for quantity, color, odor, and thickness.

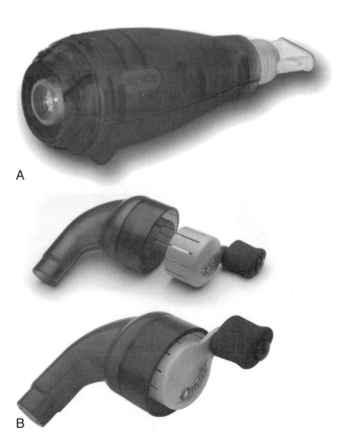

Figure 10-23 Examples of oscillatory positive expiratory pressure (OPEP) devices. **A,** One of four types of Acapella OPEP device. (Courtesy of Smiths Medical, Dublin, Ohio.) **B,** Disassembled and assembled views of the Quake OPEP device. (Courtesy of Thayer Medical, Tucson, AZ.)

b. Recommend a treatment be terminated (code: IIIE1) [difficulty: R, Ap, An]

It is unlikely that a patient will have an adverse reaction from any device. However, it is possible that some patients will not like the feeling of increased pressure in the lungs. In this case, it may be better to stop the treatment and switch to another method of secretion management.

During the treatment, ask the patient if he or she feels dyspnea, pain, or chest discomfort. Also monitor the patient's breath sounds, blood pressure, heart rate, and breathing pattern and rate. Monitor oxygenation by pulse oximetry, mental clarity, and skin color. Be prepared to stop the treatment if necessary. Review the contraindications listed in Box 10-6 and hazards listed in Box 10-7. If a bronchodilator or mucolytic medication is being delivered with the OPEP treatment, monitor the patient for any adverse reactions to the medication.

c. OPEP therapy equipment

1. Assemble the necessary equipment for the procedure (code: IIA16) [difficulty: R, Ap]

The Flutter (Fig. 10-22) is a pipe-shaped device with a steel ball nesting loosely inside the bowl. The device has been used with cystic fibrosis patients to help them loosen their secretions. It is believed that the high-frequency oscillations of backpressure on the airway caused by the fluttering steel ball help to dislodge thick (viscous) secretions. The Flutter must be kept upright during the patient's exhalation to work properly. The device is preassembled by the manufacturer. A perforated cap should be over the bowl to keep the ball from falling while letting exhaled air escape. There are no accessories for pressure monitoring or adding medications.

The Acapella (Fig. 10-23, A) uses an adjustable counterweighted lever and magnet to produce variable frequency and amplitude of the expiratory pressure. It has the same clinical indications as the Flutter device. The original Acapella is available with a choice of two models based on the patient's expiratory flow. The green DH model is indicated for patients with an expiratory flow >15 L/min (>0.25 L/s). The blue MD model is indicated for patients with an expiratory flow <15 L/min (<0.25 L/s). This allows for a better match of the unit with the patient's pulmonary function. The newer Choice model can be disassembled for easier cleaning. A possible advantage of the Acapella devices over the Flutter is that they can be used in any patient position.

All Acapella models with its adult mouthpiece are preassembled by the manufacturer. Each has an adjustable knob at the end of the unit opposite the patient's mouthpiece. As the knob is rotated, a magnet is moved closer to or farther from a counterweighted lever. Rotate the knob, as needed, to set the patient's expiratory frequency and amplitude pressure. The following accessories are available, if needed:
- A pressure port with tubing to connect to a pressure manometer can be added.
- A pediatric- or adult-size mask can be substituted for the mouthpiece.

- With the proper adapter, an SVN can be added for medications. In addition, a high-pressure gas source and small-bore (oxygen) tubing would also have to be connected to the nebulizer.

These accessories allow for the patient's airway pressure to be monitored, the unit to be fitted to the patient for better compliance, and therapeutic aerosols to be given.

The Quake (Fig. 10-23, B) has a main outer barrel component with the patient's mouthpiece. The handle component fits into the main component so that it can be turned. The speed at which the crank is turned determines the pressure and vibration rate. There are no accessories for adding an aerosol. Like the Acapella, the Quake can be used at any angle.

The Aerobika comes preassembled by the manufacturer. It can be disassembled into four pieces for cleaning. A breath-activated nebulizer (BAN) can be added to the expiratory port for aerosol therapy. In addition, a high-pressure gas source and small-bore (oxygen) tubing would also have to be connected to the BAN.

2. Troubleshoot any problems with the equipment (code: IIA16) [difficulty: R, Ap]

The patient must keep the Flutter in the proper position with the perforated cap in the upright position. This keeps the patient's exhaled air blowing through the device to push up the steel ball. If a patient should cough secretions into the unit, it will become clogged. Air will not flow through it. Try clearing the obstruction from the mouthpiece with a cotton swab or by running warm water through the unit. If necessary, the cap can be unscrewed from the bowl and the steel ball and cup can be removed. Wash out any secretions and reassemble.

With the Acapella, if the adjustable knob cannot move or the frequency and amplitude pressure cannot be adjusted, the unit may be obstructed by secretions or may be defective. The DM and DH models can be washed with warm, soapy water. The Choice model can be disassembled into four parts, each of which can be washed with warm, soapy water. For disinfection purposes this model is put through a dishwasher, boiled, autoclaved, or soaked in glutaraldehyde. If after cleaning and reassembly it still does not function, it is defective and must be replaced.

With the Quake, if the handle cannot be turned, it might be fouled with secretions. Separate the two components, wash out any secretions, and reassemble. With the Aerobika, if no vibrations can be felt, it might be fouled with secretions. Disassemble the four pieces, wash out any secretions, and reassemble.

Exam Hint 10-4

Expect to see at least one question about PEP therapy. Be prepared to recommend it for a patient with a secretion problem. PEP therapy may have to be modified to maximize secretion mobilization, or PEP therapy may be added to another treatment such as incentive spirometry, an SVN for medications, or HFCWO to help the patient mobilize and clear secretions.

MODULE D

High-frequency chest wall oscillation

1. Perform high-frequency chest wall oscillation (code: IIIB3) [difficulty: R, Ap, An]

High-frequency chest wall oscillation (HFCWO) is indicated to help mobilize and clear secretions. This procedure may be used in patients with cystic fibrosis, bronchiectasis, or chronic bronchitis who do not tolerate other secretion mobilization procedures. For example, a cystic fibrosis patient may have an adverse effect when put into head-down positions for postural drainage therapy.

The patient should be instructed to sit up during the treatment, put on the inflatable vest or cuirass, and connect the air hose(s) between the vest/cuirass and the pumping unit. A general recommendation is to have the patient set whatever oscillation (chest wall compression) rate that results in the greatest production of secretions. Common sense indicates that it is appropriate to start at the lowest rate and pressure and progress to a faster rate and higher pressure as the patient tolerates. However, there is laboratory evidence that an HFCWO rate of about 13-15 Hz is best at improving mucus movement. Treatments typically last 30 minutes and can be repeated up to six times per day. This procedure cannot be used in a patient with a chest wall injury such as broken ribs.

2. Recommend a treatment be terminated (code: IIIE1) [difficulty: R, Ap, An]

In general, HFCWO seems to be well tolerated. However, be prepared to stop the treatment if the vest/cuirass is causing skin irritation. With proper fitting the treatment should be well tolerated.

3. High-frequency chest wall oscillation equipment

a. Assemble the necessary equipment for the procedure (code: IIA16) [difficulty: R, Ap]

Follow the manufacturer's guidelines to assemble the components. Currently, four HFCWO devices are available: the Vest (Fig. 10-24), InCourage, and SmartVest consist of a nonstretchable inflatable vest that covers the entire torso, an electrically powered pumping and control system, and one or two connecting hoses. A variety of inflatable vests are available and one must be selected that best fits the patient's torso. With the Vest unit, the controls allow an adjustable air pulse rate of either 5 Hz (producing a vest pressure of 25 mm Hg) or 25 Hz (producing a vest pressure of 40 mm Hg).

The Hayek RTX oscillator (Fig. 10-25) consists of a flexible chest cuirass that covers the chest, an electrically powered pumping and control panel, and a connecting hose. A variety of cuirass shells are available and one must be selected that best fits the patient's anterior chest shape. This machine can deliver both positive and negative pressure to the patient's chest throughout the breathing cycle. Added negative pressure around the patient's chest will

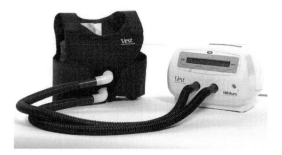

Figure 10-24 The Vest high-frequency chest wall oscillation device. The power unit has an air compressor and controls for air pulse rate and vest pressure through two hoses that connect to the vest. The inflatable vest has two ports for the hoses from the power unit. (Courtesy of Advanced Respiratory, St Paul, MN.)

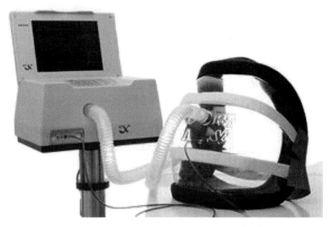

Figure 10-25 The Hayek RTX oscillator with its pumping and control unit, air hose, and patient cuirass. (Courtesy of United Hayek Industries, London, UK.)

increase inspiration. Added positive pressure around the patient's chest will increase expiration. The therapist can adjust an oscillation rate of 8-1200 oscillations/min, with an I:E ratio of 6:1 to 1:6, and inspiratory and expiratory pressures from +70 to ±50 cm water.

With any unit, it is believed that the pressure on the outside of the chest is transmitted internally to increase expiratory airflow and push secretions from small to larger airways. HFCWO has been found especially to help cystic fibrosis patients mobilize retained secretions.

b. Troubleshoot any problems with the equipment (code: IIA16) [difficulty: R, Ap]

One problem area could relate to the vest/cuirass not fitting properly. If the vest/cuirass is too large, air will leak, and the desired pressures will not be reached. Adjust the unit for a tighter fit, or place pads between the patient and the vest/cuirass to seal the leak. Too tight a vest/cuirass could rub on the skin and be uncomfortable. Loosen the vest/cuirass or add more padding over the skin. If a hose loosens from the vest/cuirass or the pumping unit, the air will leak out, and no pressure will be generated. Reattach the hose.

MODULE E

Intrapulmonary percussive ventilation

1. Perform intrapulmonary percussive ventilation (code: IIIB3) [difficulty: R, Ap, An]

Intrapulmonary percussive ventilation (IPV) provides high-frequency mini-bursts of air to oscillate the airways while an aerosolized medication is being administered. It has been advocated for patients who are at least 10 years of age and who cannot spontaneously remove their airway secretions. Patients with cystic fibrosis, bronchiectasis, or chronic bronchitis are the most likely to benefit from IPV. In addition, there is some clinical evidence that IPV will help in the prevention or treatment of atelectasis. All manufacturers of IPV devices have built their systems with an SVN for bland or medicated aerosol therapy during the IPV treatment. So, IPV effectively combines three therapeutic modalities: IPPB therapy, OPEP therapy, and aerosol therapy. An IPV treatment would typically consist of delivering a bronchodilator and/or mucolytic medication via the SVN while adjusting the inspiratory flow, peak pressure, and percussive rate to what is comfortable to the patient and results in the greatest production of secretions. With the initial treatment, a low peak pressure and low percussive rate should be set. Depending on the patient's tolerance and treatment effectiveness, the pressure and/or percussive rate can be increased. The pressure (amplitude) range is typically 10-30 cm water. Rates vary between IPV devices but have an overall range of 1-30 Hz (60-1800 cycles/min). After several IPV breaths the patient should be encouraged to perform a full cough or huff cough. Repeat the cycle of IPV breaths and coughing for 15-20 minutes, as tolerated.

2. Recommend a treatment be terminated (code: IIIE1) [difficulty: R, Ap, An]

Because IPV has aspects of IPPB, OPEP, and medicated aerosol therapy, the patient should be assessed for an adverse reaction from any of them. See the adverse reaction lists in the appropriate chapter for these therapies. Of greatest concern would be hemoptysis or pneumothorax from the high airway pressure and a tachycardia reaction from a bronchodilator medication. If any of these should be identified, the IPV treatment should be stopped and the physician notified.

3. Intrapulmonary percussive ventilation equipment

a. Assemble the necessary equipment for the procedure (code: IIA16) [difficulty: R, Ap]

As of this writing, there are four manufacturers of complex, expensive units that can be moved from patient to patient for an IPV treatment. These include a variety of models from Percussionaire and the Breas, MetaNeb, and Pegaso models. (The Pegaso A-Cough Perc can deliver IPV and mechanical insufflation–exsufflation). All models

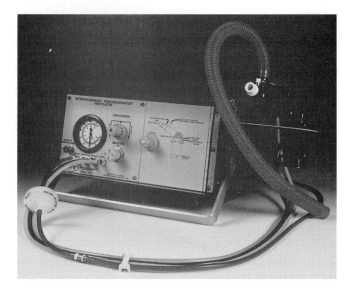

Figure 10-26 Percussionaire intrapulmonary percussive ventilator (IPV-1) with its small-volume nebulizer and associated hoses for delivering pressure and powering the nebulizer. (Courtesy of Percussionaire, Sandpoint, ID.)

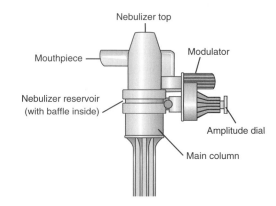

Figure 10-27 Drawing of the VORTRAN PercussiveNEB single-patient IPV device with its key features. Not shown is the small-bore (oxygen) tubing that connects a flowmeter to the unit. (Modified courtesy of VORTRAN Medical Technology, Sacramento, CA.)

have a control unit and require a high-pressure gas source or air compressor, a nebulizer, and several hoses to connect the nebulizer or other components to the gas source. Figure 10-26 shows the Percussionaire IPV-1 with its SVN and hoses. All of these units have a variety of modes and settings to control the nebulizer, percussion pressure, and percussion rate. The Percussionaire comes in models for general hospital use, for delivery of IPV to a patient receiving mechanical ventilation, and for home care.

The VORTRAN PercussiveNeb is a simpler, less expensive device that is designed for single-patient use. Figure 10-27 shows its components. In addition, it requires a high-pressure gas source, flowmeter, and small-bore (oxygen) tubing to connect the flowmeter to the Diameter Index Safety System adapter on the main column below the nebulizer.

As the flow rate is increased, the percussion rate increases. Spin the amplitude dial clockwise to increase the pressure of each percussion.

b. Troubleshoot any problems with the equipment (code: IIA16) [difficulty: R, Ap]

All IPV units require a high-pressure gas source from either piped-in air or oxygen in the hospital or an electrically powered air compressor in the home. If a unit fails to operate, check the gas source. The Percussionaire and other reusable machines have several hoses to operate the SVN and percussion pressure generator. If they are not properly connected, the gas will leak out. As discussed in Chapter 8, the SVN must be properly assembled with a patent capillary tube to draw the medication to the baffle. If secretions enter the SVN and plug the capillary tube, the SVN must be disassembled, cleaned, and reassembled.

MODULE F

Mechanical insufflation–exsufflation

1. Perform mechanical insufflation–exsufflation (code: IIIB3) [difficulty: R, Ap, An]

Mechanical insufflation–exsufflation (MIE) is also known as in–exsufflation. This form of therapy is indicated in a patient who cannot take in a large enough breath to effectively cough out secretions because of a neuromuscular disease or neurologic condition. These conditions include, but are not limited to, poliomyelitis, amyotrophic lateral sclerosis, myasthenia gravis, and spinal cord injury. The key indicator for MIE in an adult patient is a peak cough flow of <270 L/min (<4.5 L/s). A bedside peak flow measurement is the practical equivalent of a peak cough flow.

For a patient to have an effective cough, he or she must be able to deeply inspire. This requires the ability to inhale an inspiratory reserve volume to reach inspiratory capacity. (See Fig. 4-7 in Chapter 4.) The neuromuscular disease patient who cannot periodically breathe deeply cannot cough and is likely to develop atelectasis, pneumonia, and decreased chest-wall range of motion. So, a deep breath must be therapeutically provided. Insufflation refers to the controlled delivery of positive pressure to the lungs to have the patient inhale a larger than normal tidal volume. The second major component of an effective cough is a fast exhalation (the peak cough flow). A weak patient must have this fast exhalation therapeutically provided. Exsufflation is controlled sustained negative pressure that is sufficient to shear secretions from the airways and move them to the mouth for expectoration or suctioning.

As with all treatments, the insufflation and exsufflation pressures and application times should be individualized.

Most studies on adults have found that pressures of about +40/−40 cm H_2O are optimal. These pressures should initially be low and gradually increased as tolerated and until effective. Typically the pressures are maintained for 1-3 seconds. A typical MIE treatment on an experienced adult could include:

1. Pretreatment with a prescribed nebulized bronchodilator and/or mucolytic medication.
2. Gradually increasing insufflation pressure to a range of +30 to +50 cm H_2O.
3. Pressure is held for 1-3 seconds.
4. Rapid exsufflation pressure drop to a range of −30 to −50 cm H_2O.
5. Negative pressure is held for 1-3 seconds.
6. This cycle is repeated about five times.
7. The patient is encouraged to cough or is suctioned as needed.
8. After a rest period, this entire cycle is repeated until the secretions are cleared.

2. Recommend a treatment be terminated (code: IIIE1) [difficulty: R, Ap, An]

Because MIE delivers a high inspiratory pressure, like IPPB, there would be similar risks. Of greatest concern would be hemoptysis or pneumothorax. If either of these should be identified, the MIE treatment should be stopped and the physician notified. If the patient develops abdominal distension from air being forced into the stomach, the insufflation pressure should be decreased.

3. Mechanical insufflation–exsufflation equipment
a. Assemble the necessary equipment for the procedure (code: IIA16) [difficulty: R, Ap]

As of this writing, there are three types of MIE equipment: CoughAssist In-Exsufflator, Pegaso A-Cough Perc, and Nippy Clearway. Figure 10-28 shows the CoughAssist being used on a patient. Each of the devices has a central control unit for setting modes of operation and an air compressor for generating the operating pressures. They require an A/C or D/C electrical source for the control functions and air compressor. A large-bore hose and filter are connected to the control unit. The patient interface of mouthpiece, face mask, or tracheostomy adapter is connected at the other end of the hose. In addition, some units have a small-bore hose that carries the mask pressure back to the control unit for display.

b. Troubleshoot any problems with the equipment (code: IIA16) [difficulty: R, Ap]

Failure to reach the desired positive or negative pressure would indicate a leak in the system. The patient who is using a mouthpiece may be leaking through the nose. Nose clips can be applied or a face mask will need to be used. If there is a leak around the tracheostomy (or endotracheal tube), make sure the cuff is properly inflated.

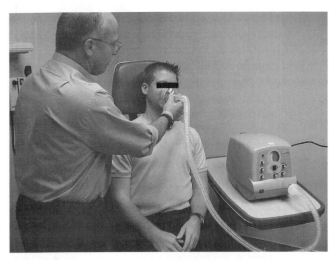

Figure 10-28 A patient being given a breathing treatment with the CoughAssist mechanical insufflation–exsufflation device. The main unit has controls for setting positive and negative pressures. Accessories include the air filter, hose, and face mask. (From Mason R, Broaddus V, Martin T, et al.: Murray & Nadel's textbook of respiratory medicine, ed 10, Philadelphia, 2010, Saunders.)

MODULE G

Respiratory care plan

1. Determine a patient's pathophysiologic state (code: IIIF1) [difficulty: R, Ap, An]

The patient's breath sounds should be auscultated before the treatment begins to determine which segments are normal or have secretions. Auscultate each segment after the treatment and after the patient has coughed. Listen for air moving into formerly silent areas or areas that are cleared of secretions.

Make a recommendation for a chest radiograph examination to find specific areas for CPT. A white shadow on a chest radiograph film over what should be normal lung may indicate areas of atelectasis or infiltrates that can be targeted for treatment. Chest radiograph examinations should be repeated to look for an improvement in the lungs. The resolution may be slow or dramatic, depending on the original problem and how it responds to the various treatments used on it.

2. Recommend starting a treatment based on the patient's response (code: IIIE2a) [difficulty: R, Ap, An]

See the previous discussions and below.

3. Recommend a change in the therapeutic plan if indicated (code: IIIF2) [difficulty: R, Ap, An]

The AARC *Clinical Practice Guideline* recommends that the following be evaluated to determine whether chest physiotherapy is needed:

- CPT is usually not indicated if an optimally hydrated patient is expectorating less than 25 mL/day with the procedure.
- A dehydrated patient should have apparently ineffective CPT continued for at least 24 hours after the patient is rehydrated. The combination of rehydration and CPT may help to mobilize previously thick secretions.
- CPT is not indicated in a patient producing more than 30 mL of secretions per day if the treatments do not increase the sputum production. The patient is already able to expectorate the sputum effectively.

For any of the previously discussed procedures, be prepared to measure the patient's blood pressure, heart rate, and respiratory rate before, during, and after a change in therapy. Minor changes (less than 20%) can be expected. The patient's oxygenation should improve as secretions and mucous plugs are removed and atelectatic areas open. The patient's breath sounds should be auscultated before and after any treatment procedure. Listen for air moving into formerly silent areas and for secretions being cleared.

Ask the patient how he or she feels before, during, and after the treatment. CPT should not be performed for at least 1 hour after a patient has eaten to minimize the chances of nausea from the head-down position.

PEP therapy has been indicated in patients who have retained secretions that are difficult to expectorate. Increase or decrease the PEP level to help the patient without causing fatigue or complications. If PEP therapy does not increase the amount of sputum produced per day in a patient who already produces more than 30 mL, PEP may not be needed. It does not make sense to continue an ineffective treatment.

4. Initiate and conduct patient and family disease management education (code: III I5) [difficulty: Ap, An]

The previously discussed procedures are used primarily with cystic fibrosis or chronic bronchitis patients. All have been shown to help in the mobilization of secretions. However, each patient may find that one procedure works better than another. Teach the patient and/or family members about the ordered procedure. CPT can be performed by family members on the patient. Many patients, even older children, can be taught to self-administer PEP and OPEP therapy. Be prepared to make recommendations to change the type of procedure and the way each procedure is conducted. In addition, other respiratory care procedures (e.g., O_2 therapy) and inhaled bronchodilators and mucolytic medications may have to be modified as the patient's condition warrants.

5. Recommend a treatment be terminated (code: IIIE1) [difficulty: R, Ap, An]

See the previous discussion with each therapeutic modality.

6. Recommend discontinuing a treatment based on the patient's response (code: IIIE2h) [difficulty: R, Ap, An]

Review the previous discussion for indications that the patient has recovered and no longer needs ACT procedures. For example, the secretions have decreased or can be easily expectorated by the patient, or both.

The patient's breath sounds should improve if retained secretions are expectorated. Review Boxes 10-2 and 10-3 for contraindications and hazards/complications of postural drainage and percussion and vibration. Review Boxes 10-6 and 10-7 for contraindications and hazards/complications of PEP therapy.

BIBLIOGRAPHY

Alves LA, Pitta F, Brunetto AF: Performance analysis of the Flutter VRP1 under different flows and angles, *Respir Care* 53(3):316, 2008.

American Association for Respiratory Care: Clinical practice guideline: postural drainage therapy, *Respir Care* 36:1418, 1991. Retired.

American Association for Respiratory Care: Clinical practice guideline: use of positive airway pressure adjuncts to bronchial hygiene therapy, *Respir Care* 38(5):516, 1993. Retired.

American Association for Respiratory Care: Clinical practice guideline: directed cough, *Respir Care* 38(5):495, 1993. Retired.

American Association for Respiratory Care: Clinical practice guideline: effectiveness of nonpharmacologic airway clearance therapies in hospitalized patients, *Respir Care* 58(12):2187, 2013.

Andrews J, Sathe NA, Krishnaswami S, McPeeters MI: Nonpharmacologic airway clearance techniques in hospitalized patients: a systematic review, *Respir Care* 58(12):2160, 2013.

Berlinski A, Willis JR: Albuterol delivery via intrapulmonary percussive ventilator and jet nebulizer in a pediatric ventilator model, *Respir Care* 55(12):1699, 2010.

Branson RD, Hess DR, Chatburn RL: *Respiratory care equipment*, ed 2, Philadelphia, 1999, Lippincott Williams & Wilkins.

Cairo JM: Lung expansion therapy devices. In Cairo JM, editor: *Mosby's respiratory care equipment*, ed 9, St Louis, 2014, Mosby.

Campbell TC, Ferguson N, McKinlay RGC: The use of a simple self-administered method of positive expiratory pressure (PEP) in chest physiotherapy after abdominal surgery, *Physiotherapy* 72(10):498, 1986.

Chatburn RL: High-frequency assisted airway clearance, *Respir Care* 52(9):1224–1235, 2007.

Chatwin M, Simonds AK: The addition of mechanical insufflation/exsufflation shortens airway-clearance sessions in neuromuscular patients with chest infections, *Respir Care* 54(11):1473, 2009.

Davidson KL: Airway clearance strategies for the pediatric patient, *Respir Care* 46(7):823, 2002.

Eid N, Buchheit J, Neuling M, et al.: Chest physiotherapy in review, *Respir Care* 36(4):270, 1991.

Eubanks DH, Bone RC: *Comprehensive respiratory care*, ed 2, St Louis, 1990, Mosby.

Fink JB: Volume expansion therapy. In Burton GC, Hodgkin JE, Ward JJ, editors: *Respiratory care: a guide to clinical practice*, ed 4, Philadelphia, 1997, Lippincott-Raven.

Fink JB: Bronchial hygiene therapy and lung expansion. In Fink JB, Hunt GE, editors: *Clinical practice in respiratory care*, Philadelphia, 1999, Lippincott-Raven.

Fink JB: Positive pressure techniques for airway clearance, *Respir Care* 47(7):786, 2002.

Fink JB: Positioning versus postural drainage, *Respir Care* 47(7):769, 2002.

Fink JB: Forced expiratory technique, directed cough, and autogenic drainage, *Respir Care* 52(9):1210, 2007.

Fink JB, Hess DR: Secretion clearance techniques. In Hess DR, MacIntyre NR, Mishoe SC, et al.: *Respiratory care principals and practice*, Philadelphia, 2002, Saunders.

Fink JB, Mahlmeister MJ: High-frequency oscillation of the airway and chest wall, *Respir Care* 47(7):797, 2002.

Flume PA, Robinson KA, O'Sullivan BP, Finder JD, Vender RL, Willey-Courand DB, et al.: Cystic fibrosis pulmonary guidelines: airway clearance therapies, *Respir Care* 54(4):522, 2009.

Frownfelter DL: Chest physical therapy and airway care. In Barnes TA, editor: *Core textbook of respiratory care practice*, ed 2, St Louis, 1994, Mosby.

Hass CF, Loik PS, Gay SE: Airway clearance applications in the elderly and in patients with neurologic and neuromuscular compromise, *Respir Care* 52(10):1362, 2007.

Hess DR: Sputum collection, airway clearance, and lung expansion therapy. In Hess DR, MacIntyre NR, Mishoe SC, Galvin WF, Adams AB, editors: *Respiratory care principles and practice*, ed 2, Burlington, MA, 2012, Jones & Bartlett Learning.

Hess DR, Branson RD: Chest physiotherapy, incentive spirometry, intermittent positive-pressure breathing, secretion clearance, and inspiratory muscle training. In Branson RD, Hess DR, Chatburn RL, editors: *Respiratory care equipment*, ed 2, Philadelphia, 1999, Lippincott Williams & Wilkins.

Hill KV: Bronchial hygiene therapy. In Aloan CA, Hill TV, editors: *Respiratory care of the newborn and child*, ed 2, Philadelphia, 1997, Lippincott-Raven.

Hirsch CA: Airway clearance therapy. In Kacmarek RM, Stoller JK, Heuer AJ, editors: *Egan's fundamentals of respiratory care*, ed 10, St Louis, 2013, Mosby.

Hoffman GL, Cohen NH: Positive expiratory pressure therapy, *NBRC Horizons* 19(2):1, 1993.

Homnick DN: Mechanical insufflation-exsufflation for airway mucus clearance, *Respir Care* 52(10):1296, 2007.

Johnson NT, Pierson DJ: The spectrum of pulmonary atelectasis: pathophysiology, diagnosis, and therapy, *Respir Care* 31(11):1107, 1986.

Kacmarek RM, Dimas S, Mack CW: *The essentials of respiratory care*, ed 4, St Louis, 2005, Mosby.

Kempainen RR, Milla C, Dunitz J, Savik K, Hazelwood A, Williams C, et al.: Comparison of settings used for high-frequency chest-wall compression in cystic fibrosis, *Respir Care* 55(6):695, 2010.

Lapin CD: Airway physiology, autogenic drainage, and active cycle of breathing, *Respir Care* 47(7):778, 2002.

Lester MK, Flume PA: Airway-clearance therapy guidelines and implementation, *Respir Care* 54(6):733, 2009.

Malmeister MJ, Fink JB, Hoffman GL: Positive-expiratory-pressure mask therapy: theoretical and practical considerations and a review of the literature, *Respir Care* 36(11):1218, 1991.

Myslinski MJ, Scanlan CL: Bronchial hygiene therapy. In Wilkins RL, Stoller JK, Kacmarek RM, editors: *Egan's fundamentals of respiratory care*, ed 9, St Louis, 2009, Mosby.

Myers TR: Positive expiratory pressure and oscillatory positive expiratory pressure therapies, *Respir Care* 52(10):1308, 2007.

Oberwaldner PT, Evans JC, Zach MS: Forced expirations against a variable resistance: a new chest physiotherapy method in cystic fibrosis, *Pediatr Pulmonol* 2(6):358, 1986.

Paneroni M, Clini E, Simonelli C, Bianchi L, Degli Antoni F, Vitacca M: Safety and efficacy of short-term intrapulmonary percussive ventilation in patients with bronchiectasis, *Respir Care* 56(7):984, 2011.

Rutkowski JA: Pulmonary hygiene and chest physical therapy. In Wyka KA, Mathews PJ, Rutkowski J, editors: *Foundations of respiratory care*, ed 2, Clifton Park, NY, 2012, Delmar.

Rutkowski JA: Hyperinflation therapy. In Wyka KA, Mathews PJ, Rutkowski J, editors: *Foundations of respiratory care*, ed 2, Clifton Park, NY, 2012, Delmar.

dos Santos AP: Guimaraes RC, de Carvalho EM, Gastaldi AC: Mechanical behaviors of Flutter VRP1, Shaker, and Acapella devices, *Respir Care* 58(2):298, 2013.

van der Schans CP: Conventional chest physical therapy for obstructive lung disease, *Respir Care* 52(9):1198, 2007.

Schechter MS: Airway clearance applications in infants and children, *Respir Care* 52(10):1382, 2007.

Scott AA, Koff PB: Airway care and chest physiotherapy. In Koff PB, Eitzman D, Neu J, editors: *Neonatal and pediatric respiratory care*, ed 2, St Louis, 1993, Mosby.

Shapiro BA, Kacmarek RM, Cane RD, et al.: *Clinical application of respiratory care*, ed 4, St Louis, 1991, Mosby.

Silva CEA, Eng JGS, Jansen JM, de Melo Eng PL: Laboratory evaluation of the Acapella device: pressure characteristics under different conditions, and a software tool to optimize its practical use, *Respir Care* 54(11):1480, 2009.

Sobush DC, Hilling L, Southorn PA: Bronchial hygiene therapy. In Burton GC, Hodgkin JE, Ward JJ, editors: *Respiratory care: a guide to clinical practice*, ed 4, Philadelphia, 1997, Lippincott-Raven.

Toussaint M, Guillet MC, Paternotte S, Soudon P, Haan J: Intrapulmonary effects of setting parameters in portable intrapulmonary percussive ventilation devices, *Respir Care* 57(5):735, 2012.

Volsko TA: Airway clearance therapy: finding the evidence, *Respir Care* 58(10):1669, 2013.

Walsh BK: Airway clearance techniques and lung volume expansion. In Walsh BK, Czervinske MP, DiBlasi RM, editors: *Perinatal and pediatric respiratory care*, ed 3, St Louis, 2010, Saunders.

White GC: *Equipment theory for respiratory care*, ed 4, Albany, NY, 2005, Thomson Delmar Learning.

Wojciechowski WV: Incentive spirometers, secretion evacuation devices, and inspiratory muscle training devices. In Barnes TA, editor: *Core textbook of respiratory care practice*, ed 2, St Louis, 1994, Mosby.

SELF-STUDY QUESTIONS

See Appendix for answers.

1. A 15-year-old female patient with cystic fibrosis has copious amounts of secretions. She cannot tolerate postural drainage therapy because she gets a headache when tipped head-down. Aerosolized bronchodilators and mucolytic agents are ordered every 4 hours by SVN. What else should be recommended?
   A. Add incentive spirometry.
   B. Aerosolized medications by IPPB
   C. Add PEP therapy.
   D. Modify the PDT positions so her head is not lower than her body.

2. To get the best patient results, manual percussion should be performed with
   1. The hand cupped
   2. A tight, fixed-wrist position
   3. The elbows relaxed
   4. The hand flat
   5. The wrist relaxed
   A. 3, 4, and 5 only
   B. 2, 3, and 4 only
   C. 2 and 4 only
   D. 1, 3, and 5 only

3. How should manual vibration be performed as part of CPT?
   1. On inspiration
   2. At a rate of 20-30 cycles/s
   3. On expiration
   4. At a rate of 3 cycles/s
   5. Throughout the breathing cycle
   A. 2 and 4 only
   B. 1 and 4 only
   C. 3 and 4 only
   D. 4 and 5 only

4. When a patient's chart is reviewed, it is important to look for contraindications to CPT. These would include all of the following EXCEPT:
   A. Increased intracranial pressure
   B. Recent stroke
   C. Small VC in a bedridden patient
   D. The patient has just eaten

5. A stroke patient has been admitted and is in a coma. The physician is concerned that the patient may develop atelectasis and pneumonia. What should be recommended to help prevent these problems?
   A. Regular turning
   B. PEP therapy
   C. IPPB
   D. CPAP

6. An order is received to perform postural drainage, percussion, and vibration on a patient. No segments are specified. On reviewing the chest X-ray film, the therapist notices infiltrates in the lower right

lung field. Which of the following segments should be treated?
1. Apical
2. Lateral basal
3. Superior
4. Medial
5. Posterior basal
A. 2 and 5 only
B. 3, 4, and 5 only
C. 1 and 4 only
D. 2, 3, and 5 only

7. A physician has ordered PEP therapy with albuterol (AccuNeb). All of the following are needed to start the treatment EXCEPT:
A. Variable orifice resistor
B. Pressure manometer
C. Bedside spirometer
D. Nebulizer with reservoir

8. All of the following are contraindications to percussion and vibration EXCEPT:
A. Performing the procedure over the kidneys
B. Mobilizing large amounts of secretions
C. Performing the procedure over bare skin
D. Performing the procedure over or near a surgical site

9. A patient is positioned on the left side with the foot of the bed raised 18 inches. The patient would be draining which lung segment?
A. Anterior basal
B. Superior
C. Lateral and medial lingular
D. Posterior basal

10. A patient has been ordered to start PEP therapy. During the initial instruction and patient practice, it is noticed that the pressure is 25 cm H_2O and the patient's I:E ratio is 1:5. How should the procedure be revised?
A. Adjust the PEP device to have the patient exhale through a larger hole.
B. Have the patient continue but coach the patient to exhale faster.
C. Adjust the PEP device to have the patient exhale through a smaller hole.
D. Add a bronchodilator medication to the PEP device.

11. A respiratory therapist is reviewing a patient's chart and looking for indications for postural drainage. All of the following would be included EXCEPT:
A. A patient with bronchiectasis and retained secretions
B. A patient with cystic fibrosis who has retained secretions
C. Draining of an empyema
D. Removal of an aspirated foreign body

12. The respiratory therapist has received an order to perform postural drainage, percussion, and vibration on a 23-year-old female patient. The lateral and medial segments of the right middle lobe are among those that need to be treated. How should the procedure be performed?
A. Drain, percuss, and vibrate the segments.
B. Drain and vibrate the segments.
C. Drain but not percuss or vibrate those segments.
D. Drain and use a mechanical percussor.

13. A patient is using the Flutter and coughs productively. Later, the patient tries to use the device but finds that no air will go through it. What should be done?
A. Have the patient breathe in harder.
B. Check for an obstruction.
C. Remove the steel ball to reduce the backpressure.
D. Have the patient blow out harder.

14. A patient with bilateral pneumonia is positioned for drainage of the lateral and medial segments of the right middle lobe. After 5 minutes in this position, the patient complains of SOB. The electrocardiogram shows the patient to be having premature ventricular contractions. The most likely cause of this is:
A. Hypoxemia from the position
B. A full stomach is causing vagal stimulation
C. Increased intracranial pressure
D. Increased venous return to the heart

15. The respiratory therapist is using a pneumatically powered mechanical percussor on a patient receiving CPT. The unit is powered by an E cylinder of O_2 because piped-in O_2 is unavailable. After a few minutes of operation, it is noticed that the percussor begins to slow down and then stops. What should be done?
A. Switch to an electrically powered percussor.
B. Make sure the cylinder is completely turned on.
C. Check the unit's batteries.
D. Check the electrical cord.

16. A mechanical percussor is ordered to assist with secretion clearance in a patient receiving CPT. The patient is positioned to drain the posterior basal segments of both lower lobes. The percussor is activated and applied to the patient's lower back. After 1 minute, the patient complains of skin discomfort. What should the respiratory therapist do?
A. Have the patient sit up.
B. Apply oxygen and check the pulse oximeter value.
C. Increase the speed on the percussor.
D. Change to another type of pad on the percussor.

17. Which of the following can be successfully used with a 6-year-old child?
1. Autogenic drainage
2. Chest physiotherapy
3. Oscillatory positive expiratory pressure

   4. ACBT
   5. IPV
   A. 1 and 3 only
   B. 4 and 5 only
   C. 2, 3, and 4 only
   D. 1, 2, and 5 only

18. A patient who is being instructed in PEP therapy complains that it is taking too long to breathe out. What should be done?
   A. Tell the patient to blow out harder.
   B. Change the expiratory resistance to a larger diameter orifice.
   C. Change the expiratory resistance to a smaller diameter orifice.
   D. Increase the flow of oxygen to the system.

19. IPV has been ordered for an adult patient with bronchiectasis. An aerosolized bronchodilator has also been ordered. How should the two treatments be delivered?
   1. Bronchodilator given before the IPV
   2. Low pressure setting
   3. Bronchodilator with IPV
   4. High pressure setting
   5. Bronchodilator after IPV
   A. 2 and 3 only
   B. 1 and 2 only
   C. 3 and 5 only
   D. 4 and 5 only

20. A 56-year-old patient has been in the Trendelenburg position for 10 minutes receiving percussion and vibration. Tachycardia and dyspnea develop. Which of the following actions should be completed by the respiratory therapist?
   A. Continue for 5 minutes with gentle percussion.
   B. Turn the patient to the other side.
   C. Give the patient oxygen.
   D. Have the patient sit up.

21. A 12-year-old patient with cystic fibrosis had PEP therapy started at 5 cm water. After a few minutes of use, the patient has a strong but unproductive cough. What should be done now?
   A. Increase the PEP level to 10 cm water.
   B. Increase the PEP level to 15 cm water.
   C. Change to incentive spirometry.
   D. Discontinue the treatment.

22. After several days of receiving postural drainage and percussion therapy to all lobes in the left lung, the patient's chest radiograph shows improvement except for the lateral basal segment of the left lower lobe. In what position should the patient now be placed for postural drainage?
   A. Right side down with the head of the bed down 30 degrees
   B. Right side down with the bed flat
   C. Left side down with the head of the bed down 30 degrees

   D. Flat on his back with the bed flat and a pillow beneath the knees

23. For drainage of the superior and inferior lingula segments, the patient should be positioned:
   1. With the foot of the bed elevated 14 inches
   2. One-fourth turn up from the front-down position on the bed
   3. One-fourth turn up from the back-down position on the bed
   4. With the foot of the bed elevated 30 degrees
   5. Flat on his or her back
   A. 1 and 3 only
   B. 4 and 5 only
   C. 1 and 2 only
   D. 1 and 5 only

24. The patient benefits from using the Flutter by which of the following?
   1. Increased transpleural pressure
   2. Airway vibrations
   3. Increased intrapleural pressure
   4. Rapid variation in airway pressure
   A. 1 and 2 only
   B. 2 and 3 only
   C. 3 and 4 only
   D. 2 and 4 only

25. A 48-year-old woman had her gallbladder removed. What is most effective in preventing postoperative atelectasis?
   A. Blow bottles
   B. PEP therapy
   C. Mechanical chest percussor
   D. Inspiratory muscle training

26. A patient is starting HFCWO to help mobilize secretions. Which of the following instructions should the patient be given for the initial treatment?
   1. Lie on the side with secretions.
   2. Sit up straight.
   3. Set the controls at a low pressure.
   4. Set the controls at a high pressure.
   5. Set the unit for nebulization.
   A. 2 and 3 only
   B. 1 and 3 only
   C. 2, 4, and 5 only
   D. 1, 3, and 5 only

27. A 70-year-old patient who had a stroke has aspirated and now has a fever and pulmonary secretions. The respiratory therapist notices on the anteroposterior and right lateral chest radiographs that the posterior segment of the right upper lobe is opaque. What postural drainage position should be used with this patient?
   A. On the right side, head down 30 degrees, one-fourth turn up from face down
   B. Sitting upright and leaning forward 30 degrees

C. Head down 15 degrees, pillow behind the right side to turn one-fourth turn up from flat

D. Head down 15 degrees, pillow behind the left side to turn one-fourth turn up from flat

28. The respiratory therapist is working with a patient who begins to expectorate blood after being positioned for drainage of the superior segment of the left lower lobe. Percussion was provided with a mechanical device. After the patient has expectorated 50 mL of blood, what should be recommended as the best action?

A. Continue the treatment because the patient has not lost a great deal of blood.

B. Continue the treatment on only the upper and middle lobes.

C. Stop the treatment, sit the patient up, and call the physician.

D. Continue the treatment with manual percussion only.

29. CPT (postural drainage, percussion, and vibration) has been performed for 5 days on a cooperative patient with bronchiectasis. During that time, the patient has been treated with antibiotics, well fed, and hydrated. The patient has produced a total of 20 mL of sputum during the past 24 hours. What should be recommended?

A. Continue the current treatment program for 48 hours and evaluate the patient again.

B. Add ultrasonic nebulizer treatments to the CPT to better liquefy the secretions.

C. Add nasotracheal suctioning to the CPT to remove the secretions.

D. Discontinue the CPT and follow the patient's progress.

30. A 10-year-old male patient with cystic fibrosis has large amounts of secretions. He cannot tolerate postural drainage because of nausea when he is tipped down. He is receiving aerosolized bronchodilator and mucolytic medications. To improve his condition, the respiratory therapist could recommend all of the following EXCEPT:

A. OPEP therapy

B. Quake unit

C. HFCWO

D. Continuous positive airway pressure

31. A 12-year-old patient does not tolerate postural drainage for secretion clearance. The physician wishes to consider high-frequency airway oscillation. Which of the following options should be recommended first?

A. HFCWO

B. Acapella

C. IPV

D. ACBT

32. A 27-year-old patient with an unstable T-1 spinal cord injury has been admitted for treatment of bronchitis. A bedside assessment is performed and it is found that the patient cannot cough out the secretions. Bedside spirometry reveals the patient has a peak flow of 200 L/min (3.3 L/s). What treatment should be recommended?

A. HFCWO

B. Chest physiotherapy

C. Mechanical insufflation–exsufflation

D. Positive expiratory pressure

11 | Cardiac Monitoring and Cardiopulmonary Resuscitation

Note: It can be anticipated that the Therapist Multiple-Choice Examination (TMC) will include an *average of 5 of 140 actual questions* (4% of the exam) on cardiac monitoring and cardiopulmonary resuscitation (CPR). (This is based on the question mix typically found on the National Board of Respiratory Care's (NBRC's) previous Entry Level Examinations and Written Registry Examinations.)

Remember that the TMC version you take will include 20 additional questions being evaluated for possible inclusion in other versions of the TMC. So, there will be a total of 160 questions taken. There is no way to differentiate between the 140 actual questions and the 20 questions being evaluated for future use. Please go to the Introduction for detailed information on the TMC and the Clinical Simulation Examination.

MODULE A

Evaluate data in the patient record.

1. Evaluate cardiac enzyme laboratory results (code: IA4) [R, Ap]

There are five blood marker studies to help determine if a patient has had a myocardial infarction (MI). The most sensitive and specific markers for an MI are creatine kinase–MB (CK-MB; also known as creatine phosphokinase), troponin I (cardiac troponin I, cTnI), and troponin T (cardiac troponin T, cTnT). Troponin I is felt to be a more specific marker of heart damage than troponin T. Less useful markers for an MI are lactate dehydrogenase (LDH) and aspartate aminotransferase (AST; also known as serum glutamic–oxaloacetic transaminase).

The CK-MB and troponin I and T tests should be done if an MI is suspected. The LDH can be done to help confirm the CK-MB findings or if the patient has delayed coming to the hospital after experiencing heart attack signs and symptoms. The AST may be done if another confirming test is needed. All five MI markers have predictable onset, peak, and return to normal timelines:

CK-MB timeline

Increase: 4-6 hours after MI
Peak: 12-24 hours after MI
Return to normal: 3 days after MI

Note: Although the CK-MB test is the best marker for an acute MI, a similar pattern will be seen if the patient had recent cardiac surgery or a coronary angioplasty or was defibrillated.

Troponin I timeline

Increase: 2-4 hours after MI
Initial peak: 15-24 hours after MI
Lower peak: 60-80 hours after MI
Return to normal: 7 days after MI

Troponin T timeline

Increase: 2-4 hours after MI and remains elevated
Return to normal: 7 days after MI

LDH timeline

Increase: 12-48 hours after MI
Peak: 48-72 hours after MI
Return to normal: 7-14 days after MI

AST timeline

Increase: 8-12 hours after MI
Peak: 24-48 hours after MI
Return to normal: 5-7 days after MI

2. Evaluate trends in cardiac catheterization results (code: IA14c) [R, Ap]

Right-heart catheterization is done to measure right-heart pressures, evaluate the function of the pulmonic and tricuspid valves, sample blood oxygen content from the right heart chambers, and measure cardiac output. The catheter is inserted via the right basilic vein in the arm and superior vena cava or the femoral vein and inferior vena cava.

Left-heart catheterization is done to measure left-heart pressures, evaluate the function of the mitral and aortic valves, and evaluate the function of the left ventricle. The catheter is inserted via the femoral artery and aorta. This approach is also used when the coronary arteries are catheterized to assess blood flow and treat a blockage with angioplasty or placement of a stent.

Many patients known or suspected of having a valve problem or narrowed coronary artery will have cardiac catheterization performed. After a treatment has been performed (valve replacement or removing a blockage), cardiac catheterization is often performed again to help determine if the treatment was successful.

3. Evaluate trends in echocardiography results (code: IA14d) [R, Ap]

Echocardiography (also called Doppler echocardiography) uses very high frequency sound waves that are sent through the chest wall to detect blood flow through the heart, heart valve regurgitation, the size of the right or left ventricle, and the function (pumping) of the right and left ventricles. During a basic echocardiogram, the sound waves reflect off of internal structures to show blood flow or heart movement. These reflected sound waves are converted to an electrical signal to give a two-dimensional image on a video screen. There are three more advanced variations on the echocardiogram.

The *color Doppler* uses applied colors to demonstrate blood flow and the heart's function. These color changes enhance the basic two-dimensional image to a three-dimensional image and show the velocity of blood flow.

The *stress echocardiogram* is done to increase the accuracy of a standard exercise test (see Chapter 18). As soon as possible after a patient finishes a treadmill or bicycle exercise test, an echocardiogram is performed. This shows the functioning of the heart at its maximum performance. These findings are then compared to a previously performed resting echocardiogram. If a patient cannot exercise, the drug dobutamine (Dobutrex) is given intravenously to stimulate the heart to its peak performance.

The *transesophageal echocardiogram* is done to evaluate the heart's performance with an internal view. In this procedure, a special flexible endoscope with a piezoelectric crystal is advanced down the esophagus of a sedated patient. When the endoscope tip has reached the stomach, its tip is flexed to touch the stomach wall. From this internal vantage point, the heart's functioning can be viewed very accurately. As the endoscope is withdrawn through the esophagus, additional views of the heart can be taken.

Many patients having a known or suspected valve problem or decreased right- or left-ventricle function will have an echocardiogram performed. After treatment has been performed, an echocardiogram is performed again to help determine if the treatment was successful.

MODULE B

Electrocardiogram monitoring and diagnostic electrocardiogram

1. Review the patient record for trends in electrocardiogram monitoring (code: IA14a) [R, Ap]

Review the chart of any patient admitted with a significant cardiopulmonary problem for a record of previous cardiac monitoring. Look for a record of rhythm disturbances.

2. Recommend an electrocardiogram (code: IE10) [R, Ap]

a. Cardiac monitoring

Recommend electrocardiogram (ECG) monitoring in any patient with a significant cardiopulmonary problem or who could have significant changes in heart rate and rhythm. This could include, but is not limited to, congestive heart failure, previous MI, suspicion of current MI, pulmonary embolism, pneumonia, or other problem that could result in serious hypoxemia. In addition, ECG monitoring should be done on a patient with an electrolyte disturbance or who is receiving replacement electrolytes intravenously, especially potassium. The patient care setting could be the Emergency Department, Intensive Care Unit, a general care unit, or when the patient is being transported.

To perform ECG monitoring, it is necessary to select the proper cardiac electrodes and monitoring unit. Cardiac electrodes, or leads, pick up the electrical signal from the heart and conduct it to the monitor. They are usually called *chest leads* (or *chest electrodes* or *precordial leads*) and consist of four parts: (1) a conducting wire coated with an electrically neutral plastic, (2) an adapter at one end of the wire that plugs into the electrocardiograph machine, (3) a different adapter at the opposite end of the wire that attaches to a patient electrode, and (4) the patient electrode (Fig. 11-1, A). Conducting jelly is added to the surface of the electrode to reduce the skin's resistance to the heart's electrical signal. An adhesive ring holds the electrode tightly to the skin. The conducting wire snaps or clips onto the back of the electrode. Typically, three to five of these chest leads are used for a period of hours or days for basic rhythm monitoring or Holter monitoring. Typically, three or four chest leads are used for rhythm monitoring. Holter monitoring typically involves using five chest leads.

One of the following monitoring units must be selected, based on the patient's situation:

1. Basic bedside rhythm monitoring

A bedside rhythm monitoring unit will have an oscilloscope for viewing the rhythm and additional features for counting the heart rate, setting high and low heart rate alarms, and recording the rhythm on standard ECG paper for a permanent record. The unit receives input from three or four chest leads (Fig. 11-1, B). That collective signal is sent to the oscilloscope (video display terminal) for a real-time display of the patient's rhythm. If the high or low rate setting is reached, an audible and visual alarm is triggered. The patient's heart rhythm will then be recorded on ECG paper. Or, manually push the record button for an ECG paper record of an unusual event. These units are often seen mounted at the patient's bedside in the Intensive Care Unit.

The most common chest electrode pattern used for rhythm monitoring is called *lead II*. The three chest electrodes are placed as shown in Figure 11-1, B. The negative

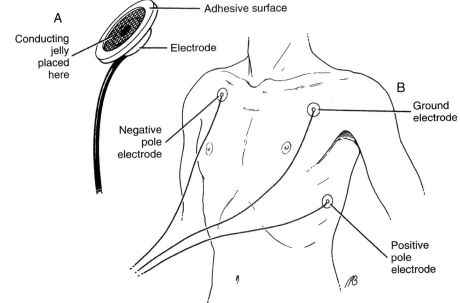

Figure 11-1 **A,** Close-up of the features of a prepackaged monitoring electrode or lead. **B,** Standard electrode placements for lead II monitoring. This results in the traditional-looking electrocardiogram waveform with upright P, QRS, and T waves. (*Note:* The electrodes are often labeled as right arm (RA) instead of negative pole, left arm (LA) instead of ground electrode, and left leg (LL) instead of positive electrode.) (From Eubanks DH, Bone RC: Comprehensive respiratory care, ed 2, St Louis, 1990, Mosby.)

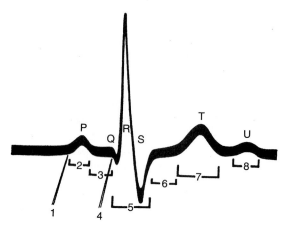

Figure 11-2 Sequence of electrical events of the cardiac cycle during normal sinus rhythm. (See Table 11-1 for the description of each event.) (From Phillips RE, Feeney MK: The cardiac rhythms: a systematic approach to interpretation, ed 3, Philadelphia, 1990, Saunders.)

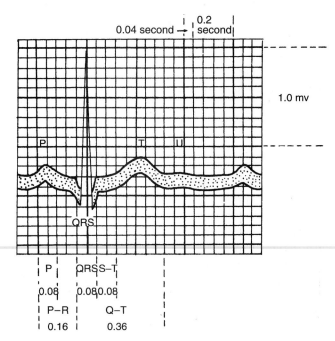

Figure 11-3 Timing of the electrical events of the cardiac cycle during normal sinus rhythm. (From Spearman CB, Sheldon RL, Egan DF: Egan's fundamentals of respiratory therapy, ed 4, St Louis, 1982, Mosby.)

(right arm) electrode is on the right upper chest. The positive (left leg) electrode is placed on the left lateral chest. The ground (left arm) electrode is placed on the left upper chest. With this electrode configuration, known as the Einthoven triangle, the heart's electrical signal is followed as it flows from the right atrium to the left ventricle. This results in the so-called normal ECG tracing with upright P, R, and T waves, as shown in Figures 11-2 and 11-3. Table 11-1 shows the sequential electrical events of the normal cardiac rhythm that correspond to those in Figure 11-2.

2. CPR cart

A CPR "crash" cart will have electrocardiograph leads and a monitor mounted on it. These are connected to

the defibrillator to allow synchronous defibrillation (cardioversion) or asynchronous defibrillation. Typically, three or four chest leads are used for rhythm monitoring (Fig. 11-1, B). Crash carts have other features that are similar to those seen on bedside rhythm monitoring units. Portable versions of these units are used when the patient must be transported. A portable unit operates by battery power when unplugged from the wall electrical outlet.

3. Holter monitoring

Holter ECG monitoring is done to evaluate noncritical home care patients with a suspected cardiac problem. Because the patient will be mobile for 1-3 days while being monitored, the limb leads are placed on the upper and lower chest area. Precordial leads are placed normally. The patient wears a tight-fitting undershirt or netlike dressing to keep the leads in place. The patient cannot bathe while the leads are on. In addition, the patient keeps a diary of any episodes of chest pain, dyspnea, and so forth. The whole system includes the portable, battery-powered recording device for the patient's ECG, a set of chest leads, a carrying bag for the recording device, and a patient activity diary (Fig. 11-4).

Successful ECG monitoring requires that the correct electrodes be chosen, put together properly, attached to

TABLE 11-1	Electrophysiologic Events Represented by the Electrocardiogram
Sequential Electrical Events of the Cardiac Cycle	**Electrocardiographic Representation**
1. Impulse from the sinus node	Not visible
2. Depolarization of the atria	P wave
3. Depolarization of the atrioventricular node	Isoelectric
4. Repolarization of the atria	Usually obscured by the QRS complex
5. Depolarization of the ventricles	QRS complex
a. Intraventricular septum	a. Initial portion
b. Right and left ventricles	b. Central and terminal portions
6. Quiescent state of the ventricles immediately after depolarization	ST segment: isoelectric
7. Repolarization of the ventricles	T wave
8. Afterpotentials following repolarization of the ventricles	U wave

From Phillips RE, Feeney MK: The cardiac rhythms: a systematic approach to interpretation, ed 3, Philadelphia, 1990, Saunders.

the patient as indicated, and connected to the correct ECG machine. Any errors will result in an electrical signal that is distorted or absent. With all types of cardiac leads, bad skin contact, dried conducting jelly, or a disconnected wire results in a distorted or absent electrical signal. Recheck all patient electrodes and wire connections if a problem is seen.

Connect the patient's chest leads cable into the proper monitor. Turn on the monitor, and select the desired electrical signal from the heart (usually lead II). Confirm that the electrical signal is displayed on the monitor, and set any alarm limits.

b. Perform a diagnostic ECG (code: IC1) [difficulty: R]

A diagnostic ECG (also called a *12-lead ECG*) test is indicated if the patient is suspected of having a serious cardiac problem such as an MI (or acute myocardial infarction, AMI). Symptoms such as syncope, angina pectoris, sudden crushing chest pain, or shortness of breath or signs such as unstable heart rate and blood pressure point to a heart problem. Growing evidence indicates that men and women have different signs and symptoms during an MI. Men tend to have crushing central chest pain that may radiate down the left arm or the left side of the neck, diaphoresis, cold extremities, shortness of breath, and a feeling of impending doom. Women tend to experience pain in the lower back and the abdominal area. A diagnostic ECG is needed to document the nature of the cardiac problem or rule out the heart as a source of the symptoms.

To perform a diagnostic (12-lead) ECG, get the proper cardiac electrodes and recording ECG machine. These electrodes will be used for only a few minutes as the recording of the heart's electrical activity is being done. They come in two sets, one for the limbs and one for the chest.

A 12-lead ECG test requires a machine capable of receiving electrical input from the four limb leads and six precordial leads (Figs. 11-5 and 11-6). The operator can manually select the lead combinations needed to

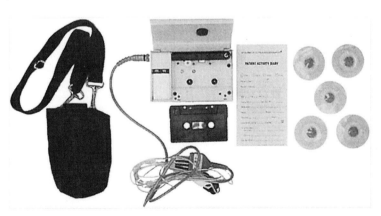

Figure 11-4 Holter monitoring system for ambulatory electrocardiography. (From Pagana K, Pagana TJ: Mosby's manual of diagnostic and laboratory tests, ed 4, St Louis, 2010, Mosby.)

get the 12 different combinations for a 12-lead ECG tracing. However, modern units do this automatically when the operator turns them on. The various ECG combinations are printed out on ECG paper. Modern units also store the patient's information on a self-contained computer.

The limb leads come as a group of four with one for each arm and leg (Fig. 11-5). Precordial leads come in a group of six and are placed on the chest in the positions shown in Figure 11-6. A conducting and adhesive jelly is used to reduce the skin's resistance and to hold the lead in place. The limb leads are longer, and they may need to be held in place by a rubber strap.

The 12-lead ECG involves the use of an electrocardiograph machine with heat-sensitive ECG recording paper, four limb leads, and six precordial leads (see Figs. 11-5 and 11-6). Table 11-2 describes the locations of the precordial leads and the positive and negative electrode combinations that are used to record the heart's electrical signal through the 12 different leads. Each lead individually records the heart's electrical activity, but it does so from a different position in relation to the heart. These 12 leads give the physician a three-dimensional impression of how the cardiac conduction system and the myocardium are functioning. Abnormal functioning can be diagnosed. Review the normal anatomy and physiology of the heart and its conduction system, if necessary.

Clinical experience is important in performing a diagnostic ECG. Improper placement of the precordial or limb leads can easily result in a misleading ECG tracing and a misdiagnosis. For example, reversing the arm leads causes the QRS to be reversed in lead I. Technical errors in grounding the patient and not keeping the patient still during the ECG also result in useless tracings because of electrical interference and an unstable baseline.

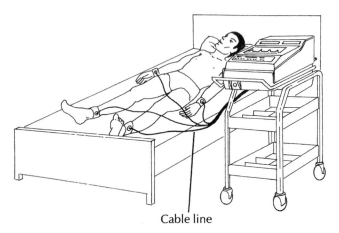

Figure 11-5 Limb electrodes or leads properly placed on all four of the patient's limbs. Make sure that the right leg lead is placed on the right leg, the right arm lead is placed on the right arm, and so forth. The electrode cables are then plugged into the electrocardiograph machine to record the electrocardiogram tracings. (From Eubanks DH, Bone RC: Comprehensive respiratory care, ed 2, St Louis, 1990, Mosby.)

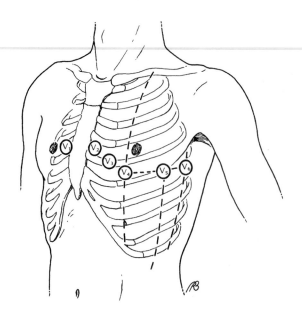

Figure 11-6 Proper placement of the six precordial leads. (See Table 11-2 for a description of the locations.) (From Eubanks DH, Bone RC: Comprehensive respiratory care, ed 2, St Louis, 1990, Mosby.)

TABLE 11-2		Standard Electrocardiogram Leads	
	Leads	**Positive Electrode**	**Negative Electrode**
Bipolar	1. I	Left arm	And right arm
	2. II	Left leg	And right arm
	3. III	Left leg	And left arm
Unipolar	4. aV$_R$	Right arm	Central terminal*
	5. aV$_L$	Left arm	
	6. aV$_F$	Left leg	
Precordial	7. V$_1$	Right of sternum in 4th ICS	Central terminal*
	8. V$_2$	Left of sternum in 4th ICS	
	9. V$_3$	Midway between V$_2$ and V$_4$	
	10. V$_4$	Midclavicular line in 5th ICS	
	11. V$_5$	Midway between V$_4$ and V$_6$	
	12. V$_6$	Lateral chest in 5th ICS	

aV, augmented voltage; ICS, intercostal space.

*The central terminal is a combination of electrode potentials producing a summation effect. This serves as the single negative or indifferent electrode. The specific combination of electrodes for each lead is automatically determined in the lead selector switch.

From Phillips RE, Feeney MK: The cardiac rhythms: a systematic approach to interpretation, ed 3, Philadelphia, 1990, Saunders.

Exam Hint 11-1

Usually one or two questions require the respiratory therapist to recognize possible signs of a MI and recommend either ECG monitoring or the performance of a diagnostic 12-lead ECG.

MODULE C

Evaluate the results of a diagnostic electrocardiogram. (code: ID1) [difficulty: R, Ap]

Before discussing diagnostic electrocardiogram (12-lead ECG) interpretation, it is important to review how ECG paper is designed so that the heart's electrical signal traced on it can be understood. This special paper is heat sensitive and, after exiting the ECG machine, shows a black line from the heated stylus. Figure 11-7 shows the grid markings on the paper and how to interpret the ECG tracing for voltage and time. Each large square box is 5 mm in height and represents 0.5 mV of the heart's electrical force. The large square box is divided into five smaller boxes that are 1 mm in height and represent 0.1 mV. Timing of the ECG tracing is determined by the speed with which the paper passes under the heated stylus. Normally, this is 25 mm/s. At this speed, each large square box is 20 seconds, and each of the five small boxes is 0.04 second; 300 large boxes comprise 1 minute (0.20 second × 300 = 60 seconds).

The following 10 features should be examined and time-interval measured in every ECG:

1. Heart rate
2. Rhythm
3. P wave
4. PR interval
5. QRS interval
6. QRS complex
7. ST segment
8. T wave
9. QT interval
10. U wave

The systematic evaluation of these factors usually results in a clear understanding of the patient's cardiac function. All of these factors are discussed and illustrated in this chapter. Before evaluating the ECG paper tracing for possible cardiac dysrhythmias, first rule out any artifacts and determine the patient's heart rate.

1. Artifacts

An ECG *artifact* is an artificially made electrical signal that does not relate to the patient's heart activity. An artifact can usually have one of three causes. First, the ECG electrodes are not in good contact with the skin or are placed in the wrong area. For example, a chest lead has come off or the limb leads are reversed. Second, wires from another monitoring system are in contact with the ECG leads and there is electrical interference. Third, unusual electrical activity is coming from the patient. For example, the patient is shivering, having muscle tremors, or having seizures. The respiratory therapist can cause an artifact by performing chest percussion over a patient's chest ECG lead. In many cases, an artifact can be eliminated by the filtering systems built into the recording unit. In other cases, the underlying problem will have to be corrected to get an accurate electrical signal showing cardiac activity.

2. Heart rate

The *heart rate* can be most accurately found by counting it for 1 minute; however, this time-consuming method is not always practical. An approximate heart rate can be quickly found. First, find a heartbeat tracing in which the R wave is on a heavy vertical line. Then count the number of large boxes between this first R wave and the next R wave. Approximate heart rates can be estimated as follows:

- Two large boxes = 150 beats/min (300 divided by 2)
- Three large boxes = 100 beats/min (300 divided by 3)
- Four large boxes = 75 beats/min (300 divided by 4)
- Five large boxes = 60 beats/min (300 divided by 5)
- Six large boxes = 50 beats/min (300 divided by 6)

For example, in Figure 11-8, during inspiration there are three large boxes between R waves for a heart rate of about 100/min. During exhalation there are four large boxes between R waves for a heart rate of about 75/min. The heart rate can also be estimated by counting the number of beats in 6 seconds and multiplying by 10.

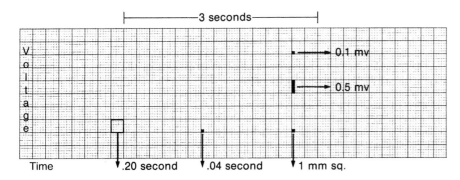

Figure 11-7 Electrocardiogram paper with added details on how to interpret time and voltage. (From Patel JM, McGowan SG, Moody LA: Arrhythmias: detection, treatment, and cardiac drugs, Philadelphia, 1989, Saunders.)

3. Normal sinus rhythm

Obviously, the normal cardiac rhythm must be understood to distinguish it from abnormal rhythms. The normal adult's cardiac rhythm is usually called normal sinus rhythm (NSR) and has these characteristics:

- Heart rate between 60 and 100 beats/min while at rest
- Rhythm that varies by no more than ±10% between QRS complexes
- P wave before every QRS complex and upright in lead II
- A QRS complex follows every P wave
- Proper timing of the components of the ECG rhythm Figure 11-3 shows the timing of the components of an NSR.

4. Abnormal cardiac rhythms

The following list of abnormal cardiac rhythms (usually called arrhythmias or dysrhythmias) includes many of those that are commonly encountered in clinical practice. It is beyond the scope of this text to discuss all possible dysrhythmias. Instead, those that are either frequently seen or dangerous are described. Each of the following cardiac irregularities is (1) defined, (2) exemplified, (3) described, (4) discussed in terms of its clinical significance, and (5) accompanied by a treatment (if any) description.

a. Arrhythmias with a sinoatrial node origin

The following three arrhythmias all originate from the sinoatrial (SA) node. The electrical signal follows the normal pathway and results in contraction of both atria and ventricles, as expected. They are distinguished from NSR by the differences in rate and regularity of the impulses.

1. Sinus arrhythmia

This arrhythmia is characterized by normal complexes but is a heart rate that varies with the respiratory cycle (see Fig. 11-8 for an example). Notice how the QRS complexes are closer together on inspiration than on expiration. This is because the increased venous return to the heart during inspiration causes the heart to fill more quickly, so that the pulse rate quickens. The opposite rhythm effect is sometimes seen with a patient on a positive pressure ventilator. No cardiac treatment is needed. Every attempt should be made to lower the intrathoracic pressure in the mechanically ventilated patient.

2. Sinus tachycardia

Sinus tachycardia in the adult is defined as a heart rate of more than 100 beats/min while at rest. All complexes are normal, and the rate is seldom more than 140 (see Fig. 11-9 for an example). Causes include hypoxemia, caffeine, anxiety, fever, pain, or hypotension. Correction of the problem results in the heart rate decreasing to the normal range. Cardiac drugs are not needed to correct the rhythm if the patient does not have clinically significant symptoms.

3. Sinus bradycardia

Sinus bradycardia is defined as a heart rate of less than 60 beats/min while at rest (Fig. 11-10). All complexes remain normal. This is commonly seen in well-trained athletes during rest and in patients receiving digitalis or morphine. Cardiac drugs are not needed.

If sinus bradycardia is associated with a myocardial infarct, it may result in fainting or congestive heart failure

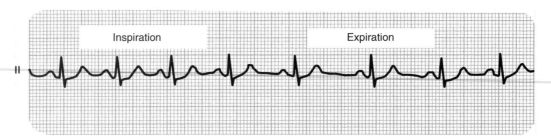

Figure 11-8 Sinus arrhythmia showing slightly increased heart rate during inspiration and slightly decreased heart rate during exhalation. (From Goldberger AL: Clinical electrocardiography: a simplified approach, ed 7, St Louis, 2006, Mosby.)

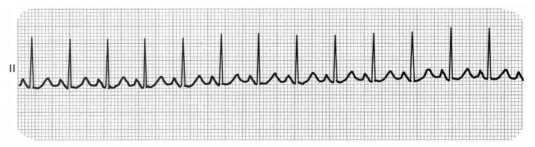

Figure 11-9 Sinus tachycardia. (From Goldberger AL: Clinical electrocardiography: a simplified approach, ed 7, St Louis, 2006, Mosby.)

(pulmonary edema). The patient must be treated not only for the heart attack but also to increase the heart rate. Atropine is the first medication given to speed the heart rate. A pacemaker is needed if the patient does not respond to medications and continues to have symptoms.

b. Arrhythmias with an abnormal atrial origin

The following three arrhythmias originate in either one or both atria from a source other than the SA node. The electrical signal travels through the atria, which contract. It then moves on to the atrioventricular (AV) node and the ventricles, which contract normally. All of these arrhythmias result in faster than normal atrial contraction and often in a faster than normal ventricular contraction.

1. Paroxysmal atrial tachycardia

Paroxysmal atrial tachycardia (PAT; also known as paroxysmal supraventricular tachycardia) is a series of three or more premature atrial contractions. It is characterized by a heart rate between 140 and 250 beats/min with an average rate of 180. The ECG tracing will show a normal QRS complex after each P wave (Fig. 11-11). Notice the abnormal origin of the P wave seen during the PAT episode. The recommended term for any abnormal origin of a heartbeat is *focus*. The term *foci* refers to more than one abnormal site for a heartbeat.

Patients with long runs of PAT usually complain of a sudden onset of pounding or fluttering in the chest. This is often associated with breathlessness, weakness, and angina pectoris in patients with coronary artery disease. Because of these problems, long runs of PAT must be treated. Treatment usually progresses in the following sequence: (1) give a sedative, (2) stimulate the vagus nerve

by rubbing the carotid sinus (Fig. 11-12), (3) give the medication propranolol (Inderal) or another beta-adrenergic receptor blocking agent, and (4) perform synchronized cardioversion. (This last procedure is described in Chapter 18.) Obviously, if the patient responds to one treatment method, no need exists to go on to the next.

2. Atrial flutter

Atrial flutter is characterized by a single, fast, abnormal atrial focus that fires at a rate of about 250-350 beats/min. This rate is so fast that the AV node does not pass all of them along to the ventricles. On an ECG, a ratio between the fast flutter waves and the QRS complex is seen. Usually this ratio is 2:1, but it may be 3:1, 4:1, or more. (See Fig. 11-12 for several example ECG tracings of atrial flutter.) As with PAT, the fast ventricular rate found in atrial flutter is not well tolerated. An attempt must be made to suppress the abnormally fast atrial focus. Carotid sinus pressure, digoxin (Lanoxin), and synchronized cardioversion are the preferred treatments to slow the heart rate.

3. Atrial fibrillation

This condition is identified by the variably shaped fibrillation waves and the irregular spacing between the QRS complexes. Each focus is seen on the ECG as a separately shaped wave. As with atrial flutter, the AV node does not pass the electrical current from each fibrillation wave through to the ventricles. However, with atrial fibrillation, the ratio is not set, and variable spacing is seen between the QRS complexes, with an inconsistent rate (Fig. 11-13). Patients with atrial fibrillation do not completely empty their atria. Often this results in the formation of blood clots that become pulmonary or cerebral emboli. Digitalis

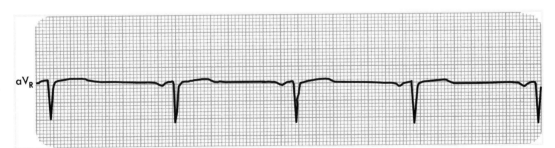

Figure 11-10 Sinus bradycardia. (From Goldberger AL: Clinical electrocardiography: a simplified approach, ed 7, St Louis, 2006, Mosby.)

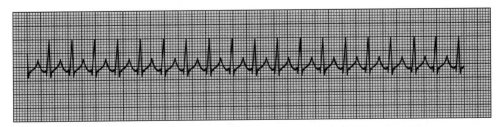

Figure 11-11 A short run of paroxysmal atrial tachycardia. Although a short run is probably not dangerous, a long run should be treated. (From Heuer AJ, Scanlan CL: Wilkins' clinical assessment in respiratory care, ed 7, St Louis, 2014, Mosby.)

Atrial flutter

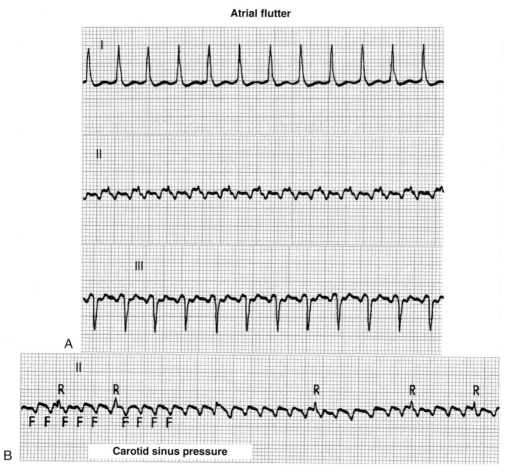

Figure 11-12 Two examples of atrial flutter. **A,** Note the variable appearance of the flutter waves in different leads. This example shows a 2:1 ratio between atrial contractions and ventricular contractions. **B,** This shows how the ventricular rate is decreased after carotid sinus pressure is applied. "F" shows flutter waves from a single focus. "R" marks R waves when the electrical signal traveled through the atrioventricular node to stimulate the ventricles. (From Goldberger AL: Clinical electrocardiography: a simplified approach, ed 8, Philadelphia, 2013, Saunders.)

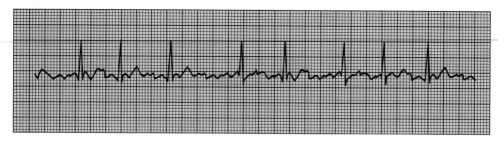

Figure 11-13 Atrial fibrillation. Note the variable shapes to the fibrillation waves, indicating their different origins. Also note how the distances between the R waves change considerably. This depends on when an electrical signal from the atria passes through the atrioventricular node to the ventricles. (From Heuer AJ, Scanlan CL: Wilkins' clinical assessment in respiratory care, ed 7, St Louis, 2014, Mosby.)

and synchronized cardioversion usually are effective treatments. Heparin or Coumadin may be added to prolong the blood-clotting time.

c. Arrhythmias with an atrioventricular node origin

Both of the following arrhythmias originate in the atrioventricular (AV) node. The patient may or may not have a normal SA node, atria, and ventricles.

1. Atrioventricular block

AV block is most commonly caused by digitalis toxicity, arteriosclerosis, or MI. The last two may result in scarring, inflammation, or edema. These slow or prevent the transmission of the electrical signal from the SA node through the AV node and to the ventricles. *First-degree* AV block is seen with an increased PR interval of at least 0.20 second. Each P wave is followed by a normal QRS complex

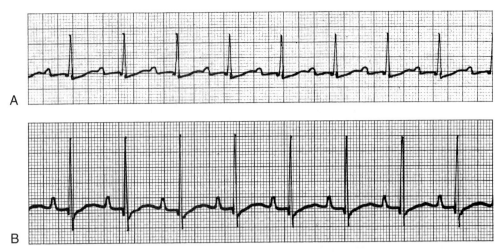

Figure 11-14 First-degree atrioventricular block results in a PR interval that is longer than the normal interval of five small blocks or 20 seconds. **ECG strip A** shows a PR interval of 0.30 second. **ECG strip B** shows a PR interval of 0.24 second. (A From Conover MB: Understanding electrocardiography, arrhythmias, and the 12-lead ECG, ed 4, St Louis, 1984, Mosby. B From Conover MB: Understanding electrocardiography, ed 8, St Louis, 2003, Mosby.)

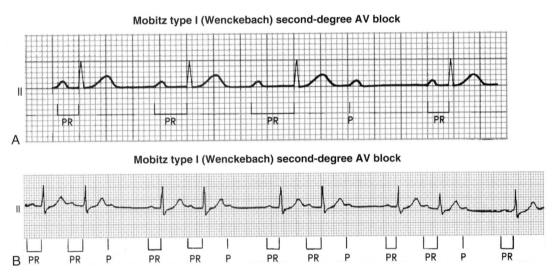

Figure 11-15 Two examples of Wenckebach (Mobitz type I) second-degree atrioventricular block. Note how the PR interval progressively lengthens with each beat until one P wave is not conducted through at all. The cycle then repeats itself. (From Goldberger AL: Clinical electrocardiography: a simplified approach, ed 8, Philadelphia, 2013, Saunders.)

(Fig. 11-14). It does not require any treatment. *Second-degree* AV block results in some P waves being blocked out completely with no ventricular response. This more serious condition comes in two different variations. Wenckebach (also known as Mobitz type I) is characterized by a progressively longer PR interval until a P wave is not conducted through at all. Then the cycle starts over again and continues to repeat itself (refer to Fig. 11-15 for examples.) Medications such as atropine or isoproterenol may be used to increase the heart rate. Mobitz type II is seen on the ECG as a rhythm in which the PR interval is normal for those that result in a QRS complex, but some P waves

are completely blocked (Fig. 11-16). The ratio between those P waves that conduct and those that are blocked off may be 2:1, 3:1, or 4:1. Mobitz type II is a sign of severe conduction-system disease. The usual treatment is to place a cardiac pacemaker into the patient. *Third-degree* AV block also is known as complete heart block (Fig. 11-17). No P waves are conducted through to the ventricles. The ventricles beat about 40 times per minute based on the intrinsic rate of the bundle of His and Purkinje fibers. Obviously, a heartbeat this slow is not normal or healthy. Patients have no stamina and frequently faint. A cardiac pacemaker must be placed into these patients.

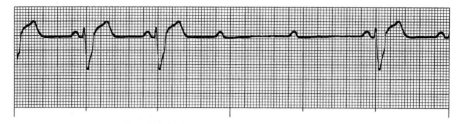

Figure 11-16 Mobitz type II second-degree heart block. Note how some P waves are conducted through the atrioventricular node with a resulting QRS complex and other P waves are not conducted. (From Aehlert B: ECGs made easy, ed 3, St Louis, 2006, Mosby.)

Third-degree (complete) AV block

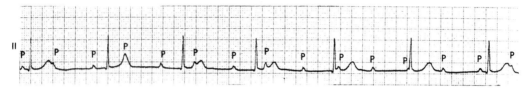

Third-degree (complete) AV block

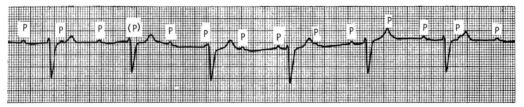

Figure 11-17 Two examples of third-degree (complete) heart block. Both show P waves that have no relation to the QRS complexes. The top example has QRS complexes of the normal width, indicating that the atrioventricular (AV) junction is acting as the pacemaker. The bottom example has QRS complexes that are wider than normal because the ventricles are being paced from below the AV junction. Instead, an idioventricular pacemaker is determining the patient's heart rate. (Top, from Goldberger AL: Clinical electrocardiography: a simplified approach, ed 8, Philadelphia, 2013, Saunders; Bottom, from Goldberger AL: Clinical electrocardiography: a simplified approach, ed 7, St Louis, 2006, Mosby.)

2. Junctional premature beats

A junctional premature beat is also known as a premature AV nodal contraction, nodal beat, or junctional beat (Fig. 11-18). This arrhythmia involves the AV node sending out a premature electrical signal and becoming the primary pacemaker instead of the SA node. The ventricles contract normally with the expected QRS complex.

d. Arrhythmias with a ventricular origin

1. Myocardial infarction

A myocardial infarction (MI) or acute myocardial infarction (AMI), commonly known as a heart attack, is an occlusion of a coronary artery that results in the death of some segment of the heart muscle. Often the patient with partial or complete coronary artery occlusion has symptoms of shortness of breath, central chest pain, pain that radiates down the left arm or up the left side of the neck, or a feeling of stomach upset. If an ECG is performed, it may show ST segment depression as a sign of myocardial hypoxia (Fig. 11-19). If the patient is quickly treated, heart muscle damage may be prevented by opening the blocked artery.

Often, however, the patient comes to the hospital too late, and an MI with muscle damage is present. If the damaged area is large enough, the heart fails to pump adequately, and the patient dies. A smaller infarct weakens the heart. In addition, the damaged or dying tissue acts as an abnormal focus for the arrhythmias discussed next. The ECG changes that occur during the acute stage of an MI and as the heart heals are shown in Figure 11-20 and are listed here:

1. The initial ECG may be normal. This happens about 15% of the time. The patient should be admitted for observation and cardiac enzyme studies performed if symptoms are present.
2. The first sign of an MI is an elevated ST segment. This occurs within a few hours of the injury.
3. Next the T wave inverts. This happens within hours to days of the infarct.
4. The ST segment returns to the normal baseline position within days to weeks.

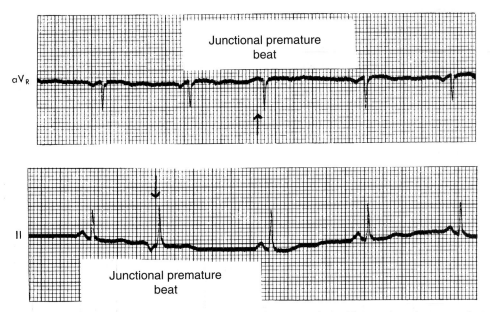

Figure 11-18 Two electrocardiogram tracings of junctional premature beats. They are from the same patient but from different leads. Arrows, retrograde P waves of opposite polarity from normal. (From Goldberger AL, Goldberger E: Clinical electrocardiography, St Louis, 1981, Mosby.)

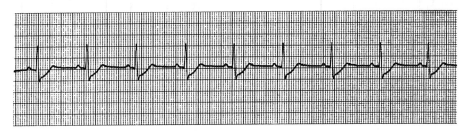

Figure 11-19 An electrocardiogram tracing showing ST segment depression. This is usually caused by myocardial hypoxia and can lead to a myocardial infarction if not promptly treated. (From Wilkins RL, Dexter JR, Heuer AJ: Clinical assessment in respiratory care, ed 6, St Louis, 2010, Mosby.)

5. After a period of weeks to months, the T wave becomes upright again. A lasting ECG change is an enlarged Q wave as shown.

2. Premature ventricular contraction

A premature ventricular contraction (PVC) is an abnormal, fast contraction of the ventricles that originates from a focus below the AV node (Fig. 11-21). This is usually a sign of a diseased or hypoxic ventricle. Pathologic causes include arteriosclerotic heart disease or MI. An example of an isolated PVC is shown in Figure 11-22 and has these traits:

- It is premature and happens before the normal heartbeat.
- No P wave is present.
- The QRS complex is bizarre looking and more than 0.12 second wide.
- The T wave is inverted.
- Usually, a fully compensatory pause occurs before the next normal heartbeat.

A single PVC is not dangerous unless it originates during the T wave, when the heart is especially vulnerable to electrical stimulation. Then, it can cause ventricular fibrillation (VF).

If all PVCs look the same, they originate from the same area (focus) and are called *unifocal*. All patients with PVCs should be watched more closely and probably treated when their PVCs are seen more frequently than 1 in 10 beats, seen in groups of two or three, or seen in multiple configurations. For example, two different-looking PVCs mean that two different ventricular foci are firing prematurely (Fig. 11-23). These different-looking PVCs would be called *multifocal*. *Bigeminy* occurs when every second beat is a PVC; *trigeminy* is when every third beat is a PVC. These dangerous situations must be rapidly treated. Lidocaine (Xylocaine) is given intravenously if the heart rate is more than 60 beats/min. If that does not work, procainamide hydrochloride (Pronestyl) is added. Additionally, the patient is given supplemental oxygen to improve oxygenation to the irritable heart.

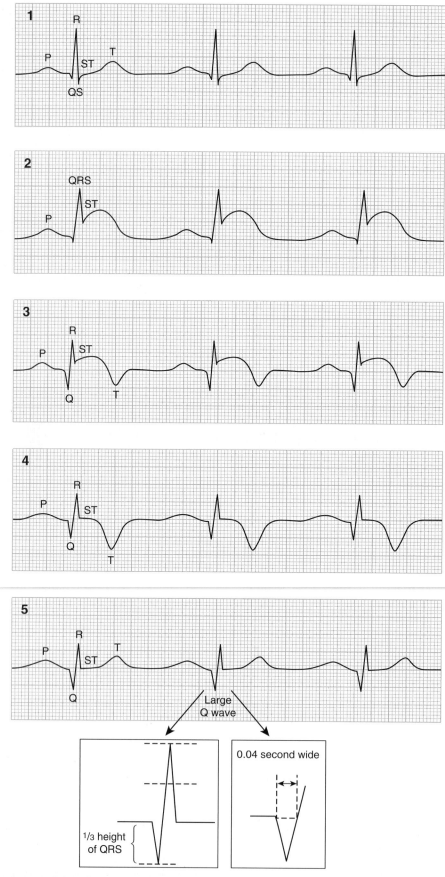

Figure 11-20 The sequence of electrocardiogram rhythms commonly seen after a myocardial infarction. See the text for a description of each step in the sequence.

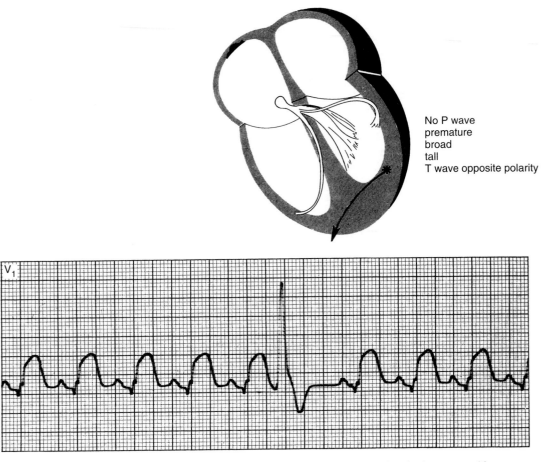

No P wave
premature
broad
tall
T wave opposite polarity

Figure 11-21 Premature ventricular contraction (PVC; arrow) is detected when an impulse is propagated from a ventricular focus before the next normal beat is due. The QRS complex is commonly widened and not preceded by a P wave. A longer than usual (compensatory) pause follows. Retrograde activation of the atria may occur after a premature contraction, or the normal sinus P waves may continue. The sinus P waves after the PVC are blocked by conduction-system refractoriness. (From Conover MB: Understanding electrocardiography, ed 8, St Louis, 2003, Mosby.)

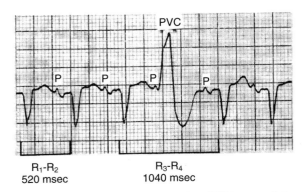

R_1-R_2
520 msec

R_3-R_4
1040 msec

Figure 11-22 Premature ventricular contractions (PVCs) cause a fully compensatory pause. Note that the interval between the two sinus beats that surround the PVC (R_3 and R_4 in this case) is exactly two times the normal interval between the sinus beats R_1 and R_2. Notice that the P waves come on time, except that the third P wave is interrupted by the PVC and therefore does not conduct normally through the atrioventricular junction. The next (fourth) P wave also comes on time. The sinus node continues to pace despite the PVC, resulting in the fully compensatory pause. (From Goldberger AL: Clinical electrocardiography: a simplified approach, ed 7, St Louis, 2006, Mosby.)

3. Ventricular tachycardia

Ventricular tachycardia (VT or V tach) is a serious consequence of untreated PVCs. VT is defined as a series of three or more consecutive PVCs (Fig. 11-24). Runs of VT may be fairly short or prolonged. The rate counted during VT is between 110 and 250 beats/min. Cardiac output decreases dramatically during this arrhythmia. If the patient has a stable blood pressure, VT is treated with lidocaine as an antiarrhythmic. Synchronized cardioversion is needed if the lidocaine is ineffective. If the VT is sustained and the patient is unresponsive, pulseless, or hypotensive or in pulmonary edema, defibrillation (also called asynchronous cardioversion) is necessary. The medication amiodarone HCl (Pacerone) may also be used to help stop VT. If left untreated, VT usually progresses to either ventricular flutter (Fig. 11-25) or VF (discussed next). Ventricular flutter looks similar to VT on the ECG except that the rate is usually faster and the rhythm less regular. Its treatment is the same as that for VT and, if left

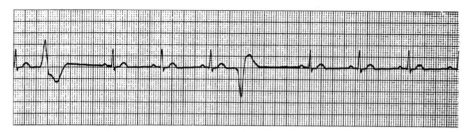

Figure 11-23 An electrocardiogram tracing showing multifocal premature ventricular contractions (PVCs). Counting from the left, after the normal beat, note that the next beat and the sixth beat are PVCs. Because they look different, they do not originate at the same abnormal focus. Therefore the patient has multifocal PVCs. This dangerous situation should be quickly corrected. (From Wilkins RL, Dexter JR, Heuer AJ: Clinical assessment in respiratory care, ed 6, St Louis, 2010, Mosby.)

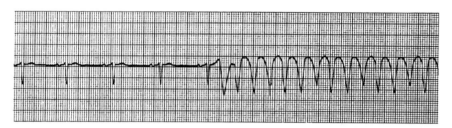

Figure 11-24 Electrocardiogram tracing showing normal sinus rhythm that suddenly converts to ventricular tachycardia (VT). This can happen if a premature ventricular contraction occurs early in the heart's repolarization process and is called the R-on-T phenomenon. If VT is not treated promptly, it will deteriorate into ventricular flutter or ventricular fibrillation. (From Heuer AJ, Scanlan CL: Wilkins' clinical assessment in respiratory care, ed 7, St Louis, 2014, Mosby.)

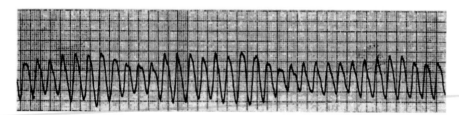

Figure 11-25 Example of an electrocardiogram showing ventricular flutter. If this arrhythmia is not treated promptly, it will deteriorate into ventricular fibrillation. (From Kacmarek RM, Mack CW, Dimas S: The essentials of respiratory care, ed 3, St Louis, 1990, Mosby.)

untreated, it will progress to VF. Both of these arrhythmias originate from a single fast ventricular focus, as shown in Figure 11-21.

4. Ventricular fibrillation

Ventricular fibrillation (VF or V fib) is caused when multiple, fast ventricular foci are firing (refer to Fig. 11-26 for the electrical pathways). When several ventricular foci are firing in an uncoordinated manner, the rhythm is chaotic and without any pattern. Virtually no cardiac output occurs. The patient is pulseless and without any blood pressure. This is a true medical emergency. If it is not treated immediately, brain death will occur within minutes. CPR must be started to provide oxygen to the brain.

The treatment of choice for VF is defibrillation as quickly as possible. No attempt is made to synchronize the electrical shock. Figure 11-27 shows the usual position of the defibrillator paddles. It is hoped that with prompt CPR efforts and electrical defibrillation, the patient's heartbeat will return to a normal sinus rhythm (see Fig. 11-2).

5. Ventricular asystole

Ventricular asystole (or asystole) occurs when no cardiac electrical signal and no myocardial activity are present. The ECG tracing shows a flat line, indicating the absence of cardiac electrical activity. The presence of this arrhythmia is ominous. When seen after a full attempt at CPR, it indicates a nonfunctioning heart. The patient will almost

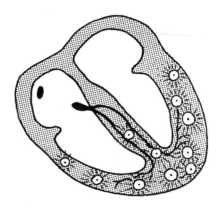

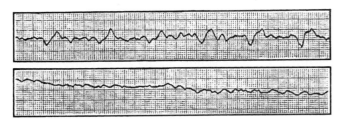

Figure 11-26 Multiple disorganized contractions of the ventricles characterize ventricular fibrillation and represent cardiac arrest. It may be of sudden onset or may follow premature ventricular contractions, ventricular tachycardia, or ventricular flutter. (From Stein E: Clinical electrocardiography: a self-study course, Philadelphia, 1987, Lea & Febiger.)

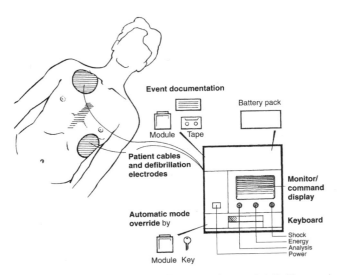

Figure 11-27 Schematic drawing of automated external defibrillator and its attachment to the patient. (Modified from Cummins RO: Advanced cardiac life support, Dallas, TX, 1994, American Heart Association.)

assuredly die. Some physicians may elect to defibrillate the patient in asystole in an attempt to generate some sort of rhythm. Because of the dire consequences of ventricular asystole, it is wise to double-check all the equipment. This includes the ECG leads or defibrillator paddles being used to check the rhythm, all electrical connections, and the functioning of the ECG monitor to be sure that no technical error can be found.

Exam Hint 11-2

There is usually at least one CPR-related question that includes an ECG tracing. Usually it is of *VT* or *VF*. The question usually involves the patient being pulseless or without a blood pressure. The therapist must realize that the situation is life threatening and requires CPR or defibrillation.

MODULE D

Provide respiratory care techniques in cardiac arrest situations (Code: IIIG1a) [R, Ap, An].

Note: Starting in 2015, the NBRC will no longer be testing basic cardiac life support, advanced cardiac life support, pediatric advanced life support, or neonatal resuscitation program steps or procedures. This is because respiratory therapists are already tested by the American Heart Association or other organizations in these important activities. However, as the module heading states, respiratory care techniques used during CPR and other emergency situations will still be tested. The first item below is included because it has been tested on previous NBRC exams. The other items are listed on the current Detailed Content Outline.

1. Observe the size of the patient's pupils and their reaction to light

Normally the pupils constrict when a light is shined into them. The pupils dilate within 30-40 seconds after cardiac arrest and do not constrict normally when the brain is hypoxic. If CPR is being done properly to deliver oxygen to the brain, the pupils should constrict normally. Fixed (nonreactive) and dilated pupils are ominous signs. Even if the heart can be restarted, the brain has probably had irreversible damage.

In several conditions, the pupils do not react as expected. The pupils remain constricted if the victim has received morphine sulfate or other opiates. The pupils are dilated if the victim has received atropine, quinidine, or epinephrine. Hypothermia also causes the pupils to dilate.

2. Arterial blood gases

a. Recommend an arterial blood gas analysis (code: IE9) [difficulty: R, Ap, An]

Blood for arterial blood gas (ABG) determination is usually drawn in any hospital-based CPR effort. It should not be done at the expense of time that should be spent starting effective ventilations and chest compressions or defibrillating the heart. The blood gas values give important information on the patient's oxygenation and help to determine whether the patient is acidotic. Changes in the ventilation efforts and medications such as bicarbonate are based on information from the ABGs. See Chapter 3 for the discussion on arterial blood sampling.

b. Draw an ABG sample (code: IC6) [difficulty: R, Ap]

The femoral site is usually the best to draw from in a CPR situation because it is the largest artery and the easiest to hit. It is far enough from the chest that blood can be drawn without interfering in the chest compression efforts. See Chapter 3 for the general steps in drawing an ABG sample.

c. Evaluate the results of the ABG analysis (code: IC6) [difficulty: R, Ap]

The full discussion of ABG interpretation is presented in Chapter 3. During a CPR attempt, the key things to look for are the patient's PaO_2 and $PaCO_2$, because they relate to the adequacy of ventilations and chest compressions. If the patient has an acidotic pH and a normal or low $PaCO_2$, the patient has an uncorrected metabolic acidosis. Intravenous (IV) sodium bicarbonate is indicated.

3. Perform endotracheal intubation (code: IIIA3e) [difficulty: R, Ap, An]

Oral endotracheal intubation is usually performed during a CPR attempt. See Chapter 12 for a complete discussion of endotracheal tubes, intubation equipment, and the process of performing intubation. Current CPR guidelines indicate that if an endotracheal tube cannot be placed into a patient, a laryngeal mask airway or Combitube may be inserted to provide a secure airway.

4. Assist the physician/provider in performing defibrillation (code: IIIH8) [difficulty: R, Ap]

Defibrillation sends a specific amount of direct electrical current (DC) through the patient's chest wall and heart. Its purpose is to stimulate the entire cardiac muscle and electrical system so that the source of an abnormal signal will be suppressed. The SA node usually then takes over as the normal pacemaker. Chapter 18 includes a table listing the stepped progression of power used in defibrillation.

Synchronized defibrillation (cardioversion) (see Chapter 18) should be performed in cases of atrial flutter, PAT, atrial fibrillation, and VT, unless the patient is pulseless, unresponsive, or hypotensive or in pulmonary edema.

Unsynchronized defibrillation should be performed as soon as possible under the following circumstances: VF or VT when the patient is pulseless, unresponsive, or hypotensive or in pulmonary edema.

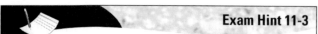

Exam Hint 11-3

Usually one question requires the therapist to identify the indications for defibrillation and recommend the procedure.

5. Recommend cardiovascular drugs (code: IIIE4e) [difficulty: R, Ap]

a. Cardiotonic (positive inotropic) drugs

Positive inotropic agents are used to increase the contractility of the heart muscle. Two classes of drugs do this, and both are used in patients who have a weak or damaged myocardium. They increase the patient's myocardial contractility. This results in increased cardiac output, increased blood pressure, and increased urine output. The best-known, older group consists of cardiac glycosides and is commonly referred to as "digitalis." The cardiac glycosides increase the level of intramuscular sodium and calcium to increase the contraction of the heart muscle. Of these, Lanoxin (digoxin) is the preferred medication for a patient with congestive heart failure.

The newer group includes synthetic catecholamine agents. The catecholamine agents are similar to adrenaline and stimulate beta receptors in the heart. Dobutamine hydrochloride (Dobutrex) is used as a short-term agent in adult patients who have organic heart disease or who have had heart surgery. Its use results in an increase in contraction with only a minor increase in heart rate. Epinephrine (adrenaline) is used during a cardiac arrest to increase heart rate and contractility.

b. Antiarrhythmic drugs

Bradycardia is defined as a heart rate of less than 60 beats/min in an adult at rest. If the patient has symptoms such as light-headedness or low blood pressure, the heart rate should be increased. Common medications that increase the heart rate include atropine (atropine sulfate), isoproterenol (Isuprel), and epinephrine (adrenalin chloride).

Tachycardia (a resting adult heart rate of greater than 100 beats/min) and abnormal, fast heartbeats originating from the atria or ventricles are potentially very dangerous. Fast tachycardia and dangerous arrhythmias must be controlled with medications that slow the heart's conduction system or suppress the generation of abnormal electrical signals. Common medications that do this include propranolol (Inderal), lidocaine (Xylocaine), and procainamide (Pronestyl).

c. Vasoconstricting drugs

Vasoconstrictors are medications that cause the peripheral blood vessels to constrict so that blood flow is reduced through them. Many medications do this by stimulating the α_1 receptors on the vessels. They are chiefly used in a hypotensive patient. Hypotension is usually defined as a systemic blood pressure of less than 80 mm Hg in an adult and less than 70 mm Hg in a child. A pressure of less than this does not adequately perfuse the kidneys. Urine output decreases dramatically or stops altogether. Cerebral blood flow also is greatly reduced. When hypotension is caused by vasodilation, as in allergic anaphylaxis or sepsis, it usually has to be treated by inducing vasoconstriction. Hypotension from heart failure or an

MI often also must be treated with a vasoconstrictor. Common examples of medications that cause vasoconstriction to increase blood pressure include dopamine hydrochloride (Intropin) and norepinephrine (Levophed, Levarterenol).

The effects of dopamine are dose related. At relatively low doses, an increase in renal blood flow is noted, and urine output increases, with no change in blood pressure. At medium doses, an increase in myocardial contractility and a progressive peripheral vasoconstriction is found. These effects increase the blood pressure without decreasing renal blood flow. At high doses, the total systemic vascular resistance further increases. However, renal blood flow and urine output both decrease. Current practice indicates that dopamine works best in patients with moderate hypotension. A patient who does not respond to dopamine probably needs norepinephrine (Levophed or Levarterenol) to increase the blood pressure. Any time a hypotensive patient is given a vasoconstricting agent, the blood pressure, peripheral blood flow, and urine output must be watched closely. The prognosis is grim for patients who do not respond to these medications or attempts to correct the underlying condition.

d. Vasodilating drugs

Hypertension in the adult is defined as a blood pressure of greater than 140/90 mm Hg. The higher the blood pressure, the greater the strain on the heart. It also increases the risk of vessel rupture and stroke.

A wide variety of medications in a number of drug categories are used to reduce blood pressure. They range from diuretics to reduce blood volume, to calcium and sympathomimetic blockers that reduce heart rate and vasodilate, to angiotensin-converting enzyme inhibitors. Medications in these categories are used to treat moderate, chronic hypertension.

The patient in a hypertensive crisis (blood pressure greater than 200/120 mm Hg) must be treated quickly and effectively. The following medications are commonly given by the IV route to control severe hypertension:
- Nitroprusside (Nipride)
- Diazoxide (Hyperstat)
- Trimethaphan (Arfonad)

Nitroprusside also is given to reduce the afterload in a patient with left-ventricular failure after an MI. Any patient who is receiving a powerful vasodilator must have frequent blood pressure monitoring.

e. Bicarbonate (sodium bicarbonate)

According to the most recent guidelines, bicarbonate (sodium bicarbonate) should be used, if at all, only after all other CPR procedures have been instituted. Bicarbonate may then be used if a diagnosis has been made and ABG results document that the patient has a metabolic acidosis. Additionally, bicarbonate is given to help treat the patient with hyperkalemia, or tricyclic or phenobarbital overdose. Bicarbonate also may be beneficial if the patient has been in prolonged arrest or if CPR has been performed for an extended time.

When used, bicarbonate should be given initially at a dose of 1 mEq/kg; a half dose is then given every 10 minutes. If available from ABG results, use the calculated base deficit or bicarbonate concentration as a guideline for giving more bicarbonate. Do not completely correct the base deficit to avoid accidentally making the patient alkalotic.

6. Administer medications by endotracheal instillation (code: IIID3) [difficulty: R, Ap]

Cardiac medications may be instilled down the endotracheal tube when a resuscitation attempt is under way and the patient does not have a functional central or peripheral intravenous line. The following medications may be instilled into adult patients: naloxone (Narcan), atropine, vasopressin (Arginine), epinephrine, and lidocaine (Xylocaine). (Hint: Use "NAVEL," from the first letters of the generic name of these medications, to help remember them.) In the case of a known or suspected opioid (morphine, heroin) overdose, Narcan can be administered into a nostril for absorption by the nasal sinuses. Narcan should only be given intravenously to a newborn infant.

The dose of any medication is based on the patient's size and may be larger than that given intravenously. This is because the medication is diluted through the airways and must be absorbed through the mucous membrane. Previous adult guidelines indicated that the endotracheal dose should be 2 to 2.5 times greater than the normal iv amount. The medication should be diluted by adding 10 mL of normal saline or distilled water.

The following steps for instillation are recommended:
1. Disconnect the manual resuscitator from the endotracheal tube, and stop the chest compressions.
2. (Optional) Pass a suction catheter or feeding tube past the distal tip of the endotracheal tube.
3. Quickly inject the drug solution down the endotracheal tube or catheter.
4. If used, withdraw the suction catheter.
5. Reconnect the manual resuscitator to the endotracheal tube and give the patient several deep breaths. This helps to force the medication down to the alveolar level or causes aerosolization so that faster absorption occurs.
6. Resume chest compressions and ventilation.

Exam Hint 11-4

Epinephrine (adrenaline) is a first-line drug used in a CPR attempt. It is used during bradycardia, asystole, and VF because it increases the heart rate, stroke volume, and vasoconstriction to raise blood pressure. (In addition, it is a bronchodilator.)

7. Capnometry

a. Recommend capnometry (code: IE8) [difficulty: R, Ap, An]

See below.

b. Perform capnography (code: IC2) [difficulty: R, Ap]

See below.

c. Evaluate the results of the procedure (code: ID2) [difficulty: R, Ap, An]

The general discussion of capnography was presented in Chapter 5, and exhaled carbon dioxide monitoring is presented in Chapter 12. Either can be used to help confirm that the endotracheal tube is properly located within the trachea and the patient is exhaling carbon dioxide. It also is helpful if the patient is being transported or the endotracheal tube is being repositioned. In addition, clinical evidence suggests that monitoring the exhaled carbon dioxide level during a CPR attempt is helpful in evaluating the patient's metabolic response. In general, if chest compressions and assisted ventilation are effective, carbon dioxide will be removed from the tissues and circulated to the lungs for exhalation. If the CPR efforts are ineffective, little exhaled carbon dioxide is measured. The absence of exhaled carbon dioxide, despite a proper CPR effort, is a grave sign.

Exam Hint 11-5

There is usually one question related to advanced CPR procedures such as life-threatening arrhythmia recognition, intubation and airway management issues, and defibrillation.

MODULE E

Resuscitation devices

1. Manual resuscitator (bag-valve or bag-mask)

a. Assemble the necessary equipment (code: IIA7) [difficulty: R, Ap]

The first consideration when deciding which manual resuscitation bag to select is the size of the patient. Although the volume of the reservoir bag and the tidal volume expelled from it vary among the types of bags, three basic sizes are available. An infant or newborn unit typically has a reservoir bag volume of about 250 mL. A pediatric unit usually has a reservoir bag volume of about 250-500 mL, and an adult unit typically has a reservoir bag volume of 1500-2000 mL. In addition to all of these reusable units, a number of disposable units are thrown away after one patient use. They also come in comparable infant, pediatric, and adult reservoir bag volumes. The bag's gas outlet port to the patient has a 22-mm outer diameter to fit into a face mask (Fig. 11-28) and a 15-mm inner diameter that an endotracheal tube adapter fits into (see Fig. 12-24 in Chapter 12).

Any unit should deliver 100% oxygen at the flow rate of 15 L/min. An oxygen reservoir system must be added to the basic unit to achieve these oxygen percentages. The valve to the patient must be clearable within 20 seconds if it becomes fouled by vomitus, sputum, or blood.

Neonatal and pediatric units must have a pressure release (pop-off) valve that opens at 40 cm H_2O pressure. The pressure may be adjustable. If an adult unit has a pressure release valve, it must have an override system that is easy to operate. If the unit has an add-on positive end-expiratory pressure (PEEP) valve, it must be easy to operate.

Figure 11-28 shows images of a complete set of Laerdal infant, pediatric, and adult manual resuscitators. The following steps should be taken when the function of a manual resuscitator is evaluated:

1. Squeeze and release the bag to see if the nonrebreathing valve and air/oxygen reservoir intake valve open and close properly.
2. Feel the air leave the outlet port of the nonrebreathing valve when the bag is squeezed.
3. Occlude the outlet port, and squeeze the bag. No gas should leak out. If present, the pop-off valve should open at the correct pressure.
4. The face mask should fit onto the 22-mm outer diameter fitting and have its cushion properly inflated. The mask is selected based on the size of the patient's face. As Figure 11-28 shows, the masks come in pediatric, infant, and adult sizes.

Connect the correct manual resuscitator and mask so that the patient can be "bagged" with room air. Supplemental oxygen will need to be provided by one of two ways: (1) Plug an oxygen flowmeter with nipple adapter into the wall oxygen outlet. Connect small-bore oxygen tubing to the flowmeter's nipple adapter and the oxygen inlet nipple adapter on the resuscitator bag. (2) Get an E-size tank of oxygen with regulator and oxygen nipple adapter (see Fig. 6-6 in Chapter 6.) Connect small-bore oxygen tubing to the regulator's nipple adapter and the oxygen inlet nipple adapter on the resuscitator bag. With either system, turn on the oxygen flow to 15 L/min so that the patient can be bagged with 100% oxygen. After the patient has had an endotracheal tube (or laryngeal mask airway or esophageal obturator airway) inserted, disconnect the resuscitator from the mask and attach it to the tube.

If the physician orders an impedance threshold device (ITD) (also known as an impedance threshold valve) to be used, it is connected between the resuscitator bag and either the endotracheal tube or the mask. The ResQPOD is an example. An ITD has been shown to increase negative intrathoracic pressure. This decrease in pressure on the upstroke of a chest compression causes increased venous return to the heart with increased coronary perfusion

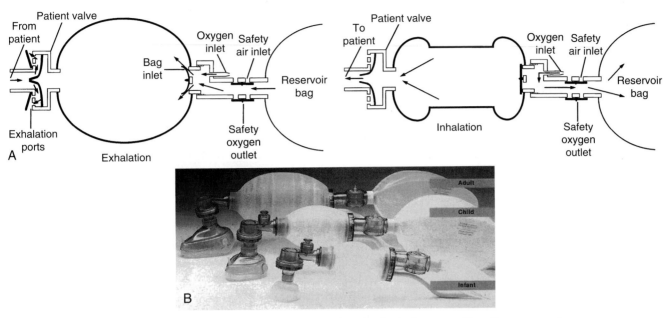

Figure 11-28 **A**, Cutaway drawings of a resuscitation bag showing its features and how the one-way valves open and close during exhalation and inhalation. Note that during exhalation, the patient's breath is vented to the room and supplemental oxygen is drawn from the reservoir bag into the main bag. To deliver a breath to the patient, the operator squeezes the main bag. This opens the valve to the patient and closes the valve from the reservoir bag. **B**, Photograph showing an adult, child, and infant resuscitation bag with attached face mask and oxygen reservoir bag. These features are found on all modern units: a self-filling main bag, exhalation valve that does not jam at an oxygen flow of 15 L/min or in subfreezing temperatures (it must be clearable of debris within 20 seconds), intake valve for adding draw room air or supplemental oxygen into the reservoir bag, transparent mask that easily conforms to the patient's face, pressure relief (pop-off) valve that is set to open at 40 cm water, standard 15-mm inner diameter/22-mm outer diameter connector for the endotracheal tube or face mask, and oxygen enrichment/reservoir system. In addition, some units have an adjustable positive end-expiratory pressure valve (not shown) attached to the exhalation valve. (A from Cairo JM: Mosby's respiratory care equipment, ed 9, St Louis, 2014, Mosby. B courtesy of Laerdal Medical, Wappingers Falls, NY.)

pressure. An ITD is contraindicated in patients with pulmonary edema or congestive heart pressure.

b. Troubleshoot any problems with the equipment (code: IIA7) [difficulty: R, Ap]

Check for a reversed or improperly seated one-way valve (spring-loaded, duckbill, or leaf type) if the gas does not enter or exit the unit as it should. In clinical use, mucus, vomitus, and blood can foul the expiratory one-way valve system. By regulation, the valve must be clearable within 20 seconds. Do this by disconnecting the unit from the patient, aiming the adapter into a neutral area, and squeezing the bag to blow out the obstruction. Replace a unit that cannot be promptly cleared of any debris.

2. Mouth-to-valve mask resuscitator

a. Assemble the necessary equipment (code: IIA7) [difficulty: R, Ap]

The following are important considerations when selecting the best mouth-to-valve device (also called a mouth-to-mask device or pocket mask) for the victim:

- The mask must fit the victim's face so that no air leak is present. Infant, child, and adult sizes should be available.
- The mouthpiece should be designed so that it fits only one way into the mask. Some units include a short length of aerosol tubing between the mouthpiece and the mask for greater flexibility.
- The one-way (nonrebreathing) valve should be designed to ensure that all of the rescuer's breath is directed into the victim and the victim's exhaled breath is vented to room air rather than back at the rescuer. Some units include a bacteria filter in the one-way valve between the rescuer and the victim.
- It should be possible to add supplemental oxygen through a T-piece or nipple on the mask. This is important for hospital or ambulance use. If a T-piece is added, it must be designed to easily fit between the mouthpiece and the face mask. An oxygen-administration nipple should have a cap over it when not in use to prevent any leakage of the delivered breath.

Mouth-to-valve resuscitators are relatively simple devices. Most have only two or three pieces: a face mask, a mouthpiece with a one-way valve, and possibly an oxygen

T-piece (Fig. 11-29). The "male" and "female" connections are designed to fit together in only one way. When they are properly assembled, no air should leak out when the breath is delivered to the victim.

b. Troubleshoot any problems with the equipment (code: IIA7) [difficulty: R, Ap]

If the breath cannot be delivered, check the one-way valve to make sure that it has not been put together backward. Reverse it, if necessary, and ventilate the victim's airway. Keep the oxygen nipple on the mask or T-piece capped off if it is not being used. Air will leak out during the delivered breath if the cap is left off the nipple.

Exam Hint 11-6

Usually an exam question deals with a malfunctioning manual resuscitator or mouth-to-valve resuscitator. Often the question involves identifying that the patient's chest does not rise despite the ventilating device being used to deliver a breath. Fixing the problem can involve clearing an obstruction or properly assembling a one-way valve. If the unit cannot be quickly repaired, it should be replaced.

Exam Hint 11-7

An endotracheal tube should be inserted into the patient as soon as possible during a CPR attempt. If an endotracheal tube cannot be placed, a laryngeal mask airway or Combitube can be inserted. Then, a manual resuscitation bag with 100% oxygen should be used to ventilate the patient. Less effective ventilation methods include a mouth-to-mask valve or bag-mask system. A gas-powered pneumatic (demand valve) resuscitator should not be used because the delivered tidal volume is unpredictable and too large a volume can cause barotrauma.

MODULE F

Respiratory care plan

1. Determine a patient's pathophysiologic state (code: IIIF1) [difficulty: R, Ap, An]

The respiratory therapist must be able to recognize life-threatening arrhythmias. It is critical for the respiratory therapist to be able to recognize the need to start CPR and perform advanced life-support procedures.

2. Recommend starting a treatment based on the patient's response (code: IIIE2a) [difficulty: R, Ap, An]

Be prepared to start the advanced CPR-related procedures listed in Module D.

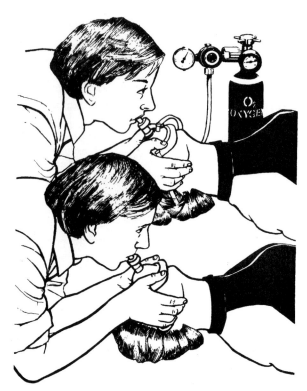

Figure 11-29 Proper positioning to use a mouth-to-valve mask resuscitator. The top rescuer has added supplemental oxygen to the device. The bottom rescuer is ventilating without the use of added oxygen. (Courtesy of Laerdal Medical Corporation, Wappingers Falls, NY.)

3. Recommend a change in the therapeutic plan if indicated (code: IIIF2) [difficulty: R, Ap, An]

Be prepared to recommend a change in CPR activities if the patient's cardiac arrhythmia should change in response to treatment such as defibrillation.

4. Recommend a treatment be terminated (code: IIIE1) [difficulty: R, Ap, An]

The practitioner should make a recommendation to the physician to stop a procedure being performed as an adjunct to CPR if the patient is having an adverse reaction to it. For example, bag-and-mask ventilation may force air into the stomach; recommend intubation. Always notify the physician of any change in the patient's condition or if a complication to any CPR-related procedure is seen.

5. Recommend discontinuing a treatment based on the patient's response (code: IIIE2h) [difficulty: R, Ap, An]

The physician will make the decision to stop futile CPR activities that are taking place in the hospital.

BIBLIOGRAPHY

American Association for Respiratory Care: Clinical practice guideline: resuscitation in acute care hospitals, *Respir Care* 38(11):1179, 1993.

American Association for Respiratory Care: Clinical practice guideline: defibrillation during resuscitation, *Respir Care* 40(7):744, 1995.

American Association for Respiratory Care: Clinical practice guideline: management of airway emergencies, *Respir Care* 40(7):749, 1995.

American Association for Respiratory Care: Clinical practice guideline: capnography/capnometry during mechanical ventilation—2-3 revision & update, *Respir Care* 48(5):534, 2003.

American Association for Respiratory Care: Clinical practice guideline: resuscitation and defibrillation in the health care setting: 2004 revision and update, *Respir Care* 49(9):1085, 2004.

Barnes TA: Emergency cardiovascular life support. In Wilkins RL, Stoller JK, Kacmarek RM, editors: *Egan's fundamentals of respiratory care*, ed 9, St Louis, 2009, Mosby.

Barnes TA: Emergency cardiovascular life support. In Kacmarek RM, Stoller JK, Heuer AJ, editors: *Egan's fundamentals of respiratory care*, ed 10, St Louis, 2013, Mosby.

Bevis R, Moore CJ: Cardiopulmonary resuscitation. In Hess DR, MacIntyre NR, Mishoe SC, Galvin WF, Adams AB, editors: *Respiratory care principles and practice*, ed 2, Burlington, MA, 2012, Jones & Bartlett Learning.

Cairo JM: Assessment of cardiovascular function. In Cairo JM, Pilbeam SP, editors: *Mosby's respiratory care equipment*, ed 8, St Louis, 2010, Mosby.

Cairo JM: Assessment of cardiovascular function. In Cairo JM, editor: *Mosby's respiratory care equipment*, ed 9, St Louis, 2014, Mosby.

Cox GG, Mathews PJ: Radiology for the respiratory therapist. In Wyka KA, Mathews PJ, Rutkowski J, editors: *Foundations of respiratory care*, ed 2, Clifton Park, NY, 2012, Delmar.

Davis D: *Differential diagnosis of arrhythmias*, Philadelphia, 1991, Saunders.

Durbin CG: Airway management. In Cairo JM, Pilbeam SP, editors: *Mosby's respiratory care equipment*, ed 7, St Louis, 2004, Mosby.

Eubanks DH, Bone RC: *Comprehensive respiratory care*, ed 2, St Louis, 1990, Mosby.

Fink JB, Hunt GE, editors: *Clinical practice in respiratory care*, Philadelphia, 1999, Lippincott-Raven.

Fluck RR: Emergency medicine. In Wyka KA, Mathews PJ, Clark WF, editors: *Foundations of respiratory care*, Albany, NY, 2002, Delmar.

Fluck Jr RR: Emergency respiratory care. In Wyka KA, Mathews PJ, Rutkowski J, editors: *Foundations of respiratory care*, ed 2, Clifton Park, NY, 2012, Delmar.

Goldberger AL, Goldberger ZD, Shvilkin A: *Goldberger's clinical electrocardiography*, ed 8, Philadelphia, 2013, Saunders.

Goldberger AL: *Clinical electrocardiography*, ed 6, St Louis, 1999, Mosby.

Govert JA, Hess DR: Hemodynamic monitoring. In Hess DR, MacIntyre NR, Mishoe SC, Galvin WF, Adams AB, editors: *Respiratory care principles and practice*, ed 2, Burlington, MA, 2012, Jones & Bartlett Learning.

Hall ML: Echocardiography, radioisotope studies, electron beam computed tomography, magnetic resonance imaging, and phonocardiography. In Woods SL, Sivarajan Froelicher ES, Underhill Motzer S, editors: *Cardiac nursing*, ed 4, Philadelphia, 2000, Lippincott.

Hess D, Goff G, Johnson K: The effect of hand size, resuscitator brand, and use of two hands on volumes delivered during adult bag-valve ventilation, *Respir Care* 34:805, 1989.

Heuer AJ: Interpreting the electrocardiogram. In Kacmarek RM, Stoller JK, Heuer AJ, editors: *Egan's fundamentals of respiratory care*, ed 10, St Louis, 2013, Mosby.

Heuer AJ: Interpretation of electrocardiogram tracings. In Heuer AJ, Scanlan CL, editors: *Clinical assessment in respiratory care*, ed 7, St Louis, 2014, Mosby.

Hinski ST: Electrocardiogram interpretation. In Hinski ST, editor: *Respiratory care clinical competency lab manual*, St Louis, 2014, Mosby.

Kacmarek RM, Dimas S, Mack CW: *The essentials of respiratory care*, ed 4, St Louis, 2005, Mosby.

Leeuwen AM, Poelhuis-Leth DJ, Bladh ML: *Davis's comprehensive handbook of laboratory diagnostic test with nursing implications*, ed 5, Philadelphia, 2013, FA Davis.

Ludwig B, Mathews M: Cardiac and hemodynamic monitoring. In Wyka KA, Mathews PJ, Rutkowski J, editors: *Foundations of respiratory care*, ed 2, Clifton Park, NY, 2012, Delmar.

Madama VC: Safe mouth-to-mouth resuscitation requires adjunct equipment, caution, *Occup Health Saf* 60(1):56, 1991.

Marshak AB: Emergency life support. In Wilkins RL, Stoller JK, Scanlan CL, editors: *Egan's fundamentals of respiratory therapy*, ed 8, St Louis, 2003, Mosby.

McMahon Busch M, Juel R, Newton KM: Cardiac catheterization. In Woods SL, Sivarajan Froelicher ES, Underhill Motzer S, editors: *Cardiac nursing*, ed 4, Philadelphia, 2000, Lippincott.

Pagana K, Pagana TJ: *Mosby's diagnostic and laboratory test reference*, ed 9, St Louis, 2009, Mosby.

Patel JM, McGowan SG, Moody LA: *Arrhythmias: detection, treatment, and cardiac drugs*, Philadelphia, 1989, Saunders.

Phillips RE, Feeney MK: *The cardiac rhythms: a systematic approach to interpretation*, ed 3, Philadelphia, 1990, Saunders.

Shapiro BA, Kacmarek RM, Cane RD, et al.: *Clinical application of respiratory care*, ed 4, St Louis, 1991, Mosby.

Shilling AM, Durbin Jr CG: Airway management devices and advanced cardiac life support. In Cairo JM, editor: *Mosby's respiratory care equipment*, ed 9, St Louis, 2014, Mosby.

Simmons KF, Scanlan CL: Airway management. In Wilkins RL, Stoller JK, Kacmarek RM, editors: *Egan's fundamentals of respiratory care*, ed 9, St Louis, 2009, Mosby.

Sorensen KA, Wilkins RL: Interpretation of the electrocardiogram. In Wilkins RL, Stoller JK, Kacmarek RM, editors: *Egan's fundamentals of respiratory care*, ed 9, St Louis, 2009, Mosby.

Thigpen K, Davis SP, Basol R, Lange P, Jain SS, Olsen JD, et al.: Implementing the 2005 American heart association guidelines, including use of the impedance threshold device, improves hospital discharge rate after in-hospital cardiac arrest, *Respir Care* 55(8):1014–1019, 2010.

White GC: *Equipment theory for respiratory care*, ed 4, Albany, NY, 2005, Delmar.

Wooding Baker M: Laboratory tests using blood. In Woods SL, Sivarajan Froelicher ES, Underhill Motzer S, editors: *Cardiac nursing*, ed 4, Philadelphia, 2000, Lippincott.

1. A fully compensatory pause is seen after which type of heartbeat?
   A. NSR
   B. PVC
   C. PAT
   D. VT

2. All the following are acceptable ways to ventilate a patient during CPR EXCEPT:
   A. Endotracheal tube
   B. Pneumatic (demand-valve) resuscitator
   C. Mouth-to-valve resuscitator
   D. Manual resuscitator

3. A male patient comes into the Emergency Department appearing ashen gray and complaining of sudden, severe pain beneath his sternum and shortness of breath. He says this began after he exercised vigorously for 45 minutes. After putting an O_2 mask on the patient, what should be done?
   A. Start ECG monitoring.
   B. Recommend that he begin a supervised exercise program at the hospital.
   C. Perform a peak flow test to check on exercise-induced asthma.
   D. Immediately draw an ABG sample.

4. Upon entering a patient's room, the respiratory therapist notices that the ECG monitor shows VT. A carotid pulse cannot be felt and the nurse says that he cannot find a blood pressure. What should be recommended?
   A. Check the other arm for a blood pressure.
   B. Defibrillate the patient.
   C. Intubate the patient and start the patient on a ventilator.
   D. Initiate synchronized cardioversion of the patient.

5. Counting from the left, the first and sixth rhythms on the ECG strip shown here represent:
   A. Atrial flutter
   B. Second-degree heart block
   C. Unifocal PVCs
   D. Multifocal PVCs

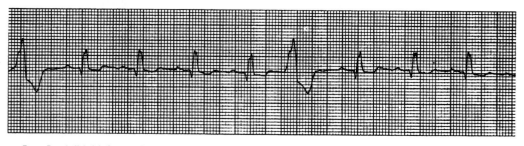

From Patel JM, McGowan SG, Moody, LA: Arrhythmias: detection, treatment and cardiac drugs, Philadelphia, 1989, Saunders.

6. A 65-year-old patient has been successfully resuscitated in the Emergency Department after suffering an MI. The patient is still unstable with frequent PVCs and needs to be transported to the cardiac care unit for management. Which of the following would be most important for monitoring the patient during the transportation?
   A. Pulse oximeter
   B. Portable capnography unit
   C. Portable ECG machine with defibrillator
   D. 12-lead ECG unit to record any arrhythmias

7. Two respiratory therapists are performing chest compressions, manually ventilating an intubated patient during a resuscitation attempt. The nurse and physician are both unable to start an IV line to give medications. What should be recommended?
   A. Instill the medications down the endotracheal tube.
   B. Keep trying new sites from which to start the IV line.
   C. Nebulize the medications.
   D. Give the medications by subcutaneous injection.

8. A respiratory therapist notices that a patient with a 28% air-entrainment mask is unresponsive to questions. The ECG rhythm seen below is noticed on the monitor. What should be recommended as a first reaction?
   A. Check the calibration on the ECG machine.
   B. Replace the ECG leads.
   C. Increase the O_2 percentage because the patient is hypoxic.
   D. Defibrillate the patient.

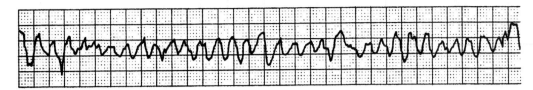

From Patel JM, McGowan SG, Moody, LA: Arrhythmias: detection, treatment and cardiac drugs, Philadelphia, 1989, Saunders.

9. It is noticed during a diagnostic ECG that the QRS complex is inverted on lead II. What would most likely cause this?
   A. An electrode is loose.
   B. The patient is shivering.
   C. The arm electrodes are reversed.
   D. The unit is out of calibration.

10. A 64-year-old woman was admitted with a diagnosis of MI. She was treated with a clot-dissolving medication and recovered quickly. What procedure should be performed to evaluate the condition of her coronary arteries?
    A. Left-heart catheterization
    B. Stress echocardiogram
    C. Right-heart catheterization
    D. 12-lead electrocardiogram

11. The physician has heard a heart murmur on a 24-year-old patient. A mitral valve regurgitation is suspected. What procedure should be performed to determine if that is the case?
    A. Right-heart catheterization
    B. Posteroanterior chest radiograph
    C. Echocardiogram
    D. Stress test

12. A 48-year-old male patient has been admitted with a suspected MI. What blood tests should be performed to determine if he has had an MI?
    1. CK-MB
    2. Troponin I
    3. D-Dimer
    4. BUN
    5. LDL
    A. 1 and 2 only
    B. 3 and 5 only
    C. 2, 3, and 4 only
    D. 1, 2, 3, and 5 only

13. While doing O_2 equipment rounds, the respiratory therapist comes upon a cyanotic patient who is not breathing. After repositioning the patient and hyperextending the neck, it is noticed that the patient has open lip ulcers. What would be the best way to ventilate this patient?

A. Perform mouth-to-mouth ventilation.
B. Use a mouth-to-valve device stored in the room for this purpose.
C. Run to the CPR crash cart and get a manual resuscitation bag and mask.
D. Wait for the anesthesiologist to intubate the patient's airway, then use a manual resuscitation bag.

14. To ensure that a manual ventilator is ready for use, what should be done?
    1. Make sure that no gas escapes through the outlet port when it is closed off and the bag is squeezed.
    2. Squeeze the bag, and make sure that the air/O_2 reservoir intake valve closes properly.
    3. Squeeze the bag, and make sure the nonrebreathing valve opens properly.
    4. Feel for air leaving the outlet port when the bag is squeezed.
    5. Squeeze the bag, and make sure that the air/O_2 reservoir intake valve opens properly.
    A. 4 and 5 only
    B. 2 and 3 only
    C. 1, 2, and 5 only
    D. 1, 2, 3, and 4 only

15. Blood for an ABG measurement needs to be drawn during a CPR attempt. Which site should be recommended for this?
    A. Carotid
    B. Radial
    C. Brachial
    D. Femoral

16. A mouth-to-valve resuscitation device is being used on an apneic patient. The respiratory therapist delivers a breath, but the patient's chest does not rise. What should be done next?
    A. Begin chest compressions.
    B. Request a lateral neck radiograph.
    C. Check the valve for proper position.
    D. Perform abdominal thrusts.

17. An NSR can be identified by:
    1. A resting rate of 60-100 beats/min in an adult
    2. A P wave before every QRS complex
    3. A regular rhythm
    4. A QRS complex after every P wave
    5. An upright T wave in lead II
    A. 2 and 4 only
    B. 2, 3, and 4 only
    C. 1, 2, 3, and 5 only
    D. 1, 2, 3, 4, 5

18. A ventilator-dependent patient is set up for routine ECG monitoring. Because of refractory hypoxemia, the physician orders 10 cm water of PEEP. Shortly after the PEEP therapy is added, it is noticed that sinus arrhythmia has developed. Which of the following is the best course of action to follow?
    A. Recommend the administration of atropine.
    B. Recommend synchronized cardioversion.
    C. Recommend decreasing the PEEP from 10 to 5 cm water.
    D. Make a record of the rhythm, and inform the nurse and physician of your observation.

19. Electrocardiogram monitoring is justified with a patient in the Intensive Care Unit in all of the following situations EXCEPT:
    A. If it is used to evaluate peripheral perfusion.
    B. If the patient has an electrolyte disturbance.
    C. If the patient has a history of arrhythmias.
    D. If the patient is being given a rapid infusion of potassium.

20. After an exercise routine, a 59-year-old man experiences sudden chest pain with shortness of breath. ECG monitoring in the Emergency Department reveals the following rhythm strip. What should the respiratory therapist recommend?
    1. Synchronized cardioversion
    2. 12-lead ECG
    3. Defibrillation
    4. Administer oxygen
    5. Angioplasty
    A. 1 and 5 only
    B. 2 and 4 only
    C. 2, 3, and 4 only
    D. 1, 2, 3, 4, 5

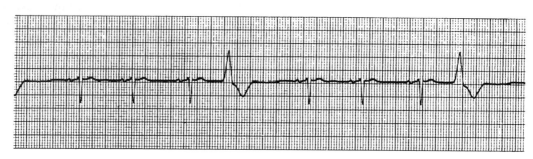

From Wilkins RL, Krider, SJ, Sheldon, RL: Clinical assessment in respiratory care, ed 4, St Louis, 2000, Mosby.

21. Which of the following medications can be administered down the endotracheal tube during a CPR attempt on an adult?
    1. Epinephrine
    2. Potassium chloride
    3. Atropine
    4. Lidocaine
    A. 1 only
    B. 2 and 3 only
    C. 1 and 4 only
    D. 1, 3, and 4 only

22. A paramedic and a respiratory therapist are performing CPR procedures on an adult patient. Upon looking at the ECG monitor, the following rhythm strip is seen. What should be recommended in this situation?
    A. Defibrillate the patient.
    B. Increase the oxygen flow to the manual resuscitation bag and mask.
    C. Change ventilation and chest compression duties.
    D. Intubate the patient.

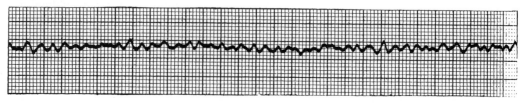

From Goldberger AL: Clinical electrocardiography, ed 6, St Louis, 1999 Mosby.

23. CPR steps have been under way for 15 minutes when an ABG sample is drawn and sent off for analysis. The following results are obtained with 100% oxygen being used to ventilate the patient:

    pH, 6.97

    $PaCO_2$, 30 torr

    PaO_2, 210 torr

    HCO_3^-, 8 mEq/L

    What should the therapist recommend at this time?
    A. Decrease the oxygen percentage.
    B. Decrease the respiratory rate.
    C. Administer IV sodium bicarbonate.
    D. Add mechanical dead space to the manual resuscitator.

24. During a CPR attempt on a 50-year-old patient, the respiratory therapist successfully intubates the patient and begins ventilating with a manual resuscitator. The physician is unable to start an IV line. How should the CPR drugs be given?
    A. Intraosseous injection
    B. Endotracheal instillation
    C. Intracardiac injection
    D. Nasal spray

25. A 59-year-old patient is brought to the hospital with a complaint of sudden, severe substernal chest pain and dyspnea. What initial thing should the respiratory therapist recommend?
    A. Begin ECG monitoring.
    B. Draw an ABG sample.
    C. Get a chest radiograph.
    D. Get a capnometer value.

26. Defibrillation should be done immediately in which of the following patient situations?
    A. Second-degree heart block
    B. Atrial flutter
    C. Pulseless VT
    D. Sinus tachycardia

27. An infant daughter has just been delivered by cesarean section to an anesthetized mother. Because she is not breathing adequately, an endotracheal tube has been inserted. What can be done to improve the infant's condition and get her to breathe?
    A. Give IV epinephrine.
    B. Give IV naloxone (Narcan).
    C. Begin bag/mask ventilation with oxygen.
    D. Give endotracheal atropine (atropine sulfate).

28. Bag/mask ventilation with oxygen is being provided to a 57-year-old adult at a rate of 12/min. The patient's other vital signs include heart rate of 52/min and blood pressure 95/55 mm Hg. What can be done to improve the patient's vital signs?
    A. Administer endotracheal lidocaine (Xylocaine).
    B. Begin chest compressions.
    C. Intubate the patient.
    D. Administer intravenous epinephrine (adrenaline).

12 Airway Management

Note: It can be anticipated that the Therapist Multiple-Choice Examination (TMC) will include an *average of 10 of 140 actual questions* (7% of the exam) on airway management. (This is based on the question mix typically found on the National Board of Respiratory Care's (NBRC's) previous Entry Level Examinations and Written Registry Examinations.)

Remember that the TMC version you take will include 20 additional questions being evaluated for possible inclusion in other versions of the TMC. So, there will be a total of 160 questions taken. There is no way to differentiate between the 140 actual questions and the 20 questions being evaluated for future use. Please go to the Introduction for detailed information on the TMC and the Clinical Simulation Examination.

MODULE A

General airway management topics

1. Evaluate data in the patient record about artificial airways (code: IA3) [difficulty: R, Ap]

Check the patient's record for any information on an artificial airway such as an endotracheal or tracheostomy tube. A change in the type of airway should also be noted.

2. Inspect the patient to assess the characteristics and patency of the airway (code: IB2b) [difficulty: R, Ap, An]

Look at the patient's facial area and throat for signs of a congenital defect or traumatic injury. See below.

3. Recognize a difficult airway (code: IIIA2) [difficulty: R, Ap, An]

Often a difficult airway can be visually identified. A congenital defect or traumatic injury to the face or neck can compromise the patient's airway.

Macroglossia is an example of a congenital defect that can cause a partial airway obstruction with inspiratory stridor. A child with this condition has an excessively large tongue that is often seen to protrude out of the mouth (Fig. 12-1). Macroglossia is associated with Down syndrome, Beckwith-Wiedemann syndrome, and several metabolic disorders. Immediate treatment may require (1) manually moving the mandible forward to pull the large tongue out of the airway, (2) inserting an oropharyngeal

airway or nasopharyngeal airway, and (3) placing the infant in the prone position. If the infant has a life-threatening airway obstruction that is not corrected by these procedures, an endotracheal tube or tracheostomy tube must be inserted. Long-term management may require a tracheostomy or corrective facial surgery.

It is standard practice for emergency medical personnel to place a neck brace on a trauma victim (for example, an automobile crash) to stabilize a cervical spine injury. In some cases, the patient is strapped on a body board in addition to wearing a neck brace. Usually the neck brace is not removed until after neck radiographs are taken and a physical exam is performed to disprove a cervical spine injury. If a patient wearing a neck brace has an upper-airway obstruction, it may be possible to insert an oropharyngeal airway or nasopharyngeal airway to push the tongue forward to ease breathing. If these devices are not effective, and the neck cannot be hyperextended to open the airway, an emergency airway is needed. It is possible that a laryngeal mask airway (LMA) or Combitube could be inserted by an emergency medical technician, paramedic, or respiratory therapist. If these devices are not able to provide a secure airway, a physician will need to perform nasotracheal intubation or a tracheostomy (see Chapter 18).

4. Properly position the patient to maintain a patent airway (code: IIIA1) [difficulty: R, Ap]

The head-tilt/chin-lift maneuver is the procedure of choice for opening the airways of all patients except those with a known or suspected cervical (neck) spine injury. The victim is gently positioned on his or her back. In an adult, the head is firmly pushed back with one hand, and the jaw is pulled upward with the fingers of the other hand (Fig. 12-2). A small pad can be placed behind the neck and head to put the patient in the "sniffing position." In an infant, it is not necessary to tilt the head back beyond a neutral position. Children may need to have the head pushed back slightly beyond neutral.

The jaw-thrust maneuver is the procedure of choice for opening the airway of all patients with a known or suspected cervical spine injury. The rescuer's elbows are rested on the ground, and the hands are placed on either side of the victim's jaw. Keep the head in line with the body. Lifting of the jaw usually opens the airway and eliminates the need to tilt the head back. See Figure 12-3 for the adult maneuver.

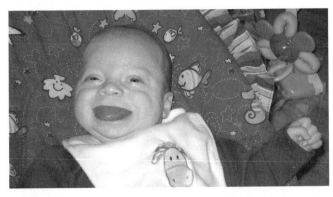

Figure 12-1 Close-up photograph of an infant with macroglossia. Note the larger than normal tongue that can obstruct the upper airway. (From Zitelli and Davis, 1992; courtesy of Dr. Christine L. Williams, New York Medical College.)

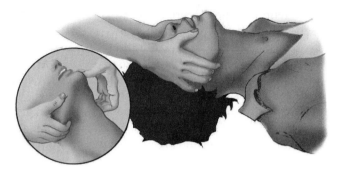

Figure 12-3 The jaw-thrust maneuver can be used to open the airway of an unconscious, supine person with a suspected or known cervical spine injury. The head is not tilted back. (From Barnes TA: Emergency cardiovascular life support. In Kacmarek RM, Stoller JK, Heuer AJ, editors: Egan's fundamentals of respiratory care, ed 10, St Louis, 2013, Mosby.)

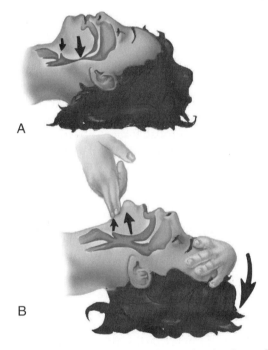

Figure 12-2 Head-tilt/chin-lift method for opening the airway. **A,** In an unconscious, supine adult the tongue and epiglottis can block the posterior pharynx. **B,** Careful tilting of the head and lifting of the chin can open the airway. *Note:* This procedure should not be performed on a person with a suspected or known cervical spine injury. (From Kacmarek RM, Stoller JK, Heuer AJ, editors: Egan's fundamentals of respiratory care, ed 10, St Louis, 2013, Mosby.)

The patient may be supine during the airway-opening procedures just mentioned. Frequently, however, the patient is positioned with the head and body elevated. An unconscious patient is less likely to vomit and aspirate in either Fowler's or semi-Fowler's position. The combination of either of these body positions with the head and neck hyperextended into the sniff position will probably keep the airway open and minimize the risk of aspiration of vomitus. Turning the patient's head to one side may also reduce the risk of aspiration. Placing the patient into either Fowler's or semi-Fowler's position will also minimize the patient's work of breathing (WOB) and help to reduce hypoxemia.

5. Perform respiratory care-related procedures in a cardiopulmonary emergency such as an obstructed or lost airway (code: IIIG1a) [difficulty: R, Ap, An]

An artificial airway is indicated in any patient who cannot protect his or her airway. The patient may be at risk of upper-airway obstruction from the tongue falling back, may have facial trauma or be undergoing surgery, may be at risk of vomiting and aspirating, or may need mechanical ventilation for assisted breathing. Select the best one based on the patient's needs. These airways are presented in the remainder of this chapter.

Exam Hint 12-1

Identify that the patient has an airway problem. Know the uses, advantages, and disadvantages of the various airway devices. Be prepared to make a recommendation for which device to use or when to change to a different airway device, as necessary.

6. Humidify an artificial airway

a. Recommend a change in humidification (code: IIIE3c) [difficulty: R, Ap]

See below.

b. Assemble and troubleshoot humidifiers (code: IIA3) [difficulty: R, Ap]

Patients with an oropharyngeal or nasopharyngeal airway may also be given supplemental humidity by a simple aerosol mask to help prevent drying of secretions. If a patient is given more than 4 L/min of oxygen, supplemental humidity should be provided. Patients with an endotracheal or tracheostomy tube in place should ideally be provided 100% relative humidity at body temperature. If not, secretions in the airway may dry and result in mucous plugs. Depending on the patient situation, a heat–moisture exchanger (HME) or heated humidifier may be used. However, it may be necessary to change from a HME to a cascade-type or wick-type humidifier if the patient has thick secretions that are difficult to remove by coughing or suctioning. Humidification is discussed with the various oxygen delivery systems. See Chapter 8 for a complete discussion of humidity and aerosol therapy and administrative devices.

MODULE B

Oropharyngeal airways

1. Recommend the insertion or change of an artificial airway (code: IIIE2e) [difficulty: R, Ap, An]

An oropharyngeal airway is typically used in one of the three following situations: (1) in an unconscious patient at risk of obstructing the airway with his or her tongue, (2) in an unconscious seizure patient who may bite his or her tongue during another seizure, or (3) in an orally intubated patient to prevent the endotracheal tube from being bitten. An oropharyngeal airway should not be used in a conscious patient because it may cause gagging.

2. Oropharyngeal airway equipment

a. Assemble the necessary equipment (code: IIA10) [difficulty: R, Ap]

The oropharyngeal airway (or bite block) is made of plastic that is hard enough to withstand any patient's biting force. A properly sized and placed oropharyngeal airway lifts the tongue forward from the posterior portion of the oropharynx to keep a patent airway and make suctioning oral secretions easier. An oropharyngeal airway is poorly tolerated in a conscious patient and can cause gagging and even vomiting. Oropharyngeal airways are available in a variety of sizes that fit infants or adults. The proper size is found by holding the airway against the patient's face with the flange against the lips. The end of the airway should reach the angle of the jaw (Fig. 12-4). Too large an airway can block the oropharynx by extending past the tongue. An airway that is too small can push the tongue back into the oropharynx rather than pulling the tongue forward, as intended. Figure 12-5 shows a properly placed and sized oropharyngeal airway.

A number of manufacturers make oropharyngeal airways, which fall into two basic types: hollow center and I-beam (Fig. 12-6).

1. Hollow center

Hollow-center types (Guedel is a common brand) have an oval or rectangular shape in cross-section and are hollow in the center. A suction catheter can be easily placed through the hollow center so that the back of the throat

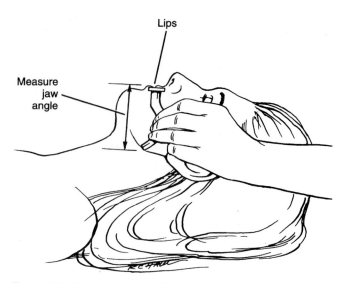

Figure 12-4 Procedure for measuring the proper size of the oropharyngeal airway. (From Eubanks DH, Bone RC: Comprehensive respiratory care, ed 2, St Louis, 1990, Mosby.)

can be cleared of secretions. Some types have an outer tube that can be attached by a practitioner to provide a mouthpiece for rescue breathing. If rescue breathing must be performed, it is probably more effective to ventilate with a mask and manual resuscitator when one becomes available.

2. I-beam

I-beam types (Berman is a common brand) are shaped like an I-beam in cross-section. A suction catheter can easily be guided along the groove on either side of the I-beam to the back of the throat so that secretions can be removed.

Most oropharyngeal airways are single units. There is nothing to assemble. There are some hollow-center types that have an attachable outer part. The outer part is snapped onto the oropharyngeal airway when the practitioner must perform rescue breathing. It has a wide flange so that the lips can be covered and sealed to prevent a leak.

b. Troubleshoot any problems with the equipment (code: IIA10) [difficulty: R, Ap]

Make sure that the channel in the hollow-center types is patent. If a unit is plugged by secretions, blood, or a foreign substance, the patient cannot breathe through the opening. A suction catheter cannot be passed through either. Remove an airway that is not patent.

3. Establish and manage the patient's airway (code: IIIA3b) [difficulty: R, Ap]

There are three widely used methods to insert an oropharyngeal airway.

a. First method (antianatomic approach)

1. Open the patient's mouth with the cross-finger technique. Insert the airway upside down into the patient's

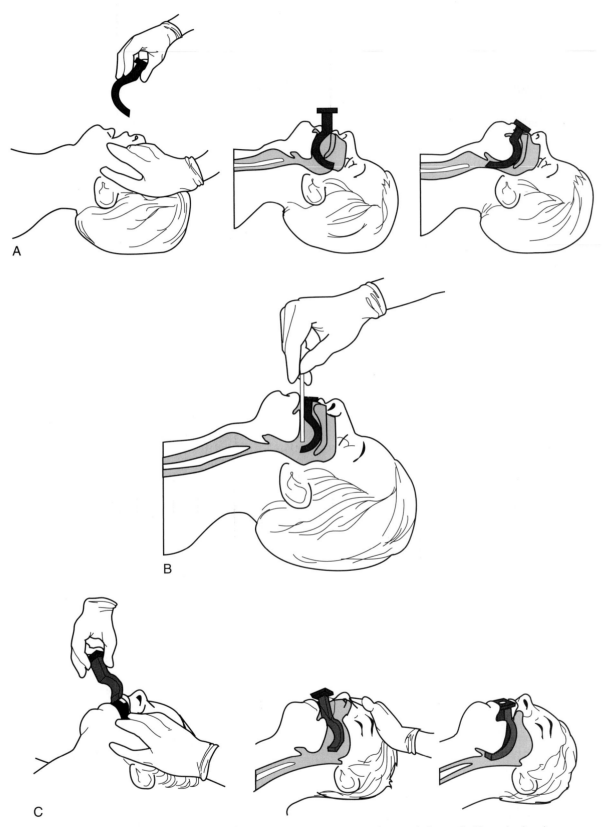

Figure 12-5 Three different possible procedures for inserting an oropharyngeal airway. **A,** Airway is placed with the tip pointing toward the palate. Then it is rotated 180 degrees to support the tongue. **B,** A tongue depressor is used to move the tongue toward the jaw. The airway is then slid behind the tongue to support it, and the tongue depressor is removed. **C,** A cheek is gently pulled aside to make room to place the airway behind the tongue. (From Shilling A, Durbin CG: Airway management devices and advanced life support. In Cairo JM: Mosby's respiratory care equipment, ed 9, St Louis, 2014, Mosby.)

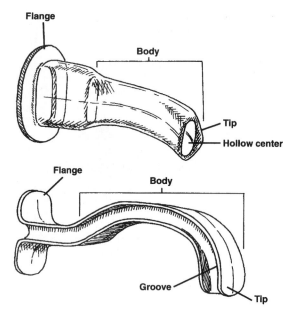

Figure 12-6 Close-ups of hollow and I-beam types of oropharyngeal airways.

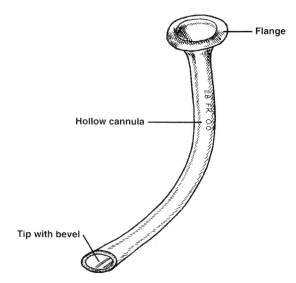

Figure 12-7 Typical nasopharyngeal airway.

mouth until it reaches the palate. Some authors recommend inserting it past the uvula.

2. Twist the airway 180 degrees, and insert it the rest of the way until the tongue is supported by the curved body.
3. The flange should rest at the lips (Fig. 12-5, A).

b. Second method (anatomic approach)

1. Insert a tongue blade into the mouth and push the tongue toward the jaw.
2. The curved body of the airway is directed into the mouth to support the tongue.
3. The flange should rest at the lips (Fig. 12-5, B).

c. Third method (side approach)

1. Open the patient's mouth with the cross-finger technique. Insert the airway into the mouth with the curved body rotated toward a cheek.
2. Twist the airway 90 degrees, and insert it the rest of the way so that the tongue is supported by the curved body.
3. The flange should rest at the lips (Fig. 12-5, C).

MODULE C

Nasopharyngeal airways

1. Recommend the insertion or change of an artificial airway (code: IIIE2e) [difficulty: R, Ap, An]

A nasopharyngeal airway has three indications. First, it is used to keep the tongue from blocking the airway when an oropharyngeal airway cannot be used. This would include conscious supine patients or patients with oral trauma or jaw surgery. Second, it is also used as a guide to

pass a catheter for tracheal suctioning or to pass a flexible fiberoptic bronchoscope. The nasopharyngeal airway protects the patient's mucous membranes from the trauma of repeatedly passed catheters. Third, a nasopharyngeal airway is used in a patient currently having a seizure with a tightly closed jaw. In this case, an oropharyngeal airway cannot be used. The nasopharyngeal airway can be passed into the patient's oropharynx to push the tongue forward and maintain an airway. The nasopharyngeal airway is probably not as effective in keeping the tongue forward as the oropharyngeal airway. However, it is better tolerated in a semiconscious or alert patient.

2. Nasopharyngeal airway equipment

a. Assemble the necessary equipment (code: IIA10) [difficulty: R, Ap]

Nasopharyngeal airways (also known as nasal airways, nasal trumpets, or nasal stents) are made of a relatively soft and pliable plastic or rubber. This decreases the chances of damaging the delicate mucous membranes of the nasal turbinate opening as it passes through the nasopharynx.

Several manufacturers make the two basic types of nasopharyngeal airways—the *blunt tip* and the *beveled tip*. The beveled-tip types are available with right-sided and left-sided cut bevels. If possible, open the airway with the bevel cut opening toward the patient's oropharynx (toward the nasal septum). For example, if the airway is going to be inserted into the left naris, the bevel should be cut on the right side of the tube so that it is open to the patient's oropharynx. If you were inserting the tube into the right nostril, you would want the bevel cut on the left side of the tube.

See Figure 12-7 for a close-up of a nasopharyngeal airway. All nasopharyngeal airways have a wide flange that fits close to the patient's nostril. This prevents the entire tube from being pushed into the patient. All nasopharyngeal

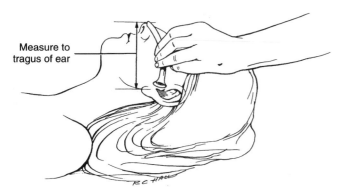

Figure 12-8 Procedure for measuring the proper size of the nasopharyngeal airway. (From Eubanks DH, Bone RC: Comprehensive respiratory care, ed 2, St Louis, 1990, Mosby.)

airways have a cannula with a channel for breathing or suctioning. Nasopharyngeal airways are available in a variety of sizes for adults. They can be properly sized by measuring from the tip of the nose to the tragus of the ear and adding 2-3 cm (Fig. 12-8). All nasopharyngeal airways are made up of a single piece. There is nothing to assemble.

b. Troubleshoot any problems with the equipment (code: IIA10) [difficulty: R, Ap]

Make sure that the tube is not plugged by dried secretions, blood, or a foreign body. If plugged, the patient cannot breathe through it, and a suction catheter cannot be passed through it. Remove a plugged nasopharyngeal airway.

3. Establish and manage the patient's airway (code: IIIA3a) [difficulty: R, Ap]

The following steps are taken to insert a nasopharyngeal airway:

1. Select the most patent nostril. Check the patient's electronic medical record for a history of a broken nose, deviated septum, or current head cold. Interview the conscious patient to determine whether one nostril is more open than the other. Place your finger in front of the patient's nostrils to feel which one has greater airflow. Avoid forcing the airway into a nostril and nasal passage that may be damaged by the procedure.
2. Lubricate the properly sized airway with a sterile, water-soluble lubricant such as K-Y jelly. Place the lubricant on a sterile, 4 × 4-in gauze pad, and then smear it over the length of the airway.
3. Tell the patient what you are going to do.
4. Gently place the airway into the nostril. It should be directed straight back parallel to the hard palate. Stop if you feel any resistance. Try a different angle if resistance is felt. Do not force the airway. Try the other nostril if necessary.
5. Secure the airway by sticking a safety pin through the flange and taping the pin to the bridge of the patient's

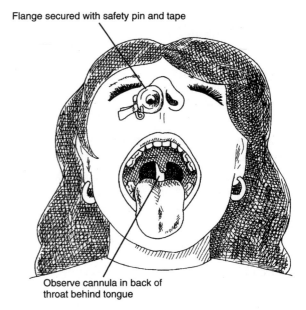

Figure 12-9 Proper position of the nasopharyngeal airway behind the tongue can be determined by looking into the mouth. The tube is also secured by placing a safety pin through the flange and taping it to the cheek.

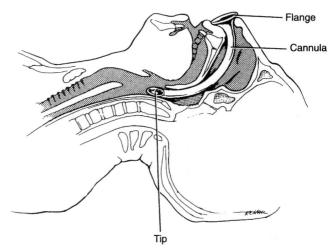

Figure 12-10 Cross-section of the head showing the proper position of the nasopharyngeal airway. (From Ellis PD, Billings DM: Cardiopulmonary resuscitation: procedures for basic and advanced life support, St Louis, 1980, Mosby.)

nose or cheek (Fig. 12-9). This helps prevent the airway from being accidentally dislodged or inserted further.

6. Rotate the airway to the other nostril, if possible, on a regular basis. This helps prevent ulceration of the mucous membrane. Some authors recommend rotation at least every 48 hours, whereas others recommend rotation at much shorter time intervals.

Check the placement by looking into the patient's mouth with a flashlight and tongue depressor. A properly placed nasopharyngeal airway can be seen in the oropharynx and extends behind the tongue (Figs. 12-9 and 12-10). The placement should be checked each time a tube is replaced or moved from one nostril to the other. If a nasopharyngeal tube is inserted too deeply, it can block the glottis opening into the trachea.

MODULE D

Laryngeal mask airways

1. Recommend the insertion or change of an artificial airway (code: IIIE2e) [difficulty: R, Ap, An]

A laryngeal mask airway (LMA) is a type of supraglottic airway that is composed of a modified endotracheal tube with a standard 15-mm-outer diameter (OD) adapter (for attaching a resuscitation bag or ventilator circuit) at the proximal end and a silicone laryngeal mask at the distal end. The mask is inflated by attaching a syringe to the one-way valve and pilot balloon on an inflation tube, in the same manner as an endotracheal tube cuff (Fig. 12-11). When the mask is inflated, it surrounds and seals the larynx. LMAs were first used in the operating room by anesthesiologists. Currently, emergency medical personnel and respiratory therapists use LMAs as an alternative to endotracheal tubes or Combitubes in patients with a difficult airway or

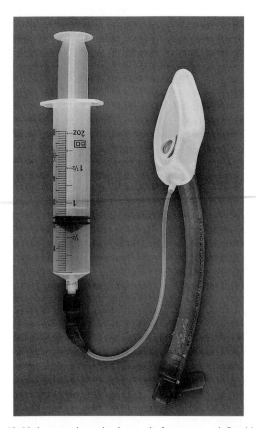

Figure 12-11 Laryngeal mask airway. It features an inflatable mask that creates a seal around the patient's larynx. A syringe is attached to the one-way valve to deflate and inflate the mask. The proximal end of the tube can be connected to a resuscitation bag, anesthesia machine, or mechanical ventilator. (From LMA International, Henley-on-Thames, England.)

during a CPR effort. Experience has shown that an LMA can be easily and quickly inserted without any additional equipment. Patients with asthma or irritable airways will have less coughing or bronchospasm than if an endotracheal tube were inserted. It has been shown that ventilating a patient with a resuscitation bag to an LMA is as effective as or better than bag/mask ventilation. See Box 12-1 for indications and contraindications for and limits to an LMA.

Remember that an LMA does not provide as secure an airway as an endotracheal tube. There are two limitations to using an LMA. First, the LMA does not absolutely protect against aspiration. Second, tidal volume gas can leak if ventilation pressures are greater than 20 cm H_2O. This can lead to a smaller than desired tidal volume and/or gas being forced into the stomach. Excessive air in the stomach can cause vomiting. If either of these possibilities is of paramount clinical concern, the patient should have an endotracheal tube inserted rather than an LMA.

2. Laryngeal mask airway equipment

a. Assemble the necessary equipment (code: IIA10) [difficulty: R, Ap]

The LMA is available in eight sizes for insertion into patients ranging in weight from a small child to a large adult. Selected sizes include mask size 1 for a neonate or child up to 5 kg (up to 11 lb), mask size 2½ for children weighing between 20 and 30 kg (44 and 66 lb), mask size 4 for adults weighing 50-70 kg (110-154 lb), and mask size 5 for large adults weighing 70-100 kg (154-220 lb). Other mask sizes are available for patients within these weight ranges or for very large adults.

BOX 12-1 Laryngeal Mask Airway: Indications, Contraindications, and Limits

Indications

Patient has undergone a CPR effort or has a difficult airway and cannot have an endotracheal tube or Combitube.

Patient needs a patent airway and cannot have his or her neck hyperextended for endotracheal intubation.

A channel is needed through which to pass an endotracheal tube into the trachea.

Contraindications

Patient is conscious or resists placement of the LMA.

Patient is known to have or might have food in the stomach.

Patient will require high pressure to ventilate (because of low lung compliance and/or high airway resistance).

Patient has severe gastroesophageal reflux disease (GERD).

Limits

Aspiration is possible if the patient's stomach is not empty or the patient has GERD.

There is tidal volume leakage out of the mouth or into the stomach if the ventilating pressure is >20 cm H_2O.

Several manufacturers make standard LMAs like that shown in Figure 12-11. In addition, there are two commonly seen modifications. The first is an LMA that facilitates tracheal intubation by easily allowing an endotracheal tube to slide through its lumen. The second is an LMA that includes a port for gastric suction to vent any air in the stomach. Adjunct supplies include a water-soluble lubricant for the laryngeal mask, syringe to inflate the mask, and protective gear for the practitioner, such as a goggles, face mask, gown, and gloves.

Make sure that the proximal end has a 15-mm-OD adapter attached. Check the laryngeal mask to be sure it is functioning. Inflate the cuff with a syringe, disconnect the syringe to make sure the one-way valve works, reattach the syringe, and deflate the mask.

b. Troubleshoot any problems with the equipment (code: IIA10) [difficulty: R, Ap]

Do not use an LMA that does not have a proximal adapter or if the mask will not inflate properly.

3. Establish and manage the patient's airway (code: IIIA3c) [difficulty: R, Ap, An]

Figure 12-12 shows the procedure for inserting an LMA and how the inflated mask covers the laryngeal inlet (glottis opening into the trachea). When the properly sized LMA is being placed, it is gently advanced until resistance is felt. (If the LMA is too small, no resistance will be felt because it will slide into the esophagus.) The distal tip of the mask will stop at the upper esophageal sphincter. The cuff is then inflated to cover the tracheal opening and seal off the esophagus. (Later, the cuff pressure can be measured; it should not exceed 60 cm H_2O.) Manually ventilate the patient's lungs with a resuscitation bag. The following steps should be taken to ensure that the LMA is properly placed to cover the opening to the trachea: (1) when the LMA mask is inflated, the tube will move out of the mouth about 1-2 cm; (2) auscultate for equal, bilateral breath sounds; (3) auscultate for the absence of sounds over the stomach; (4) an end-tidal carbon dioxide monitor should show exhaled CO_2.

Once the LMA is properly located, it needs to be stabilized. This is usually done by taping the tube to the patient's upper lip or using a manufactured tube-holding device. Observe that the black line that runs the length of the tube, and marks its center, is not twisted. If the tube is twisted, the tracheal mask may not cover the glottis. This would cause a leak and loss of tidal volume.

4. Measure the tracheal tube cuff pressure and/or volume (code: IC20) [difficulty: R, Ap]

See below.

5. Evaluate the tracheal tube cuff pressure and/or volume (code: ID19) [difficulty: R, Ap, An]

A standard cuff measuring device (such as the Cufflator) can be used to measure the mask pressure. It should not be

greater than 60 cm H_2O to seal the airway. (See the later discussion on managing an endotracheal tube for more information on securing the tube and measuring cuff pressure.)

MODULE E

Esophageal–tracheal tubes

1. Recommend the insertion or change of an artificial airway (code: IIIE2e) [difficulty: R, Ap, An]

The Combitube (also known as the esophageal–tracheal Combitube or ETC) is a double-lumen tube that can be used to ventilate a patient whether the tube is placed into the esophagus (as intended) or the trachea (Fig. 12-13). The Combitube is one version of a series of tubes called esophageal obturator airways (EOAs) that are designed to be placed into the esophagus of an unconscious adult patient. Clinical experience has shown that a Combitube provides a reasonably secure airway in emergency situations, such as when performing CPR. It can be used as an alternative to an LMA. At the time this book was being published, there were at least five different types of EOAs that provide the same two functions: ensure a stable airway for artificial ventilation and prevent vomiting and aspiration. Clinical experience with the various types of esophageal obturator airways is highly recommended because they do not appear or operate like standard endotracheal tubes. See Box 12-2 for more information.

2. Esophageal–tracheal airway equipment

a. Assemble the necessary equipment (code: IIA10) [difficulty: R, Ap]

The Combitube is available in two sizes. The longer, larger size (41 Fr) is used for patients who are more than 16 years of age and more than 60 in (5 feet) in height. The Combitube SA is smaller (37 Fr) and intended for smaller patients. Neither size is intended for small pediatric patients. Both Combitube types are included in a kit with a 140-mL syringe to inflate the larger, proximal cuff in the patient's oral pharynx and a 20-mL syringe to inflate the smaller, distal cuff in the patient's esophagus (or trachea). The practitioner should have protective gear such as goggles, face mask, gown, and gloves.

Before placing either Combitube version into the patient, check that each cuff will inflate, hold air, and deflate properly. Each of the tubes should have a standard 15-mm-OD ventilator adapter inserted into its proximal end.

b. Troubleshoot any problems with the equipment (code: IIA10) [difficulty: R, Ap]

Do not use a unit that has a defective cuff(s) or missing adapters. If a cuff should fail during patient use, the Combitube should be removed. It can be replaced by another unit, another type of secure airway can be inserted, or bag/mask ventilation can be performed.

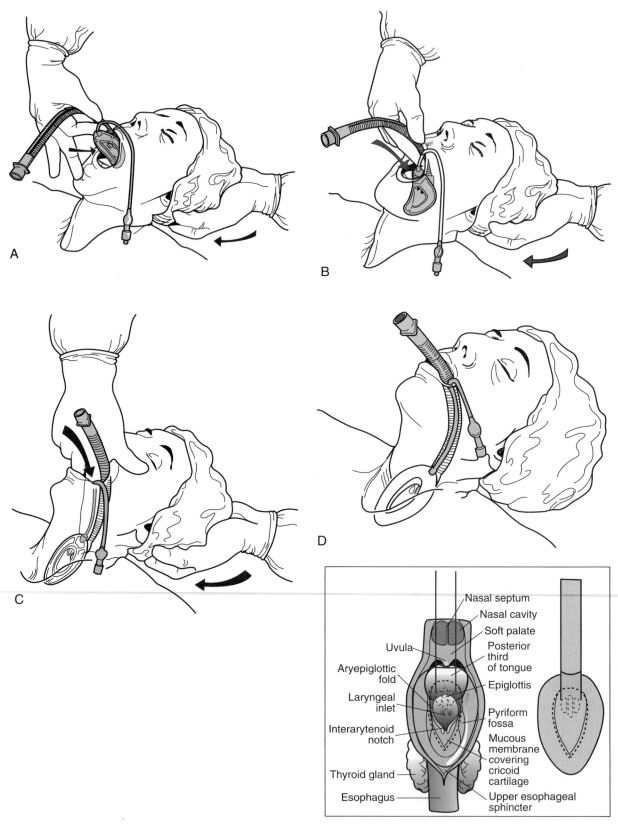

Figure 12-12 Steps to insert an Laryngeal mask airway to make sure that it seals the patient's larynx. **A,** The lubricated mask is deflated and manually inserted into the mouth. **B,** The mask should easily slide behind the tongue into the oral pharynx. **C,** The mask is gently advanced until resistance is felt as the mask lodges at the opening of the larynx. **D,** The syringe is attached to the one-way valve and air is pumped into the mask to seal the larynx. Attach a resuscitation bag to the proximal end of the tube and inflate the patient's lungs. Listen for bilateral breath sounds. See the inset for the anatomic structures related to the larynx, glottis, and esophagus. (Redrawn from Gensia Automedics, San Diego, CA. In Cairo JM, Pilbeam SP, editors: Mosby's respiratory care equipment, ed 8, St Louis, 2010, Mosby)

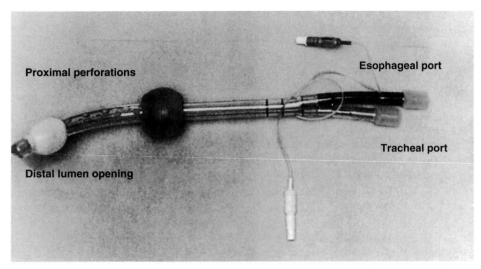

Figure 12-13 Combitube with its component features. Note that the Combitube has two lumens and two cuffs. The lumen with the distal cuff is inserted into the patient's esophagus (or occasionally the trachea). The proximal cuff is inserted into the patient's pharynx. Each cuff has its own inflating tube with one-way valve. There are perforations in the esophageal tube between the two cuffs that allow ventilation through the esophageal port. The proximal end of both tubes has a standard 15-mm-OD adapter for attachment of a resuscitation bag. Depending on the placement of the Combitube in the esophagus (as intended) or trachea, the patient's lungs can be ventilated through the esophageal or the tracheal port when both cuffs are inflated. (Courtesy Covidien, Mansfield, Massachusetts.)

BOX 12-2   Combitube: Indications, Contraindications, Advantages, and Disadvantages

General Indications

Emergency personnel are not trained in endotracheal intubation.

Attempted endotracheal intubation has not been successful.

Patient is apneic, without reflexes, and unconscious.

General Contraindications

Endotracheal intubation can be performed.

Patient is responsive with an intact gag reflex.

Patient is too small for the Combitube.

Esophageal obturator device would be needed for more than 1-2 hours.

Patient is known to have esophageal trauma or pathology or to have ingested a corrosive substance.

Advantages

Rapidly controls the airway.

Can be inserted into the patient in an awkward position without the head or neck being hyperextended.

Prevents the insufflation of gas into the stomach during bag/mask ventilation.

Prevents the movement of stomach contents into the pharynx.

Has esophageal gastric tube airway (EGTA) advantages.

The stomach can be emptied by passing a Levin tube through the esophageal tube.

The patient's lungs can be ventilated whether the tube is placed into the esophagus (as intended) or the trachea.

Prevents aspiration of blood or secretions from the upper airway.

Disadvantages

Accidental and unrecognized tracheal intubation is possible.

The possibility of upper-airway tear and hemorrhage during tube insertion exists.

Incomplete cuff seals result in air leak during ventilation.

The airway cannot be reliably kept open.

---

3. Establish and manage the patient's airway (code: IIIA3d) [difficulty: R, Ap, An]

Proper placement of the Combitube is needed to ensure that it can be correctly maintained in the airway. Figure 12-14 shows the procedure for inserting a Combitube. When the tube enters the esophagus as intended, both cuffs are inflated, and the patient is ventilated through the longer, colored tube, bilateral breath sounds will be heard (see Fig. 12-14, C). Continue to ventilate the patient's lungs and tape the tube in place. If breath sounds are not heard, the tube has accidentally entered the patient's trachea. Now, ventilate through the shorter, clear tube and listen for bilateral breath sounds. If they are heard, continue to ventilate and tape the tube in place to the patient's upper lip (see Fig. 12-14, D).

4. Measure the tracheal tube cuff pressure and/or volume (code: IC20) [difficulty: R, Ap]

See below.

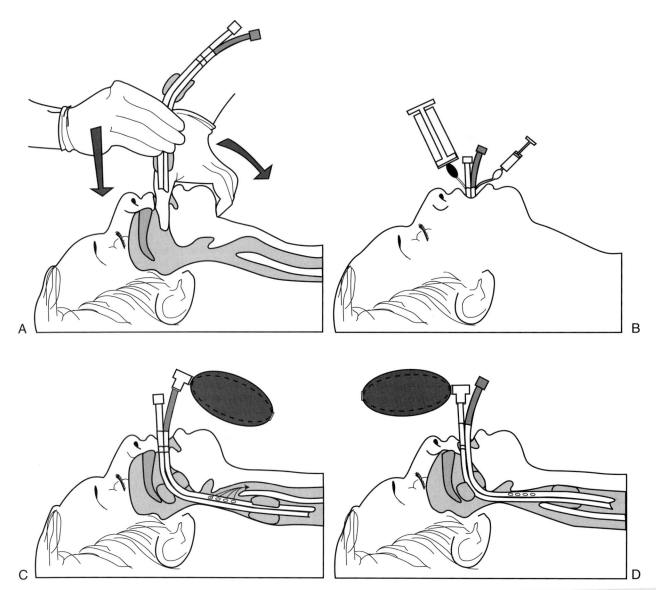

Figure 12-14 Steps in the insertion of a Combitube to make sure that it seals the patient's airway. **A,** One hand is used to grasp the jaw and pull it forward. With both cuffs deflated and the patient's head in a neutral position, the Combitube is inserted into the center of the mouth. **B,** Outer view of the Combitube after it has been gently inserted until the black rings on the tube are at the teeth. **C,** Inner view of the *usual* location of the tube in the patient's esophagus. Both cuffs are inflated. The resuscitation bag is attached to the longer, colored esophageal tube and the patient's lungs are ventilated. Listen for bilateral breath sounds. **D,** Inner view of the *occasional* location of the tube in the patient's trachea. Both cuffs are inflated. The resuscitation bag is attached to the shorter, clear tracheal tube and the patient's lungs are ventilated. Listen for bilateral breath sounds. (From Cairo JM: Mosby's respiratory care equipment, ed 9, St Louis, 2014, Mosby)

5. Evaluate the tracheal tube cuff pressure and/or volume (code: ID19) [difficulty: R, Ap, An]

Follow the manufacturer's recommendation for cuff volumes. With the original Combitube, the large, pharyngeal cuff is designed to hold 100 mL of air; the smaller cuff is designed to hold 15 mL of air. Put enough air into the cuffs so that there is no air leak when manual ventilation is performed.

MODULE F

Tracheostomy tubes

1. Recommend the insertion or change of an artificial airway (code: IIIE2e) [difficulty: R, Ap, An]

The tracheostomy tube offers the same uses as the endotracheal tube, such as maintaining a secure airway, providing

TABLE 12-1	Endotracheal and Tracheostomy Tube Sizes Based on Patient Age*		
Age	ID (mm)	Approximate OD (mm)	Fr Size (OD)
Newborn			
<1000 g	2.5	4.0	12
1000-2000 g	3.0	5.0	14
2000-3000 g	3.5	5.5	16-18
3000 g to 6 months of age	3.5-4.0		
Pediatric			
18 months	4.0	6.0	18
3 years	4.5	6.5	20
5 years	5.0	7.0	22
6 years	5.5	8.0	24
8 years	6.0	9.0	26
Adult			
16 years	7.0	10.0	30
Normal-sized woman	7.5-8.0	11.0	32-34
Normal-sized man	8.0-8.5	12.0	34-36
Large adult	9.0-10.0	13.0-14.0	38-42

Fr, French; ID, internal diameter; OD, outer diameter.

*Two notes: First, it is important to always use the largest tube that can be placed into the patient without causing any harm during the intubation. This is because the larger the ID of the tube, the less airway resistance it causes. Be prepared to insert a tube that is one size larger or smaller than anticipated based on individual variances. Second, the mathematical relationship between the OD in millimeters and Fr size can be easily calculated. The Fr size is determined by multiplying the OD in millimeters by 3. The OD in millimeters is found by dividing the Fr size by 3.

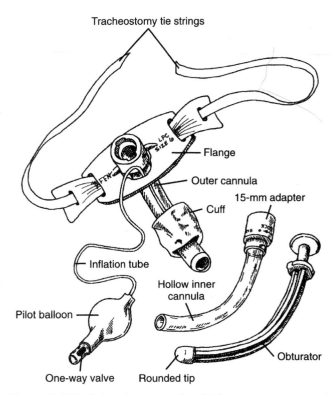

Figure 12-15 Typical tracheostomy tube with its component parts and features.

a direct suctioning route to the lungs, preventing aspiration, and ensuring a safe route to provide mechanical ventilation. In addition, it is placed in the patient who has an upper-airway obstruction or facial trauma that makes intubation impossible. A tracheostomy tube is often placed in a patient who requires long-term mechanical ventilation. Some patients with a permanent neurologic problem that limits their breathing will have a tracheostomy performed. By not breathing through the upper airway, their anatomic dead space is reduced. In the long term, a tracheostomy is said to be more comfortable than an endotracheal tube, even though it requires a surgical procedure for its placement. An additional advantage of a tracheostomy tube over an endotracheal tube is that it allows the patient to eat and drink.

2. Standard and fenestrated tracheostomy tube equipment

a. Assemble the necessary equipment (code: IIA10) [difficulty: R, Ap]

These tubes are available in a variety of sizes for patients of all ages from neonate to adult. See Table 12-1 for tracheostomy tube sizes (this also applies to tracheostomy buttons and endotracheal tubes) based on patient age. It is common practice to refer to the needed tube size by its inner diameter (ID). For example, a tracheostomy tube for an adult female would be 7.5- or 8.0-mm ID.

Most modern tracheostomy tubes are constructed of a hard polyvinyl chloride plastic and have a high-volume, low-pressure cuff. There are now tracheostomy tubes that feature an added cannula for suctioning out any oral secretions that have accumulated above the cuff. (See Fig. 12-32 for an endotracheal tube with this feature.) Some specialty tubes are made of silver, rubber, or latex. The older, silver tubes may not have a cuff or the cuff may be removed. A syringe is needed to inflate the tube cuff.

The following are commonly seen examples of tracheostomy tube styles:

1. Single-cannula tube

The single-cannula tracheostomy tube has a single channel that the patient breathes through, a cuff to seal the airway, and a flange at the base of the neck. See below for the general discussion that applies to this and dual-cannula tubes.

2. Dual-cannula tube

A dual-cannula tracheostomy tube has a main outer cannula and an inner cannula that is placed into the outer cannula. Refer to Figure 12-15 for these features of a typical dual-cannula tracheostomy tube:

a. The proximal end is outside of the patient's stoma and attached to an adjustable flange. The angle of the flange can be adjusted so that the distal end of the cannula fits properly into the patient's trachea. Soft, cloth tracheostomy tie strings are attached to the ends of the flange. The loose ends are tied behind the patient's neck to hold the tube in place. Or, the strings end in Velcro and are connected together to hold the tube. The distal end of the cannula has a small area where radiopaque material is embedded. As with an endotracheal tube, this allows the end of the cannula to be seen on a chest radiograph. The cuff is a high-residual-volume, low-pressure type. Air is inserted and withdrawn from the cuff by an inflation tube with a pilot balloon and one-way valve.

b. The obturator is slid into the outer cannula's opening before it is inserted into the patient's stoma. The obturator has a rounded end that protrudes from the end of the cannula. This prevents any tissue trauma during the insertion. The obturator is removed as soon as the cannula is in place.

c. The hollow inner cannula is slid into the outer cannula's opening and locked into place with a clockwise twist. This completes the airway for the patient to breathe through. The proximal end has a standard 15-mm-OD adapter so that all respiratory care equipment fits onto it. The distal end is flush with the end of the outer cannula. Some practitioners believe that the inner cannula should be periodically removed and cleaned so that secretions do not accumulate. Other practitioners believe that this is unnecessary if the airway is properly humidified and suctioning is performed as needed.

3. Fenestrated dual-cannula tracheostomy tube

Dual-cannula fenestrated tubes allow the patient to breathe through either the inner cannula lumen or the fenestration when the inner cannula is removed. A fenestrated tube is often placed in a patient who can breathe spontaneously and who is being considered for a complete removal of the tracheostomy tube. If the patient does well with this tube, it can probably be removed safely. If the patient has difficulty, the plug can be removed, the inner cannula can be replaced, and the patient's airway can be suctioned or mechanically ventilated.

Refer to Figure 12-16 when reviewing these features of the fenestrated tracheostomy tube:

a. The outer cannula has an opening called the fenestration (window). The rest of the cannula, cuff, inflation tube, and flange are the same as already discussed.

b. The inner cannula functions as discussed earlier. When the cuff is inflated, mechanical ventilation can be provided.

c. The outer cannula plug is used to prevent the patient from breathing through the proximal end of the tube. The plug does not cover the fenestration;

therefore the patient is able to breathe through the upper airway. The patient can now talk and expectorate any secretions. The cuff is usually deflated to further open the upper airway.

> **Exam Hint 12-2**
>
> A single-cannula tracheostomy tube should be replaced with a fenestrated tube when a patient is improving and can breathe spontaneously (off of the ventilator) for an extended time. Remove the inner cannula and deflate the cuff so that the patient can breathe through the upper airway. Replace the inner cannula and inflate the cuff when mechanical ventilation is resumed.

b. Troubleshoot any problems with the equipment (code: IIA10) [difficulty: R, Ap]

Before a tracheostomy (or endotracheal) tube is inserted into a patient, the cuff must be tested. Do this by attaching a syringe to the one-way valve and inflating the cuff. Remove the syringe. The cuff must stay inflated to show that it and the one-way valve work properly. Then reattach the syringe and deflate the cuff. Do not use a tube with a leaking cuff or leaking one-way valve. Make sure that the obturator, inner cannula, and plug all fit properly into the outer cannula. They all should easily snap into place and be easily removable. Check this before inserting the tube into the patient's tracheotomy.

Secretions, blood, or foreign matter can plug the lumen of the tube. Suction to remove any obstruction. It is also possible for the cuff to herniate and cover the end of the tube. If the catheter cannot be inserted beyond the tube and the patient is having respiratory distress, the tube will have to be removed. Replace the defective tracheostomy tube with another as soon as possible.

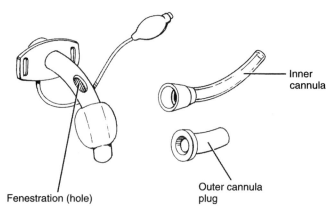

Figure 12-16 Fenestrated tracheostomy tube with its component parts and features. (From Eubanks DH, Bone RC: Comprehensive respiratory care, ed 2, St Louis, 1990, Mosby.)

4. Establish and manage the patient's airway (code: IIIA3f) [difficulty: R, Ap, An]

The practitioner should follow the appropriate infection control procedures when working with a patient's tracheotomy stoma and a tracheostomy tube. This can include wearing gloves, goggles, mask, and cover gown if indicated. See Chapter 2 if needed.

The first step in assessing tube placement is knowing that it was properly inserted. With the cuff deflated and the obturator inserted into the cannula, the tube should be gently slid through the stoma. The natural curvature of the tube should result in the distal tip being placed within the trachea and the flange being against the neck of the patient. If left out too far, the cuff may be seen at the stoma. An air leak may be heard or secretions may be seen to bubble out of the stoma. Correct the problem by deflating the cuff, inserting the tube so that the flange is against the base of the neck, and reinflating the cuff. Forcing should be avoided as this may indicate that the tip of the tube is entering the surrounding tissues. Also, the proper size tube will not need to be forced through the stoma. Inflate the cuff. All of the patient's breathing should pass through the tube. Auscultate for equal and bilateral breath sounds. No breath sounds should be heard over the patient's stomach area. An exhaled carbon dioxide monitor can also be attached to the proximal end of the tube to measure the concentration of carbon dioxide being exhaled by the patient.

After being assured that the tracheostomy tube is properly located, wrap the tie strings behind the patient's neck and tie them with a bowknot or fasten the Velcro straps. Securing the strings should help to prevent the tube from being misplaced or pulled out.

5. Review the chest radiograph to assess the position of the tracheostomy tube (code: IB7b) [difficulty: R, Ap, An]

The physician should have an upper-airway or chest radiograph taken to confirm that the distal tip of the tube is positioned midline within the trachea. It should not be twisted laterally because the tip can cause damage to the tracheal wall. All modern tracheostomy tubes (and endotracheal tubes) contain a strip of radiopaque material near the distal tip of the tube. This is easily noticed as the white line seen on the chest radiograph and confirms the location of the tip of the tube in the airway (see Fig. 12-24).

6. Measure the tracheal tube cuff pressure and/or volume (code: IC20) [difficulty: R, Ap]

See below.

7. Evaluate the tracheal tube cuff pressure and/or volume (code: ID19) [difficulty: R, Ap, An]

The cuff pressure should be measured on a regular basis to make sure that it is being kept at a safe level. In most patients, a safe cuff pressure is no more than 20-25 mm Hg (25-35 cm H_2O). (A more complete discussion of cuff pressure measurement follows in the discussion on endotracheal tubes.)

8. Change the tracheostomy tube (code: IIIA5) [difficulty: R, Ap, An]

A tracheostomy tube may have to be changed because of a ruptured cuff or because of another problem. In addition, patients with a permanent tracheostomy have the tube changed on a routine schedule as part of tracheostomy care. These two different situations are discussed separately.

a. Emergency tube change

Several factors can cause the clinical emergency of obstruction, such as the cuff herniating over the end of the tube, a mucous plug blocking the lumen, or the end of the tube being forced into the tracheal tissues. Unfortunately, these problems cannot be seen from the outside. If the patient experiences a sudden partial or complete airway obstruction, quickly deflate the cuff to rule it out as a cause of the obstruction. If the obstruction is still present, attempt to pass a suction catheter. If it can be passed though the tube, perform suctioning to remove any mucous plug. If the tube has an inner cannula and the catheter cannot be passed, remove the inner cannula. If it is plugged with mucus, remove the mucus and replace the inner cannula. If none of these procedures opens the patient's airway, it is likely that the distal tip of the tracheostomy tube is misplaced into the soft tissues. Withdraw the tube and let the patient breathe through the stoma. An apneic patient must be temporarily ventilated with mouth-to-stoma breaths. As rapidly and carefully as possible, insert another tracheostomy tube. Inflate the cuff and check that the patient can breathe normally.

However, if loose tracheal mucosa is blocking the airway, an endotracheal tube must be inserted past the tissue and deeper into the trachea. Call the physician as soon as possible to evaluate the patient's condition.

b. Routine tube change

If possible, the tube should not be changed until 7-14 days after a fresh tracheostomy procedure. This allows time for the stoma site to form granulomatous tissue as it begins to heal. The site is then less likely to bleed as the tube is changed. When the tracheostomy tube is changed, it is usually part of tracheostomy wound care. The following are typical steps in changing the tracheostomy tube:

1. Gather the necessary equipment: a new tracheostomy tube of the same size and the next size smaller, its inner cannula, its obturator, tracheostomy tie strings to secure the tube in the patient (see Fig. 12-15), a sterile tracheostomy dressing pad (4 × 4 in for an adult), sterile scissors, a 10-mL syringe to inflate the cuff, sterile water-soluble lubricant, sterile gloves, and mask and goggles. Make sure the cuff inflates and deflates properly.
2. Put on the gloves, mask, and goggles.
3. Maintaining sterile technique, make sure the obturator easily fits into and can be withdrawn from the tracheostomy tube.
4. Open the tracheostomy dressing pad (it has a slit in the center of the gauze pad).
5. Apply some lubricant to the tip of the tracheostomy tube.
6. Tell the patient what you are going to do.
7. Remove the oxygen and/or aerosol from the patient.
8. Suction the patient's trachea. Reoxygenate the patient.
9. Untie the tracheostomy strings or separate the Velcro straps.
10. Deflate the cuff.
11. Remove the current tracheostomy dressing pad.
12. Remove the tracheostomy tube by pulling it in a curved motion toward the patient's chest.
13. Inspect the tracheostomy opening for signs of infection such as redness, pus, or swelling.
14. Clean the stoma site with hydrogen peroxide or according to protocol. Report signs of infection to the nurse or physician.
15. Carefully insert the new tracheostomy tube with obturator into the stoma. The motion should be opposite that used to remove the original tube. Make sure not to force the tube into the tissues of the trachea.
16. Remove the obturator and insert the inner cannula. Lock it in place.
17. Give the patient oxygen and/or aerosol as before the tube change.
18. Inflate the cuff to a safe pressure.
19. Listen for bilateral breath sounds.
20. Slide the new tracheostomy dressing pad around the tube so that the slit fits around it.
21. Tie the tracheostomy tie strings or fasten the Velcro straps behind the patient's neck.

9. Perform tracheostomy care (code: IIIA4) [difficulty: R, Ap, An]

Routine tracheostomy care generally includes the steps previously described, except the removal of the tracheostomy tube. While performing tracheostomy care, inspect the stoma for possible signs of infection, clean the stoma site with hydrogen peroxide or according to protocol, apply a topical antibiotic, if indicated, and replace the 4 × 4-in tracheostomy dressing pad.

10. Extubate the patient

a. Recommend extubation (code: IIIE2g) [difficulty: R, Ap, An]

Tracheostomy extubation should be performed only after correction of the causes that led to insertion of the tracheostomy tube. (Endotracheal tube extubation is discussed below.) If the patient has required mechanical ventilation, review the discussion in Chapter 15 that relates to weaning the patient and extubation.

b. Perform extubation (code: IIIA8) [difficulty: R, Ap, An]

Tracheostomy extubation should be performed only by trained personnel and under the proper conditions to ensure the patient's safety. See Box 12-3 for a list of complications that can occur after extubation. The generally recommended steps in extubation include the following:

1. Evaluate the patient's cardiopulmonary status. The reason(s) for the tube being placed should be corrected. The most recent blood gas results should be acceptable. Tracheal secretions should be minimal and not so thick that they cannot be expectorated by the patient. Bedside spirometry results should show an acceptable tidal volume, vital capacity, and maximal inspiratory pressure.
2. Inform the patient about the removal of the tube and the follow-up care that is needed.

BOX 12-3   Complications after Extubation

Tracheostomy Tube Removal
Difficult tube removal from a tight stoma
Granuloma or scar at the stoma
Unhealed, open stoma
Hypoxemia and/or hypercapnia secondary to hypoventilation

Endotracheal Tube Removal
Reflex laryngospasm
Bronchospasm
Regurgitation and aspiration of stomach contents
Aspiration of oral secretions
Sore throat
Dysphagia
Postintubation laryngeal edema (croup)
Hoarseness from vocal cord edema or paralysis
Hypoxemia and/or hypercapnia secondary to hypoventilation

Cuff-Related Complications
Granuloma
Tracheomalacia
Tracheal stenosis
Tracheal web formation
Tracheoesophageal fistula
Tracheoinnominate artery fistula

3. The patient's inspired oxygen percentage may be kept the same or increased before the extubation. If increased, it should be done at least 5-10 minutes before the tube is removed.
4. Suction the trachea until all secretions are removed.
5. Suction the oral pharynx to remove all saliva. Be prepared to suction additional oral secretions and mucus after extubation.
6. In rapid succession:
   a. Give a deep sigh breath.
   b. Deflate the cuff. Cut the inflation tube to the cuff to ensure its collapse.
   c. Pull out the tube when the lungs are full.

Alternatively, in rapid succession:
   a. Give a deep sigh breath.
   b. Place a suction catheter through the tube into the trachea. This works best with a self-contained catheter and sheath system.
   c. Deflate the cuff. Cut the inflation tube to the cuff to ensure its collapse.
   d. Pull out the tube when the lungs are full.
   e. Apply suction as the tube is withdrawn.
7. Have the patient cough vigorously to remove any secretions.
8. Depending on the physician's order, do one of the following:
   • Apply a bland aerosol by tracheostomy mask to the stoma site with the previous amount of oxygen.
   • Cover the stoma site with a sterile 4 × 4-in dressing. Tape it in place. Apply a bland aerosol by face mask with the previous amount of oxygen.
9. Monitor and evaluate the patient every 30 minutes for several hours. Encourage deep breathing and coughing. Check the vital signs and breath sounds. Be prepared to reintubate the patient if necessary. Measure pulse oximetry continuously or arterial blood gases after 10-20 minutes.

After extubation, the following are usually done every shift to ensure healing of the stoma:
1. Remove the dressing. Inspect the stoma for signs of infection such as pus, redness, and swelling.
2. Clean the stoma site with hydrogen peroxide on a sterile gauze pad.
3. Apply antibiotic ointment to the stoma site, if indicated.
4. Reapply a sterile dressing.

MODULE G

Tracheostomy buttons

1. Recommend the insertion or change of an artificial airway (code: IIIE2e) [difficulty: R, Ap, An]

A tracheostomy button is a hard plastic tube that is placed into the patient's stoma to keep it open after the tracheostomy tube has been removed (Fig. 12-17). A button is inserted because the physician has determined that the stoma must be kept open in case the tracheostomy tube must be reinserted. Advantages of the button include the patient being able to eat, talk, and cough normally. Yet, in case the patient has difficulty or needs a breathing treatment, a secure airway can be quickly reestablished.

2. Tracheostomy button equipment
a. Assemble the necessary equipment (code: IIA10) [difficulty: R, Ap]

In general, the patient sizes for tracheostomy buttons match the sizes for tracheostomy tubes listed in Table 12-1. Refer to Figure 12-17 when reviewing these features of the tracheostomy button and accessories:

• The hollow outer cannula has a slightly flared proximal end. This keeps the button from slipping entirely into the patient. The distal end is flanged and split into several flexible "grippers."
• A closure plug fits into the outer cannula and snaps into the flexible grippers on the end of the outer cannula. This seals the button so that the patient breathes through the upper airway.
• A hollow inner cannula can be inserted into the outer cannula instead of the plug. This inner cannula has a standard 15-mm OD so that a T-piece/Briggs adapter or other respiratory care equipment can be attached if needed. The patient's secretions can also be suctioned.
• Spacers of various lengths are used to make sure that the inner cannula is placed at the right depth. The end of the tube should enter the trachea but not

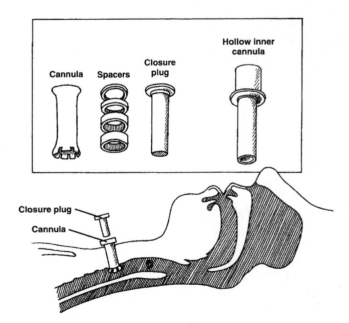

Figure 12-17 Typical tracheostomy button properly positioned in patient. The inset shows its component parts.

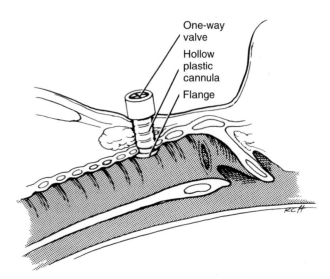

Figure 12-18 Kistner tracheostomy button. The addition of a one-way valve causes the patient to breathe in through the button and exhale through the upper airway. (From Eubanks DH, Bone RC: Comprehensive respiratory care, ed 2, St Louis, 1990, Mosby.)

obstruct it. See the airway picture in Figure 12-17 for the proper position.

A one-way valve may be added to the button. This would be used for patients who must not inspire through their upper airway but may exhale through it. In patients with a very small tidal volume, inhaling through one of these valves reduces the patient's upper-airway anatomic dead space. Because expiration is through the upper airway, the patient can speak normally. Refer to Figure 12-18 when reviewing these features of the Kistner tracheostomy button with an attached one-way valve:

- The hollow plastic cannula keeps the stoma open. The distal end is flanged so that it is not likely to be pulled out of the trachea accidentally.
- The proximal end of the cannula is capped with a one-way valve. The valve allows the patient to inhale room air or an oxygen- and aerosol-enriched gas source. Expiration is through the upper airway. The patient can talk, eat, and cough normally.

The newer Passy-Muir and Mallinckrodt speaking valves (presented below) function the same way.

b. Troubleshoot any problems with the equipment (code: IIA10) [difficulty: R, Ap]

Make sure that all component pieces of these tracheostomy buttons fit together properly and can be easily disconnected if necessary. The cannula must be kept clear of any secretions, blood, or foreign debris. A suction catheter should be passable through the hollow opening in the cannula. If the button is obstructed and the patient is having trouble breathing through the upper airway, the button should be removed and replaced with another button or a tracheostomy tube.

3. Establish and manage the patient's airway (code: IIIA3f) [difficulty: R, Ap, An]

After the physician removes the tracheostomy tube, the depth of the stoma is measured. Based on that depth, spacers are added to the cannula to obtain the appropriate depth. Once the button is placed, the patient should not have any added resistance to breathing. If the button becomes misplaced and the patient has difficulty breathing, the button should be removed. A tracheostomy tube can then be inserted.

MODULE H

Speaking tubes and valves

1. Recommend the insertion or change of an artificial airway (code: IIIE2e) [difficulty: R, Ap, An]

A speaking tracheostomy tube is indicated in a patient who requires full breathing support on a mechanical ventilator but is conscious and wishes to speak. In some instances a speaking valve can be added to a standard tracheostomy tube in a mechanically ventilated patient. In this situation, the cuff must be deflated for the exhaled tidal volume gas to pass through the vocal cords for speaking. These patients should be able to do some spontaneous breathing and safely tolerate the variable ventilator tidal volume resulting from the leak around the deflated cuff. Remember to reset the ventilator's exhaled low tidal volume alarm because no exhaled gas will return through the ventilator circuit. This loss of a critical alarm system means that other alarms such as tachycardia, bradycardia, and low pulse oximeter value are even more important for patient safety.

Usually, a speaking valve is added to a tracheostomy button in a patient who is not ventilator-dependent. This patient cannot or should not be inhaling through the nose or mouth but can exhale through the natural upper airway. Commonly, these are patients with a neuromuscular disease or high cervical spine injury. Their condition causes them to have a small tidal volume, which results in a large percentage of dead space ventilation. Placing a tracheostomy tube or button into these patients improves their dead space to tidal volume ratio and improves their blood gas values.

2. Speaking tube or speaking valve equipment

a. Assemble the necessary equipment (code: IIA10) [difficulty: R, Ap]

Table 12-1 lists the standard sizes of tracheostomy tubes. A speaking tracheostomy tube should match the same size as the current tracheostomy tube or button. At the time of writing, speaking tracheostomy tubes are available only in older child and adult sizes. See Figure 12-19 for the features of the Pitt speaking tracheostomy tube. (The Vocalaid tube is similar in function.) In addition to

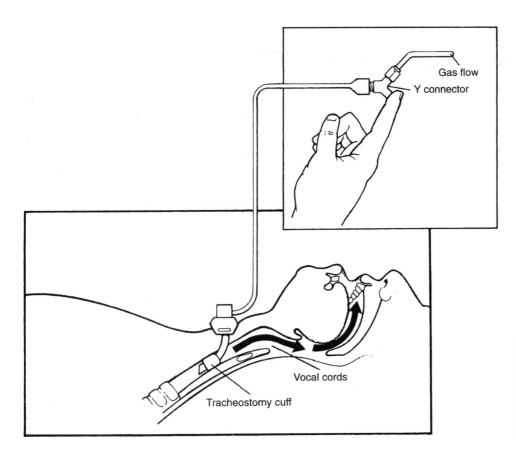

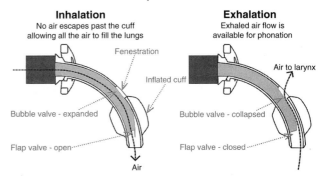

Figure 12-19 Pitt tracheostomy tube permits the patient to speak. Note its special feature that directs outside gas flow past the vocal cords. (From Wilkins RL, Stoller JK, Kacmarek, RM: Egan's fundamentals of respiratory care, ed 9, St Louis, 2009, Mosby.)

the standard breathing cannula, there is a small-diameter tube that carries compressed gas through a hole in the posterior curve of the cannula. A Y-connector is added to the compressed gas tube. Usually about 4-6 L/min of compressed air or oxygen is set on a flowmeter to run to the Y. Closing off the other opening in the Y with a finger diverts the gas into the patient's larynx for speaking. A little experimentation will help the patient find the flow that works best. The patient's voice may not be as strong as normal but should be understandable. If the patient cannot speak at all, check that the gas is turned on and that the tubing is properly connected. With the Pitt speaking tube, all of the patient's exhaled tidal volume is returned to the ventilator. So, all alarm systems are fully functional.

The Blom tracheostomy tube and Blom speech cannula are a newer system that enables the ventilator-dependent patient to speak (Fig. 12-20). The Blom tracheostomy tube functions as a standard fenestrated tube with an inner cannula (as shown in Fig. 12-16). However, when the standard inner cannula is replaced with the Blom speech cannula, the mechanically ventilated patient is able to speak. The speech cannula has a unique design that separates the directional flow of the inspiratory and expiratory gases. During inspiration, the fenestration is closed and the patient receives the full tidal volume. During expiration, the main cannula is closed and the tidal volume is directed out through the fenestration. The patient can now speak with the full exhaled tidal volume.

Figure 12-20 The Blom tracheostomy tube and Blom speech cannula function like a fenestrated tracheostomy tube. When set up properly, this system lets the mechanically ventilated patient speak. See the text for the complete discussion. (Courtesy of Pulmodyne, Indianapolis, IN.)

When the Blom speech cannula is used, several ventilator adjustments must be made. First, a heated humidifier must be used instead of an HME to humidify the tidal volume gas. This is because no exhaled air passes through the HME to humidify it before the next inhalation. Second, the ventilator's low tidal volume/low minute volume alarms must be set to their minimum level to avoid a nuisance alarm situation. Third, the Blom exhaled volume reservoir (EVR) needs to be added into the ventilator circuit. The purpose of the EVR is to provide a small volume of gas to the ventilator's volume or flow sensors to in effect "trick" them into not alarming. During inspiration some tidal volume gas inflates the EVR bellows. During expiration the bellows empties into the ventilator's sensors. Insert the EVR between the end of the expiratory circuit and the exhalation inlet port if the ventilator measures tidal volume at the ventilator. Insert the EVR between the flow sensor and the patient if the ventilator measures tidal volume through a proximal flow sensor. It will not be possible to use the Blom speech cannula if the EVR cannot be incorporated into the patient circuit or the volume alarms cannot be adjusted to avoid constant nuisance alarming. Last, the EVR must be removed when the Blom speech cannula is not being used. All alarm systems should then be readjusted to their normal settings. An HME can also be used now.

The improved oral communication provided by a speaking tube is a great help to the patient's psychological well-being. Because the cuff remains inflated, the patient can still be mechanically ventilated. The tracheostomy tube provides the added benefit of a route for suctioning secretions. The patient can continue to eat and drink as usual.

There are several versions of speaking valves including the Passy-Muir (Fig. 12-21), Blom low-profile valve, and Mallinckrodt Phonate. All speaking valves are available in a standard size to fit onto a 15-mm-OD tracheostomy tube or tracheostomy button. (See Fig. 12-18 for how the speaking valve is positioned on a tracheostomy button or tube.) If a speaking valve is added to a standard tracheostomy tube, the *cuff must be deflated*. If the cuff is left inflated, the patient will *not be able to exhale*. If a speaking valve is added to a fenestrated tracheostomy tube, the cuff may be left inflated but the *inner cannula must be removed* (see Fig. 12-16). If the cuff is left inflated and the inner cannula is left in place, the patient will *not be able to exhale*. This is a *life-threatening* situation.

All speaking valves feature a one-way valve that opens when the patient inspires to allow room air or supplemental oxygen to be inhaled. Mechanical ventilation may also

be provided. When the patient exhales, the valve closes. This causes exhaled tidal volume gas to pass through the vocal cords for speech. Aerosol therapy may be provided either by a tracheostomy mask over the valve or by a T-piece attached to it. The speaking valve may be removed when a medication is nebulized to keep it from becoming fouled with the medication. (See Chapter 6 for a discussion of these aerosol/oxygen delivery systems.) If the patient is breathing spontaneously and needs low-flow supplemental oxygen, use the valve that includes a small-bore oxygen tubing nipple (see Fig. 12-21).

As an alternative, the Olympic Trach-Talk combines an elbow adapter to the tracheostomy tube and a T-piece with a one-way valve (Fig. 12-22). This device provides the patient with aerosol and/or oxygen with humidity through the one-way valve during inspiration. On exhalation, the valve closes and the patient exhales through the vocal cords for speech.

Be aware that for a speaking valve to work with a ventilator-dependent patient, the cuff must be deflated. This will result in some loss of delivered tidal volume. Make sure that the patient can tolerate this. Also adjust the ventilator's alarm settings accordingly.

b. Troubleshoot any problems with the equipment (code: IIA10) [difficulty: R, Ap]

For a speaking tracheostomy tube, see the preceding discussion on care of standard or fenestrated tracheostomy tubes. The same problems can occur with speaking tracheostomy tubes. Assess the patient's ability to speak in an

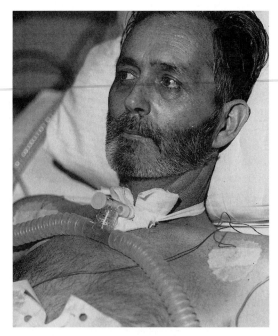

Figure 12-22 A patient with a tracheostomy tube and attached Olympic Trach-Talk speaking device. It features a one-way valve so that the patient breathes in through the valve and exhales through the upper airway for speech. (From Cairo JM, Pilbeam SP: Mosby's respiratory care equipment, ed 8, St Louis, 2010, Mosby.)

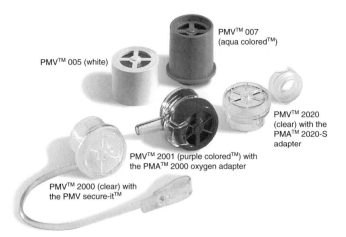

Figure 12-21 Photograph of a variety of speaking valves made by Passy-Muir. When the one-way valve is attached to a tracheostomy tube or tracheostomy button, the patient breathes in through the valve and exhales through the upper airway for speech. (Courtesy of Passy-Muir, Inc., Irvine, CA.)

understandable way. Enough gas must pass through the vocal cords for this to happen.

With a speaking valve, make sure that the one-way valve opens and closes properly. If a spontaneously breathing patient's valve was to become plugged with secretions, the patient would have to inhale through the natural upper airway rather than the valve. Depending on the type of tracheostomy tube, the cuff must be deflated and/or the inner cannula removed for the patient to be able to exhale.

3. Establish and manage the patient's airway (code: IIIA3h) [difficulty: R, Ap, An]

The assessment of the placement of a speaking tracheostomy tube would be the same as discussed previously with standard tracheostomy tubes.

MODULE I

Laryngectomy tubes

1. Recommend the insertion or change of an artificial airway (code: IIIE2e) [difficulty: R, Ap, An]

A laryngectomy tube is inserted into the patient who has had his or her larynx surgically removed (laryngectomy) because of cancer. As part of the surgical procedure, the patient will have a permanent tracheostomy opening and the upper airway will be surgically sealed off. Because air will no longer pass through the nose or mouth, the patient will no longer be able to speak, have a sense of smell, or be able to blow his or her nose. Often, a tracheostomy tube is placed into the surgical opening immediately after the operation. A laryngectomy tube is inserted into the stoma when appropriate.

Eventually, some patients will no longer need a laryngectomy tube. They will simply breathe though the stoma. If the patient should need any future respiratory therapy procedures, they must be provided through the stoma or an added laryngectomy or tracheostomy tube because the upper airway is permanently closed.

2. Laryngectomy tube equipment

a. Assemble the necessary equipment (code: IIA10) [difficulty: R, Ap]

There are two main types of laryngectomy tube (Fig. 12-23). The original laryngectomy tube is inserted after the surgical procedure and prevents any stenosis (narrowing) of the tracheostomy stoma. To help with esophageal phonation, some patients will have a voice prosthesis surgically placed between the trachea and the esophagus. These patients need the fenestrated laryngectomy tube so that exhaled air can pass through the voice prosthesis. Both types of tube come in a variety of sizes to fit the patient's anatomy. Neck straps with Velcro ends can be placed through two holes in the flange of the tube to hold it in place. Many patients will cover the tube opening with a sterile gauze for cleanliness and to provide some humidification. However, if the patient needs more humidified air, a small HME can be placed into the flange. A scarf or other clothing item can be placed over everything for cosmetic purposes. A downward-angled adapter should be inserted into the flange when the patient is showering to prevent any water from being aspirated.

b. Troubleshoot any problems with the equipment (code: IIA10) [difficulty: R, Ap]

There should be few problems with a laryngectomy tube because all types are a single channel without a cuff. As

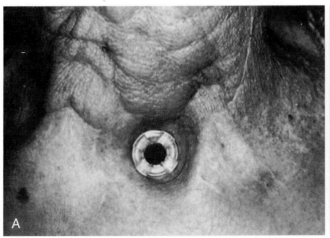 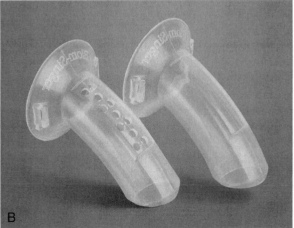

Figure 12-23 A laryngectomy tube is used to keep an open stoma and channel for breathing after a patient has had a surgical laryngectomy. **A,** Close-up photo of a patient's throat area. The flange of the laryngectomy tube and its open channel can be seen. **B,** Photo showing the posterior curve of two Blom-Singer laryngectomy tubes. The tube on the left is fenestrated with openings to allow air to pass through a voice prosthesis for esophageal phonation. The tube on the right is the standard original tube that does not have any fenestrations. (A from Black J, Hawks J: Medical-surgical nursing, ed 7, St Louis, 2005, Mosby; B image Courtesy of InHealth Technologies, Carpinteria, CA.)

with any other type of tracheostomy tube, the laryngectomy tube must be kept clear of secretions.

3. Establish and manage the patient's airway (code: IIIA3g) [difficulty: R, Ap, An]

The home-bound patient must be trained to remove the tube, inspect the stoma for any sign of infection, clean the tube, and place it back into the stoma opening.

MODULE J

Endotracheal tubes and intubation equipment

1. Recommend the insertion or change of an artificial airway (code: IIIE2e) [difficulty: R, Ap, An]

An endotracheal tube is indicated when a secure, patent airway is required for endotracheal suctioning or mechanical ventilation. Aspiration is also prevented when the cuff is inflated. It is generally accepted that an endotracheal tube provides for a more secure airway than an LMA or Combitube. In most emergency situations an oral endotracheal tube is indicated over a nasal endotracheal tube because the oral route is faster and easier. A nasal endotracheal tube is indicated when the patient has oral trauma or when a cervical spine injury prevents the neck from being hyperextended for placing the oral tube.

2. Endotracheal tube equipment

a. Assemble the necessary equipment (code: IIA10) [difficulty: R, Ap]

An endotracheal tube is the best emergency device for maintaining a secure airway. It also provides a direct suctioning route to the lungs and prevents aspiration. Mechanical ventilation can easily be provided through it. See Table 12-1 for a list of endotracheal tube sizes (this also applies to tracheostomy tubes and buttons) based upon the patient's age. It is common practice to refer to the needed tube size by its ID. For example, an endotracheal tube for an adult male would be 8.0- or 8.5-mm ID.

An endotracheal tube is meant to be a temporary airway; however, it can stay in a patient for weeks if necessary. Virtually all endotracheal tubes used clinically now are made of pliable plastic. Always select a tube that has a large residual volume and low-pressure cuff unless there is a specific contraindication. For the most part, oral and nasal endotracheal tubes can be used interchangeably. The nasal endotracheal tube is longer and more curved than an oral endotracheal tube. The greater curve of the nasal tube should result in less pressure on the nasal mucosa. An anesthesiologist requests a nasal tube if he or she is going to place it by the nasal route. Oral tubes are used in the majority of patients.

The tubes are available in sizes from 4-mm OD through 14-mm OD so that patients of all ages and sizes can be intubated. The OD size increments are 0.5 mm. The thickness of the outer wall of the tube varies from 0.5 to 1 mm, which results in a reduction of the ID of the tube by about 1-2 mm. Table 12-1 lists the approximate ID of an endotracheal tube to place into a patient based on age. As stated above, it is common practice to refer to the size of endotracheal tube (or tracheostomy tube) needed by its ID. Once the tube has been confirmed as properly placed into the patient, the excess tube, beyond 3-4 cm past the teeth, should be removed. This reduces the airway resistance and mechanical dead space.

Most endotracheal tubes have the standard features shown in Figure 12-24. There are a number of specialty endotracheal tubes that can be found in limited use. They all share the same characteristics except for some special feature. These tubes are worth considering if available.

1. Pediatric endotracheal tubes

Pediatric endotracheal tubes are available in two basic types. One type has a constant diameter. During intubation, the tube should be inserted until the black mark about 2 cm from the tip is at the vocal cords. The second type has a body with a relatively wide proximal part that narrows at the distal end. The design is supposed to allow the smaller diameter tip to be passed through the vocal cords but prevent the wide "shoulder" from passing into the trachea. The distal ends of both types of tube have a single opening with a bevel cut (Fig. 12-25). It is recommended that children less than 8 years of age have a tube without a cuff.

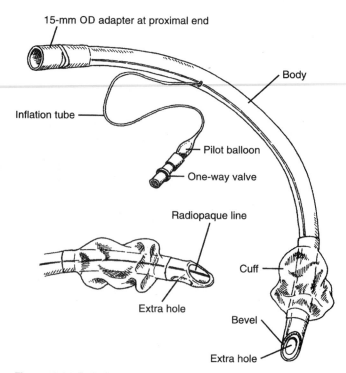

Figure 12-24 Typical, modern endotracheal tube with its component parts. The inset shows important features found at the distal end of the tube.

2. Wire-reinforced tubes

Wire-reinforced (also called armored) tubes have a steel spring coiled through them (Fig. 12-26). An advantage of these tubes over regular tubes is that they are more resistant to collapse if the patient bites on them. Furthermore, the tube may be bent for shape and does not kink if the patient's head is turned at an angle that might kink an ordinary tube.

3. Preformed tubes

Preformed tubes have been preshaped for surgical procedures on the head and neck. One style has a forward bend so that the tube can be taped to the chin (Fig. 12-27). This shape keeps the tube and anesthesia circuit away from the patient's nose, eyes, and top of the head. There are also tubes with a backward bend so that they can be taped to the forehead (Fig. 12-28). This shape keeps the tube and anesthesia circuit away from the patient's throat area.

4. Guidable (trigger) tubes

Guidable tubes have a string embedded within the wall of the tube (Fig. 12-29). When the ring at the proximal end is pulled, the distal tip is flexed up to shorten the radius of the curve. This allows the tube to be directed into the anterior trachea. Guidable trigger tubes make it easier to

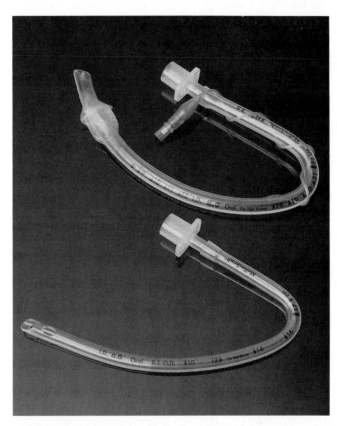

Figure 12-27 Photograph of cuffed and uncuffed SAE endotracheal tubes with an anterior bend to allow access to the upper part of the patient's face and head. (From Cairo JM, Pilbeam SP: Mosby's respiratory care equipment, ed 8, St Louis, 2010, Mosby.)

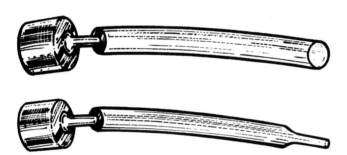

Figure 12-25 Comparison of the two different types of pediatric endotracheal tubes. The top type of tube is made by several manufacturers and has a uniform diameter. The bottom tube is made by Cole and features a narrowing of the distal tip to pass through the vocal cords. Note that neither has a cuff. (From Burgess WR, Chernick V: Respiratory therapy in newborn infants and children, ed 2, New York, 1986, Thieme.)

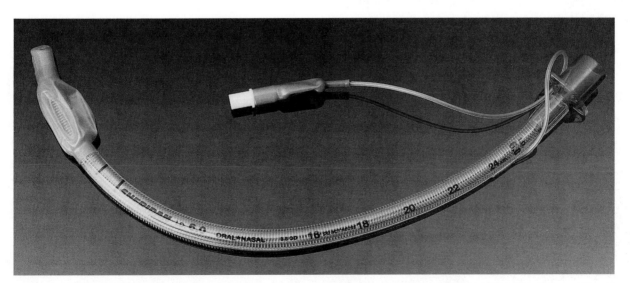

Figure 12-26 Photograph of a spiral wire-reinforced (also called an armored) endotracheal tube. (Courtesy Covidien, Mansfield, Massachusetts.)

intubate a patient with an anterior larynx or to perform a blind nasal intubation.

5. Double-lumen endotracheal tubes

Double-lumen endotracheal tubes are used to allow independent lung ventilation. A double-lumen tube is also used during special procedures performed on one lung such as bronchoscopy, bronchoalveolar lavage, lobectomy, and pneumonectomy. The other lung may be mechanically ventilated to maintain the patient's blood gas values

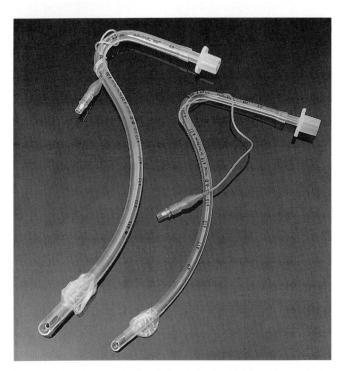

Figure 12-28 Photograph of cuffed endotracheal tubes with a posterior bend to allow access to the patient's neck area. (From Cairo JM, Pilbeam SP: Mosby's respiratory care equipment, ed 8, St Louis, 2010, Mosby.)

(Fig. 12-30). An adapter can be added to join the two proximal ends of the channels so that a single ventilator can be used to ventilate both lungs. The Carlens tube is used to preferentially intubate the left bronchus. The White tube is used to preferentially intubate the right bronchus (Fig. 12-31 shows both). Robertshaw makes tubes for either right or left bronchial intubation.

Several limitations are inherent in all double-lumen tubes. First, they can be used only on adults because the smallest size is 8-mm OD. Second, the small internal diameter of the two lumens results in a high airway resistance. Third, a much smaller than normal suction catheter must be used to remove any tracheal secretions.

6. Tubes for high-frequency jet ventilation

These special-purpose tubes have a main lumen for a standard ventilator and an additional lumen to which a jet ventilator is attached. See Chapter 15 for more discussion and a photograph.

7. Oropharyngeal suctioning tubes

In response to the concern about oropharyngeal secretions leaking around the endotracheal tube cuff and causing ventilator-associated pneumonia (VAP), an endotracheal tube with a built-in suctioning catheter has been invented (Fig. 12-32). The catheter runs down the outer curve of the tube to just above the cuff. When vacuum is applied to the catheter, any secretions that have accumulated above the cuff are suctioned out of the area. It functions like a standard, cuffed endotracheal tube in all other aspects.

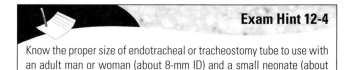

Exam Hint 12-4

Know the proper size of endotracheal or tracheostomy tube to use with an adult man or woman (about 8-mm ID) and a small neonate (about 3-mm ID).

Figure 12-29 Photograph of an Endotrol guidable (trigger) endotracheal tube. A wire is embedded within the wall of the tube. When the ring at the proximal end is pulled, the distal tip is flexed up to shorten the radius of the curve. This allows the tube to be directed into the anterior trachea. (From Cairo JM: Mosby's respiratory care equipment, ed 9, St Louis, 2014, Mosby.)

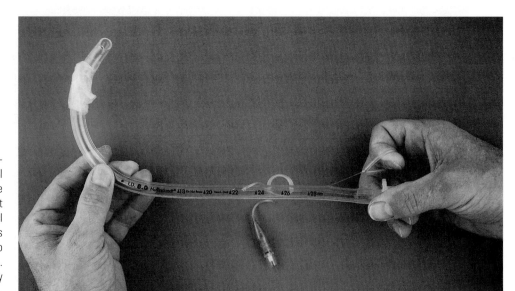

Refer to Figure 12-24 for these components of a standard endotracheal tube:

- The hollow curved body is the main part of the tube through which the patient can breathe, or a suction catheter can be placed. The OD and ID sizes are printed on the side of the tube. Make sure that the central channel is not plugged by dried secretions, blood, or foreign debris.
- The proximal end is left outside of the patient's nose or mouth. An adapter with a 15-mm-OD equipment connector is inserted into the tube. The other end of the adapter narrows and is individually sized to fit snugly into the ID of the endotracheal tube. The adapters cannot be cross-fitted to different sizes of endotracheal tubes.
- The distal end is inserted into the patient's trachea. The tip is cut with either a right- or left-sided bevel. The bevel cut creates an oval-shaped opening that is less likely to become plugged with secretions than is a round opening. An extra hole (the Murphy eye) is cut in the tube on the opposite side of the bevel.
- A line of radiopaque material is embedded in the tube from the tip back to the cuff. It is seen as a white line on the chest radiograph, showing the location of the tube's tip in the trachea (see the inset in Fig. 12-24).
- A cuff (balloon) is located a few centimeters from the tip of the tube. It is inflated with air to seal the trachea so that mechanical ventilation can be performed and aspiration is prevented. Most modern tubes have a large-residual-volume, low-pressure cuff.

- *Note:* Most tubes that are 4.0-mm ID/6.0-mm OD or larger have cuffs. However, there are cuffless tubes larger than this for pediatric patients. Pediatric and neonatal tubes smaller than 4.0-mm ID/6.0-mm OD will not have a cuff.
- A cuff-filling inflation tube is connected about halfway down the tube. The proximal end is left out of the patient's mouth, and the distal end goes to the cuff so that it can be inflated and deflated. A pilot balloon that inflates and deflates with the cuff is found in the middle of the capillary tube or connected with the one-way valve at the distal end. The one-way valve has an end that connects to any syringe. When the syringe is

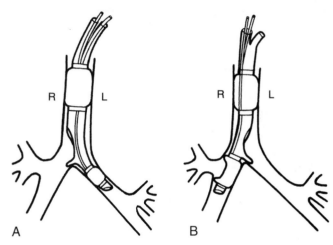

Figure 12-31 Two types of double-lumen endotracheal tubes. **A,** Carlens tube: Its distal end enters the left mainstem bronchus. **B,** White tube: Its distal end enters the right mainstem bronchus. Note how both tubes have a cuff that seals the trachea and a cuff that seals a bronchus. Each has its own inflation tube, pilot balloon, and one-way valve. (From Miller RD, editor: Anesthesia, New York, 1981, Churchill Livingstone.)

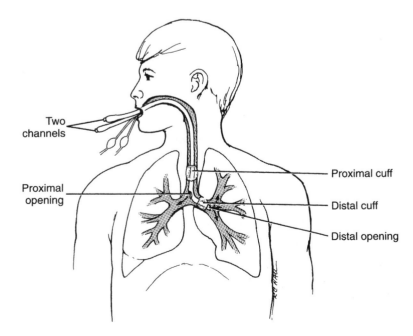

Figure 12-30 Double-lumen endotracheal tube properly positioned in patient so that both lungs can be independently ventilated or suctioned or to have special procedures performed. (From Eubanks DH, Bone RC: Comprehensive respiratory care, ed 2, St Louis, 1990, Mosby.)

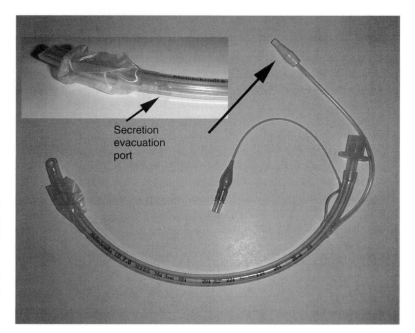

Figure 12-32 Photographs of a Hi–Low Evac endotracheal tube that has an added channel to suction oral secretions from the subglottic area. The removal of these secretions should help to reduce the possibility of the patient developing ventilator-associated pneumonia. The small arrow points to the secretion removal channel above the cuff. The large arrow points to the catheter at the other end of the channel. It is connected to the continuous vacuum system. (From Cairo JM: Mosby's respiratory care equipment, ed 9, St Louis, 2014, Mosby.)

disconnected, the one-way valve seals to prevent the air in the cuff from escaping.

- With a double-lumen endotracheal tube, each lumen has its own 15-mm adapter, cuff, one-way valve, pilot balloon, and inflation tube to inflate the cuff. As with traditional endotracheal tubes, both cuffs should be test-inflated. They should hold the air without a leak and then be easily deflated. One additional piece of equipment, a plastic wye (Y), can be used with a double-lumen tube. The plastic Y can be used to connect the proximal ends of both tubes. Both 15-mm adapters are removed and one branch of the Y is inserted into each of the proximal ends of the tubes. The open end of the Y has a 15-mm adapter so that it can be connected to a ventilator or oxygen source.

b. Troubleshoot any problems with the equipment (code: IIA10) [difficulty: R, Ap]

The cuff(s) should be inflated and the syringe should be disconnected from the one-way valve before the tube is placed in the patient. This ensures that the system works properly. The cuff(s) should hold the air. Do not use any tube with a leaking cuff or leaking one-way valve. Deflate the cuff before placing the tube into the patient.

3. Intubation equipment: laryngoscope and blades

a. Assemble the necessary equipment (code: IIA9) [difficulty: R, Ap]

A laryngoscope and blade are used for traditional line-of-sight endotracheal intubation. The laryngoscope is made up of two basic parts: a handle and a blade. The most commonly seen handle is made of stainless steel; some newer units are made of plastic. The handle contains two C-cell batteries to power the light source in the blade. They all

have a common base with a hooking bar so that the blades can be attached (Figs. 12-33 and 12-34).

Blades are available in a variety of sizes from pediatric to adult. They all have a common hook so that they can be snapped and locked in place on the handle. The stainless-steel handles use stainless-steel blades. The newer plastic handles use plastic blades. The two different sets of handles and blades are not interchangeable. The blades are available in two different shapes. The Miller blades are straight and the MacIntosh blades are curved (see Fig. 12-33). The person performing the intubation may specify a particular style of blade as well as blade size. See Figure 12-34 for the steps in fastening any blade to the handle:

1. Hold the handle in the left hand and the blade in the right hand.
2. Place the hook on the blade over the hooking bar on the base of the handle.
3. Pull the blade down so that it snaps into place on the handle. The handle and blade should fit together at a 90-degree angle.
4. Make sure that the light bulb in the stainless-steel blade is tight.

b. Troubleshoot any problems with the equipment (code: IIA9) [difficulty: R, Ap]

The light source shines when the handle and blade are properly connected because an electrical circuit has been completed. Failure of the light source to shine may result from any of the following problems:

- The handle and blade are not properly connected and snapped into place. Disconnect them by performing the opposite motions and reconnect them properly.
- There are cross-connected stainless-steel and plastic components. Stainless-steel handles go only with

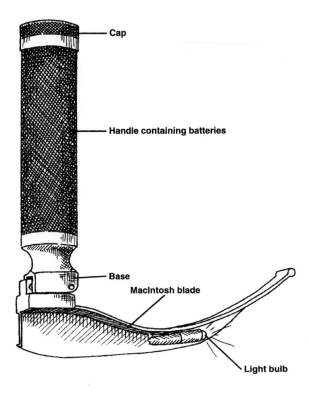

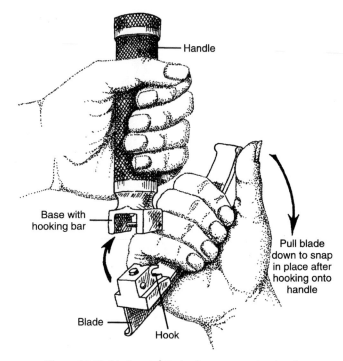

Figure 12-34 Motions to attach a laryngoscope to a handle.

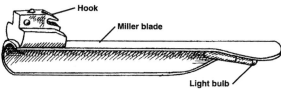

Figure 12-33 Laryngoscope handle with a MacIntosh (curved) blade attached. A Miller (straight) blade is shown below for comparison. Note component parts and features.

stainless-steel blades, and plastic handles go with plastic blades.

- The batteries are low, as shown by the bulb failing to glow or glowing with a yellow instead of a white light. Unscrew the cap from the handle. Replace the old batteries with two new C-cell batteries. When reassembled, the bulb should glow with a white light.
- The batteries are not placed properly. It does not matter if a positive or negative pole touches the base of the handle. Be sure that a positive pole touches a negative pole or vice versa so that electrical current will flow properly. When reassembled, the bulb should glow with a white light.
- The light bulb in the stainless-steel blade is loose or defective. Tighten the light bulb by turning it clockwise. It should glow if it was just loose. Unscrew and throw away a defective light bulb. Replace it with a light bulb of the same size. When reassembled, the bulb should glow with a white light. The newer plastic laryngoscopes use a fiberoptic bundle as the light source. There is no light bulb to tighten or replace.

BOX 12-4   Equipment for Oral and Nasal Intubation

Pediatric and adult laryngoscope handles with batteries
Straight and curved pediatric and adult laryngoscope blades
Variety of nasal and oral endotracheal tubes
Water-soluble, sterile lubricant
Metal stylet
Magill forceps for nasal intubation
Hemostat
Tongue depressors
Oropharyngeal airways
Bite block
Nasopharyngeal airways
10-mL syringe with three-way stopcock
Manometer to measure intracuff pressure
Tape or tube-restraining device
Yankauer or other oral suction device
Sterile suction catheter for tracheal suctioning
Stethoscope for listening to breath sounds

In addition to the laryngoscope handle and blades, there are a number of additional items that are typically needed to ensure a smooth, safe intubation procedure. These are listed in Box 12-4.

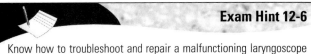

Exam Hint 12-6

Know how to troubleshoot and repair a malfunctioning laryngoscope and blade.

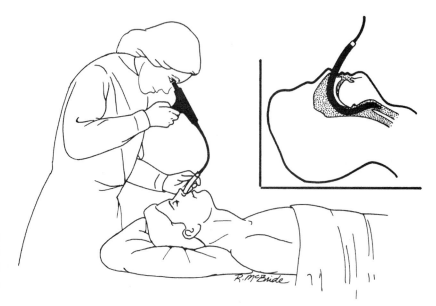

Figure 12-35 A fiberoptic laryngoscope that is being used to insert an endotracheal tube through the nasal passage. (From Kacmarek RM, Stoller JK, Heuer AJ: Egan's fundamentals of respiratory care, ed 10, St Louis, 2013, Mosby.)

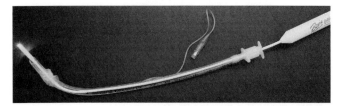

Figure 12-36 Photograph of a light wand inserted through the lumen of an endotracheal tube. The light wand's light will shine through the laryngeal structures to show that the tip of the tube has entered the patient's trachea. (From Cairo JM: Mosby's respiratory care equipment, ed 9, St Louis, 2014, Mosby.)

4. Intubation equipment: fiberoptic devices

a. Assemble the necessary equipment (code: IIA9) [difficulty: R, Ap]

Indirect or video laryngoscopy is used when the physician expects a difficult intubation where line-of-sight intubation will not be possible. A physician may use a short fiberoptic laryngoscope (Fig. 12-35) or traditional fiberoptic bronchoscope (see Fig. 18-3 in Chapter 18) to visualize the larynx and trachea during a difficult intubation. Either can be used during a nasal or oral endotracheal intubation procedure.

A fiberoptic lighted stylet or light wand (Fig. 12-36) can be placed through the lumen of the endotracheal tube so that the lighted distal tip is at the end of the tube. When the room is darkened and the tube enters the trachea, a bright light will shine through the tissues over the throat.

A closed-circuit video system could be used to replace direct visualization of the larynx. These devices employ a laryngoscope handle and blade with a tiny lens at the tip of the blade (Fig. 12-37). A fiberoptic bundle carries the image of the patient's larynx from the blade tip to a monitor in the handle for viewing. Other video systems utilize a monitor that is separated from the intubation

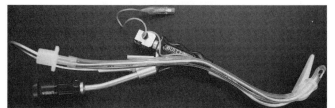

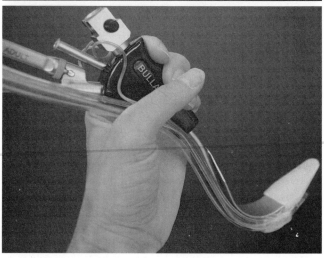

Figure 12-37 The Bullard video laryngoscope and blade features a self-contained video monitor to see the patient's larynx during an intubation attempt. Note that the endotracheal tube and its stylet are held in a groove for placement into the trachea. (From Cairo JM: Mosby's respiratory care equipment, ed 9, St Louis, 2014, Mosby.)

instrument. The separate monitor allows the intubation procedure and the patient's laryngeal area to be viewed by other people for teaching purposes.

b. Troubleshoot any problems with the equipment (code: IIA9) [difficulty: R, Ap]

Review the discussion on bronchoscopy in Chapter 18 for the details on the equipment. The fiberoptic tube should be lubricated so that it will easily slide through the lumen of the endotracheal tube (see Fig. 12-35). After the physician has confirmed that the distal end of the fiberoptic tube has entered the trachea, the endotracheal tube is gently pushed into the trachea. The fiberoptic tube is then withdrawn, the cuff is inflated, and the endotracheal tube is secured. If the endotracheal tube will not slide into the patient's trachea, either it is too large or there is not enough lubricant on the fiberoptic tube. It may be necessary to withdraw them, correct the problem, and start over again.

The light wand needs functioning batteries in the proximal handle in order to glow. Replace any nonfunctioning batteries. The unit should have a water-soluble lubricant added so that it easily passes in and out of the endotracheal tube's channel.

The closed-circuit laryngoscope handle and monitor need to have functioning batteries. Units with a separate video monitor need to be plugged into an electrical outlet and properly assembled. If the lens at the tip of the fiberoptic bundle becomes fogged over or blocked by secretions or blood, nothing can be seen. The blade will have to be removed and the lens cleared of debris.

MODULE K

Endotracheal intubation and tube management

1. Establish the patient's airway (code: IIIA3e) [difficulty: R, Ap, An]

Oral endotracheal intubation is the recommended procedure for securing the airway during an emergency such as a CPR attempt. In uncomplicated cases, the patient can be quickly intubated with an apneic period of no more than 20 seconds. This procedure is explained for a team of two respiratory therapists. (See Chapter 18 for the discussion of a respiratory therapist assisting a physician with the intubation procedure.) It is difficult, if not impossible, for a single therapist to perform this important task without placing the patient at great risk. Usually the therapist who intubates is considered the leader and the other therapist acts as the assistant. Therapists must feel comfortable in both roles. See Box 12-5 for a list of indications and contraindications for oral intubation and Box 12-6 for a list of complications.

Steps in an emergency oral endotracheal intubation include the following:
1. Prepare the patient. The assistant should:
   a. Place the head and neck in the sniff position.
   b. Ventilate the patient's lungs with 100% oxygen by a face mask and manual resuscitation (bag/mask ventilation).
2. The intubator should put on a surgical mask, goggles, and clean gloves on both hands and then perform the following.

BOX 12-5 Indications and Contraindications for Oral Endotracheal Intubation

General Indications for Endotracheal Intubation
Provides a secure, patent airway.
Provides a route for mechanical ventilation.
Prevents aspiration of stomach or mouth contents.
Provides a route for suctioning the lungs.
Patient is undergoing general anesthetic.

Indications for Oral Intubation
Is the fastest, easiest method to secure the airway.
A simpler, less invasive method cannot ensure an open airway.

Contraindications for Oral Intubation
Cervical spine injury such that the patient's neck cannot be hyperextended.
Lower facial injury.
Oral surgery.

BOX 12-6 Complications of Endotracheal Intubation

General Complications
Reflex laryngospasm
Perforation of the esophagus or pharynx
Esophageal intubation
Bronchial intubation
Reflex bradycardia
Tachycardia or other dysrhythmias from hypoxemia
Hypotension
Bronchospasm
Aspiration of tooth, blood, gastric contents, laryngoscope bulb
Laceration of pharynx or larynx
Nosocomial infection
Vocal cord injury
Laryngeal or tracheal injury from the tube or excessive cuff pressure

Complications of the Oral Route
Cervical spine injury
Tooth trauma from the blade being pulled back
Eye trauma from the handle or the operator's hand

Complications of the Nasal Route
Bleeding
Ulceration
Sinusitis

---

3. Prepare the endotracheal tube.
   a. Select the proper endotracheal tube. (See Table 12-1 for the recommended tube sizes based on the patient's age. It is common practice to select the tube size based on its ID. For example, a premature neonate would need a 2.5-mm-ID tube.) If time permits, the next smaller and larger tube sizes should also be selected.

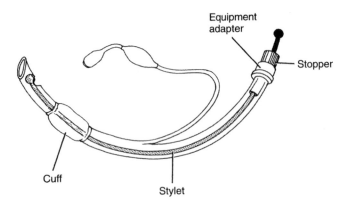

Figure 12-38 Stylet with stopper properly placed in standard endotracheal tube to maintain its curved shape. (From Eubanks DH, Bone RC: Comprehensive respiratory care, ed 2, St Louis, 1990, Mosby.)

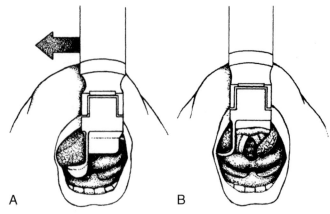

A   B

Figure 12-39 Proper placement of the laryngoscope blade to move the patient's tongue. **A,** Proper placement of the laryngoscope blade to the right of the patient's tongue to move it to the left. This should give a clear view of the glottis. **B,** Tongue partially obstructs the view if it is not moved to the left. (From Shapiro BA et al: Clinical application of respiratory care, ed 4, St Louis, 1991, Mosby.)

  b. Inflate the cuff using a 10- or 20-mL syringe. Remove the syringe from the one-way valve. Make sure that it holds the air and then deflate the cuff completely.

  c. Lubricate the last few centimeters of the endotracheal tube with a water-soluble lubricant.

  d. (Optional step) Lubricate a stylet with the sterile water-soluble lubricant. Place the stylet into the tube so that the natural curve of the tube is maintained. The tip of the stylet should not go past the end of the tube (Fig. 12-38). Some practitioners may prefer not to use a stylet. Many believe that the stylet offers the advantage of being able to bend the tube to match the patient's anatomy if a second attempt is needed.

4. Prepare the laryngoscope and blade.

  a. Select a laryngoscope handle.

  b. Select a laryngoscope blade. The blades are available in several sizes from pediatric to adult. There are two main classes of blades: straight and curved (see Fig. 12-33). The straight blades (Miller) are designed to lift the epiglottis to expose the tracheal opening. The curved blades (MacIntosh) are designed to fit into the vallecula (between the base of the tongue and the epiglottis). As the blade is lifted, the epiglottis is raised and the tracheal opening can be seen. Personal experience and training lead the intubator to select between the two styles.

  c. Attach the blade to the handle (see Fig. 12-34). Make sure that the light bulb shines brightly.

5. The intubator should tell the assistant to stop ventilating the patient and stand clear so that an intubation can be attempted. The assistant should check his or her watch to silently count off 30 seconds. The intubator should be told when 30 seconds has passed so that the patient can be reventilated if the intubation is proving to be difficult.

6. Open the victim's mouth as widely as possible without using force. Remove any dentures or foreign material. Suction any saliva, blood, or vomitus.

7. Grasp the laryngoscope handle in the left hand. Carefully advance the blade between the teeth or gums along the right side of the mouth. Move the tongue to the left side of the mouth to allow a clear view of the oropharynx (Fig. 12-39). Advance the blade along the base of the tongue until the epiglottis is seen.

8. With a *straight* blade:

  a. Advance the blade so that it barely passes the epiglottis.

  b. Do not advance the blade too far or it will enter the esophagus or larynx.

With a *curved* blade:

  a. Advance the blade tip into the vallecula.

  b. Lift the blade tip into this space.

9. With either blade, lift the laryngoscope handle and blade toward the patient's chest at a 45-degree angle (Fig. 12-40). The straight blade lifts the epiglottis. The curved blade lifts the soft tissues of the vallecula and the epiglottis lifts with them. Do *not* pull back on the patient's upper teeth.

10. The vocal cords and glottis should be clearly seen (Fig. 12-41). If needed, tell the assistant to put gentle, downward pressure on the patient's larynx. This may help to bring the glottis into better view.

11. Tell the assistant to place the endotracheal tube into your right hand.

12. Place the tube into the right side of the patient's mouth and direct it into the trachea. (The assistant may feel over the larynx as the tube enters the trachea. If necessary, the assistant may need to apply gentle pressure over the larynx to move it more posterior.) In the adult, advance the tube until the proximal end of the cuff is 3-4 cm past the vocal cords (Fig. 12-42). In children less than 6 months of age, with an uncuffed endotracheal tube, advance the tube until the tip is about 1 cm past the vocal cords.

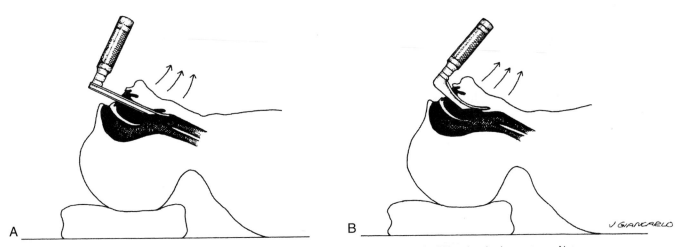

Figure 12-40 Proper use of the laryngoscope blade to expose the larynx by lifting the glottic structures. Note how the lifting is at a 45-degree angle toward the patient's chest. *Never* pull back on the blade against the teeth. **A,** A straight blade is used to lift the epiglottis to expose the trachea. **B,** A curved blade is used to lift soft tissues of the vallecula to expose the trachea. (From Shapiro BA et al: Clinical application of respiratory care, ed 4, St Louis, 1991, Mosby.)

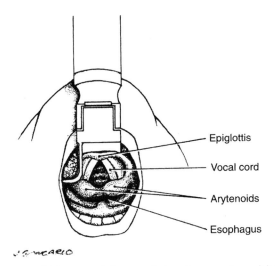

Figure 12-41 Major anatomic features that can be seen when epiglottis is lifted. Opening to trachea can be seen between vocal cords. (From Shapiro BA et al: Clinical application of respiratory care, ed 4, St Louis, 1991, Mosby.)

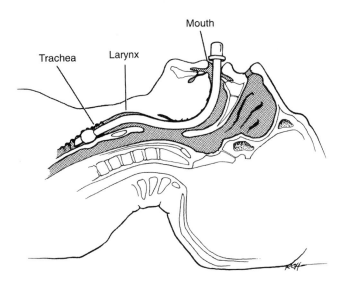

Figure 12-42 Oral endotracheal tube properly positioned within the trachea. (From Eubanks DH, Bone RC: Comprehensive respiratory care, ed 2, St Louis, 1990, Mosby.)

13. Hold the tube in place.
14. Withdraw the laryngoscope blade.
15. Tell the assistant to inflate the cuff. Place about 10 mL of air into the cuff (of an adult's tube; less in a pediatric tube) so that some resistance can be felt. The cuff pressure can be measured and adjusted later.
16. Pull out the stylet (if used).
17. The assistant should ventilate the patient's lungs with the manual resuscitator bag or a demand valve.
18. The intubator should listen to both lung fields in the upper lobes and bases. Bilateral breath sounds should be heard.
19. If the breath sounds are equal and bilateral, the assistant can secure the tube in place with tape or a tube holder. If the breath sounds are unequal or absent

on one side, the tube has been placed into a bronchus (usually the right mainstem). The cuff should be deflated and the tube then withdrawn 1-2 cm in an adult, less in a child. The cuff should be reinflated and breath sounds assessed again. When the breath sounds are equal, the tube can be secured.
20. If no breath sounds are heard, listen over the stomach area. If air is heard bubbling into the stomach, the tube has been placed into the esophagus. Immediately remove the tube. Ventilate the patient's lungs and prepare to attempt reintubation.

The practitioner should perform only those procedures for which he or she has been trained. If the patient cannot be intubated with the standard equipment and procedure, an anesthesiologist or trained physician should be requested. Be prepared to assist as necessary.

2. Manage the patient's airway (code: IIIA3e) [difficulty: R, Ap, An]

Clinical experience has shown that there is no single fool-proof procedure that can confirm that the endotracheal tube is within the trachea. Current guidelines recommend that several of the following procedures be done to confirm proper tube placement within the trachea.

a. Palpate the patient to determine asymmetric chest movements and/or tracheal deviation (code: IB3c) [difficulty: R, Ap, An]

As discussed previously, the first step to confirm tube placement during the intubation procedure is to palpate it passing through the larynx and entering the trachea. Most often the endotracheal tube can be palpated in an infant as it is being inserted. This is because the laryngeal structures are so pliable. Feeling the tube being inserted through the larynx indicates that it is properly located within the trachea. If the tube cannot be palpated through the larynx, it has probably been inserted into the esophagus. It is more difficult to use this technique with confidence in adults because their laryngeal structures are stiffer.

If the tube is advanced and cannot be palpated within the trachea, there are two other possible locations. First, the endotracheal tube could have been placed into the esophagus. Breath sounds will be heard over the epigastric area rather than the lungs. The abdominal area would be felt to move rather than the chest during an inspiration. Deflate the cuff, withdraw the tube, and bag/mask ventilate the patient's lungs. Second, the tube could have entered the trachea but deviated through the tracheal wall to enter one or the other lung field. Assess the patient for a possible pneumothorax, including findings of asymmetric chest movements, crepitus, and/or tracheal deviation. Withdraw the tube and begin bag/mask ventilation. Call a physician for help.

b. Auscultate to assess the patient's breath sounds (code: IB5a) [difficulty: R, Ap, An]

Respiratory efforts without breath sounds indicate that a complete obstruction exists in the patient's airway. Inspiratory stridor or wheezing indicates that a partial obstruction exists in the patient's airway. Listen for stridor over the larynx and wheezing over the major airways. The restoration of the normal airway should result in the return of normal breath sounds over all areas of both lung fields (unless there is another, unrelated problem).

After intubation, deliver a breath and listen over the epigastric area to rule out tube placement in the esophagus. After ruling out esophageal placement, check for bilateral breath sounds. Confirm equal bilateral breath sounds by first listening over the apical areas and then the lateral areas. If the tube has been inserted too far, it usually enters the right mainstem bronchus because it separates from the trachea at a less acute angle than the left mainstem bronchus. No breath sounds will be heard over the

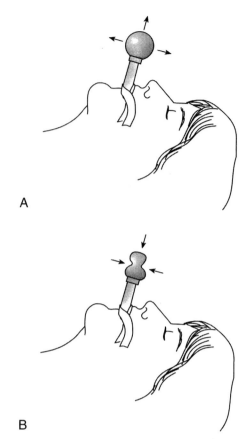

A

B

Figure 12-43 Esophageal detection device. This squeeze-bulb device is attached to the proximal end of the patient's endotracheal tube and air is squeezed out. **A,** The bulb is reinflated with air from the patient's lungs when the endotracheal tube has been properly placed. **B,** The bulb fails to reinflate when the endotracheal tube has been accidentally placed into the patient's esophagus. (From Scanlan C, Simmons K: Airway management. In Scanlan CL, Wilkins RL, Stoller JK, editors: Egan's fundamentals of respiratory care, ed 7, St Louis, 1999, Mosby.)

left lung field. If both lung fields cannot be auscultated, at least listen to the right apical area. This one site can be checked because the segmental bronchus to the right upper lobe separates from the right mainstem bronchus in such a way that if the right mainstem bronchus is intubated, the upper lobe segmental bronchus will be blocked.

While listening to the patient's breath sounds, look at the endotracheal tube. The condensation of moisture on the inside of the tube during exhalation would also confirm that the tube is in the trachea (or a bronchus) instead of the esophagus.

c. Esophageal detection device

The esophageal detection device (EDD) is able to show that the endotracheal tube has been placed within an airway by pulling a small sample of gas from the patient's lungs. If the endotracheal tube has been accidentally put into the esophagus, the deflated bulb will stay collapsed (Fig. 12-43). A limitation of the EDD is that it inflates whether the endotracheal tube is placed into the trachea or either mainstem bronchus. Remember to auscultate for bilateral breath sounds.

d. Detect exhaled carbon dioxide

1. Evaluate capnography data in the patient record (code: IA13f) [difficulty: R, Ap]

It is now common clinical practice to check for the presence of exhaled carbon dioxide to confirm endotracheal intubation. In the operating room the anesthesiologist will attach a capnography system to a patient's endotracheal tube or add one into a ventilator circuit. In most other intubation situations, a simple, inexpensive colorimeter device is used. With either device, if the patient is not in cardiopulmonary arrest and the tube is within the trachea or a major bronchus, exhaled CO_2 will be found. If none is detected, the tube has been placed into the esophagus. Deflate the cuff and remove the tube. Begin bag/mask ventilation until the patient is stable and then insert a new endotracheal tube.

2. Assemble exhaled carbon dioxide detectors (code: IIA21) [difficulty: R, Ap]

Most exhaled carbon dioxide detectors are inexpensive, single-patient-use, disposable devices. They are called colorimetric units because they change color when exhaled carbon dioxide passes through the sensitive material within the capsule (Fig. 12-44). The units are placed onto an endotracheal tube's 15-mm-OD adapter to monitor the proper placement of the endotracheal tube. This is often done if a patient is being transported and there is a possibility that the tube could be dislodged. Exhaled carbon dioxide detectors are also used during CPR attempts to help determine if resuscitation attempts are being performed on a viable patient. If the patient is not producing exhaled CO_2, there is no metabolic activity. The physician may then decide to stop CPR efforts.

As of this writing, available disposable units include the Nelcor Easy Cap II for adults and Pedi-Cap for children, the Mercury Medical Neo-Stat CO_2 neonatal patients, and the A.C.E. StatCheck II, which is integrated with neonatal, pediatric, and adult manual resuscitation bags. The Easy Cap II CO_2 detector (see Fig. 12-44) is the original unit and very widely used. It is available in a pediatric size for infants weighing 1-15 kg and in a standard size for larger children and adults. Its carbon dioxide indicator changes color from dark purple to yellow when CO_2 is exhaled through it. The other disposable units also indicate the presence of exhaled CO_2 by an indicator turning yellow.

The MiniCAP III CO_2 detector is a reusable capnometer that has a mainstream type of infrared carbon dioxide detector. The unit is powered by a battery pack. Its light-emitting diode signals the presence of carbon dioxide with each exhalation. A capnometer should be selected if it is necessary to obtain a more accurate CO_2 reading. Remember that capnometry cannot confirm that the tube

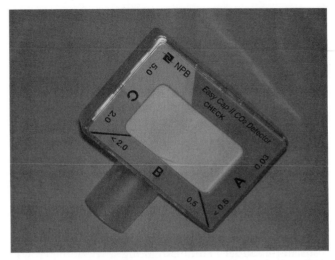

Figure 12-44 Easy Cap II CO_2 detector. This disposable device is available in adult and pediatric sizes and is able to detect exhaled carbon dioxide. A color change from dark purple to yellow indicates exhaled CO_2 to confirm tracheal placement of an endotracheal tube or effective efforts at cardiopulmonary resuscitation. (Courtesy of Nellcor Puritan Bennett, Pleasanton, CA, part of Covidien.)

is properly placed into the trachea rather than a bronchus. Check for equal, bilateral breath sounds. See Chapter 5 for a full discussion on capnometry.

The following discussion applies to the Easy Cap II and Pedi-Cap units. Each is a single unit within a sealed foil container. Remove the unit from the container and compare the initial purple color of the indicator with the purple color labeled CHECK on the product dome. Do *not* use a unit whose color is not the same or darker than that on the product dome. Attach the unit to the patient's endotracheal tube by its 15-mm-ID connector port. The unit's 15-mm-OD circuit end is connected to the manual resuscitator to ventilate the patient's lungs. If a heat and moisture exchanger is used, it should be placed between the patient's endotracheal tube and the Easy Cap II or Pedi-Cap unit and manual resuscitator. The Easy Cap II or Pedi-Cap should not be used with a heated humidifier or nebulizer because too much humidity affects its accuracy. Neither unit is intended to be used for more than 2 hours because the color change will fade.

The MiniCAP III has a disposable adapter that connects the mainstream CO_2 detector to the patient's endotracheal tube. The adapter has a 15-mm-ID end for attachment to the endotracheal tube and a 15-mm-OD end to which the manual resuscitator can be attached. The assembly and operation of a capnometer are discussed in Chapter 5. Review this material if necessary.

3. Troubleshoot any problems with the equipment (code: IIA21) [difficulty: R, Ap]

Because the Easy Cap II and Pedi-Cap are self-contained single-piece units, there is nothing to repair. The following items can contaminate either unit and cause a patchy yellow or white discoloration of the indicator: stomach contents, mucus, pulmonary edema fluid, and intratracheal epinephrine. If the color does not change with the breathing cycle, the unit should be discarded. The 15-mm-ID patient connector port fits only over the endotracheal tube adapter. The 15-mm-OD circuit connector port fits only into the manual resuscitator or demand-valve adapter. An Easy Cap II or Pedi-Cap should not be used during mouth-to-mouth resuscitation, to detect right mainstem bronchus intubation, to detect hypercarbia, or to determine the placement of an esophageal obturator airway.

The adapter is the only removable part in the MiniCAP III. It fits only in one direction into the CO_2 detection unit. The other end of the adapter fits only into a manual resuscitator outlet. Troubleshooting a capnometer was presented in Chapter 5.

e. Recommend a chest radiograph (code: IE3) [difficulty: R, Ap, An]

A chest radiograph should always be taken to confirm the location of a newly placed endotracheal or tracheostomy tube. The chest radiograph should be repeated if there has been a significant change in the patient's condition or if the tube has been pulled back or pushed deeper into the trachea. Ideally the tip of the tube is in the middle third of the trachea. In the adult this would be several centimeters above the carina.

A chest radiograph also confirms the presence and location of an opaque foreign body in the airway. Metallic objects, stones, and coins can be clearly seen. Less radiopaque objects can be barely seen, if at all. The chest radiograph also detects a pneumothorax related to the tracheostomy procedure or other pulmonary conditions. If needed, an upper-airway radiographic examination can be performed to look for a foreign body or to check the position of the tracheostomy tube.

f. Review the chest radiograph to assess the position of the endotracheal tube (code: IB7b) [difficulty: R, Ap, An]

All modern endotracheal and tracheostomy tubes contain a strip of radiopaque material near the distal tip of the tube. This is easily noticed as the white line seen on the chest radiograph and confirms the location of the tip of the tube in the airway (see Fig. 12-24). The ideal location of the tip of the endotracheal tube is the middle third of the trachea. When the tube is positioned properly, it is less likely for the tip to be pushed into the carina when the patient bends his or her head forward or for the cuff to hit the vocal cords if the patient's head is bent back. Both endotracheal and tracheostomy tubes should be positioned midline within the trachea. They should not be twisted laterally because the tip can cause damage to the tracheal wall.

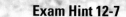

Exam Hint 12-7

Be prepared to determine the proper placement of the endotracheal tube by any of the following: (1) palpation of the larynx and neck, (2) auscultation of bilateral breath sounds, (3) determination of moisture condensation within the tube during exhalation, (4) detection of exhaled carbon dioxide, (5) observation of bilateral symmetric chest movement on inspiration, (6) visualization of the tip of the tube on a chest radiograph, or (7) observation that the 24-cm mark on the tube will be at an adult's front teeth (incisors).

Check the chest radiograph for positioning. If the tube is too high within the trachea, it may be pulled up through the vocal cords if the patient's head is hyperextended. An air leak may be heard at the larynx if the patient is using a mechanical ventilator. In this case, the cuff should be deflated and the tube inserted deeper into the trachea.

Conversely, if the tip of the tube is inserted too deeply into the trachea, it may be pushed into a mainstem bronchus if the patient's head is moved toward the chest. In this situation no breath sounds would be heard in the opposite lung (usually the left). The patient's throat should be suctioned, the cuff deflated, and the tube pulled up into the middle third of the trachea. Reinflate the cuff after the tube is repositioned. A chest radiograph should be taken to confirm the tube's position after it has been moved.

g. Secure the endotracheal tube

Before the endotracheal tube is secured, its depth in the airway should be determined. The endotracheal tube body has centimeter marks inscribed on it, starting at the distal end and finishing at the proximal end. Check and record the centimeter mark present at the patient's teeth or gums. The average adult's distance from the midtrachea to the teeth is about 23-25 cm. The practitioner can determine if the tube has been accidentally pulled out a little or pushed further into the patient by looking at the current centimeter mark. If the tube is intentionally adjusted, the new centimeter mark should be checked and recorded.

A wide variety of handmade, as well as manufactured, devices are available to secure the endotracheal tube in the correct position. Figure 12-45 shows one way to make a tube holder from adhesive tape. This is flexible when the patient moves and is inexpensive. Tincture of benzoin can be applied to the patient's cheeks to make the tape hold more securely without tearing the skin. An oropharyngeal airway may or may not be needed.

The manufactured tube holders are made of plastic with cloth ties and usually include a built-in bite block. Make sure that it is sized properly to the patient's mouth. Too large a bite block can injure the tongue, lips, and mouth. Watch for a gag reflex. This type of holder is useful in the patient who is prone to seizures.

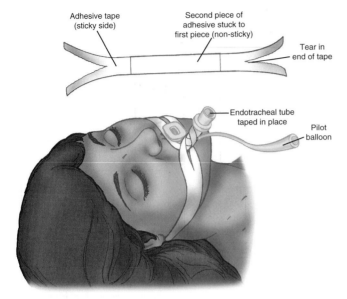

Adhesive tape (sticky side)

Second piece of adhesive stuck to first piece (non-sticky)

Tear in end of tape

Endotracheal tube taped in place

Pilot balloon

Figure 12-45 Taping the endotracheal tube to secure it in the airway. (From Kacmarek RM, Stoller JK, Heuer AJ: Egan's fundamentals of respiratory care, ed 10, St Louis, 2013, Mosby.)

Exam Hint 12-8

There is usually a question that addresses understanding that the lack of breath sounds over the left lung indicates that the endotracheal tube has been placed into the right mainstem bronchus. Suction the patient's throat, deflate the cuff, withdraw the tube into the trachea, and reinflate the cuff. The typical NBRC question focuses on withdrawing the tube. Note that the 24-cm mark on the tube is at the average adult patient's front teeth (incisors).

---

3. Determine the tracheal tube cuff pressure and/or volume (code: IC20) [difficulty: R, Ap]

All of the adult and larger pediatric endotracheal and tracheostomy tubes have a cuff for sealing the airway. Most brands of modern tubes have cuffs that are designed to have a relatively large reservoir volume that fills at a relatively low pressure. The soft, flexible balloon seals the airway by having a large surface area that conforms to the shape of the trachea.

There are two slightly different ways to inflate the cuff and maintain a safe cuff pressure. Both methods can be used only with patients on a positive-pressure ventilator.

a. Minimal leak

1. Connect the cuff pressure measuring device (see next discussion) to the one-way valve on the cuff-inflating tube.
2. Listen with a stethoscope over the patient's larynx.
3. Inflate or deflate the cuff as necessary while listening for an air leak.
4. Stop changing the air volume when a minimal leak is heard at the peak airway pressure in the breathing

cycle. The tidal volume should still be delivered except for this minor leak.
5. Note the cuff pressure when the minimal leak was heard. Note the cuff volume, if possible.
6. Disconnect the cuff pressure measuring device.
7. It may be necessary to add more volume and pressure to the cuff if the leak gets worse when the peak airway pressure increases.

b. Minimal occluding volume

The purpose is to find the cuff pressure that results in *no leak* at the cuff when the patient's airway pressure is greatest. The following are the steps in the procedure:

1. Connect the cuff pressure measuring device (see next discussion) to the one-way valve on the cuff-inflating tube.
2. Listen with a stethoscope over the patient's larynx.
3. Inflate or deflate the cuff as necessary while listening for an air leak.
4. Stop changing the air volume when no leak is heard at the peak airway pressure in the breathing cycle.
5. Note the cuff pressure when the seal was heard. Note the cuff volume, if possible.
6. If the patient is on a ventilator with a monitor, check the volume–time curve to confirm that the inhaled volume and exhaled volume match with a return to the baseline pressure.
7. Disconnect the cuff pressure measuring device.
8. It may be necessary to add more volume and pressure to the cuff if a leak results when the peak airway pressure increases.

This discussion relates only to those tubes that must be actively filled with air and have variable intracuff pressures. Several manufacturers have developed endotracheal and tracheostomy tubes that have built-in cuff pressure limitations. Follow the manufacturer's guidelines when inflating these cuffs. This discussion would not be complete without mentioning systems designed to raise the cuff pressure to match the peak airway pressure of a patient using a mechanical ventilator. A tube connects the inspiratory circuit to the one-way valve on the cuff-inflating tube. As a positive-pressure breath is delivered, the pressure in the circuit is also applied to the patient's cuff. There should be no loss of tidal volume. When the patient exhales and the airway pressure drops to normal, the cuff pressure also drops back to its normal level.

c. Select a cuff pressure and/or volume measuring system

A cuff pressure manometer is needed to measure the air pressure within an endotracheal or tracheostomy tube cuff. When a tracheal tube is first inserted, the volume of air that is injected into the cuff should be measured and charted. The pressure within the cuff should also be noted. After that, if more air is inserted or any air is removed

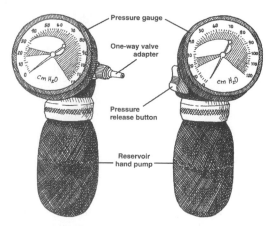

Figure 12-46 Cufflator device used to measure cuff pressure with its component parts.

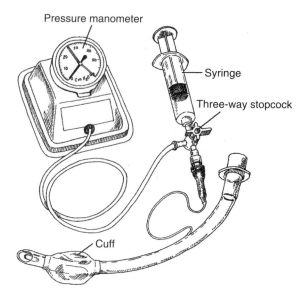

Figure 12-47 Cuff measuring device made from pressure manometer, three-way stopcock, and 10-mL syringe.

from the cuff, it should be measured and recorded in the chart. The resulting final cuff pressure must also be recorded. A number of manufactured units are available for measuring cuff pressure. The Cufflator (Fig. 12-46) is discussed here because it is widely used. This system consists of a pressure gauge calibrated in centimeters of water, a hand-pumped reservoir, an internal one-way valve, a pressure-release valve, and an adapter to fit into the one-way valve on the cuff-inflating tube. A three-way stopcock can be added to the one-way valve adapter. This can be used to prepressurize the system before attaching it to the patient's one-way valve on the cuff-inflating tube. The pressure in the cuff can be measured as air is added by squeezing the hand pump or as air is removed by the pressure-release valve. The volume of air added or removed cannot be measured.

A second system can be "homemade," although it is also commercially available. It consists of a 5- to 10-mL syringe, a three-way stopcock, and a pressure gauge (either millimeters of mercury or centimeters of water). The syringe and pressure gauge are attached to two of the ports on the stopcock. The third port on the stopcock is connected to the one-way valve on the cuff-inflating tube. When the stopcock handle is opened to all three ports, the pressures throughout the system and the cuff are the same. Air can be added or removed with the syringe. The pressure gauge shows the system and cuff pressure as the air volume is adjusted (Fig. 12-47). One advantage of this system over the Cufflator is that the volume of air that is added or subtracted can be measured. This system can also be prepressurized so that its pressure matches the pressure anticipated in the cuff. With any of these systems, it is necessary to keep airtight connections. If the pressure drops unexpectedly, an air leak will be noticed. Tighten the connections to create a seal so that the pressure is maintained.

It is commonly recommended that the cuff pressure be monitored at least every 8 hours or whenever air is injected or withdrawn from the cuff.

4. Evaluate the tracheal tube cuff pressure and/or volume (code: ID19) [difficulty: R, Ap, An]

All manufacturers (except Kamen-Wilkenson) have designed cuffs that must be actively filled with air by way of a one-way valve and syringe. These cuffs have greater than atmospheric pressure within them. That pressure is placed against the wall of the trachea. There are two, possibly conflicting, goals related to finding the best cuff pressure (reflecting cuff volume) for an endotracheal tube or tracheostomy tube. First, there needs to be enough cuff pressure to prevent supraglottic saliva from leaking past the cuff and into the trachea and lungs. The goal here is to prevent ventilator associated pneumonia (VAP)/health-care-associated pneumonia. There is clinical evidence that a cuff pressure of less than 15 mm Hg (30 cm H_2O) is an independent risk factor for developing VAP.

Second, the cuff pressure must be kept low enough to allow blood to flow through the tracheal mucosa. It is clear that a cuff pressure greater than the patient's mucosa capillary pressure prevents the flow of blood through the area covered by the cuff. Tissue ischemia (hypoxia) results. If the ischemia is severe enough, tissue necrosis follows. The higher the cuff pressure and the longer the high cuff pressure is maintained, the greater the likelihood of tissue necrosis or tracheomalacia. If the necrosis is circumferential (all the way around) to the trachea, tracheal stenosis may occur. Tracheal stenosis is found when the diameter of the trachea is narrowed because of scar tissue buildup after the normal mucosa and underlying tissues have died. The patient's airway is permanently narrowed and, if serious, must be surgically corrected. Another severe complication of high cuff pressures and tracheal necrosis is the development of a tracheoesophageal fistula. This is an opening between the trachea and the esophagus. This is more likely when the patient also has a nasogastric tube in place. The fistula permits food and liquids to pass into the airway and lungs, causing pneumonia. Mechanical ventilation is more difficult because of the air leak from the lungs to the esophagus. Surgical repair of the fistula is required. The most serious complication relates to erosion of the anterior tracheal wall. This will lead to the innominate artery being damaged. Massive hemorrhage and death can occur if the artery is not quickly surgically repaired. If sudden, massive bleeding is seen, the cuff must be hyperinflated to tamponade the artery before calling the physician.

To try to accomplish both goals of preventing VAP and maintaining tracheal blood flow, the following guidelines are given:

1. Maintain cuff pressure between 15 and 22 mm Hg (20 and 30 cm H_2O).
2. If a mechanically ventilated patient requires high-pressure breaths to deliver the tidal volume, there may be a significant air leak. In this situation, it may be necessary to keep a higher cuff pressure than the ideal maximum of 22 mm Hg (30 cm H_2O). However, Shapiro and associates have stated that if the cuff pressure must be greater than 20 mm Hg, the endotracheal or tracheostomy tube is too small. Ideally, the tube should be replaced with a larger one. However, some patients are too unstable to tolerate reintubation and must simply have the cuff pressure increased temporarily.

Exam Hint 12-9

There is usually a question about adjusting the cuff pressure to a safe level of 15-22 mm Hg (20-30 cm H_2O). If that results in an air leak, recommend replacing a small tracheal tube with a larger one to have a lower cuff pressure.

MODULE L

Endotracheal extubation

1. Exchange the endotracheal tube (code: IIIA5) [difficulty: R, Ap, An]

There are usually only two reasons to replace a patient's endotracheal tube. First, the tube should be changed if it is too small and the cuff must be overfilled to seal the airway. Excessive pressure results in damage to the tracheal wall.

Second, the tube should be replaced if the cuff is leaking or ruptured and the airway cannot be sealed. The patient may be reintubated by the procedure described earlier. Alternatively, a tube-changing stylet may be used (Fig. 12-48). The stylet is a hollow, flexible plastic tube that can be bent and holds its shape. It has a center mark and 1-cm markings counting out to each end. These are to help keep the proper depth for inserting the replacement

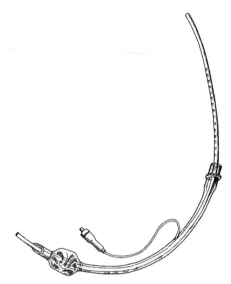

Figure 12-48 Endotracheal tube changer (guide) inserted through an endotracheal tube. The JEM 400 unit can be inserted through a tube that is 7.5-mm ID or larger. The tube changer is used to aid in replacement of an esophageal obturator airway or a defective endotracheal tube with a functional endotracheal tube. See text for how to use the tube changer instead of traditional intubation equipment. (Modified from Heffner JE: Respir Manage 19(3):53, 1989.)

endotracheal tube. It can be used on an endotracheal tube that has at least a 7.5-mm ID. The procedure for changing the endotracheal tube with a tube-changing stylet includes the following:

1. Obtain the needed equipment: replacement endotracheal tube and one that is a size smaller, 10-mL syringe to inflate the cuff, sterile gloves, goggles, and sterile water-soluble lubricant. Make sure the cuff inflates and deflates properly.
2. Tell the patient what you are going to do. Put on the gloves, goggles, and mask.
3. Remove the patient's oxygen equipment.
4. Suction the secretions from the patient's trachea and oral pharynx.
5. Reoxygenate and ventilate the patient's lungs.
6. Place some lubricant on the outside of the stylet.
7. Remove the oxygen equipment and pass the stylet through the endotracheal tube into the patient's trachea.
8. Insert it to about the same depth as marked on the distal end of the endotracheal tube. For example, if the distal end of the endotracheal tube is 22 cm, insert the tube changer to 22 cm.
9. Deflate the cuff on the endotracheal tube.
10. While holding the distal tip of the tube changer in place, pull the defective endotracheal tube over the tube changer and out of the patient.
11. Advance the new endotracheal tube over the stylet. Hold the distal end of the stylet and push the new tube into the patient to the same depth mark on the stylet at which the old tube had been positioned.

12. Hold the endotracheal tube in place and remove the stylet.
13. Ensure that the tube has been placed into the trachea to the proper depth by listening for bilateral breath sounds.
14. Inflate the cuff to a safe pressure.
15. Secure the tube in place and note the depth marking at the patient's teeth or gums.
16. Obtain a chest radiograph.

A defective one-way valve or severed cuff-inflating tube may not necessarily lead to a reintubation; often it can be bypassed. This is done by slipping a small-diameter blunt needle (usually about 21 gauge) into the inflating tube, attaching a three-way stopcock to the hub of the needle, and screwing a 10-mL syringe into one of the stopcock ports (Fig. 12-49). The cuff pressure can be measured by attaching a pressure manometer to the other port on the stopcock. Air can be added by the 10-mL syringe and the pressure measured simultaneously (Fig. 12-50). There is

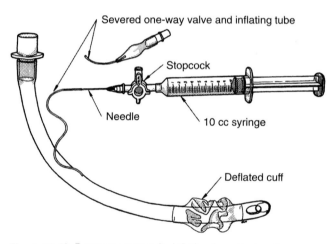

Figure 12-49 Emergency system for inflating the cuff when the one-way valve and inflating tube are severed. (From Sills JR: Respir Care 31:199-201, 1986.)

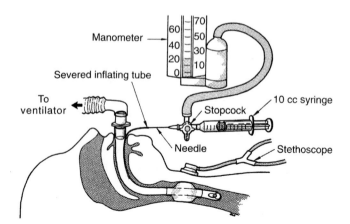

Figure 12-50 Measuring intracuff pressure as the cuff is reinflated with an emergency system. The stethoscope is used to listen for the presence of a leak at the larynx. (From Sills JR: Respir Care 31:199-201, 1986.)

now a commercially available system to bypass a severed cuff-inflating tube.

2. Recommend extubation (code: IIIE2g) [difficulty: R, Ap, An]

Extubation should be considered only after it has been determined that the original problem(s) that necessitated the endotracheal tube has been corrected. It should be reasonably anticipated that once the endotracheal tube has been removed it will not have to be replaced. The patient should be able to sustain a patent airway, expectorate secretions effectively, and maintain acceptable arterial blood gas values. Supplemental oxygen may be needed. Also see the discussion in Chapter 15 that relates to weaning from mechanical ventilation and readiness for extubation. (The only exception to the preceding general guidelines would be when terminal extubation is performed. In this situation, it has been determined that further medical intervention is futile and the patient and/or family want extubation.)

If extubation is planned, make sure that all needed personnel, supplies, and equipment are available in case the patient needs to be reintubated. This includes, but is not limited to, someone trained to perform intubation, intubation equipment and endotracheal tubes, alternative airways such as an LMA suctioning equipment, bag/mask resuscitator, ECG monitor, and pulse oximeter.

3. Perform extubation (code: IIIA8) [difficulty: R, Ap, An]

Extubation should be performed only by trained personnel and under the proper conditions to ensure the patient's safety. See Box 12-3 for a list of complications that can occur after extubation. The generally recommended steps in extubation include the following:

1. Evaluate the patient's cardiopulmonary status. The reason(s) for the tube being placed should be corrected. The most recent blood gas results should be acceptable. Tracheal secretions should be minimal and not so thick that they cannot be expectorated by the patient. Bedside spirometry results should show an acceptable tidal volume, vital capacity, and maximal inspiratory pressure.
2. Inform the patient about the removal of the tube and the follow-up care that is needed.
3. The patient's inspired oxygen percentage may be kept the same or increased before the extubation. If increased, it should be done at least 5-10 minutes before the tube is removed.
4. Suction the trachea until all secretions are removed.
5. Suction the oral pharynx to remove all saliva. Be prepared to suction additional oral secretions and mucus after extubation.
6. In rapid succession:
   a. Give a deep sigh breath from the ventilator or resuscitation bag.

b. Deflate the cuff. Cut the inflation tube to the cuff to ensure its collapse.

c. Pull out the tube following its natural curve when the lungs are full.

Alternatively, in rapid succession:

a. Give a deep sigh breath from the ventilator or resuscitation bag.

b. Place a suction catheter through the tube into the trachea. This works best with a self-contained catheter and sheath system.

c. Deflate the cuff. Cut the inflation tube to the cuff to ensure its collapse.

d. Pull out the tube when the lungs are full.

e. Apply suction as the tube is withdrawn.

7. Have the patient cough vigorously to remove any secretions.

8. Apply a cool, bland aerosol by face mask with the previous amount of oxygen.

9. Monitor and evaluate the patient every 30 minutes for several hours. Encourage deep breathing and coughing.

10. Check the vital signs.

11. Measure pulse oximetry or arterial blood gases after 20 minutes.

12. Listen to the breath sounds and larynx. Inspiratory stridor is a sign of laryngeal edema.

Exam Hint 12-10

Inspiratory stridor after endotracheal extubation is a sign of serious laryngeal edema. Administer oxygen and nebulize racemic epinephrine (MicroNephrin, AsthmaNefrin, Nephron) as a topical vasoconstrictor. Be prepared to reintubate a patient who does not respond.

MODULE M

Respiratory care plan

1. Determine a patient's pathophysiologic state (code: IIIF1) [difficulty: R, Ap, An]

Be able to recognize an airway obstruction problem in a patient and recommend or place the proper airway device to correct the problem. A chest radiograph should always be taken to confirm the location of a newly placed endotracheal or tracheostomy tube. All modern endotracheal and tracheostomy tubes contain a strip of radiopaque material near the distal tip of the tube. This is easily noticed as the white line seen on the chest film and confirms the location of the tip of the tube in the airway (see Fig. 12-24). The chest radiograph should be repeated if a significant change has occurred in the patient's condition or if the tube has been pulled back or pushed more deeply into the trachea. The chest film would also show a pneumothorax related to the tracheostomy procedure or other pulmonary condition.

2. Recommend starting a treatment based on the patient's response (code: IIIE2a) [difficulty: R, Ap, An]

See below.

3. Recommend a change in the therapeutic plan if indicated (code: IIIF2) [difficulty: R, Ap, An]

The indications or uses for the various airways are listed with the information on that airway. In general, the airway should be removed when it is no longer needed. Typically, an oropharyngeal airway should be removed from a patient who has regained consciousness. A nasopharyngeal airway should be removed if the patient no longer needs it as an airway or for a suctioning route. If an LMA is employed in the operating room, it is typically removed when the patient has recovered from the anesthesia. If an LMA or Combitube is used as a temporary emergency airway, they are typically removed when the patient has recovered. Or, if a longer duration and more secure airway is needed, these tubes are replaced with an endotracheal tube. Endotracheal and tracheostomy tubes can be removed when the patient does not need mechanical ventilation or a suctioning route, is no longer in danger of aspiration, or does not need a permanent artificial airway.

Effective communication is important for good patient care. The conscious patient with an endotracheal tube or tracheostomy is unable to speak. Alternative ways to communicate must be provided. A speaking tracheostomy tube or valve may be tried. Other examples of communication adjuncts include alphabet boards and picture boards for pointing and pencil and paper for notes. Head nods for yes and no and lip reading are often used. It is important that questions are worded so that they can be answered with a *yes* or *no*. Avoid questions that require a lengthy written answer unless the patient seems ready and willing to do so.

It is not possible to predict how a patient may react to the placement of an artificial airway or its prolonged need. Some patients react with relief and relax when the WOB is reduced. Others may become angry at the limitations imposed on them. Still others may become depressed. Be prepared to deal with these reactions or changes in the patient's emotional response to this very stressful situation.

4. Recommend a treatment be terminated (code: IIIE1) [difficulty: R, Ap, An]

See below.

5. Recommend discontinuing a treatment based on the patient's response (code: IIIE2h) [difficulty: R, Ap, An]

Be prepared to stop or to recommend the discontinuation of a particular airway and initiate the use of another, as needed. The indications for each type of airway have been presented earlier in the chapter.

BIBLIOGRAPHY

Altobelli N: Airway management. In Kacmarek RM, Stoller JK, Heuer AJ, editors: *Egan's fundamentals of respiratory care*, ed 10, St Louis, 2013, Mosby.

American Association for Respiratory Care: clinical practice guideline: management of airway emergencies, *Respir Care* 40(7):749, 1995 (Retired).

American Association for Respiratory Care: clinical practice guideline: removal of the endotracheal tube—2007 revision & update, *Respir Care* 52(1):81, 2007.

Anesthesia: *Practice guidelines for management of the difficult airway* 98(5):1269–1277, May 2003.

Artime CA, Hagberg CA: Tracheal extubation, *Respir Care* 59(6):991–1005, 2014.

Barnes TA: Emergency cardiovascular life support. In Kacmarek RM, Stoller JK, Heuer AJ, editors: *Egan's fundamentals of respiratory care*, ed 10, St Louis, 2013, Mosby.

Bolzan DW, Gomes WJ, Faresin SM, de Camargo Carvalho AC, De Paola AAM, Guizilini S: Volume–time curve: an alternative for endotracheal tube cuff management, *Respir Care* 57(12):2039–2044, 2012.

Branson RD, Gomaa D, Rodriquez D: Management of the artificial airway, *Respir Care* 59(6):974–990, 2014.

Cairo JM: *Pilbeam's mechanical ventilation*, ed 5, St Louis, 2012, Mosby.

Cheung NH, Napolitano LM: Tracheostomy: epidemiology, indications, timing, technique, and outcomes, *Respir Care* 59(6):895–919, 2014.

Circulation 2005: *Adjuncts for airway control and ventilation* 112, IV-51-IV-51; originally published online November 28, 2005.

Collins SR: Direct and indirect laryngoscopy: equipment and techniques, *Respir Care* 59(6):850–864, 2014.

Collins SR, Blank RS: Fiberoptic intubation: an overview and update, *Respir Care* 59(6):865–880, 2014.

Davies JD, Costa BK, Asciutto AJ: Approaches to manual ventilation, *Respir Care* 59(6):810–824, 2014.

Davies JD, May RA: Bortner: airway management. In Hess DR, MacIntyre NR, Mishoe SC, Galvin WF, Adams AB, editors: *Respiratory care principles & practice*, ed 2, Burlington, MA, 2012, Jones & Bartlett Learning.

Desai TR, Statter MB, Aresnman RM: Surgical management of the airway. In Goldsmith JP, Karotkin EH, editors: *Assisted ventilation of the neonate*, ed 3, Philadelphia, 1996, Saunders.

Deutsch ES: Tracheostomy: pediatric considerations, *Respir Care* 55(8):1082–1090, 2010.

Durbin CG, Perkins MP, Moores LK: Should tracheostomy be performed as early as 72 hours in patients requiring prolonged mechanical ventilation? *Respir Care* 55(1):76–87, 2010.

Durbin CG: Tracheostomy: why, when, and how? *Respir Care* 55(8):1056–1068, 2010.

Durbin CG, Bell CT, Shilling AM: Elective intubation, *Respir Care* 59(6):825–849, 2014.

Fisher DF, Kondili D, Williams J, Hess DR, Bittner EA, Schmidt UL: Tracheostomy tube change before day 7 is associated with earlier use of speaking valve and earlier oral intake, *Respir Care* 58(2):257–263, 2013.

Gros A, Holzapfel L, Marque S, Perard L, Demingeon G, Piralla B, et al.: Intra-individual variation of the cuff-leak test as a predictor of post-extubation stridor, *Respir Care* 57(12):2026–2031, 2012.

Haas CF, Eakin RM, Konkle MA, Blank R: Endotracheal tubes: old and new, *Respir Care* 59(6):933–955, 2014.

Hess DR: Managing the artificial airway, *Respir Care* 44:759, 1999.

Hess DR: Tracheostomy tubes and related appliances, *Respir Care* 50(4):497–510, 2005.

Hess DR, Altobelli NP: Tracheostomy tubes, *Respir Care* 59(6):956–973, 2014.

Hess DR, Branson RD: Airway and suctioning equipment. In Branson RD, Hess DR, Chatburn RL, editors: *Respiratory care equipment*, ed 2, Philadelphia, 1999, Lippincott Williams & Wilkins.

Hurford WE: The video revolution: a new view of laryngoscopy, *Respir Care* 55(8):1036–1045, 2010.

Jacobs IN, Pettignano MM, Pettignano R: Airway management. In Walsh BK, Czervinske MP, DiBlasi RM, editors: *Perinatal and pediatric respiratory care*, ed 3, St Louis, 2010, Saunders.

JEM 400 Endotracheal Tube Changer (Guide), product literature, Instrumentation Industries Inc, Bethel Park, PA.

Kacmarek RM, Dimas S, Mack CW: *The essentials of respiratory care*, ed 4, St Louis, 2005, Mosby.

Kunduk M, Appel K, Tunc M, Alanoglu Z, Alkis N, Dursun G, et al.: Preliminary report of laryngeal phonation during mechanical ventilation via a new cuffed tracheostomy tube, *Respir Care* 55(12):1161–1670, 2010.

Lewis RM: Airway care. In Fink JB, Hunt GE, editors: *Clinical practice in respiratory care*, Philadelphia, 1999, Lippincott-Raven.

May RA, Bortner PL: Airway management. In Hess DR, MacIntyre NR, Mishoe SC, et al.: *Respiratory care principles & practice*, Philadelphia, 2002, Saunders.

McIntyre D: Airway management. In Wyka KA, Mathews PJ, Rutkowski J, editors: *Foundations of respiratory care*, ed 2, Clifton Park, NY, 2012, Delmar.

Mechlin MW, Hurford WE: Emergency tracheal intubation: techniques and outcomes, *Respir Care* 59(6):881–894, 2014.

Menon N, Joffe AM, Deem S, Yanez ND, Grabinski A, Dagal AHC, et al.: Occurrence and complications of tracheal reintubation in critically ill adults, *Respir Care* 57(10):1555–1563, 2012.

O'Connor HH, White AC: Tracheostomy decannulation, *Respir Care* 55(8):1076–1081, 2010.

Pacheco-Lopez PC, Berkow LC, Hillel AT, Akst LM: Complications of airway management, *Respir Care* 59(6):1006–1021, 2014.

Part 4: adult basic life support, *Circulation* 112:IV18–IV34, 2005.

PressureEasy Cuff Pressure Controller, ReviveEasy PtL Airway, and Endotracheal/Trach Tube Pilot Tube Repair Kit, product literature, Respironics, Monroeville, PA.

Ramachandran SK, Kumar AM: Supraglottic airway devices, *Respir Care* 59(6):920–932, 2014.

Shilling AM, Durbin Jr CG: Airway management devices and advanced life support. In Cairo JM, editor: *Mosby's respiratory care equipment*, ed 9, St Louis, 2014, Mosby.

Shimizu T, Mizutani T, Yamashita S, Hagiya K, Tanaka M: Endotracheal tube extubation force: adhesive tape versus endotracheal tube holder, *Respir Care* 56(11):1825–1829, 2011.

Sills JR: An emergency cuff inflation technique, *Respir Care* 31(3):199, 1986.

White AC, Kher S, O'Connor HH: When to change a tracheostomy tube, *Respir Care* 55(8):1069–1075, 2010.

White AC, Purcell E, Urquhart B, Joseph B, O'Connor HH: Accidental decannulation following placement of a trachestomy tube, *Respir Care* 57(12):2019–2025, 2012.

White GC: *Equipment theory for respiratory care*, ed 4, Albany, NY, 2005, Delmar.

1. A respiratory therapist is preparing a stainless-steel-type laryngoscope handle and blade for an anesthesiologist. The light does not shine. Which of the following should be done to fix the problem?
     1. Get a smaller blade to fit the handle.
     2. Get a larger blade to fit the handle.
     3. Tighten the light bulb.
     4. Replace the handle with a plastic one.
     5. Replace the batteries.
   A. 4 only
   B. 2 only
   C. 3 and 5 only
   D. 1 and 4 only

2. An oropharyngeal airway would be indicated under which of the following conditions?
     1. Maintain the airway before a tracheostomy.
     2. Seizure activity is expected or present.
     3. Supine unconscious patient with an upper-airway obstruction
     4. Patient with a traumatic jaw injury
     5. An orally intubated patient is biting the tube.
   A. 3 and 5 only
   B. 4 and 5 only
   C. 1 and 4 only
   D. 2, 3, and 5 only

3. A respiratory therapist has just assisted with the endotracheal intubation of a normotensive adult patient. To minimize the risk of soft-tissue injury to the trachea, the tube cuff pressure should be:
   A. Less than 20 cm H_2O
   B. Less than 25 cm H_2O
   C. Less than 30 cm H_2O
   D. Less than 35 cm H_2O

4. A 50-year-old male patient with throat cancer will be having a laryngectomy tomorrow with the placement of a voice prosthesis. What type of airway would best serve the patient's long-term needs?
   A. Fenestrated laryngectomy tube
   B. Single-cannula tracheostomy tube
   C. Fenestrated tracheostomy tube
   D. Tracheostomy button

5. A respiratory therapist replaces a patient's tracheostomy tube with another one of the same size and inflates the cuff with 5 mL of air as was previously. Immediately, the patient has difficulty breathing and no air can be felt coming from the tube. What could be the problem?
   A. The tip of the tube has been placed into the subcutaneous tissues.
   B. The patient has closed the epiglottis over the trachea.
   C. More air must be added to the cuff to form a seal.
   D. The tube has accidentally been placed into the esophagus.

6. While assisting with a CPR attempt, the anesthesiologist asks for a properly sized endotracheal tube so that the patient's airway can be quickly intubated. The patient is a large, physically fit man. What tube would be best?
   A. A 7.0-mm-ID oral endotracheal tube
   B. A 10.0-mm-ID nasal endotracheal tube
   C. An 8.0-mm-ID nasal endotracheal tube
   D. A 9.0-mm-ID oral endotracheal tube

7. A spontaneously breathing patient's tracheostomy tube cuff pressure has been measured at 10 mm Hg. What would be recommended?
   A. Leave the cuff pressure as it is.
   B. Increase the cuff pressure to 15 mm Hg.
   C. Increase the cuff pressure to 30 cm water.
   D. Replace the tube with a larger one.

8. A 45-year-old female patient is brought into the Emergency Department from an automobile accident. She has facial trauma, including a broken nose and jaw. Because of heavy bleeding into her mouth, she is having difficulty breathing. Which of the following should be recommended to ensure a safe, effective airway?
   A. Place an oral airway.
   B. Place a tracheostomy tube.
   C. Place a nasopharyngeal airway.
   D. Place a nasal endotracheal tube.

9. While working in the neonatal Intensive Care Unit, a respiratory therapist is called to assist in the care of a 900-gram premature newborn. The neonatologist asks you to get the proper endotracheal tube for intubation. What would be the correct size tube?
   A. 1.5-mm ID
   B. 2.5-mm ID
   C. 3.5-mm ID
   D. 4.0-mm ID

10. A 59-kg (130-lb) woman must be intubated to initiate mechanical ventilation. What size tube should be used?
   A. 6.0-mm ID
   B. 6.5-mm ID
   C. 7.5-mm ID
   D. 9.0-mm ID

11. A respiratory therapist is going to assist in the ambulance transport of a 25-year-old patient. The patient has an oral endotracheal tube, and bag/mask ventilation will be performed during the trip. Which of the following should be chosen to help ensure that the endotracheal tube stays properly placed within the trachea?
   A. Pulse oximeter
   B. Capnograph
   C. Colorimetric CO_2 detector
   D. Electrocardiogram

12. All of the following should be monitored after a patient returns from having a tracheostomy tube placed EXCEPT:
    A. Cuff pressure
    B. Bowel sounds
    C. Breath sounds
    D. Excessive bleeding

13. Auscultation of a recently intubated patient in respiratory failure reveals absent breath sounds on the left side of the chest. The most likely cause of this finding is:
    A. Placement of the endotracheal tube into the right mainstem bronchus
    B. Placement of the endotracheal tube into the left mainstem bronchus
    C. Placement of the endotracheal tube into the esophagus
    D. A pneumothorax on the right side

14. While working the night shift, a respiratory therapist is called to intubate an apneic patient. Which of the following would be needed for an emergency oral intubation?
    1. Laryngoscope handle
    2. Stylet
    3. Proper laryngoscope blade
    4. 10-mL syringe
    5. Magill forceps
    A. 1 and 3 only
    B. 2 and 4 only
    C. 1, 2, 3, and 4 only
    D. 2, 3, 4, and 5 only

15. A respiratory therapist is assisting with the extubation of an adult patient. At what point in the procedure should the tube be removed?
    A. At the end of a peak inspiratory effort
    B. At the end of a normal exhalation
    C. At the start of a peak inspiratory effort
    D. During a forced vital capacity effort

16. A patient with a tracheostomy has just returned from a series of radiography procedures. Suddenly, the patient develops respiratory distress and cannot breathe. A suction catheter cannot be passed through the tracheostomy tube. What should be done?
    A. Attempt to pass a smaller suction catheter.
    B. Remove the tracheostomy tube.
    C. Ventilate with a manual resuscitation bag.
    D. Insert an endotracheal tube.

17. After a successful CPR attempt, a patient with an oral endotracheal tube is placed on a mechanical ventilator in the Intensive Care Unit. The respiratory therapist notices that the exhaled CO_2 monitor is appropriately changing color with each breath cycle. The patient's breath sounds are present on the right side but diminished on the left side. What is the most likely cause of this situation?
    A. Left-sided pneumothorax
    B. Right bronchial intubation

C. Malfunctioning exhaled CO_2 monitor
D. Delivered tidal volume is too small.

18. An 18-year-old woman has been admitted after being found unconscious from a drug overdose. She has severe atelectasis of the left lung caused by lying on her left side for 2 days. Her right lung is normal. She is going to require mechanical ventilation to open the atelectatic areas. What endotracheal tube should be suggested to properly treat the abnormal lung?
    A. Double lumen
    B. Standard
    C. Fenestrated tracheostomy
    D. Wire reinforced

19. An adult patient with epilepsy has been having unpredictable seizure activity. What oral endotracheal tube should be suggested to provide a secure airway?
    A. Double lumen
    B. Preformed
    C. Wire reinforced
    D. Guidable

20. A conscious patient is recovering from Guillain-Barré syndrome and is able to breathe spontaneously off of the mechanical ventilator for several hours. The patient currently has a single-cannula 7.5-mm-ID tracheostomy tube. To help the patient's weaning process but enable the patient to be ventilated at night, what should be done?
    A. Remove the tracheostomy tube when the patient is off of the ventilator.
    B. Substitute a speaking-type tracheostomy tube.
    C. Replace the current tracheostomy tube with one that is 6.0-mm ID.
    D. Substitute a fenestrated tracheostomy tube.

21. A semiconscious patient with many tracheal secretions will need frequent nasotracheal suctioning. What can be done to minimize trauma from the procedure?
    A. Insert a tracheostomy button with a speaking valve.
    B. Insert a nasopharyngeal airway.
    C. Sedate the patient and insert an oropharyngeal airway.
    D. Suction through a fenestrated tracheostomy tube.

22. An adult patient with a tracheostomy button and an attached speaking valve is complaining that it is difficult to breathe. You find that a 12-Fr suction catheter cannot be passed through the button. What should be done?
    A. Place a transtracheal oxygen catheter through the tracheostomy button.
    B. Force a larger suction catheter through the button.
    C. Remove the button and orally intubate the patient.
    D. Remove the speaking valve and assess the patient.

23. During a surgical procedure, the anesthesiologist wishes to protect the patient's airway and provide mechanical ventilation, but does not want to place an endotracheal tube. What airway should be used?
    A. Combitube
    B. Laryngeal mask airway
    C. Oropharyngeal airway
    D. Nasopharyngeal airway in each nostril

24. An unconscious 17-year-old patient has arrived in the Emergency Department. The patient was involved in an automobile accident, has a neck injury, and is wearing a neck brace. If the patient were to show signs of an upper-airway obstruction, all of the following could be used to maintain the airway EXCEPT:
    A. Oral endotracheal tube
    B. Nasopharyngeal airway
    C. Laryngeal mask airway
    D. Oropharyngeal airway

25. Immediate complications of an oral intubation include all of the following:
    1. **Tooth trauma**
    2. **Esophageal intubation**
    3. **Tracheoesophageal fistula**
    4. **Bronchial intubation**
    A. 3 and 4 only
    B. 2 and 3 only
    C. 1, 2, and 4 only
    D. 1, 2, 3, 4

26. A hospitalized patient rapidly develops ventilatory failure because of an accidental overdose of morphine sulfate for pain control. The preferred way to quickly provide a safe, secure airway is to:
    A. Place an oropharyngeal airway.
    B. Hyperextend the patient's neck.
    C. Place a nasal endotracheal tube.
    D. Place an oral endotracheal tube.

27. Indications for oral intubation include all the following EXCEPT:
    A. The patient requires mechanical ventilation.
    B. The patient has a cervical spine injury.
    C. The patient requires frequent tracheal suctioning.
    D. The patient is at risk for vomiting and aspirating.

28. A 2-year-old child admitted with severe croup has just been extubated after 2 days with an oral endotracheal tube. The child is given oxygen and aerosolized water through a heated large-volume nebulizer. Thirty minutes later, mild inspiratory stridor is heard over the child's throat area. What should be done *first*?
    A. Deliver nebulized racemic epinephrine.
    B. Reintubate the child.
    C. Perform a cricothyrotomy.
    D. Perform a tracheostomy.

29. A 55-year-old, 77-kg (170-lb) ventilator-dependent male patient has returned from the operating room with a 6.0-mm-ID tracheostomy tube. The respiratory therapist determines the cuff pressure to be 35 mm Hg. The ventilator is delivering a tidal volume of 750 mL and returning a tidal volume of 650 mL, and a leak can be heard at the tracheostomy site. What should be done?
    A. Increase the tidal volume by 100 mL to restore the delivered tidal volume.
    B. Increase the cuff pressure to stop the tidal volume leak.
    C. Replace the tracheostomy tube with one that is 8.5-mm ID.
    D. Deflate the cuff enough to reduce the cuff pressure to 20 mm Hg.

30. An intubated and mechanically ventilated adult patient has been returned to the long-term care unit after being transported to the radiology department for an abdominal radiograph examination. The respiratory therapist observes that the patient's trachea is midline; however, the patient's left chest area does not rise with inspiration as much as the right chest area. The endotracheal tube is at the 28-cm mark at the patient's teeth. What should be done now?
    A. Check the abdominal radiograph for signs of vomiting and aspiration.
    B. Pull the endotracheal tube back about 4 cm.
    C. Check the patient's end-tidal carbon dioxide level.
    D. Deliver a larger tidal volume breath to inflate the left lung better.

31. A patient is about to have an oral endotracheal tube inserted. What can be done during and/or after the procedure to determine its position within the trachea?
    1. **Get a chest radiograph.**
    2. **Palpate the larynx during insertion.**
    3. **Auscultate bilateral breath sounds.**
    4. **Attach an EDD after the tube is placed.**
    5. **Check for exhaled carbon dioxide.**
    A. 1 and 4 only
    B. 2 and 3 only
    C. 1, 3, and 5 only
    D. 1, 2, 3, 4, 5

32. A patient who suffered facial burns and smoke inhalation has recovered enough to be extubated. Although the patient is receiving 40% oxygen with a bland aerosol, significant inspiratory stridor is noticed within 15 minutes. Following the inhalation of a vasoconstricting medication, the patient's breath sounds are improved. Thirty minutes later the patient's SpO_2 level is 80% and the inspiratory stridor is more serious. The patient is very anxious and is pulling off the oxygen mask. What should the respiratory therapist recommend to best manage the patient's problem?
    A. Draw an arterial blood gas sample for measurement.
    B. Increase the patient's oxygen to 50%.
    C. Intubate the patient.
    D. Administer a sedative medication.

33. During a CPR attempt, a pediatric patient had an oral endotracheal tube placed. To ensure that the endotracheal tube is placed properly, all of the following should be recommended EXCEPT:
    A. Listen to the right upper lobe for breath sounds.
    B. Listen for bilateral lung sounds.
    C. Have a lateral neck radiograph taken.
    D. Have a chest radiograph taken.

34. A patient in the recovery room is found to have a tracheostomy tube cuff pressure of 35 mm Hg. If left unchanged, this cuff pressure could cause which of the following?
    1. Tracheomalacia
    2. Tracheoesophageal fistula
    3. Innominate artery erosion
    4. Damage to the vocal cords
    5. Loss of venous flow through the tracheal soft tissues
    A. 2 and 4 only
    B. 3 and 5 only
    C. 1, 2, and 4 only
    D. 1, 2, 3, and 5 only

35. A properly inserted Combitube will usually:
    1. Intubate the trachea
    2. Intubate the esophagus
    3. Prevent vomiting
    4. Maintain the airway
    A. 1 and 4 only
    B. 1 and 3 only
    C. 2 and 4 only
    D. 2, 3, and 4 only

36. A newborn child with macroglossia is having moderate airway obstruction episodes. What could be done to help manage the current situation?
    1. Place a nasopharyngeal airway.
    2. Place a tracheostomy button.
    3. Place the newborn in the prone position.
    4. Place an oral endotracheal tube.
    A. 2 only
    B. 1 and 3 only
    C. 3 and 4 only
    D. 1, 2, and 4 only

37. A 28-year-old patient is brought into the Emergency Department. The patient has a cervical spine injury from a diving accident and is wearing a neck brace. The patient is unconscious and inspiratory stridor can be heard. Arterial blood gases on 40% oxygen show the following: PaO_2 57 mm Hg, $PaCO_2$ 56 mm Hg, and pH 7.30. The physician has decided to establish a secure airway. What device should be recommended?
    A. 7.0-mm nasotracheal tube
    B. Berman oral airway
    C. 8.5-mm Carlens orotracheal tube
    D. 9.0-mm nasotracheal tube

38. An adult female patient is recovering from her neuromuscular disease. She has a standard tracheostomy tube and requires mechanical ventilation only during the night when sleeping. The physician asks the respiratory therapist for a recommendation about what can be done to enable her to communicate during the day but be put on the ventilator at night. What should be recommended?
    A. Change her to a fenestrated tracheostomy tube.
    B. Put a tracheostomy button into her during the day.
    C. Put an uncuffed tracheostomy tube into her.
    D. Put the obturator into her current tracheostomy tube during the day.

39. The Combitube has advantages over the standard LMA because:
    1. It can be placed nasally.
    2. A gastric tube can be placed through it to empty the stomach.
    3. It is available in small pediatric sizes.
    4. The patient can be ventilated whether it is placed into the esophagus or the trachea.
    A. 2 and 4 only
    B. 1 and 2 only
    C. 3 and 4 only
    D. 1 and 4 only

13 Suctioning the Airway

Note: It can be anticipated that the Therapist Multiple-Choice Examination (TMC) will include an *average of 4 of 140 actual questions* (3% of the exam) on suctioning the airway. (This is based on the question mix typically found on the National Board of Respiratory Care's previous Entry Level Examinations and Written Registry Examinations.)

Remember that the TMC version you take will include 20 additional questions being evaluated for possible inclusion in other versions of the TMC. So, there will be a total of 160 questions taken. There is no way to differentiate between the 140 actual questions and the 20 questions being evaluated for future use. Please go to the Introduction for detailed information on the Therapist Multiple-Choice Examination and the Clinical Simulation Examination.

MODULE A

Secretion removal and collection devices

1. Oropharyngeal suctioning catheters

a. Assemble oropharyngeal suctioning equipment (code: IIA11) [difficulty: R, Ap]

Oropharyngeal suctioning is considered a clean (not sterile) procedure. The suctioning device is often originally packaged sterile but may be used more than once. The Yankauer suction catheter is widely used, although several types are available. The Yankauer suction catheter is made of hard plastic and is angled to reach into the back of the mouth. One large opening or several medium-sized openings may be found at the tip of the catheter. The openings are large enough to permit easy suctioning of saliva, food, or vomit. Some handles include a thumb control valve so that suction can be applied to the tip only when wanted. Covering the opening with a thumb creates a vacuum at the tip for suctioning the patient's mouth (Fig. 13-1). The Yankauer may be discarded when no longer needed or sterilized for use with another patient.

A flexible plastic or rubber catheter also can be used. It should be the largest diameter possible to reduce the chance of it becoming plugged. If available, the opening at the catheter tip should be cut straight (perpendicular) across instead of at an angle. Side openings are not needed (Fig. 13-2). The catheter is discarded when no longer needed.

The catheter and Yankauer come preassembled. The proximal end must be attached to a vacuum source by a length of soft rubber tubing. With clean gloves on both hands, attach the Yankauer, plastic, or rubber catheter to the vacuum tubing. The vacuum must be applied to the tip of the catheter for oral secretions to be removed. Check for a vacuum at the tip by any of the following methods:

- Listen for the sound of air being drawn into the tip.
- Put the tip into a container of sterile water. Close the thumb control opening. The water must be drawn up the catheter.
- Place a clean-gloved hand over the tip if no water is available. Close the thumb control opening. The glove should be sucked onto the catheter.

b. Troubleshoot any problems with the equipment (code: IIA11) [difficulty: R, Ap]

If no vacuum is felt at the catheter tip, the following possible causes must be investigated.

1. The vacuum is not turned on

Check the following:
a. Some centralized vacuum systems have a single dial that turns the system off and on and sets the vacuum level. Other centralized vacuum systems have an ON and OFF switch and a dial for the vacuum level.
b. Freestanding vacuum systems must be plugged into a working electrical outlet. The ON and OFF switch must be turned on. Simple suctioning systems have a preset vacuum level. The more sophisticated systems have a variable vacuum level that must be set with a dial.

2. The system is not sealed, and the vacuum is lost to the atmosphere

Check the following:
a. Make sure the rubber vacuum tubing fits tightly over the connectors on the catheter and on the vacuum system.
b. Make sure the catheter and vacuum tubing are not cracked or cut. Replace a Yankauer, plastic, or rubber catheter or vacuum tubing that is defective.
c. Close the thumb control if it has been left open.

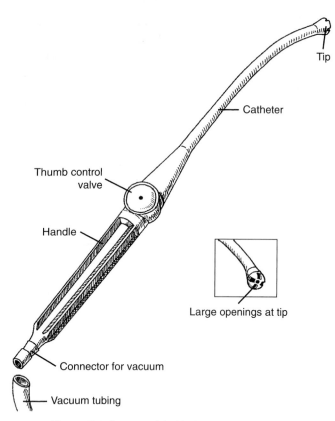

Figure 13-1 Features of the Yankauer suction catheter.

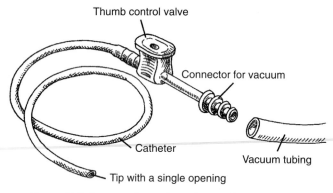

Figure 13-2 Features of a suction catheter with a cross-cut tip.

d. Check the central or freestanding vacuum system to make sure the secretion collection bottle is sealed properly.

3. The system is blocked, and no vacuum can get through to the tip

Check the following:
a. Check for a pinch in the vacuum tubing or soft catheter.
b. Check for a blockage in the catheter or vacuum tubing. Try to suction some sterile water to clear the blockage into the secretion collection bottle. Replace the catheter or vacuum tubing, or both, if the blockage cannot be cleared.
c. Empty a full collection bottle.

2. Tracheal suctioning catheters
a. Assemble tracheal suctioning equipment (code: IIA11) [difficulty: R, Ap]

Suction catheters are used to remove secretions and foreign material from the trachea. They come sterile and individually packaged. For adults and children, it is highly recommended that the outer diameter (OD) of the catheter be no more than one-half (50%) of the inner diameter (ID) of the artificial airway it is passing through. For infants, it is highly recommended that the OD of the catheter be no more than 70% of the ID of the artificial airway it is passing through. This guideline serves two purposes. First, a smaller catheter removes less air from the patient's lungs. This will help to minimize hypoxemia and atelectasis. Second, a smaller catheter minimizes obstruction of the airway so that the patient will be able to breathe around the catheter.

Exam Hint 13-1

Remember that for adults and children the outer diameter of the suction catheter should be no more than one-half (50%) of the inner diameter of the endotracheal tube or tracheostomy tube.

Table 13-1 presents the recommended suction catheter sizes for the various endotracheal tubes (ETs) or tracheostomy tubes (TTs). The practitioner also can easily compare the relative sizes of the tube and suction catheter at the bedside before suctioning. Suction catheters are sized by the French (Fr) scale of the OD. ETs and TTs are sized by ID and OD in millimeters and often by OD in French. Review Table 12-1 in Chapter 12 if necessary.

b. Calculations related to catheter size (math review)

The following formula can be used to calculate the OD of any suction catheter to determine the ET or TT size with which the suction catheter may be used:

EXAMPLE 1

Calculate the OD of a 12-Fr suction catheter:
This size of catheter, therefore, could be used with an 8-mm ID ET. Figure 13-3 shows the relative sizes of this ET and catheter.

Use the following formula to estimate the maximum suction catheter French size for the ID of an ET or TT:

$$\frac{\text{ID of endotracheal tube} \times 3}{2} = \text{Maximum diameter (Fr) of catheter}$$

EXAMPLE 2

Calculate the largest suction catheter size that should be used with a size 8 (ID) ET:

$$\frac{8 \times 3}{2} = \frac{24}{2} = 12 \text{ Fr suction catheter}$$

TABLE 13-1	Recommended Suction Catheter French Sizes for Endotracheal and Tracheostomy Tubes*	
Age	**Tube Inner Diameter (mm)**	**Size of Suction Catheter (Fr)**
Infant		
1000 g	2.5	5
1000-2000 g	3	6
2000-3000 g	3.5	8
3000 g to 6 months	3.5-4	8
Child		
18 months	4	8
3 years	4.5	8
5 years	5	10
6 years	5.5	10
8 years	6	10
Adult		
16 years	7	10
Normal-size woman	7.5-8	12
Normal-size man	8-8.5	14
Large adult	9-10	16

*For suctioning of endotracheal tubes (ETs) and tracheostomy tubes (TTs) of an adult or child, the suction catheter's outer diameter should be no more than one-half (50%) of the inner diameter of the ET or TT. For suctioning an infant's ET or TT, the suction catheter's outer diameter should be no more than 70% of the inner diameter of the artificial airway.

Therefore, a 12-Fr suction catheter could be used with an 8-mm ID ET (or TT) (see Fig. 13-3).

Knowing the ID of a suction catheter is helpful because it relates to the maximum particle size that can pass through it. The following formula can be used to interconvert from French OD to millimeters ID:

$$mm = \frac{Fr - 2}{4}$$

EXAMPLE 3

What is the ID in millimeters of a 12-Fr suction catheter?

$$mm = \frac{12 - 2}{4}$$

$$mm = \frac{10}{4}$$

$$mm = 2.5 \quad \text{(see Figure 13-3)}$$

Therefore, a 12-Fr suction catheter (with a 4-mm OD) can be used to suction particles up to 2.5 mm in diameter.

c. Open-airway suctioning

The term *open-airway suctioning* (open suctioning technique) is used here to refer to a suctioning procedure on a patient who is spontaneously breathing room air after being disconnected from the source of supplemental

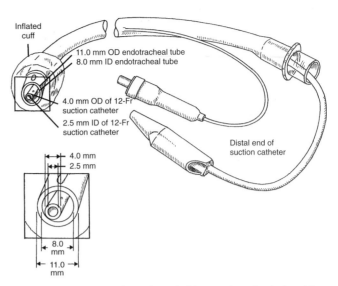

Figure 13-3 A 12-Fr suction catheter inside an endotracheal tube with an 8-mm inner diameter (ID). The outer diameter (OD) of the suction catheter should be no more than one-half the ID of the tube so that the patient can breathe around it.

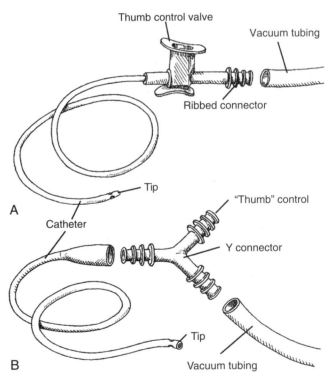

Figure 13-4 Two types of suction catheters with angle-cut tips and side holes. **A,** This catheter has its own thumb control valve. **B,** This catheter must have a thumb control valve constructed from a Y-connector.

oxygen. For example, in a patient with a normal upper airway, the oxygen mask is removed for nasotracheal suctioning. Also, in a patient with an ET or TT, the aerosol T-piece (Briggs adapter) or ventilator circuit is removed to allow suctioning.

These types of catheters have been in use for many years. The two basic types are shown in Figure 13-4. Closing the

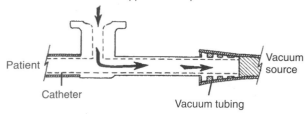

An open thumb control valve lets room air enter
so that no vacuum is applied to the patient

Figure 13-5 Close-up of a thumb control valve showing how room air is drawn into the vacuum tubing when the valve is left open. Closing the valve creates a vacuum at the catheter tip, allowing secretions to be suctioned.

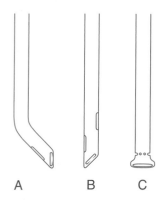

Figure 13-6 Close-ups of the ends of three suction catheters. **A,** Coudé (curved-tip) catheter. The curve may help guide the catheter into either the left or the right mainstem bronchus. **B,** Bevel-cut tip with two offset side holes. **C,** Ring tip with several side holes around it.

thumb control, as shown in Figure 13-5, allows the vacuum to be selectively applied to the secretions when desired. The tips of the catheters can vary greatly. A considerable amount of effort has been spent trying to develop a catheter tip that most effectively removes secretions without damaging the tracheal mucosa. Figure 13-6 shows some of the catheter tips that have been developed to minimize mucosal damage. Note that all feature at least one opening in the catheter that is back from the opening at the tip. Compare this with the single end opening found on the oral suction catheter (see Fig. 13-2). The side openings are designed to prevent the vacuum from being applied to the tip when it makes contact with the mucosa.

Figure 13-4 shows the attachment of an open-airway suction catheter to the vacuum tubing. The other end of the vacuum tubing is attached to the vacuum regulator system. Notice in Figures 13-4 and 13-6 that most catheters are straight throughout their length. All of these catheters tend to enter the right mainstem bronchus during deep suctioning. This is because the right mainstem bronchus's angle off of the trachea is less acute than that of the left mainstem bronchus. Therefore, it is difficult, if not impossible, to use any of these catheters to suction the left mainstem bronchus. The Coudé catheter has an angled tip to make it easier to guide into the left (or right) mainstem bronchus (see Fig. 13-6, C). When these catheters are

used, the direction of the thumb control valve can help the therapist determine the direction of the bent catheter tip.

Use of these traditional types of catheters during open-airway suctioning always results in some level of hypoxemia. The newer, insufflating suction catheter is designed to provide either oxygen through the catheter or vacuum for suctioning. The thumb control end of the catheter is modified with two male-type tubing connectors and a way to switch the lumen of the catheter between them. The thumb control is set to direct the oxygen through the catheter and into the patient's airway as the catheter is advanced. After the catheter has been deeply placed into the trachea for suctioning, the thumb control is switched from delivering oxygen to applying suction.

With open-airway suctioning, only the hand covered by a sterile glove can touch the sterile catheter. A clean glove can be on the practitioner's other hand because it does not touch the catheter.

While holding the body of the catheter, the thumb control valve, and the vacuum connector with the sterile-gloved hand and the vacuum tubing with the clean-gloved hand, slip the vacuum tubing over the catheter's vacuum connector. The seal should be tight so that no vacuum leak occurs. From now on, only the sterile-gloved hand may touch the part of the catheter that makes contact with the patient. The clean-gloved hand may touch only the thumb control valve and vacuum tubing. If the catheter is contaminated, it must be discarded.

The catheter can be tested for patency and vacuum at the tip by the three methods described earlier in the discussion on oropharyngeal suction devices. Note that only a *sterile* glove may be touched against the tip of the suction catheter to check for a vacuum.

d. Closed-airway suctioning

The term *closed-airway suctioning* (closed suctioning technique) is used here to refer to a suctioning procedure in which the patient remains connected to the original source of oxygen. This is the preferred method of suctioning any intubated patient receiving mechanical ventilation who is likely to become hypoxic when disconnected from the oxygen source. The closed suctioning technique should be used with those who are receiving a high oxygen percentage, have positive end-expiratory pressure (PEEP), or are at risk of lung derecruitment. In addition, closed-airway suctioning may reduce the risk of ventilator-associated pneumonia.

In closed-airway suctioning systems, a flexible, clear plastic sheath covers the catheter to maintain its sterility (Fig. 13-7). Because of this, the practitioner should wear clean rather than sterile gloves. When used for patients who need frequent suctioning, self-contained systems have a financial advantage over the traditional disposable catheter and gloves suctioning kits. Closed-system suction catheters come with either the traditional straight tip or the Coudé tip for selective bronchial suctioning.

Another device used to create a sealed system for ET suctioning consists of an elbow adapter that has an inner

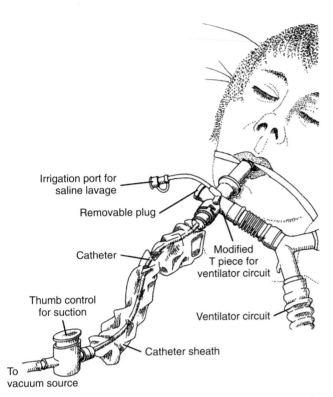

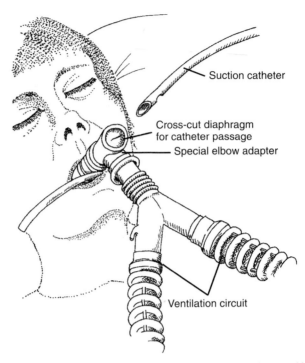

Figure 13-8 Features and placement of a special elbow adapter, which allows closed-airway suctioning without loss of tidal volume or pressure during mechanical ventilation.

Figure 13-7 Self-contained catheter and sheath suctioning system for closed-airway suctioning. Based on the Kimberly–Clark/Ballard Trach Care closed endotracheal suction device.

plastic sleeve or diaphragm. As the traditional catheter is inserted into the opening on the elbow adapter, the sleeve or diaphragm conforms to the catheter so that no air leakage occurs (Fig. 13-8). This ensures that the ventilator-delivered volumes and pressures are not lost through a leak.

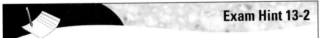

Exam Hint 13-2

Remember that endotracheal suctioning is a sterile procedure. Gloves or a catheter that has become contaminated must be replaced with new sterile equipment.

e. Troubleshoot any problems with the equipment (code: IIA11) [difficulty: R, Ap]

The three common causes of an equipment failure and how to troubleshoot them are described in the earlier discussion on oropharyngeal suction devices. Remember to completely withdraw the closed-airway suctioning catheter from the ET into the sheath, or it will partially obstruct the tube.

3. Specimen collectors

a. Assemble specimen collection equipment (code: IIA11) [difficulty: R, Ap]

A variety of specimen collectors (commonly called *Lukens traps*) are available. They are packaged as sterile so that no contamination of the sputum sample with nonpatient organisms occurs. Figures 13-9 through 13-12 show the key features and functions of several sputum sample collectors. The sputum sample is obtained through a suction catheter or bronchoscope.

The specimen container (jar) has volume markings. It screws into either a special lid used to suction the specimen or a regular lid. The regular lid is used for shipment to the laboratory. The special lids used in the systems featured in Figures 13-9 and 13-10 must have a short length of rubber vacuum tubing connected between the lid and a sterile catheter. Figure 13-11 shows a system with its own catheter. The vacuum source is provided to these specimen collectors by a length of vacuum tubing, as in the previously described suction catheter systems. Figure 13-12 shows a DeLee system, which is sometimes used in the delivery room. The physician, nurse, or practitioner uses mouth suction to remove secretions from the newborn. In all of these examples, after the sample has been collected, the special lid is replaced with the regular specimen jar lid.

A properly working specimen collection system provides a vacuum to the tip of the suction catheter when the thumb control valve or mouthpiece is sealed and vacuum is applied. This is tested by dipping the catheter tip into a container of sterile water or saline solution. The liquid is drawn up the catheter and deposited in the specimen jar. (The water can be discarded from the jar.)

b. Troubleshoot any problems with the equipment (code: IIA11) [difficulty: R, Ap]

Failure to have a vacuum at the tip of the suction catheter may be caused by any of the previously mentioned problems. Each can be checked and corrected by the methods

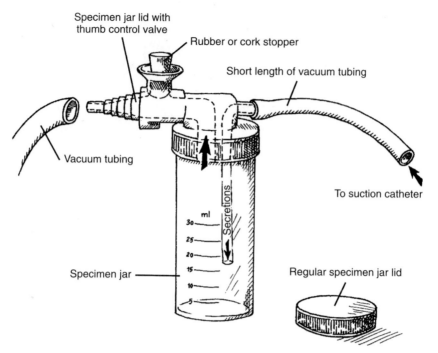

Figure 13-9 Features of a collection system for sputum specimens that includes a thumb control valve.

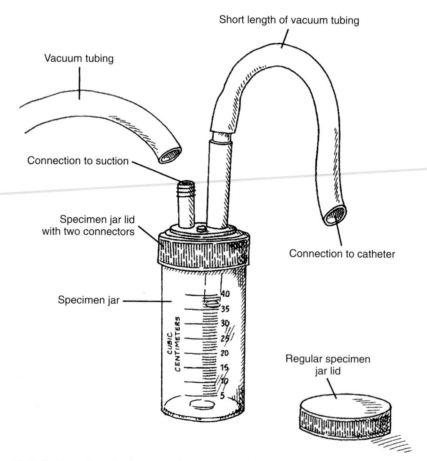

Figure 13-10 Features of a collection system for sputum specimens that does not have a thumb control valve.

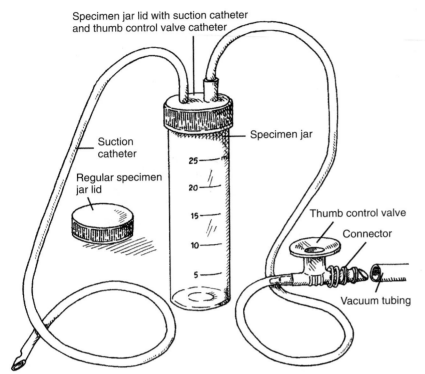

Specimen jar lid with suction catheter and thumb control valve catheter

Suction catheter

Regular specimen jar lid

Specimen jar

Thumb control valve

Connector

Vacuum tubing

Figure 13-11 Features of a collection system for sputum specimens that has a thumb control valve built into the catheter.

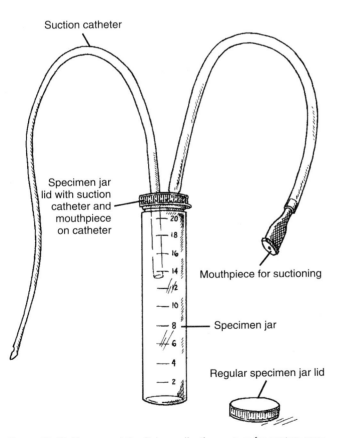

Suction catheter

Specimen jar lid with suction catheter and mouthpiece on catheter

Mouthpiece for suctioning

Specimen jar

Regular specimen jar lid

Figure 13-12 Features of the DeLee collection system for sputum specimens, showing the mouthpiece through which the practitioner can apply suction.

listed earlier. There are two causes of an inability to suction secretions. First, the jar is not tightly connected into the special lid, allowing room air to be drawn in. Simply attach the lid tightly. Second, the secretion channel is plugged. Discard it and replace it with a new specimen collector.

MODULE B

Vacuum regulator systems

1. Assemble the necessary vacuum regulator system: vacuum pump, regulator, and collection bottle (canister) (code: IIA11) [difficulty: R, Ap]

Vacuum regulators are preassembled by the manufacturer. The two basic types are described here. Components must be added to make them fully functional.

a. Portable vacuum systems

Portable units are designed to be moved with the patient. They may be mounted on a small platform (Fig. 13-13) or on a wheeled cart. The portable systems generally include an electrically powered vacuum pump with an ON/OFF switch and a collection bottle. Some units have a control valve for adjusting the level of negative pressure. A negative-pressure gauge is used to determine how much vacuum is being applied. A length of rubber vacuum tubing is used to pass the negative pressure from the pump to the collection bottle. Another length of vacuum tubing is used to pass the vacuum to the suction catheter. Portable

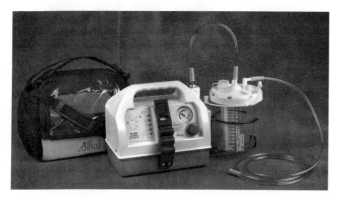

Figure 13-13 Portable suction machine, showing the electrically powered motor, collection bottle and cap, and connecting tubing. (Courtesy of Allied Health Care Products, St Louis, MO.)

systems are not as powerful as central vacuum systems. They are less effective at suctioning out large amounts of thick secretions.

In general, the following steps are followed to make the unit operational:

1. Plug the vacuum pump into a working electrical outlet. Battery-operated units should have fully charged batteries.
2. Place a clean, empty collection bottle into its holder on the cart. The bottle should be able to hold at least 500 mL of fluid.
3. Slip the rubber lid onto the open top of the collection bottle. Both vacuum tubing connectors on the lid must be patent.
4. Slip one end of a short length of vacuum tubing over the connector on the vacuum pump and the other end over one of the tubing connectors on the collection bottle lid.
5. Slip one end of vacuum tubing over the other tubing connector on the collection bottle lid. The vacuum tubing should be no more than 3 feet long. The other end of the vacuum tubing is connected to the suction catheter.
6. Turn on the unit and determine the negative pressure as follows:
   • Pinch closed the long vacuum tubing
   • Turn on the vacuum pump
   • Observe the pressure on the negative-pressure gauge
7. If the unit has a fixed vacuum level, the observed negative pressure should match that listed by the manufacturer.
8. If the unit has a variable vacuum level, adjust the vacuum control knob to the desired level.

b. Central vacuum systems

Central (wall) vacuum systems usually are available at each patient's bedside in all special care units. Each of the wall outlets is connected through a hospital-wide piping system to a large, electrically powered vacuum pump. It is capable of generating a negative pressure far greater than that needed in most patient care situations. A regulator is used to reduce the vacuum to the desired clinical level

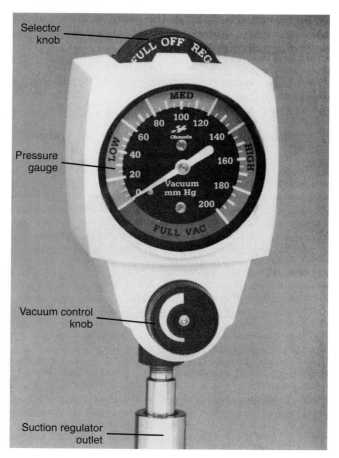

Figure 13-14 Features of the Ohmeda central vacuum regulator with a three-position selector knob. (Courtesy of Ohmeda Medical, Columbia, MD.)

(Fig. 13-14). Either a Quick Connect or a Diameter Index Safety System connector is used to attach the regulator to the central vacuum system.

Most regulators have a selector knob that allows the user to turn the vacuum off (OFF setting) or to switch between full vacuum (FULL setting) and a regulated level of vacuum (REG setting). The FULL setting opens the unit to the maximum level of vacuum available from the central pump. The REG setting allows the user to adjust the vacuum level through a wide range.

In general, the following steps are followed to make the unit operational:

1. Connect the regulator to a working suction outlet.
2. Screw a clean, empty collection bottle onto its connector on the regulator. The bottle must be able to hold at least 500 mL of fluid.
3. Slip one end of a length of vacuum tubing over the tubing connector on the collection bottle. The vacuum tubing should be no more than 3 feet long. The other end of the vacuum tubing is connected to the suction catheter.
4. Determine the negative pressure as follows:
   • Pinch closed the vacuum tubing (Fig. 13-15)
   • Turn the selector knob to REG
   • Observe the pressure on the negative-pressure gauge

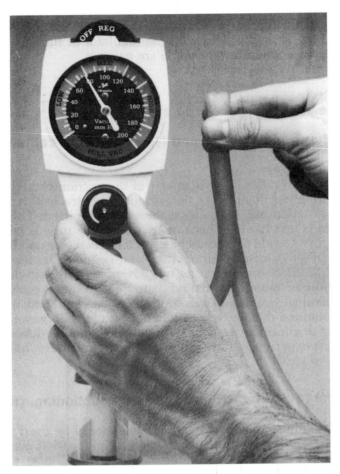

Figure 13-15 The negative pressure level is set on the Ohmeda central vacuum regulator by pinching the vacuum tubing and adjusting the vacuum control knob. The vacuum pressure is displayed on the pressure gauge. (Courtesy of Ohmeda Medical, Columbia, MD.)

5. Adjust the vacuum control knob to the desired level. If the secretions are too thick to be drawn up the suction catheter, the negative pressure must be increased.

2. Troubleshoot any problems with the equipment (code: IIA11) [difficulty: R, Ap]

a. Portable vacuum systems

With a portable vacuum system, check the following when trying to determine the cause of a loss of vacuum:
- The vacuum pump is plugged into a working electrical outlet.
- The vacuum pump is turned on.
- The vacuum control valve is set at the desired negative pressure.
- The lid to the collection bottle is tightly sealed.
- The vacuum tubing tightly connects the pump to the collection bottle and the collection bottle to the suction catheter.
- No knots or obstructions are present in the vacuum tubing or catheter.
- The collection bottle is not filled above its maximum level.

Correct any potential problems. Do not use a portable vacuum system that will not generate the negative pressure it is supposed to generate.

b. Central vacuum systems

With a central vacuum system, check the following when trying to determine the cause of a loss of vacuum:
- The regulator is plugged into a working vacuum outlet.
- The vacuum control valve is set at the desired negative pressure.
- The collection bottle is tightly screwed onto the suction-regulator outlet.
- The vacuum tubing tightly connects the collection bottle to the suction catheter.
- No knots or obstructions are present in the vacuum tubing or catheter.
- The collection bottle is not filled above its maximum level.

Correct any potential problems. Do not use a central vacuum system outlet that will not generate the negative pressure it should generate. Occasionally, less negative pressure than expected is found when the central vacuum system is being heavily used. No problem exists with the regulator or tubing. The vacuum pressure will increase when fewer people are suctioning.

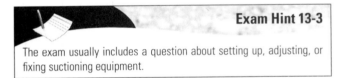

Exam Hint 13-3

The exam usually includes a question about setting up, adjusting, or fixing suctioning equipment.

MODULE C

Initiate suctioning procedures to remove tracheal and oral secretions.

Tracheal or oral secretions must be actively removed by suctioning whenever the patient cannot clear them out and there is a risk of aspiration or airway obstruction. Suctioning may be needed in patients who are unconscious and lack swallowing or coughing reflexes or in patients who may be too weak to cough effectively to remove tracheal secretions. Often the physician writes a standing order to suction the patient as needed. However, in many institutions, a protocol exists to suction any patient who is at risk of obstruction of the airway. For example, a comatose patient who vomits should have the mouth suctioned out even if no specific order is written.

1. Hazards and complications associated with suctioning

Suctioning secretions from a patient's trachea, by any method, places the patient at risk. The respiratory therapist must be prepared to auscultate breath sounds and check the patient's vital signs. Additional equipment may

---

BOX 13-1   Hazards and Complications of Endotracheal Suctioning

---

Cardiac arrest
Respiratory arrest
Hypoxemia
Cardiac dysrhythmias
Bronchoconstriction/bronchospasm
Increased intracranial pressure
Hypertension
Hypotension
Apnea from interruption of mechanical ventilation
Pulmonary hemorrhage
Mechanical trauma to tracheal and bronchial mucosa
Cross-infection between the patient and the respiratory therapist
Atelectasis

BOX 13-2   Contraindications for, Hazards of, and Complications of Nasotracheal Suctioning

---

Contraindications
Absolute
Epiglottitis
Laryngotracheobronchitis (croup)
Basilar skull fracture

Relative
Blocked nasal passages
Nasal bleeding
Acute facial, neck, or head injury
Bleeding disorder
Upper respiratory tract infection
Irritable airway
Laryngospasm

Hazards and Complications
Cardiac arrest
Respiratory arrest
Hypoxemia
Cardiac dysrhythmias
Bronchoconstriction/bronchospasm
Increased intracranial pressure
Hypertension
Hypotension
Pulmonary hemorrhage
Cross-infection between the patient and the respiratory therapist
Atelectasis
Pain
Catheter misdirected into esophagus
Gagging and/or vomiting
Uncontrolled coughing
Mechanical trauma (nasal turbinates, perforation of pharynx, nasal bleeding, bleeding of the tracheal and bronchial mucosa)

---

be needed, such as a pulse oximeter, electrocardiogram monitor, and manual resuscitation bag and mask. Box 13-1 presents the hazards and complications of endotracheal suctioning. Box 13-2 presents the contraindications, hazards, and complications of nasotracheal suctioning. In addition, the respiratory therapist must protect himself or herself from the patient's secretions by wearing eye goggles, a face mask, and gloves. The following two complications can occur during the suctioning procedure. They must be prevented if possible and corrected if they happen.

a. Minimize hypoxemia during the suctioning procedure (code: IIIC1) [difficulty: R, Ap, An]

Suctioning the trachea removes air (including oxygen), as well as secretions, from the lungs. However, hypoxemia can be minimized by hyperoxygenating the patient for 1-2 minutes before suctioning. It is generally recommended that the patient receive 100% oxygen, if possible. Infants younger than 6 months should be given a fractional concentration of inspired oxygen (F_IO_2) only 10%-20% greater than their base level to minimize the risk of retinopathy of prematurity, also known as *retrolental fibroplasia*.

Before beginning the procedure, check the patient's arterial blood gas results or SpO_2 to see whether the patient is hypoxic. The SpO_2 also can be monitored throughout the suctioning procedure to evaluate for hypoxemia (review the chapter for guidelines on oxygenation and limiting hypoxemia). After suctioning, the patient can be given supplemental oxygen until the SpO_2 reaches the baseline level, typically at least 90%. The patient's chart also should be checked for any history of cardiac problems. Sudden hypoxemia from suctioning can result in life-threatening dysrhythmias, such as premature ventricular contractions. Check the patient's pulse rate and rhythm before and after suctioning. If the patient is using a cardiac monitor, it should be watched for rate and rhythm changes that are

related to the suctioning procedure. Tachycardia is frequently seen with hypoxemia. Check the blood pressure of any patient who has suctioning-related dysrhythmias. The patient's vital signs should return to normal when oxygenation is restored.

Any modern mechanical ventilator can be set to deliver 100% oxygen. The most current ventilators have a 100% oxygen button designed just for this purpose. Pushing it results in the patient receiving pure oxygen for 1-2 minutes (depending on the manufacturer). Several sigh breaths also can be delivered. A closed-airway suction catheter can be used with the ventilator, as discussed earlier, to minimize hypoxemia.

For a spontaneously breathing patient, a nonrebreathing mask can be applied and set to deliver close to 100% oxygen. If a nonrebreathing mask is not available, turn up the oxygen flow or percentage on whatever appliance the patient is using. A spontaneously breathing patient with an ET or TT can have 100% oxygen delivered through a Briggs adapter/aerosol T-piece. A manual resuscitation bag also can be used to give the patient several sigh breaths.

All patients must be reoxygenated before another attempt at suctioning is made. Giving 100% oxygen after the suctioning procedure helps the patient to reoxygenate faster. Giving several sigh breaths also helps reoxygenation to occur faster than normal tidal volume breathing does.

b. Vagus or vagal nerve stimulation

Vagal nerve endings are found in the hypopharynx and trachea. When they are mechanically stimulated by a suction catheter, any of the following may be seen:

- The patient may have an induced bronchospasm.
- The patient may become bradycardic.
- The patient's blood pressure may decrease secondary to the bradycardia.

Listen to the patient's breath sounds before and after suctioning to determine whether an increase in wheezing is present, which could indicate bronchospasm. Check the heart rate and rhythm by palpation or cardiac monitor to determine whether the patient is becoming bradycardic. The blood pressure also can be measured to check for hypotension.

Further suctioning should be delayed, if possible, until the patient's wheezing and vital signs have returned to normal. It may be necessary to modify the suctioning procedure by not going as deeply and striking the carina, not twisting the catheter, or not suctioning for as long to reduce the risk of vagal stimulation. A local anesthetic, such as lidocaine (Xylocaine), can be nebulized (with a physician's order) to reduce the local reaction to the catheter.

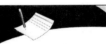

Exam Hint 13-4

There is usually a question about safety issues related to suctioning. Understand the importance of hyperoxygenating a patient before and after a tracheal suctioning procedure. Hypoxemia can result in unstable vital signs. Be prepared to stop suctioning, give extra oxygen, or get help. Vagal stimulation can cause bradycardia and/or bronchospasm.

2. Perform endotracheal tube or tracheostomy tube suctioning on the patient (code: IIIB2) [difficulty: R, Ap, An]

The American Association for Respiratory Care (AARC) Clinical Practice Guidelines listed in the Bibliography section at the end of the chapter present all the suctioning indications. Key indications include:

- Removing accumulated secretions, blood, or other debris from the breathing tube or the patient's airways
- Obtaining a sputum sample for microbiology or cytology examination
- Stimulating the patient's cough to help mobilize pulmonary secretions

- Clinical indications of retained secretions, such as breath sounds demonstrating rhonchi (crackles), increased tactile fremitus, worsening oxygenation, or worsening mechanical ventilation parameters (e.g., increased peak inspiratory pressure and/or decreased tidal volume)

The procedure for ET or TT suctioning is the same for both types of tubes, except that the catheter does not need to be inserted as far into the TT before hitting the carina. The generally accepted steps in the procedure are as follows:

1. Check the chart for specific orders, an order to suction as needed, or any special patient considerations, such as unstable vital signs, cardiopulmonary conditions, oxygenation, and the types and amounts of secretions.
2. Gather the necessary equipment:
   - Suction catheter for an adult or child no larger than one-half (50%) the ID of the patient's ET or TT. An infant's suction catheter outer diameter should be no more than 70% of the ID of the artificial airway. See Table 13-1 for recommendations.
   - Two sterile gloves to wear for open-airway suctioning or two procedure (clean) gloves for closed-airway suctioning.
   - Specimen collector if ordered.
   - Vacuum system and vacuum tubing.
   - Sterile water or normal saline in a sterile basin.
3. Explain the procedure to the patient.
4. If possible, place the patient in the semi-Fowler's and sniffing positions.
5. Give the adult patient 100% O_2 for 30-60 seconds before suctioning and for at least 1 minute afterward until the patient is no longer hypoxemic. (For an infant younger than 6 months, increase the F_IO_2 by 0.1.)
6. Get help if necessary.
7. Set the desired vacuum level. The AARC Clinical Practice Guidelines suggest that the vacuum be set at the lowest possible level that still effectively removes secretions. The following ranges for vacuum are appropriate:
   - Adults: −100 to −150 mm Hg
   - Children: −100 to −120 mm Hg
   - Infants: −80 to −100 mm Hg
   - Neonates: −80 to −100 mm Hg

   To prevent tissue trauma, hypoxemia, and atelectasis, negative pressures greater than −150 mm Hg should not be used.
8. Wash your hands.
9. Using sterile technique, put on the gloves, remove the catheter from its packaging, and connect the vacuum tubing to the catheter.
10. Test that the vacuum is reaching the tip of the catheter.
11. Disconnect the ventilator circuit or O_2 appliance from the tube (except with a closed-airway suctioning system).

12. Suction the tube:
   (a) Without any vacuum, quickly and gently pass the catheter down the tube until an obstruction is felt. Withdraw the catheter 2 cm.
   (b) Withdraw the catheter with a twisting motion while suctioning intermittently. Suction to clear out any secretions. Typically, in an adult, suctioning may be applied for 5-10 seconds. In an infant, suctioning may be applied for no longer than 5 seconds.
   (c) Turning the patient's head to the right might help direct the catheter down the left mainstem bronchus. The catheter tends to enter the right mainstem bronchus if the head is in a neutral position or twisted to the left.
   (d) The entire procedure of disconnection of the O_2, suctioning, reconnection of the O_2, and normal breathing should done in less than 15 seconds.

13. Reoxygenate the patient for at least 1 minute before suctioning again. Giving 100% O_2 (or 10% more than the base level in an infant) and several sigh breaths helps accomplish this faster.

14. Monitor the patient's vital signs, SpO_2 level, and breath sounds before suctioning again. Suction again, if needed, when the patient is stable.

15. Saline should *not* be routinely instilled into the patient's tracheal tube. However, normal saline solution may be instilled to lubricate the tube or if the secretions are too thick to be suctioned out easily. The saline solution may help to loosen the secretions. The patient also is likely to cough vigorously. The amount of saline solution to be instilled varies with the size of the patient and the thickness of the secretions. The general guidelines for instillation of normal saline solution are as follows:
   - Neonate: 0.5-1.0 mL
   - Child: 2-5 mL
   - Adults: about 5 mL at a time or in divided doses
   - A physician's order may be needed to instill saline solution.

16. Dispose of the catheter and glove by pulling the glove inside out over the catheter. If a self-contained system is part of the ventilator circuit, it should be replaced when the circuit is replaced, if not sooner. Current guidelines recommend replacement when visibly soiled or malfunctioning.

17. Rinse sterile water or sterile saline through the vacuum tubing to clear it of secretions.

18. Turn off the suction unit.

3. Perform nasotracheal suctioning on the patient (code: IIIB2) [difficulty: R, Ap, An]

See the AARC Clinical Practice Guidelines listed in the Bibliography section at the end of the chapter for all of the suctioning indications. Key indications include:
- Removing accumulated secretions, blood, or other debris from the patient's airways
- Obtaining a sputum sample for microbiology or cytology examination
- Stimulating the patient's cough to help mobilize pulmonary secretions
- Clinical indications of retained secretions, such as breath sounds revealing rhonchi (crackles), increased tactile fremitus, or worsening oxygenation

The nasotracheal suctioning procedure is performed on a patient who does not have an ET or TT. Significant clinical practice is needed to become proficient.

The generally accepted steps in the procedure are as follows:

1. Check the chart for specific orders, an order to suction as needed, or any special patient considerations, such as a deviated nasal septum, unstable vital signs, cardiopulmonary conditions, supplemental oxygenation, and type and amount of secretions.

2. Gather the needed equipment:
   - Suction catheter no larger than one-half the diameter of the patient's nostril
   - Appropriate size and type of nasopharyngeal airway to minimize nasal mucosal damage (see Chapter 12 for information on nasopharyngeal airways and their insertion)
   - Sterile, water-soluble lubricant jelly
   - Sterile 4 × 4-in gauze pad
   - Sterile gloves for both hands or one sterile glove to hold the catheter and one clean glove for the other hand
   - Specimen collector if ordered
   - Vacuum system and vacuum tubing
   - Sterile water or normal saline in a sterile basin

3. Prepare the patient for the procedure
   - Explain the procedure to the patient.
   - Put lubricating jelly on the nasopharyngeal airway and insert it into the selected nostril.
   - If possible, place the patient in the semi-Fowler's and sniffing positions.

4. Give the patient 100% O_2 for 30-60 seconds before suctioning and for at least 1 minute afterward until the patient is no longer hypoxemic. (For an infant younger than 6 months, increase the F_IO_2 by 0.1.)

5. Get help if necessary.

6. Wash your hands. (This may be skipped in an emergency.)

7. Set the desired vacuum level. The AARC Clinical Practice Guidelines suggest that the vacuum be set at the lowest possible level that still effectively removes secretions. The following ranges for vacuum are appropriate:
   - Adults: −100 to −150 mm Hg
   - Children: −100 to −120 mm Hg
   - Infants: −80 to −100 mm Hg
   - Neonates: −80 to −100 mm Hg

To prevent tissue trauma, hypoxemia, and atelectasis, negative pressures greater than −150 mm Hg should not be used.

8. Using sterile technique, put on the gloves, remove the catheter from its packaging, apply lubricant jelly to the catheter tip, and connect the vacuum tubing to the catheter.

9. Test that the vacuum is reaching the tip of the catheter.

10. If the patient is wearing an O_2 appliance, remove it so that the nose can be reached. If supplemental oxygen was being used, directing the end of the O_2 tubing or nasal cannula prongs toward the patient's mouth may help to prevent hypoxemia.

11. Suction the trachea:

    (a) Without any vacuum, advance the catheter into the nasopharyngeal airway. If no nasopharyngeal airway is available, without any vacuum, advance the catheter into the most open nasal passage. The catheter should be advanced parallel to the turbinates to minimize tissue trauma. Never force the catheter. (The most patent nasal passage can be determined by checking the chart for a history of deviated septum, asking the patient if one side feels more open, or feeling which nostril has more airflow through it.)

    (b) Have a cooperative patient stick out his or her tongue. With an uncooperative patient, the practitioner or assistant can grasp the tongue with a 4 × 4-in gauze pad or gloved hand.

    (c) Advance the catheter as the patient inspires. The epiglottis and vocal cords are open at this time, and it is easiest to slip the catheter into the trachea. A cooperative patient should be told to inhale slowly and deeply. Some practitioners find it helpful to disconnect the catheter from the vacuum tubing and listen to the end of the catheter for the sound of air movement. The patient will cough vigorously when the catheter is in the trachea (Fig. 13-16).

    (d) Advance the catheter until an obstruction is felt. Then pull the catheter back about 2 cm.

    (e) Withdraw the catheter with a twisting motion while suctioning intermittently. Suction to clear out any secretions. Typically, in an adult, suctioning may be applied for 5-10 seconds. Suctioning in an infant should be applied for no longer than 5 seconds. If the secretions are cleared, the catheter is pulled out. Practitioners disagree on whether the catheter should be withdrawn or left in place if the patient still has secretions. Some prefer to withdraw the catheter, let the patient rest and reoxygenate, and reinsert the catheter for more suctioning. Others prefer to leave the catheter in place to minimize tissue trauma from a reinsertion, let the patient rest and reoxygenate, and then suction again.

    (f) The entire procedure usually takes longer than 20 seconds; therefore the O_2 tubing must be kept directed toward the patient's mouth.

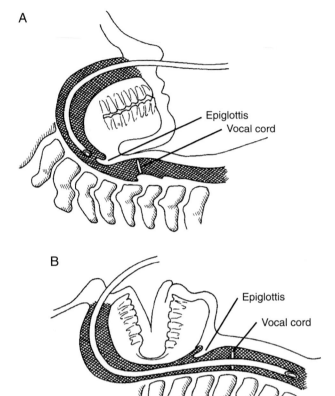

Figure 13-16 Cross-section through the airway showing nasotracheal suctioning. **A,** The patient's head may be kept in a neutral position as the catheter is advanced through a nostril to the back of the throat. **B,** The patient's head is carefully moved to the sniff position. During inspiration, the catheter is advanced into the trachea. The patient will cough, and the secretions can be suctioned out.

    (g) Turning the patient's head to the right may help direct the catheter down the left mainstem bronchus. The catheter will tend to enter the right mainstem bronchus if the head is in a neutral position or twisted to the left.

12. Reoxygenate the patient for at least 1 minute before suctioning again. Giving 100% O_2 (or 10% more than the base level in an infant) helps accomplish this faster.

13. Monitor the patient's vital signs, SpO_2 level, and breath sounds before suctioning again. Suction again, if needed, when the patient is stable.

14. If normal saline solution is needed, it may be instilled down the suction catheter by pulling off the vacuum tubing, inserting the tip of the syringe (not needle) into the end of the catheter, covering the thumb control valve, and squirting the saline solution into the catheter. The other considerations listed earlier would apply here.

15. Dispose of the catheter and glove by pulling the gloves inside out over the catheter.

16. Rinse water or saline through the vacuum tubing to clear it of secretions.
17. Turn off the suction unit.

4. Perform oropharyngeal suctioning on the patient (code: IIIB2) [difficulty: R, Ap, An]

If a patient is unable to swallow saliva or food properly or has vomitus in the mouth, it must be removed. Signs of improper swallowing may include drooling, gagging, retching, and coughing. Oropharyngeal suctioning is performed on intubated and unintubated patients. In many institutions, the suctioning device may be used more than once.

The generally accepted steps for oropharyngeal suctioning of an unintubated patient are as follows:

1. Check the chart for specific orders, an order to suction as needed, or any special patient considerations.
2. Gather the needed equipment:
   - Yankauer or regular suction catheter
   - Two clean gloves
   - Vacuum system
   - Water or normal saline solution in a basin
3. Explain the procedure to the patient.
4. If possible, place the patient in the semi-Fowler's and sniffing positions.
5. If the patient is not using supplemental oxygen, it is probably not necessary to give it. Keep a nasal cannula in place during the procedure. Remove an oxygen mask only long enough to perform the suctioning procedure and then replace the mask.
6. Get help if necessary.
7. Set the desired vacuum level. The AARC Clinical Practice Guidelines suggest that the vacuum be set at the lowest possible level that still effectively removes secretions. The following ranges for vacuum are appropriate:
   - Adults: −100 to −150 mm Hg
   - Children: −100 to −120 mm Hg
   - Infants: −80 to −100 mm Hg
   - Neonates: −80 to −100 mm Hg
8. Wash your hands. (This may be skipped in an emergency.)
9. Using clean technique, put on the gloves, remove the catheter from its packaging, and connect the vacuum tubing to the catheter.
10. Test that the vacuum is reaching the tip of the suctioning device.
11. If the patient is wearing an O_2 mask, it must be removed so that the mouth may be reached. If necessary, an assistant may be able to direct the end of the O_2 tubing toward the patient's mouth to help prevent hypoxemia. Alternatively, a nasal cannula can be put on the patient with the same liter flow.
12. Suction the oropharynx:
    (a) Gently insert the Yankauer or catheter along one side of the mouth between the cheek and tongue and advance it toward the throat. Apply vacuum to remove any secretions, vomitus, or food. Repeat the procedure on the other side of the mouth.
    (b) A spontaneously breathing patient should be able to tolerate several seconds of suctioning.
    (c) Try to avoid stimulating the patient's gag reflex by not striking the oropharynx. Retching, gagging, and vomiting can result from a stimulated gag reflex. An unintubated patient would be at risk of aspirating vomitus.
    (d) After suctioning, allow the patient to recover. Replace the oxygen mask if it was removed.
    (e) Monitor the patient's vital signs and oxygenation.
    (f) Open the patient's mouth and look for additional secretions that need to be removed.
    (g) If necessary, repeat the oral suctioning procedure and reevaluate the patient.
13. Pull the gloves inside out over each other and dispose of them.
14. Suction some water or saline through the device and vacuum tubing to rinse the secretions clear.
15. Turn off the suction unit.

MODULE D

Respiratory care plan

1. Determine a patient's pathophysiologic state (code: IIIF1) [difficulty: R, Ap, An]

Coarse, intermittent expiratory crackles (rhonchi) indicate that secretions are in the airway. The amount and consistency of sputum a patient produces depends on the lung disorder and whether it is worsening or improving. For example, if pneumonia or bronchitis is worsening, secretion production is increased. If the patient is dehydrated, the sputum contains less water than normal and will become thicker (more viscous). Tracheal suctioning should clear these secretions and result in the return of normal breath sounds (or at least an improvement). As the patient's condition improves, a return to normal sputum consistency should occur, and less should be produced. Pneumonia and bronchitis result in chest radiograph changes that show areas of infiltrate. Disease involvement of the right or left lung (or both), individual lobes, and segments can be determined. As the patient's condition improves, the chest radiograph should show clearing of infiltrates.

When there are clinical signs that the lumen of the ET or TT is partially obstructed, every effort should be made to clear the obstruction. If the mucus is too thick (viscous) to be removed through a suction catheter, the tracheal tube may need to be removed and replaced. Obviously, this places the patient at risk without a secure airway as the exchange is made. However, there are two devices that are designed to clear a lumen obstruction. The mucus shaver is a balloon-tipped catheter that can be used to pull biofilm out of the interior of the tracheal tube. The rescue cath is another balloon-tipped catheter that has been shown to be effective at pulling out thick mucus and mucus plugs from the lumen of the tracheal tube. In all cases in which there is a complete obstruction of the tracheal tube and the patient cannot breathe, the tube must be removed. A manual resuscitation bag and mask can be used to ventilate the patient until a new tube can be inserted.

2. Recommend starting a treatment based on the patient's response (code: IIIE2a) [difficulty: R, Ap, An]

See below.

3. Recommend a change in the airway clearance procedures (code: IIIE3d) [difficulty: R, Ap, An]

See below.

4. Recommend a change in the therapeutic plan if indicated (code: IIIF2) [difficulty: R, Ap, An]

The standard physician's order for suctioning usually states that suctioning should be done as needed (PRN). The respiratory therapist, the nurse, or both should be able to evaluate the patient and perform suctioning when it is justified. The physician should *not* order that the patient be suctioned on a set schedule (e.g., every hour). This could result in the patient being suctioned when it is not needed. Also, such a restrictive order would prevent the therapist and nurse from suctioning more often if needed. The respiratory care plan should allow the therapist to make the following changes.

a. Make a change in the size and type of suction catheter

As discussed earlier, for an adult or child the OD of the suction catheter should be no more than one-half (50%) the ID of the patient's ET. With a neonate, the OD of the catheter should not be more than 70% the ID of the ET. If the secretions are easy to suction out, a smaller catheter may be used. A smaller catheter is advantageous because it will remove less air from the patient's lungs during suctioning. So, the patient is less likely to become hypoxic.

A catheter with a Coudé tip should be used if the catheter must be directed into one or the other mainstem bronchus (usually the left). Closed-airway catheters, such as those made by Ballard Medical Products, offer two advantages over single-use catheters. First, they are more economical if the patient needs frequent suctioning. Second, a patient using a mechanical ventilator continues to be ventilated and oxygenated and PEEP can be maintained during the suctioning episode. The newer catheters that offer intermittent or continuous insufflation of oxygen may reduce the hypoxemia that many patients experience during the suctioning procedure. However, they can be difficult to use and costly.

b. Change the depth of suctioning

The most recent AARC Clinical Practice Guidelines recommend that *shallow suctioning* be done to prevent trauma to the tracheal mucosa. Shallow suctioning is defined as passing the suction catheter to a predetermined depth. This is usually only to the tip of the ET or TT. This procedure will remove secretions only from the tube, not from the patient's trachea.

Deep suctioning is defined as insertion of the catheter until resistance is met (the carina) and then withdrawal of the catheter 1 cm before applying negative pressure. Traditionally, deep suction has been performed to stimulate the patient to cough and to directly remove secretions from the trachea and possibly mainstem bronchi.

c. Change the level of vacuum used when suctioning

In general, the lowest possible vacuum level that adequately removes secretions should be used. The AARC Clinical Practice Guidelines on suctioning list appropriate negative pressure ranges for patients based on their age. These are listed in the suctioning procedures given earlier. Be prepared to reduce the suctioning pressure if the patient has low viscosity (more watery, thinner) secretions that are easy to remove. Conversely, be prepared to increase the suctioning pressure if the patient's secretions are more viscous (thicker) and difficult to remove.

d. Instill an irrigating solution into the trachea

The current recommendation is *not* to routinely instill normal saline before suctioning. Historically, sterile normal saline solution (0.9%) was instilled into the trachea to dilute and mobilize pulmonary secretions. Patients would also have their cough stimulated. However, the most recent AARC guideline on suctioning states that the majority of references do not find saline instillation to be beneficial. In some cases this practice may be harmful. Possible adverse effects of saline instillation include excessive coughing, dyspnea, bronchospasm, tachycardia, hypoxemia, increased intracranial pressure, and displacement of biofilm from the inside of the ET into the lower airway.

Current literature does support instilling normal saline in these situations: (1) to lubricate the suction catheter or (2) to help in the removal of a mucous plug or thick, tenacious secretions. These saline volumes have been reported: (1) 0.5-1.0 mL in a neonatal patient, (2) 2-5 mL in an older child, and (3) about 5 mL in an adult.

e. Change the frequency of suctioning

Suctioning should be performed only when secretions are present. Patients should not be routinely suctioned. Listen to the patient's breath sounds for coarse expiratory crackles (rhonchi) or palpate the chest for secretions (tactile fremitus) between suctioning efforts. Signs seen during mechanical ventilation include: (1) sawtooth pattern on a flow-volume loop seen on the monitor screen, (2) increase in the peak inspiratory pressure during volume-controlled ventilation, (3) decrease in the tidal volume during pressure-controlled ventilation.

Secretions obstruct the airways and should be removed if possible. Often this requires more than one suctioning attempt. The patient is unlikely to be harmed with repeated suctioning as long as proper technique is followed and the patient is reoxygenated between sessions. Watch for any of the complications listed in Boxes 13-1 and 13-2. Stop suctioning when it is no longer indicated.

f. Change the duration of suctioning

The entire procedure should take no longer than 15 seconds. Actual suctioning should be 5-10 seconds in an adult and no more than 5 seconds in a neonate. However, some patients may not be able to tolerate suctioning this long because of hypoxemia or unstable vital signs. Be prepared to suction for a shorter period. It is safer to suction repeatedly than to increase the suctioning time.

5. Recommend a treatment be terminated (code: IIIE1) [difficulty: R, Ap, An]

Stop the procedure if the patient becomes hypoxic or has tachycardia, bradycardia, arrhythmias, hypotension, bronchospasm, or any of the other hazards or complications listed in Boxes 13-1 and 13-2. Bloody secretions indicate possible mucosal damage and justify stopping the procedure. Hypoxemia can cause unstable vital signs, and vagal stimulation can cause bradycardia and bronchospasm. Be prepared to stop suctioning, provide extra oxygen, or get help.

Conscious patients should be able to report how they feel after the suctioning procedure. Hopefully, a patient reports less dyspnea. Inform the patient's nurse or physician and the supervising therapist if the patient has any serious questions or problems. Routine communication should occur as needed between these people and any other caregiver.

6. Recommend discontinuing a treatment based on the patient's response (code: IIIE2h) [difficulty: R, Ap, An]

Life-threatening complications of suctioning include hypoxemia, tachycardia, bradycardia, arrhythmias, hypotension, bronchospasm, pneumothorax, and pulmonary hemorrhage. If any of these problems arise, contact the physician and discuss discontinuing the suctioning procedure. Once the underlying problem has been corrected and safe suctioning can be performed, the order may be reinstated.

Suctioning should also be discontinued when the patient has recovered to the point at which it is no longer needed. Either the patient's secretions have decreased in volume or the patient now is able to cough them out.

Exam Hint 13-5

Be prepared to recognize the need for suctioning, adjust the suctioning equipment, or adjust the procedure based on the patient's reaction to it.

BIBLIOGRAPHY

Altobelli N: Airway management. In Kacmarek RM, Stoller JK, Heuer AJ, editors: *Egan's fundamentals of respiratory care*, ed 10, St Louis, 2013, Mosby.

American Association for Respiratory Therapy: Guidelines for the prevention of nosocomial infections, *AARC Times* 7(9):49–52, 1983.

American Association for Respiratory Care (AARC): Clinical practice guideline: nasotracheal suctioning, *Respir Care* 37:898, 1992.

American Association for Respiratory Care (AARC): Clinical practice guideline: endotracheal suctioning of mechanically ventilated adults and children with artificial airways, *Respir Care* 38:500, 1993.

American Association for Respiratory Care (AARC): Clinical practice guideline: suctioning of the patient in the home, *Respir Care* 44:99, 1999 (Retired).

American Association for Respiratory Care (AARC): Clinical practice guideline: nasotracheal suctioning: 2004 revision and update, *Respir Care* 49:1080, 2004.

American Association for Respiratory Care (AARC): Clinical practice guideline: removal of the endotracheal tube—2007 revision & update, *Respir Care* 52:81, 2007.

American Association for Respiratory Care (AARC): Clinical practice guideline: endotracheal suctioning of mechanically ventilated patients with artificial airways, *Respir Care* 55:758, 2010.

Butler TJ: Suctioning. In Butler TJ, editor: *Laboratory exercises for competency in respiratory care*, Philadelphia, 2013, FA Davis.

Denunzio C, Heuer AJ: Fundamentals of physical examination. In Heuer AJ, Scanlan CL, editors: *Clinical assessment in respiratory care*, ed 7, St Louis, 2014, Mosby.

Eubanks DH, Bone RC: *Comprehensive respiratory care*, ed 2, St Louis, 1990, Mosby.

Fink JB, Hess DR: Secretion clearance techniques. In Hess DR, MacIntyre NR, Mishoe SC, et al.: *Respiratory care principles and practice*, Philadelphia, 2002, Saunders.

Hess DR, Branson RD: Airway and suctioning equipment. In Branson RD, Hess DR, Chatburn RL, editors: *Respiratory care equipment*, ed 2, Philadelphia, 1999, Lippincott Williams & Wilkins.

Hess DR: Sputum collection, airway clearance, and lung expansion therapy. In Hess DR, MacIntyre NR, et al.: *Respiratory care: principles and practice*, ed 2, Burlington, MA, 2012, Jones & Bartlett Learning.

Jacobs IN, Pettignano MM, Pettignano R: Airway management. In Walsh BK, Czervinske MP, DiBlasi RM, editors: *Perinatal and pediatric respiratory care*, ed 3, St Louis, 2010, Saunders.

Lewis RM: Airway care. In Fink JB, Hunt GE, editors: *Clinical practice in respiratory care*, Philadelphia, 1999, Lippincott Williams & Wilkins.

McIntyre D: Airway management. In Wyka KA, Mathews PJ, Rutkowski J, editors: *Foundations of respiratory care*, ed 2, Clifton Park, NY, 2012, Delmar.

Plevak DJ, Ward JJ: Airway management. In Burton GG, Hodgkin JE, Ward JJ, editors: *Respiratory care*, ed 4, Philadelphia, 1997, Lippincott-Raven.

Rarey KP, Youtsey JW: *Respiratory patient care*, Englewood Cliffs, NJ, 1981, Prentice Hall.

Roth P: Airway care. In Aloan CA, Hill TV, editors: *Respiratory care of the newborn and child*, ed 2, Philadelphia, 1997, Lippincott.

Russian CJ, Gonzales JF, Henry NR: Suction catheter size: an assessment and comparison of 3 different calculation methods, *Respir Care* 59(1):32–38, 2014.

Scott AA, Koff PB: Airway care and chest physiotherapy. In Koff PB, Eitzmann DV, Neu J, editors: *Neonatal and pediatric respiratory care*, ed 2, St Louis, 1993, Mosby.

Shapiro BA, Kacmarek RM, Cane RD, et al.: *Clinical application of respiratory care*, ed 4, St Louis, 1991, Mosby.

Shilling AM, Durbin Jr CG: Airway management devices and advanced cardiac life support. In Cairo JM, editor: *Mosby's respiratory care equipment*, ed 9, St Louis, 2014, Mosby.

Simmons KF, Scanlan CL: Airway management. In Wilkins RL, Stoller JK, Kacmarek RM, editors: *Egan's fundamentals of respiratory care*, ed 9, St Louis, 2009, Mosby.

Stone RH, Bricknell SS: Experience with a new device for clearing mucus from the endotracheal tube, *Respir Care* 56:520, 2011.

White GC: *Equipment theory for respiratory care*, ed 4, Clifton Park, NY, 2005, Thomson Delmar Learning.

Wilkins RL, Hodgkin JE, Lopez B: *Fundamentals of lung and heart sounds*, ed 3, St Louis, 2004, Mosby.

Wojciechowski WV: Incentive spirometers and secretion evacuation devices and inspiratory muscle training devices. In Barnes TA, editor: *Core textbook of respiratory care practice*, ed 2, St Louis, 1994, Mosby.

SELF-STUDY QUESTIONS

See Appendix for answers.

1. All of the following statements about the use of a Lukens trap are true EXCEPT:
   A. A vacuum source is needed.
   B. All connections must be tight for it to work properly.
   C. Either a suction catheter or a bronchoscope is needed.
   D. It is indicated for a patient with a strong, productive cough.

2. A patient is being mechanically ventilated with 60% oxygen and 8 cm H_2O of PEEP. The patient's SpO_2 and blood pressure have decreased twice when removed from the ventilator for suctioning. What should be recommended to prevent this from happening again?
   A. Switch to a smaller suction catheter.
   B. Switch to a larger suction catheter.
   C. Increase the PEEP to 10 cm H_2O before and after suctioning.
   D. Use a closed-system suction catheter.

3. The proper-size suction catheter should be no larger than what fraction of an adult ET's inner diameter?
   A. ¼
   B. ½
   C. ⅔
   D. ¾

4. It is difficult to remove the tracheal secretions from an adult patient using −60 mm Hg of vacuum pressure. What should be done?
   A. Suction for 20 seconds.
   B. Suction more frequently.
   C. Increase the vacuum pressure to −80 mm Hg.
   D. Change from the central vacuum system to a portable one.

5. If a patient has a PaO_2 of 65 mm Hg, the most important step to take to prevent hypoxemia during suctioning is to

   A. Give the patient 100% O_2 before and after the procedure.
   B. Use a large catheter to remove the secretions quickly.
   C. Hyperextend the patient's neck and head.
   D. Use a small catheter so that the patient can breathe around it.

6. The best positions in which to place a patient before nasotracheal suctioning are:
   1. **Supine**
   2. **Trendelenburg**
   3. **Sniff (neck and head hyperextended)**
   4. **Semi-Fowler's**
   A. 1 and 4 only
   B. 1 and 3 only
   C. 2 and 3 only
   D. 3 and 4 only

7. When preparing to suction a patient, all of the following should be done EXCEPT:
   A. Set the vacuum control to FULL.
   B. Screw a 500-mL collection bottle tightly onto the vacuum connector.
   C. Attach 3 feet of vacuum tubing to the tubing connector on the collection jar.
   D. Pinch closed the vacuum tubing when the vacuum is turned on to measure the vacuum level.

8. A 40-year-old patient has pneumonia in the left lower lobe with a large amount of secretions. What should be recommended for better suctioning?
   A. Use the largest diameter suction catheter available.
   B. Use a suction catheter with a Coudé tip.
   C. Use the longest suction catheter available.
   D. Suction for a longer period.

9. A respiratory therapist notices that a patient's Yankauer suction catheter is cracked. The best thing to do is:
   A. Continue to use it.
   B. Tape over the crack.
   C. Put lubricating jelly in the crack to seal it.
   D. Replace the catheter.

10. While a respiratory therapist is preparing to suction a patient for a mucus sample it is noticed that the vacuum is not reaching the end of the catheter. Which of the following are possible causes?
    1. **The vacuum is not turned on.**
    2. **All connections are airtight.**
    3 **The catheter is plugged with foreign matter.**
    4. **The specimen jar is not screwed tightly into the special lid.**
    A. 2 and 3 only
    B. 2 and 4 only
    C. 1, 3, and 4 only
    D. 1, 2, 3, 4

11. A patient is receiving mechanical ventilation through an 8-mm oral ET. Over the course of the shift, the patient is seen to have more tracheal secretions. What is the best course of action?
    A. Suction more often.
    B. Suction for longer periods.
    C. Change to the closed-suctioning technique.
    D. Administer nebulized atropine.

12. An intubated patient has thick secretions. The nurse has recommended that normal saline be instilled into the patient's trachea. What are the possible adverse effects of doing this?
    1. **Endotracheal tube biofilm is displaced**
    2. **Hypoxemia**
    3. **Bronchospasm**
    4. **Excessive coughing**
    A. 1 and 4 only
    B. 2 and 3 only
    C. 2, 3, and 4 only
    D. 1, 2, 3, 4

13. A ventilator-dependent patient required a vacuum pressure of −120 mm Hg to remove thick secretions. After treatment with a mucolytic drug, the patient's secretions are much easier to remove. What should be recommended?
    A. Reduce the vacuum pressure to −100 mm Hg and monitor the ease of secretion removal.
    B. Maintain the present vacuum level and suction less often.
    C. Increase the vacuum pressure to −140 mm Hg and suction less often.
    D. Reduce the vacuum pressure to −60 mm Hg and suction more often.

14. A conscious patient requires nasotracheal suctioning. During the procedure, the patient's blood pressure decreases to 100/60 mm Hg, and the heart rate decreases from 110 to 60 beats/min. What should be done?
    A. Change to a catheter with a larger diameter.
    B. Shorten the suctioning time.
    C. Insert an oropharyngeal airway before suctioning.
    D. Squirt 5 mL of saline down the suction catheter into the patient's trachea.

15. The respiratory therapist is called to set up a suctioning system for a new patient in the Intensive Care Unit. To measure the vacuum pressure, what should be done?
    A. Check the manometer while occluding the catheter tip.
    B. Set the vacuum control to maximum.
    C. Close the thumb control valve on the catheter.
    D. Check the manometer while pinching off the connecting tubing.

16. An intubated patient has pneumonia, and a sputum sample must be sent to the laboratory for culture and sensitivity testing. What is the most appropriate way to obtain a sample?
    A. Place a Lukens trap between the suction catheter and the vacuum tubing.
    B. Suction the oropharynx with a sterile Yankauer suction catheter.
    C. Place a Lukens trap between the vacuum tubing and the collection bottle.
    D. Suction the patient and place the catheter inside the Lukens trap.

17. A 30-year-old postoperative patient with clear breath sounds is receiving mechanical ventilation. The patient was suctioned 2 hours ago with scant results. The nurse wants to suction the patient again before the shift change. What should be recommended?
    A. Shallow suctioning
    B. Suction with a Coudé tip catheter.
    C. Instill 5 mL of normal saline.
    D. Deep suctioning

18. Placing a suction catheter into a patient's trachea and applying vacuum pressure causes:
    1. **Transient hypoxemia**
    2. **Removal of secretions**
    3. **Stopping of the hypoxic drive because of vagal stimulation**
    4. **Removal of air from the lungs**
    A. 3 only
    B. 3 and 4 only
    C. 2 and 4 only
    D. 1, 2, and 4 only

19. When a catheter OD is selected for suctioning through an infant's TT, it is important that the OD be:
    A. No more than 25% the ID of the tube
    B. No less than 40% the ID of the tube
    C. No less than 50% the ID of the tube
    D. No more than 70% the ID of the tube

20. During nasotracheal suctioning, it is important to:
    A. Lubricate the catheter with sterile water.
    B. Lubricate the catheter tip with a sterile, water-soluble lubricant jelly.
    C. Place the catheter in the refrigerator to make it firmer and easier to pass.
    D. Lubricate the catheter with a sterile, normal saline solution.

21. While connecting the suction catheter to the vacuum tubing, a respiratory therapist accidentally touches the tip of the catheter with the clean-gloved hand. What should be done?
    A. Discard the clean glove and start over.
    B. Suction the patient.
    C. Put a sterile glove over the clean glove and suction the patient.
    D. Discard the catheter and start over.

22. A 17-year-old patient with an oral ET has just had open-airway suctioning performed. The respiratory therapist notes that bright red blood is removed, along with some clear secretions. What should be done?
    A. Stop the suctioning procedure and monitor the patient.
    B. Change to a closed-airway suctioning system.
    C. Instill 5 mL of normal saline and suction again to remove the saline and blood.
    D. Change to a nasal ET and suction normally.

23. A 67-year-old woman who suffered a stroke is having difficulty swallowing her oral secretions. An order is written to perform oropharyngeal suctioning. What risks or hazards are associated with this procedure?
    A. Bradycardia
    B. Gagging
    C. Hypoxemia
    D. Tachycardia

24. A 16-year-old young woman is receiving mechanical ventilation via a 7-mm ET. After she is suctioned with a 14-Fr catheter, the electrocardiograph monitor shows that she is bradycardic. What should be recommended?
    A. Administer 10 cm H_2O PEEP.
    B. Limit suctioning to twice a shift.
    C. Change to a 10-Fr catheter.
    D. Use a catheter with a Coudé tip.

25. An adult patient receiving mechanical ventilation with 80% oxygen and 10 cm H_2O PEEP experiences hypoxemia, tachycardia, and hypotension every time open-airway suctioning is performed. What should the respiratory therapist recommend to the physician?
    A. Increase the PEEP level to 15 cm H_2O before suctioning.
    B. Reduce the duration of suctioning but do it more often.
    C. Discontinue suctioning until a closed-airway suctioning system can be set up.
    D. Turn up the oxygen level to 100% before the patient is suctioned.

26. A 47-year-old woman with chronic obstructive pulmonary disease and pneumonia has copious amounts of thick secretions. Nasotracheal suctioning is being initiated because of her weak, ineffective cough. What is the maximum suctioning pressure that may be used?
    A. −100 mm Hg
    B. −125 mm Hg
    C. −150 mm Hg
    D. −175 mm Hg

14 Intermittent Positive-Pressure Breathing

Note: It can be anticipated that the Therapist Multiple-Choice Examination (TMC) will include an *average of 3 of 140 actual questions* (2% of the exam) on intermittent positive-pressure breathing (IPPB). (This is based on the question mix typically found on the National Board of Respiratory Care's previous Entry Level Examinations and Written Registry Examinations.)

Remember that the TMC version you take will include 20 additional questions being evaluated for possible inclusion in other versions of the TMC. So, there will be a total of 160 questions taken. There is no way to differentiate between the 140 actual questions and the 20 questions being evaluated for future use. Please go to the Introduction for detailed information on the TMC and the Clinical Simulation Examination.

MODULE A

Perform hyperinflation by IPPB therapy (code: IIIB5) [difficulty: R, Ap].

1. Description

The Respiratory Care Committee of the American Thoracic Society published the following definition in its 1980 *Guidelines for the Use of Intermittent Positive Pressure Breathing (IPPB):* "'IPPB treatments' refers to the use of a pressure-limited respirator to deliver a gas with humidity and/or aerosol to a spontaneously breathing patient for periods of time that are generally no greater than 15 to 20 minutes each."

The patient's tidal volume (V_T) should be greater than normal when enhanced by IPPB. This large V_T is caused by the use of positive pressure against the lungs. Pressure is also directed against the airways and, through contact with the airways and lungs, the entire chest. The patient's exhalation is usually passive but can be slowed through modification of the exhalation valve.

Shapiro and associates (1991) list the following as the physiologic effects of IPPB:

a. Increased mean airway pressure

By definition of IPPB, the patient is receiving a positive airway pressure instead of generating a negative intrathoracic pressure to create the V_T. Most authors recommend that patients with heart disease be monitored closely for the effects of increased mean airway pressure. Decreasing the normal return of venous blood to the heart, thereby decreasing the cardiac output, is possible. Shapiro and associates (1991) recommend an expiratory time that is long enough to allow for normal venous return before the next positive-pressure breath is given. The patient's heart rate and blood pressure can be monitored to ensure that they stay in the normal range.

Pulmonary barotrauma is the second concern raised by the use of positive airway pressure. It is possible for patients with small-airways disease to trap air in the alveoli. This can lead to the rupture of a bleb, thus causing a pneumothorax. Care must be taken with the patient with bullous emphysema to ensure that the V_T is exhaled completely.

b. Increased V_T

The primary goal of IPPB is to increase the patient's assisted V_T to greater than the spontaneous V_T. Indeed, if the spontaneous V_T is greater than the assisted V_T, IPPB is not needed for lung expansion. However, incentive spirometry (IS) may still be indicated.

c. Decreased work of breathing

A properly coached passive treatment with the controls set to meet the patient's inspiratory needs causes a decrease in the work of breathing (WOB). This necessitates considerable skill on the part of the practitioner. Sensitivity, inspiratory flow, and peak pressure must be frequently adjusted to minimize the patient's work. The patient must be asked if the control adjustments make it easier or harder to inhale. Failure to tailor the breathing treatment to the patient's needs may actually increase the WOB.

d. Alteration of the inspiratory/expiratory ratio

Patients with high airway resistance or low lung compliance often change their breathing patterns to reduce the WOB (see Chapter 1). These new breathing patterns may lead to worsening of the patient's condition. Alteration of normal ventilation and perfusion ratios in the lungs may worsen hypoxemia. Properly administered and coached IPPB can be used to adjust the inspiratory/expiratory (I:E) ratio to the benefit of the patient. The patient can be taught how to breathe in a more physiologically normal pattern.

2. Indications

The following indications and guidelines are listed in the American Association for Respiratory Care (AARC) *Clinical Practice Guidelines* (1991, 2003) on IPPB:

a. To treat atelectasis when other deep-breathing methods are ineffective

Patients who are uncooperative, unconscious, or physically incapable of being coached in deep-breathing and coughing techniques or in performing IS may be helped by IPPB. An inspiratory pause at the end of the IPPB breath helps to better distribute the gas to open areas of atelectasis. The AARC guidelines on IPPB list the following poor pulmonary function values as supporting the need for IPPB, rather than IS, because the patient would have an ineffective cough:

- Vital capacity (VC) less than 10 mL/kg of ideal body weight
- Forced vital capacity (FVC) less than 70% of predicted
- Forced expiratory volume in 1 second less than 65% of predicted
- Maximum voluntary ventilation less than 50% of predicted

The following have been listed as *initial* clinical goals for an IPPB delivered V_T:

1. At least 25% larger than the spontaneous V_T.
2. 10-15 mL/kg of ideal body weight.
3. At least 1/3 (33%) of the patient's predicted inspiratory capacity (IC). (Predicted IC = 50 mL/kg of ideal body weight.)

The first option will result in the lowest goal. The third option will result in the highest goal. Option 2 will provide a goal that ranges between the first and the third options. Remember that these can be used to set an initial goal. This initial goal should be increased as the patient tolerates and as his or her condition warrants.

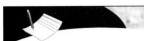

Exam Hint 14-1

It is important to understand the indications of IPPB versus IS in the treatment of a patient with atelectasis. In general, IPPB would be indicated in a patient who is not able to properly perform IS.

b. To more effectively deliver aerosolized medications

If the patient cannot coordinate his or her breathing pattern to make use of a metered-dose inhaler or hand-held nebulizer, IPPB may be used. Examples of when IPPB is preferable include any situation in which the patient is unconscious, uncooperative, or physically incapable. These patients are physically unable to make effective use of simpler methods of lung inflation (IS) or to take an aerosolized medication (metered-dose inhaler or hand-held nebulizer). Examples of these types of patients include the elderly, the chronically debilitated, patients with neuromuscular diseases, and patients with kyphoscoliosis. It may also be used to provide temporary support to home care patients.

c. To enhance the patient's cough effort and sputum clearance

The combination of aerosolized saline, with or without a bronchodilator or mucolytic, and deeper V_T may help the patient to cough more productively. The practitioner must stop the treatment periodically to coach the patient's cough effort.

The following additional indications were listed in the *Guidelines for the Use of Intermittent Positive Pressure Breathing (IPPB)* published by the Respiratory Care Committee of the American Thoracic Society (1980).

d. To treat impending ventilatory failure as seen by an increased arterial carbon dioxide partial pressure ($PaCO_2$)

It may be possible to delay or avoid intubation and mechanical ventilation in the deteriorating chronic obstructive pulmonary disease (COPD) patient. The patient is able to relax and reduce the WOB during a passive IPPB treatment. It may be necessary to give IPPB for 5-10 minutes as often as every 30 minutes to 1 hour. The treatment should also be given with the intention of helping the patient's cough and sputum clearance. (An alternative to frequent IPPB treatments is noninvasive positive-pressure ventilation. This is discussed in Chapter 15.)

e. To help manage the patient with acute pulmonary edema

IPPB can help in the management of this patient by temporarily increasing mean airway pressure. This reduces the venous return to the heart, which may reduce pulmonary edema. The IPPB procedure does not correct the underlying cardiac problem, which must be treated by other means.

f. To induce a sputum sample for culture and sensitivity or other diagnostic studies

Inducing a sputum sample by IPPB is indicated only if simpler methods have failed.

g. To deliver medications for special purposes when simpler methods are ineffective

IPPB should be used to deliver medication when simpler methods fail, for example, to deliver a local anesthetic such as lidocaine (Xylocaine) before a bronchoscopy procedure.

3. Contraindications

a. An *untreated pneumothorax* is listed by all authors and the AARC guidelines as an absolute contraindication. An increased intrathoracic pressure converts a simple pneumothorax into a tension pneumothorax. The consequences can be fatal. Once a chest tube has been inserted into the pleural space and a pleural drainage system set up, IPPB can be administered. There may be an increase in the air leak, but it will not be life-threatening.

The AARC guidelines list the following as relative contraindications. Any patient with one of the following contraindications should be evaluated carefully before a decision about the clinical use of IPPB is made:

b. Active hemoptysis

Expectoration of blood indicates that a tear has occurred in the airway or lung tissues. The IPPB treatment should be stopped if there is a large amount of hemoptysis. Certainly massive hemoptysis (defined as greater than 600 mL of blood expectorated in a 16-hour period) contraindicates IPPB.

c. Hemodynamic instability
d. Intracranial pressure greater than 15 mm Hg
e. Chest radiograph that shows a bleb
f. Tracheoesophageal fistula
g. Recent surgery on the esophagus, skull, face, or mouth
h. Untreated, active tuberculosis (hazard to the practitioner)
i. Nausea, air swallowing, or hiccups (singultation)

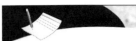

Exam Hint 14-2

Past examinations have included questions about the contraindications for IPPB, especially untreated pneumothorax or hemoptysis.

4. Hazards and precautions

The AARC guidelines list the following hazards and precautions for IPPB therapy:
  a. Pneumothorax
  b. Barotrauma
  c. Increased airway resistance from a bronchospastic reaction to the positive pressure or an adverse reaction to a medication. This can result in alveolar over-distension and air trapping.
  d. Hyperoxia when 100% oxygen is delivered to the patient. Some COPD patients who are hypercarbic and breathing on hypoxic drive may hypoventilate as a result. In this situation, use room air to power the IPPB unit.
  e. Secretions that may become impacted when the inhaled gas is not humidified adequately
  f. Nosocomial infection
  g. Decreased venous return
  h. Increased ventilation-to-perfusion mismatch. This may worsen any hypoxemia.
  i. Hyperventilation
  j. Psychologic dependence. This may be seen in the long-term home care patient who does not want to switch to another method of taking inhaled medications.
  k. Hypocarbia
  l. Hemoptysis
  m. Gastric distension
  n. Air trapping, auto-positive end-expiratory pressure (PEEP), or overdistended alveoli

5. Initiation of therapy

a. Steps in the basic procedure

1. Check for a complete and proper order specifying the patient, oxygen percentage, frequency of treatment, medication, and any special considerations.
2. Gather the necessary IPPB unit (powered by either compressed gas or electricity), patient circuit, medication, and patient interface (mouthpiece, lip seal, or face mask).
3. Assemble the equipment outside of the patient's room.
4. Introduce yourself and the department you represent, and state your purpose to the patient.
5. Confirm the patient's identity.
6. Have the patient sit up in bed or in a chair; an obese patient may stand.
7. Interview the patient and explain the IPPB procedure.
8. Assess the patient's vital signs.
9. Assess the patient's breath sounds.
10. Prepare the IPPB unit for operation:
    A. If the unit is electrical, plug it into a working outlet.
    B. If the unit is pneumatic, plug it into either a compressed air or an oxygen outlet, as ordered. *Note:* If the Vortran-IPPB unit is directly connected to the gas outlet, it will deliver a set flow of 40 L/min. To adjust the gas flow, a 0-75 L/min flowmeter needs to be connected to the gas source. The unit comes with a 7-foot length of oxygen tubing with a Diameter Index Safety System (DISS) spin nut at each end. This is used to connect the gas source to the unit.
    C. Set the following controls:
       i. Set sensitivity at −1 cm H_2O pressure.
       ii. If a Bennett PR-2 is being used, set the nebulizer to run on inspiration only.
       iii. Adjust the flow as necessary.
       iv. Set the peak pressure at about 10-15 cm H_2O.
    D. Add the medication or saline solution to the nebulizer. Test the nebulizer by turning on the machine.
    E. Cover the mouthpiece with a clean tissue to ensure that it cycles off at the preset pressure.
11. Instruct the patient to sip on the mouthpiece like a straw to turn the machine on. Have the patient relax and let the machine fill his or her lungs with air until the set peak pressure is reached and the unit cycles off. Then the patient should hold his or her breath in for 2-3 seconds and exhale slowly.
12. Adjust the flow for patient comfort. In general, the inspiratory time should be about 1-2 seconds and the I:E ratio about 1:3.
13. Adjust the pressure for patient comfort while delivering a large V_T breath. Use a hand-held spirometer (Wright respirometer) to measure the exhaled V_T.
14. Limit the time of the treatment to about 15 minutes.

b. Giving a passive treatment

Most authors describe the patient taking a passive treatment. In a passive treatment, the patient relaxes and lets the machine fill the lungs until the preset pressure is reached.

As mentioned earlier, the patient is then told to hold in his or her breath before exhaling passively. This treatment is given with the intent of minimizing the patient's WOB. A slow flow rate is used so that any nebulized medication is deposited deeply into the small airways and lungs. Most importantly, this slow deep breath will maximize air delivery to the low lung compliance areas with atelectasis.

c. Giving an active treatment

Several authors advocate having the patient take an active treatment in which he or she interacts with the IPPB machine to obtain as deep a breath as possible.

Welch and colleagues (1980) have found that the patient's posttreatment IC is greatest when the practitioner

(1) uses as high a peak pressure as the patient can tolerate and (2) coaches the patient to inhale as deeply as possible with the IPPB machine. They and others believe that this is the best way to treat or prevent atelectasis. Monitor the patient for signs of barotrauma/volutrauma.

6. Initial settings on the Bird Mark 7

The older version of the Mark 7 is used as the model respirator of the Bird series. The current Mark 8 has similar features. Other Bird units have slightly different controls and features. Refer to Figure 14-1 for the following:

- Adjust the *air-mix* knob to the desired gas mix. (See the inspired oxygen percentage discussion below.)

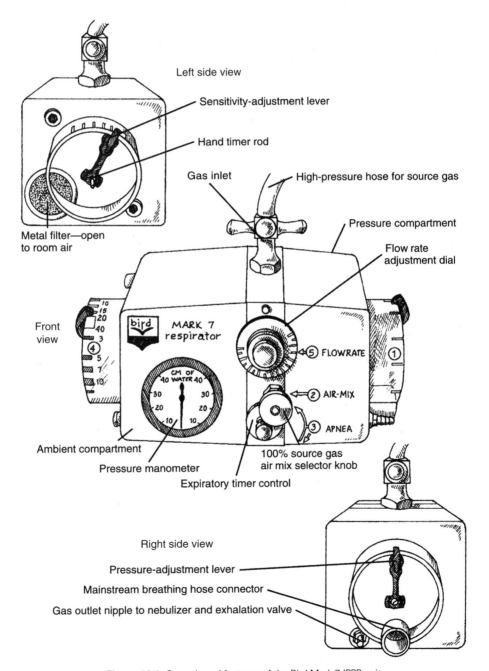

Figure 14-1 Controls and features of the Bird Mark 7 IPPB unit.

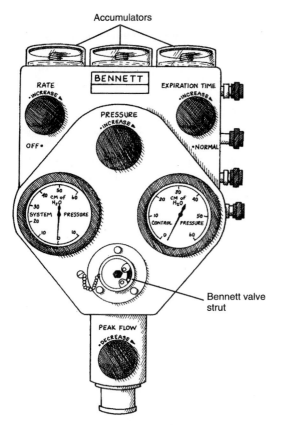

Figure 14-2 Front controls and features of the Bennett PR-II IPPB unit.

- Sensitivity should be set so that the patient has to generate about –1 cm H_2O pressure to cycle the unit on. Set the *sensitivity* control (on the left-hand side of the unit when facing it) to the reference number 15. This is at approximately the 2 o'clock position. Turning the control lever counterclockwise makes the unit more sensitive. Push in the hand timer rod to note that the unit cycles on easily.

- Flow should be set so that the patient feels comfortable with the inspiratory time. Set the *flow rate* knob so that the reference number 15 is at the 12 o'clock position; the *off* sign will be at the 8 o'clock position. Turning the *flow rate* knob counterclockwise increases the flow.

- Peak pressure should be set at about 10-15 cm H_2O pressure. Set the *pressure* control (on the right-hand side of the unit when facing it) to the reference number 15. This is at approximately the 10 o'clock position. Turning the control lever more clockwise increases the peak pressure. Hold a clean tissue against the patient's mouthpiece to see that the unit cycles off at the desired peak pressure.

7. Initial settings on the Bennett PR-2

The PR-2 is used as the model respirator of the Bennett series. (Although the PR-2 is no longer being manufactured, many are still in clinical use.) Other Bennett units have slightly different controls and features. Refer to Figures 14-2 and 14-3 for the following:

- Adjust the *air dilution* knob to the desired gas mix. (See the inspired oxygen percentage discussion below.)

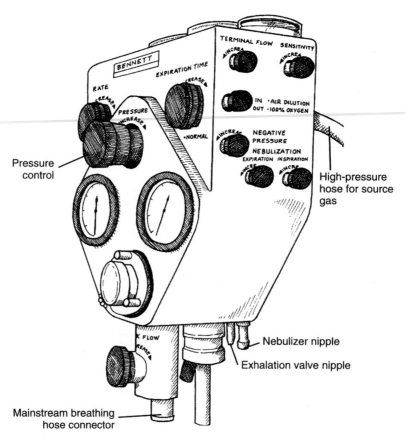

Figure 14-3 Right-side controls and features of the Bennett PR-II IPPB unit.

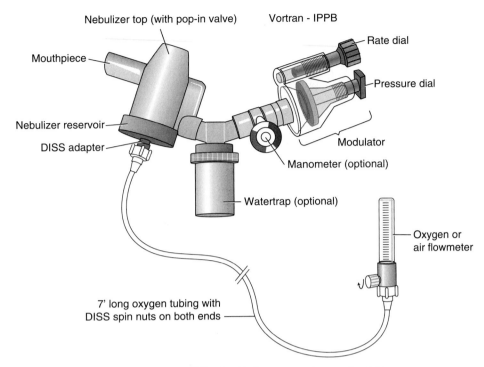

Figure 14-4 Vortran-IPPB unit with flowmeter and connecting tubing.

- Sensitivity should be set so that the patient has to generate about −1 cm H_2O pressure to cycle the unit on. Turning the control lever counterclockwise makes the unit more sensitive. Push up on the Bennett valve strut to note that the unit cycles on easily.
- Flow should be set so that the patient feels comfortable with the inspiratory time. The Bennett valve is designed to automatically open and close itself to allow the patient as much flow as desired. Set the *peak flow* control knob as counterclockwise as possible so that it is at the maximum setting. Turning the *peak flow* knob more clockwise will decrease the patient's peak flow.
- Peak pressure should be set at about 10-15 cm H_2O pressure. Dial the *pressure* control clockwise until the *control pressure* gauge shows the desired peak pressure. Hold a clean tissue against the patient's mouthpiece to see that when the unit cycles off the *system pressure* gauge reads the same as the *control pressure* gauge.
- Turn the *inspiration nebulization* control counterclockwise for medication to be nebulized only during an inspiration. Some practitioners believe that the *expiration nebulization* control should be turned on slightly so that the mouthpiece and circuit dead space are filled with medication before the next breath. Others are opposed to this because it wastes medication when the patient stops the treatment.
- A small leak in the circuit, mouthpiece, or face mask can be overcome by adding some additional flow by turning on the *terminal flow* control. It is normally left off. Turn the control counterclockwise to add as much additional flow as necessary to overcome the leak.

Details on the design and control specifications for the various Bird and Bennett models can be found in the manufacturers' literature and books on respiratory therapy equipment.

8. Initial settings on the Vortran-IPPB

The Vortran-IPPB unit is designed for use by a single patient and is disposable (Fig. 14-4). It consists of a modulator (for adjusting peak pressure and rate of exhalation) and a nebulizer. Optional components include a water trap and pressure manometer. These steps are recommended for an ideal treatment:

- Set the air or oxygen flowmeter at 30 L/min. The range for flow is 15-40 L/min.
- Peak pressure should be set at about 10-15 cm H_2O pressure. *Note:* The Vortran will automatically add PEEP at about 1/10 the peak pressure. The range of PEEP is 2-5 cm H_2O pressure.
- Hold a clean tissue against the patient's mouthpiece to see that the unit cycles off at the desired peak pressure.

MODULE B

Recommend changes in IPPB therapy (code: IIIE3e) [difficulty: R, Ap, An].

1. Change the patient–machine interface
a. Mouthpiece

A conscious, cooperative patient can take a treatment with a mouthpiece. He or she must be instructed to place the

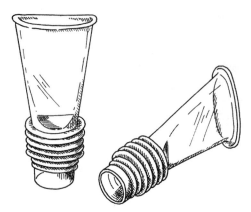

Figure 14-5 Universal IPPB mouthpiece with a tapered 22- to 18-mm machine connector.

mouthpiece between the teeth (or gums) and seal the lips around it so that there is no leak. Instruct the patient to sip gently on it to turn the IPPB machine on. As long as the lips are sealed and there are no other leaks, the positive-pressure breath will stop when the preset pressure is reached. Nose clips are often helpful to prevent a leak through the nose as the patient is learning how to take the treatment. The nose clips can be removed after the patient has learned how to seal the nasopharynx with the soft palate.

A variety of mouthpieces are available. All share two common features: a raised edge so that the teeth do not slip off and a 22-mm-outer diameter (OD) connector end to insert into the IPPB circuit (Fig. 14-5).

b. Mouth seal (Bennett seal)

An unconscious, uncooperative, or aged patient who cannot seal his or her lips can be aided by placing a soft rubber seal around the mouthpiece. The practitioner gently holds the seal around the patient's lips to seal the airway so that the patient can trigger the breath and cycle the machine off (Fig. 14-6). Nose clips are also commonly needed.

c. Face mask

The face mask can be used if the mouth seal does not provide an airtight seal. This might be because of the patient's facial structure or lack of teeth. Mouth trauma, surgery, or lip sores are other reasons to use a face mask.

The mask should be clear and properly sized to fit comfortably over the patient's nose and mouth. The practitioner should be able to get a seal with a minimum amount of hand pressure (Fig. 14-7). The equipment connection opening in the mask has a 22-mm inner diameter (ID) so that it connects directly to the IPPB circuit. A 22-mm-OD male adapter and short length of aerosol tubing can be added for flexibility and patient comfort. The clear mask is important so that the practitioner can see whether the patient has vomited or has a large amount of secretions or saliva in his or her mouth. The mask should never be strapped to the patient's face so that the practitioner can attend to another patient.

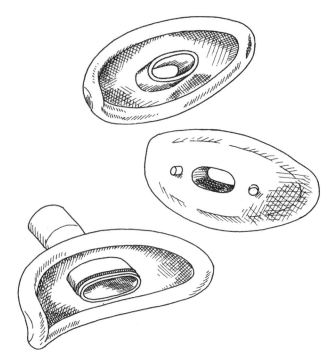

Figure 14-6 Top, Bennett or mouth flange seal. Bottom, IPPB mouthpiece inserted into the seal.

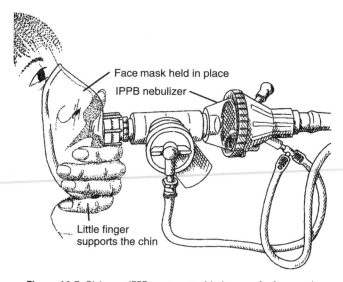

Face mask held in place
IPPB nebulizer
Little finger supports the chin

Figure 14-7 Giving an IPPB treatment with the use of a face mask.

This is the least effective patient attachment device if the therapeutic goal is to deliver an aerosolized medication. Much of the medication drains out on the patient's face or in the nasal passages if he or she is a nose breather.

d. Tracheostomy/endotracheal tube (elbow) adapter

The elbow adapter is designed to connect the patient's tracheostomy or endotracheal tube to the IPPB circuit (or other respiratory care equipment). The IPPB end has a 22-mm-ID connector. The tracheostomy/endotracheal tube end has a 15-mm-ID connector (Fig. 14-8). If the

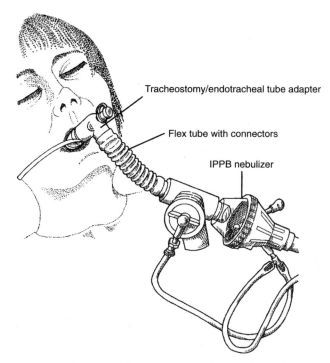

Figure 14-8 Giving an IPPB treatment with the use of a tracheostomy/endotracheal tube adapter.

Tracheostomy/endotracheal tube adapter

Flex tube with connectors

IPPB nebulizer

tube's cuff has been deflated, it must be reinflated to seal the airway. An unsealed cuff results in an air leak, and the gas flow will not turn off.

2. Correct patient–ventilator dyssynchrony (code: IIIC5) [difficulty: R, Ap, An]

Synchrony refers to the patient breathing in a coordinated pattern with the IPPB unit. Because the patient has to interact with the unit, some practice is required. The respiratory therapist must coach the patient to alter his or her breathing pattern as well as adjust the controls on the IPPB unit. Usually this involves adjusting sensitivity and flow.

a. Adjust the sensitivity

The sensitivity of the IPPB unit refers to how much effort or work the patient must perform to turn the unit on for a breath. Commonly, the sensitivity is set so that the patient has to generate a negative pressure of only about −1 cm H_2O pressure to begin an inspiration. This can be seen by the needle deflecting into the negative range on the pressure manometer. Ask the patient whether the machine can be easily turned on to get a breath. The IPPB unit should not be set at a level so sensitive that it self-cycles.

The sensitivity range on the Bird series is −0.01 to −5 cm H_2O. Turning the *sensitivity/starting effort* adjustment lever counterclockwise toward the smaller reference numbers makes the unit more sensitive. The sensitivity range on the Bennett series is −0.5 to −1 cm H_2O. Turning the *sensitivity* control counterclockwise makes the unit easier to turn on.

b. Adjust the flow

The patient should initially feel comfortable with the flow rate and the inspiratory time. Ideally, the flow should result in a smooth, steady rise in the pressure up to the preset maximum pressure. Reduce the flow if the pressure rises too quickly. Increase the flow if the pressure wavers higher and lower; this indicates the patient is breathing in faster than the gas is being delivered. Ask the patient a simple question such as, "Is the breath coming too fast or too slow?" He or she can give you a short answer or even a hand gesture in response. As the treatment progresses, the practitioner may be able to adjust the flow to modify the patient's breathing pattern to better achieve the therapeutic goal, for example:

- Anxious patients may initially need a fast flow. As they are coached to relax and become accustomed to the treatment, the practitioner should try to reduce the flow.
- Slower flows result in medications being deposited deeper into the lungs. This is important if the patient is having a bronchodilator, mucolytic, or antibiotic nebulized.
- Faster flows result in the deposition of medications in the upper airways. This is important if the patient is receiving racemic epinephrine for laryngeal edema or lidocaine for a local anesthetic of the upper airway before bronchoscopy.

Turning the *inspiratory time/flow rate* control counterclockwise increases the flow rate on the Bird series. Pulling the *air-mix* knob out from the center body increases the total flow by allowing room air to be entrained along with the source gas. Flow rate in the PR-II is determined by the patient's inspiratory effort and the degree to which the Bennett valve is open. Flow can be decreased somewhat by turning the *peak flow* control clockwise. Flow is not affected by the position of the *air dilution* knob.

3. Initiate and adjust the inspired oxygen percentage (code: IIIC1) [difficulty: R, Ap, An]

Compressed air or oxygen can power both the Bird and the Bennett units. The patient's condition determines the oxygen percentage administered. The physician may include the oxygen percentage in the treatment order. Some departments have oxygen protocols in their treatment procedure. Generally, compressed air (21% oxygen) should be used whenever the patient does not need supplemental oxygen.

A patient with COPD who is retaining carbon dioxide and breathing on hypoxic drive should also be given room air via the IPPB unit. The patient may be allowed to keep wearing a nasal cannula with oxygen during the treatment so that the blood oxygen level is kept normal. The unavailability of piped-in compressed air should not be an excuse to give a patient a high oxygen percentage when it may be harmful. IPPB can be given through a gas-powered unit driven by a compressed air cylinder or through an electrically powered unit.

Supplemental oxygen is given if any unit is powered by oxygen. With the Mark 7 and PR-II, the *air-mix/air dilution* knobs are set to dilute the source gas with room air. The Vortran-IPPB will add room air to the source gas. This is appropriate for patients who require supplemental oxygen and are not at risk of stopping their spontaneous ventilation. Most practitioners use this method of giving IPPB because piped oxygen is usually available in all patient rooms.

Pure oxygen should be given to the patient who is severely hypoxemic. Examples include acute pulmonary edema, respiratory failure, and carbon monoxide poisoning. The *air-mix/air dilution* knobs must be set so that only the source gas (oxygen) is delivered to the patient.

For varying oxygen percentages on the Mark 7, note the following guidelines:

- Pushing the *air-mix* knob into the center body results in pure source gas. This can be either air or oxygen.
- Pulling the *air-mix* knob out of the center body results in a dilution of the source gas with room air. If oxygen is the source gas, the room air will dilute the delivered gas to between 60% and 90% (or more) oxygen.

For varying oxygen percentages on the PR-II, note the following guidelines:

- Pulling the *air dilution* knob out of the body results in pure source gas. This can be either air or oxygen.
- Pushing the *air dilution* knob into the body results in a dilution of the source gas with room air. If oxygen is the source gas, the room air will dilute the delivered gas to between 40% and 80% oxygen.
- Turning on the *terminal flow* control results in the dilution of source gas with room air. This dilutes the final percentage if the source gas is oxygen.

4. Adjust the volume, pressure, or both

A review of the current respiratory care textbooks reveals that all authors agree that the basic goal of IPPB is to increase how deeply the patient inspires. Unfortunately, there is considerable difference about what inspiratory volume is being measured or by how much that breath should be increased for therapeutic goals to be achieved. The AARC has released the following guidelines on the subject:

- The *AARC Clinical Practice Guideline* (2011) on IS: IPPB, rather than IS, is indicated to treat atelectasis if (1) the patient's IC is less than 33% of predicted or (2) the patient's VC is less than 10 mL/kg of ideal body weight.
- Therefore IPPB would be indicated only when the patient cannot perform IS or is unable to reach the above clinical goals.
- The *AARC Clinical Practice Guideline* (1993) on IPPB: The V_T delivered during an IPPB-assisted breath should be at least 25% greater than the patient's spontaneous breaths.

Calculate the minimum IPPB-delivered V_T goal for a 35-year-old 150-lb ideal body weight male with pneumonia. He has a spontaneous V_T of 500 mL. Steps in the calculation include:

Minimum IPPB-assisted tidal volume
$$= \text{spontaneous tidal volume} \times 1.25$$

Minimum IPPB-assisted tidal volume $= 500 \text{ mL} \times 1.25 = 625 \text{ mL}$

- The 2003 revision and update of the 1993 *AARC Clinical Practice Guideline* on IPPB states that the V_T delivered during an IPPB-assisted breath should be at least one-third (0.33) of the patient's predicted IC.

Calculate the minimum IPPB-delivered V_T goal for a 35-year-old 150-lb ideal body weight male with pneumonia. He has a spontaneous V_T of 500 mL. Steps in the calculation include:

1. Convert the patient's body weight in pounds (lb) to kilograms (kg):

$$\frac{150 \text{ lb}}{2.2 \text{ lb/kg}} = 68.18 \text{ kg} \text{ (use 68 kg for this calculation)}$$

2. Calculate the patient's predicted IC:

Predicated $IC = 50 \text{ mL} \times \text{kg of ideal body weight}$

Therefore predicated $IC = 50 \text{ mL} \times 68 \text{ kg} = 3400 \text{ mL}$

3. Calculate the patient's minimum IPPB-assisted V_T goal:

Minimum IPPB goal $= 0.33 \times \text{predicated IC}$
$$= 0.33 \times 3400 \text{ mL} = 1122 \text{ mL}$$

Therefore the patient should receive an IPPB-assisted V_T of at least 1122 mL.

If the therapeutic goal is to prevent or treat atelectasis, having the patient inspire a deeper than spontaneous V_T breath should help. It seems reasonable to follow the AARC guidelines as clinical goals. Following the 2003 updated guidelines would provide the patient with a larger IPPB-assisted V_T. However, depending on the patient's tolerance, it may be necessary to begin with a smaller initial V_T goal (1993 guidelines) and then increase the goal as tolerated.

Because all of the current IPPB units are pressure cycled, the only way to increase the inspired volume during a passive treatment is to increase the peak pressure. Coaching the patient during an active treatment results in a larger volume without the need for as great a peak pressure. Decrease the peak pressure if the patient complains of discomfort or cannot hold that much pressure without losing the lip seal.

5. Recommend changes to reduce auto-PEEP (code: IIIE3f) [difficulty: R, Ap, An]

PEEP is pressure added through a mechanical ventilator at the end of an exhalation to prevent the patient from exhaling fully. PEEP keeps the patient's airway pressure greater than atmospheric (commonly given as the baseline pressure of zero). The clinical effect of PEEP is to increase a patient's residual volume (RV) and functional residual capacity (FRC) to improve oxygenation. It is used when the patient has a clinical condition, such as atelectasis or acute respiratory distress syndrome, that results in small lung volumes. The Vortran-IPPB unit will automatically add PEEP that is about 1/10 of the set peak pressure. The PEEP range is 2-5 cm H_2O.

Auto-PEEP is end-expiratory pressure in the lungs that cannot be seen on the IPPB unit's (or ventilator's) pressure manometer. Auto-PEEP is caused by air trapping because the patient does not have enough time to exhale completely. In other words, the patient starts another inspiration before the previous breath was completely exhaled. This problem is most commonly seen in patients with small-airways disease such as asthma and COPD.

Over the course of an IPPB treatment, patients who have small-airways disease can develop air trapping. This can lead to an increased RV and FRC, which is seen as auto-PEEP. This unwelcome lung overinflation increases the risk of pulmonary barotrauma. If auto-PEEP is known or suspected during an IPPB treatment, *expiratory retard* can be added to help ensure a complete exhalation. Adding expiratory retard to the treatment increases backpressure on the airways and has the same effect as pursed-lip breathing. The clinical effect of adding some backpressure on the smallest airways is to keep them open longer so that the more distal air can be exhaled.

The following two procedures can be used to help identify the presence of auto-PEEP:

1. Measure the exhaled volumes during the treatment and monitor the patient's response to the inspired breath. If the patient is exhaling less V_T with succeeding breaths or the patient complains of fullness, it is likely that air trapping is taking place.
2. Listen to the patient's breath sounds for a pause at the end of exhalation before the next inspiration begins. If there is no end-expiratory pause before the next breath, it is likely that the patient is air trapping.

If auto-PEEP is identified, expiratory retard can be added to reduce it. Too little retard results in some air trapping and an incompletely exhaled V_T. Too much retard results in an uncomfortably long expiratory time and additional air trapping. This would cause an increased mean intrathoracic pressure. The proper amount of expiratory retard should result in the patient feeling comfortable with the breathing cycle and being able to completely exhale the delivered V_T. Listen to the patient's breath sounds for a silent pause at the end of exhalation. If wheezing is present, it should be minimized when the proper amount of retard is added. This is because the backpressure is properly adjusted to minimize small-airway collapse and distal gas is fully exhaled.

Bird makes a retard cap that fits over the exhalation valve port on their permanent circuit. The cap has a series of different-sized holes through which the exhaled gas can pass (Fig. 14-9). By rotating the cap progressively from the largest to the smallest opening and evaluating the patient at each setting, the proper size of opening and amount of retard can be determined. The largest hole results in the least expiratory retard, and the smallest hole results in the greatest retard.

Bennett makes a retard exhalation valve that can be substituted for the regular exhalation valve on their permanent circuit (Fig. 14-10). The valve consists of a spring attached to a nut and a diaphragm. As the nut is turned counterclockwise, the spring pushes the diaphragm closer to the exhalation valve opening. This causes resistance to the exhalation of the V_T and a backpressure is created against the airways. Start with the least amount of expiratory retard and evaluate the patient before increasing the amount of expiratory retard. Be aware that if too much pressure is placed against the exhalation valve opening, the patient will not be able to exhale back to atmospheric pressure. This would create PEEP and should not be done without an order from the physician.

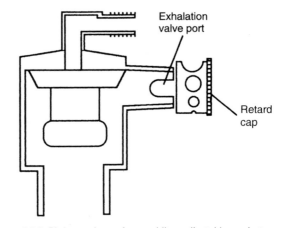

Figure 14-9 Bird retard cap for providing adjustable expiratory resistance. (From McPherson SP, Spearman CB: Respiratory care equipment, ed 5, St Louis, 1995, Mosby.)

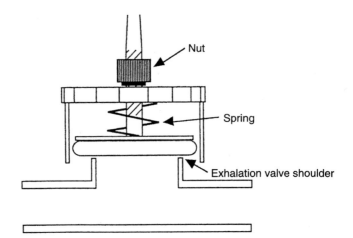

Figure 14-10 Bennett retard exhalation valve for providing adjustable expiratory resistance. (From McPherson SP, Spearman CB: Respiratory care equipment, ed 5, St Louis, 1995, Mosby.)

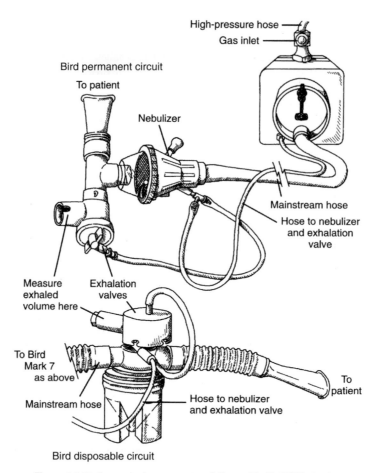

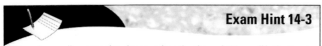

Figure 14-11 Features of permanent and disposable Bird IPPB circuits.

Be sure to ask the patient's opinion about the use of expiratory retard. The conscious, cooperative patient can tell you if he or she feels like more air is getting out by the use of the retard or if the lungs feel more full because too much retard is being used. Too much retard may also make the expiratory time uncomfortably long.

Exam Hint 14-3

There is usually a question that requires the therapist to modify the treatment. Increase the pressure to give a larger V_T; decrease the pressure to give a smaller V_T. If the patient wants a faster breath, increase the flow.

MODULE C

Assemble and troubleshoot the patient breathing circuit.

1. Assemble an IPPB breathing circuit (code: IIA14) [difficulty: R, Ap] and nebulizer (code: IIA4) [difficulty: R, Ap]

The Vortran-IPPB device does not have a separate patient circuit. The basic unit consists of the modulator (for adjusting peak inspiratory pressure and rate of exhalation) and nebulizer (with a reservoir and top) that fit together.

To know what pressure is being delivered to the patient, a pressure manometer and water trap need to be added (see Fig. 14-4). A 7-foot length of oxygen tubing with a DISS spin nut at each end is used to connect the source gas to the nebulizer. If the unit is directly connected to a regulator, a set flow of 40 L/min will be delivered. To adjust the gas flow, a 0-75 L/min flowmeter needs to be connected by the oxygen tubing to the gas source. This is a disposable unit used for only one patient.

Historically, the two most widely used pneumatically powered IPPB machines are the Bird Mark 7/8 (or a variation of it found in the series) and the Bennett PR-2. They have been widely used in hospitals. Historically, the most widely used electrically powered IPPB machines are the Bennett AP-4 and AP-5. They have been mainly used in the home. The Bird and Bennett units require a circuit that is designed specifically for them. Figure 14-11 shows a drawing of a permanent (reusable after cleaning) and a disposable circuit for a Bird machine. Figure 14-12 shows a drawing of a permanent (reusable after cleaning) and a disposable circuit for a Bennett machine.

a. General setup procedures

1. Check for plentiful source gas (usually piped air or oxygen). If an oxygen or air tank is used, make sure that it has

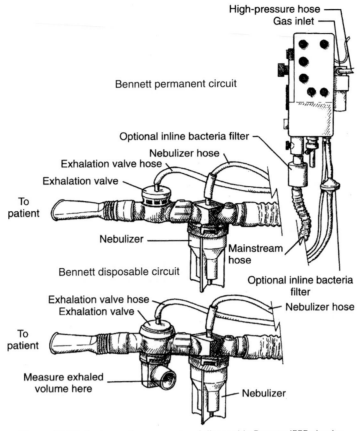

Figure 14-12 Features of permanent and disposable Bennett IPPB circuits.

the proper regulator. A flowmeter can be added if the Vortran unit is used. Check the pressure in the gas cylinder.

2. Attach the high-pressure hose to the source gas and the IPPB unit at the gas inlet. Make sure that the connections are tight.

3. Bacteria filters are optional. They are inserted between the IPPB unit gas outlets and the mainstream and nebulizer hoses.

4. A cascade-type humidifier is optional. Some practitioners prefer to warm and humidify the mainstream gas before it reaches the patient.

5. Check to see that the IPPB circuit is assembled properly and that all of the connections are tight.

6. Set the initial treatment parameters for sensitivity, flow, air mix, and peak pressure. Manually cycle the unit on. Cover the mouthpiece to see that the unit cycles off at the preset pressure.

7. Add any medication to the nebulizer. Check to see that the nebulizer is producing a mist.

b. Bird setup

1. One end of the mainstream (large-bore) hose is connected to the mainstream breathing hose connector on the right side of the unit. The other end is connected to the nebulizer.

2. One end of the nebulizer (small-bore) hose is connected to the small nipple on the right-hand side of the unit. The other end is connected to a T-piece at the nebulizer.

3. A piece of small-bore hose is used to connect one limb of the T-piece and the exhalation valve. Gas flowing through this hose powers both the nebulizer and the exhalation valve.

c. Bennett setup

1. One end of the mainstream (large-bore) hose is connected to the mainstream breathing hose connector on the underside of the unit. The other end is connected to the nebulizer.

2. One end of the nebulizer (medium-bore) hose is connected to the larger of two nipples on the underside of the unit. The other end is connected to the nebulizer nipple.

3. One end of the exhalation (small-bore) hose is connected to the smaller of two nipples on the underside of the unit. The other end is connected to the exhalation valve nipple.

2. Troubleshoot any problems with the breathing circuit (code: IIA14) [difficulty: R, Ap] and nebulizer (code: IIA14) [difficulty: R, Ap]

Fixing a problem is possible only after the problem has been identified. The practitioner should be familiar with both permanent and disposable types of Bird and Bennett circuits and the Vortran-IPPB unit. Leaks of any sort prevent the unit from cycling off so that the patient can exhale. Tighten any friction-fit or screw-type connections to stop the leak. A leak at the source-gas connection or high-pressure hose gas inlet connection results in a rather loud hissing sound. When connections are tightened properly, the hissing and leak will stop.

Debris such as mucus or blood can plug the nebulizer capillary tube and prevent any mist from being formed. Disassemble the nebulizer and rinse it under running water to try to clear the capillary tube. Replace the nebulizer if necessary.

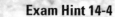

Exam Hint 14-4

Past examinations have included questions regarding the reasons that an IPPB machine would fail to cycle off. Identify the following leaks and know how to seal them: around the patient's mouthpiece (use a Bennett seal or face mask), within the circuit (tighten all connections), cuff on a tracheostomy or endotracheal tube (inflate the cuff), defective exhalation valve (replace the circuit).

MODULE D

Respiratory care plan

1. Determine a patient's pathophysiologic state (code: IIIF1) [difficulty: R, Ap, An]

Atelectasis is determined by characteristic chest radiograph findings and decreased or absent breath sounds over the affected area. Wheezing breath sounds would indicate small-airway closure. The patient may be experiencing bronchospasm. Pulmonary edema has characteristic chest radiograph findings and cardiovascular indicators. Crackles are often heard. Review the discussion on these conditions and their findings in Chapters 1 and 5. IPPB has been used in the management of patients with these conditions if other methods are not effective.

2. Recommend starting a treatment based on the patient's response (code: IIIE2a) [difficulty: R, Ap, An]

IPPB should be used for hyperinflation therapy only when less expensive options (such as IS) are shown to be impractical or ineffective. One of the goals of IPPB is to give the patient larger V_T than normal. The larger V_T should result in breath sounds being heard more clearly at the bases of the lungs. Additional secretions may be heard in the airways if the larger V_T result in their mobilization. However, if deeper breaths enable the patient to cough more effectively, additional secretions should be expectorated. Wheezing should be diminished if a bronchodilator medication is nebulized to a patient with bronchospasm.

Ask about the patient's feelings about the treatment, and write them in the chart. Note any significant comments made by the patient. Note the patient's preferred flow and pressure or volume settings.

3. Recommend a change in the therapeutic plan if indicated (code: IIIF2) [difficulty: R, Ap, An]

For the patient to receive the best care possible, the respiratory therapist must know the indications, contraindications, complications, and hazards of the respiratory care procedures the patient will receive. The patient must be assessed before, during, and after the treatment or procedure to determine if it was effective. The key goal of an appropriate care plan is that the patient's condition be treated in the best way possible. Modifications to the care plan must be made, as needed, as the patient's condition changes.

The respiratory therapist should be a member of the patient care team of the physician, nurse, and others in deciding how best to care for the patient. The following steps are necessary in developing the respiratory care plan for any patient:

1. Determine an expected outcome or goal(s).
2. Develop a plan to achieve success.
3. Decide how to measure if the goal(s) has been achieved.
4. Plan a timeline to measure the patient's progress.
5. Document the patient's response to care and the final outcome.

The patient should be fully cooperative to make the best use of IPPB. It may be counterproductive to try to force an IPPB treatment on a combative or uncooperative patient. A patient who has a neuromuscular deficit may need assistance in holding the IPPB circuit or keeping a good lip seal on the mouthpiece. A flexible mouth seal or face mask treatment may have to be given. Be prepared to make a recommendation to have a patient use IS, short-term continuous positive airway pressure, or IPPB for hyperinflation therapy. Also be prepared to make a recommendation for a patient to use a metered-dose inhaler, small-volume nebulizer, or IPPB for the delivery of an aerosolized medication.

4. Recommend a treatment be terminated (code: IIIE1) [difficulty: R, Ap, An]

Patient safety should always be an important consideration during the treatment. The respiratory therapist should know the complications and hazards of any patient care activity that is performed. Be prepared to stop the treatment if the patient has a sudden adverse reaction to it (for example, hemoptysis or signs and symptoms of a pneumothorax). Additionally, be prepared to recommend to the physician that the treatment be discontinued if it is likely to result in additional serious adverse reactions.

However, some adverse reaction may require only a pause or adjustment in the IPPB treatment. For example:

- If a patient hyperventilates and feels nauseated or faint, a short pause for normal breathing will help the patient feel normal again. Then IPPB can be restarted but with a slower respiratory rate or smaller V_T.
- The general treatment length of 15-20 minutes may cause fatigue. This is often seen in aged or debilitated patients. Provide a shorter but still effective treatment.
- Stop the treatment if the patient has a pulse rate change of 20% per minute or more. It is most common to see the pulse rate increase because of a nebulized bronchodilator drug. Wait for the heart rate to drop to normal before resuming the treatment. If tachycardia occurs again, discuss decreasing the medication dose with the physician.
- IPPB may cause a decreased venous return to the heart that may be shown by an increased heart rate or drop in blood pressure. Stop the treatment and monitor

the patient's vital signs. If they return to normal, give the IPPB treatment with a lower peak pressure and smaller V_T.

5. Recommend discontinuing a treatment based on the patient's response (code: IIIE2h) [difficulty: R, Ap, An]

The contraindications, hazards, and precautions to IPPB were discussed earlier in Module A under the sections "Contraindications" and "Hazards and precautions." The treatment should be discontinued if the patient has an untreated pneumothorax or massive hemoptysis. Other serious problems could also justify the cancellation of the order.

The IPPB treatments can be discontinued if the patient's atelectasis is resolved. If atelectatic areas have been opened, normal breath sounds should be heard. Or, IPPB can be discontinued if another, less expensive treatment, such as IS, can be properly performed by the patient.

BIBLIOGRAPHY

AARC clinical practice guideline: incentive spirometry, *Respir Care* 30:1402, 1991.

AARC clinical practice guideline: intermittent positive pressure ventilation, *Respir Care* 38:1189, 1993.

AARC clinical practice guideline: intermittent positive pressure ventilation—2003 revision & update, *Respir Care* 48:540, 2003.

AARC: clinical practice guideline: incentive spirometry *Respir Care* 56(10):1600–1604, 2011.

Branson RD, Hess DR, Chatburn RL, editors: *Respiratory care equipment*, ed 2, Philadelphia, 1999, Lippincott Williams & Wilkins.

Butler TJ: *Laboratory exercises for competency in respiratory care*, ed 3, Philadelphia, 2013, FA Davis.

Cairo JM: Lung expansion devices. In Cairo JM, Pilbeam SP, editors: *Mosby's respiratory care equipment*, ed 8, St Louis, 2010, Mosby.

Cairo JM: Lung expansion therapy devices. In Cairo JM, editor: *Mosby's respiratory care equipment*, ed 9, St Louis, 2014, Mosby.

Eubanks DH, Bone RC: *Comprehensive respiratory care*, ed 2, St Louis, 1990, Mosby.

Fink JB: Volume expansion therapy. In Burton GG, Hodgkin JE, Ward JJ, editors: *Respiratory care*, ed 4, Philadelphia, 1997, Lippincott.

Fink JB: Bronchial hygiene and lung expansion. In Fink JB, Hunt GE, editors: *Clinical practice in respiratory care*, Philadelphia, 1999, Lippincott Williams & Wilkins.

Fink JB, Hess DR: Secretion clearance techniques. In Hess DR, MacIntyre NR, Mishoe SC, editors: *Respiratory care principles & practices*, Philadelphia, 2002, Saunders.

Fisher DF: Lung expansion therapy. In Kacmarek RM, Stoller JK, Heuer JK, editors: *Egan's fundamentals of respiratory care*, ed 10, St Louis, 2013, Mosby.

Fluck RJ Jr: Intermittent positive-pressure breathing devices and transport ventilators. In Barnes TA, editor: *Respiratory care practice*, ed 2, St Louis, 1994, Mosby.

Hess DR: Sputum collection, airway clearance, and lung expansion therapy. In Hess DR, MacIntyre NR, Mishoe SC, Galvin WF, Adams AB, editors: *Respiratory care: principles and practice*, ed 2, Burlington, MA, 2012, Jones & Bartlett Learning.

McPherson SP: *Respiratory care equipment*, ed 5, St Louis, 1995, Mosby.

Miller WF: Intermittent positive pressure breathing (IPPB). In Kacmarek RM, Stoller JK, editors: *Current respiratory care*, Philadelphia, 1988, BC Decker.

Respiratory Care Committee of the American Thoracic Society: Guidelines for the use of intermittent positive pressure breathing (IPPB), *Respir Care* 25:365, 1980.

Rutkowski JA: Pulmonary hygiene and chest physical therapy. In Wyka KA, Mathews PJ, Rutkowski J, editors: *Foundations of respiratory care*, ed 2, Clifton Park, NY, 2012, Delmar.

Shapiro BA, Kacmarek RM, Cane RD, et al.: *Clinical application of respiratory care*, ed 4, St Louis, 1991, Mosby.

Weizalis CP: Intermittent positive-pressure breathing. In Barnes TA, editor: *Respiratory care practice*, ed 2, St Louis, 1994, Mosby.

Welch MA Jr, Shapiro BJ, Mercurio P, Wagner W, Hiravama G: Methods of intermittent positive pressure breathing, *Chest* 78:463, 1980.

White GC: *Equipment theory for respiratory care*, ed 4, Albany, NY, 2005, Delmar.

Wilkins RL: Lung expansion therapy. In Wilkins RL, Stoller CL, Kacmarek RM, editors: *Egan's fundamentals of respiratory care*, ed 9, St Louis, 2009, Mosby.

1. If a patient complains of difficulty in starting the IPPB treatment, which control should be adjusted?
   A. Pressure
   B. Flow
   C. Sensitivity
   D. Terminal flow

2. A patient is having difficulty keeping a tight seal around the mouthpiece. The patient complains that the breath is too long and takes out the mouthpiece. To help cycle off the PR-2, what should be adjusted?
   A. Pressure
   B. Flow
   C. Terminal flow
   D. Expiratory retard

3. A patient with pulmonary edema has cyanotic lips and nail beds. What O_2 percentage should be recommended for IPPB treatment?
   A. 21%
   B. 40%
   C. 80%
   D. 100%

4. All of the following indicate the need for IPPB EXCEPT:
   A. A patient who cannot coordinate the use of a metered-dose inhaler or a hand-held nebulizer
   B. A comatose patient with atelectasis
   C. A patient with an IC of 8 mL/kg
   D. A cooperative patient with atelectasis

5. A respiratory therapist is ordered to give an IPPB treatment to a comatose patient who has lip ulcers. What patient–machine connection should be used?
   A. Mouthpiece
   B. Face mask
   C. Bennett seal with mouthpiece
   D. Nose clips and mouthpiece

6. At the start of IPPB treatment, at what level should the sensitivity control be set at on a Bird unit?
   A. 0 cm H_2O
   B. –1 cm H_2O
   C. –3 cm H_2O
   D. –5 cm H_2O

7. A respiratory therapist is giving an IPPB treatment with a Bird Mark 7 unit. To give the patient 100% O_2, the *air-mix* control knob is pushed in. What effect does this adjustment have on the flow rate to the patient?
   A. Decreases the flow of gas
   B. Increases the flow of gas
   C. No effect
   D. Increases the sensitivity

8. In the Emergency Department, a respiratory therapist is giving an IPPB treatment with albuterol (AccuNeb) to an asthmatic male patient. During a break in the treatment, the patient complains that his lungs feel too full and he does not feel like all the IPPB volume is getting out. What should be done?
   A. Increase the flow.
   B. Add expiratory retard.
   C. Increase the system pressure.
   D. Change to 100% oxygen.

9. While giving an IPPB treatment with a Vortran unit, a hissing sound is heard and the patient complains that the inspiratory time is too long. What is the most likely problem?
   A. The nebulizer hose is attached to the exhalation valve.
   B. The nebulizer medication jar is loose.
   C. The bacteria filter is missing.
   D. The inspiratory and expiratory hoses are reversed.

10. A respiratory therapist is giving an IPPB treatment when the patient complains of a sharp chest pain. After a few more deep breaths, the patient is short of breath. The therapist notices that the patient's breath sounds are now diminished on the left side. What should be done?
    A. Continue the treatment for the next 5 minutes to finish the ordered time.
    B. Decrease the peak pressure and complete the ordered treatment.
    C. Stop the treatment and notify the physician of the patient's complaints.
    D. Monitor the patient closely for the duration of the treatment.

11. An IPPB treatment should be stopped under which of the following conditions?
    1. You suspect the patient has a pneumothorax.
    2. The patient has difficulty keeping the lips sealed.
    3. The patient feels faint and dizzy.
    4. The patient coughs up blood.
    A. 1 and 4 only
    B. 2 and 3 only
    C. 1, 2, and 3 only
    D. 2, 3, and 4 only

12. A respiratory therapist is about to give an asthmatic 16-year-old female patient her second IPPB treatment with a bronchodilator medication. When checking the equipment, it is noticed that the equipment is set with a rather fast inspiratory flow. Her chart had a note that she was very anxious when first admitted. She seems calmer now. How should the treatment be started?
    A. Increase the pressure setting to deliver a larger breath.
    B. Keep the flow the same to deliver a larger breath.

C. Make the machine as sensitive as possible to easily trigger it.
D. Decrease the flow on the machine.

13. A 45-year-old female 50-kg (110-pound) patient is recovering after abdominal surgery. The physician has ordered IPPB to help correct her atelectasis after IS was found to be ineffective. Her spontaneous V_T is 350 mL. Based on this information, at what level should her minimum initial IPPB V_T be set?
    A. 350 mL
    B. 450 mL
    C. 700 mL
    D. 900 mL

14. Atelectasis has been diagnosed by chest radiograph in an unconscious patient who had recent open heart surgery. Before surgery, the patient's best FVC value was 55% of the predicted. What should be recommended to treat the patient's atelectasis problem?
    A. IPPB
    B. IS
    C. Nasotracheal suctioning
    D. Flutter

15. A patient with COPD has been receiving IPPB treatments on a Bird Mark 7 for 5 days. Expiratory retard was added 4 days ago. Because the retard has not been evaluated since then, the physician asks that it be done. The respiratory therapist proceeds to make the following adjustments in the retard cap settings and makes the following observations:

Retard Cap Setting	Exhaled Tidal Volume (mL)	Wheezing	Patient's Impression
1 (smallest)	850	None	Exhalation too long
2	825	Some in bases	Exhalation too long
3	800	Some in bases	Comfortable
4	700	All lobes	Lungs feel full

Based on this information, which retard cap setting should be recommended?
    A. 1
    B. 2
    C. 3
    D. 4

16. A 13-year-old patient with cystic fibrosis is receiving IPPB to deliver an aerosolized bronchodilator and mucolytic. The respiratory therapist notices that the pressure gauge needle is bouncing higher and lower as the patient takes a breath. What should be done?
    A. Increase the target pressure.
    B. Increase the sensitivity setting.
    C. Increase the flow.
    D. Tell the patient to inhale more quickly.

17. A patient has an IPPB V_T goal of 900 mL but is exhaling only 700 mL. There is no air leak. What should be done to deliver a larger volume?
    A. Increase the delivered pressure.
    B. Decrease the flow.
    C. Add expiratory retard.
    D. Have the patient inhale more forcefully.

18. An 82-kg (180-pound) male is recovering after an accidental drug overdose. Because of hypoventilation and being semicomatose, he has developed bilateral atelectasis. Calculate the ideal minimum IPPB-delivered V_T goal for him. His spontaneous V_T is 600 mL.
    A. 700 mL
    B. 900 mL
    C. 1400 mL
    D. 3000 mL

15 | Mechanical Ventilation of the Adult

Note: It can be anticipated that the Therapist Multiple-Choice Examination (TMC) will include an *average of 36 of 140 actual questions* (26% of the exam) on mechanical ventilation of the adult. (This is based on the question mix typically found on the National Board of Respiratory Care's (NBRC's) previous Entry Level Examinations and Written Registry Examinations.) *This is the most heavily tested content area of the exam.*

Remember that the TMC version you take will include 20 additional questions being evaluated for possible inclusion in other versions of the TMC. So, there will be a total of 160 questions taken. There is no way to differentiate between the 140 actual questions and the 20 questions being evaluated for future use. Please go to the Introduction for detailed information on the TMC and the Clinical Simulation Examination.

MODULE A

Evaluate monitoring trends in the patient record.

1. Work of breathing (code: IA13b) [difficulty: R, Ap]

Work of breathing (WOB) normally refers to how much energy the patient has to expend to inhale. Patients with stiff lungs, high inspiratory airway resistance, or both have an increased WOB. Exhalation normally is passive and requires no work. However, some patients with high expiratory airway resistance (discussed below) have increased WOB to exhale. Look in the patient's electronic medical record for information on patient complaints of shortness of breath and easy tiring as signs of increased WOB.

A patient who has been intubated and placed on a modern mechanical ventilator with a microprocessor and graphics software can have WOB measured. See Figure 15-1 for a pressure/volume loop tracing that shows a patient's WOB. WOB is minimized when the ventilator is set to minimize the negative pressure and inspiratory flow the patient has to generate.

If the breathing of an intubated and ventilated patient appears to be unsynchronized with the ventilator, his or her WOB should be evaluated. Ask the conscious patient simple questions to try to determine what the problem is. Observe the patient for use of accessory muscles as a sign of increased WOB. If the ventilator is capable, program it to perform a pressure/volume loop of the patient's WOB.

Be prepared to adjust parameters such as the machine's sensitivity and inspiratory flow to minimize the patient's workload.

2. Airway resistance (code: IA13b) [difficulty: R, Ap]

Airway resistance (Raw) may have been measured earlier in the pulmonary function laboratory or on the ventilator. Compare any earlier values with new measurements. This is important for understanding the patient's trends toward an improving or a worsening pulmonary condition.

Airway resistance is measured in units of centimeters of water per liter per second at a standard flow rate of 0.5 L/s (30 L/min). The normal spontaneously breathing adult's Raw is 0.6-2.4 cm water/L/s; the normal 3-kg infant's Raw is 30 cm water/L/s. Do not forget that this procedure is being performed on a patient with an intubated airway on a ventilator. The endotracheal tube adds to the patient's total Raw. The smaller the tube is, the greater is the resistance that it offers to gas flowing through it. Altering inspiratory flow has an influence on the peak pressure measured for the calculation. As flow is reduced, gas turbulence is reduced and peak pressure is reduced. Conversely, a higher flow creates more turbulence and a higher peak pressure is seen.

3. Pulmonary compliance (code: IA13b) [difficulty: R, Ap]

This value may have been measured earlier in the pulmonary function laboratory or on the ventilator. Compare any earlier values with new values. This is important for determining the patient's trends toward an improving or a worsening pulmonary condition.

The compliance values indicate how easily the tidal volume can be delivered into the lungs. Static compliance (Cst) is the measurement of work required to overcome the elastic resistance to ventilation. It is a measurement of the compliance of the lungs and thorax (C_{LT}). Static compliance is measured in units of milliliters per centimeters of water pressure. The normal adult's static compliance is 100 mL/cm water; the normal 3-kg infant's static compliance is 5 mL/cm water.

Dynamic compliance (Cdyn), sometimes called *dynamic characteristic*, is the measurement of the combination of the patient's static compliance and airway resistance. As was discussed previously, airway resistance is the pressure required to move a tidal volume through the airways. It also is known as *nonelastic resistance to ventilation.*

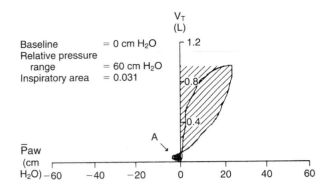

Baseline = 0 cm H_2O
Relative pressure
range = 60 cm H_2O
Inspiratory area = 0.031

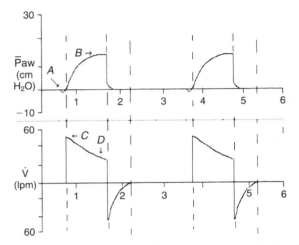

Figure 15-1 Two graphic tracings of pressure support ventilation. *Top graphic* shows the pressure/volume loop of a patient triggering a breath. The arrow marked A shows the work of breathing provided by the patient. The shaded area on right indicates how much work was provided by ventilator. *Bottom graphic* shows airway pressure ($\bar{P}aw$) versus time and flow ($\dot{V}$) versus time tracings. Arrows: **A,** where the patient initiated a breath; **B,** where the ventilator cycled off when the pressure support level of 15 cm water was reached; **C,** high peak flow at the start of the breath; **D,** how flow rate decreases as the pressure support level is reached. (Reprinted by permission of Nellcor Puritan Bennett, Inc., LLC, Boulder, CO, part of Covidien.)

MODULE B

Perform and evaluate procedures to gather clinical information.

1. Utilize ventilator graphics (e.g., waveforms, scales to support oxygenation and ventilation) (code: IIIC6) [difficulty: R, Ap, An]

A patient who has been intubated and placed on a modern mechanical ventilator with a microprocessor and graphics software can have ventilator flow, volume, and pressure waveforms visualized on the monitor, stored in memory, or printed out. Look for this information and compare it with the patient's current situation. See Figure 15-2 for examples of pressure, volume, and flow tracings. See Figure 15-3 for key points of information available from a flow versus time graph.

Follow the ventilator manufacturer's steps to direct the unit to create flow, volume, and pressure waveforms. The patient can be instructed, based on the breathing test, to perform a breathing maneuver actively or to lie passively as the ventilator delivers a breath.

The operator typically can select any two of the following for display on the monitor: time, flow, pressure, and volume. Certain combinations are selected to best present the needed information. For example, air trapping is best shown by comparing flow versus time (Fig. 15-4), peak and plateau pressures are best shown by comparing pressure versus time (Fig. 15-5), and lung inflection points are best shown by comparing volume versus pressure (discussed later). Note examples of ventilator graphics throughout this chapter.

A number of flow, volume, and pressure waveforms have been included in this chapter for practice. In addition, review Figures 4-1 and 4-11 in Chapter 4 for examples of pulmonary function test waveform tracings. The examples in this chapter include common clinical situations and are accompanied by explanations to help with interpretation.

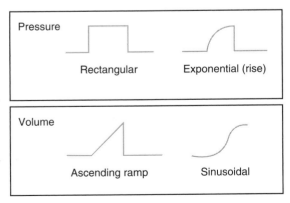

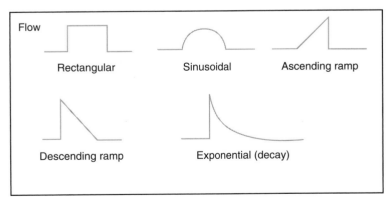

Figure 15-2 Examples of waveforms for pressure, flow, and volume that can be seen on the graphics monitor of a microprocessor-type ventilator. The practitioner can select from these and other options to display needed graphs to help guide patient care. See examples throughout the chapter. (From Cairo JM: Pilbeam's mechanical ventilation: physiological and clinical applications, ed 5, St. Louis, 2012, Mosby.)

2. Determine the patient's airway resistance (code: IC12) [difficulty: R, Ap]

This calculation is important because it provides valuable information on the patient's pulmonary condition. The Raw value indicates how difficult it is to move the tidal volume through the patient's airways and whether aerosolized bronchodilating medications are effective.

It is reasonable to recommend an airway resistance measurement on any patient who has an increased airway resistance problem such as chronic obstructive pulmonary disease (COPD), asthma, bronchospasm, or wheezing breath sounds. It also is reasonable to measure airway resistance before and after a bronchodilator medication is given to determine whether it had any benefit.

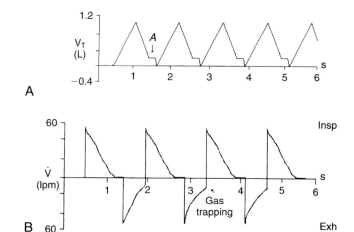

Figure 15-4 Two graphic tracings of expiratory air trapping. **A,** Volume versus time. Arrow *A* shows that the exhaled tidal volume tracing does not reach the baseline. Inspiratory tidal volume is greater than expiratory tidal volume, indicating air trapping. **B,** Flow versus time. Inspiratory flow is the tracing above the horizontal baseline of zero flow. Expiratory flow is the tracing below the horizontal baseline. The patient's expiratory flow does not return to zero; this indicates air trapping. The higher the flow rate, the more air trapping is present. Air trapping leads to auto-positive end-expiratory pressure. It can be minimized by increasing expiratory time, giving an aerosolized bronchodilator to treat bronchospasm, or suctioning out any secretions. (Reprinted by permission of Nellcor Puritan Bennett LLC, Boulder, CO, part of Covidien.)

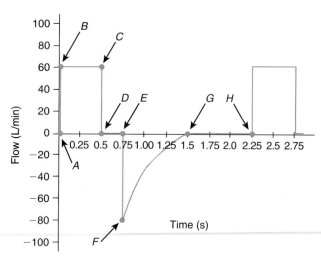

Figure 15-3 Analysis of key points in a flow/time graph. Shown is the inspiratory rectangular waveform during volume ventilation and exhalation of the tidal volume. Arrows: **A,** start of inspiratory flow; **B,** peak inspiratory flow of 60 L/min (1 L/s); **C,** end of inspiratory flow. Total inspiratory flow time is found between points *B* and *C* (0.5 s) when the tidal volume is delivered. The tidal volume can be calculated at 500 mL (1 L/s of flow × 0.5 s of inspiratory time = 0.5 L [500 mL] tidal volume). **D** and **E,** inspiratory hold (inflation hold) of 0.25 second after the end of inspiration. Without inspiratory hold, the patient would begin exhalation at point *D.* Total inspiratory time is 0.75 second (0.5 second inspiratory flow time +0.25 second inspiratory hold time = 0.75 second). **F,** peak expiratory flow of −80 L/min (−1.33 L/s); **G,** end of expiratory flow. Expiratory flow time is 0.75 second. **H,** start of the next inspiration. **G** and **H,** 0.75 second of zero flow time. Total expiratory time is 1.5 seconds (0.75 second expiratory flow time +0.75 second zero flow time). Inspiratory/expiratory ratio is 1:2 (0.75 second of total inspiratory time/1.5 seconds of total expiratory time). (Modified from Pilbeam SP: Ventilator graphics. In Pilbeam SP, Cairo JM (editors): Mechanical ventilation: physiologic and clinical applications, ed 4, St Louis, 2006, Mosby.)

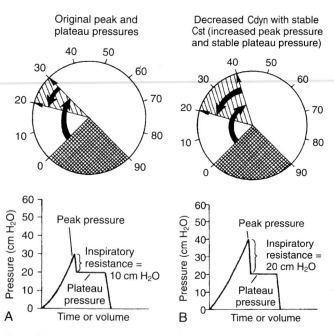

Figure 15-5 Decreased dynamic compliance (Cdyn) with a stable static compliance (Cst). **A,** Original pressure manometer reading and pressure/volume curve. **B,** Altered pressure manometer reading and pressure/volume curve.

Most of the microprocessor ventilators offer software for calculating these values. However, in other situations, airway resistance must be calculated manually as follows.

1. Cycle a tidal volume. The patient should be breathing passively; fighting the breath will result in an erroneously high peak pressure, and assisting with the breath will result in an erroneously low peak pressure.
2. Note the peak airway pressure on the manometer.
3. Briefly prevent the tidal volume from being exhaled. No air should be moving. Note that the pressure manometer shows a peak pressure and then a static or plateau pressure that is stable as long as the tidal volume is held in the lungs. Record the plateau pressure.
4. Calculate the flow in liters per second by taking the flow in liters per minute and dividing it by 60 seconds.
5. Place the peak airway pressure, plateau pressure, and flow into the following formula and solve for airway resistance:

$$Raw = \frac{\text{Peak airway pressure} - \text{Plateau pressure}}{\text{Flow in L/s}}$$

Exam Hint 15-2

The airway resistance calculation has been tested on previous examinations, so review the math.

EXAMPLE

A mechanically ventilated patient has a peak airway pressure of 30 cm water and a plateau pressure of 20 cm water. The peak flow is set at 60 L/min.

Calculate peak flow in liters per second:

$$\frac{60 \text{ L/min}}{60 \text{ s}} = 1 \text{ L/s}$$

Calculate airway resistance:

$$Raw = \frac{\text{Peak airway pressure} - \text{Plateau pressure}}{\text{Flow in L/s}}$$

$$Raw = \frac{30 \text{ cm H}_2\text{O} - 20 \text{ cm H}_2\text{O}}{1 \text{ L/s}} = 10 \text{ cm H}_2\text{O/L/s}$$

This value is greater than normal for a patient who is breathing spontaneously. However, remember that the patient's airway is intubated. This results in a smaller airway diameter and greater resistance. Some practitioners use the calculated airway resistance as the basis for setting the pressure support ventilation level (discussed later). Increased airway resistance may indicate bronchospasm or secretions in the airways. Delivering an aerosolized bronchodilator or suctioning should result in the return of airway resistance to the original level.

3. Auto-positive end-expiratory pressure

a. Perform the procedure to detect auto-positive end-expiratory pressure (code: IC15) [difficulty: R, Ap]

Auto-positive end-expiratory pressure (auto-PEEP) is PEEP in the lungs that cannot be seen on the ventilator's pressure manometer. (The terms *inadvertent PEEP* and *intrinsic PEEP* also are used.) Auto-PEEP is caused by air trapping resulting from an inadequate expiratory time. It becomes more likely when the inspiratory time is increased or the expiratory time is decreased or in patients with long time constants of ventilation. Simply put, the next breath is delivered before the patient has exhaled completely (see Fig. 15-4). This problem is seen frequently in patients with status asthmaticus or COPD because of early small-airway closure. In patients with acute respiratory distress syndrome (ARDS) who are receiving pressure-controlled inverse ratio ventilation, the long inspiratory times used increase the risk of expiratory air trapping. Auto-PEEP is more likely to be found when the inspiratory/expiratory (I:E) ratio becomes 2:1 or greater.

The level of auto-PEEP can be determined in different ways, depending on the type of ventilator that is being used. It can be measured on the pressure manometer of most ventilators. The trapped expiratory gas also can be seen on the graphic display of all current-generation microprocessor-type ventilators. The following procedure can be followed for determining the presence or level of auto-PEEP:

1. Note the delivery of a tidal volume.
2. Watch the pressure gauge as it decreases to zero (or the level of therapeutic PEEP) at the end of exhalation. Make sure that the patient is exhaling passively to obtain an accurate reading.
3. Reduce the rate control to delay the next breath.
4. Occlude the expiratory tubing (or push the expiratory hold button or add inflation hold on other ventilators) to prevent any further exhalation for about 3-5 seconds (Fig. 15-6).
5. If the pressure gauge is being monitored, note any pressure increase above the baseline pressure, or, if the ventilator has a graphics monitor, note the failure of the exhaled tidal volume or expiratory flow to return to baseline to confirm the presence and amount of auto-PEEP (see Fig. 15-5).
6. Listen to the patient's breath sounds during a standard breath and during the prolonged exhalation. It is likely that during the standard breath, expiratory sounds will be heard until inspiratory sounds begin. During prolonged exhalation, the expiratory sounds continue for a longer time and then end with silence. This silent pause time indicates that no more expiratory airflow is occurring.

It is important to add any auto-PEEP to the amount of therapeutic PEEP the patient has. This should be recorded as the total PEEP. For example, the patient

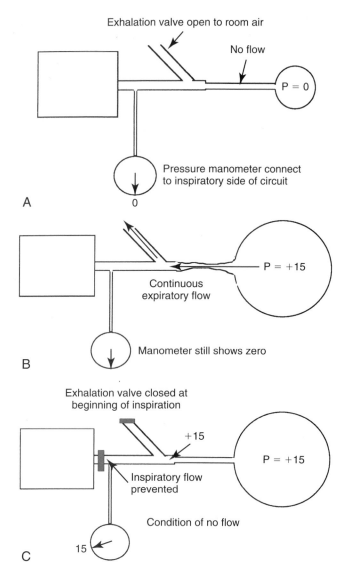

Figure 15-6 Identification of auto–positive end-expiratory pressure (auto-PEEP) from air trapping. **A,** A normal patient will completely exhale before the next tidal volume breath is delivered. The manometer shows a pressure of zero (ambient, atmospheric pressure), which matches the patient's airway and lung pressures. **B,** A patient with increased airway resistance (asthma or chronic obstructive pulmonary disease [COPD]), who is not able to exhale completely before the next breath is started. Even though the manometer shows zero pressure, pressure from the trapped gas is increased within the airways and lungs. **C,** Auto-PEEP can be measured by closing the exhalation valve at the end of inspiration and stopping the next tidal volume breath. During this prolonged expiratory time, flow and pressure equilibrate. The manometer pressure now shows the actual increased pressure with the patient's airways and lungs. Reduce auto-PEEP by reducing airway resistance and increasing the expiratory time. (From Pilbeam S, Cairo J [editors]: Mechanical ventilation, ed 4, St Louis, 2006, Mosby.)

has 5 cm of therapeutic PEEP and 2 cm of auto-PEEP for 7 cm of total PEEP. It may be thought that the total PEEP level places the patient at risk for volutrauma or decreased venous return and lowered cardiac output (CO). The amount of auto-PEEP can be reduced by

TABLE 15-1	Reasons/Solutions for Air Trapping and Auto-PEEP
Problem	**Solution(s)**
a. Bronchospasm causing slow expiratory flow	Administer a bronchodilator medication.
	Increase expiratory time by decreasing inspiratory time.
	Add expiratory retard.
b. Secretions causing slow expiratory flow	Suction the patient's airway.
c. Large tidal volume that is not fully exhaled	Reduce the tidal volume. Increase the expiratory time by decreasing inspiratory time.

PEEP, positive end-expiratory pressure.

decreasing the inspiratory time, increasing the expiratory time, or decreasing the tidal volume. Lack of auto-PEEP can be confirmed by this procedure. If the auto-PEEP cannot be eliminated, therapeutic PEEP can be added to match it. By increasing the baseline pressure, the patient can more easily trigger an assisted or synchronous intermittent mandatory ventilation (SIMV) breath. It is especially important to decrease auto-PEEP and therapeutic PEEP levels as the patient's C_{LT} improves and airway resistance returns to normal.

b. Evaluate the auto-PEEP procedure results (code: ID14) [difficulty: R, Ap, An]

Figure 15-4 demonstrates two ways that air trapping on exhalation can be identified as auto-PEEP. Note in Figure 15-4 (bottom) that the patient's expiratory flow does not reach the baseline pressure before another breath is delivered. This proves that air trapping has occurred. The larger the gap between the pressure at the end of expiration and at baseline, the greater is the air trapping.

If a patient has auto-PEEP, every attempt should be made to determine why the patient is air trapping. Although the basic problem is an expiratory time that is too short for full exhalation of the tidal volume, a more specific reason should be found, and then a solution can be found. Table 15-1 shows possible reasons for air trapping and auto-PEEP and solutions.

Not every possible solution can be used. The patient's situation must be considered. For example, increasing the expiratory time will reduce the inspiratory time if the same rate is to be kept. Increasing the expiratory time and keeping the same inspiratory time will reduce the patient's respiratory rate. This will reduce the minute volume and will increase the patient's carbon dioxide level. Additionally, reducing the tidal volume will reduce the minute volume and will increase the patient's carbon dioxide level.

4. Plateau pressure

a. Determine the patient's plateau pressure (code: IC14) [difficulty: R, Ap]

The plateau pressure on the ventilator is determined for evaluation of the patient's C_{LT}. A change in the patient's C_{LT} will correlate with changes in the patient's lung condition. The following two areas of discussion cover C_{LT}, performing the C_{LT} procedure, and interpreting the results.

There are two ways to determine the plateau pressure. First, have the patient lie passively and set the ventilator to prevent a delivered tidal volume from being exhaled (inflation hold). Second, have the patient lie passively, and manually cover the end of the expiratory tubing to prevent a delivered tidal volume from being exhaled. The hold should be for about 2 seconds so that the pressure manometer value is stable.

b. Evaluate the plateau pressure procedure results (code: ID13) [difficulty: R, Ap, An]

An accurate plateau pressure can be measured only if the patient cooperates and does not interact with the ventilator. Note the stable airway pressure as the plateau pressure (see Fig. 15-5, A). After the plateau pressure has been determined, the patient must exhale completely. It may be necessary to delay the next timed ventilator tidal volume breath to avoid "stacking" a new breath when the first has not yet been exhaled. It is recommended that the plateau pressure procedure be repeated to ensure that the measured pressure is accurate.

5. Determine the patient's pulmonary compliance (code: IC12) [difficulty: R, Ap]

It is reasonable to recommend that C_{LT} should be measured on any patient who has clinical evidence of a significant change in C_{LT}. This may occur in conditions such as acute respiratory distress syndrome (ARDS), pneumonia, pulmonary edema, or pulmonary fibrosis. Compliance can be measured to document worsening of the patient's condition or to determine whether compliance is improving with treatment. Most microprocessor ventilators offer software that can be used for calculating all of these values. However, in other situations, they must be calculated manually, as follows.

a. Procedure for calculating the tubing compliance factor

Before the actual calculation of the patient's static and dynamic compliance can be performed, the compliance of the breathing circuit should be determined. During positive-pressure ventilation, some of the set tidal volume never reaches the patient because it is "lost" in the circuit. Remember that when a positive-pressure breath is delivered, the ventilator circuit will be expanded and the gas within the tubing will be compressed. The term *compressed volume* is commonly used to describe this lost volume. Subtract the compressed volume from the exhaled volume coming from the ventilator to determine the patient's actual tidal volume. (Some of the current generation of

microprocessor ventilators will calculate the compressed volume. The therapist can have the ventilator compensate for the lost volume and deliver a tidal volume that meets the set volume on the ventilator.)

For greatest accuracy in the calculation of static and dynamic compliance and the calculation of actual tidal and sigh volumes, any lost volume must be subtracted from the exhaled tidal volume to find the actual tidal volume. The tubing compliance factor is used in the calculation to determine the compressed volume, through the following procedure:

1. Remove the patient from the ventilator and manually ventilate him or her during this procedure.
2. Set the pressure limit as high as possible.
3. Block the breathing circuit at the patient connector. Make sure there are no leaks.
4. Cycle a tidal volume. If possible, set inflation hold for 2 seconds to see a stable pressure.
5. Perform either of the following: (1) note the pressure developed in the circuit as the tidal volume stretches out the circuit or (2) if the ventilator's peak pressure hits the pressure limit, note the delivered tidal volume and the pressure limit. In both cases, measure the exhaled tidal volume.

Note: If the patient is receiving PEEP therapy, subtract the PEEP level from the measured pressure to find the true pressure.

6. The compliance factor is found by dividing the exhaled tidal volume by the pressure.
7. Return the patient to the ventilator.

EXAMPLE

The patient has a set tidal volume of 600 mL. By using step 5b, the pressure is found to be 80 cm water, and the measured tidal volume is found to be 320 mL.

$$\text{Compliance factor} = \frac{320 \text{ mL}}{80 \text{ cm}} = 4 \text{ mL/cm water}$$

The compressed volume is found by multiplying the compliance factor by either the peak or the plateau pressure when a tidal volume is delivered. The compressed volume is then subtracted from the exhaled tidal volume to determine the patient's actual tidal volume.

Exam Hint 15-3

Commonly, examinations have had a question requiring the calculation of static compliance or dynamic compliance or both. Be able to perform the following calculations.

b. Procedure for calculating static compliance

1. Determine the compliance factor of the breathing circuit (as described previously).
2. Reattach the patient to the ventilator. Reset all controls to their ordered or preset positions.
3. Cycle a tidal volume. The patient should be breathing passively; fighting the breath will result in an

erroneously high peak pressure, and assisting with the breath will result in an erroneously low peak pressure.

4. Briefly prevent the tidal volume from being exhaled. No air should be moving. Note that the pressure manometer shows a peak pressure and then a static or plateau pressure that is stable as long as the tidal volume is held in the lungs. Note the *plateau* pressure.

5. Calculate the Cst by using the formula

$$Cst = \frac{\text{Exhaled tidal volume} - \text{Compressed volume}}{\text{Plateau pressure} - \text{PEEP}}$$

in which compressed volume is the compliance factor × plateau pressure.

c. Procedure for calculating dynamic compliance

1. Determine the compliance factor of the breathing circuit (as described previously).

2. Reattach the patient to the ventilator. Reset all controls to their ordered or preset positions.

3. Cycle a tidal volume. The patient should be breathing passively; fighting the breath will result in an erroneously high peak pressure, and assisting with the breath will result in an erroneously low peak pressure.

4. Note the *peak pressure* on the manometer. If the pressure at the end of inspiration is less than the peak pressure, the pressure at the end of inspiration should be used in the calculation.

5. Calculate the Cdyn using the formula

$$Cdyn = \frac{\text{Exhaled tidal volume} - \text{Compressed volume}}{\text{Peak pressure} - \text{PEEP}}$$

in which compressed volume is compliance factor × peak pressure.

EXAMPLE

Calculate the static and dynamic compliance on a ventilated patient *without PEEP* therapy.

The patient has an exhaled tidal volume of 600 mL. The peak pressure is 30 cm water, and the static or plateau pressure is 20 cm water. The compliance factor has been determined to be 4 mL/cm water. The compressed volume at the plateau pressure is determined to be 80 mL (4 mL/cm compliance factor × 20 cm). The compressed volume at the peak pressure is determined to be 120 mL (4 mL/cm compliance factor × 30 cm).

$$Cst = \frac{600 \text{ mL} - 80 \text{ mL}}{20 \text{ cm} - 0}$$
$$= \frac{520 \text{ mL}}{20 \text{ cm}}$$
$$= 26 \text{ mL/cm water}$$

$$Cdyn = \frac{600 \text{ mL} - 120 \text{ mL}}{30 \text{ cm} - 0}$$
$$= \frac{480 \text{ mL}}{30 \text{ cm}}$$
$$= 16 \text{ mL/cm water}$$

EXAMPLE

Calculate the static and dynamic compliance on a ventilated patient *with PEEP* therapy.

The same patient has an exhaled tidal volume of 600 mL. Because of refractory hypoxemia, 10 cm of PEEP therapy is started. The peak pressure is now 36 cm water, and the static or plateau pressure is now 25 cm water. The compliance factor has been determined to be 4 mL/cm water. The compressed volume at the plateau pressure is determined to be 60 mL (4 mL/cm compliance factor × 15 cm [25 cm – 10 cm PEEP]). The compressed volume at the peak pressure is determined to be 104 mL (4 mL/cm compliance factor × 26 cm [36 cm – 10 cm PEEP]).

$$Cst = \frac{600 \text{ mL} - 60 \text{ mL}}{25 \text{ cm} - 10 \text{ cm}}$$
$$= \frac{540 \text{ mL}}{15 \text{ cm}}$$
$$= 36 \text{ mL/cm water}$$

$$Cdyn = \frac{600 \text{ mL} - 104 \text{ mL}}{36 \text{ cm} - 10 \text{ cm}}$$
$$= \frac{496 \text{ mL}}{26 \text{ cm}}$$
$$= 19 \text{ mL/cm water}$$

6. Evaluate the results of the airway resistance and pulmonary compliance procedures (code: ID11) [difficulty: R, Ap, An]

Any increase in airway resistance or decrease in C_{LT} or both creates an increase in the patient's WOB. Examples of conditions or situations in which an increased airway resistance is found include bronchospasm, secretions, mucosal edema, airway tumor, placement of a small endotracheal tube, and biting or kinking of the endotracheal tube. C_{LT} is decreased by pneumonia, pulmonary edema, ARDS, pulmonary fibrosis, atelectasis, consolidation, hemothorax, pleural effusion, air trapping, pneumomediastinum, and pneumothorax. Examples of chest wall and abdominal conditions that reduce compliance include various chest wall deformities, circumferential chest or abdominal burns, enlarged liver, pneumoperitoneum, peritonitis, abdominal bleeding, herniation, and advanced pregnancy. Correction of the problem should return the patient's ventilator pressure(s) to baseline and normalize the patient's WOB.

There are six possible combinations of increasing or decreasing static and dynamic C_{LT}. Each has its own possible causes and is discussed in turn. The patient must be passive on the ventilator for the measured values to be accurate. Check two or three breaths for increased accuracy. Let the patient have a normal breath or two between each of the peak and plateau pressure measurement breaths.

a. Decreased dynamic compliance with stable static compliance

Decreased dynamic compliance with stable static compliance is noticed as an *increase* in the peak pressure with an

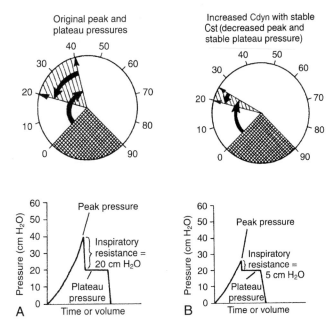

Figure 15-7 Increased dynamic compliance (Cdyn) with a stable static compliance (Cst). **A,** Original pressure manometer reading and pressure/volume curve. **B,** Altered pressure manometer reading and pressure/volume curve.

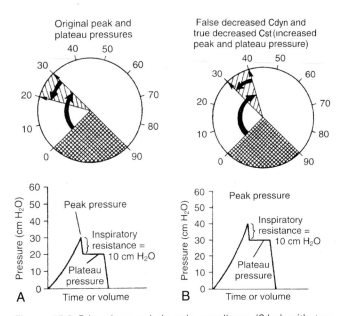

Figure 15-8 False decreased dynamic compliance (Cdyn) with true decreased static compliance (Cst). **A,** Original pressure manometer reading and pressure/volume curve. **B,** Altered pressure manometer reading and pressure/volume curve.

unchanged plateau pressure (see Fig. 15-5). It is caused by increased airway resistance (for example, bronchospasm, secretions, water in the circuit, kinked circuit or endotracheal tube). Correction of the underlying problem results in return of the peak pressure to the original level.

Note that the inspiratory resistance has doubled from the original 10-20 cm, whereas the plateau pressure has not changed. This confirms that the problem originates in the airway or breathing circuit. The patient's C_{LT} has not changed.

b. Increased dynamic compliance with stable static compliance

Increased dynamic compliance with stable static compliance is noticed as a *decrease* in peak pressure with an unchanged plateau pressure (Fig. 15-7). This represents an improvement in the patient's airway resistance from the original condition. Secretions can be diminished, mucous plugs cleared, bronchospasm corrected, and so forth.

Note that the peak pressure has decreased from the original level of 20 cm to just 5 cm. This confirms that the patient's airway resistance has decreased. The patient's C_{LT} has not changed.

c. False decreased dynamic compliance with true decreased static compliance

False decreased dynamic compliance with true decreased static compliance is noticed as an *increase* in *both* peak and plateau pressures (Fig. 15-8). This is seen when the patient's lung/thoracic compliance worsens. The plateau pressure is elevated, and the static compliance is decreased.

As an artifact of the stiffer lungs, the peak pressure also is elevated and the dynamic compliance is decreased. However, the difference between peak and plateau pressures remains the same. This demonstrates that no real increase in the patient's airway resistance has occurred.

d. True decreased dynamic compliance with true decreased static compliance

True decreased dynamic compliance with true decreased static compliance also is noticed as an *increase* in *both* peak and plateau pressures (Fig. 15-9). This is seen with the combination of decreased C_{LT} and increased airway resistance. Causes of both of these problems were discussed earlier.

e. False increased dynamic compliance with true increased static compliance

False increased dynamic compliance with true increased static compliance is noticed as a *decrease* in *both* peak and plateau pressures (Fig. 15-10). This is seen when the patient's lung/thoracic compliance improves. The plateau pressure decreases and, as an artifact, the peak pressure also decreases. Notice that the difference between peak and plateau pressures remains the same. This indicates that the patient's airway resistance is unchanged.

f. True increased dynamic compliance with true increased static compliance

True increased dynamic compliance with true increased static compliance also is noticed as a *decrease* in *both* peak and plateau pressures (Fig. 15-11). This is seen when the patient's airway resistance and his or her lung/thoracic

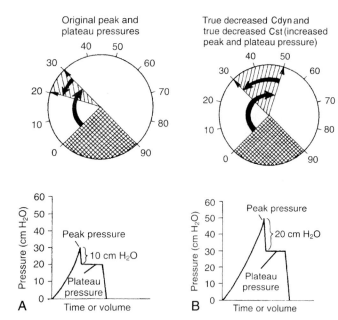

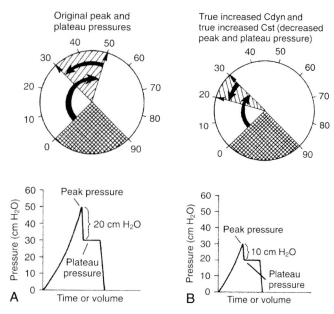

Figure 15-9 True decreased dynamic compliance (Cdyn) with true decreased static compliance (Cst). **A,** Original pressure manometer reading and pressure/volume curve. **B,** Altered pressure manometer reading and pressure/volume curve.

Figure 15-11 True increased dynamic compliance (Cdyn) with true increased static compliance (Cst). **A,** Original pressure manometer reading and pressure/volume curve. **B,** Altered pressure manometer reading and pressure/volume curve.

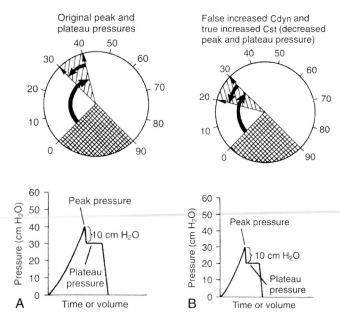

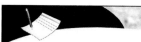

Figure 15-10 False increased dynamic compliance (Cdyn) with true increased static compliance (Cst). **A,** Original pressure manometer reading and pressure/volume curve. **B,** Altered pressure manometer reading and pressure/volume curve.

practitioners advocate using several different tidal volumes (e.g., 6, 8, 10, and 12 mL/kg of ideal body weight) when measuring dynamic and static pressures. The measured values are plotted on a graph to find the patient's optimal tidal volume that results in the highest static compliance value. Figure 15-12 shows a series of these graphs. The curves for diseased lungs and airways are quite different from those of a normal person or a patient with a pulmonary embolism. Because of this, a pulmonary embolism should be considered if the patient's condition deteriorates rapidly and no change in dynamic or static compliance values is observed.

Exam Hint 15-4

Every examination has had questions that deal with the interpretation of increasing or decreasing peak pressure (changing airway resistance) or increasing or decreasing plateau pressure (changing C_{LT}). Be able to identify a clinical change, possible causes of the change, and corrective actions.

---

compliance improve. Notice that the plateau pressure has decreased, thus indicating more compliant lungs. Also notice that the difference between peak and plateau pressures has decreased. This demonstrates that the airway resistance also has decreased.

All six examples of increasing or decreasing static or dynamic C_{LT} or both make use of a single tidal volume that is analyzed for peak and plateau pressures. Some

MODULE C

Provide conventional mechanical ventilation to adequately oxygenate and ventilate the patient.

Conventional mechanical ventilation is defined here as the use of a single ventilator that can provide the customary modes and options needed by the large majority of patients. This ventilatory support is provided through an endotracheal tube or a tracheostomy tube. Several physiologic

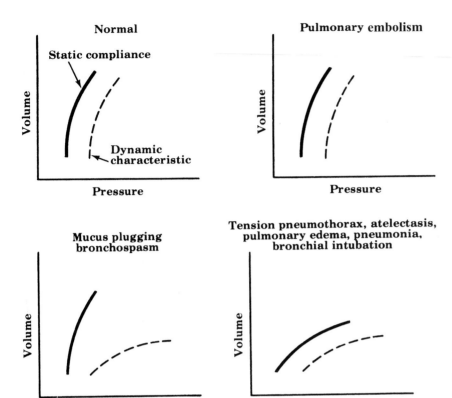

Figure 15-12 Pressure/volume curves for normal airways and lungs, pulmonary embolism (no change in airway resistance or lung compliance (C_{LT})), increased airway resistance, and decreased C_{LT}. (Source: Bone RC: Respir Care 28[5]:597, 1983.)

criteria have been compiled to help the clinician determine when a patient is in respiratory or ventilatory failure (Box 15-1) and needs breathing support. Remember that the patient may not fail each and every criterion. However, the patient will often fail one or more criteria in each category.

1. Recommend changes in mechanical ventilation parameters and settings (code: IIIE3f) [difficulty: R, Ap, An]

See below.

2. Initiate and adjust continuous mechanical ventilation (code: IIIC4a) [difficulty: R, Ap, An]

The NBRC will ask questions about specific indications and applications of conventional mechanical ventilators. Questions will be asked about which parameters and settings to recommend and the initiation and adjustment of those settings. The discussion below includes specific items listed on the Detailed Content Outline. Also included are other topics within the broader scope of conventional mechanical ventilation that are found in clinical practice. See below for the discussion.

3. Support oxygenation

a. Recommend oxygen therapy (code: IIIE3b) [difficulty: R, Ap, An]

Any patient who is hypoxic and suffering its clinical effects should be given supplemental oxygen. In most cases the goal of O_2 administration is to keep the PaO_2 between 60 and 90 torr and the SpO_2 level at greater

---

BOX 15-1   Indications for Ventilatory Support

Ventilation
Apnea
$PaCO_2$ ≥55 torr in a patient who is not ordinarily hypercapneic
Dead space: tidal volume (V_D/V_T ratio) of >0.55-0.6 (55%-60%)

Oxygenation
PaO_2 <80 torr on 50% oxygen or more
$P(A–a)O_2$ <300-350 torr on 100% oxygen
Intrapulmonary shunt >15%-20%

Pulmonary Mechanics
Spontaneous tidal volume 3-4 mL/lb or 7-9 mL/kg of ideal body weight
Vital capacity <10-15 mL/kg
Maximum inspiratory pressure (MIP) less than –20 to –25 cm water
Forced expiratory volume in 1 second (FEV_1) <10 mL/kg
Respiratory rate <12 breaths/min or >35 breaths/min in an adult
Rapid, shallow breathing index (breaths/minute divided by tidal volume in liters) >105

Miscellaneous
Unconscious patient with worsening neurological condition
Unstable and unacceptable vital signs
Unstable cardiac rhythm caused by hypoxemia and/or acidosis
Worsening cardiopulmonary or other major organ system

---

than 90%. Exceptions are patients who are breathing on hypoxic drive and who are in a cardiac arrest situation. The patient with COPD who has a chronically low PaO_2 level and a chronically high $PaCO_2$ level may be allowed to have a PaO_2 value as low as 50-55 torr and an SpO_2

value as low as 85%. The patient who is extremely hypoxic must be given up to 100% O_2. Those patients who have refractory hypoxemia (e.g., ARDS) do not respond with a normal increase in the PaO_2 level as the O_2 percentage is increased.

b. Initiate and adjust oxygen therapy (code: IIIC1) [difficulty: R, Ap, An]

Most ventilators have very accurate oxygen delivery systems. Many also incorporate an internal oxygen analyzer. However, it is common practice to use a calibrated, external oxygen analyzer to confirm the oxygen percentage. It is vital to know the patient's inspired oxygen percentage to correctly assess oxygenation.

The following formula can be used to help guide the use of supplemental oxygen in most stable patients:

$$\text{Desired } F_IO_2 = \frac{\text{Desired } PaO_2 \times \text{Current } F_IO_2}{\text{Current } PaO_2}$$

EXAMPLE

A patient has a PaO_2 level of 55 mm Hg on 30% oxygen. The clinical goal is a PaO_2 level of 90 mm Hg. What oxygen percentage should the patient have?

$$\text{Desired } F_IO_2 = \frac{\text{Desired } PaO_2 \times \text{Current } F_IO_2}{\text{Current } PaO_2}$$

$$\text{Desired } F_IO_2 = \frac{90 \text{ mm Hg} \times 0.3}{55 \text{ mm Hg}}$$

$$\text{Desired } F_IO_2 = \frac{27}{55}$$

$$\text{Desired } F_IO_2 = 0.49 \text{ or } 49\% \text{ oxygen}$$

Those patients who have refractory hypoxemia (e.g., ARDS) will not respond with a normal increase in PaO_2 level as the oxygen percentage is increased. In the short term, use whatever oxygen percentage is needed to achieve the clinical goal. The risk of oxygen toxicity increases when the F_IO_2 is greater than 0.5 for periods of longer than 48 hours. Always recheck the patient's arterial oxygen level after a change in the F_IO_2 has been made.

Either of the following formulas can be used in the special situation of determining the flows of air and oxygen into a "bleed-in" type of intermittent mandatory ventilation (IMV) or continuous positive airway pressure (CPAP) system to obtain an ordered F_IO_2. Either version can be used for determining gas flows, total flow, and oxygen/air ratio through an air entrainment (Venturi) mask.

The first formula follows:

$$(\text{L/min air} \times F_IO_2 \text{ of air}) + (\text{L/min } O_2 \times F_IO_2 \text{ pure } O_2) =$$
$$\text{Total flow} \times \text{Unknown } F_IO_2$$

The second formula follows:

$$F_1C_1 + F_2C_2 = F_TC_T$$

in which F_1 is the flow of the first gas (oxygen), C_1 is the concentration of oxygen in the first gas (1.0 for pure oxygen), F_2 is the flow of the second gas (air), C_2 is the concentration of oxygen in the second gas (0.21 for air), F_T is the total flow of both gases, and C_T is the concentration of oxygen in the mix of both gases. Use algebraic manipulation to solve for the unknown.

EXAMPLE

Determine the oxygen percentage through a bleed-in system that has an oxygen flow of 10 L/min and an airflow of 15 L/min. Determine the total flow through the system. Determine the ratio of oxygen to air.

$$(\text{L/min air} \times F_IO_2 \text{ of air}) +$$
$$(\text{L/min } O_2 \times F_IO_2 \text{ pure } O_2) = \text{Total flow} \times \text{Unknown } F_IO_2$$
$$(15 \times 0.21) + (10 \times 1.0) = (15 + 10) \times \text{Unknown } F_IO_2$$
$$(3.15) + (10) = (25) \times \text{Unknown } F_IO_2$$
$$13.15 = 25 \, F_IO_2$$
$$(\text{Divide both sides by 25})$$

$$0.526 \text{ or } 52.6\% = F_IO_2$$

$$\text{Total flow} = 15 + 10 = 25 \text{ L/min}$$

$$\text{Ratio} = \frac{10 \text{ L/min oxygen}}{15 \text{ L/min air}}$$

c. Minimize hypoxemia by positioning the patient properly (code: IIIC2) [difficulty: R, Ap, An]

Many patients who receive mechanical ventilation will be in the supine position. However, if a patient is short of breath when lying supine, he or she should be repositioned to sit more upright in a Fowler's or semi-Fowler's position. This seems to work best in patients with bilateral pulmonary problems such as congestive heart failure or pneumonia. If the patient cannot sit up and the lung problem is one-sided, roll the patient so that the more functional lung is *down*. The good lung should be positioned *up* in the following exceptions:

- Undrained pulmonary abscess that should not be drained into the good lung
- Neonatal congenital diaphragmatic hernia in which the good lung should not be compressed by the bowel in the chest cavity
- Pulmonary interstitial emphysema in which, by lying on the bad lung, the air leak and functional residual capacity can be reduced.

In either case, always ask the patient whether the new position helps to make breathing easier. If not, reposition the patient until breathing is more comfortable with less shortness of breath. In general, Trendelenburg is not well tolerated. A patient with a closed head injury and brain edema should not be put into the Trendelenburg position.

Prone positioning has been shown to improve oxygenation in some patients with ARDS. However, this position creates patient care challenges and has not been shown to improve patient outcomes. At the time of this writing, prone positioning is considered to be a rescue therapy for some patients with an acute lung injury or ARDS.

d. Minimize hypoxemia during suctioning or other ventilator procedures (code: IIIC2) [difficulty: R, Ap, An]

Ensuring adequate oxygenation during suctioning is discussed in Chapter 13. In brief, remember to give the adult patient 100% oxygen for at least 30 seconds before suctioning. With open-airway suctioning, perform the task as quickly and safely as possible to minimize time off the ventilator. Leave the patient on 100% oxygen for at least 1 minute after the procedure is completed, or until he or she returns to a stable condition as before the procedure. Children younger than 6 months can have the F_IO_2 increased by 10% for the procedure. See Chapter 13 for the complete discussion on suctioning.

In an adult, it is acceptable to increase the inspired oxygen up to 100% before and after a procedure that requires disconnection from the ventilator. The goal is to prevent hypoxemia. The patient should be ventilated manually with a resuscitation bag if indicated. Always remember to return the patient to the original oxygen percentage when clinically indicated.

4. Initiate and adjust continuous mechanical ventilation settings (code: IIIC4a) [difficulty: R, Ap, An]

a. Sensitivity

Sensitivity is the term used to describe the amount of work or effort the patient must perform to trigger the ventilator to deliver a tidal volume breath. Many older ventilators required the patient to generate a *negative pressure* to trigger the unit. The term *pressure triggering* is used often to describe this type of sensitivity. With these machines, the sensitivity usually is set at about −1 to −2 cm water pressure.

Newer ventilators also have the sensitivity option in which the patient generates an *inspiratory flow* to trigger a ventilator tidal volume breath. The term *flow triggering* often is used to describe this sensitivity option on the ventilator. With a ventilator using flow-triggering sensitivity, the patient initiates a tidal volume when his or her inspiratory flow is about 2 L/min (33 mL/s) less than the set baseline flow through the circuit. Very weak patients find that flow sensitivity requires less work than pressure sensitivity to initiate a ventilator breath. However, patients with severe obstructive airflow problems (COPD, asthma) may have difficulty triggering a breath with flow sensitivity. They may find pressure sensitivity requires less work. The newest generation of ventilators can have both pressure and flow sensitivity set. Whichever is triggered first results in a ventilator-delivered breath.

b. Flow

Flow is adjusted to set the inspiratory time and the I:E ratio. In addition, flow is set to meet the patient's needs.

Inspiratory flow should be great enough to minimize the WOB. Increase flow if the patient has signs of greater demand, such as using accessory muscles of inspiration or lack of synchrony with the ventilator, or if the pressure manometer deflects greatly below the baseline pressure or shows a low initial increase in inspiratory pressure. On a microprocessor-type ventilator with a monitor, look at the inspiratory flow curve (see Fig. 15-2) for signs of deviation from what is expected. When a patient is initially placed on a ventilator in the Volume Control, Assist/Control (VC, A/C) mode, a flow of about 60 L/min (1 L/s) (with a range of 40-80 L/min) is commonly set.

In addition, most current-generation ventilators offer more than one inspiratory flow pattern (see Fig. 15-2). The sine wave is most physiologically like a normal, spontaneous inspiration. The other waveforms can be compared with the sine wave to determine which one best meets the patient's needs. Typically, the rectangular (square) wave or descending ramp (decreasing) wave is selected when a patient is first put on a volume-cycled ventilator in the A/C mode. Ideally, the best flow pattern is one in which the patient's peak and mean airway pressures ($\overline{Paw}$) are lowest, exhalation is complete, breath sounds are improved bilaterally, heart rate and blood pressure are stable, and the patient feels most comfortable.

If the Pressure Support (PS) or Pressure Control (PC) mode is used, the patient is able to interact with the ventilator to receive whatever flow is needed. Many patients find these modes to be very comfortable because of this. An additional feature of the PS and PC modes on many ventilators enables the respiratory therapist to further modify how quickly the ventilator reaches its peak inspiratory flow. This feature is variously called inspiratory rise time, rise time, inspiratory pressure rise time, or pressure slope. If the patient is short of breath, a short rise time should be set so that the peak flow is quickly reached. A calm patient would probably be more comfortable with a longer rise time to the peak flow. Look at the ventilator's monitor for the flow tracing for help in adjusting the rise time to minimize patient–ventilator dyssynchrony (see below for more discussion).

c. I:E ratio

The I:E ratio is adjusted to ensure that the patient can inhale in as physiologically appropriate a manner as possible and completely exhale the inspired tidal volume. Typically, the initial I:E ratio is set at 1:2. Be watchful of an incomplete exhalation, which will cause air trapping and auto-PEEP (see Fig. 15-4). If the ventilator does not display the I:E ratio, it can be calculated from the inspiratory time and expiratory time. See Table 15-2 for the calculation of time variables in mechanical ventilation.

Increasing expiratory time to eliminate auto-PEEP was discussed above. This discussion will focus on the need to increase the inspiratory time. This is done to improve oxygenation by holding the tidal volume in the

TABLE 15-2	Time Variables in Mechanical Ventilation	
Term	**Symbol**	**Formula for Calculation**
Frequency (rate)	f	Count breaths/min or 60/ $t_I + t_E$
Cycle time	$t_I + t_E$	Add $t_I + t_E$ or 60/f
Inspiratory time	$t_I(I)$	$t_I = 60/f - t_E$ or $t_I = \%t_I \times (t_I + t_E)$
Expiratory time	$t_E(E)$	$t_E = 60/f - t_I$
Inspiratory/expiratory ratio	I:E or t_I/t_E	I:E = t_I/t_E
Percentage inspiratory time	$\%t_I$	$\%t_I = (t_I/t_E + t_E) \times 100$

lungs for longer than normal. When the inspiratory time is longer than the expiratory time (e.g., 2:1), the patient is said to have an *inverse I:E ratio* and *inverse ratio ventilation* (IRV). This technique has been used successfully in low-C_{LT} adult patients who do not respond to pressure control ventilation (PCV). Increased inspiratory time and decreased expiratory time should be used in any condition in which the patient has a small time constant of ventilation (T_C) ($T_C = C_{LT} \times Raw$). This would be observed clinically as a normal Raw but a low C_{LT} in such conditions as ARDS, pulmonary edema, pneumonia, or an enlarged abdomen. Increasing the inspiratory time to create an inverse I:E ratio keeps the alveoli inflated longer to provide more time for O_2 to diffuse, prevent atelectasis, and maintain the functional residual capacity (FRC). Typically patients being considered for IRV are already being ventilated in the PC mode. Therefore the merging of the two modes is called *pressure-controlled inverse ratio ventilation* (PCIRV). The following have been recommended as initial PCIRV settings:

1. If the patient is being switched from volume-cycled ventilation to PCIRV, set the PCV level at the patient's static C_{LT} pressure. However, if the patient was already on PCV at a higher pressure, keep this higher pressure.
2. Set the O_2 at 100%.
3. Keep the current respiratory rate.
4. Keep the I:E ratio at 1:1 for now.
5. PEEP should be removed if it is currently less than 8 cm H_2O. Cut the PEEP level in half if it is currently more than 8 cm H_2O. As the I:E ratio is made inverse, air trapping increases the patient's FRC.

Draw a set of arterial blood gas (ABG) samples after 15 min on PCIRV, and check the patient's vital signs. Monitor the exhaled tidal volume (V_T) for a decrease. If the ventilator gives a real-time graph of pressure, volume, and flow, these should be monitored for air trapping (auto-PEEP). (See Fig. 15-3 for an auto-PEEP flow/time tracing.)

If the initial set of blood gases on PCIRV does not show adequate oxygenation, the inspiratory time will have to be increased. The inspiratory time must be increased progressively and expiratory time decreased if the patient's C_{LT} worsens. It is also possible to alternate a 2- to 3-cm H_2O increase in PCV level with small increases in inspiratory time. Blood gases must be analyzed with each increase in inspiratory time, decrease in expiratory time, or increase in PCV. Once an acceptable PaO_2 is established, it usually is not necessary to make additional increases in inspiratory time if the patient's pulmonary condition does not worsen. Look for an increase in $PaCO_2$ or end-tidal CO_2 as a sign of inadequate V_T. It may be necessary to increase the PCV level to increase the V_T. Also monitor the patient's vital signs and CO, if possible, to look for a decrease in CO. PCIRV ratios as inverse as 3:1 or 4:1 have been reported. When this happens, the pressure/volume curve takes on a characteristic "square-wave" shape (as is shown later in Fig. 15-14, B). The I:E ratio must be returned to normal as the patient's C_{LT} improves through a gradual decrease in inspiratory time or increase in expiratory time. The patient's blood gas result should be evaluated with each step to be sure that oxygenation is maintained at a safe level.

Exam Hint 15-5

Usually two questions are related to modifying the inspiratory flow to meet the patient's need for a faster breath or modifying the I:E ratio. Remember that if the patient has auto-PEEP, an adjustment, such as increased expiratory time, must be made to allow a complete exhalation.

d. Correct patient–ventilator dyssynchrony (code: IIIC5) [difficulty: R, Ap, An]

Except for the rare instances in which a patient is apneic, there are numerous patient–ventilator interactions. They occur when the patient initiates a breath, during inspiration when a ventilator breath is delivered, and during the cycling from inspiration to expiration. Any time the patient's efforts and the ventilator's reaction do not match there is dyssynchrony (asynchrony). There are three types of interaction problems: (1) In *trigger dyssynchrony* the patient's breathing efforts do not result in a ventilator-delivered breath. The pressure or flow sensitivity setting must be adjusted to correct this problem. (2) In *flow dyssynchrony* the patient's inspiratory flow demand is not matched by the ventilator's flow delivery. The flow must be increased or decreased to meet the patient's needs. (3) In *cycling dyssynchrony* the patient's inspiratory to expiratory breathing does not match the ventilator's settings. The inspiratory time or I:E ratio should be adjusted.

Signs that the patient is breathing out of phase with the ventilator (dyssynchrony) include:

- The use of inspiratory accessory muscles (see Figs. 1-18 and 1-23)
- Chest and abdominal wall not moving at the same time (see Fig. 1-22)
- Nasal flaring (see Fig. 1-22)

- Distressed look on the patient's face with nasal flaring and diaphoresis
- Tachycardia and increased respiratory rate
- Mismatching of patient breathing attempts and delivered ventilator breaths
- Active exhalation while the ventilator is still delivering a breath

Dyssynchrony can cause increased WOB and patient anxiety. Look at the ventilator's graphic display for pressure, flow, and volume changes that do not match. A pressure/volume loop graphic display (see Fig. 15-1) will show the patient's WOB. Speak to the conscious, cooperative patient to try to determine the problem. Because a patient with an intubated airway cannot speak, it is necessary to communicate about the patient's feelings by asking simple questions that can be answered by a *yes* nod or *no* shake of the head. Other methods of communication include a pad of paper and pencil and picture boards. It is not possible to predict how a patient will react to the initiation of mechanical ventilation or its prolonged need. Some patients react with relief and relax when the WOB is reduced. Others may become angry at the limitations imposed on them. Still others may become depressed. The issue of a patient's emotional reaction to illness is discussed in detail in Chapter 1.

If sensitivity, flow, and timing adjustments are not effective at restoring patient–ventilator synchrony, a change of ventilator mode may correct the problem. Many patients report that breathing on the PS mode is very comfortable. It allows the patient to trigger each breath and the inspiratory flow and time. See the discussion below.

e. Medications to improve patient tolerance of mechanical ventilation

1. Recommend sedatives and hypnotics (code: IIIE4g) [difficulty: R, Ap]

See below.

2. Recommend analgesics (code: IIIE4h) [difficulty: R, Ap]

See below.

3. Recommend neuromuscular blocking agents (code: IIIE4i) [difficulty: R, Ap]

An adult who is attempting to inhale or exhale out of sequence with the ventilator is considered to be "bucking" or "fighting" the ventilator. This causes dyssynchrony and is seen most commonly in the Control and Assist/Control modes. If the dyssynchrony between the patient's efforts and the ventilator is too great, the risks of hypoxemia, air trapping, and pneumothorax are increased. Carefully evaluate the patient to determine whether he or she is breathing rapidly because of pain, anxiety, or improper adjustment of the ventilator. Make sure that the settings (sensitivity, inspiratory flow, respiratory rate, inspiratory time, pressure limit) are set correctly for the patient's condition. Sedation or paralysis should be considered only

after all other causes of dyssynchrony have been ruled out. The following patient questions and conditions must be considered before a medication is selected to control the patient's breathing efforts:

- *Is the patient in pain?* If so, an opiate analgesic such as morphine sulfate is commonly administered intravenously for fast onset. Morphine has the additional effects of reducing anxiety and inducing sleep. The synthetic opioid fentanyl citrate (Sublimaze) is given intravenously and is preferred in patients with renal insufficiency or hemodynamic instability. Because all opiates are central nervous system depressants, make sure that the ventilator alarm systems are functioning properly in case the patient becomes disconnected.
- *Is the patient agitated?* Asynchrony with the ventilator for no known physical reason often can be attributed to anxiety or fear. Benzodiazepines, including diazepam (Valium) and midazolam (Versed), are the drugs of choice for the treatment of agitation. They have a sedating effect within minutes when given intravenously.
- *Does the patient need to be paralyzed?* If total muscular relaxation along with apnea is necessary, a skeletal muscle paralyzing agent should be used. Usually a short-term, depolarizing neuromuscular blocker such as succinylcholine (Anectine) is used during a difficult intubation. A single intravenous dose paralyzes a combative patient for about 10 minutes. For paralysis during mechanical ventilation, one of the following long-term, nondepolarizing neuromuscular blocking agents is used commonly: pancuronium (Pavulon), atracurium (Tracrium), or vecuronium (Norcuron). These are given intravenously and cause paralysis that lasts 2-4 hours.

Remember that these paralyzing agents have no effect on the patient's ability to feel pain or on fear of what is happening. Pain medications such as morphine must be given as necessary. A sedating agent such as Valium is also given to counteract the emotional stress of being awake but unable to move. Review related medication discussions in Chapter 9, if needed.

Exam Hint 15-6

Expect to see questions requiring the therapist to recommend a medication for sedating an agitated patient or addressing the need to paralyze a patient receiving mechanical ventilation.

---

f. Initiate and adjust alarms (code: IIIC4d) [difficulty: R, Ap]

Alarm systems are different for each type of ventilator. Generally speaking, they are set with a safety margin of ±10% from the patient's normal ventilator settings. A variation of greater than 10% results in an audible or visual alarm condition. Most ventilators alarm if the I:E ratio is

1:1 or less. All audible and visual alarm systems must be tested and function properly. The practitioner should be familiar with the most widely used adult and infant ventilators and their alarm systems. Following are examples of alarms with a ±10% setting:

- The tidal volume is 500 mL. Set the low-volume alarm at 450 mL and the high-volume alarm at 550 mL.
- The minute volume is 5000 mL. Set the high-volume alarm at 5500 mL and the low-volume alarm at 4500 mL.
- The oxygen percentage is set at 40%. Set the high-percentage alarm at 45% and the low-percentage alarm at 35%.
- The low-pressure or disconnection alarm is set to sound if the ventilator-delivered pressure is about 5 cm water below the peak pressure. For example, if the peak pressure has been at about 40 cm water, the low-pressure or disconnection alarm should be set at 35 cm water. If a leak or disconnection occurs, the alarm sounds when the peak pressure does not reach 35 cm water. If the patient is on a CPAP system, the low-pressure or disconnection alarm should be set to sound if the pressure decreases about 2-3 cm water below the set level. For example, if the patient is on 10 cm water CPAP, the alarm should be set at 8 cm water.

Many types of alarms have a timer that can be set to delay when the alarm sounds. If the alarm is on a ventilator, the delay should be set for about 3-5 seconds longer than the cycling time. For example, if the patient has a backup rate of 10 times/min, the cycling time between mandatory breaths is 6 seconds. Set the timer to delay the alarm sounding for about 10 seconds. If the patient is disconnected from the ventilator and the peak pressure does not reach 35 cm water, the alarm will sound in 10 seconds. If the patient is on a CPAP system, the timer may be set for no delay or for a short delay. Adjust all the alarms to fit the clinical setting and the patient's condition. Some may need tighter limits, and others may need wider limits than those just discussed.

When the VC, A/C mode is used, a high-pressure alarm should be set. Commonly this is about 10 cm water higher than the peak pressure. For example, the patient's peak pressure is 30 cm water. Set the high-pressure alarm at 40 cm water. If the patient should cough and the peak pressure hits 40 cm water, the alarm will sound and tidal volume will be stopped.

Exam Hint 15-7

Be able to troubleshoot an alarm situation, correct the problem, and reset the alarm settings as needed. For example, the high-pressure alarm will go off and the tidal volume will be stopped if the peak pressure hits the alarm setting. This could be caused by an increase in airway resistance or a decrease in C_{LT}. A disconnection alarm is probably the most important to set because the patient will not be mechanically ventilated if disconnected from the ventilator.

---

g. Humidification

1. Recommend a change in humidification (code: IIIE3c) [difficulty: R, Ap]

The 2012 American Association for Respiratory Care (AARC) guidelines on humidification state that all patients with an artificial airway who are receiving mechanical ventilation should breathe humidified gases. Other guidelines are summarized here: If passive humidification (heat-moisture exchanger, HME) is used, it should provide a minimum humidity level of 30 mg water/L. An HME is not recommended for noninvasive ventilation (NIV). An HME should not be used to help prevent ventilator-associated pneumonia (VAP). If active humidification (heated wick-type or cascade-type humidifier) is used, it should provide a humidity level between 33 and 44 mg water/L at a gas temperature of 34-41° C (93-106° F) with 100% relative humidity at the ventilator circuit Y-piece. Although some patients receiving NIV may not need to breathe humidified gas, active humidification is suggested to improve the patient's comfort and adherence.

2. Maintain adequate humidification (code: IIIA6) [difficulty: R, Ap]

The goal for most patients is to minimize their humidity deficit by using gas that is humidified and warmed to near body temperature. This can be accomplished by a heated wick-type or cascade-type humidifier or by an HME. The patient should breathe humidified gases warmed to close to body temperature. This decreases the patient's humidity deficit to a minuscule level and reduces the "rain out" of water vapor condensing in the ventilator circuit. When a heated humidifier is used, a temperature probe should be placed in the inspiratory tubing close to the patient to monitor the inspired gas temperature.

Passive humidification (an HME) is indicated in the following situations:

- The patient has few, if any, secretions.
- The patient probably will be weaned from the ventilator within 96 hours.
- The patient is being transported on mechanical ventilation.

Passive humidification is contraindicated in the following situations:

- The patient has thick, bloody, or copious secretions.
- The patient has a large air leak such that the exhaled volume is less than 70% of the inhaled V_T. This causes a relatively dry hygroscopic filter. (Patients with uncuffed or torn cuffs on their endotracheal tubes or large bronchopleural fistulas would have large V_T leaks.)
- The patient's temperature is less than 32° C.
- The patient's spontaneous minute volume ($\dot{V}_E$) is greater than 10 L/min, because the filter's ability to hold moisture will be exceeded, and the patient will breathe in some dry air.

Active humidification (heated wick-type or cascade-type humidifier) is indicated in these situations:

- The patient has thick or copious secretions. An increase in the amount or thickness of secretions or a change from white to yellow or green justifies the switch to a cascade-type humidifier.
- The patient probably will require mechanical ventilation for longer than 96 h.
- The patient cannot have mechanical dead space added to the breathing circuit. If the patient's V_T is small, an HME should not be used because of its added dead space.
- An HME should not be used with a patient receiving a very large V_T because the filter's ability to hold moisture will be exceeded, and the patient will breathe in some dry air. Check the manufacturer's literature for the maximum recommended V_T.
- If the patient has a large air leak, as may be seen with a deflated cuff or a bronchopleural fistula, an HME should not be used. With a large air leak, more air is inspired than expired, and the exchanger cannot fully humidify the inspired V_T.

5. Modes of ventilation

Mode can be defined as the *type of breath* and the *pattern of breath* that a patient receives during mechanical ventilation. When choosing the type of breath to deliver, the respiratory therapist is selecting the primary control variable. Based on what is controlled, other factors will be adjustable. There are two main control variables from which to choose: *volume control* (VC) or *pressure control* (PC). (Special modes such as noninvasive ventilation and high-frequency ventilation are discussed in Module D.) VC Ventilation will deliver a known tidal volume to the patient regardless of changes in airway resistance or C_{LT}. Using older terminology, this would be called volume-cycled ventilation. This known tidal volume (with a set respiratory rate) will provide a known minute volume and result in a desired $PaCO_2$. The main limitations or drawbacks of VC are a high peak pressure and possible patient–ventilator dyssynchrony. PC utilizes a set pressure to deliver a tidal volume. Using older terminology, this would be called pressure-cycled ventilation. As with VC, the pressure-controlled tidal volume and rate will produce a minute volume and achieve a desired $PaCO_2$. The main disadvantage of PC is an unstable tidal volume if the patient has a change in airway resistance or C_{LT}.

After choosing VC or PC, the respiratory therapist must select the patient's pattern of breathing. The chosen pattern controls how much breathing support is provided by the ventilator and how much breathing is done by the patient. There are three main patterns of breathing (and numerous variations) from which to choose: assist/control, synchronous intermittent mandatory ventilation, and pressure support. Each is discussed in some detail below.

Briefly, A/C has the greatest control by providing a set rate, SIMV has less control by providing some breaths but allowing the patient to breathe independently, and PS has the least control by requiring the patient to initiate all breaths.

Exam Hint 15-8

There is a great variety of proprietary terms for ventilator modes (and their abbreviations) used by manufacturers. However, the NBRC has adopted a simplified list of abbreviations for mechanical ventilation modes: *NPPV* (noninvasive positive pressure ventilation; the same thing as NIV, noninvasive ventilation), *PS* (pressure support), *CPAP* (continuous positive airway pressure), *HFOV* (high-frequency oscillatory ventilation), *PC* (pressure control), *VC* (volume control), *A/C* (assist/control), and *SIMV* (synchronous intermittent mandatory ventilation). The last four modes can be combined: PC, A/C; PC, SIMV; VC, A/C; and VC, SIMV.

Historically, the NBRC has limited questions to the most widely used modes of ventilation as listed above. However, other newer modes (and their abbreviations) should be understood if possible. It is beyond the scope of this text to cover every possible mode of ventilation.

The current generation of microprocessor-type ventilators offers the physician and respiratory therapist numerous options for tailoring how the breath will be delivered—the mode—to best meet the patient's needs. With most patients either VC or PC may be used as long as it is properly managed. However, most respiratory therapists will select VC during the initial application of mechanical ventilation to deliver a set tidal volume. A/C is selected to provide a set respiratory rate while enabling the patient to breathe more often if desired. So, most practitioners will initially select VC, A/C for the majority of patients. After the patient has been stabilized, or if there is a need to limit inspiratory pressure, a change to PC or another mode may be made. In addition, the following should be considered when one is deciding what mode(s) to use.

a. Increased WOB

Patients who show increased WOB may have a very high airway resistance, as in status asthmaticus, or may have a very low lung/thoracic compliance, as in ARDS. Many practitioners believe that the A/C mode, when applied properly to a sedated patient, is best for these problems because the patient's WOB is almost eliminated. Other practitioners believe that SIMV is a physiologically superior mode of ventilation. Pressure support ventilation (PSV) has been shown to be beneficial to patients with increased WOB from the high airway resistance caused by a small-diameter endotracheal tube.

b. Hypercapnia

A patient may have hypercapnia (a high carbon dioxide level) because of sedation from a morphine or heroin overdose or may have COPD with worsening of the chronic hypercapnia. In either case, the patient becomes progressively more

---

BOX 15-2   Indications for Intermittent Mandatory Ventilation (IMV)/Synchronous Intermittent Mandatory Ventilation (SIMV) Tolerance

---

Indications That IMV/SIMV Is Being Well Tolerated

Stable spontaneous respiratory rate
Stable heart rate
Stable spontaneous tidal volume
Stable vital capacity, maximum inspiratory pressure (MIP), and/or FEV_1
No use or stable use of accessory muscles of ventilation
Patient indicates that he or she is comfortable
Stable blood gases

Indications That IMV/SIMV Is Not Being Well Tolerated

Increased spontaneous respiratory rate
Tachycardia or dysrhythmias such as premature ventricular contractions
Decrease in spontaneous tidal volume
Decrease in vital capacity, MIP, and/or FEV_1
Beginning or increased use of accessory muscles of ventilation
Patient complains of dyspnea
Deterioration of blood gases as seen by a falling PaO_2 or SpO_2 and a rapidly falling or rising $PaCO_2$

BOX 15-3   Patient Monitoring during CPAP/PEEP Therapy

Good Tolerance of CPAP/PEEP Therapy

Increased PaO_2
Increased static C_{LT}
Stable cardiac output (CO) as shown by the following:
    Stable heart rate without rhythm disturbances
    Stable blood pressure
The following can be measured only through a pulmonary artery/
    Swan-Ganz catheter:
    Stable or increased $P\overline{v}O_2$ (mixed venous oxygen)
    Stable CO
    Decreased pulmonary vascular resistance
    Decreased intrapulmonary shunt

Poor Tolerance of CPAP/PEEP Therapy

Increased PaO_2 (this can be deceiving if it is the only information observed)
Decreased static C_{LT}
Decreased cardiac output (CO) as shown by the following:
    Increased heart rate or rhythm disturbances
    Decreased blood pressure
The following can be measured only through a pulmonary artery/
    Swan-Ganz catheter:
    Decreased $P\overline{v}O_2$
    Decreased CO
    Increased pulmonary vascular resistance
    Increased intrapulmonary shunt

CPAP, continuous positive airway pressure; PEEP, positive end-expiratory pressure.

---

hypoxemic (unless given supplemental oxygen) as the carbon dioxide level increases. Control or A/C mode is best for setting a minimum minute volume to determine the maximum carbon dioxide level. As the patient recovers, SIMV or PSV allows the gradual reduction of ventilatory support. See Box 15-2 for indications for SIMV tolerance.

c. Hypoxemia

If hypoxemia is secondary to a decreased FRC, as in ARDS or atelectasis, the treatment of choice for hypoxemia is CPAP on a free-standing system or PEEP on a conventional volume-cycled ventilator. If the problem results from an increased intrapulmonary shunt, the patient may need PEEP or CPAP, as well as up to 100% oxygen. See Box 15-3 for patient monitoring during PEEP and CPAP. PCIRV and high-frequency ventilation have been used with success in hypoxemic patients with a pulmonary air leak for whom conventional volume ventilation has failed.

The following modes of ventilation are delivered through most types of electrically powered and microprocessor-type ventilators.

d. Control

Control (C) sets the ventilator with a mandatory respiratory rate and tidal volume. It is the simplest method of providing ventilatory support and may be used on an apneic patient. With the Control mode the machine is incapable of allowing any patient interaction. For example, the ventilator might be set to deliver a tidal volume of 700 mL at a rate of 14 times/min. Because the patient

cannot trigger any breaths, this mode would be used only when the patient must be kept sedated or pharmacologically paralyzed (Fig. 15-13, A shows the pressure/time curve).

e. Assist/control

The A/C mode has a set backup respiratory rate and tidal volume. However, A/C allows the patient to trigger additional machine-delivered breaths. A sensitivity control is adjusted to allow the patient to easily start a breath as needed. (Fig. 15-13, B shows the pressure/time curve).

f. Intermittent mandatory ventilation

IMV has a set backup respiratory rate and tidal volume. In addition, between mandatory breaths, the patient can breathe spontaneously as frequently as desired. The patient also can take in as large a spontaneous tidal volume as needed. However, these patient breaths are not synchronized with the ventilator breaths. IMV was used in older ventilators before there was a way to synchronize the patient and ventilator breaths. The sensitivity control is set so that the patient cannot trigger any extra ventilator tidal volume breaths (Fig. 15-13, C shows the pressure/time curve). The IMV mode has been replaced in modern adult patient ventilators with the SIMV mode, as discussed below. (The IMV mode is still used

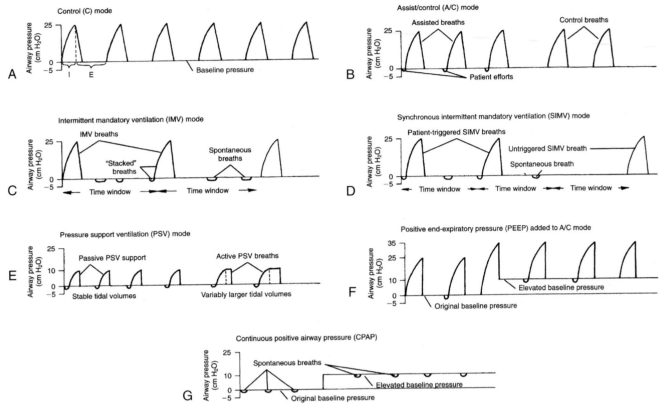

Figure 15-13 Pressure versus time waveforms for various modes of mechanical ventilation. **A,** Control (C) mode shows no patient effort and consistent inspiration/expiration ratios. **B,** Assist/control (A/C) mode shows that patient's initial effort triggers machine tidal volume breath. **C,** Intermittent mandatory ventilation (IMV) mode shows spontaneous tidal volume breaths occurring between predetermined machine tidal volume breaths. Note "stacked" breaths that happen when patient takes in a breath that then is supplemented by a machine breath. **D,** Synchronous intermittent mandatory ventilation (SIMV) mode shows that a patient effort within a time window results in delivery of machine tidal volume. Any other patient efforts within the time window result in a spontaneous tidal volume. If no patient efforts occur within the time window, machine tidal volume will be delivered automatically. **E,** Pressure support ventilation (PSV) mode shows how patient must initiate all breaths that then are supported to the predetermined airway pressure. Stable tidal volumes are seen if the patient inhales passively. Variably larger tidal volumes result if the patient inhales more actively. **F,** Positive end-expiratory pressure therapy can be added to A/C mode (as shown) or any other mode. The elevated baseline pressure prevents alveolar collapse. The sensitivity control must be set at –1 to –2 cm water so that the patient is able to trigger a breath without undue effort. **G,** Continuous positive airway pressure (CPAP) shows that the patient takes spontaneous tidal volumes while exhaling against an elevated baseline pressure.

with some neonatal ventilator patients and is discussed in Chapter 16.)

g. Synchronous intermittent mandatory ventilation

SIMV has a set backup respiratory rate and tidal volume. SIMV is similar to IMV in allowing spontaneous breathing except that the sensitivity control is functional. The patient can trigger a machine-delivered tidal volume during a preset time interval. The timing of the backup rate is such that the patient can get only as many ventilator breaths as are set. Spontaneous tidal volumes vary with the patient's efforts. For example, the ventilator might be set to deliver a 700-mL tidal volume 8 times/min. Let us say that the patient breathes spontaneously 10 more times and has an average tidal volume of 400 mL.

The total rate is counted at 18. The total minute volume is the combination of the machine's minute volume and the patient's minute volume (Fig. 15-13, D shows the pressure/time curve).

h. Pressure support ventilation

PS, or PSV, is similar to intermittent positive-pressure breathing (IPPB) in that when the patient initiates a ventilator breath, a preset pressure is delivered to the airway. With PSV the patient must have an intact respiratory center and stable breathing. The PSV breaths are time cycled and pressure limited. The physician orders a PS level for one of two reasons, depending on the clinical goal. First, enough PS is ordered to overcome the patient's calculated airway resistance. This usually is done when the patient has an increased WOB from a smaller than ideal endotracheal tube. Second, PS is ordered to deliver a targeted tidal volume. In most cases, the tidal volume will be stable if the patient passively takes the PS breath, or it can be larger if the patient interacts actively with the pressure that is delivered (see Figs. 15-5 and 15-13, E for the pressure/time curve).

Because PS utilizes a set delivered pressure, the patient's tidal volume can vary with changing C_{LT} and/or airway resistance. To bring stability to the tidal volume under changing patient conditions, several ventilator manufacturers have developed automatic compensation systems. See the Dual-Control mode discussion below.

When the PS level is adjusted to deliver a V_T, this is called maximum PSV (PSV_{max}). The clinical guidelines for PSV_{max} are as follows:

- Use enough pressure to deliver a desired V_T as discussed below.
- The patient should not have to assist the ventilator at a rate greater than 20 times/min to achieve acceptable ABG values.

PSV_{max} has been used in patients with resolving acute respiratory failure. Usually these patients have been maintained on the A/C mode for several days to minimize their WOB while they are undergoing treatment for their condition. PSV_{max} is considered ideal for reconditioning the diaphragm and other respiratory muscles. Reconditioning occurs when the assist or "trigger" pressure for the breath is kept as low as possible (–1 to –2 cm H_2O pressure) and the V_T is kept large. This pattern results in a low respiratory muscle workload. As the patient continues to improve, the PS level is reduced.

The patient's V_T is stable as long as the patient passively takes in the PS-supported breath; the V_T can be larger if the patient interacts actively with the delivered pressure. (See Fig. 15-5, B for a pressure/flow curve and Fig. 15-13, E for a pressure/time curve.)

The PSV level also has been used to overcome the Raw caused by the patient's endotracheal tube. (See the example calculated earlier in the chapter.) Too small an endotracheal tube may prevent some patients from successfully weaning using the SIMV mode. The addition of enough PSV to overcome the additional WOB caused by the tube enables the patient to wean successfully and the airway to be extubated.

The PS level is reduced, as tolerated, when the patient's C_{LT} or Raw improves. As both return to normal, the only barrier to extubation is the resistance offered by the endotracheal tube. Some practitioners advocate extubation when the PS level is 10 cm H_2O or less, which is probably the pressure level needed to overcome the tube's resistance. Thus the patient should tolerate extubation without any increase in WOB.

i. Pressure control ventilation

PC, or PCV, involves the delivery of tidal volume breaths that are pressure limited and time cycled. It has been advocated for patients with bilateral low-compliance conditions (e.g., ARDS) and patients with a pneumothorax secondary to volutrauma/barotrauma. A ventilator rate can be set and the patient can trigger additional breaths. As the inspiratory time is increased, it can become longer than the expiratory time. This results in PCIRV. Figure 15-14 shows the volume, flow, and pressure tracings.

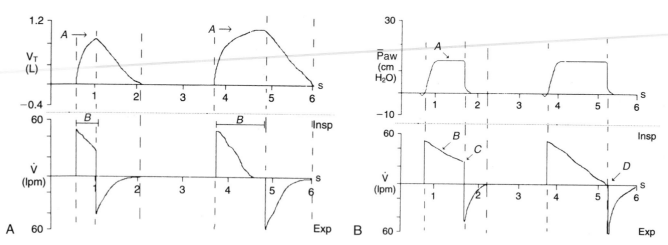

Figure 15-14 Two sets of graphic tracings of pressure control ventilation. **A,** Two tracings show volume (V_T) versus time and flow ($\dot{V}$) versus time. Arrow *A* shows tidal volume, *B* shows inspiratory flow. Note how tidal volume increases as inspiratory time is increased. However, as is shown in the lower right tracing, as flow decreases to zero, no more volume is delivered. **B,** Two tracings show pressure versus time and flow versus time. Arrow *A* shows the pressure control level being reached with an inspiratory plateau or "square wave" appearance, *B* shows declining inspiratory flow, and *C* shows final flow when inspiration is time cycled off and exhalation begins. This graphic can be used to help adjust a longer inspiratory time. If the Pressure Control Inverse Ratio Ventilation (PCIRV) were being optimally adjusted, the inspiration time could be increased until inspiratory flow reached zero (indicated by arrow *D*). (Image used by permission from Nellcore Puritan Bennett, LLC, Boulder, CO, part of Covidien.)

Because PC utilizes a set delivered pressure, the patient's tidal volume can vary with changing C_{LT} and/or airway resistance. To bring stability to the tidal volume under changing patient conditions, several ventilator manufacturers have developed automatic compensation systems. See the Dual-Control mode discussion below.

The PC level is set as low as possible to achieve an adequate V_T for gas exchange. The exhaled volume must be monitored continuously because the V_T will decrease if the patient's C_{LT} or Raw worsens. If either or both improve, the V_T will increase. The patient with a pulmonary air leak loses variable amounts of V_T from the chest tube, depending on changes in compliance and resistance. An ABG sample must be evaluated with a change in the PCV level or V_T. The PC mode is well tolerated by many patients because of the freedom they have to set the rate, inspiratory flow through the demand valve, and minute volume ($\dot{V}_E$). PC also may be combined with SIMV and PS as the clinical situation indicates. Following are some suggestions for initial PC settings:

1. Set the PEEP to the same level used on the constant volume ventilator to maintain the patient's FRC.
2. Set the PC level at the patient's static C_{LT} pressure. Be prepared to increase this pressure. The clinical goal is to give a V_T close to that delivered previously.
3. Set the rate the same as before.
4. Set the inspired O_2 the same as before. Some may prefer to set it at 100% until blood gas results show that it can be lowered.
5. Set the inspiratory time under pressure control so that the I:E ratio is the same as before.

Check the patient's vital signs for tolerance, and get an ABG sample in about 15 minutes. If the Raw or C_{LT} worsens, the PC level must be increased to maintain or increase the V_T. Obviously, as the patient's Raw and C_{LT} improve (or pulmonary air leak decreases), the PC level must be decreased to maintain the desired V_T.

j. Airway pressure release ventilation

The Airway Pressure Release Ventilation (APRV) mode has been used with success in patients with ARDS who have not responded well to constant volume ventilation. APRV can be described simply as a mode in which the patient can breathe spontaneously at two different levels of CPAP. A difference from conventional CPAP is that the two levels are held for set periods. The ventilator options for this mode are simple. The practitioner sets the low pressure (P_{low}), the high pressure (P_{high}), and the times at which the patient will be at those pressure levels. Low pressure sometimes is referred to as *CPAP* and high pressure as *release pressure*. The timing changes from low pressure to high pressure and back to low pressure effectively deliver a tidal volume. (See Fig. 15-15 for a pressure/time tracing. Compare this to the tracings of Fig. 15-13, F and G.)

When APRV is compared with other modes of ventilation, several similarities are evident between it and PCIRV with PEEP and bilevel ventilation. All have an elevated baseline pressure that allows the patient to breathe

spontaneously. All have variable inspiratory times for the higher pressure level. None delivers a set tidal volume to the patient. The only real difference seems to be that the patient can breathe spontaneously at the higher pressure level only with APRV. If the patient does not make any respiratory efforts, APRV functions like PC or bilevel ventilation.

A set of blood gases, vital signs, pulmonary artery catheter values, and so forth should be obtained on the current constant volume ventilator settings as a baseline before APRV is started. The following suggestions for initiating APRV are similar to those listed earlier for starting PCIRV:

1. Set the high pressure (release pressure) at the patient's optimal PEEP/CPAP level. Often this is in a range between the patient's static C_{LT} pressure and peak pressure (Fig. 15-16). The clinical goal is to safely maximize the patient's FRC.
2. Set the low pressure (CPAP) at the level of PEEP that was used on the constant volume ventilator. This is done to maintain the patient's FRC. See point *A* of Figure 15-16.
3. Set the inspired oxygen in the same way as before. Some may prefer to set it at 100%, as with PCIRV, until blood gas results show that it can be lowered.
4. Set the timing of the high pressure and low pressure values so that more time is spent at the high pressure than at the low pressure. Often the low pressure time is limited to 1-1.5 seconds. Keep the same respiratory rate as before. Even if the patient is apneic, as the ventilator switches from high pressure to low pressure, the patient exhales a tidal volume to blow off carbon dioxide.

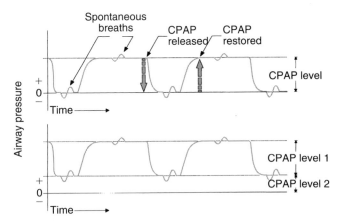

Figure 15-15 Airway pressure release ventilation (APRV) involves spontaneous breathing under one or two elevated baseline pressures. In the *top graph*, the patient can breathe during ambient pressure and during continuous positive airway pressure (CPAP). In the *bottom graph*, the patient breathes during a lower CPAP level and a higher CPAP level. In both situations, the patient breathes spontaneously at a high pressure level for a prolonged, adjustable length of time. Then, for a short, adjustable time, the higher pressure drops to the lower pressure level. This allows the patient to exhale a larger than usual volume. The higher pressure then is restored. This causes a large tidal volume to be inhaled. (From Dupuis Y: Ventilators: theory and clinical applications, ed 2, St Louis, 1992, Mosby.)

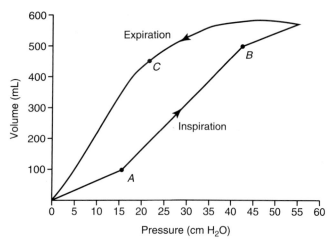

Figure 15-16 Pressure/volume loop showing lower and upper inflection points in a patient with acute respiratory distress syndrome (ARDS). Point *A*, lower inflection point during inspiration that indicates the opening pressure of alveoli (15 cm water). This is the minimum positive end-expiratory pressure level needed to maintain a patient's functional residual capacity. Point *B*, upper inflection point during inspiration that indicates that the lungs are being overstretched (40 cm water). This should be the upper limit of peak airway pressure to avoid overdistention and volutrauma. Flattening of the pressure/volume loop to the right of point *B* shows that little volume is delivered despite increased pressure. Point *C*, upper inflection point of expiration (20 cm water). As the airway pressure drops below this point, alveolar collapse can occur.

Monitor the patient's ventilator-delivered and spontaneous tidal volumes and rates. Check vital signs. Get an ABG sample in about 15 minutes.

If the patient's initial blood gas results on APRV show hypoxemia, the following options are available: (1) increase the inspired oxygen percentage if it is not already at 100%, (2) increase the low-pressure level, (3) increase the high-pressure level, or (4) increase the time the patient is kept at the high-pressure level. Reducing any or all of these options will decrease the patient's PaO_2 if it is too high.

If the blood gas results show hypoventilation, the following options are available: (1) increase the high-pressure level or (2) decrease the time at the high-pressure level to increase the respiratory rate. Do the opposite to increase the $PaCO_2$ if the patient is being hyperventilated.

As with the previous ventilator modalities, the patient should be monitored closely and should have an ABG drawn for evaluation of every change.

Exam Hint 15-9

Expect questions that require selecting or changing the mode of ventilation depending on the patient's condition. Select the A/C mode if the patient needs full breathing support. Select the SIMV mode if the patient needs to be partially supported. Select the PS mode to overcome the resistance of the endotracheal tube. Change a patient receiving volume-cycled ventilation to pressure-cycled ventilation because of a plateau pressure of greater than 30 cm H_2O.

---

6. Recommend, initiate, and adjust variations and combinations of modes of ventilation

Often, when a patient has more than one problem, more than one solution may be needed. The following are combinations of modes from which to choose.

a. Mandatory minute ventilation

Mandatory Minute Ventilation (MMV) is a variation on the SIMV mode. It has been used as a weaning mode that limits the increase in carbon dioxide if the patient should tire. With MMV, the patient is assured of a preset minute volume regardless of his or her spontaneous breathing. It has been proposed as an effective way to ventilate and wean patients who can breathe spontaneously but who have an unreliable respiratory drive and unstable tidal volume. Examples include patients who have received narcotic, sedative, anesthetic, or neuromuscular blocking medications. Patient conditions for which MMV is indicated include encephalopathy and cerebral disorders such as stroke. In addition, MMV may be used during the recovery period of a neuromuscular disease. Ventilators that include the MMV mode all are controlled by a microprocessor that monitors the ventilator's and the patient's tidal volume and rate. The following guidelines have been recommended for the initiation of MMV:

1. Set the ventilator tidal volume according to established guidelines as discussed below.
2. Spontaneous breaths may be taken through a demand valve or may be pressure supported.
3. Determine the minimum minute volume according to the patient's preexisting condition and the clinical goals:

The patient who has been on SIMV should have the MMV set at 90% of the SIMV-delivered minute volume. For example, the patient has an SIMV rate of 5 breaths/min and a tidal volume of 500 mL. Therefore the ventilator is delivering 2.5 L of minute volume (5 × 500 mL), and the MMV would be set at 2250 mL (90% of 2.5 L).

The patient who has been on A/C should have the mandatory minute volume set at 80% of the A/C-delivered minute volume. For example, the patient has an A/C rate of 10 breaths/min and a tidal volume of 500 mL. Therefore the ventilator is delivering 5 L of minute volume (10 × 500 mL), and the MMV would be set at 4 L (80% of 5 L).

Ideally MMV establishes a minimum safe volume of ventilation. If the patient inhales less than this volume, the ventilator delivers as many breaths as necessary at the preestablished tidal volume to make up the difference. Be aware that a patient who is breathing rapidly with a small tidal volume may move enough gas to exceed the minimum minute volume. Because of this risk, it is important to set a low tidal volume alarm or a high respiratory rate alarm or both to give warning. Do not let the programming of an MMV create a false sense of security with these patients.

b. Pressure control/pressure control inverse ratio ventilation, synchronous intermittent mandatory ventilation, and PEEP

PC or, if necessary, PCIRV has been used with success in patients with low compliance (ARDS) or a pulmonary air leak. When the peak pressure is limited, less air seems to leak out and the tissues are more likely to heal. Therapeutic PEEP is applied to increase the patient's FRC to correct hypoxemia. The SIMV feature is added to let the patient breathe spontaneously if desired and to stay more synchronized with the ventilator. With lung healing, the PEEP level is decreased and the inspiratory time is shortened. SIMV with a constant tidal volume may be used during the weaning phase. See Figure 15-14 for pressure and flow tracings during PC.

c. Synchronous intermittent mandatory ventilation with pressure support ventilation and PEEP

SIMV is used to give the patient a controlled number of deep tidal volume breaths. The patient can breathe as often as desired between the mandatory breaths. The patient's total minute volume can be determined by adding the combination of SIMV and pressure-supported breaths. A maximum acceptable $PaCO_2$ can be established with the proper combination of SIMV breaths and PS level. A PS level of more than 10 cm water may be needed. In addition, the PS ensures that the airway resistance of the endotracheal tube is overcome. (See the airway resistance calculation earlier in the chapter.) PEEP therapy is applied to the level necessary to obtain a clinically safe PaO_2 at the lowest possible F_IO_2. Figure 15-17, A shows the pressure/time curve.

Patients who have both a ventilation problem and an oxygenation problem benefit from these modes of ventilation. They have the desire to breathe on their own but a very limited ability to do so. All three modes can be adjusted independently for more or less support, as indicated by the patient's clinical condition and blood gas results.

d. Synchronous intermittent mandatory ventilation with PEEP

IMV/SIMV and PEEP therapy are applied as indicated. Pressure support is not needed if the patient is strong enough to overcome the airway resistance of the endotracheal tube and breathe with a clinically acceptable tidal volume. Figure 15-17, B shows the pressure/time curve.

e. Synchronous intermittent mandatory ventilation with pressure support ventilation

SIMV and PS levels are increased or decreased on the basis of the factors discussed earlier. This patient has the ability to provide some, but not all, of his or her own ventilation. The PaO_2 is clinically acceptable at an oxygen percentage probably no higher than 40%.

A fairly common clinical situation is seen in which the recovering patient does well on a gradually decreasing number of SIMV breaths until he or she can go no lower.

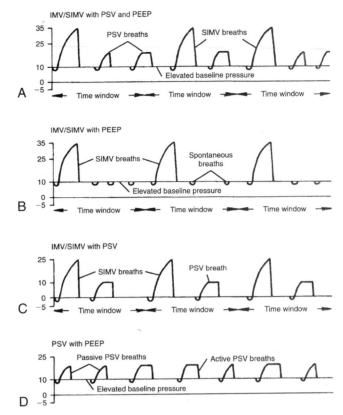

Figure 15-17 Modification of combinations of intermittent mandatory ventilation (IMV)/synchronous intermittent mandatory ventilation (SIMV), pressure support ventilation (PSV), and positive end-expiratory pressure (PEEP). **A,** IMV/SIMV with PSV and PEEP. **B,** IMV/SIMV with PEEP. **C,** IMV/SIMV with PSV. **D,** PSV with PEEP. See text for descriptions of various combinations and their clinical applications.

The barrier seems to be the airway resistance of the endotracheal tube. (See the airway resistance calculation earlier in this chapter.) The addition of some PS overcomes that resistance so that the SIMV level can be reduced further. When the SIMV frequency is down to four or less, the patient is providing almost all of his or her minute volume. The greatest barrier to breathing is likely to be the resistance of the endotracheal tube. The decision then can be made to extubate the patient. Figure 15-17, C shows the pressure/time curve.

f. Pressure support ventilation with positive end-expiratory pressure

PSV and PEEP are applied as discussed earlier. This patient has the drive to breathe on his or her own; however, he or she has some limitation in the ability to overcome the resistance of the endotracheal tube or to generate a consistently large enough tidal volume. (See the airway resistance calculation earlier in the chapter.) In addition, the patient has a significant oxygenation problem and needs some PEEP therapy. With recovery, both PS and PEEP can be reduced. They may be reduced individually or simultaneously as the patient's strength and/or oxygenation improves. Figure 15-17, D shows the pressure/time curve.

g. Dual-control

Several current-generation ventilators provide Dual-Control mode ventilation. Dual-Control mode combines the best features of pressure ventilation and volume ventilation. Simply put, the ventilator will automatically increase or decrease the airway pressure to deliver the desired tidal volume despite decreases or increases in C_{LT}. Dual-Control is designed to provide additional support if the patient's C_{LT} and/or airway resistance should worsen. Conversely, Dual-Control will automatically reduce the set pressure when the patient is easier to ventilate so that too large a tidal volume is not delivered. All manufacturers have their own name for this compensation system and have developed different ways to accomplish the goal of a stable tidal volume. Examples include *pressure augmentation* on the Bear 1000, *volume-assured pressure support* on the Bird 8400, *dual-control pressure ventilation* on the Puritan Bennett 840, *volume support* on the Servo-i, and *AutoFlow* on the Dräger Evita 4, XL, and V500. It is beyond the scope of this text to cover each of these. However, the practitioner is encouraged to understand their essential features and to know that they are added to the Pressure Support mode to ensure a stable, ordered tidal volume.

7. Initiate and adjust the tidal volume and sigh volume
a. Tidal volume

Historical Note: For many years clinical practice and the NBRC exams used a *set* initial tidal volume of 10 mL/kg of ideal body weight (IBW; same as predicted body weight). Because of compressed volume loss (circuit stretch and gas compression), the *delivered* tidal volume was less than what was set. Two recent advances have changed the clinical practice of selecting the tidal volume. The first is the advent of microprocessor ventilators that can calculate compressed volume loss and automatically compensate for it. For example, the physician wants the patient to have an actual tidal volume of 500 mL. If the compressed volume loss is 50 mL, the ventilator delivers 550 mL so that the patient receives an actual 500-mL tidal volume. Second, research has shown that patients with an acute lung injury (ALI) or ARDS should receive a much smaller tidal volume than a person with normal lungs. This lung-protective strategy or open lung strategy employs a smaller tidal volume, a high PEEP level, and a high respiratory rate. A patient with an obstructive lung problem such as COPD or asthma may also need a smaller than normal lung tidal volume to lessen the chance of air trapping and auto-PEEP. The following presentation attempts to summarize the key recommendations for tidal volume selection.

1. Spontaneous tidal volume

A spontaneously breathing person exhales a large enough tidal volume (at the necessary respiratory rate) to remove carbon dioxide as fast as it is produced by his or her metabolism. This results in a normal carbon dioxide level and acid–base balance. The spontaneously breathing person being weaned from a ventilator or breathing with the assistance of CPAP or Pressure Support should have a predicted tidal volume that follows the Radford nomogram (Fig. 15-18). It uses body weight and respiratory rate to predict tidal volume. The Radford nomogram can also be used to help select an initial target for the ventilator tidal volume for many patients with normal lungs. For example, a 70-kg (154-lb) adult with normal lungs and metabolism needs a tidal volume of about 5-7 mL/kg (about 3 mL/lb) of ideal body weight to adequately remove carbon dioxide. So, with a respiratory rate of 12-15/min, this person would have a tidal volume of about 450 mL.

As discussed in the Historical Note above, because compressed volume within the ventilator circuit causes some of the set tidal volume to not reach the patient's lungs, a larger set tidal volume is usually needed with nonmicroprocessor ventilators. (Review "Procedure for calculating the tubing compliance factor" earlier in the chapter.) If a patient is on a ventilator that does not compensate for compressed volume, calculate a *set* tidal volume using 10 mL/kg. For example, a 70-kg (154-lb) adult with normal lungs would have an initial *set* tidal volume of 700 mL (70 kg × 10 mL/kg). Because of compressed volume, the *delivered* tidal volume would be less than 700 mL. This has been the protocol on previous versions of the NBRC exams.

It is presumed in the following discussion that a microprocessor-type ventilator is used and the patient will receive the desired tidal volume. These guidelines are a composite of the current tidal volume recommendations put forward by leading respiratory care researchers and authors and are based on the patient's pulmonary condition:

2. Normal lungs: ventilator tidal volume of 6-8 mL/kg of IBW

This might be a patient with a normal cardiopulmonary system who is receiving mechanical ventilation because of a neurologic problem. For example, the previously mentioned 70-kg (154-lb) adult with normal lungs needs a *set* mechanical ventilator tidal volume in the following range:

$$6 \text{ mL} \times 70 \text{ kg} = 420 \text{ mL}$$

$$8 \text{ mL} \times 70 \text{ kg} = 560 \text{ mL}$$

3. Restrictive lung disease: ventilator tidal volume of 4-6 mL/kg of IBW

Conditions when a small tidal volume would be indicated include:

- ALI or ARDS when the lung-protective strategy is being employed
- Chronic restrictive lung disease such as pulmonary fibrosis
- Surgically reduced lung structure such as lobectomy or pneumonectomy

For example, the previously mentioned 70-kg (154-lb) adult with stiff lungs needs a mechanical ventilator tidal volume in the following range:

$$4 \text{ mL} \times 70 \text{ kg} = 280 \text{ mL}$$

$$6 \text{ mL} \times 70 \text{ kg} = 420 \text{ mL}$$

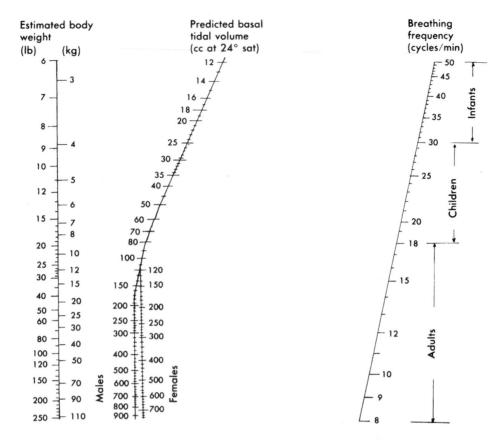

Corrections of predicted basal tidal volumes.
    For patients not in coma: add 10%
    Fever: add 5% for each °F above 99 (rectal)
        add 9% for each °C above 37 (rectal)
    Altitude: add 5% for each 2000 feet above sea level
        add 8% for each 1000 meters above sea level
    Intubation: subtract volume equal to one-half body weight in pounds
            subtract 1 cc/kg of body weight
    Dead space: add equipment dead space

Figure 15-18 Radford nomogram. To use the nomogram, place the left edge of a ruler on the patient's estimated body weight and move the right edge to the patient's breathing frequency. The predicted basal tidal volume now can be found. For example, a 150-lb male who is breathing 12 times per minute will have a predicted tidal volume of 500 cc (mL). (From Radford EP Jr: Ventilation standards for use in artificial respiration. J Appl Physiol 7[4]:451, 1955.)

After the tidal volume has been set, it is very important to check the plateau pressure (P_{plat}). (See the above discussion for the technique.) Current guidelines on lung-protection strategy indicate that a plateau pressure of <30 cm water should reduce the risk of barotrauma to the lungs. If the patient with ALI or ARDS still has a high plateau pressure, the tidal volume should be further reduced. If the patient has a high $PaCO_2$ value and a low plateau pressure, the tidal volume can be increased.

4. Obstructive lung disease: set ventilator tidal volume of 8-10 mL/kg of IBW

This might be a patient with COPD or status asthmaticus. The respiratory rate should be low enough to allow for complete exhalation. For example, the previously mentioned 70-kg (154-lb) adult with overstretched lungs needs a mechanical ventilator tidal volume in the following range:

$$8 \text{ mL} \times 70 \text{ kg} = 560 \text{ mL}$$

$$10 \text{ mL} \times 70 \text{ kg} = 700 \text{ mL}$$

If the patient has an air-trapping problem, the tidal volume should be reduced. See the above discussion on auto-PEEP for more options on reducing air trapping.

5. Tidal volume adjustment

It is common practice to get a set of ABG values after the patient is stable on the ventilator. The tidal volume can then be adjusted depending on whether the patient's $PaCO_2$ value is too high or too low for the therapeutic goal. The most direct way to change alveolar ventilation is to modify the delivered tidal volume. If everything else remains the same, a larger tidal volume results in a lower $PaCO_2$ value. Conversely, a smaller tidal volume results in a higher $PaCO_2$ value.

The following formula can be used to help predict what tidal volume produces a desired $PaCO_2$ value:

$$(V_T - [VD_{anat} + VD_{mech}]) \times f \times PaCO_2 = \\ (V_T' - [VD_{anat} + VD_{mech}]) \times f \times PaCO_2'$$

in which

- V_T = current tidal volume
- VD_{anat} = anatomic dead space (this is calculated at 1 mL/lb or 2.2 mL/kg of ideal body weight)
- VD_{mech} = added mechanical dead space
- f = respiratory (ventilator) rate
- $PaCO_2$ = actual patient $PaCO_2$ value
- V_T' = desired tidal volume
- $PaCO_2'$ = desired patient $PaCO_2$ value

Note that other, simpler formulas are available for calculating a change in minute volume or tidal volume. This one is presented because it takes into account more factors and can be used to calculate a change in tidal volume, rate, or mechanical dead space.

EXAMPLE

The patient is a febrile 70-kg (154-lb) man who is being ventilated on the Control mode (he is apneic). His ventilator settings are tidal volume 1000 mL, rate 12 times/min, fractional inspired oxygen concentration (F_IO_2) 0.3, and no added mechanical dead space. His ABG values are pH 7.48, $PaCO_2$ 30 torr, PaO_2 90 torr, SaO_2 95%, and base excess (BE) 0. The clinical goal is to adjust the patient's tidal volume as needed to produce a $PaCO_2$ value of 40 torr. In summary,

- V_T = 1000 mL, current tidal volume
- VD_{anat} = 154 mL of anatomic dead space (this is calculated at 1 mL/lb or 2.2 mL/kg of ideal body weight)
- VD_{mech} = no added mechanical dead space
- f = 12 times/min for the ventilator rate
- $PaCO_2$ = 30 torr, actual patient $PaCO_2$ value
- V_T' = desired tidal volume
- $PaCO_2'$ = 40 torr, desired patient $PaCO_2$ value

Placing the data and goal into the formula results in the following:

$$(V_T - [VD_{anat} + VD_{mech}]) \times f \times PaCO_2 = \\ (V_T' - [VD_{anat} + VD_{mech}]) \times f \times PaCO_2'$$
$$(1000 - [154 + 0]) \times 12 \times 30 = (V_T' - [154 + 0]) \times 12 \times 40$$

Simplifying produces the following:

$$(846) \times 12 \times 30 = (V_T' - 154) \times 480$$

$$304,560 = 480 \, V_T' - 73,920$$
$$378,480 = 480 \, V_T'$$
$$788 \, mL = V_T'$$

The solution is to reduce the patient's tidal volume from 1000 to 788 mL.

Exam Hint 15-10

Every available NBRC examination has had several problems that require the test taker to determine an original ventilator tidal volume or a new tidal volume to correct for overventilating (low carbon dioxide level) or underventilating (high carbon dioxide level) a patient. On previous exams, an initial tidal volume of 10 mL/kg of ideal body weight would be selected. More recent guidelines would point to selecting a tidal volume of about 8 mL/kg. A patient with ALI or ARDS should have a smaller tidal volume. Increase or decrease the tidal volume, as needed, from this starting point. Often the patient's height and weight are given. Be careful to not overventilate a patient who is obese.

b. Sigh volume

An additional consideration is whether to give the patient a sigh breath, which is a volume larger than the normal V_T. People normally spontaneously sigh (yawn) every few minutes. It serves the purpose of opening up atelectatic alveoli and reorienting the surfactant in the alveoli so that they are stable. It is controversial to add sighs to a patient who is receiving mechanical ventilation. With the current clinical practice of giving most patients a low level of PEEP to prevent atelectasis, there is little need for sighs to be given.

Historically, many patients who were ventilated in the VC, A/C mode received a ventilator sigh volume just as they did a V_T. A sigh volume is typically 1.5 to 2 times the V_T if the V_T is in the low range. If the patient has a problem of atelectasis or consolidation, a sigh volume may be indicated. The patient may not need a sigh volume if the set V_T is at the middle to upper limit. When a sigh is given, compare the inspired and expired volumes to ensure that no air trapping occurs. Most current ventilators allow the clinician to tailor the sigh frequency to best meet the patient's clinical needs. The sigh frequency should be increased in patients with atelectasis or consolidation. The sigh frequency may have to be decreased or eliminated in patients who are air trapping the V_T or sigh volume. Sighs usually are not given in any mode other than A/C.

A patient with COPD or asthma, pneumothorax, or cardiac status that is sensitive to high peak pressures may be contraindicated for a sigh volume. The patient with air trapping of the V_T should have a smaller (possibly no) sigh volume. Sighs are not recommended when a patient is receiving a tidal volume at the upper end of the normal range and the plateau pressure is >30 cm water. This patient is at risk for barotrauma/volutrauma.

8. Initiate and adjust the inspiratory hold

Inspiratory hold (also known as *inflation hold*) is a technique whereby the patient is temporarily prevented from exhaling the ventilator-delivered V_T. Figure 15-19 shows the pressure/time waveform. The pressure found during the inspiratory hold period is called the *inspiratory plateau* or *plateau pressure*. Inspiratory hold is added therapeutically to improve distribution of the V_T. Patients with ARDS and pulmonary edema can benefit from it. Oxygenation should improve in direct proportion to the duration of the inspiratory plateau. The duration of the inspiratory plateau is measured in different ways, depending on the ventilator. For example, some ventilators add inspiratory hold in steps of 0.1 second up to several seconds total. Other ventilators add it as a variable percentage of the total duration of the breathing cycle.

Notice that the use of an inspiratory plateau increases the inspiratory phase of the breathing cycle. For example, adding 0.5 second of inspiratory hold to 1 second of inspiratory time results in a total inspiratory phase of 1.5 seconds. This will cause a shorter expiratory time if the rate is kept the same (or the rate must be reduced to keep the same I:E ratio). Because of the shortened expiratory time, it is very important to make sure that the V_T is exhaled completely. If the expiratory time is too short, the patient will have air trapping and auto-PEEP (see Fig. 15-3). The patient's condition should be monitored closely to determine whether the level of inspiratory plateau is appropriate. The inspiratory plateau must be reduced as the patient's ventilation and C_{LT} improve. Patients with normal ventilation and compliance should not receive any inspiratory plateau.

Nontherapeutic inspiratory plateau is added temporarily to determine the plateau pressure on the ventilator. This is considered to be the pressure needed to deliver the V_T. With this information, the patient's effective Cst can be calculated. Its calculation and interpretation were discussed earlier in this chapter. An inspiratory plateau of 1.0 second usually is long enough to find the plateau pressure. Remember to turn off the inspiratory plateau afterward.

9. Initiate and adjust the respiratory rate

See Table 1-2 in Chapter 1 for a listing of the normal resting respiratory frequencies based on age. If the patient is apneic and has a normal temperature and metabolic rate with an appropriately set tidal volume, respiratory rates in the indicated ranges will produce a normal $PaCO_2$ level. This must be confirmed by an ABG measurement. If the tidal volume cannot be changed, adjusting the respiratory rate will modify alveolar ventilation. A higher respiratory rate, with everything else remaining the same, will result in a lower $PaCO_2$ level. Conversely, a lower respiratory rate, with everything else remaining the same, will result in a higher $PaCO_2$ level.

See Figure 15-18 for the Radford nomogram for use in predicting a normal respiratory rate and tidal volume based on weight. It can be used to establish an initial rate for most patients with normal lung function: about 15/min. A chronically hypercapneic patient (COPD) must be ventilated with some caution. Giving this type of patient a higher ventilator-delivered rate and a larger tidal volume will result in blowing off too much carbon dioxide and cause a respiratory alkalosis. An initial rate of 8-10/min is recommended. Adult patients with a chronic restrictive lung disease, a pneumonectomy, or ARDS may need a respiratory rate of 20-30 per minute to meet their minute volume needs. This is because their condition requires a smaller tidal volume than normal.

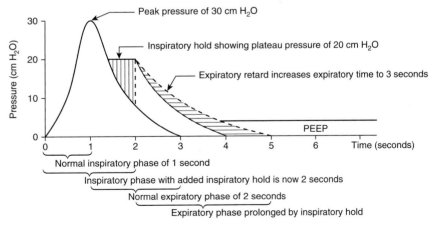

Figure 15-19 Pressure/time waveform showing how exhalation can be modified. An inspiratory plateau (inspiratory hold) is seen when the tidal volume is held within the lungs for a period of time. With expiratory retard, the gas is exhaled more slowly than during a passive breath. These two modifications of exhalation may or may not be combined with positive end-expiratory pressure.

The same formula that was used to predict a tidal volume change can be used to help predict what *respiratory rate* will produce a desired $PaCO_2$ value:

$$(V_T - [VD_{anat} + VD_{mech}]) \times f \times PaCO_2 =$$
$$(V_T - [VD_{anat} + VD_{mech}]) \times f' \times PaCO_2'$$

EXAMPLE

The patient is the same febrile 70-kg (154-lb) man who is being ventilated on the Control mode (he is apneic). His ventilator settings are tidal volume 1000 mL, rate 12 times/min, F_IO_2 0.3, and no added mechanical dead space. His ABG values are pH 7.48, $PaCO_2$ 30 torr, PaO_2 90 torr, SaO_2 95%, and BE 0. The clinical goal is to adjust the patient's rate as needed to produce a $PaCO_2$ value of 40 torr. In summary,

- V_T = 1000 mL, current tidal volume
- VD_{anat} = 154 mL of anatomic dead space (this is calculated at 1 mL/lb or 2.2 mL/kg of ideal body weight)
- VD_{mech} = no added mechanical dead space
- f = 12 times/min for the ventilator rate
- f′ = desired ventilator rate
- $PaCO_2$ = 30 torr, actual patient $PaCO_2$ value
- $PaCO_2'$ = 40 torr, desired patient $PaCO_2$ value

Placing the data and goal into the formula results in the following:

$$(V_T - [VD_{anat} + VD_{mech}]) \times f \times PaCO_2 =$$
$$(V_T - [VD_{anat} + VD_{mech}]) \times f' \times PaCO_2'$$

$$(1000 - [154 + 0]) \times 12 \times 30 = (1000 - [154 + 0]) \times f' \times 40$$

$$[846] \times 12 \times 30 = [846] \times f' \times 40$$

$$304{,}560 = 33{,}840f'$$

$$9 = f'$$

The solution is to reduce the patient's respiratory rate from 12 to 9 breaths/min.

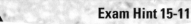

Exam Hint 15-11

Every available NBRC examination has had several problems that require the test taker to determine an original ventilator respiratory rate or a new respiratory rate to correct for hyperventilating (low carbon dioxide level) or hypoventilating (high carbon dioxide level) a patient. Typically start with a respiratory rate of about 15 in an adult with normal lungs. The patient with ARDS would need a faster rate. Increase or decrease the rate as needed from this starting point.

10. Choose and adjust the minute ventilation

The subjects of minute ventilation and alveolar minute ventilation were covered in Chapter 4. Minute volume is the product of tidal volume and rate. Review the calculations as needed. An adult with a normal metabolism will need a minute volume of about 100 mL/kg of IBW per minute. Blood gases must always be evaluated for the $PaCO_2$

level to tell whether the patient's minute ventilation is adequate. A high carbon dioxide level indicates a need to increase the tidal volume, respiratory rate, or both. A low carbon dioxide level indicates a need to decrease the tidal volume, respiratory rate, or both. In both cases, the key to modifying the carbon dioxide level is to modify the alveolar ventilation. This is best accomplished by changing the tidal volume rather than the rate. The following formula can be used to calculate a change in the minute volume:

$$\dot{V}_E' = \frac{PaCO_2 \times \dot{V}_E}{PaCO_2'}$$

in which

$$\dot{V}_E' = desired \text{ minute volume}$$
$$\dot{V}_E = current \text{ minute volume}$$
$$PaCO_2 = current \text{ carbon dioxide level}$$
$$PaCO_2' = desired \text{ carbon dioxide level}$$

EXAMPLE

The patient is the same febrile 70-kg (154-lb) man who is being ventilated on the Control mode (he is apneic). His ventilator settings are tidal volume 1000 mL, rate 12 times/min, F_IO_2 0.3, and no added mechanical dead space. His ABG values are pH 7.48, $PaCO_2$ 30 torr, PaO_2 90 torr, SaO_2 95%, and BE 0. The clinical goal is to adjust the patient's minute volume as needed to produce a $PaCO_2$ value of 40 torr. Placing the data and the goal into the formula results in the following:

$$\dot{V}_E' = \frac{PaCO_2 \times \dot{V}_E}{PaCO_2'}$$

$$\dot{V}_E' = \frac{30 \times 12{,}000}{40\,\dot{V}_E'}$$

$$\dot{V}_E' = \frac{360{,}000}{40\,\dot{V}_E'}$$

$$\dot{V}_E' = 9000 \text{ mL}$$

The goal can be accomplished by reducing the minute volume from 12,000 to 9000 mL. As was mentioned earlier, this is best done by reducing the tidal volume. Remember that the tidal volume should not be less than the guidelines listed above to avoid the development of atelectasis. The respiratory rate may be decreased, if necessary, to provide this reduced minute volume.

11. Mechanical dead space

Mechanical dead space (VD_{mech}) should be recommended when the mechanically ventilated patient is hyperventilating, and attempts to reduce the tidal volume and/or rate have not increased the $PaCO_2$ to the desired goal.

Mechanical dead space is added to increase the patient's $PaCO_2$ level. This is done by having the patient rebreathe gas from his or her anatomic dead space. This high-CO_2 gas then is inhaled back to the alveolar level and increases the patient's $PaCO_2$ level. The more dead space tubing there is, the more carbon dioxide is retained. It is important to realize that this same rebreathed volume of gas is lower in oxygen because of its diffusion into the patient's pulmonary circulation. If a large amount of mechanical dead space is added, it will be necessary to increase the F_IO_2 to keep the ordered level. Measure the oxygen percentage between the dead space and the endotracheal or tracheostomy tube adapter.

Mechanical dead space is used only in the C and A/C modes. It should not be used in SIMV, pressure support, or CPAP mode. Typically, a length of large-bore or aerosol tubing is added into the breathing circuit between the Y and the patient's endotracheal or tracheostomy tube (see Fig. 15-29).

The following formula can be used to predict what amount of *mechanical dead space* (VD_{mech}') will produce the desired $PaCO_2$ level. It can be used to calculate how much dead space should be added or subtracted.

$$([V_T - VD_{anat}] - VD_{mech}) \times f \times PaCO_2 =$$
$$([V_T - VD_{anat}] - VD_{mech}') \times f \times PaCO_2'$$

in which

V_T = current tidal volume

VD_{anat} = anatomic dead space This is calculated at 1 mL/lb or 2.2 mL/kg of ideal body weight

VD_{mech} = current mechanical dead space

f = ventilator rate

$PaCO_2$ = actual patient $PaCO_2$ value

VD_{mech}' = desired mechanical dead space

$PaCO_2'$ = desired patient $PaCO_2$ value

EXAMPLE

Your patient is a febrile 70-kg (154-lb) man who is being ventilated on the Control mode (he is apneic). His ventilator settings are tidal volume 1000 mL, rate 12/min, F_IO_2 0.3, and no added mechanical dead space. His ABGs are pH 7.48, PaO_2 90 torr, SaO_2 95%, and BE 0. The clinical goal is to adjust the patient's mechanical dead space as needed to produce a $PaCO_2$ of 40 torr. In summary,

V_T = 1000 mL current tidal volume

VD_{anat} = 154 mL anatomic dead space This is calculated at 1 mL/lb or 2.2mL/kg of ideal body weight

VD_{mech} = no added mechanical dead space

f = 12 for ventilator rate

$PaCO_2$ = 30 torr actual patient $PaCO_2$ value

VD_{mech}' = the desired amount of mechanical dead space

$PaCO_2'$ = 40 torr desired patient $PaCO_2$ value

Placing the data and the goal into the formula results in the following equation:

$$([V_T - VD_{anat}] - VD_{mech}) \times f \times PaCO_2 =$$
$$([V_T - VD_{anat}] - VD_{mech}') \times f \times PaCO_2'$$

$$([1000 - 154] - 0) \times 12 \times 30 = ([1000 - 154] - VD_{mech}') \times 12 \times 40$$

Simplifying produces the following:

$$(846) \times 12 \times 30 = (846 - VD_{mech}') \times 480$$
$$304,560 = (846 \times 480) - (VD_{mech}' \times 480)$$
$$304,560 = 406,080 - 480\,VD_{mech}'$$
$$-101,520 = -480\,VD_{mech}'$$
$$211.5\text{ mL} = VD_{mech}'$$

The solution is to increase the patient's mechanical dead space from 0 to 212 mL.

Exam Hint 15-12

Usually one question deals with recommending the addition of mechanical dead space when ABG results show that the patient is being hyperventilated. Recommend the removal of mechanical dead space when the carbon dioxide level is too high.

12. Initiate and adjust PEEP therapy

The most effective way to enhance oxygenation is to increase the patient's baseline pressure above atmospheric. Positive end-expiratory pressure (PEEP) is a mechanically elevated baseline pressure. In other words, the patient's end-expiratory pressure is above atmospheric. PEEP is administered through a mechanical ventilator and is not a mode by itself. Rather, it is used in conjunction with any of the previously mentioned modes. (All of the considerations for PEEP apply to CPAP except that the patient must be able to breathe adequately to maintain a normal CO_2 level. CPAP is discussed below.)

Therapeutic PEEP generally is indicated in any acute, bilateral, generalized pulmonary condition in which the FRC is decreased. Usually the patient has been diagnosed with an ALI or ARDS. Other examples of small FRC conditions helped by PEEP include generalized atelectasis, pulmonary edema, and infant respiratory distress syndrome (RDS). All of these patients show decreased C_{LT} as measured by their Cst. When the FRC is decreased, shunt is increased, and the patient has refractory hypoxemia. The higher the level of PEEP, the more progressively the patient's FRC is increased. The therapeutic goal of this is to increase the PaO_2. (Fig. 15-13, F shows the pressure/time curve.) Patients with chronically small FRC, such as those with pulmonary fibrosis and kyphoscoliosis, are not helped by the application of PEEP.

Specific indications for PEEP include the following:
- Intrapulmonary shunt >15%
- Refractory hypoxemia (PaO_2 <60 mm Hg despite an F_IO_2 of up to 0.8-1.0)
- The patient has had an F_IO_2 >0.5 for 48-72 hours and shows no indication of a rapidly improving PaO_2. PEEP is added so that the F_IO_2 can be lowered to a safer level.

Before PEEP is begun, the patient should be monitored carefully with blood gas analysis and vital sign checks to establish the baseline conditions. Watch for side effects of barotrauma or decreased cardiac output (CO) from too much pressure. The same parameters should be monitored after each change in the PEEP level to determine how the patient is tolerating it. (CPAP has the same indications and physiologic effects as PEEP and is discussed below.)

The best or optimal level of PEEP is the level that results in the best delivery of oxygen to the tissues (not necessarily the arterial blood). Often, a secondary goal is to reduce the inspired oxygen to a safe level. The patient is at risk for oxygen toxicity if more than 50% oxygen is inhaled for longer than 48-72 hours. See Box 15-3 for recommendations on what to monitor during the application of PEEP and how to evaluate the data.

The application of PEEP has risks. Clinically, these risks must be weighed against the potential benefit to the patient. In the profoundly hypoxic patient, PEEP can be lifesaving. Some clinicians use low levels of PEEP (up to 5 cm water) in patients with normal lungs or overly compliant lungs (emphysema) to maintain the baseline level of FRC. Hazards of PEEP include the following:
- Pulmonary barotrauma: pneumothorax, tension pneumothorax, mediastinal emphysema, pulmonary interstitial emphysema in the neonate, subcutaneous emphysema
- Decreased venous return to the heart, causing decreased CO and tachycardia, decreased blood pressure, decreased tissue perfusion as measured by a decreased mixed venous oxygen ($P\overline{v}O_2$) level, decreased urine output

a. Increasing PEEP

PEEP therapy is usually begun at an initial level of 5 cm water. After the patient's response has been determined, 2-5 cm more PEEP may be applied. The patient is reevaluated. This process goes on until the desired clinical benefit is reached. Figure 15-20 shows a number of physiologic parameters that can be measured and evaluated.

Different approaches to the application of PEEP are used to find the best level. One approach could be called minimum PEEP. It involves the application of PEEP to the minimum level that allows the inspired oxygen percentage to be lowered to a safer level. A clinical goal is to minimize the risk of oxygen toxicity. In this approach, PEEP is raised until the PaO_2 is greater than 60 torr or the SpO_2 is greater than 90% on 60% oxygen or less. Usually no more

than 10-15 cm water of PEEP is needed. A patient with an ALI is more likely to need a low to moderate level of PEEP.

Another approach could be called *best PEEP* or *optimum PEEP*. This approach has the clinical goal of reducing the patient's shunt fraction to less than 15% by keeping the lungs ideally inflated. Often this requires more pressure than the minimal PEEP approach. Because this higher pressure level is more likely to cause hemodynamic problems, the patient should have a pulmonary artery catheter inserted. With it, the patient's CO, mixed venous oxygen level, pulmonary capillary wedge pressure, and pulmonary vascular resistance can be measured (see Fig. 15-20). In addition, the patient may need increased intravenous fluids, dopamine (Intropin), and digitalis (Digoxin) for cardiovascular support. The higher PEEP levels increase the risk of pulmonary barotrauma. Therefore the patient must be watched closely for signs of a pneumothorax. A patient with ARDS is more likely to need a high level of PEEP. This higher, optimal level of PEEP is a critical part of the open lung strategy employed to protect the lung and prevent ventilator-induced lung injury.

b. Decreasing PEEP

As the patient begins to recover, the PEEP level may be reduced in steps of 2-5 cm water. Again, the patient is evaluated after every change in the PEEP level. If the patient's cardiovascular status is normal, the following are recommendations for how to decrease PEEP and oxygen levels:
- Decrease PEEP first if the PaO_2 level is greater than 60 torr and the F_IO_2 is less than 0.5.
- Decrease oxygen first if the PaO_2 level is greater than 60 torr and the F_IO_2 is greater than 0.5.

If the patient is showing an adverse reaction to the PEEP level, such as decreased CO or barotrauma, the PEEP level should be decreased before the oxygen percentage. Clinical judgment must be used to decide whether a high oxygen percentage or a high PEEP level is a greater danger to the patient. Minimize or remove the element that puts the patient at greater risk.

Exam Hint 15-13

Typically, several questions deal with the clinical application and modification of PEEP. Know to increase PEEP if the patient is hypoxic, is receiving a high oxygen percentage, and is hemodynamically stable. Know to decrease PEEP if the patient is well oxygenated and is receiving a moderate oxygen percentage, is not hemodynamically stable, or has a PEEP-related complication. A decrease in the patient's CO is a key indicator of excessive PEEP causing hemodynamic problems.

---

13. Initiate and adjust expiratory retard

Expiratory retard is backpressure that prevents the collapse of the smallest airways. It is shown in the Figure 15-19 pressure/time waveform. Some ventilators have a control that adjusts both inspiratory hold and expiratory retard, so care must be taken when a change is made in either. As was discussed in Chapter 14, expiratory retard is indicated in any patient who has air trapping and is not exhaling completely. It functions similar to pursed-lip breathing in the spontaneously breathing patient.

Expiratory retard may be indicated in a patient with an air-trapping condition such as asthma, emphysema, or bronchitis. It is important with these types of patients to measure the inspiratory and expiratory V_T. Air trapping is confirmed when the expiratory volume is less than the

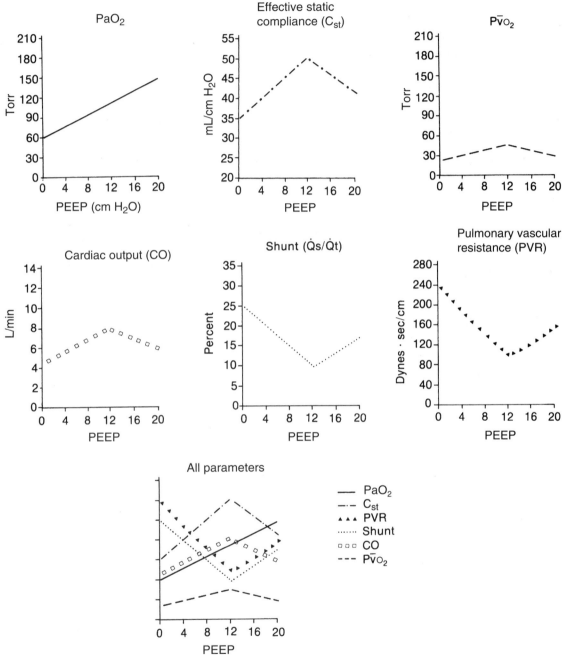

Figure 15-20 Optimal or best positive end-expiratory pressure (PEEP) level is determined by monitoring some or all of the following parameters: PaO_2, effective static compliance (Cst), pressure of mixed venous oxygen ($P\bar{v}O_2$), cardiac output (CO), shunt ($\dot{Q}s/\dot{Q}t$), and pulmonary vascular resistance (PVR). Ideally, as functional residual capacity (FRC) is increased by PEEP, lung compliance is improved, and ventilation and perfusion are better matched. CO should remain stable. It can be measured by the use of a pulmonary artery (Swan-Ganz) catheter or indirectly followed by monitoring the patient's heart rate and blood pressure. As can be seen, the optimal PEEP is found at 12 cm water pressure. Excessive PEEP is seen by the resulting decrease in static compliance and CO.

inspiratory volume. When one is listening to the patient's breath sounds, it will be noted that no pause occurs at the end of exhalation before the next inspiration is started. In extreme cases, the pressure manometer does not return to the baseline level. These patients should be checked for the presence and level of auto-PEEP. The proper level of expiratory retard is determined by trial and error. The following parameters should be monitored to find the proper amount:

- Inspiratory and expiratory V_T's should be the same.
- The patient's breath sounds should reveal wheezing to be absent or minimal and a silent pause should be noted at the end of exhalation before the next V_T is delivered.
- Auto-PEEP should not occur.
- The patient should feel subjectively that he or she has exhaled completely before the next breath is given.

The patient must be monitored frequently when expiratory retard is being used. As the patient is treated with bronchodilating medications, the bronchospasm should diminish. Expiratory retard should not be necessary when the airway resistance has returned to normal.

14. Assess the patient's response to mechanical ventilation

a. Auscultate to assess breath sounds (code: IB5) [difficulty: R, Ap, An]

Check for equal, bilateral breath sounds after a patient has been intubated. Also, auscultate the patient's breath sounds after any significant change in the ventilator or in the patient's condition. Review the discussion on breath sounds in Chapter 1, if necessary.

b. Monitor airway pressures

Other than plateau pressure, these topics are not specifically listed on the Detailed Content Outline. However, airway pressure changes have been previously tested. Modern microprocessor-type ventilators allow the operator to monitor the patient's sensitivity pressure, peak pressure, plateau pressure, and mean airway pressure.

1. Sensitivity

If pressure sensitivity is used, it should be set so that the patient has to generate only −1 to −2 cm water pressure to trigger a ventilator breath. If the ventilator is insensitive to the patient's needs, WOB will be increased (see Fig. 15-1).

2. Peak pressure (P_{peak})

The peak pressure reached during delivery of a tidal volume is the pressure required to push the gas through the circuit, the endotracheal tube, and the patient's airways, and to expand the lungs. The sigh volume requires greater pressure because it is a larger volume. These pressures should be recorded regularly whenever the patient and the machine are checked. The importance of peak pressure in

calculating dynamic compliance was discussed earlier in the chapter.

3. Plateau pressure (P_{plat}) (code: ID13) [difficulty: R, Ap, An]

The plateau pressure is found when the tidal volume has been delivered to the lungs and is held within them temporarily. The importance of plateau pressure in calculating static compliance was discussed earlier in the chapter.

4. Baseline pressure

The baseline pressure is the pressure measured at the end of exhalation. Normally it is seen as zero on the ventilator's pressure manometer. (Remember that in this case, zero is actually local barometric pressure.) If the patient has therapeutic PEEP or CPAP, the baseline pressure will be greater than zero.

5. Mean airway pressure

Mean airway pressure ($\overline{Paw}$, MAP, $\overline{Paw}$) is the average pressure over an entire breathing cycle. Most current neonatal and adult ventilators are able to calculate and display the value (Fig. 15-21). $\overline{Paw}$ is influenced by the patient's C_{LT}, Raw, and ventilator settings such as the I:E ratio. If a volume-cycled ventilator is being used, a decrease in compliance or an increase in resistance results in an increase in the $\overline{Paw}$ because it takes more pressure to deliver the tidal volume; a higher peak pressure is seen. Conversely, if the patient's compliance increases or resistance decreases, the $\overline{Paw}$ decreases. It is important to evaluate the patient further when a change in $\overline{Paw}$ is noticed. This is because the new pressure, by itself, does not clarify whether a change in compliance, resistance, or both has occurred. Any treatments that improve C_{LT} and reduce airway resistance result in reduced $\overline{Paw}$. It is important to calculate both dynamic and static compliance (discussed earlier) when trying to determine how the patient's condition has changed.

In general, an increase in $\overline{Paw}$ increases the patient's oxygenation because the alveoli are kept open longer, allowing more time for diffusion and preventing alveolar collapse. (Fig. 16-12 shows how several ventilator adjustments can

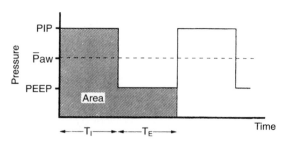

Figure 15-21 Pressure/time tracing showing mean airway pressure ($\overline{Paw}$). PEEP, positive end-expiratory pressure; PIP, peak inspiratory pressure; T_E, expiratory time; T_I, inspiratory time. (From Chatburn RL: Classification of mechanical ventilators, Respir Care 36(6):569, 1991.)

change the $\overline{Paw}$. See the related discussion in Chapter 16.) If alveolar ventilation is improved, the $PaCO_2$ also may be reduced.

If the $\overline{Paw}$ is too high, risk of pulmonary barotrauma is increased and CO is decreased. This is especially true if PEEP is increased to raise the $\overline{Paw}$. Watch the patient closely whenever a ventilator change is made that increases the $\overline{Paw}$. A sudden deterioration in cardiopulmonary function may be caused by a pneumothorax. Reduced urine output, increased heart rate, and decreased blood pressure often are seen when CO is reduced. The $\overline{Paw}$ should be reduced if any of these situations is seen. To prevent these complications, it is necessary to reduce the $\overline{Paw}$ whenever the patient's pulmonary condition improves. As compliance increases toward normal, it is not necessary to use as high a $\overline{Paw}$ to maintain acceptable blood gases.

c. Blood gas analysis and monitoring

1. Evaluate data on blood gas analysis results in the patient record (code: IA5) [difficulty: R, Ap]

An arterial blood sample should be taken for analysis in the following situations: (1) after the patient is first established on the ventilator, (2) when there is a significant change in ventilator settings (inspired oxygen percentage, rate, tidal volume, PEEP level), and (3) when the patient's condition changes significantly.

2. Evaluate the results of blood gas analysis (code: ID6) [difficulty: R, Ap, An]

Interpretation of the ABG results will provide vital information to guide additional ventilator changes. Chapter 3 provides a complete discussion on interpretation.

d. Noninvasive monitoring

1. Evaluate trends on capnometry, pulse oximetry, and transcutaneous oxygen and carbon dioxide monitoring results in the patient record (code: IA5) [difficulty: R, Ap]

See below.

2. Perform noninvasive monitoring: capnometry, pulse oximetry, and transcutaneous oxygen and carbon dioxide monitoring (code: IC2) [difficulty: R, Ap]

See below.

3. Evaluate the results of capnography, pulse oximetry, and transcutaneous oxygen and carbon dioxide monitoring (code: ID2) [difficulty: R, Ap, An]

Capnography is widely used to evaluate the patient's ability to exhale carbon dioxide and to evaluate certain conditions in which dead space can change. Changes in tidal volume, rate, and mechanical dead space will affect carbon dioxide removal. See the capnography discussion and examples of exhaled carbon dioxide waveforms in Chapter 5. Pulse oximeter values are monitored routinely for

oxygenation. Chapter 3 provides a complete discussion. Transcutaneous oxygen and carbon dioxide monitoring is used primarily with neonatal patients. See Chapter 3 for the discussion of interpretation.

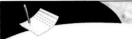

Exam Hint 15-14

Expect to see many ABG values and blood gas monitoring values incorporated into questions about adjusting the ventilator. Review Chapter 3, if necessary, for interpretation guidelines. Hypoxemia should be treated by increasing the oxygen percentage or increasing the PEEP level. As the patient improves, these can be reduced. If the patient's carbon dioxide level is too high, increase the rate or the tidal volume. If too much carbon dioxide is being blown off, decrease the rate or the tidal volume.

MODULE D

Provide unconventional mechanical ventilation to adequately oxygenate and ventilate the patient.

1. Recommend changes in mechanical ventilation parameters and settings (code: IIIE3f) [difficulty: R, Ap, An]

See below.

2. Initiate and adjust continuous mechanical ventilation (code: IIIC4a) [difficulty: R, Ap, An]

Unconventional mechanical ventilation is defined here as the use of specialized ventilators that can provide unique modes and options needed by special populations of patients. This ventilatory support may or may not be provided through an endotracheal tube or a tracheostomy tube. See below for the discussion.

The NBRC may ask questions about specific indications and applications of unconventional mechanical ventilators. Questions may be asked about which parameters and settings to recommend and the initiation and adjustment of those settings. The discussion below includes specific items listed on the Detailed Content Outline. Also included are other topics within the broader scope of unconventional mechanical ventilation that are found in clinical practice.

3. High-frequency ventilation (code: IIIC4c) [difficulty: R, Ap, An]

High-frequency ventilation (HFV) is needed whenever the patient's condition calls for a higher respiratory rate or a smaller tidal volume than usually is delivered on a conventional volume-cycled ventilator. A high-frequency ventilator can deliver a respiratory rate far higher than the limit of 150/min set by the U.S. Food and Drug Administration (FDA) on all conventional adult and neonatal/pediatric ventilators.

The FDA has approved HFV for use on adults during bronchoscopy and laryngoscopy procedures and when a patient with a bronchopleural fistula cannot be managed on a conventional ventilator. Although patients with ARDS have not been officially approved for HFV, the procedure has been used when a patient is hypoxic despite maximum settings on a conventional ventilator. (Box 16-5 in Chapter 16 lists clinical uses for HFV with infants and children.)

Currently HFV can be delivered in three different ways. The first involves the use of a conventional ventilator set at a rate of up to the FDA maximum of 150/min. This method is called high-frequency positive-pressure ventilation (HFPPV). With it, the set tidal volume is decreased to something less than standard (<8 mL/kg). The second involves the use of high-frequency jet ventilation (HFJV). This method of ventilation can be provided by a specific jet ventilator (Bunnell Life Pulse) that is used in conjunction with a conventional ventilator set on the SIMV or CPAP mode. To do this, the standard endotracheal tube adapter is replaced with a special jet adapter (see Figs. 15-26 and 16-16). The HFJV unit is connected to the long catheter on the adapter. The conventional ventilator is connected to the main lumen on the adapter. Gas from the HFJV unit entrains additional gas through the main lumen to create the patient's tidal volume. HFJV units can deliver a small tidal volume several hundred times per minute. The third method involves a high-frequency oscillation (HFO) ventilator. HFO makes use of a conventional endotracheal tube (as does HFPPV). However, the delivered tidal volume is the smallest, and the respiratory rate can be the fastest of all three methods. Table 16-2 in Chapter 16 presents a comparison of all three methods. The equipment used for HFJV and for HFO is described later in Module E.

Table 15-3 lists considerations for the initial settings and for adjustment of HFV delivered to infants and adults by a jet ventilator or an oscillator ventilator.

Current clinical experience is recommended for any HFV method. Although adult patients have been treated successfully with HFV, far greater use of these techniques has occurred with infants and children. Therefore, Chapter 16 provides further discussion.

4. Noninvasive ventilation (code: IIIC4b) [difficulty: R, Ap, An]

NIV is also known as noninvasive positive-pressure ventilation (NPPV). (*Note:* The Detailed Content Outline states "NIV" whereas the validation study TMC used the abbreviation "NPPV.") Most of the time, patients receiving NIV are ventilated with the aid of a nasal mask similar to that used to deliver mask CPAP. A full face mask often is needed if the patient leaks through the mouth with a nasal mask.

Most patients who are candidates for NIV are fairly stable, are not intubated and can protect their airway, can breathe spontaneously, and should need only short-term ventilator support. There is strong clinical evidence for the use of NIV in the following situations:

- COPD exacerbation to avoid intubation and mechanical ventilation
- Avoiding reintubation of a weaned and extubated COPD patient
- Cardiogenic pulmonary edema
- Pulmonary infiltrates in an immunocompromised patient
- Sleep apnea from upper-airway obstruction

TABLE 15-3	High-Frequency Ventilation Operational Considerations			
	Infant Jets	**Adult Jets**	**Infant Oscillators**	**Adult Oscillators**
Initial recommended frequency	7 Hz (IMV background rate of 2)	5 Hz	15 Hz	3-5 Hz
Initial tidal volume and pressures	Jet-drive pressure to produce 90% of CV peak pressure; I time 0.02 s	Jet drive pressure of 25-35 psi; I:E = 1:2-1:1	Amplitude to create chest vibration visually; I:E = 1:1 Mean pressure = CV mean + 5 cm H_2O	Amplitude to create chest vibration visually; I:E = 1:2-1:1 Mean pressure = CV mean + 5 cm H_2O
To change effective V_A	Alter drive pressure*; alter inspiratory time[†]; alter frequency[‡]	Alter drive pressure*; alter inspiratory time[†]; alter frequency[‡]	Alter pressure amplitudes*; alter inspiratory time[†]; alter frequency[‡]	Alter pressure amplitudes*; alter inspiratory time[†]; alter frequency[‡]
To change mean $\overline{P}_{aw}$ (for $\dot{V}/\dot{Q}$ effects on PaO_2)	Alter applied PEEP; alter inspiratory time[†]	Alter applied PEEP (if available); alter inspiratory time	Alter bias flow; alter outflow resistor; alter inspiratory time[†]	Alter bias flow: alter outflow resistor; alter inspiratory time[†]

CV, conventional ventilation; I, inspiratory; I:E, inspiratory:expiratory ratio; IMV, intermittent mandatory ventilation; PaO_2, arterial oxygen pressure; $\overline{P}aw$, airway pressure; PEEP, positive end-expiratory pressure; V_A, alveolar ventilation; V_T, tidal volume; $\dot{V}/\dot{Q}$, ventilation/perfusion ratio.

*↑pressure = ↑tidal volume = ↑V_A.

[†]↑Inspiratory time = ↑tidal volume = ↑V_A *unless* air trapping develops, in which case, tidal volume may ↓.

[‡]Frequency response may be variable: ↑ frequency may increase total ventilation *but* ↑ frequency can ↓ tidal volume through shorter inspiratory time and pulse attenuation through narrow endotracheal tubes.

From MacIntyre NR: High-frequency ventilation. In: MacIntyre NR, Branson RD, editors: Mechanical ventilation, ed 2, St Louis, 2009, Saunders.

There is weaker evidence for the use of NIV in the following situations:

- Asthma exacerbation
- Obesity hypoventilation syndrome
- Postsurgical period

NIV should not be used with a patient who is critically ill and unstable. This patient must be intubated and placed on a standard volume-cycled ventilator.

Often patients receiving NPPV are ventilated with two different levels of positive pressure. This is referred to as *bilevel ventilation*. The baseline pressure is greater than zero for setting a CPAP or PEEP level. The peak pressure is set to deliver a desired tidal volume (similar to PS ventilation). Both levels can be adjusted independently. If only the baseline pressure is elevated, the patient is receiving CPAP. If only the peak pressure is elevated, the patient is receiving PS ventilation. Respironics (Carlsbad, CA) has pioneered the development of ventilators for conventional ventilation or noninvasive bilevel ventilation.

As was stated above, the patient must have a properly fitting nasal or face mask to receive NIV. These ventilation masks are similar to CPAP masks and are referred to as such. CPAP masks are available in different sizes for children older than 3 years and for adults. Nasal masks are designed to cover only the nose. They allow the patient to eat, drink, speak, and use the mouth as a second airway for breathing in case a malfunction of the CPAP system occurs. The mouth also acts as a pressure relief route should the CPAP pressure become too great. Pressures of up to 10-15 cm water usually can be maintained (Fig. 15-22). Usually, the mask is made of a transparent plastic. Face masks are designed to cover the nose and mouth. They are similar in design to the masks used during bag/mask ventilation and also are made of a transparent plastic. The face mask must be used if the patient has persistent mouth breathing and cannot use a nose mask. With a good seal, pressures of greater than 15 cm water can be maintained.

In recent years, a wide variety of NIV mask systems have been developed (Fig. 15-23). In any situation, the clinical goal is to find a CPAP/NIV mask with a soft, very compliant seal that closely fits the contours of the patient's face. A strapping system is needed to hold the mask in place. Too large a mask will not seal and will allow gas to leak and pressure to decrease. The patient may show increased snoring or airway obstruction with periods of apnea. A mask that is too small or misfitting can cause an uneven distribution of pressure on the face. This can lead to abrasions or pressure sores and ulcers on the face.

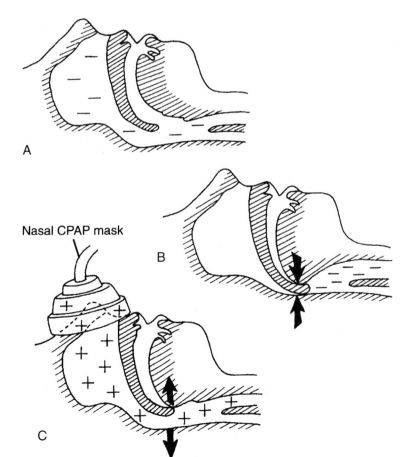

Nasal CPAP mask

A

B

C

Figure 15-22 Effects of a nasal continuous positive airway pressure (CPAP) mask. **A,** Normal upper airway remains patent during sleep. **B,** Abnormal upper airway of patient with obstructive apnea collapses on inspiration during sleep. **C,** Pressure from nasal CPAP mask keeps abnormal upper airway patent during sleep. (Modified from Scanlan CL, Spearman CB, Sheldon RL, editors: Egan's fundamentals of respiratory care, ed 5, St Louis, 1990, Mosby.)

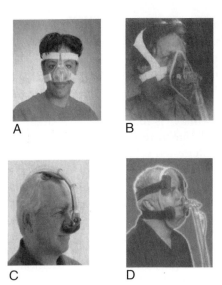

Figure 15-23 Examples of types of masks used to deliver continuous positive airway pressure or noninvasive positive-pressure ventilation. **A,** Nasal mask designed to cover the entire nose. **B,** Full face mask (oronasal mask) designed to cover the nose and mouth. **C,** Nasal pillows that fit into the nostrils. **D,** Total face mask that covers the entire facial area. The key elements to consider in deciding which mask to use are patient fit without leaks and comfort. (**A, C,** and **D** from Hess DR, Kacmarek RM: Essentials of mechanical ventilation, ed 2, New York, 2002, McGraw-Hill. **B** from Hill NS: Complications of noninvasive positive pressure ventilation, Respir Care 42(12):432-442, 1997.)

The bilevel settings must be determined at the bedside by asking for the patient's subjective opinion, listening to breath sounds, checking vital signs, and evaluating ABG values. If supplemental oxygen is needed, it can be added at a port on the patient's mask, at the humidifier, or at the outlet from the bilevel unit. Up to 15 L/min can be added without affecting the performance of the bilevel system. It is not possible to know the delivered oxygen percentage until after the bilevel ventilation settings have been determined. The oxygen flow then should be increased gradually while the patient's SpO$_2$ value increases to the desired saturation level.

The function of the Respironics Esprit system is reviewed briefly. The respiratory therapist can choose from two modes of operation and can select from the following:

- Expiratory positive airway pressure (EPAP) for an elevated baseline pressure. This is functionally similar to CPAP.
- Inspiratory positive airway pressure (IPAP) to deliver a tidal volume. This is functionally similar to setting the peak pressure on a pressure-cycled ventilator.
- Spontaneous ventilation mode (SPONT) requires the patient to initiate each assisted breath. The respiratory therapist can set IPAP and EPAP levels. This delivers bilevel ventilation.
- Spontaneous/timed ventilation mode (SPONT/T) allows the patient to breathe spontaneously while having a time-cycled minimum respiratory rate set by the therapist. IPAP and EPAP levels also are set to deliver bilevel ventilation.

When bilevel ventilation is started, set the EPAP level, if needed, to elevate the patient's baseline pressure. The EPAP level establishes the patient's FRC to improve oxygenation. Increase or decrease EPAP as you would adjust PEEP or CPAP. Review Box 15-3 for patient monitoring with EPAP. Next, set the IPAP level to achieve the desired tidal volume.

With bilevel ventilation, the difference between IPAP and EPAP is called *pressure boost* and delivers the tidal volume. If a larger tidal volume is needed, increase the IPAP level. Conversely, decrease the IPAP level to obtain a smaller tidal volume. It is important to remember that the delivered tidal volume varies depending on changes in the patient's airway resistance and lung/thoracic compliance, as well as in the machine settings.

5. Initiate and adjust mask or nasal continuous positive airway pressure (code: IIIC3) [difficulty: R, Ap, An]

Continuous positive airway pressure (CPAP) is a pressure above atmospheric that is maintained at the airway opening throughout the respiratory cycle during spontaneous breathing. (See Fig. 15-13, G for the pressure/time curve.) CPAP is similar to PEEP in purpose and effect. Remember that with CPAP, the patient does not receive any ventilator-delivered tidal volume breaths. The patient must be capable of providing *all* ventilation for carbon dioxide removal. When CPAP is delivered through the mechanical ventilator, the respiratory rate is turned off. However, alarm systems are still functioning for patient safety. Most modern ventilators can be programmed to deliver a set tidal volume and rate if a period of apnea is detected. For this to occur, an apnea time must be set. For example, if the patient does not breathe for 10 seconds, the ventilator will deliver a tidal volume of 500 mL at a rate of 12/min with the Assist/Control mode. Review the Mandatory Minute Ventilation discussion above for more information.

Some hospitals will make use of a free-standing system for delivering CPAP. This patient must have a stable drive to breathe because there is no ventilator backup system if apnea occurs. Typically these patients are ventilated with a nasal mask or face mask rather than through an endotracheal tube. See the discussion under "NIV" on the importance of selecting the best mask for the patient. Figures 15-22 and 15-23 show CPAP masks. See Figures 15-29 and 16-4 for free-standing CPAP systems.

Before a patient receives CPAP therapy, the respiratory therapist and the physician must be assured that the patient has the ability to breathe adequately to eliminate carbon dioxide. CPAP is contraindicated in an apneic patient or in one who may become apneic. (This patient must be fully supported on the ventilator.) The patient must have an adequate respiratory rate, tidal volume, and minute volume. The heart rate and blood pressure should be stable. Maximum inspiratory pressure and vital capacity values may be acceptable or low. Blood gas analysis typically shows refractory hypoxemia but a normal or low $PaCO_2$ level. This shows that the patient would benefit from an elevated baseline pressure to increase the FRC but is capable of ventilating.

CPAP involves the same indications, hazards, and patient evaluation processes as were discussed earlier for PEEP therapy. One possible physiologic benefit of CPAP over PEEP is that less reduction in venous return to the heart is seen. This occurs because with CPAP, the patient is breathing spontaneously. Therefore patients treated with CPAP may be able to tolerate higher pressure levels than those being ventilated with PEEP therapy.

CPAP usually is increased and decreased in steps of 2-5 cm water. As with PEEP, the patient is evaluated before CPAP is begun and again after each pressure change is made. See Box 15-3 for recommendations on what to monitor during the application of CPAP and how to evaluate the data.

The patient must be monitored carefully for fatigue because the patient is providing all of the minute ventilation. Signs of fatigue include increasing respiratory rate, decreasing tidal volume or vital capacity, decreasing maximum inspiratory pressure, and tachycardia. Blood gas measurement may show a stable or decreasing PaO_2 value. An increasing $PaCO_2$ level is a definite sign of fatigue. The patient may complain of dyspnea. The practitioner may notice that the patient is working harder than normal to breathe, as shown by increased use of the accessory muscles of ventilation and heavy perspiration. When these signs occur, CPAP therapy should be discontinued and mechanical ventilation instituted in a mode that best fits the patient's needs.

Exam Hint 15-15

Know that CPAP can be used and increased if the patient's carbon dioxide level is normal and hypoxemia is present. Increase or decrease CPAP by following the same parameters used to evaluate a change in PEEP. Know to switch to mechanical ventilation when (1) the maximum level of CPAP is being used and the patient is still hypoxemic or (2) the patient is hypoventilating.

Note: Independent lung ventilation and external negative-pressure ventilation are not specifically listed as testable by the NBRC. However, they have been tested on previous examinations.

6. Independent (differential) lung ventilation

Independent lung ventilation (ILV) involves the use of a separate mechanical ventilator for each lung. A double-lumen endotracheal tube must be placed into the patient to allow this procedure. (See Figs. 12-30 and 12-31 in Chapter 12 and the related discussion.) Box 15-4 lists indications for double-lumen endotracheal tubes and ILV. In all cases, the patient has one normal lung and one

---

BOX 15-4 Indications for Double-Lumen Endotracheal Tubes and Independent Lung Ventilation

Thoracic surgery
  Pneumonectomy
  Some lobectomies
  Thoracic aortic surgery
  Thoracoscopy
  Some esophageal surgery
Selective airway protection
  Secretions (tuberculosis, bronchiectasis, or abscess)
  Whole-lung lavage
  Massive hemoptysis
Bronchopleural fistula
Unilateral lung disease
  Unilateral parenchymal injury
  Aspiration
  Pulmonary contusion
  Pneumonia
  Massive pulmonary embolism
  Reperfusion edema
  Asymmetric ARDS
  Asymmetric pulmonary edema
  Atelectasis
Unilateral airflow obstruction
  Single-lung transplant for chronic airflow obstruction
  Unilateral bronchospasm
Severe bilateral lung disease
  ARDS
  Aspiration
  Pneumonia

ARDS, acute respiratory distress syndrome.
From Tuxen D: Independent lung ventilation. In: Tobin MJ, editor: Principles and practice of mechanical ventilation, New York, 1994, McGraw-Hill, pp 571-588.

abnormal lung. Overriding concerns with ILV are to ventilate the patient adequately through the normal lung and to allow the injured lung to heal.

A common initial approach is to select two identical ventilators that allow synchronization of the patient's respiratory rate. The Servo and Dräger ventilators are suited to this. They allow one unit to be designated the "primary" ventilator to set the respiratory rate for it and the "secondary" unit. Each unit then can have the same mode and I:E ratio. This synchronized ILV method still allows the independent setting of tidal volume, oxygen percentage, and PEEP for each lung.

For example, an 80-kg adult man normally receives an initial tidal volume of about 800 mL (10 mL × 80 kg). If both lungs functioned normally, each would receive 400 mL. However, with unilateral lung disease, the bad lung receives little tidal volume and the normal lung receives too much and becomes overdistended. It is therefore important to set the initial tidal volume to the good lung at *half* the normal volume for both lungs. For this patient example, the normal lung's initial tidal volume should be set at 400 mL (5 mL × 80 kg). To avoid changing too many parameters at once, the same oxygen percentage and PEEP level as originally set are kept. The abnormal lung is ventilated on the basis of its pathologic condition or may be left unventilated.

After 15 min, check the patient's ABG values. Depending on the results, adjust the ventilator settings for the good lung as would be done typically to remove carbon dioxide and maintain oxygenation. The ventilator settings for the diseased lung must be adjusted carefully to allow healing and prevent complications such as atelectasis and pneumonia.

When the patient has a bronchopulmonary fistula, the air leak through the bad lung can be so great that a high-frequency ventilator must be used rather than a conventional ventilator. In this situation, no synchronization of rate or any other parameters can be set. The good lung is ventilated conventionally to maintain the patient's blood gas values. The HFV is set to provide some support with a small tidal volume and low ventilating pressures. The clinical goal is to prevent excessive lung pressure so that the lung tear heals.

The patient can be converted back to breathing through one conventional ventilator when normal functioning returns to the injured lung. This can be done when the peak pressure, plateau pressure, and MAP for both lungs are about the same. When these values match or are close, similar C_{LT} and airway resistance values are indicated. The first step in converting from ILV to conventional ventilation involves combining the proximal ends of the double-lumen endotracheal tube with a Y adapter. When this is done, one ventilator can deliver tidal volume breaths to each lung. It is suggested that the PC mode be used so that excessive pressure is not applied to the healing lung. Set the peak pressure at or just below the previous peak pressure used with the healing lung. Set the PEEP level at the previous pressure used with the healing lung. Check the patient's ABG values after 15 minutes. Be prepared to adjust the conventional ventilator as needed to get the desired blood gas values. Watch for problems with the healing lung, and be prepared to go back to independent lung ventilation if necessary. When it appears certain that the patient is tolerating conventional ventilation, the double-lumen endotracheal tube should be removed and replaced with an appropriate single-lumen tube. This allows better suctioning and results in less airway resistance through the tube. Wean and extubate the patient when appropriate.

7. External negative-pressure ventilation

These ventilators have proved useful in patients with the following characteristics: (1) normal, intact upper airway, (2) ability to swallow, (3) normal airway resistance, (4) normal lung/thoracic compliance, and (5) ability to ventilate until respiratory muscle fatigue becomes too great.

Patients with the following disease conditions have been ventilated successfully by a negative-pressure ventilator:

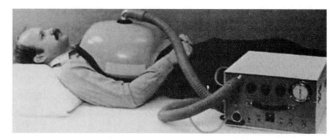

Figure 15-24 Patient in chest cuirass (LifeCare). Note control box on right that contains a vacuum motor. Hose connects vacuum motor to patient inside chest shell. (From Hill NS: Clinical application of body ventilators, Chest 90[6]:897, 1986.)

(1) neuromuscular defects such as poliomyelitis, post-polio syndrome, muscular dystrophy, and high spinal cord injury; (2) kyphoscoliosis with resulting restrictive lung disease; and (3) COPD during an acute worsening.

Negative-pressure ventilators work by creating negative pressure around the patient's whole body or over the anterior chest and abdomen. The negative pressure expands the thorax, and a tidal volume is inhaled. If the patient needs supplemental oxygen, it must be given by nasal cannula or face mask. Three basic types of external negative-pressure ventilators are available: Drinker body respirator (so-called "iron lung"), body wrap, and chest cuirass (Fig. 15-24).

The following steps are used to initiate ventilation:

1. Select a ventilator rate that meets the patient's needs. This can be about 5-10 breaths less than the patient's own rate in a patient with some breathing ability. In an apneic patient, the rate can be varied between 14 and 24 per minute.
2. Gradually increase the negative pressure until the patient cannot speak during the inspiratory phase. A pressure of −7 to −15 cm water is enough for most patients. A maximum pressure of −35 cm water often can be achieved. It is possible to create a positive pressure during exhalation, if needed, by closing a valve. This usually is limited to times when an assisted cough is called for.
3. Use a hand-held spirometer to measure the patient's tidal volume.
4. After a few minutes, ask the patient, "Does the breath feel deep enough, too deep, or not enough? Do you have tingling fingers or feel dizzy (signs of hyperventilation)?"
5. Adjust the negativity or rate or both to meet the patient's needs.
6. Draw an ABG sample after about 15 minutes. Speed is important because the unit must be opened for collection of the sample. Interpret the ABG results as usual.
7. If the carbon dioxide level is higher than desired, increase the rate or set a more negative pressure to increase the minute volume. Do the opposite if the patient is being hyperventilated. If the patient is hypoxic, provide supplemental oxygen by nasal cannula or face mask.

MODULE E

Mechanical ventilation equipment

Note: The literature produced by the manufacturers and the descriptions used in many standard texts break down the various ventilators into more categories than are used by the NBRC. To avoid confusion, this text uses the more simplified terminology of the NBRC.

A *pneumatically powered ventilator* is defined here as a ventilator powered by compressed gas. Older units operate without any electrically powered control systems (electrically powered alarm systems may or may not be added). More recent units will also have electrically powered controls and alarm systems.

Electrically powered ventilators are defined here as ventilators that are electrically powered or controlled. Most volume-cycled ventilators fall into this category.

Microprocessor ventilators are electrically powered but are controlled by one or more microprocessors (computers). Many of the most current volume-cycled ventilators have microprocessors to control their functions.

Fluidic ventilators typically make use of electrical circuits with flip-flops to respond to changes in gas flow and pressure throughout the system. Fluidic ventilators are powered by compressed gas.

Noninvasive ventilators are designed for home use or short-term hospital use and are electrically powered and controlled. They have fewer controls and alarms than hospital-based critical care ventilators. A nasal or full-face mask, rather than an endotracheal tube, is used to attach the ventilator to the patient.

High-frequency ventilators are used in a limited population of critically ill patients who are doing poorly despite all attempts at conventional mechanical ventilation. These units are designed to deliver very rapid respiratory rates and very small tidal volumes.

1. Assemble and troubleshoot mechanical ventilators

a. Pneumatic ventilators

1. Assemble the necessary equipment (code: IIA8) [difficulty: R, Ap, An]

Historically, the most commonly used pneumatically powered ventilators include the Bird series and the Bennett PR-2. A control or backup rate can be set on these units in case the patient is apneic. All other controls and functions are the same as those discussed in Chapter 14

for IPPB treatments. The following equipment and procedures are necessary:

- Bennett PR-2 or Bird ventilator with an air/oxygen blender and hoses
- Bennett or Bird breathing circuit
- Bacteria filters
- Proper humidification system: a pass-over- or cascade-type humidifier or an HME (discussed later). Put sterile, distilled water into the pass-over- or cascade-type humidifier.
- One or two water traps for condensation from the circuit
- Add an alarm system(s) such as a low-volume bellows spirometer or a low-pressure/disconnection alarm.
- If a low-volume bellows spirometer alarm is used, a length of large-bore tubing is needed to connect the exhalation valve to the bellows.

Most modern pneumatically powered ventilators require electricity by battery or wall outlet to operate properly. They are used for patient transportation within or between hospitals or at the scene of a disaster. The Impact Uni-Vent 750 is an example. It has been included in the Strategic National Stockpile for rapid shipment to the site of a natural disaster or terrorist attack.

Refer to Figures 14-11 and 14-12 in Chapter 14 for the IPPB circuits. The ventilator and circuits are similar to those used in IPPB therapy with the following exceptions:

- Set the ordered oxygen percentage on the blender; set the Bird *air-mix* and Bennett *air dilution* selection controls to pure source gas from the blender. Analyze the F_1O_2 through a port in the inspiratory limb of the circuit.
- If a pass-over or cascade-type humidifier is used, a short length of large-bore tubing is connected between the outlet of the mainstream inline bacteria filter and the inlet of the humidifier. The inspiratory limb of the circuit is connected to the outlet of the humidifier (see Fig. 16-13 in Chapter 16). If an HME is used, it is added between the circuit and the tracheostomy/endotracheal tube adapter.
- A tracheostomy/endotracheal tube adapter is always used to connect the circuit to the patient.
- Add at least one disconnection alarm to the circuit. It could be a low-pressure or disconnection alarm added into the inspiratory limb of the circuit with a Briggs adapter/T-piece.
- Water traps are placed in the lowest part of the inspiratory and expiratory limbs of the circuit to hold any condensed water vapor.

2. Troubleshoot any problems with the equipment (code: IIA8) [difficulty: R, Ap, An]

Both of these types of ventilators send gas through the circuit during an inspiration and do not cycle off until the preset pressure is reached. Test the tightness of the circuit, backup rate, and delivered tidal volume by placing a test lung on the patient connection of the circuit. Set the controls to deliver the prescribed order. Be prepared to make final adjustments once either unit has been placed on the patient. The patient's airway resistance and C_{LT} greatly affect the functioning of both units.

Troubleshooting problems with these units was discussed in Chapter 14. Make sure that all connections are tight; more are available now with the addition of the humidification system and expiratory limb to the spirometer.

A defective exhalation valve will allow gas to pass through the circuit rather than go to the patient. A pressure-cycled ventilator will not cycle to exhalation.

b. Electrical ventilators

1. Assemble the necessary equipment (code: IIA8) [difficulty: R, Ap, An]

Many mechanical ventilators are powered or controlled electrically. They function primarily as volume-cycled units, meaning that a preset volume is delivered from the ventilator with each breath regardless of the patient's condition. Each ventilator is unique in its abilities, modes, and so forth. It is beyond the scope of this book to discuss each and every volume-cycled ventilator. They are presented in a generic manner. The learner should become familiar with the function of the Maquet Servo-i (Maquet, Inc., Wayne, NJ), an electrically powered microprocessor ventilator, and other widely used machines. (See Fig. 16-14 in Chapter 16.)

Each ventilator must be learned for its specifics. Generally speaking, the following steps should be taken to ensure that the ventilator is functioning properly:

1. Select the proper ventilator for the physician's orders and the patient's needs.

2. Attach the circuit properly, and make sure that all connections are tight (Fig. 15-25).
3. Select the appropriate humidification device: a pass-over type, cascade type, or HME. Put sterile, distilled water into the pass-over or cascade unit.
4. Preset all of the physician-ordered parameters and any other settings that are needed to make the ventilator fully functional.
5. Place a test lung on the circuit at the patient connection.
6. Make sure that the ventilator delivers the preset rate, volume, oxygen percentage, I:E ratio, and so forth.

2. Troubleshoot any problems with the equipment (code: IIA8) [difficulty: R, Ap, An]

A low volume can be caused by a leak; check all connections, and tighten them as needed. The volume can be measured directly as it leaves the ventilator and at the exhalation valve to help determine the source of the wrong volume. If the unit shows a volume entering the exhalation valve and spirometer instead of the test lung during inspiration, the exhalation valve is broken. All alarms must be working properly. Batteries must be replaced when discharged.

c. Microprocessor ventilators

1. Assemble the necessary equipment (code: IIA8) [difficulty: R, Ap, An]

The microprocessor ventilators (e.g., Maquet Servo-i, Maquet, Inc., Bridgewater, NJ, Fig. 16-14; Hamilton-C3, Hamilton Medical AG, Bonaduz, Switzerland, Fig. 16-13) are the most advanced generation of mechanical ventilators. They are powered electrically but are controlled by

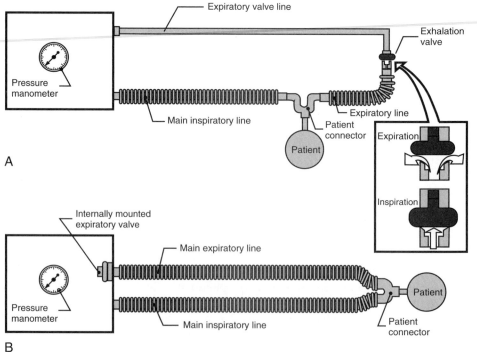

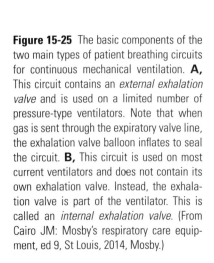

Figure 15-25 The basic components of the two main types of patient breathing circuits for continuous mechanical ventilation. **A,** This circuit contains an *external exhalation valve* and is used on a limited number of pressure-type ventilators. Note that when gas is sent through the expiratory valve line, the exhalation valve balloon inflates to seal the circuit. **B,** This circuit is used on most current ventilators and does not contain its own exhalation valve. Instead, the exhalation valve is part of the ventilator. This is called an *internal exhalation valve.* (From Cairo JM: Mosby's respiratory care equipment, ed 9, St Louis, 2014, Mosby.)

one or more microprocessors (computers). They offer all commonly found modes of ventilation. In addition, many of these machines offer computer software for measuring bedside spirometry for weaning, WOB, and other parameters that give the clinician much valuable information. Airway resistance and static and dynamic C_{LT} can be calculated automatically. Flow, volume, and pressure tracings are displayed graphically on the computer screen. Auto-PEEP can be documented and measured. These units offer the greatest quantity of patient data and the best clinical flexibility of all currently available ventilators. The most challenging patients probably can be best cared for on one of these machines.

2. Troubleshoot any problems with the equipment (code: IIA8) [difficulty: R, Ap, An]

All of the previous general discussion on electrically powered ventilators applies to the microprocessor ventilators as well. An additional advantage of these units is that they self-diagnose most problems and display the problem for you. If a microprocessor should fail, the unit should be removed from the patient. The biomedical department or manufacturer has to replace the computer chip.

d. Fluidic ventilators

1. Assemble the necessary equipment (code: IIA8) [difficulty: R, Ap, An]

An example of a fluidic ventilator is the Bio-Med MVP-10 (Bio-Med Devices, Guilford, CT). It is a neonatal/pediatric unit that can be used in the hospital or for patient transport. Make sure that high-pressure gas hoses between the unit and the wall outlets are connected tightly to prevent leaks. The patient circuit and humidification system must be installed properly and must be operating.

2. Troubleshoot any problems with the equipment (code: IIA8) [difficulty: R, Ap, An]

Typically, fluidic ventilators are powered pneumatically and have fluidic controls. Make sure that the oxygen and air sources are up to the required pressure (usually 50 psig). Fluidic controls are very sensitive to any obstruction and to changes in other settings. Make sure that gas inlet and outlet filters are kept clear of obstructions.

e. Noninvasive ventilators

1. Assemble the necessary equipment (code: IIA8) [difficulty: R, Ap, An]

A noninvasive ventilator is intended for an adult patient who is capable of some spontaneous breathing for a limited period. The unit typically is used for bilevel ventilation with a patient who is having breathing difficulty but does not require intubation and full ventilatory support. Current ventilators include the Respironics Focus (Philips Respironics, Inc., Murrysville, PA) and the Puritan-Bennett GoodKnight 425 (Covidien-Puritan Bennett, Boulder, CO).

2. Troubleshoot any problems with the equipment (code: IIA8) [difficulty: R, Ap, An]

Follow the manufacturer's guidelines for putting the circuit on the unit and adding a humidifier, if needed. A nasal or full-face mask of proper size is needed to attach the circuit to the patient. Check carefully for any leakage between the mask and the patient's face.

f High-frequency jet ventilators (HFJVs)

1. Assemble the necessary equipment (code: IIA8) [difficulty: R, Ap, An]

The Bunnell Life Pulse high-frequency jet ventilator (Bunnell, Inc., Salt Lake City, UT) is designed for use with neonatal patients with infant RDS who have failed with conventional ventilation. The Bunnell ventilator (see Fig. 16-15 in Chapter 16) is unique in that it must be used in conjunction with a conventional ventilator. This second ventilator is placed in the CPAP or SIMV mode during use of the jet.

In addition, the standard endotracheal tube adapter must be replaced with the Bunnell LifePort endotracheal tube adapter (Bunnell, Inc.) See Figures 15-26, B and 16-16. The jet ventilator is attached to the long catheter. The traditional ventilator is attached to the main lumen of the endotracheal tube. Based on the physical principles that govern jets, additional gas is entrained through the main lumen. This entrained gas must be humidified if the jet gas is dry. All exhaled gas passes out through this main lumen, where it can be measured through the traditional ventilator's spirometry system. This ventilator's alarm systems also can be used, and SIMV breaths and PEEP can be added if needed. Figure 15-27 shows a schematic drawing of a jet ventilator. Make sure that the jet ventilator and conventional ventilator are operating properly. The following are general considerations with setting up the HFJV system:

- 50 psig source gas(es) of oxygen or oxygen and air is needed to generate a driving pressure.
- A patient circuit is specifically suited to the jet ventilator.
- A drive pressure control lets the operator set the peak pressure of the jet.
- An inspiratory time control sets the I:E ratio.
- Rate can be varied within the limits set by the unit.
- The inspired oxygen percentage can be dialed on the unit itself or on an external air/oxygen blender before going into the unit.
- Humidification must be provided by the Bunnell ventilator and/or the conventional ventilator.
- Both ventilators must be attached to the special endotracheal tube adapter.

2. Troubleshoot any problems with the equipment (code: IIA8) [difficulty: R, Ap, An]

As with any ventilator, make sure that all connections are tight. Leaks are a particular problem because of the high

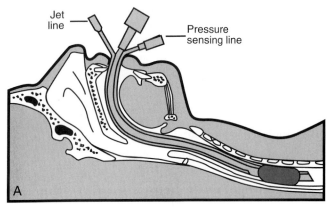

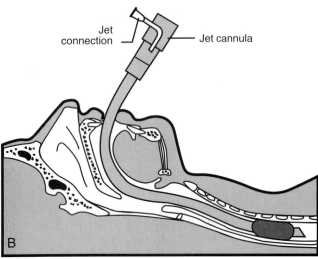

Figure 15-26 Special airways needed for high-frequency jet ventilation (HFJV). **A,** A special multiple-channel endotracheal tube used for HFJV. The jet gas enters the patient through the jet line. The pressure-sensing line is used to monitor pressures at the end of the endotracheal tube. The main channel is used to entrain additional tidal volume gas from a standard ventilator and to perform suctioning. *Note:* At the time of printing, the manufacturer of the Hi-Lo Jet Tube had stopped production. It is not known if another manufacturer will begin production. **B,** The patient with a standard endotracheal tube can receive HFJV by replacing the adapter with a special jet adapter. Jet gas enters through the jet connection. The main channel (jet cannula) is used to entrain additional tidal volume gas from a conventional ventilator and to perform suctioning. See Figure 16-16 for a photograph of the actual jet adapter. (From Cairo JM: Mosby's respiratory care equipment, ed 9, St Louis, 2014, Mosby.)

pressures leaving the unit and the small tidal volumes that are delivered.

g. High-frequency oscillator ventilators (HFOVs)

1. Assemble the necessary equipment (code: IIA8) [difficulty: R, Ap, An]

The SensorMedics 3100A (Viasys Healthcare, Yorba Linda, CA; Fig. 16-17 in Chapter 16) is used with neonates and children, and the SensorMedics 3100B (Viasys Healthcare) is used with adults. Both units require a special circuit.

2. Troubleshoot any problems with the equipment (code: IIA8) [difficulty: R, Ap, An]

Experience with the equipment is recommended for assembly of the specific circuit, as needed. Any humidification system can be added. Both ventilators' circuits are designed to combine two separate flows of gas for the patient's tidal volume. As with any circuit, make sure that all connections are tight.

2. Ventilator breathing circuits

a. Assemble the necessary equipment (code: IIA14) [difficulty: R, Ap]

A permanent or a disposable circuit may be selected, based on the type of ventilator on which it must be placed. A circuit with an external exhalation valve must be used with older ventilators such as the Bennett MA-1 (Covidien-Puritan Bennett) and the Bear 2 (Cardinal Health, Viasys Bear Medical Systems, Palm Springs, CA). In addition, if a Bird-series unit is used as a ventilator, its circuit has an external exhalation valve (see Fig. 15-25, A). All modern electrical and microprocessor ventilators feature an internal exhalation valve and do not need one included in the circuit (see Fig. 15-25, B). If the patient must receive aerosolized medications, the circuit should include a nebulizer or should be able to accept one. If not included, the nebulizer or metered-dose inhaler adapter must be added into the inspiratory limb of the circuit (Fig. 15-28).

Also consider whether it is better to use an unheated or a heated circuit. Usually the circuit is unheated. With these, a cascade-type humidifier or an HME is used to warm and humidify the inspired gas. However, some practitioners prefer to use a heated circuit for the care of neonates. These circuits may have heated wires loosely running through the lumen of the tubing or may have a wire embedded within the tubing itself. A heated-wire circuit offers finer control over the temperature of the inspired gas and minimizes condensation. Follow the manufacturer's guidelines to make sure that the system can adequately humidify the minute volume that is being used.

Noninvasive ventilators, such as the Respironics series, have specific circuits designed only for the unit. Traditional ventilator circuits cannot be placed on a noninvasive ventilator. Assemble the circuit with the features needed to manage the patient. Common, but not universal, features of the inspiratory limb of the circuit include a water trap, a humidification system, a nebulizer, a thermometer or temperature probe, a pressure-monitoring port, and an oxygen-monitoring port. Common, but not universal, features of the expiratory limb of the circuit include an exhalation valve and a water trap.

The heated-wire circuits must be used only with the humidifier with which they are specifically designed to work. The humidifier has a thermostat that regulates warming of the humidifier water and heated wires to the same temperature. Never cover a heated-wire circuit with

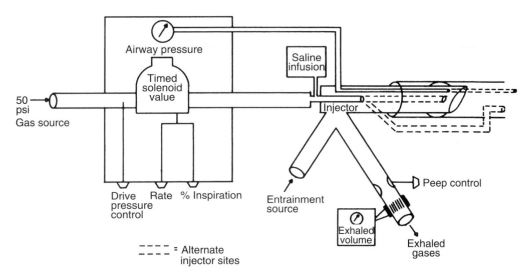

Figure 15-27 Schematic diagram of a high-frequency jet ventilator concept. From MacIntyre NR: Jet ventilation in the adult with breathing rates up to 150 bpm, Riverside, CA, 1985, Bear Medical Systems. Courtesy of Viasys Respiratory Care, Inc.

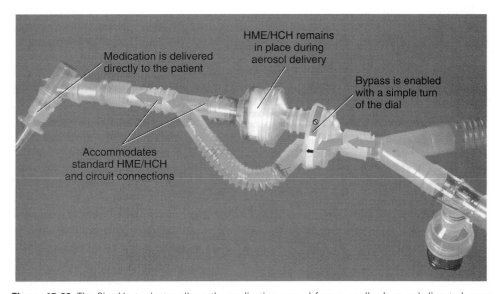

Figure 15-28 The CircuVent adapter allows the medication aerosol from a small-volume nebulizer to bypass an heat-moisture exchanger (HME). After treatment, remember to reset the adapter so that the patient's tidal volume passes though the HME normally. The HME is located properly between the Y of the ventilator circuit and the patient's endotracheal tube. Try to select an HME that has the smallest internal volume to minimize mechanical dead space and rebreathed carbon dioxide. Mechanical dead space in this system includes all tubing between the Y of the circuit and the endotracheal tube. This includes the CircuVent adapter and its bypass tubing, when used, or the HME and its large-bore tubing during normal breathing. (From Smiths Medical North America, Norwell, Massachusetts.)

a patient's sheets or blanket or any other material. Do not rest the circuit on anything such as the bed rail, patient's body, or medical equipment. These circuits should always be supported on a boom arm or tube-tree.

Noninvasive ventilator circuits must be set up as specified for the ventilator. Depending on the unit, an HME or cascade-type humidifier is added to add moisture to the patient's tidal volume gas.

All circuits use a Y-connector to tie the inspiratory and expiratory limbs together and attach the circuit to the patient. See Figure 16-13 in Chapter 16 for a ventilator circuit attached to the Hamilton-C3. Make sure that the water level is maintained properly in the humidifier.

b. Troubleshoot any problems with the equipment (code: IIA14) [difficulty: R, Ap]

Check the circuit and connections for leaks if the volume returned from the patient is less than what was set or delivered. The set volume should be measured with a hand-held spirometer as it exits the ventilator, at connection points through the circuit, and at the exhalation valve or ventilator spirometer or both. The VC or ventilator spirometer may be out of calibration. If the unit shows a volume entering the spirometer instead of the test lung during inspiration, the exhalation valve is broken. Replace a circuit with a leak or a defective exhalation valve that cannot be fixed.

A circuit must be replaced if it is damaged in a way that prevents the patient from being ventilated. This is seen most commonly in circuits with external exhalation valves (see Fig. 15-25, A). If the balloon-type valve is damaged and will not close, the tidal volume will leak out rather than enter the patient. The circuit must be replaced. If the expiratory valve line is pulled off at the ventilator or exhalation valve, it must be replaced or the valve will not close.

3. Initiate protocols to prevent ventilator associated pneumonia (code: IIIA7) [difficulty: R, Ap]

The AARC Clinical Practice Guideline on ventilator circuit changes and their relation to ventilator associated pneumonia (VAP) (2003) included the following guidelines:

- The circuit should not be changed routinely for infection control purposes.
- Change the circuit when it is obviously soiled (e.g., blood, sputum).
- Passive humidifiers (HMEs) do not need to be changed daily.
- An HME can be used for at least 48 hours and possibly for up to a week.
- Change an HME when it is obviously soiled (e.g., blood, sputum).
- A closed-airway suction catheter should be considered part of the VAP prevention plan and does not need to be changed on a daily basis.

It is reasonable to expect the 2003 guidelines to be tested by the NBRC.

4. Ventilator PEEP valves

a. Assemble the necessary equipment (code: IIA2) [difficulty: R, Ap, An]

A variety of PEEP systems can be added to a ventilator or CPAP circuit. Consult an equipment book for the details of their operation. Many of the newer ventilators have internal exhalation valves and PEEP-generating Venturi systems with nothing to assemble at the bedside. Failure to generate PEEP indicates that the exhalation valve or the PEEP-generating Venturi system has failed in some manner (see Fig. 15-25, B).

Most older ventilators (Bird series, Bennett MA-1, and Bear 2) use a balloon-like exhalation valve. A direct relationship exists between the volume of gas that is kept in the balloon, the pressure and resistance that it creates, and the PEEP level that is generated (see Fig. 15-25, A).

The key thing to check with any PEEP-generating system is that the proper level of PEEP is generated and maintained. Once the ordered PEEP level is set, it should be seen as stable on the pressure manometer throughout the respiratory cycle. Sensitivity should be set at no more than −1 to −2 cm water. That way, the PEEP level is maintained at close to the ordered level even during an assisted breath. For example, PEEP is set at 10 cm, and the sensitivity is set at −1 cm. When the patient triggers a breath, it will occur at 9 cm PEEP.

b. Troubleshoot any problems with the equipment (code: IIA2) [difficulty: R, Ap, An]

Malfunctioning internal exhalation valves or PEEP-generation Venturi systems cannot be repaired easily at the bedside. The ventilator must be replaced. Balloon-type exhalation valves (see Fig. 15-25, A) are prone to the following two problems:

1. The small-bore tube carrying gas from the ventilator to the balloon valve is pulled off. Reconnect the tubing to the ventilator nipple connection or to the exhalation valve nipple connection.
2. The balloon is torn, and the gas leaks out. This can be confirmed by disassembling the exhalation valve assembly. If possible, replace the balloon, and reassemble the exhalation valve. If the balloon cannot be repaired, replace the entire circuit with a new exhalation valve.

Both of these problems are exhibited when the inspiratory tidal volume flows past the patient and directly into the exhaled tidal volume spirometer. Little or no airway pressure is generated. The patient is poorly ventilated, if at all. This problem must be corrected immediately while the patient is ventilated manually.

5. Continuous positive airway pressure (CPAP) breathing circuits

a. Assemble the necessary equipment (code: IIA14) [difficulty: R, Ap]

Most current-generation ventilators have a built-in CPAP mode. No additional circuitry is needed. After switching to the CPAP mode, set the desired level by adjusting the PEEP/CPAP dial and watching the reading on the pressure manometer.

Several manufacturers make CPAP systems for home use in the treatment of patients with obstructive sleep apnea. These CPAP systems typically include an air pump to generate flow to the patient, a CPAP-generating device, a circuit designed to work with the system, a patient mask(s), and an alarm system.

Free-standing CPAP breathing circuits used in hospitals vary considerably. No manufacturer has developed a system that dominates the marketplace. Most commonly, each respiratory care department develops its own breathing circuit to meet its own needs.

Figure 15-29 and Figure 16-4 in Chapter 16 show the typical components used in a free-standing CPAP breathing circuit. Components include the following:

- Air/oxygen blender
- Pediatric or adult flowmeter on the blender

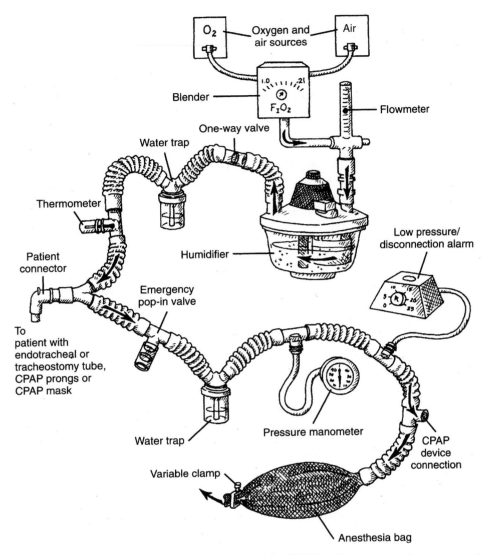

Figure 15-29 Sample free-standing patient breathing circuit for CPAP. Note the components that are commonly added into the circuit.

- Humidifier
- Inspiratory circuit of large-bore or aerosol tubing with the following additions: port for an oxygen analyzer, water trap, one-way valve, and thermometer
- Y connector to connect the inspiratory and expiratory limbs of the circuit
- Patient connector (elbow adapter) to endotracheal or tracheostomy tube, CPAP prongs, or CPAP mask
- Expiratory circuit of large-bore or aerosol tubing with the following additions: water trap, high-pressure pop-off valve (not shown), pressure manometer for measuring the CPAP level, low-pressure or disconnection audible alarm, anesthesia bag as a reservoir, variable resistance clamp on the tail of the anesthesia bag, Briggs adapters/T-pieces for connecting the various features, emergency pop-in (antiasphyxia) valve in case gas flow is stopped, and CPAP device.

The CPAP level is adjusted by means of a variety of devices collectively called *threshold resistors*, which include the following:
- A column of water with a length of expiratory tubing inserted the needed depth below the surface (so-called "bubble CPAP").
- A vertically mounted ball bearing. It creates a resistance as gas flows up past it. These ball-bearing resistors come in weights of 2.5, 5, and 10 cm water.
- A spring-loaded resistor that is adjusted to apply the desired CPAP level against the airway.
- A free-standing Venturi PEEP system. Gas from the Venturi jet creates backpressure against the escaping patient tidal volume.

Air exits through each of these devices when they are working properly. All CPAP systems must be adjusted by checking the pressure level on the manometer. Set the low-pressure or disconnection audible alarm to sound at a few centimeters below the CPAP level. For example, if

10 cm CPAP is ordered, set the alarm to sound if the pressure drops below 8 cm of CPAP.

b. Troubleshoot any problems with the equipment (code: IIA14) [difficulty: R, Ap]

Flow through the CPAP breathing circuit must be sufficient to meet the patient's needs. Adjust the flowmeter setting and clamp on the anesthesia bag so that it is somewhat inflated, with excess air escaping out past the clamp. With all of the devices, gas escapes through the path of least resistance. All or some may escape through the anesthesia bag, the CPAP device, or both. The bag should collapse somewhat during the patient's inspiration and expand somewhat during the expiration. The CPAP level should not decrease by more than 1 or 2 cm from baseline during an inspiration.

Make sure that the water level is maintained properly in the humidifier. Fill it with sterile, distilled water as often as necessary.

A sudden decrease in the CPAP level to zero indicates a disconnection at the patient or somewhere in the breathing circuit. Check all connections, and reassemble the break. The patient may have to be ventilated manually while the problem is corrected.

If the CPAP level decreases by more than 2 cm water during an inspiration, the flow is inadequate and should be increased. Flow also is inadequate if the patient shows increased use of accessory muscles of respiration or complains of increased WOB. Too high a flow is revealed by an inadvertently high level of CPAP or the patient complaining of difficulty exhaling.

Water column systems must be monitored frequently because of water loss caused by evaporation. The actual CPAP level is progressively less than desired as the water is lost gradually. This system must have water added to it regularly or must have the expiratory tubing inserted deeper to keep the desired CPAP level.

The ball-bearing resistor system must be mounted vertically for gravity to keep the desired weight against the circuit. If it falls over and is horizontal, the CPAP pressure will be lost.

6. CPAP systems: face mask, nasal mask

a. Assemble the necessary equipment (code: IIA2) [difficulty: R, Ap, An]

A CPAP mask and breathing circuit are used primarily for patients who have obstructive sleep apnea. CPAP, by means of the mask, forces soft tissues open to the point that the airway is never obstructed (see Fig. 15-22). The patient now is able to sleep normally and remain oxygenated. The patient should have the CPAP mask, breathing circuit, and proper CPAP level determined by a sleep study in the hospital. The patient can use the system at home once it is set up properly and he or she has been trained in its use.

In recent years, a CPAP mask has been used as an alternative to NIV to temporarily assist the breathing of a patient with respiratory distress. The hope is to support the patient's breathing long enough to treat the underlying problem(s). The Boussignac CPAP valve (Vygon, Edouen, France) offers a way for first responders/paramedics to easily provide CPAP to a patient with cardiogenic pulmonary edema while being transported to the hospital. The valve is connected to a standard face mask. An oxygen source is connected to oxygen tubing that is then connected to the Boussignac valve. With a tight fit of the mask on the patient's face, the oxygen flow rate (about 20-30 L/min) determines the CPAP level and oxygen percentage. Limitations of the Boussignac valve are an uncertain CPAP level and the delivery of dry gas. However, if this is successful, the patient may not need to be intubated. These patients require careful assessment and monitoring.

The two main categories of CPAP masks come in different sizes for children older than 3 years to adults. (See Fig. 15-23 for examples.) Nasal mask and pillow systems are designed to cover only the nose. These allow the patient to speak and offer the mouth as a second airway for breathing in case a malfunction of the CPAP system occurs. The mouth also acts as a pressure relief route if the CPAP pressure should become too great. Pressures of up to 15 cm water usually can be maintained in an adult. Pressures of up to 10 cm water usually can be maintained in a child.

Full-face mask and total-face mask systems are designed to cover the nose and mouth. These are transparent and are similar to the mask used during bag/mask ventilation. The face mask must be used if the patient has persistent mouth breathing and cannot use a nose mask. With a good seal, pressures of greater than 15 cm water can be maintained.

All types of CPAP masks have a soft, very compliant seal to closely fit the contours of the face. Straps are needed to hold the mask in place. It is imperative that the mask properly fit the patient's face.

Several companies manufacture CPAP mask systems for home care. These are relatively simple circuits that do not have a humidification system or the other attachments seen in the hospital. Check the manufacturer's literature for specific directions on their application to the patient. As is shown in Figure 15-23, the straps must be tight enough to seal the mask to the face but not so tight as to cut off circulation to the skin. Any CPAP mask system must be able to generate enough flow to meet the patient's minute volume and peak flow needs. The CPAP level must be stable throughout the breathing cycle.

b. Troubleshoot any problems with the equipment (code: IIA2) [difficulty: R, Ap, An]

Too large a mask does not seal and allows gas to leak out. This is seen as decreased CPAP pressure on the manometer. The patient may show increased snoring or airway obstruction with periods of apnea. A mask that is too small or misfitting can cause an uneven distribution of pressure on the face. This can lead to abrasions or pressure sores and ulcers on the face.

A sudden decrease in the CPAP level to zero indicates a disconnection at the patient or somewhere in the breathing circuit. Check all connections, and reassemble the break. If the CPAP level decreases by more than 2 cm water during an inspiration, the flow is inadequate and should be increased. Flow also is inadequate if the patient shows increased use of accessory muscles of respiration or complains of increased WOB. Too high a flow is seen by an inadvertently high level of CPAP or by the patient's complaining of difficulty exhaling.

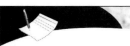

Exam Hint 15-17

Two or more questions usually relate to troubleshooting equipment problems. Expect a question that involves a leak with the loss of delivered tidal volume. If the source of the leak is a loose CPAP or NIV mask, it must be adjusted or replaced. Be prepared to troubleshoot problems with a leak in the circuit tubing or the exhalation valve. Change a ventilator circuit that is obviously fouled with blood or secretions.

7. Humidifiers

a. Assemble the necessary equipment (code: IIA3) [difficulty: R, Ap]

A cascade-type, wick-type, etc., humidifier is indicated in these situations:

- The patient has thick or copious secretions. An increase in the amount or thickness of secretions or a change from white to yellow or green justifies the switch to a cascade-type humidifier.
- The patient probably will require mechanical ventilation for longer than 96 hours.
- The patient cannot have mechanical dead space added to the breathing circuit. If the patient's (especially a neonate's or child's) tidal volume is smaller than the HME dead space, the HME should not be used. SIMV systems typically are set up without mechanical dead space, so an HME should not be used.
- An HME should not be used for a patient receiving very large tidal volumes because the filter's ability to hold moisture is exceeded, and the patient will breathe in some dry air. Check the manufacturer's literature for the maximum recommended tidal volume.
- If the patient has a large air leak, as seen with a deflated cuff or bronchopleural fistula, an HME should not be used. With a large air leak, more air is inspired than expired, and the exchanger will not be able to fully humidify the inspired tidal volume.

A general discussion of this equipment was presented in Chapter 8. (See Fig. 15-29 for a setup in a CPAP breathing circuit.) The selected humidifier must be capable of providing 100% relative humidity. Pass-over humidifiers are preferred in neonates.

The humidifier's temperature usually is maintained at between 31° C and 35° C. Normally, the temperature at the patient's airway should never be greater than 37° C. An exception to this rule is the hypothermic patient. Inhaled gas that is warmed to a few degrees above normal body temperature speeds the rewarming process.

Typically, a temperature probe is added into the inspiratory limb of the circuit near the Y. If a heated-wire circuit is being used with an infant, the temperature probe should be outside of the incubator and away from a radiant warmer's direct heat. The humidifier should provide at least 30 mg/L of water vapor.

Make sure that the water level is kept in the recommended range to humidify the gas properly. Avoid being sprayed with any circuit water during disconnections from the patient. It is considered contaminated and should be disposed of similar to any other contaminated fluid from the patient.

An AARC Clinical Practice Guideline on ventilator circuit changes (1994) recommends that a cascade-type or wick-type humidifier and the patient circuit be changed at least every 5 days for infection control purposes. The guideline also recommends that a nebulizer used for humidification purposes and the patient circuit should be changed every 24 hours for infection control purposes.

More recently, the AARC Clinical Practice Guideline on care of the ventilator circuit and its relation to ventilator-associated pneumonia (2003) included the following guidelines:

- The circuit should not be changed routinely for infection control purposes.
- Change the circuit when it is obviously soiled (e.g., blood, sputum).
- Passive humidifiers (HMEs) do not need to be changed daily.
- An HME can be used for at least 48 hours and possibly for up to a week.
- Change an HME when it is obviously soiled (e.g., blood, sputum).

b. Troubleshoot any problems with the equipment (code: IIA3) [difficulty: R, Ap]

A loose connection at the humidifier (or anywhere else in the circuit) results in loss of volume or pressure or both to the patient. Check the entire circuit. When the leak is fixed, the volume and pressure are restored. The humidifier should warm to the desired temperature. Do not use a humidifier that does not warm properly.

8. Heat and moisture exchangers

a. Assemble the necessary equipment (code: IIA3) [difficulty: R, Ap]

An HME is designed to be warmed by the patient's exhaled breath and to absorb the water vapor from the gas (see Fig. 8-9 in Chapter 8). The next inspired volume then is warmed and humidified by evaporation. The key element in the exchanger is a hygroscopic filter medium. Under ideal conditions, the units can achieve up to 70%-90% body humidity. They should provide minimally 30 mg/L of water at 30° C. A general discussion of this equipment is presented in Chapter 8. See Figure 15-28 for a setup in a ventilator breathing circuit.

An HME is indicated in the following situations:
- The patient has few, if any, secretions.
- The patient probably will be weaned from the ventilator within 96 hours.
- The patient is being transported on mechanical ventilation.

An HME is contraindicated in the following situations:
- The patient has thick, bloody, or large amounts of secretions.
- The patient has a large air leak such that the exhaled volume is less than 70% of the inhaled tidal volume. This results in a relatively dry hygroscopic filter. (Patients with uncuffed or torn cuffs on their endotracheal tubes or large bronchopleurocutaneous fistulas have large tidal volume leaks.)
- The patient's temperature is less than 32° C.
- The patient's spontaneous minute volume is greater than 10 L/min.

Consider the following when selecting an HME:
- Select a unit with the smallest possible dead space volume. Watch for an increase in the patient's $PaCO_2$ if the HME adds too much dead space or the patient's tidal volume is too small.
- Pick the unit that provides the greatest percentage of body humidity. Do not use one that cannot meet these minimum standards.
- If the patient has a known pulmonary infection, select an HME that is also a bacteria filter.
- Should the unit be disposable or reusable? Staffing, infection control, and equipment processing considerations make a difference in unit selection.

Remember to always remove or bypass the HME when delivering nebulized medications through the circuit. If not, the HME will trap all of the nebulized medication and none will be delivered to the patient.

Most of these units are preassembled by the manufacturer, with nothing to add. It may be necessary to attach a length of large-bore or aerosol tubing or an elbow adapter to make the unit fit onto the Y or endotracheal tube. All come with standard 15- or 22-mm connector ends. Air should flow easily through them with little resistance.

An AARC Clinical Practice Guideline on circuit changes (1994) states that HMEs can be used for up to 4 days if the patient does not have a major secretion problem. Each individual HME can be used for at least 24 hours unless it is obviously fouled. The whole patient circuit should be changed at least every 5 days for infection control purposes. The AARC Clinical Practice Guideline on care of the ventilator circuit and its

relation to ventilator-associated pneumonia (2003) included the following guidelines:
- Passive humidifiers (HMEs) do not need to be changed daily.
- An HME can be used for at least 48 hours and possibly for up to a week.
- Change an HME when it is obviously soiled (e.g., blood, sputum).

b. Troubleshoot any problems with the equipment (code: IIA3) [difficulty: R, Ap]

Any disconnections can be easily noticed and reconnected. Replace any unit that has a mucous plug or other debris obstructing the channel. This might be demonstrated by a sudden increase in the patient's peak airway pressure.

Exam Hint 15-18

When secretions are coughed into an HME, it becomes obstructed. This is demonstrated by a rapid increase in the peak pressure during an inspiration. Remove the obstructed HME. Replace it or change to a wick-type humidifier.

---

9. Perform quality control procedures on mechanical ventilators (code: IIC5) [difficulty: R, Ap]

Follow the manufacturer's guidelines for quality control procedures on a mechanical ventilator. Microprocessor ventilators usually have a software package that performs self-diagnostic tests on the unit. Obviously, the ventilator should deliver the volume, flow, and pressure that are set on the controls. Do not use a unit that fails a quality control check.

MODULE F

Weaning the patient from the ventilator and extubation

1. Weaning parameters

a. Evaluate weaning parameters in the patient record (code: IA13d) [difficulty: R, Ap]

Review the clinical data if the patient had a previous, unsuccessful weaning attempt. Before another weaning attempt is made, the bedside spirometry tests listed below should be performed.

b. Tidal volume, minute volume, and vital capacity

1. *Measure tidal volume, minute volume, and vital capacity (code: IC4) [difficulty: R, Ap].*
2. *Evaluate the results of the tidal volume, minute volume, and vital capacity procedures (code: ID4) [difficulty: R, Ap, An].*

c. Maximum inspiratory and expiratory pressures

1. *Measure maximum inspiratory pressure and maximum expiratory pressure (code: IC13) [difficulty: R, Ap].*

BOX 15-5   Indications That the Patient Probably Can Be Weaned from the Ventilator

Oxygenation
PaO_2 ≥80 torr or SpO_2 >90% on 50% oxygen or less
$P(A–a)O_2$ <300-350 torr on 100% oxygen
Intrapulmonary shunt of <15%

Ventilation
$PaCO_2$ <55 torr in a patient who is not ordinarily hypercapneic
Dead space/tidal volume (V_D:V_T) ratio <0.55-0.6 (55%-60%)
Rapid, shallow breathing index (breaths/min divided by tidal volume in liters) <105

Pulmonary Mechanics
Spontaneous tidal volume of 3-4 mL/lb or 7-9 mL/kg of ideal body weight
Vital capacity of ≥10-15 mL/kg
Maximum inspiratory pressure (MIP) more than –20 to –25 cm water pressure
FEV_1 >10 mL/kg
Respiratory rate of 12-35/min (adult)

Miscellaneous
Conscious and cooperative patient who wants to breathe spontaneously
Stable and acceptable normal blood pressure and temperature
Stable cardiac rhythm; heart rate should not increase by >15%-20%
Corrected underlying problem that led to ventilatory support
Normal fluid balance and electrolyte values
Proper nutritional status

---

2. Evaluate the results of the maximum inspiratory pressure and maximum expiratory pressure procedures (code: ID12) [difficulty: R, Ap, An]

Indications that the patient can tolerate weaning should include some, if not all, of the criteria listed in Box 15-5. The patient need not pass each and every criterion. However, the more the patient can attain, the more likely he or she is to wean successfully. Individual physicians and practitioners may favor some of these conditions over others and may include other factors not listed. Review the discussion on pulmonary mechanics and bedside spirometry in Chapter 4, if needed.

2. Recommend liberating (weaning) the patient from mechanical ventilation (code: IIIE2h) [difficulty: R, Ap, An]

After evaluating all of the patient's clinically pertinent data, be prepared to recommend whether a patient should be weaned or not. Some patients do not wean successfully even though objective criteria indicate that they should. Conversely, some patients wean successfully even when objective criteria indicate otherwise. Keep in mind that each patient must be evaluated individually. Look at the objective criteria and how the patient actually performs during weaning.

3. Liberate (wean) the patient from mechanical ventilation (code: IIIC8) [difficulty: R, Ap, An]

Each of the five methods presented here has its advocates and a body of clinical evidence to show that it is a valid weaning technique. The practitioner must evaluate the patient before recommending any particular weaning method. The patient also must be evaluated during the weaning trial to determine whether the method chosen is meeting his or her needs. The practitioner must be prepared to discontinue weaning if the patient is failing and must be ready to try another weaning approach to help ensure success.

a. Spontaneous breathing trial

1. Perform a spontaneous breathing trial (code: IC16) [difficulty: R, Ap]

A spontaneous breathing trial (SBT) is used widely with patients who have been ventilated for a short period and now appear ready to breathe on their own. When the patient is stable, awake, and alert and meets the criteria listed in Box 15-5, he or she can be prepared for weaning. The patient should have sedation stopped, be instructed about weaning, be suctioned, and be put into a Fowler's or semi-Fowler's position if possible. Current recommendations are to try a daily SBT and evaluate the patient's performance. During an SBT, ventilator discontinuance and weaning begin at the same moment (Fig. 15-30, A). The patient goes from having the ventilator provide up to 100% of the minute volume to providing none of it. The patient should be watched continuously because he or she is now breathing totally independently. Pulse oximetry and, if possible, end-tidal carbon dioxide should be monitored. Vital signs and pulmonary mechanics should be measured every 5-10 minutes throughout the procedure. If the patient's condition deteriorates, mechanical ventilation is reestablished. If the patient is stable, an ABG sample should be taken after about 20 minutes. There are four ways to set up an SBT:

(1) T-piece (Briggs adapter) with reservoir (see Fig. 6-34 in Chapter 6). The ventilator circuit is disconnected, and the patient breathes an aerosol and oxygen mix through a T-piece. The oxygen percentage should be the same as originally inspired or up to 10% higher, depending on the patient's PaO_2 level on the ventilator.

(2) CPAP through the ventilator or a free-standing system (see Figs. 15-29 and 16-4). The CPAP supports the FRC and oxygenation while the patient breathes spontaneously. If the ventilator is used, its alarm systems will need to be adjusted so that if an apnea period is detected, the ventilator will resume delivering programmed tidal volume breaths.

(3) Pressure support through the ventilator. The PS level needs to be set high enough to overcome the airway resistance of the endotracheal tube while the patient breathes spontaneously. As stated above, the ventilator needs to be programmed to deliver tidal volume breaths if the patient becomes apneic.

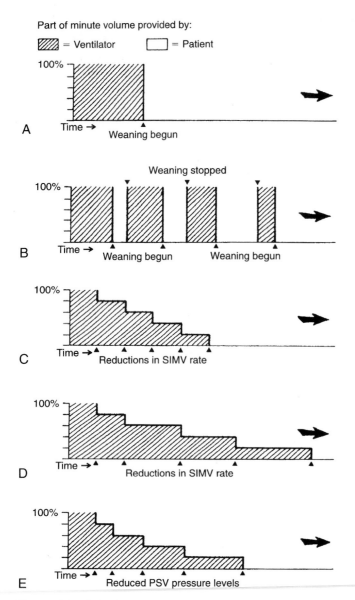

Figure 15-30 A–E, Options for weaning a patient from a mechanical ventilator. See the text for a description of each option. PSV, pressure support ventilation; SIMV, synchronous intermittent mandatory ventilation.

(4) Automatic tube compensation (ATC) through the ventilator. Similar to pressure support, the level of ATC must be set to overcome the airway resistance of the endotracheal tube. Again, the ventilator needs to be programmed to deliver tidal volume breaths if the patient becomes apneic.

2. Evaluate the results of a spontaneous breathing trial (code: ID15) [difficulty: R, Ap, An]

If the blood gas, pulse oximetry, and end-tidal carbon dioxide results are acceptable and the patient's pulmonary mechanics and vital signs are stable, the SBT has been successful. At this point, the decision can be made to extubate the patient. Approximately 75% of patients who tolerate the SBT can be successfully extubated. If the patient failed the SBT, full ventilatory support should be resumed for 24 hours before trying another. If the patient fails several SBT attempts, a more gradual weaning method can be tried as discussed below.

b. Intermittent ventilator discontinuance.
This method is used after the SBT method proves less than successful. The patient is started on a schedule of intermittent weaning periods and rest periods (Fig. 15-30, B). One intermittent SBT method has a cycle of lengthening weaning periods and reduced rest periods. This goes on until the patient is weaning for an extended period. Another method involves a cycle of set rest periods (commonly 0.5-1 hour) and lengthening weaning periods as the patient becomes stronger. Again, blood gas values should be monitored after about 20 minutes of weaning. The weaning period can be extended as long as the patient is stable or until extubated.

c. Regular steps in SIMV weaning.
As was discussed earlier, SIMV was developed originally as a ventilating mode and has become a widely used weaning mode. It allows the patient a more gradual transition toward totally providing all of the WOB. SIMV seems to work especially well in weaning patients who have been ventilator dependent for an extended period. By gradually taking over more of the WOB, the patient reconditions respiratory muscles that may have atrophied through lack of use. The patient also is gaining self-confidence that complete weaning will occur. An additional benefit is that all ventilator alarm systems are functional, and the patient does not need to be watched directly as closely as in the two previously mentioned weaning methods.

This particular SIMV weaning pattern can be applied to a patient who is stable and is making rapid progress (Fig. 15-30, C). The weaning pattern might involve reducing the SIMV rate in increments of about two per minute on a set time schedule. About 20 minutes after the SIMV rate is reduced, blood gas values should be monitored. The patient's respiratory mechanics are monitored closely. It is important to calculate the patient's spontaneous minute volume (rate × tidal volume). It should be approximately the same volume as was subtracted from the ventilator-delivered minute volume. The process continues as long as the patient tolerates each decrease in the SIMV rate. The stable, strong patient can be weaned rather quickly down to an SIMV rate of two to four times per minute. The decision often is made at this point to use a T-piece, as was discussed earlier, or to extubate the airway.

d. Irregular steps in SIMV weaning.
This method is applied when the regular SIMV method is unsuccessful. Often the patient starts out on a cycle of regular reductions in SIMV rate. This goes on until a point is reached at which the patient has a setback and cannot tolerate any further reduction in the SIMV rate. The rate may be kept at that level for an extended period until the patient is ready for

a further decrease (Fig. 15-30, D). Additional decreases in the IMV rate proceed as the patient tolerates them. No attempt is made to set up a regular pattern of reducing the rate.

It may be necessary to increase the rate to higher previous levels if the patient has a serious setback. One possible cause that may prevent the SIMV rate from decreasing is resistance to breathing through the demand valve and breathing circuit. A trial on a T-piece (which offers no resistance) may prove to be the final step in weaning. If this fails for the patient, the reason is probably the resistance caused by the endotracheal tube. The pressure support weaning method then should be tried on the patient.

e. Weaning by pressure support ventilation. The PSV mode is available on most modern electrically powered and microprocessor ventilators (Fig. 15-30, E). When it is used as a weaning method, the pressure support level is reduced gradually. Decreasing pressure support steps of 2-5 cm water are made commonly. The patient has to increase his or her WOB gradually to inspire a tidal volume. Blood gas values and pulmonary mechanics should be evaluated after each decrease in the pressure support level. A modest pressure support level of 2-5 cm water is maintained to overcome any resistance of the endotracheal tube. If the patient does well during an extended trial of minimum pressure support, extubation is performed unless the endotracheal tube is needed for other reasons.

The criteria listed in Box 15-5 can be used in evaluating any patient who is being weaned by any of these methods. General signs that the patient is not tolerating weaning include anxiety, agitation, a large increase or decrease in respiratory rate, angina, tachycardia, an increase in premature ventricular contractions or other serious dysrhythmias, bradycardia, hypertension, hypotension, cyanosis, hypoxemia, and hypercarbia with acidemia. The patient probably will not exhibit all of these signs. Some tend to be seen together because they relate to the patient's WOB. Others appear to give conflicting signals of success or failure. It is the practitioner's responsibility to evaluate the patient's condition to determine whether weaning should be continued or ventilatory support resumed.

Exam Hint 15-19

Expect to see several questions that relate to evaluating a patient's ability to wean. These will include such information as initial bedside spirometry, arterial blood gas results, and vital signs. If a patient is able to wean, expect to make recommendations on which method(s) to use. Finally, expect to see questions related to evaluating a patient who is weaning. You will need to evaluate current bedside spirometry, arterial blood gas results, and vital signs. Make a decision to continue weaning, to change the weaning procedure, or to put the patient back on the ventilator. Review the content of Box 15-5.

5. Extubation

a. Recommend extubation (code: IIIE2g) [difficulty: R, Ap, An]

Extubation usually can be safely accomplished when the patient meets the following criteria:

- Has the desired pulmonary mechanics and vital signs listed in Box 15-5
- Has demonstrated the ability to breathe effectively for a clinically significant period as measured by the listed criteria
- Has acceptable blood gas results
- Is alert enough to protect his or her airway
- Can effectively cough out any secretions

It may be found that some patients need the endotracheal tube even though they no longer need ventilatory support. The tube provides a suctioning route if the patient is unable to cough out large amounts of secretions. The tube also protects the airway from the risk of aspiration in a comatose patient who may vomit.

b. Perform extubation (code: IIIA8) [difficulty: R, Ap, An]

The respiratory therapist must be competent at safely extubating a patient and caring for the patient's needs after extubation. Review the full discussion in Chapter 12, if needed. If the patient should have severe airway management or breathing difficulty after extubation, be prepared to insert another endotracheal tube. Review the procedure in Chapter 12, if needed. If a patient is fatigued after extubation, NIV may be used to support the patient's breathing efforts.

Exam Hint 15-20

Be prepared to recommend extubation if a patient has weaned successfully and meets all extubation criteria. More information on the extubation procedure is provided in Chapter 12.

MODULE G

Respiratory care plan

1. Determine a patient's pathophysiologic state (code: IIIF1) [difficulty: R, Ap, An]

See below.

2. Recommend starting a treatment based on the patient's response (code: IIIE2a) [difficulty: R, Ap, An]

See below.

3. Recommend a change in the therapeutic plan if indicated (code: IIIF2) [difficulty: R, Ap, An]

See below.

Be prepared to make recommendations on changing ventilator parameters based on the patient's pathologic condition, blood gas values, chest radiograph findings, breath sounds, and vital signs. Common recommendations follow.

Exam Hint 15-21

Past examinations have had questions about the management of patients with specific conditions such as increased intracranial pressure (ICP), COPD, asthma, congestive heart failure, ARDS, and pneumothorax. In addition, the Clinical Simulation Examination has at least two adult scenarios on each of the following: COPD/asthma, trauma, cardiovascular disease, and neuromuscular or neurologic disease. The management of these patients is briefly discussed next.

a. Increased intracranial pressure

Intracranial pressure (ICP) is the pressure within the cranium (skull). It is normally less than 10 mm Hg. A patient's ICP is measured by placement of a catheter into the subarachnoid space, subdural space, or ventricular space. The most common cause of increased ICP is an acute head injury in which the brain is shaken. This is caused commonly by a closed head injury. Other causes of increased ICP include craniotomy for brain tumor resection and stroke (cerebral vascular accident). Any significant increase in pressure within the skull will further injure the brain. Clinical experience has shown that when the ICP exceeds 20 mm Hg, the patient's outcome significantly worsens.

The A/C mode usually is selected with constant volume ventilation so that the patient is assured of a set minute volume if apnea occurs. It has been demonstrated that hyperventilating the patient to a $PaCO_2$ between 25 and 30 torr results in a reduced ICP. This is the result of the lowered carbon dioxide pressure causing a reduced hydrogen ion concentration and increased pH, which causes cerebral vasoconstriction. Because the cerebral blood flow is decreased by hyperventilation, it is important to maintain the patient's PaO_2 in the 90-110 torr range. Hyperventilation is used for a short period of time (usually less than 24 hours) until other therapeutic measures reduce the ICP.

b. Chronic obstructive lung disease

Patients with COPD usually are well known because of previous hospitalizations for acute exacerbations related to problems such as lung infection or heart failure. When the patient must be ventilated, it is important to maintain baseline "normal" blood gas values. This usually means accepting moderate hypoxemia and hypercarbia with a compensated respiratory acidosis. Ventilating the patient to provide textbook normal ABGs must be avoided. This is because the patient with COPD cannot maintain this level of breathing efficiency when ready to come off of the ventilator.

The A/C or SIMV mode may be used with a constant volume set or PC used to set the tidal volume. A patient with COPD must have the ventilator adjusted, including the addition of mechanical dead space, to maintain the patient's normally elevated $PaCO_2$ level. A PaO_2 of 60-70 torr usually is adequate. Keep the plateau pressure (alveolar pressure) less than 30 cm water to avoid overdistention of the patient's compliant lungs and resultant volutrauma.

If the patient has air trapping and auto-PEEP, a small amount of therapeutic PEEP may be added to help the patient exhale and to trigger the ventilator. Increase the therapeutic PEEP in 1 cm water steps until the patient is synchronized with the ventilator. Many patients with COPD need 5 cm water of PEEP or more. When the condition that caused the sudden deterioration is corrected, the patient should be weaned off of the ventilator as soon as possible to prevent atrophy of the ventilatory muscles.

c. Asthma

The patient with status asthmaticus needs mechanical ventilation when the increased airway resistance and increased WOB lead to exhaustion. This results in hypercarbia and respiratory acidosis. Air trapping (see Fig. 15-4) and auto-PEEP are also significant concerns. In these serious situations, three ventilator strategies can be implemented: (1) Small tidal volume breaths and permissive hypercapnia. If a smaller than ideal tidal volume is delivered, air trapping is less likely. A longer than normal expiratory time may also be needed. See the ARDS-Net protocol below for the permissive hypercapnia discussion. (2) Heliox (helium/oxygen) therapy. Heliox can be delivered through some ventilators and will reduce airway resistance. See the discussion in Chapter 6. (3) Inhaled bronchodilator therapy and systemic corticosteroid therapy. The specific medications are discussed in Chapter 9. An inhaled bronchodilator medication can be given through the ventilator by adding the dispenser into the inspiratory limb of the ventilator circuit. If an HME is used, it must be removed or bypassed (see Fig. 15-28). A metered-dose inhaler (MDI) can be given by adding a modified actuator into the circuit. In some cases, a reservoir is included with the actuator. Press the canister into the actuator to dispense the medication into the circuit before the next breath is delivered. A liquid medication must be given by adding a small-volume nebulizer (SVN) into the circuit. A length of small-bore oxygen tubing is connected between the nipple on the SVN and the outlet nipple on the ventilator. Turning on the ventilator's nebulizer control diverts some of the patient's tidal volume through the nebulizer. The medication is nebulized only during inspiration, and no change in delivered tidal volume or oxygen percentage is noted. Make sure that the nebulizer is turned off after the medication has been delivered. Typically the nebulizer then is removed, or bypassed, as is shown in Figure 15-28. An HME can be added back into the circuit after the treatment is completed. A vibrating mesh nebulizer (VMN) offers a second option for nebulizing liquid medications. It is electrically powered and does not need a gas source. The unit would be added into the ventilator circuit as an MDI or SVN would be. See Chapter 8 for further discussion on MDI, SVN, or VMN options for delivering aerosolized medications.

d. Congestive heart failure

Patients with congestive heart failure (CHF) usually also have a pulmonary edema problem. This results in hypoxemia and low C_{LT}. Mechanical ventilation with the A/C or SIMV mode with constant volume ventilation is needed to reduce the patient's WOB, deliver supplemental oxygen, and add therapeutic PEEP. Usually a pulmonary artery catheter is placed to measure pulmonary artery pressure, pulmonary capillary wedge pressure, and CO. If the PEEP level is increased and the patient's CO is decreased, the PEEP should be reduced to its previous level. The patient must be given a diuretic such as furosemide (Lasix) to increase urine output. The patient's heart function is improved by giving digitalis (Lanoxin, digoxin). Closely follow the patient's cardiovascular values to monitor improvement after administration of a diuretic and digitalis. Reduce the PEEP and inspired oxygen as the pulmonary edema problem is corrected. See Chapter 9 for a discussion of medications and Chapter 5 for a discussion on hemodynamic monitoring as needed.

e. Apply evidence-based guidelines: ARDS-Net protocol (code: IIIF3) [difficulty: R, Ap]

Acute respiratory distress syndrome (ARDS) is caused by a variety of pulmonary and circulatory conditions that result in nonhomogeneous damage to alveolar capillary membranes throughout the lungs. This results in noncardiac pulmonary edema with decreased pulmonary compliance and hypoxemia. Similar to the patient with CHF, the patient with ARDS needs mechanical ventilation to reduce the increased WOB, provide supplemental oxygen, and provide therapeutic PEEP. A pulmonary artery catheter is needed to follow the patient's cardiovascular status.

Unlike the patient with CHF, the patient with ARDS does not respond as favorably to diuretic and digitalis medications. The continued problem of low compliance and resulting high ventilating pressures has been linked to barotrauma/volutrauma. Recent research has led to the development of ARDS-Net lung-protective strategies to prevent ventilator-associated lung injury. Following is a summary of the key recommendations; review the full document as needed.

1. Small tidal volume ventilation

Initially, most patients with ARDS are started on the A/C or SIMV mode with constant volume ventilation. Unfortunately, many patients with severe ARDS cannot be managed in this manner. The stiff lungs result in a very

high plateau pressure and risk of pulmonary barotrauma/volutrauma (also called shear stress). Recent studies have shown that the plateau pressure found in the alveoli (P_{plat}) must be kept at <30 cm water to avoid this serious complication. To lower a dangerously high alveolar pressure, the tidal volume must be reduced. Many clinicians recommend that the patient be switched from constant volume ventilation to pressure control (PC) ventilation to do this. Recent evidence has shown a higher survival rate in patients with ARDS when the tidal volume was lowered from 12 to 6 mL/kg of ideal body weight.

If the initial set of blood gases on PC with a small tidal volume does not show adequate oxygenation, the inspiratory time must be increased. Some patients with ARDS need an increased inspiratory time such that the I:E ratio is inverse. This results in pressure control inverse ratio ventilation. The advantages of PCIRV over conventional volume ventilation include the lowered peak airway pressure and the longer inspiratory time. The lowered peak pressure is thought to reduce the risk of volutrauma. The longer inspiratory time allows alveoli with long time constants of ventilation to fill and areas of atelectasis to reopen.

2. Permissive hypercapnia

The small tidal volumes used with PCIRV can result in failure to blow off carbon dioxide to a normal level. At times, this must be clinically accepted. Permissive hypercapnia involves allowing a $PaCO_2$ of 50 torr up to 100-150 torr. It is very important to prevent the carbon dioxide level from increasing too rapidly because it causes cerebral vasodilation and increases the patient's ICP. To minimize this risk, the $PaCO_2$ should not be allowed to increase faster than 10 torr/h to a maximum of 80 torr. If the $PaCO_2$ must be allowed to increase to more than 80 torr, the rate of increase must be slower than 10 torr/h. The high $PaCO_2$ also results in a respiratory acidosis. Keep the patient's arterial pH at ≥7.25 to avoid problems related to the acidosis. It may be necessary to administer intravenous bicarbonate to correct the respiratory acidosis.

When the patient recovers, the $PaCO_2$ can be lowered gradually. If permissive hypercapnia was used for less than 24 hours, the $PaCO_2$ probably can be lowered by 10-20 torr/h. If permissive hypercapnia was used for longer than 24 hours, or if bicarbonate was given to buffer the pH, the $PaCO_2$ must be lowered more slowly. It is important to monitor the patient's arterial pH throughout this process to prevent too rapid an increase.

3. Perform lung recruitment maneuvers (code: IIIC7) [difficulty: R, Ap, An]

The purpose of a recruitment maneuver is to find the ideal amount of PEEP needed to keep the lungs open and to maintain the FRC (see Fig. 4-7 in Chapter 4). When the FRC is maintained, the tidal volume can be delivered with the least amount of pressure. A secondary benefit of setting the ideal level of PEEP is that the patient can be oxygenated at the lowest inspired oxygen percentage. A lung recruitment maneuver has similarities to a best PEEP/optimum PEEP study to find the PEEP level needed to correct the low C_{LT}, the severe hypoxemia, and the large shunt percentage that these patients have (see Fig. 15-20).

Steps in the lung recruitment maneuver include the following:

1. Inflate the lungs as much as possible by applying a series of steps of increased baseline pressure. Lung volume and pressure should be plotted with the ventilator's graphics package, if possible. Maximally, 35-45 cm water pressure is applied against the lungs for 40-60 seconds. This baseline pressure increase is intended to open up any areas of atelectasis. As the pressure is increased, the opening pressure of the lungs is found. This corresponds to point A of Figure 15-16 when areas of atelectasis open up. As the pressure is maximized, the lungs become fully inflated. More pressure does little, if anything, to add more volume. This corresponds to point B of Figure 15-16.

2. The lungs are allowed to deflate through the reduction of baseline pressure in a series of steps. The lung volumes and pressures should be graphed as this is done. The purpose of this procedure is to find the pressure when most of the lung units begin to collapse. This corresponds to point C of Figure 15-16.

3. Finally, the lung recruitment maneuver is repeated to reopen any recently closed lung units.

When the recruitment maneuver is done on a modern microprocessor ventilator with graphics software and a monitor, set the unit to display a pressure/volume loop. A loop similar to the one shown in Figure 15-16 will be seen. Point A shows the inspiratory low inflection point and is found near the FRC. This identifies the pressure needed to open up alveoli and establish the patient's FRC. Point B shows the inspiratory high inflection point and is found near the total lung capacity. This identifies the highest lung volume and highest lung pressure that should be allowed. Note the "beaking" that occurs to the right of point B. Further pressure does not greatly increase tidal volume and can result in volutrauma to any overstretched alveoli. Many clinicians use the high inflection point as the maximum pressure allowed with PCV to deliver a tidal volume. The expiratory upper inflection point, C, represents the pressure below which atelectasis may occur.

There is controversy over how to best use the above information. Some feel that the minimum level of PEEP should be applied to minimize the risk of lung injury. This would correspond with a pressure at or above point A in Figure 15-16. Some feel that a higher PEEP level should be used to minimize shunting, but less than is shown at point B in Figure 15-16. The ARDS-Net group recommends that PEEP should be set above the expiratory high inflection point. This would be greater than point C of Figure 15-16 and would prevent alveolar collapse on exhalation.

4. Auto-PEEP recognition

If PCIRV is used, the inspiratory time must be reduced toward normal as C_{LT} improves. Monitor the patient for air trapping and auto-PEEP if the expiratory time is too short (see Fig. 15-4). Full exhalation of the tidal volume must be ensured.

f. Recommend the treatment of a pneumothorax (code: IIIE2b) [difficulty: R, Ap, An]

Recognize the signs of a pneumothorax on a mechanically ventilated patient (suddenly increasing peak and plateau pressures, hypoxemia, mediastinal shift to the side opposite the pneumothorax, hyperresonant percussion noted over the pneumothorax, and asymmetric chest movement on inspiration). Chest radiograph and physical examination of the patient will reveal whether air (or fluid) is found abnormally around the lung(s) or the heart.

Common causes of pneumothorax include lung puncture during insertion of a central venous pressure line via the subclavian vein, overinflated lungs from too large a tidal volume on the ventilator, punctured lung from a sharp broken rib, and thoracentesis.

If a patient has a tension pneumothorax, a pleural chest tube must be inserted on the affected side to remove the air and relieve the pressure within the chest. In an emergency, a large-gauge needle may be placed between the second and the third ribs (second intercostal space) in the midclavicular line. These and related subjects are discussed in detail in Chapter 18. A nontension pneumothorax of greater than 10% often is treated by insertion of a pleural chest tube. In addition, a pleural chest tube is placed to remove blood or other fluid from the pleural space.

A pneumomediastinum, pneumopericardium, or pneumoperitoneum that puts the patient at risk also must be treated. A chest tube then is inserted into the area where the abnormal air is found. The same chest tube also would remove any abnormal collection of fluid. A pericardial chest tube usually is placed behind the heart to remove any blood that may leak out after open heart surgery is performed.

If the patient is being ventilated on a constant-volume ventilator, the amount of air that is lost through the pleural chest tube can be calculated. This is done by subtracting the measured exhaled volume from the measured inhaled volume (the set tidal volume). The following equation demonstrates:

Inspired tidal volume = 500 mL
Exhaled tidal volume = − 400 mL
100 mL of tidal volume is lost through the pleural chest tube.

It is not always possible to measure a consistent tidal volume when PCV or a similar mode is used. In a case like this, it is possible to make only a qualitative judgment on pleural air leak. In other words, if air is seen to bubble out through the pleural drainage system, an air leak is present. When the air stops bubbling, the pleural tear has healed. See Chapter 18 for a complete discussion on pleural drainage systems.

Remember to get an ABG after every ventilator change that could result in a different PaO_2 (pulse oximetry or transcutaneous oxygen may be substituted) or $PaCO_2$ (end-tidal CO_2 or transcutaneous carbon dioxide may be substituted). Mixed venous blood gas values should also be obtained when possible.

Exam Hint 15-22

Usually one question deals with recognizing that a patient is losing tidal volume through a pleural chest tube or that a pneumothorax has developed. Know the signs and symptoms of a pneumothorax.

---

4. Recommend a treatment be terminated (code: IIIE1) [difficulty: R, Ap, An]

See below.

5. Recommend discontinuing a treatment based on the patient's response (code: IIIE2h) [difficulty: R, Ap, An]

Physical responses to mechanical ventilation, as measured by the vital signs, can vary considerably. A patient who is anxious or angry or in pain will have an increase in vital signs. A patient who is relaxed has reduced WOB, and a patient whose blood gas values are now normal will have a return to normal vital signs. Watch carefully for the patient whose decrease in blood pressure coincides with a tachycardia. This patient may be having decreased venous return to the heart from increased intrathoracic pressure. An increased PEEP level is the most common cause of this. Be prepared to stop a treatment or procedure related to mechanical ventilation if the patient has an adverse reaction to it.

6. Assist the physician in the withdrawal of life support (code: IIIH10) [difficulty: R, Ap]

Because a mechanical ventilator is providing a vital life-support function, removing it would be done only if the patient is legally brain dead. This issue is discussed in Chapter 18.

If the life-support measures are to be stopped, the physician will usually take the patient off of the ventilator. The respiratory therapist will be called upon to turn off the alarms and turn off the ventilator. If permitted by hospital policy, the physician may write an order for the respiratory therapist to discontinue the ventilator. However, the therapist has the right to refuse to perform this task based on his or her philosophical or religious beliefs. It is very important that counseling be available and encouraged for family members and health care team members to help them cope with the passing of the patient.

BIBLIOGRAPHY

AARC clinical practice guideline: application of continuous positive airway pressure to neonates via nasal prongs, nasopharyngeal tube, or nasal mask—2004 revision and update, *Respir Care* 49(9):1100, 2004.

AARC clinical practice guideline: care of the circuit and its relation to ventilator-associated pneumonia, *Respir Care* 48:869, 2003.

AARC clinical practice guideline: endotracheal suctioning of mechanically ventilated patients with artificial airways, *Respir Care* 55(6):758–764, 2010.

AARC clinical practice guideline: evidence-based guidelines for weaning and discontinuing ventilatory support, *Respir Care* 47:69, 2002.

AARC clinical practice guideline: humidification during invasive and noninvasive mechanical ventilation, *Respir Care* 57:782–788, 2012.

AARC clinical practice guideline: humidification during mechanical ventilation, *Respir Care* 37:887, 1992.

AARC clinical practice guideline: neonatal time-triggered, pressure-limited, time-cycled, mechanical ventilation, *Respir Care* 39:808, 1994. (Retired).

AARC clinical practice guideline: patient-ventilator system checks, *Respir Care* 37:882, 1992. (Retired).

AARC clinical practice guideline: removal of the endotracheal tube—2007 revision & update, *Respir Care* 52:81, 2007.

AARC clinical practice guideline: ventilator circuit changes, *Respir Care* 39:797, 1994.

AARC clinical practice guideline: long-term invasive mechanical ventilation in the home—2007 revision & update, *Respir Care* 52(1):1056–1062, 2007.

AARC clinical practice guideline: in-hospital transport of the mechanically ventilated patient: 2002 revision and update, *Respir Care* 47(6):721, 2002.

AARC clinical practice guideline: capnography/capnometry during mechanical ventilation: 2003 revision and update, *Respir Care* 48(3):534, 2003.

AARC clinical practice guideline: selection of device, administration of bronchodilator, and evaluation of responses to therapy in mechanically ventilated patients, *Respir Care* 44(1):105, 1999.

AARC consensus statement on the essentials of mechanical ventilation, *Respir Care* 37(9):1000, 1992.

Aboussouan LS: Respiratory failure and the need for ventilatory support. In Wilkins RL, Stoller JK, Kacmarek RM, editors: *Egan's fundamentals of respiratory care*, ed 9, St Louis, 2009, Mosby.

Adams AB: Monitoring the patient in the Intensive Care Unit. In Kacmarek RM, Stoller JK, Heuer AJ, editors: *Egan's fundamentals of respiratory care*, ed 10, St Louis, 2013, Mosby.

Agarwal R, Aggarwal AN, Gupta D: Role of noninvasive ventilation in acute lung injury/acute respiratory distress syndrome: a proportional meta-analysis, *Respir Care* 55(12):1653–1660, 2012.

Altobelli N: Airway management. In Kacmarek RM, Stoller JK, Heuer AJ, editors: *Egan's fundamentals of respiratory care*, ed 10, St Louis, 2013, Mosby.

ARDS Network: Ventilation with lower tidal volumes as compared with traditional tidal volumes for acute lung injury and the acute respiratory distress syndrome patients, *N Engl J Med* 342(18):1301, 2000.

Ari A, Areabi H, Fink JB: Evaluation of aerosol generator devices at 3 locations in humidified and non-humidified circuits during adult mechanical ventilation, *Respir Care* 55(7):837–844, 2010.

Badet M, Bayle F, Richard J-C, Guerin C: Comparison of optimal positive end-expiratory pressure and recruitment maneuvers during lung-protective mechanical ventilation in patients with acute lung injury/acute respiratory distress syndrome, *Respir Care* 54(7):847–854, 2009.

Bennett S, Hurford WE: When should sedation or neuromuscular blockade be used during mechanical ventilation? *Respir Care* 56(2):168–180, 2011.

Betensley AD, Khalid I, Crawford J, Pensler RA, DiGiovine B: Patient comfort during pressure support and volume controlled-continuous mandatory ventilation, *Respir Care* 53(7):897–902, 2008.

Biehl M, Kashiouris MG, Gajic O: Ventilator-induced lung injury: minimizing its impact in patients with or at risk of ARDS, *Respir Care* 58(6):927–937, 2013.

Bone RC: Pressure–volume measurements in detection of bronchospasm and mucous plugging in acute respiratory failure, *Respir Care* 21(7):620, 1976.

Boysen PG, McGough E: Pressure-control and pressure-support ventilation: flow patterns, inspiratory time, and gas distribution, *Respir Care* 33(2):620, 1988.

Branson RD: Secretion management in the mechanically ventilated patient, *Respir Care* 52(10):1328–1347, 2007.

Branson RD, Campbell RS, Davis Jr K, et al.: Altering flowrate during maximum pressure support ventilation (PSV$_{max}$): effects on cardiorespiratory function, *Respir Care* 35(11):1056, 1990.

Branson RD, Chatburn RL: Technical description and classification of modes of ventilator operation, *Respir Care* 37(9):1026, 1992.

Branson RD, Hess DR, Chatburn RL, editors: *Respiratory care equipment*, ed 2, Philadelphia, 1999, Lippincott Williams & Wilkins.

Branson RD, Hurst JM: Laboratory evaluation of moisture output of seven airway heat and moisture exchangers, *Respir Care* 32(9):741, 1987.

Cairo JM: *Pilbeam's mechanical ventilation: physiological and clinical applications*, ed 5, St Louis, 2012, Mosby.

Cairo JM: *Mosby's respiratory care equipment*, ed 9, St Louis, 2014, Mosby.

Campbell RS, Davis BR: Pressure-controlled versus volume-controlled ventilation: does it matter? *Respir Care* 47(4):416, 2002.

Chang DW: *Clinical application of mechanical ventilation*, ed 4, Clifton Park, NY, 2014, Delmar.

Chatburn RL: A new system for understanding mechanical ventilation, *Respir Care* 36(10):1123, 1991.

Chatburn RL: Classification of mechanical ventilators, *Respir Care* 37(9):1009, 1992.

Chatburn RL, Mireles-Cabodevila E: Closed-loop control of mechanical ventilation: description and classification of targeting schemes, *Respir Care* 56(1):85–98, 2011.

Chatburn RL, Volsko TA: Mechanical ventilators: classification and principles of operation. In Hess DR, MacIntyre NR, Mishoe SC, Galvin WF, Adams AB, editors: *Respiratory care principles and practice*, ed 2, Burlington, MA, 2012, Jones & Bartlett Learning.

Daoud EG, Farag HL, Chatburn RL: Airway pressure release ventilation: what do we know? *Respir Care* 57(2):282–292, 2012.

de Wit M: Monitoring of patient-ventilator interaction at the bedside, *Respir Care* 56(1):61–72, 2011.

Dhand R: Ventilator graphics and respiratory mechanics in the patient with obstructive lung disease, *Respir Care* 50(2):246, 2005.

Drinker PA, McKhann CF III: Landmark perspective: the iron lung: first practical means of respiratory support, *JAMA* 256(11):1476, 1986.

Epstein SK: Extubation, *Respir Care* 47(4):483, 2002.

Epstein SK: Weaning from mechanical ventilation, *Respir Care* 47(4):454, 2002.

Epstein SK: Noninvasive ventilation to shorten duration of mechanical ventilation, *Respir Care* 54(2):198–208, 2009.

Epstein SK, Durbin CG Jr: Should a patient be extubated and placed on noninvasive ventilation after failing a spontaneous breathing trial? *Respir Care* 55(2):198–206, 2010.

Evidence-based guidelines for weaning and discontinuing ventilator support, *Respir Care* 47(1):69, 2002.

Fessler HE, Talmor DS: Should prone positioning be routinely used for lung protection during mechanical ventilation? *Respir Care* 55(1):88–99, 2010.

Felix WR Jr, MacDonnell KF, Jacobs L: Resuscitation from drowning in cold water, *N Engl J Med* 304(14):843, 1981.

Figueroa-Casas JB, Montoya R, Arzabala A, Connery SM: Comparison between automatic tube compensation and continuous positive airway pressure during spontaneous breathing trials, *Respir Care* 55(5):549–554, 2010.

Fink JB, Hunt GE, editors: *Clinical practice in respiratory care*, Philadelphia, 1999, Lippincott Williams & Wilkins.

Fink JB, Tobin MJ, Dhand R: Bronchodilator therapy in mechanically ventilated patients, *Respir Care* 44(1):53, 1999.

Gentile MA: Cycling of the mechanical ventilator breath, *Respir Care* 56(1):52–60, 2011.

Greer K: Hypothermia: a quiet killer, *Adv Respir Ther*, January 15, 1990.

Gregg BL: Initiation, monitoring, and discontinuing mechanical ventilation. In Wyka KA, Mathews PJ, Rutkowski J, editors: *Foundations of respiratory care*, ed 2, Clifton Park, NY, 2012, Delmar.

Gurevitch MJ: Selection of the inspiratory: expiratory ratio. In Kacmarek RM, Stoller JK, editors: *Current respiratory care*, Philadelphia, 1988, BC Decker.

Hamel DS, Cheifetz IM: Capnography to optimize and minimize mechanical ventilation. In Gravenstein JS, Jaffe MB, Paulus DA, editors: *Capnography: clinical aspects*, Cambridge, United Kingdom, 2004, Cambridge University Press.

Han J, Liu Y: Effect of ventilator circuit changes on ventilator-associated pneumonia: a systematic review and meta-analysis, *Respir Care* 55(4):467–474, 2010.

Hess DR: Approaches to conventional mechanical ventilation of the patient with acute respiratory distress syndrome, *Respir Care* 56(10):1555–1572, 2011.

Hess DR: Patient-ventilator interaction during noninvasive ventilation, *Respir Care* 56(2):153–165, 2011.

Hess DR: Noninvasive ventilation and continuous positive airway pressure. In Hess DR, MacIntyre NR, Mishoe SC, Galvin WF, Adams AB, editors: *Respiratory care principles and practice*, ed 2, Burlington, MA, 2012, Jones & Bartlett Learning.

Hess DR: The role of noninvasive ventilation in the ventilator discontinuation process, *Respir Care* 47(10):1619–1625, 2012.

Hess DR, Branson RD: Mechanical ventilation. In Hess DR, MacIntyre NR, Mishoe SC, et al.: *Respiratory care principles and practice*, Philadelphia, 2002, Saunders.

Hess DR, Kacmarek RM: *Essentials of mechanical ventilation*, ed 2, New York, 2002, McGraw-Hill.

Hess DR, MacIntyre NR: Mechanical ventilation. In Hess DR, MacIntyre NR, Mishoe SC, Galvin WF, Adams AB, editors: *Respiratory care principles and practice*, ed 2, Burlington, MA, 2012, Jones & Bartlett Learning.

Hess DR, McCurdy S, Simmons M: Compression volume in adult ventilator circuits: a comparison of five disposable circuits and a nondisposable circuit, *Respir Care* 36(10):1113, 1991.

Hill NS: Clinical application of body ventilators, *Chest* 90(6):897, 1986.

Hill NS, Eveloff SE, Carlisle CC, Goff SG: Efficacy of nocturnal nasal ventilation in patients with restrictive thoracic disease, *Am Rev Respir Dis* 145(2):365, 1992.

International Consensus Conferences in Intensive Care Medicine: Ventilator-associated lung injury in ARDS, *Am J Respir Crit Care Med* 160(6):2118, 1999.

Kacmarek RM: The role of pressure support ventilation in reducing work of breathing, *Respir Care* 33(2):99, 1988.

Kacmarek RM: Noninvasive positive pressure ventilation. In Wilkins RL, Stoller JK, Kacmarek RM, editors: *Egan's fundamentals of respiratory care*, ed 9, St Louis, 2009, Mosby.

Kacmarek RM: Initiating and adjusting invasive mechanical ventilation. In Kacmarek RM, Stoller JK, Heuer AJ, editors: *Egan's fundamentals of respiratory care*, ed 10, St Louis, 2013, Mosby.

Kacmarek RM: Discontinuing ventilatory support. In Kacmarek RM, Stoller JK, Heuer AJ, editors: *Egan's fundamentals of respiratory care*, ed 10, St Louis, 2013, Mosby.

Kacmarek RM, Dimas S, Mack CW, editors: *The essentials of respiratory care*, ed 4, St Louis, 2005, Mosby.

Kacmarek RM, Hess D: Pressure-controlled inverse-ratio ventilation: panacea or auto-PEEP? *Respir Care* 35(10):945, 1990.

Kallet RH: Patient-ventilator interaction during acute lung injury, and the role of spontaneous breathing: Part 2: airway pressure release ventilation, *Respir Care* 56(2):190–206, 2011.

Kallet RH, Diaz JV: The physiologic effects of noninvasive ventilation, *Respir Care* 54(1):102, 2009.

Keenan SP, Mehta S: Noninvasive ventilation for patients presenting with acute respiratory failure: the randomized controlled trials, *Respir Care* 54(1):116–126, 2009.

Kuhlen R, Rossaint R: The role of spontaneous breathing during mechanical ventilation, *Respir Care* 47(3):296, 2002.

MacIntyre NR: Pressure support: inspiratory assist. In Kacmarek RM, Stoller JK, editors: *Current respiratory care*, Philadelphia, 1988, BC Decker.

MacIntyre NR: Weaning from mechanical ventilatory support: volume-assisting intermittent breaths versus pressure-supporting every breath, *Respir Care* 33(2):121, 1988.

MacIntyre NR: Setting the frequency-tidal volume pattern, *Respir Care* 47(3):266, 2002.

MacIntyre NR: Patient-ventilator interactions: optimizing conventional ventilation modes, *Respir Care* 56(1):73–84, 2011.

MacIntyre NR: The ventilator discontinuation process: an expanded evidence base, *Respir Care* 58(6):1074–1082, 2013.

MacIntyre NR, Branson RD: *Mechanical ventilation*, ed 2, Philadelphia, 2009, Saunders.

Masini DE: Ethics of healthcare delivery. In Hess DR, MacIntyre NR, Mishoe SC, Galvin WF, Adams AB, editors: *Respiratory care principles and practice*, ed 2, Burlington, MA, 2012, Jones & Bartlett Learning.

Meade MO, Guyatt GH, Cook DJ: Weaning from mechanical ventilation: the evidence from clinical research, *Respir Care* 46(12):1408–1415, 2001.

Medoff BD: Invasive and noninvasive ventilation in patients with asthma, *Respir Care* 53(6):740–748, 2008.

Mehta S, Al-Hashim AH, Keenan SP: Noninvasive ventilation in patients with acute cardiogenic pulmonary edema, *Respir Care* 54(2):186–195, 2009.

Mietto C, Pinciroli R, Patel N, Berra L: Ventilator-associated pneumonia: evolving definitions and preventive strategies, *Respir Care* 58(6):990–1003, 2013.

Mistraletti G, Giacomini M, Sabbatini G, et al.: Noninvasive CPAP with face mask: comparison among new air-entrainment masks and the Boussignac valve, *Respir Care* 58(2):305–312, 2013.

Nava S: Behind a mask: tricks, pitfalls, and prejudices for noninvasive ventilation, *Respir Care* 58(8):1367–1376, 2013.

Nava S, Navalesi P, Gregoretti C: Interfaces and humidification for noninvasive mechanical ventilation, *Respir Care* 54(1):71–84, 2009.

Nava S, Schreiber A, Domenighetti G: Noninvasive ventilation for patients with acute lung injury or acute respiratory distress syndrome, *Respir Care* 56(10):1583–1588, 2011.

Nilsestuen JO, Hargett KD: Using ventilator graphics to identify patient-ventilator asynchrony, *Respir Care* 50(2):202, 2005.

Oto J, Imanaka H, Nakataki E, Ono R, Nishimura M: Potential inadequacy of automatic tube compensation to decrease inspiratory work load after at least 48 hours of endotracheal tube use in the clinical setting, *Respir Care* 57(5):697–703, 2012.

Pennock BE, Kaplan PD, Carlin BW, et al.: Pressure support ventilation with a simplified ventilatory support system administered with a nasal mask in patients with respiratory failure, *Chest* 100(5):1371, 1991.

Pezzano CJ: Physiological effects of mechanical ventilation. In Wyka KA, Mathews PJ, Rutkowski J, editors: *Foundations of respiratory care*, ed 2, Clifton Park, NY, 2012, Delmar.

Pierson DJ: Patient-ventilator interaction, *Respir Care* 56(2):214–228, 2011.

Pierson DJ: Indications for mechanical ventilation in adults with acute respiratory failure, *Respir Care* 47(3):249, 2002.

Piriyapatsom A, Bittner EA, Hines J, Schmidt UH: Sedation and paralysis, *Respir Care* 58(6):1024–1037, 2013.

Quan SF, Parides GC, Knoper SR: Mandatory minute volume (MVV) ventilation: an overview, *Respir Care* 35(9):898, 1990.

Radford EP Jr: Ventilation standards for use in artificial respiration, *J Appl Phys* 7:451, 1955.

Respironics: Guidelines for invasive applications with BiPAP systems, Carlsbad, CA, Philips Healthcare.

Respironics: Product literature on the suggested protocol for initiation of the BiPAP S/T or BiPAP S/T-D ventilatory support system, Carlsbad, CA, Philips Healthcare.

Sassoon CSH: Triggering of the ventilator in patient-ventilator interactions, *Respir Care* 56(1):39–49, 2011.

Saura P, Blanch L: How to set positive end-expiratory pressure, *Respir Care* 47(3):279, 2002.

Sehlin M, Törnell SS, Öhberg F, Johansson G, Winsö O: Pneumatic performance of the Boussignac CPAP system in health humans, *Respir Care* 56(6):818–826, 2011.

Shelledy DC: Discontinuing ventilatory support. In Wilkins RL, Stoller JK, Kacmarek RM, editors: *Egan's fundamentals of respiratory care*, ed 9, St Louis, 2009, Mosby.

Shelledy DC: Initiating and adjusting ventilatory support. In Wilkins RL, Stoller JK, Kacmarek RM, editors: *Egan's fundamentals of respiratory care*, ed 9, St Louis, 2009, Mosby.

Shelledy DC, Mikles SP: Newer modes of mechanical ventilation, I: pressure support, *Respir Manage*, July/Aug 14, 1988.

Shelledy DC, Mikles SP: Newer modes of mechanical ventilation, II: mandatory minute volume ventilation, *Respir Manage*, July/Aug 21, 1988.

Stoller JK: Establishing clinical unweanability, *Respir Care* 36(3): 186, 1991.

Strumpf DA, Carlisle CC, Millman RP, et al.: An evaluation of the Respironics BiPAP Bi-Level CPAP device for delivery of assisted ventilation, *Respir Care* 35(5):415, 1990.

The Acute Respiratory Distress Syndrome Network: *Ventilation with lower tidal volumes as compared with traditional tidal volumes for acute lung injury and the acute respiratory distress syndrome*. http://www.nejm.org/content/browser/1.asp, May 2000.

Tobin MJ: Monitoring of pressure, flow, and volume during mechanical ventilation, *Respir Care* 37(9):1081, 1992.

Tobin MJ, Lodato RF: PEEP, auto-PEEP, and waterfalls, *Chest* 96(3):449, 1989.

Tonnelier A, Tonnelier J-M, Nowak E, Gut-Gobert C, Prat G, Renault A, et al.: Clinical relevance of classification according to weaning difficulty, *Respir Care* 56(5):583–590, 2011.

Waldhorn RE: Nocturnal nasal intermittent positive pressure ventilation with bi-level positive airway pressure (BiPAP) in respiratory failure, *Chest* 101(2):516, 1992.

Waugh JB, Deshpande VM, Harwood RJ, Brown M: *Rapid interpretation of ventilator waveforms*, ed 2, Upper Saddle River, NJ, 2007, Pearson Prentice Hall.

Wellman T: Mechanics and modes of mechanical ventilation. In Wyka KA, Mathews PJ, Rutkowski J, editors: *Foundations of respiratory care*, ed 2, Clifton Park, NY, 2012, Delmar.

Wellman T: Noninvasive mechanical ventilation. In Wyka KA, Mathews PJ, Rutkowski J, editors: *Foundations of respiratory care*, ed 2, Clifton Park, NY, 2012, Delmar.

White GC: *Equipment theory for respiratory care*, ed 4, Albany, NY, 2005, Delmar.

Williams PF: Noninvasive mechanical ventilation. In Kacmarek RM, Stoller JK, Heuer AJ, editors: *Egan's fundamentals of respiratory care*, ed 10, St Louis, 2013, Mosby.

Wright J, Gong H: "Auto-PEEP": incidence, magnitude, and contributing factors, *Heart Lung* 19(4):352, 1990.

SELF-STUDY QUESTIONS

See Appendix for answers.

1. A 45-year-old female patient with sepsis is developing ARDS. She weighs 64 kg (141 lb) and has a ventilator tidal volume of 450 mL, rate of 13/min, and 10 cm water PEEP. Her arterial blood gas values are acceptable on 40% oxygen but her C_{LT} is decreasing and plateau pressure is now 35 cm water. What should be recommended to the physician?
   A. Tidal volume of 300 mL and rate of 20/min
   B. Increase PEEP to 15 cm water.
   C. Tidal volume of 600 mL and rate of 10/min
   D. Continue to monitor the patient's condition.

2. An unconscious, apneic adult male patient with a drug overdose has been admitted through the Emergency Department. He will be placed onto an older ventilator that cannot compensate for compressed volume. His ideal body weight is 80 kg (176 lb). The most appropriate uncorrected ventilator V_T would be:
   A. 950 mL
   B. 800 mL
   C. 550 mL
   D. 400 mL

3. A patient with ARDS is receiving mechanical ventilation in the PC, A/C mode with a tidal volume of 400 mL, rate of 24, 60% oxygen, and 15 cm H_2O PEEP. After performing a lung recruitment maneuver, the respiratory therapist determines the lower inflection point at 20 cm H_2O and the upper inflection point at 35 cm H_2O. Where should the PEEP level be set?
   A. <15 cm H_2O
   B. 15 cm H_2O
   C. Between 20 and 35 cm H_2O
   D. >35 cm H_2O

4. An adult male patient is on the PC, SIMV mode with a ventilator V_T of 600 mL and a backup rate of 10 times/min. His total rate is 18/min. The physician would like to evaluate the patient's readiness to wean from the ventilator. Which of the following parameters indicate that the ventilator can be discontinued?
   1. Spontaneous V_T of 5 mL/kg of ideal body weight
   2. V_D/V_T ratio of 0.4
   3. Intrapulmonary shunt of 10%
   4. VC of 9 mL/kg of ideal body weight
   5. MIP of −15 cm H_2O
   A. 1 and 2 only
   B. 3, 4, and 5 only
   C. 1, 2, and 3 only
   D. 2, 3, 4, and 5 only

5. The physician asks the respiratory therapist about which weaning method would be most successful in the patient with the weaning parameters listed in Question 4. The patient's spontaneous V_T is 400 mL. Which of the following methods should be recommended?
   A. T-piece and extubation in 30 minutes
   B. Intermittent ventilator discontinuance
   C. SIMV weaning
   D. PCV

6. A 25-year-old female postoperative patient is receiving mechanical ventilation. She is alert with a spontaneous V_T of 200 mL and the desire to breathe on her own. Because of the emergency nature of her surgery, she has a smaller than normal endotracheal tube.

Her PaO_2 is 93 torr on 40% O_2. What ventilator mode should be recommended for her?
  A. PS with PEEP
  B. MMV
  C. SIMV with PS and PEEP
  D. SIMV with PS

7. An adult patient is recovering from ARDS. The mechanical ventilator is providing CPAP at 10 cm H_2O CPAP and 40% O_2 during a spontaneous breathing trial. In evaluating the patient after 1 hour, you notice the following: SpO_2 has dropped from 95% to 90%, respiratory rate has increased from 14 to 23 breaths/min, and the patient is complaining of tiredness. What should be done?
  A. Continue for another hour and reevaluate.
  B. Raise the CPAP level to 13 cm H_2O.
  C. Decrease the CPAP to 7 cm H_2O because the patient is tired.
  D. Resume mechanical ventilation.

8. A patient has an HME in place for humidification purposes. The respiratory therapist notices that the peak pressure has increased by 10 cm H_2O in the past hour. The nurse reported to you that the patient had thick secretions when last suctioned. What should be done in this situation?
  A. Switch to a cool pass-over-type humidifier.
  B. Switch to a heated wick-type humidifier.
  C. Instill normal saline before suctioning.
  D. Turn up the temperature on the HME.

9. A mechanically ventilated female patient with pulmonary edema has the following blood gas values on 40% O_2: pH 7.43, $PaCO_2$ 35 torr, and PaO_2 75 torr. She is on the VC, A/C mode with a backup rate of 10 breaths/min and is assisting for a total rate of 18 breaths/min. Her peak airway pressure is 50 cm H_2O, and her plateau pressure is 40 cm H_2O. She developed a pneumothorax and had a chest tube inserted. What should be suggested to the physician?
  A. Switch her to the PC, A/C mode.
  B. Switch her to the APRV mode.
  C. Switch her to the CPAP mode.
  D. Sedate her so that she does not assist.

10. The respiratory therapist has started a patient on the A/C mode and will be using pressure sensitivity for patient breath triggering. What should the control be set at?
  A. 0 cm H_2O
  B. −1 to −2 cm H_2O
  C. −5 cm H_2O
  D. 1-2 cm H_2O

11. In preparing for a mode change from A/C to SIMV, the following must be done:
  1. **Turn the sensitivity control off.**
  2. **Inform the patient of the change.**
  3. Turn off the ventilator's sigh control.
  4. Add 5 cm H_2O of therapeutic PEEP.
  5. Remove any mechanical dead space.
  A. 3 and 4 only
  B. 1, 3, and 4 only
  C. 2, 4, and 5 only
  D. 2, 3, and 5 only

12. Which of the following indicates that the patient is not tolerating PEEP?
  1. Increased Cst
  2. Decreased Cst
  3. Increased intrapulmonary shunt
  4. Decreasing dead space
  5. Decreasing blood pressure
  A. 2 and 3 only
  B. 3 and 4 only
  C. 1, 3, and 5 only
  D. 2, 3, and 5 only

13. An adult mechanically ventilated patient has had a tracheostomy tube placed while in the Intensive Care Unit. When the patient coughs vigorously, about 10 mL of blood is coughed into the ventilator circuit. What should be done?
  A. Replace the circuit with a new one.
  B. Flush the blood out of the circuit with normal saline.
  C. Sedate the patient to prevent more coughing.
  D. Nebulize a local anesthetic to reduce surgical pain.

14. A patient with pneumonia is receiving mechanical ventilation, and an HME is being used for humidification. After receiving an aerosolized bronchodilator treatment, the patient coughs secretions into the HME. The high-pressure alarm begins to sound off. What should be done?
  A. Reset the high-pressure alarm.
  B. Replace the HME.
  C. Stop the bronchodilator treatment.
  D. Suction the patient.

15. A patient's breathing is being supported by a ventilator that has a circuit with an external exhalation valve. The nurse calls the respiratory therapist to evaluate the patient because the alarm is going off. Upon arrival, the therapist notices that the patient's chest is barely moving during a control breath, the peak pressure does not rise above 3 cm H_2O, and the exhaled V_T spirometer shows the set V_T when the control breath is delivered. The most likely cause of these findings is:
  A. The machine is self-cycling.
  B. The inspiratory and expiratory limbs of the circuit are reversed.
  C. The tubing to the exhalation valve is disconnected.
  D. The spirometer is out of calibration.

16. Expiratory retard would be indicated in a patient with:
    - A. Pulmonary edema
    - B. Air trapping
    - C. Pleural effusion
    - D. Pneumothorax

17. All of the following parameters indicate the need for intubation and mechanical ventilation EXCEPT:
    - A. VC of less than 10 mL/kg of ideal body weight
    - B. MIP of less than –15 cm H_2O
    - C. P(A–a)O_2 on 100% O_2 of 40 torr
    - D. V_D/V_T of 0.7

18. A patient with post-polio syndrome is being ventilated with NPPV and has an IPAP level of 15 cm water and an EPAP level of 5 cm water. The patient complains of being short of breath. The respiratory therapist checks the patient's V_T and finds that it has dropped. How should the tidal volume be restored?
    - A. Lower the IPAP level.
    - B. Lower the EPAP level.
    - C. Raise the IPAP level.
    - D. Raise the EPAP level.

19. A respiratory therapist is working with a patient with obstructive sleep apnea who is receiving bilevel NPPV through a nasal mask. During a sleep period, it is noticed that he is snoring. Which of the following ventilator adjustments should be made?
    - A. Increase the respiratory rate.
    - B. Increase the upper pressure level.
    - C. Increase the lower pressure level.
    - D. Loosen the nasal mask.

20. A respiratory therapist is working with an 80-kg (176-lb) patient who is apneic after abdominal surgery. The patient is being ventilated with the A/C mode and has the following settings:

$\dot{V}_E$	5.6 L
Rate	10/min
I:E ratio	1:3
Inspired O_2	35%
Mechanical dead space	100 mL

    The ABG results show the following:

pH	7.31
PaCO$_2$	50 torr
PaO$_2$	70 torr
HCO$_3^-$	24 mEq/L
BE	0
SaO$_2$	95%

    Which of the following should be recommended?
    - A. Remove the mechanical dead space.
    - B. Decrease the patient's $\dot{V}_E$.

    - C. Change the I:E ratio to 1:2.
    - D. Add 5 cm H_2O PEEP.

21. It is noticed that a patient's peak pressure has increased from 20 to 40 cm water without a change in static pressure. Possible causes of this include which of the following?
    1. **Retained secretions**
    2. **Pleural effusion**
    3. **Bronchospasm**
    4. **Pulmonary edema**
    - A. 2 and 4 only
    - B. 1 and 2 only
    - C. 1 and 3 only
    - D. 3 and 4 only

22. Which of the following will have the greatest impact on increasing the mean airway pressure?
    - A. Increasing the inspiratory flow
    - B. Adding 5 cm H_2O PEEP
    - C. Removing 0.5 second of inflation hold
    - D. Increasing the expiratory time by 0.25 second

23. If a ventilator-dependent patient has a large amount of thick tracheal secretions, it is best to:
    - A. Use a heated cascade-type humidifier.
    - B. Use an HME for his or her humidity needs.
    - C. Use no humidification system so that the secretions will dry.
    - D. Nebulize normal saline every 2-4 hours.

24. All of the following are needed to assemble a free-standing CPAP system EXCEPT:
    - A. Exhaled volume spirometer
    - B. Disconnect alarm
    - C. Water traps
    - D. CPAP pressure device

25. A pediatric patient is receiving volume-controlled ventilation with a tidal volume of 250 mL. The patient's breath sounds are clear, but the expiratory flow is seen on the monitor to not return to baseline before the next breath. How could this be interpreted?
    - A. Presence of auto-PEEP
    - B. Too small a tidal volume
    - C. Decreasing C_{LT}
    - D. Decreased airway resistance

26. The following values are found on an adult patient receiving volume-cycled ventilation with the VC, A/C mode:

Tidal volume	500 mL
Peak flow	45 L/min (0.75 L/s)
Peak pressure	40 cm H_2O
Plateau pressure	20 cm H_2O
PEEP	5 cm H_2O

Calculate the patient's airway resistance (cm H_2O/L/s).

A. 0.4
B. 15
C. 27
D. 800

27. A 16-year-old patient with severe asthma has been receiving nebulized albuterol (Proventil) treatments through the ventilator over the past 12 hours. What can the respiratory therapist recommend to best evaluate the patient's response?
   A. Breath sounds
   B. Chest radiograph
   C. Check airway resistance changes
   D. Check C_{LT} changes

28. A 75-year-old male with congestive heart failure has been receiving mechanical ventilation over the past 24 hours. The diuretic drug furosemide (Lasix) has been given several times. What is the best way to evaluate how the patient's lung function is responding?
   A. Compare the patient's admission weight versus current weight.
   B. Compare C_{LT} measurements at the start of therapy and now.
   C. Compare airway resistance measurements at the start of therapy and now.
   D. Evaluate breath sound changes over the past 24 hours.

29. After open heart surgery, a patient is receiving mechanical ventilation. The patient needs to have a pacemaker inserted in the cardiac procedures lab. It is expected that the patient will be back in the Intensive Care Unit within an hour or two. How should ventilatory support be provided during this time?
   A. Microprocessor-type ventilator
   B. Manual ventilation with a resuscitation bag
   C. NIV
   D. Pressure-cycled transport ventilator

30. A patient with emphysema is receiving mechanical ventilation with the following settings:

Mode	VC, A/C
Set tidal volume	600 mL
Set rate	12
Total rate	12
F_IO_2	0.30
I:E ratio	1:2

During a ventilator check, you measure the patient's exhaled tidal volume at 500 mL. What can be done to help the patient exhale more completely?
   A. Change to the Pressure Control mode.
   B. Change to a larger endotracheal tube.

C. Increase the expiratory time.
D. Decrease inspiratory flow.

31. After abdominal surgery, a female patient is awakening gradually from anesthesia. Her ventilator settings are as follows:

Mode	VC, SIMV
Set tidal volume	550 mL
Spontaneous tidal volume	400 mL when awake
Set rate	12
Total rate	16 when awake
F_IO_2	0.30
Inspiratory flow	40 L/min

When awake, she uses accessory muscles and her breathing is not synchronized with the ventilator. What can be done to improve synchrony?
   A. Increase the inspiratory flow to 50 L/min.
   B. Decrease the set tidal volume.
   C. Give her more pain medication.
   D. Give her more oxygen.

32. An adult patient with myasthenia gravis is receiving mechanical ventilation with these settings:

Mode	PC, A/C
Set tidal volume	450 mL
Set rate	10
Total rate	15
F_IO_2	0.40
Inspiratory flow	60 L/min

The patient's blood gas values are all within the normal range. While performing patient–ventilator rounds, you notice that the patient is making 24 breathing efforts/min and is using inspiratory accessory muscles. What should be done?
   A. Increase the oxygen percentage.
   B. Increase the inspiratory flow.
   C. Increase the set rate to 15.
   D. Increase the flow sensitivity.

33. An unconscious adult patient has been received in the Emergency Department after suffering a stroke. The only ventilator available is an older volume-cycled unit. The physician asks the respiratory therapist for a recommendation on the initial set ventilator tidal volume to use with the patient, who weighs 73 kg (160 lb). What should be recommended?
   A. 1000 mL
   B. 700 mL
   C. 500 mL
   D. 320 mL

34. A 6-year-old postoperative patient will be started on mechanical ventilation. What should be the initial respiratory rate?
    A. 14/min
    B. 20/min
    C. 50/min
    D. 80/min

35. A 50-year-old, 75-kg (165-lb), male patient has just returned from open heart surgery and has been placed on a microprocessor mechanical ventilator with the following settings:

Mode	VC, A/C
Set tidal volume	500 mL
Set rate	12
Total rate	12
F_IO_2	0.50
I:E ratio	1:3

After 45 minutes, he has the following arterial blood gas values:

pH	7.50
$PaCO_2$	30 torr
PaO_2	115 torr
HCO_3^-	22 mEq/L
BE	−2 mEq/L

What should be done in this situation?
    A. Decrease the tidal volume to 400 mL.
    B. Decrease the oxygen to 40%.
    C. Decrease the respiratory rate to 10/min.
    D. Increase the respiratory rate to 14/min.

36. A patient with bilateral pneumonia is receiving mechanical ventilation with the following settings:

Mode	PC, SIMV
Set tidal volume	650 mL
Set rate	14
F_IO_2	0.50
I:E ratio	1:2
PEEP	10 cm H_2O

The nurse is concerned that the patient's SpO_2 value drops from 94% to 85% when suctioned. How can this be prevented?
    A. Give 100% oxygen before suctioning.
    B. Perform suction only once an hour.
    C. Use the largest suction catheter available.
    D. Increase the PEEP level to 15 cm H_2O before suctioning.

37. A 40-year-old, 60-kg (132-lb) female patient is recovering from ARDS. Her current ventilator settings are as follows:

Mode	VC, A/C
Set tidal volume	400 mL
Set rate	12
Total rate	18
F_IO_2	0.40
I:E ratio	1:3

She has the following arterial blood gas values:

pH	7.42
$PaCO_2$	37 torr
PaO_2	85 torr
HCO_3^-	25 mEq/L
BE	+1 mEq/L

She has no complications and is conscious and cooperative. Her spontaneous tidal volume is 300 mL and vital capacity is 800 mL. What should be recommended at this time?
    A. Change to the APRV mode.
    B. Increase the set rate.
    C. Decrease the tidal volume.
    D. Change to the PS mode.

38. An adult male is recovering from a flail chest injury and the physician wants to wean him from the ventilator. The patient is intubated with a 7.0-mm-ID endotracheal tube and is breathing with support of the SIMV mode. When the set rate was decreased from 8 to 6/min, the patient became tired. How can the patient's WOB be decreased?
    A. Increase the flow through the ventilator during SIMV breaths.
    B. Nebulize a bronchodilator medication.
    C. Add automatic tube compensation.
    D. Maintain the set respiratory rate at 8.

39. A 65-year-old, 70-kg (155-lb), male patient who suffered a heart attack is receiving mechanical ventilation with the following settings:

Mode	PC, SIMV, plus Pressure Support
Set tidal volume	500 mL
Set rate	12
Total rate	18
F_IO_2	0.70

The physician is concerned that the patient may be developing pulmonary edema. These arterial blood gas values were recorded while the patient was on the ventilator:

pH	7.43
$PaCO_2$	35 torr
PaO_2	50 torr
HCO_3^-	22 mEq/L
BE	−2 mEq/L

What should be done to help manage the patient?
A. Increase the oxygen to 100%.
B. Add mechanical dead space.
C. Increase the set rate to 18/min.
D. Add 5 cm water PEEP therapy.

40. A 42-year-old patient was accidentally given an overdose of morphine for pain after surgery. Because the drug caused hypoventilation, the patient was intubated and started on mechanical ventilation in the VC, A/C mode. The morphine now has been reversed and the patient is awake. The patient has the following bedside spirometry values:

Respiratory rate	16/min
Vital capacity	2300 mL
Tidal volume	400 mL
Maximum inspiratory pressure	−55 cm H_2O

What should be done at this time?
A. Reassess the patient in 4 hours.
B. Change to the SIMV mode.
C. Remove the endotracheal tube.
D. Spontaneous breathing trial on a T-piece.

41. The PCIRV mode is indicated in which of the following conditions?
A. Asthma
B. Chronic bronchitis
C. Pulmonary contusion
D. ARDS

42. A patient is receiving CPAP at 10 cm water pressure with 40% oxygen and a flow of 6 L/min. The nurse calls the respiratory therapist because the low-pressure alarm is periodically sounding off. The therapist finds the patient to be alert and breathing comfortably. The pressure gauge shows the CPAP pressure fluctuating between 10 and 6 cm water pressure. The low-pressure alarm is set at 8 cm water with a delay of 5 seconds. What should be done about this situation?
A. Increase the flow.
B. Sedate the patient.
C. Increase the alarm delay to 10 seconds.
D. Set the low-pressure alarm at 5 cm water.

43. Which of the following clinical conditions could result in a decreased C_{LT} and increasing plateau pressure?
1. Pulmonary edema
2. Pneumonia
3. Emphysema
4. ARDS
A. 1 and 2 only
B. 2 and 3 only
C. 1, 2, and 4 only
D. 1, 2, 3, 4

44. MMV ventilation:
1. Is similar to the VC, A/C mode
2. Is indicated when a patient has an unstable respiratory drive
3. Ensures a minimum minute volume
4. Is a substitute for CPAP
A. 1 only
B. 3 only
C. 2 and 3 only
D. 1 and 4 only

45. High-frequency ventilation would be indicated for all of the following situations EXCEPT:
A. Laryngoscopy
B. Near drowning
C. Bronchopleural fistula
D. Bronchoscopy

46. A patient having a spontaneous breathing trial for weaning should be carefully assessed. Weaning should be terminated when:
1. The patient's rapid, shallow breathing index is 120
2. Cardiac dysrhythmias occur
3. The patient's $PaCO_2$ is 60 torr
4. The patient's PaO_2 is 70 torr on 40% oxygen
A. 1 and 3 only
B. 2 and 4 only
C. 2, 3, and 4 only
D. 1, 2, and 3 only

47. An adult patient was receiving a tidal volume of 500 mL on the ventilator before going to the operating room for a left pneumonectomy. How should the patient's breathing be supported after surgery?
A. Tidal volume less than before surgery.
B. The same tidal volume as before surgery.
C. A larger tidal volume than before surgery.
D. CPAP should be used.

48. A negative-pressure ventilator is indicated for all the following types of patients EXCEPT:
A. ARDS
B. Neuromuscular defects
C. Kyphoscoliosis
D. COPD in acute failure

49. An adult patient with an acute lung injury has had an optimal PEEP study performed. Which of the following parameters found during the study would help determine the best PEEP setting?
    1. Pulmonary compliance improves
    2. PaO_2 increases
    3. Shunt percentage decreases
    4. Pulmonary vascular resistance increases
    5. Pulmonary vascular resistance decreases
    6. Blood pressure decreases and heart rate increases
    A. 2, 4, and 6 only
    B. 1, 2, 3, and 5 only
    C. 2, 3, 5, and 6 only
    D. 1, 2, 3, and 4 only

50. A patient with pulmonary edema is receiving VC, A/C with the following clinical data: Set tidal volume is 700 mL. Corrected tidal volume is 600 mL. Peak pressure is 65 cm water. Plateau pressure is 48 cm water. There is 12 cm water of PEEP. Calculate the patient's static compliance.
    A. 13 mL/cm water
    B. 15 mL/cm water
    C. 17 mL/cm water
    D. 19 mL/cm water

Use the following information for questions 51 and 52: A mechanically ventilated patient has an exhaled tidal volume of 700 mL. Because of refractory hypoxemia, 6 cm of PEEP therapy is started. The peak pressure is 35 cm water, and the plateau pressure is 25 cm water. The compliance factor has been determined to be 4 mL/cm water.

51. Calculate the Cst for this patient.
    A. 19 mL/cm water
    B. 24 mL/cm water
    C. 28 mL/cm water
    D. 32 mL/cm water

52. Calculate the Cdyn for this patient.
    A. 16 mL/cm water
    B. 19 mL/cm water
    C. 24 mL/cm water
    D. 32 mL/cm water

53. When preparing to ventilate a patient with HFJV, it is necessary to have all of the following EXCEPT:
    A. Spirometer to measure tidal volume
    B. Jet injector line
    C. High-pressure oxygen source
    D. Humidifier

54. Over the course of an 8-hour shift, the respiratory therapist notices that a patient receiving constant volume ventilation has had an increase in peak pressure from 25 to 40 cm water. What could have caused this change?
    1. Airway resistance decreased
    2. C_{LT} increased
    3. Airway resistance increased
    4. C_{LT} decreased
    A. 3 only
    B. 4 only
    C. 3 and 4 only
    D. 1 and 2 only

55. A 45-year-old patient has developed pulmonary edema. The physician asks the respiratory therapist for the best ventilator adjustment to reduce the patient's intrapulmonary shunting. The therapist should recommend:
    A. Increasing the inspiratory time
    B. Increasing the sigh volume
    C. Decreasing the respiratory rate
    D. Increasing the PEEP

56. A trauma patient has a pleural chest tube to the left lung. A microprocessor-type ventilator is delivering an inspiratory tidal volume of 800 mL. The expiratory tidal volume is shown to be 600 mL. What could best explain the volume difference?
    A. Air leak through the chest tube
    B. Deflated endotracheal tube cuff
    C. Miscalibrated spirometer
    D. Bronchospasm and auto-PEEP

57. In a patient with ARDS, the indication to switch from volume-cycled ventilation to pressure-cycled ventilation is:
    A. Peak pressure of 30 cm water or greater
    B. C_{LT} less than 30 mL/cm water
    C. Plateau pressure of 30 cm water or greater
    D. Peak pressure and plateau pressure total >30 cm water

58. A 70-kg (154-lb) patient with a stroke and increased ICP is being mechanically ventilated in the A/C mode with the following settings:

Minute ventilation	6.0 L
I:E ratio	1:2
F_IO_2	0.35
Rate	12

The patient's ABG results are as follows:

pH	7.39
$PaCO_2$	43 torr
PaO_2	107 torr
BE	0
SaO_2	100%

On the basis of this information, it would be most appropriate to recommend:
- A. Decreasing the F_1O_2
- B. Decreasing the minute ventilation
- C. Increasing the respiratory rate
- D. Increasing the expiratory time

59. The chest radiograph of a patient receiving mechanical ventilation reveals atelectasis in both bases. In addition, the patient's breath sounds are diminished bilaterally, and she has a low-grade fever. Which of the following ventilator adjustments should the respiratory therapist recommend?
- A. Increase the flow rate
- B. Lengthen the expiratory time
- C. Increase the ventilator frequency
- D. Increase the ventilator sigh volume

60. A patient with ARDS is receiving a smaller than normal tidal volume with resulting hypercarbia. What guidelines should be followed with permissive hypercapnia?
1. Bicarbonate may be given to increase the pH.
2. The carbon dioxide level is allowed to increase.
3. The pH should be kept between 7.45 and 7.35.
4. The pH should be kept greater than 7.25.
5. The $PaCO_2$ should be kept between 40 and 50 torr.
- A. 3 and 5 only
- B. 2 and 4 only
- C. 2 and 5 only
- D. 1, 2, and 4 only

61. An adult female patient has the desire to breathe spontaneously and has a tidal volume that is 4 mL/kg of ideal body weight. Because of facial trauma from an automobile accident, she has a 6.5-mm-ID endotracheal tube. She also had lung contusions in the crash. Her PaO_2 is 63 torr on 55% oxygen. What ventilator mode(s) should be recommended for her?
- A. A/C with flow sensitivity for triggering the ventilator
- B. Low-level Pressure Support Ventilation with PEEP
- C. SIMV with low-level Pressure Support and PEEP
- D. SIMV with high-level Pressure Support Ventilation (PSV_{max})

62. An apneic 60-kg (132-lb) patient is being ventilated with the PC, A/C mode. The patient's ventilator settings are:

Tidal volume	400 mL
Rate	10/min
Oxygen	60%
Mechanical dead space	100 mL

The patient's ABG shows:

pH	7.32
$PaCO_2$	55 torr
PaO_2	66 torr
HCO_3^-	28 mEq/L
Base excess	+4

Considering this information, all of the following individual ventilator adjustments would improve the patient's ABG values EXCEPT:
- A. Increase the respiratory rate to 14/min.
- B. Increase the tidal volume to 500 mL.
- C. Change to SIMV with a rate of 10/min.
- D. Remove the mechanical dead space.

63. Indications that the patient is tolerating SIMV include all of the following EXCEPT:
- A. The respiratory rate is increased.
- B. The heart rate is stable.
- C. The blood gas results are stable.
- D. Accessory muscles of ventilation are not being used.

64. A 55-kg (120-lb) female patient is being ventilated with the PC, SIMV mode and a rate of 10, tidal volume of 400 mL, 10 cm water of therapeutic PEEP, and 35% inspired oxygen. She has an 8.0-mm-inner diameter tracheostomy tube. Her spontaneous tidal volume is 300 mL, with a rate of 10/min. The most recent ABG shows:

pH	7.40
$PaCO_2$	41 torr
PaO_2	95 torr
HCO_3^-	24 mEq/L
Base excess	0

What should be recommended?
- A. Reduce the SIMV rate to 3.
- B. Reduce the PEEP to 7 cm water.
- C. Increase the SIMV rate to 12.
- D. Add 10 cm of Pressure Support.

65. Five adult patients are being weaned from mechanical ventilation. After a 30-minute spontaneous breathing trial, their bedside spirometry values are shown below.

	$\dot{V}_E$ f	V_T (L)	FEV$_1$ (mL)	MIP (mL/kg)	(cm water)
Patient 1	7	2.45	350	5	−35
Patient 2	12	5.44	501	10	−30
Patient 3	15	8.25	550	15	−20
Patient 4	37	11.1	300	13	−15
Patient 5	40	17.0	425	7	−15

12 × 500

Which of the patients are ready for extubation?
A. Patients 1 and 2
B. Patients 1 and 4
C. Patients 2 and 3
D. Patients 3 and 5

66. The measurements below are obtained on a patient while the patient is being mechanically ventilated:

	6:00 PM	8:00 PM
Total respiratory rate	14	14
PEEP, cm water	8	8
P plateau, cm water	15	15
P peak, cm water	30	45
Compliance, mL/cm water	40	40

In this situation, the most appropriate action would be to:
A. Increase therapeutic PEEP.
B. Administer a bronchodilating agent.
C. Administer a diuretic agent.
D. Administer a paralyzing agent.

67. When working with a patient who recently had a bowel resection and is receiving a paralyzing medication to prevent fighting against the ventilator, it is important to:
A. Give the patient caffeine as a central nervous system stimulant.
B. Give the patient a sedative medication for pain.
C. Give the patient a medication for pain.
D. Talk quietly because the patient is probably sleeping.

68. A patient with a closed head injury and increased ICP is being ventilated mechanically in the VC, A/C mode with an F_1O_2 of 0.5, a rate of 12, and a tidal volume of 600 mL. The patient's ABG results are shown:

pH	7.43
$PaCO_2$	35 torr
PaO_2	195 torr
HCO_3^-	22 mEq/L
Base excess	−2
SaO_2	100%

The physician orders a $PaCO_2$ of 25 torr for the patient. What should the respiratory therapist change on the ventilator to accomplish this?
A. Add mechanical dead space.
B. Increase the tidal volume.
C. Decrease the oxygen percentage.
D. Decrease the ventilator rate.

69. An 80-kg (176-lb) man with bilateral pneumonia is being ventilated in the PC, A/C mode. The following data are available:

	8:00 PM	12:00 PM
Set respiratory rate	12/min	12/min
Total respiratory rate	16/min	26/min
Exhaled tidal volume	800 mL	600 mL
Inspiratory pressure	28 cm water	28 cm water

What is the most appropriate thing to do at this time?
A. Sedate the patient.
B. Increase the set respiratory rate.
C. Add Pressure Support.
D. Increase the inspiratory pressure.

70. A 17-year-old female has been admitted with status asthmaticus and placed on a microprocessor ventilator. The physician wants to know if she has any auto-PEEP. Which ventilator waveform would be best for determining this?
A. Maximum Voluntary Ventilation tracing
B. Flow/volume loop
C. Flow/time tracing
D. Pressure/time tracing

71. An adult female patient will be receiving NIV at night in her home for obstructive sleep apnea. The nasal mask has been applied and these NIV parameters have been set: IPAP 15 cm H_2O, EPAP 4 cm H_2O, rate 14/min, 30% oxygen. After trying the NIV system for 10 minutes, the patient states that she is not getting enough air. What is the first adjustment to make?
A. Increase the rate to 16 per minute.
B. Increase the oxygen to 40%.
C. Increase the IPAP to 20 cm H_2O.
D. Increase the EPAP to 8 cm H_2O.

72. After suffering multiple traumas from an automobile accident, a 43-year-old male patient is recovering. Mechanical ventilation has been needed for 5 days, and weaning is being tried for the first time. After breathing on a T-piece for 40 minutes, the patient has the following arterial blood gas values while breathing 40% oxygen:

pH	7.30
$PaCO_2$	54 torr
PaO_2	65 torr
HCO_3^-	26 mEq/L
BE	+2 mEq/L
SpO_2	91%

Bedside spirometry values are as follows:

	Start of Wean	After 40 Minutes
Vital capacity	1100 mL	700 mL
Tidal volume	400 mL	300 mL
Respiratory rate	14/min	28/min
Maximum inspiratory pressure	−26 cm H_2O	−15 cm H_2O

Based on this information, what should be recommended?

A. Return the patient to mechanical ventilation.
B. Extubate and give the patient 50% oxygen.
C. Extubate and begin PEP therapy treatments every 4 hours.
D. Continue to monitor the patient's weaning trial.

73. An adult patient with ARDS has developed a pneumothorax during volume-controlled mechanical ventilation. The physician has decided to change the patient to HFO. The following HFO parameters have been set:

Frequency	4 Hz
Amplitude	20 cm water
I:E ratio	1:2
Oxygen	60%
PEEP	8 cm water

After 50 minutes of HFO, the patient has the following blood gas values:

pH	7.31
$PaCO_2$	52 torr
PaO_2	66 torr
HCO_3^-	27 mEq/L
BE	+2 mEq/L
SpO_2	92%

What should the respiratory therapist recommend?

A. Increase the PEEP to 15 cm water.
B. Increase the amplitude to 25 cm water.
C. Change the I:E ratio to 1:1.
D. Continue to monitor the patient.

16

Mechanical Ventilation of the Neonate

Note: It can be anticipated that the Therapist Multiple-Choice Examination (TMC) will include an *average of 2 of 140 actual questions* (1% of the exam) on neonatal mechanical ventilation. (This is based on the question mix typically found on the National Board of Respiratory Care's (NBRC's) previous Entry Level Examinations and Written Registry Examinations.)

Remember that the TMC version you take will include 20 additional questions being evaluated for possible inclusion in other versions of the TMC. So, there will be a total of 160 questions taken. There is no way to differentiate between the 140 actual questions and the 20 questions being evaluated for future use. Please go to the Introduction for detailed information on the TMC and the Clinical Simulation Examination.

MODULE A

Perform continuous positive airway pressure to support oxygenation and ventilation.

1. Initiate and adjust continuous positive airway pressure (code: IIIC3) [difficulty: R, Ap, An]

a. Physiologic effects

Continuous positive airway pressure (CPAP) and positive end-expiratory pressure (PEEP) increase the patient's functional residual capacity (FRC). In neonates, the most common cause of a decreased FRC is infant respiratory distress syndrome (RDS). This condition is caused by the lack of surfactant in the lungs of the premature neonate. The neonate with RDS has relatively airless lungs with decreased compliance that are prone to atelectasis. This results in increased work of breathing and hypoxemia. Each tidal volume breath requires a greater than normal inspiratory effort (Fig. 16-1). The restoration of FRC in the neonate increases its PaO_2, decreases the percentage of shunt, narrows the alveolar-to-arterial difference in oxygen, and reduces the work of tidal volume breathing. CPAP must be used with caution in neonates with persistent pulmonary hypertension (PPHN). An excessive amount of pressure in the alveoli compresses the capillary bed. This decreases pulmonary blood flow, which in turn increases blood flow through the patent ductus arteriosus and worsens the problem.

b. Indications, contraindications, and hazards

CPAP is indicated for any condition that results in an unacceptably low PaO_2 secondary to a decreased FRC. Some neonates respond so well to CPAP that mechanical ventilation is not needed. In addition, CPAP has been used to keep open the airways of infants with tracheal malacia or other conditions in which the airways collapse abnormally. In general, contraindications include any CPAP-related condition that results in a worsening of the patient's original status. Some neonates cannot tolerate CPAP and progressively hypoventilate as the pressure level is increased. Clinical judgment is needed to decide how high the $PaCO_2$ should be allowed to rise before discontinuing the CPAP and beginning mechanical ventilation. An absolute contraindication to CPAP is apnea resulting in hypoxemia and hypotension. These infants should be mechanically ventilated. Box 16-1 gives a listing of indications, contraindications, and hazards.

Exam Hint 16-1

There is typically a question about the indications to start CPAP, the initial CPAP setting, or making a CPAP adjustment.

c. Initiation

Before starting CPAP, a set of baseline arterial blood gases should be taken. Transcutaneous oxygen monitoring or pulse oximetry may be substituted in some clinical situations if oxygenation is the only parameter that must be measured. Transcutaneous carbon dioxide ($PtcCO_2$) may be used to monitor ventilation. The neonate's vital signs should also be recorded. Assemble the CPAP circuit and pressure device. A decision must also be made to select the best patient interface. This involves choosing whether to apply the CPAP above the epiglottis (Figs. 16-2 and 16-3) or to intubate the infant and apply the CPAP within the trachea. Binasal CPAP prongs, a nasal mask, or nasopharyngeal tube CPAP are all patient interface options for applying pressure from above the epiglottis. A nasopharyngeal (NP) tube is now rarely used because

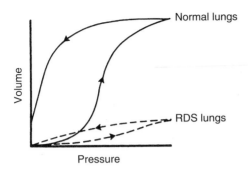

Figure 16-1 Pressure–volume curves for a normal neonate and for one with infant respiratory distress syndrome (RDS). A normal neonate's lungs inhale a relatively large tidal volume at low pressure. Note how when the same pressure is placed against the lungs of an infant with RDS, the tidal volume is much smaller. To get a normal tidal volume, the RDS infant must generate a much greater negative pressure. (From Carlo WA, Martin RJ: Pediatr Clin North Am 33:221, 1986.)

of the advances in nasal prongs. A nasal mask can be substituted if nasal prongs are not appropriate. The neonate or infant must have an endotracheal tube placed to apply CPAP within the trachea. Among the factors to be considered for the patient interface are the neonate's gestational age and weight, the amount of secretions that need to be suctioned, the pulmonary problem, and the likelihood of mechanical ventilation eventually becoming necessary. More mature and larger infants with few secretions and relatively stable pulmonary conditions will most likely have CPAP applied above the epiglottis by nasal prongs or mask. In contrast, less mature and smaller infants (less than 1000-1200 g) who need suctioning and have relatively unstable pulmonary conditions will probably be intubated. Mechanical ventilation can then be easily started if needed.

d. Clinical scenarios for CPAP use

CPAP is usually applied under one of these clinical situations:

(1) *Prophylactic application.* Many institutions now use the INSURE (INtubate, SURfactant, Extubate) protocol shortly after any premature neonate is born. The newborn is intubated and a dose of surfactant (discussed below) is given. Mechanical ventilation is started to stabilize the newborn's breathing. As soon as possible (often within an hour) the infant is weaned from the ventilator and extubated. Binasal-prong CPAP is then started.

(2) *Rescue or therapeutic application.* If a newborn is given a diagnosis of RDS after intubation and mechanical ventilation has been started, it is treated with surfactant. As the newborn improves, its ventilator support is reduced to the point of needing only CPAP. This is delivered through the endotracheal tube. The term "traditional CPAP" is often applied to using the ventilator as the delivery system.

BOX 16-1   CPAP Therapy: Indications, Contraindications, and Hazards

Indications

Infant respiratory distress syndrome (RDS)
Atelectasis
Pulmonary edema
Apnea of prematurity
Tracheal malacia
Recent extubation
Transient tachypnea of the newborn
Physical examination shows some, if not all, of the following:
  Respiratory rate 30%-40% greater than normal
  Substernal and suprasternal retractions
  Nasal flaring
  Expiratory grunting
  Cyanosis
  Chest radiograph shows atelectasis or pulmonary edema
Arterial blood gases showing:
  PaO_2 less than 50 torr on 60% or more oxygen
  Adequate ventilation with a $PaCO_2$ less than 50 torr and pH greater than 7.25
Wean from mechanical ventilation when the intermittent mandatory ventilation rate is about 4-12/min, the pulmonary condition is improved, blood gases show acceptable $PaCO_2$, and there is acceptable PaO_2 on PEEP. The CPAP level is set to match the level of PEEP used on the ventilator.

Contraindications

Prolonged apnea leading to hypoxemia and hypotension (begin mechanical ventilation)
Untreated pneumothorax or other evidence of a pulmonary gas leak
Unstable cardiovascular status such as bradycardia and hypotension
Inadequate ventilation with a $PaCO_2$ greater than 50 torr and pH less than 7.25
Unilateral pulmonary problem: untreated congenital diaphragmatic hernia
Nasal CPAP should not be used on a patient with cleft palate, choanal atresia, or tracheoesophageal fistula

Hazards

Persistent pulmonary hypertension of the newborn (PPHN)
Increased intracranial pressure that can cause intraventricular hemorrhage
Decreased cardiac output
CPAP may be ineffective if the neonate weighs less than 1000-1200 g

---

(3) *After ventilator weaning and extubation.* Many neonates will still require CPAP after being weaned from the ventilator and extubated. Binasal-prong CPAP is usually effective.

e. CPAP administration options

Depending on the clinical situation, CPAP can be administered in one of three ways:

(1) *Bubble CPAP (B-CPAP).* Respiratory therapists have delivered bubble CPAP for many years by assembling the necessary components. More recently, equipment manufacturers have offered B-CPAP systems (Fig. 16-4). One of the possible clinical advantages of B-CPAP is

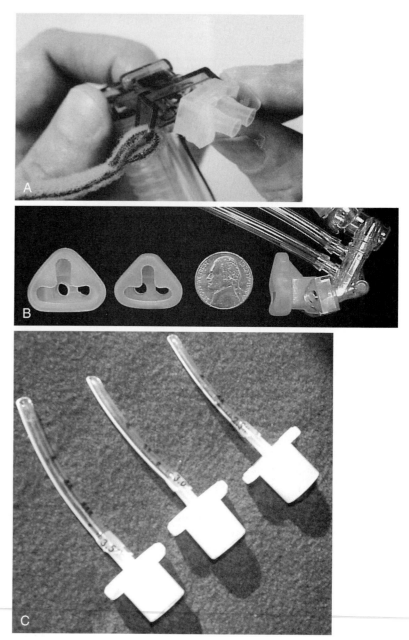

Figure 16-2 Three options for applying CPAP. **A,** Binasal CPAP can be delivered through a set of prongs and a patient circuit. **B,** Nasal masks and patient circuit. **C,** Nasopharyngeal CPAP is delivered through a shortened endotracheal tube. Shown are 2.5-, 3.0-, and 3.5-mm-ID endotracheal tubes that have been cut off at the proximal end and attached to the ventilator adapter. Always select the prongs, mask, or tube that is the proper size for the neonate. (**A** and **B** from Walsh BK, Czervinske MP, DiBlasii RM, editors: Perinatal and pediatric respiratory care, ed 3, St. Louis, 2010, Saunders; **C** from Cairo J: Mosby's Respiratory care equipment, ed 9, St Louis, 2014, Mosby.)

the rapid vibration of the lungs that results from the air/oxygen mix bubbling through the water. This has been compared to high-frequency ventilation. B-CPAP is applied by nasal prongs or mask.

(2) *Free-standing fluidic-type delivery system.* These commercially available systems are able to sense the neonate's inspiratory efforts and provide the correct amount of gas flow to maintain a consistent pressure level. The patient interface would be either nasal prongs or mask.

(3) *Ventilator CPAP (traditional CPAP).* When the ventilator is used to deliver CPAP, it is easy to begin mechanical ventilation if necessary. This is the only CPAP delivery system that includes an alarm package. Because the neonate is intubated, he or she can be suctioned if necessary. The endotracheal tube must be properly secured and cared for.

By any administration method, CPAP is usually started at about 4-6 cm water pressure whether the pressure is applied above or below the epiglottis. The inspired oxygen percentage is usually kept at the previously set level. It is important to make only one change at a time so that each adjustment can be evaluated for its own effect. For example, if you simultaneously increased the oxygen percentage by 10% and started 5 cm water of CPAP, it would not be known whether the increase in PaO_2 was from the additional oxygen, the CPAP, or both. Usually the long-term inspired oxygen is limited to 40%-50% because of concern of the possibility of pulmonary oxygen toxicity.

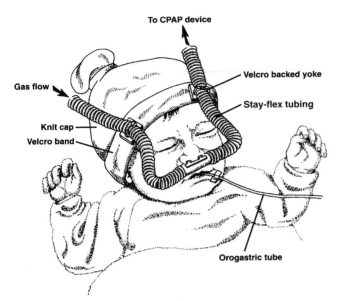

Figure 16-3 An assembly for supporting nasal CPAP prongs in an infant. (From Sills JR: Respiratory care registry guide, ed 1, St Louis, 1994, Mosby.)

f. Monitor and adjust alarm settings (code: IIIC4d) [difficulty: R, Ap]

A variety of alarms and monitoring systems should be used to ensure the patient's safety. Patient monitors should have visual and audible alarms and include the following:

- Pulse oximeter or transcutaneous oxygen monitor. Either should alarm if the patient's oxygen falls below the set, safe level.
- Transcutaneous carbon dioxide monitor. The alarm should activate if the patient's carbon dioxide level rises above a set, safe level.
- Electrocardiogram monitor. It should have alarm limits set for high and low heart rate.

Equipment should have visual and audible alarms and include the following features:

- A low-pressure alarm in case >2 cm water pressure is lost because of a leak or disconnection. For example, CPAP is set at 6 cm water and a leak drops the pressure to 3 cm water.
- A high-pressure limiting valve that prevents an accidental dangerous high pressure in the system from being applied to the patient's airways. If this pressure limit is reached, the alarm will be activated.
- An oxygen analyzer set to alarm if the patient's ordered inspired oxygen percentage is set below the ordered percentage.

g. CPAP adjustment

Blood gases and vital signs must be evaluated at the starting CPAP level. The heart rate, blood pressure, and respiratory rate should be stable or improved. Wait at least 10 minutes after a change in CPAP before getting an arterial blood gas sample. See Table 16-1 for the recommended blood gas

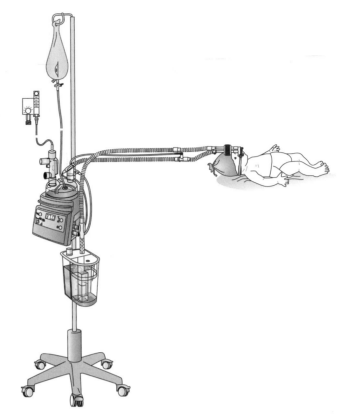

Figure 16-4 A free-standing system for delivering bubble CPAP. Key components include: (1) oxygen blender and flowmeter that deliver desired oxygen percentage to the manifold; (2) manifold mounted on the humidifier, which includes a high-pressure pop-off valve, port for an oxygen analyzer, and port for a CPAP pressure gauge; (3) servo-controlled humidifier with its reservoir bag of sterile water; (4) inspiratory limb of the patient circuit with an internal heated wire and temperature probe; (5) patient–CPAP interface of nasal prongs, nasal mask, or nasopharyngeal tube; (6) expiratory limb of the patient circuit that connects to the hollow CPAP unit probe; (7) bubble CPAP device (Fisher & Paykel Healthcare Bubble CPAP System) that is filled with sterile water (or a weak solution of acetic acid). The CPAP level is set by pushing the CPAP probe as far under water as desired. For example, pushing the end of the probe 5 cm under water creates that much CPAP. The expiratory gas passes through the hollow probe and bubbles through the water. (From Cairo J: Mosby's Respiratory care equipment, ed 9, St Louis, 2014, Mosby.)

limits. In general, the PaO_2 should be kept between 60 and 70 torr, $PaCO_2$ less than 50-55 torr, and pH at least 7.25. If the PaO_2 is too low and the patient's vital signs are acceptable, the CPAP may be increased in a step of 1-2 cm water. The vital signs and blood gases should then be reevaluated. In addition, the neonate's work of breathing can be indirectly assessed. Improved lung function will be demonstrated by seeing decreased respiratory rate, retractions, expiratory grunting, and nasal flaring and improved chest and abdominal synchrony. If necessary, the process of adding CPAP and reassessing the patient can be continued. The maximum CPAP level in a neonate is generally held to be 10 cm water; the maximum CPAP level in an infant is generally held to be 15 cm water.

TABLE 16-1	Commonly Recommended Blood Gas Goals for CPAP and Mechanical Ventilator Therapy	
	AGE OF NEONATE	
	Less Than 72 Hours	**Greater Than 72 Hours**
PaO₂ (torr)	60-70	50-70
PtcO₂ (torr)	Greater than 50,* less than 90*	Greater than 40,* less than 90*
SpO₂	92-96%	92-96%
PaCO₂ (torr)	35-45†	45-55
PtcCO₂ (torr)	May be used after correlation with PaCO₂ as discussed in Chapter 3.	
pH	7.25-7.45	7.25-7.45

PtcO₂, pressure of transcutaneous oxygen; PtcCO₂, pressure of transcutaneous carbon dioxide.

*PtcO₂ values may be used after they have been shown to correlate within 15% of the PaO₂ from an arterial blood gas.

†With CPAP, this value may be increased to 50-55 torr as long as the pH is at least 7.25.

Note: Keep the PaO₂ no greater than 80 torr in the premature neonate to reduce the risk of retinopathy of prematurity.

Mechanical ventilation is usually indicated if more than these maximum CPAP pressures are needed to correct hypoxemia. Depending on the patient, even levels less than these maximum CPAP pressures may not be well tolerated. The infant may become exhausted from exhaling against the back pressure of the CPAP system. That is seen clinically as decreased chest movement from the smaller tidal volume. The PaCO₂ will probably increase. It may be necessary to place the infant on mechanical ventilation to decrease the work of breathing and then add PEEP to maintain the FRC. When nasal prongs or an NP tube are used, CPAP pressures of greater than 8 cm water may cause the infant's mouth to open. This results in the loss of CPAP. A crying infant also opens his or her mouth and loses the CPAP. In either case, the CPAP pressure gauge drops to zero or fluctuates below the set pressure.

h. Wean the patient from CPAP (code: IIIC8) [difficulty: R, Ap, An]

As the patient improves, it is necessary to reduce the CPAP level so as not to cause pulmonary barotrauma. The pressure level can be reduced in steps of about 2 cm water. The vital signs and blood gases should be reassessed after each step. The apparatus is usually removed when the CPAP level is down to 2-4 cm water. Traditionally, the infant is then placed into an oxygen hood at the same oxygen percentage as before or 5%-15% higher. If the infant has an endotracheal tube that is needed for suctioning or a secure airway, the pressure is usually left at 2-4 cm water. After extubation, the infant is placed into an oxyhood as before. Alternatively, the neonate may be weaned to a high-flow nasal cannula and then to a traditional, low-flow nasal cannula. See Chapter 6 for more discussion on these oxygen systems.

If the infant was breathing more than 50% oxygen while on the CPAP, it may be more important to lower the oxygen before decreasing the CPAP level. The following guidelines may prove helpful when deciding whether to lower first the oxygen percentage or the CPAP level:

- If the patient has been breathing more than 50% oxygen for more than 48 hours and has stable vital signs without any pulmonary barotrauma, decrease the oxygen first. Lower the inspired oxygen in 5%-15% steps, and check the oxygenation level after each reduction. Attempt to get the oxygen down to 40%, if possible. Then decrease the CPAP level.
- If the patient is breathing 50% oxygen or less and has unstable vital signs or pulmonary barotrauma, decrease the CPAP first. After the CPAP is reduced (or removed entirely) and the patient is stable, reduce the inspired oxygen percentage.

Exam Hint 16-2

Know the indications for switching from CPAP to mechanical ventilation.

MODULE B

Perform mechanical ventilation.

1. Indications for mechanical ventilation

All authors agree that apnea is an absolute indication for mechanical ventilation. A general indication is any condition that causes respiratory failure. This is usually documented by unacceptable arterial blood gases. Box 16-2 lists indications for mechanical ventilation.

Math Review

Time Constants of Ventilation

Note: This concept has not been directly tested by the NBRC. It is hoped that understanding the concept of time constants as used here and later in the text will help the reader understand lung pathology and why certain ventilator adjustments are made.

It is important for any patient requiring mechanical ventilation to consider both the patient's lung–thoracic compliance (C_{LT}) and his or her airway resistance when setting inspiratory and expiratory times. This is especially important in neonates because, in comparison with adults, they are less compliant and have greater resistance. In addition, neonates are usually ventilated at faster rates. As a review, the respective C_{LT} and airway resistances (R_{aw}) of normal adults and infants are shown here:

Adult lung – thoracic compliance: 100 mL/cm water pressure (0.1 L/cm water pressure)

Neonatal lung – thoracic compliance: 5 mL/cm water pressure (0.005 L/cm water pressure; about 20 times stiffer than in an adult)

Adult airway resistance: 2 cm water/L/s

Neonatal airway resistance: 20 – 40 cm water/L/s (about 10 – 20 times more resistance to airflow than in an adult)

The placement of an endotracheal tube to facilitate mechanical ventilation results in a total pulmonary resistance ranging from 50 to 150 cm water/L/s. The time constant of ventilation (T_c or time constant of the respiratory system T_{RS}) is calculated as the product of compliance and resistance:

Time constant in seconds = compliance (L/cm water)
$$\times \text{ resistance (cm water/L/s)}$$

For example, using these values for a spontaneously breathing normal neonate, its time constant is calculated as

$$
\begin{aligned}
T_c &= \text{compliance (0.005 L/cm water)} \\
&\quad \times \text{resistance (30 cm water/L/s)} \\
&= 0.005 \times 30 \text{ seconds} \\
&= 0.15 \text{ seconds}
\end{aligned}
$$

Although it is technically impractical to measure the time constant of ventilation at the bedside, the concept is important because it relates to two important clinical considerations during mechanical ventilation. First, it relates to the pressure that develops at the alveolar level as the tidal volume is delivered. For each time constant, progressively more of the peak inspiratory pressure (PIP) is applied within the alveoli (Fig. 16-5). As can be seen, at three time constants, 95% of the PIP is applied to the alveoli. At five time constants, virtually the entire PIP is applied at the alveolar level. Second, the time constant relates to how rapidly the lung recoils to baseline (FRC) during an exhalation. As shown in Figure 16-5, it takes three time constants to exhale 95% and five time constants to completely exhale.

The clinical significance of this relates directly to the pulmonary condition of the patient. Infants with stiff lungs and normal resistance, as found in RDS, have a short time constant. Alveolar pressure quickly increases to match the peak inspiratory pressure. The lungs then rapidly recoil during exhalation so that there is little chance of air trapping. Infants with normal compliance and increased resistance, as found in meconium aspiration, have a long time constant. It takes a relatively long time for the alveolar pressure to reach the PIP. Also, a relatively long time is needed for the exhalation to be complete. For this reason, these infants are at risk for air trapping and auto-PEEP.

2. Select a mechanical ventilator

When selecting a ventilator, it is important to choose one that offers the features needed to ventilate the patient. For example, if real-time graphics are needed to evaluate the patient's response to a ventilator adjustment, the proper unit will be needed. Any selected ventilator must be able to meet the typical tidal volume goal for a

---

Box 16-2   Common Indications for the Initiation of Mechanical Ventilation

Respiratory Failure
PaO_2 less than 50-60 torr despite maximal CPAP therapy (about 10 cm water) and 60% or more inspired oxygen
$PaCO_2$ greater than 60 torr and pH less than 7.25

Neurologic
Complete apnea
Apneic periods leading to hypoxemia and bradycardia
Intracranial hemorrhage
Drug depression
Muscular dystrophies

Pulmonary Conditions
Infant respiratory distress syndrome (RDS)
Diffuse pneumonia
Pulmonary edema
Meconium aspiration
Diaphragmatic hernia
Cyanotic congenital cardiac defect
Persistent pulmonary hypertension of the newborn (PPHN)
Near drowning
Postoperatively after major thoracic or abdominal surgery

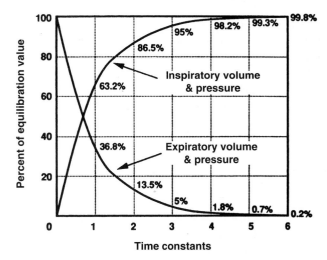

Figure 16-5 Graphic presentation of the percentages of inspiratory and expiratory volume and pressure in comparison with time constants of ventilation. (From Chatburn RL: Respir Care 36:569, 1991.)

term neonate, premature neonate, or pediatric patient. All conventional ventilators are capable of reaching the Food and Drug Administration (FDA) limited rate of 150 breaths/min.

a. Pressure ventilation

Historically, most neonatal patients requiring life support receive time-triggered, pressure-limited, time-cycled mechanical ventilation (TPTV). (This could also be called time-cycled, pressure-limited ventilation or TCPL ventilation.) These ventilators are pneumatically powered with electrical controls and alarm systems. They are used in the Intermittent Mandatory Ventilation (IMV) mode and feature a continuous flow of gas from which the neonate can breathe spontaneously. TPTV units are pressure limited to prevent an excessive peak airway pressure and can have therapeutic PEEP added. The majority of neonatal and small pediatric patients can be effectively ventilated on these types of units. This chapter focuses on TPTV ventilation. The current generation of ventilators uses pressure control (PC) or pressure support (PS) ventilation to achieve the same clinical goal of pressure-limited ventilation as TPTV. See Chapter 15 for an in-depth discussion of PC and PS.

A clinical concern with any type of pressure ventilation mode is the variable tidal volume when the patient's lung compliance changes. For example, if the patient's lungs become less compliant, the tidal volume will decrease. With improved compliance, the tidal volume will increase.

b. Volume ventilation

Volume-cycled ventilators using the Volume Control (VC) mode have been commonly used on infants who weigh more than 10 kg (22 lb). However, the most recent generation of conventional volume-cycled ventilators can be used to deliver a tidal volume as small as 2-3 mL. The use of flow sensitivity rather than pressure sensitivity has greatly improved the synchronization of the patient's breathing effort with a machine-delivered breath. Volume-oriented ventilation can also be performed with a neonatal TPTV-type ventilator if the patient is apneic. This technique is discussed later.

A clinical concern with volume ventilation is the increased airway pressure that results when the patient's lung compliance decreases. The pressure limit should be set to prevent dangerously high airway pressure.

c. Dual-control mode ventilation

Several current-generation ventilators provide Dual-Control mode ventilation. Dual-Control mode combines the best features of pressure ventilation and volume ventilation. Simply put, the ventilator will automatically increase or decrease the airway pressure to deliver the desired tidal volume despite decreases or increases in lung compliance.

d. High-frequency ventilation

High-frequency ventilation (HFV) with a small tidal volume was originally approved by the FDA for use in the rescue of neonates with RDS, a bronchopulmonary fistula, or pulmonary interstitial emphysema (PIE) who fail under conventional pressure or volume ventilation. Since then HFV has also been used in the short-term support of neonates with a variety of other conditions listed later in Box 16-5.

3. Noninvasive ventilation

a. **Recommend changes in mechanical ventilator parameters and settings (code: IIIE3f) [difficulty: R, Ap, An]**

See below.

b. **Initiate and adjust noninvasive ventilation (code: IIIC4b) [difficulty: R, Ap, An]**

Indications for noninvasive positive-pressure ventilation (NPPV) include: (1) providing ventilatory support after extubation or (2) when a patient is failing at CPAP and the physician wishes to avoid intubation and traditional mechanical ventilation. The primary causes behind the need for NPPV would include those listed in Box 16-2.

Because the patient is not intubated, the patient–ventilator interface is either nasal prongs or a nasal mask. The following discussion on pathology-based traditional mechanical ventilation would also apply to the initiation and adjustment of NPPV.

4. Continuous mechanical ventilation

a. **Recommend changes in mechanical ventilator parameters and settings (code: IIIE3f) [difficulty: R, Ap, An]**

See below.

b. **Initiate and adjust continuous mechanical ventilation (IIIC4a) [difficulty: R, Ap, An]**

> **Exam Hint 16-3**
>
> Owing to the great variety of proprietary terms for ventilator modes (and their abbreviations) used by manufacturers, the NBRC has adopted this simplified, limited number of abbreviations for mechanical ventilation modes: *NPPV* (noninvasive positive-pressure ventilation; the same thing as NIV, noninvasive ventilation), *PS* (pressure support), *CPAP* (continuous positive airway pressure), *HFOV* (high-frequency oscillatory ventilation), *PC* (pressure control), *VC* (volume control), *A/C* (assist control), and *SIMV* (synchronous intermittent mandatory ventilation). The last four modes can be combined: PC, A/C; PC, SIMV; VC, A/C; and VC, SIMV. However, other widely adopted modes (and their abbreviations) should also be understood.

1. Adjust the ventilator settings

With traditional neonatal TPTV, a set tidal volume is not ordered and cannot be measured. With volume-cycled ventilation of a pediatric or neonatal patient, the tidal volume is ordered just as it is with an adult patient. Chapter 15 focuses on volume-cycled ventilation. With any manner of ventilating the patient, the therapist is expected to set the following ventilator controls based on a protocol or the patient's condition and response to the ventilator: tidal volume, respiratory rate, oxygen percentage, sensitivity, flow, I:E ratio, alarms, and humidified gas temperature.

Specific examples of ventilator settings, based on the pathological problem, are presented in Module C.

2. Correct ventilator–patient dyssynchrony (code: IIIC5) [difficulty: R, Ap, An]

In most instances, the proper adjustment of sensitivity and/or flow will help the patient breathe in synchrony with the ventilator. There is no sensitivity control on traditional continuous-flow TPTV-type neonatal ventilators. The IMV mode is used with these units. Newer ventilators have the ability to sense a neonate's respiratory effort and trigger a machine-delivered breath. A child on a volume-cycled ventilator should have the sensitivity set at about −1 to −2 cm water pressure. Some ventilators sense a change in flow through the ventilator circuit when the neonate makes an inspiratory effort. Other ventilators make use of electrocardiogram-type leads on the neonate's chest to sense a change in electrical impedance (skin resistance) when the neonate makes an inspiratory effort. The Servo-i ventilator uses a special nasogastric tube with sensors that note diaphragm contraction and trigger a ventilator breath. No matter which method the ventilator uses to sense the patient's inspiratory effort, the neonate or child should not have to work hard to trigger a machine tidal volume.

Flow is adjusted to set the inspiratory time, set the I:E ratio, or meet the patient's needs to better synchronize breathing efforts with the ventilator. The flow should be increased if the patient appears to be attempting to inhale faster than the ventilator is delivering the tidal volume.

3. I:E ratio

The I:E ratio is adjusted to ensure that the patient can inhale in as physiologically appropriate a manner as possible and can completely exhale the inspired tidal volume. A ventilator with real-time graphics can reveal the presence of auto-PEEP (incomplete exhalation). In most situations, auto-PEEP can be reduced or eliminated by increasing expiratory time or reducing the tidal volume. In addition, suctioning out secretions and the administration of an aerosolized bronchodilator in a patient with bronchospasm can reduce air trapping and auto-PEEP.

4. Initiate and adjust alarms (code: IIIC4d) [difficulty: R, Ap]

All alarm systems must function properly, so test all audible and visual alarms. The respiratory therapist should be familiar with the most widely used neonatal ventilators and those that can be used with pediatric as well as adult patients. It is common practice to set most ventilator alarms at ±10% from the set value. A variation of greater than 10% results in an audible or visual alarm condition.

If the patient is on a CPAP system, the low-pressure or disconnection alarm should be set to alarm if the pressure drops about 2 cm water below the set level. For example,

if the patient is on 8 cm water CPAP, the alarm setting should be set at 6 cm water.

Many types of alarm systems have a timer that can be set to delay when the alarm sounds. For example, if the neonatal patient has a ventilator rate of 30/min, the cycling time between mandatory breaths is 2 seconds. The delay should be set so that the alarm sounds 1-2 seconds after a mandatory breath fails to be delivered. If the patient is on a CPAP system, the timer may be set for no delay or a short delay after the CPAP pressure drops below the set value. Always adjust all alarm systems to fit the clinical situation and the patient's condition.

5. Humidification
a. Maintain adequate humidification (code: IIIA6) [difficulty: R, Ap]
See below.
b. Recommend changes in humidification (code: IIIE3c) [difficulty: R, Ap]

The goal for most patients is to minimize their humidity deficit by giving gas that is humidified and warmed to near body temperature. It is common clinical practice to have the gas warmed to 90-95° F (about 35° C). It should be measured in the inspiratory limb of the circuit as close to the patient as possible. In some situations, a low-dead-space infant heat–moisture exchanger (HME) can be used to provide humidity. See Chapters 8 and 15 for the full discussion on humidification options.

MODULE C

Pathology-based mechanical ventilation

The initial discussion presented here is an attempt to describe what are widely accepted approaches to neonatal TPTV and related therapy. The following approaches in this discussion focus on adjusting the ventilator and treating a neonate based on its pathologic problem. The general principles for selecting tidal volume, rate, I:E ratio, and PEEP apply to VC ventilation as well as pressure control ventilation. For the most part, pediatric patients are managed on the ventilator the same as adult patients. See Chapter 15 for additional discussion.

1. Patients with normal cardiopulmonary function

Term neonatal and pediatric patients with normal cardiopulmonary function may need mechanical ventilation because of apnea from anesthesia, paralysis, or a neurologic condition. The initial TPTV ventilator parameters for this type of patient are listed in Box 16-3. Once mechanical ventilation is established, it is important to evaluate the patient's blood gases, vital signs, breath sounds, and any other pertinent clinical information before changing any ventilator parameters.

Box 16-3 Common Mechanical Ventilator Parameters for Neonatal and Pediatric Patients with Normal Lungs

Delivered tidal volume: 6-8 mL/kg (with pressure control ventilation, this may be estimated by calculation if the neonate is apneic and the pressure limit is not reached until the end of the inspiratory time)
Pressure limit (peak inspiratory pressure): 10-20 cm water
Frequency: 25-40/min
I:E ratio: 1:2 to 1:4
Inspiratory time: 0.3-0.5 second
Expiratory time: at least 0.5 second
PEEP: 3-5 cm water to replace "epiglottal PEEP"
Inspiratory flow: sufficient to see the chest move and hear bilateral breath sounds during the inspiration; 5-8 L/min is commonly used; or start with at least twice the infant's estimated minute volume (respiratory rate × estimated tidal volume of 7 mL/kg); check the blood gases for the $PaCO_2$
Oxygen percentage: 40%

As the patient recovers and begins to breathe spontaneously, it will probably be necessary to reduce the ventilator-delivered minute volume. This encourages the child to breathe more because the final goal is to completely wean and extubate the patient. The most accepted way to reduce the ventilator-delivered minute volume is to reduce the ventilator rate. A reduction of about 10% is a good starting place but must be tailored to meet the patient's needs. The tidal volume is maintained as originally set. Obtain a set of blood gases in 10-20 minutes (or follow the transcutaneous or pulse oximetry values), and check the patient's vital signs to see how well the adjustment is tolerated.

If the blood gases show an elevated $PaCO_2$, the ventilator-delivered minute volume must be raised. Do this by increasing either the alveolar ventilation or the respiratory rate. Alveolar ventilation can be increased by increasing either the inspiratory flow or the pressure limit (if it has been reached) to increase the tidal volume. The ventilator rate may be increased if the flow and pressure limit cannot be increased. An increase of about 10% is a good starting place but must be tailored to meet the patient's needs. As before, blood gases and vital signs should be monitored after every change to see if the increase is well tolerated and accomplishing what was intended.

If the blood gases show that the $PaCO_2$ is lower than desired, the ventilator-delivered minute volume must be decreased. The first parameter to adjust is usually the rate. Try decreasing the rate by about 10% and check another set of blood gas values. If other parameters need to be reduced, try decreasing the peak inspiratory pressure, inspiratory flow, or inspiratory time about 10% to decrease the tidal volume. Again, check the blood gas values after every adjustment.

If the blood gases show that the PaO_2 is higher or lower than necessary, the oxygen percentage must be adjusted.

An increase or decrease of about 5% is a good starting place but must be adjusted as needed. If the patient does not respond to the increased oxygen as expected, the patient should be reevaluated. It may be necessary to reclassify him or her into one of the following categories discussed below: decreased lung compliance, increased airway resistance, PPHN, or bronchopulmonary dysplasia.

Math Review

Calculation of Estimated Tidal Volume During TPTV Mechanical Ventilation

The NBRC examination content outline does not specifically list estimated tidal volume calculations. However, the information may be useful in understanding concepts presented later in the text.

If the neonatal patient receiving TPTV is apneic and neither assisting nor fighting against the ventilator-delivered breath, it is possible to calculate an approximate tidal volume. This is referred to as volume-oriented ventilation. The following formula is used:

$$\text{Calculated tidal volume} = (T_I \times \dot{V}) - V_c$$

in which

T_I = inspiratory time

(It is important that either the pressure limit is not reached or the pressure limit is reached at the same time inspiratory time is completed. If the pressure limit is reached before the inspiratory time limit is reached, part of the inspiratory time is spent as an inflation hold, and no additional tidal volume is delivered).

$\dot{V}$ = inspiratory flow rate on the ventilator in mL/s,

V_c = volume compressed in the circuit and ventilator

(This is found by multiplying the peak inspiratory pressure by the manufacturer's stated compliance factors for the circuit and ventilator).

For example, estimate the delivered tidal volume for an apneic 5-kg infant. The ventilator parameters are inspiratory flow 5.5 L/min, frequency 20/min, I:E ratio 1:3, inspiratory time 0.75 second, and expiratory time 2.25 seconds. PIP is 15 cm water. The internal compliance of the ventilator is 0.4 mL/cm water, and the circuit compliance factor is 1.6 mL/cm water.

$$\text{Calculated tidal volume} = (T_I \times \dot{V}) - V_c$$

in which:

T_I = 0.75 second,

$\dot{V}$ = 5.5 L/min (This is converted to mL/s by dividing the flow in L/min by 60 seconds. So, 5.5 L/min = 0.092 L/s or 92 mL/s),

V_c = 0.4 + 1.6 mL/cm water = 2 mL/cm water
   = 2 mL/cm water × 15 cm water PIP = 30 mL.

Therefore,

$$
\begin{aligned}
\text{Calculated tidal volume} &= (0.75 \text{ second} \times 92 \text{ mL/s}) - 30 \text{ mL} \\
&= (69 \text{ mL}) - 30 \text{ mL} \\
&= 39 \text{ mL (This is within the ideal} \\
&\quad \text{tidal volume range of } 30 - \\
&\quad 40 \text{ mL; based on 5 kg} \\
&\quad \text{weight} \times 6 - 8 \text{ mL/kg)}
\end{aligned}
$$

It must be emphasized that this is only a calculated tidal volume. A leak in the system, a decrease in the patient's compliance, or an increase in the patient's resistance decreases the true tidal volume. Conversely, an increase in the patient's compliance or a decrease in the patient's resistance increases the true tidal volume. Also, if the pressure limit is reached before the inspiratory time is completed, less volume than expected will be delivered. This is because part of the inspiratory time is spent as an inflation hold and no additional tidal volume is delivered (Fig. 16-6). Finally, the infant must be completely passive during the delivery of the breath.

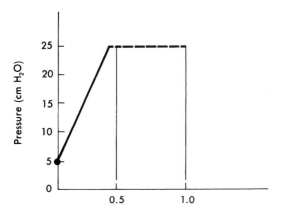

Figure 16-6 Pressure–time curve seen with pressure limit set at 25 cm water and inspiratory time being increased from 0.5 to 1 second. Pressure limit is reached when inspiratory time is about 0.5 second. As inspiratory time is increased to 1 second (or greater), the pressure limit is held at 25 cm water resulting in a square-wave pressure curve. (From Betis P, Thompson JF, Benjamin PK: Mechanical ventilation. In Koff PB, Eitzman DV, Neu J: Neonatal and pediatric respiratory care, ed 2, St Louis, 1993, Mosby.)

2. Patients with decreased lung compliance and normal airway resistance such as in infant RDS

Although premature infants weighing less than 1000 g will often have RDS, stiff lungs are also found in patients with other lung conditions such as pneumonia and pulmonary edema (Fig. 16-7). The greatest challenge presented in the care of these infants is to oxygenate them without causing oxygen toxicity or pulmonary barotrauma. Common recommendations for the initial ventilator settings are listed in Box 16-4. As discussed earlier, blood gases, vital signs, and so forth must be monitored after the infant is placed on the ventilator. Any further adjustments can then be determined and evaluated by another set of blood gases and vital signs.

The issue of time constants of ventilation helps to better explain the various options available for adjusting the ventilator. As presented earlier, the T_c (or T_{RS}) is calculated as the product of compliance and resistance. For example, using the following values for a mechanically ventilated neonate with RDS, its time constant is calculated as

T_c = compliance (0.001 L/cm water because the lungs are less compliant × resistance (100 cm water/L/s because the infant is intubated). Simplify as follows:

= 0.001 × 100 seconds

= 0.1 second (Compare this with a T_c of 0.15 for a normal, spontaneously breathing neonate)

Neonates with RDS have a relatively short time constant; therefore the tidal volume and ventilating pressure are delivered rather quickly to the lungs. However, because the lungs are so stiff, there is usually no problem with the tidal volume being fully exhaled as long as five time constants are allowed. An expiratory time of at least 0.5 second is usually

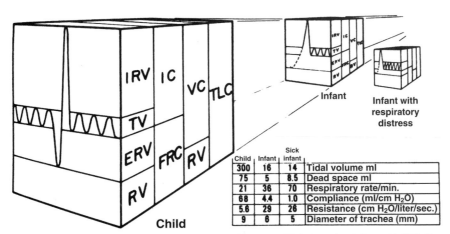

		Child	Infant	Sick Infant	
		300	16	14	Tidal volume ml
		75	5	8.5	Dead space ml
		21	36	70	Respiratory rate/min.
		68	4.4	1.0	Compliance (ml/cm H₂O)
		5.6	29	28	Resistance (cm H₂O/liter/sec.)
		9	6	5	Diameter of trachea (mm)

Figure 16-7 Comparison of the lung volumes and capacities of a 6-year-old child, a normal infant, and an infant with RDS. Note the relatively high compliance and low resistance of a normal child compared with an infant and of an infant with RDS compared with a normal infant. (From Chatburn RL, Lough MD. Mechanical ventilation. In Lough MD, Doershuk CF, Stern RC, editors: Pediatric respiratory therapy, ed 3, St Louis, 1985, Mosby.)

Box 16-4   Common Mechanical Ventilator Parameters for Neonates with Low Compliance and Normal Resistance

Delivered tidal volume: 4-6 mL/kg

Pressure limit: 20-25 cm water (this may need to be increased up to 35-40 cm water)

Frequency: 40-60/min (this may need to be raised up to 150/min)

I:E ratio: 1:2 (this may eventually need to be altered to an inverse I:E ratio)

Inspiratory time (T_I): between 0.25 and 0.5 second (this may need to be increased)

Expiratory time (T_E): at least 0.5 second (this may need to be decreased)

PEEP: 4-5 cm water initially (this may need to be increased up to 8-10 cm water)

Inspiratory flow: sufficient to see the chest move and hear bilateral breath sounds during the inspiration; 5-8 L/min is commonly used; as a general rule, the faster the rate is, the higher the flow must be to deliver an adequate tidal volume; check the blood gases for the $PaCO_2$

Oxygen percentage: 40% (this may need to be increased to keep the SpO_2 greater than 92%)

---

set initially. The various options available for increasing oxygenation are discussed on the following pages.

a. Administer oxygen

1. Initiate and adjust oxygen therapy (code: IIIC1) [difficulty: R, Ap, An]

See below.

2. Recommend changes in oxygen therapy (code: IIIE3b) [difficulty: R, Ap, An]

Up to 100% oxygen can be given to the neonate in the short term. Hypoxemia cannot be tolerated and supplemental oxygen is usually the best way to correct it. See Chapter 15 for equations that can be used to predict the oxygen percentage change needed to correct the patient's hypoxemia. Although hypoxemia cannot be tolerated, there are several limiting factors. First, it is commonly held that giving more than 50% oxygen for more than 48-72 hours increases the risk of pulmonary oxygen toxicity. Second, if more than 80% oxygen is given, some poorly ventilated alveoli will have all of the oxygen absorbed from them, leading to denitrogenation absorption atelectasis. Third, keeping the neonate's PaO_2 below 80 torr minimizes the risk of retinopathy of prematurity. Fourth, if the hypoxemia is caused by a decreased FRC because of the lack of surfactant and small lung volumes, increasing the oxygen will not markedly increase the PaO_2. Other solutions, such as adding PEEP, altering the I:E ratio to lengthen the inspiratory time, and giving surfactant, must be used. These are discussed later.

3. Minimize procedure-associated hypoxemia, for example, during patient positioning, suctioning, and equipment changes (code: IIIC2) [difficulty: R, Ap, An]

Chapter 13 discusses the suctioning procedure and steps that should be taken to prevent hypoxemia during suctioning. Older children can be given 100% oxygen during suctioning or equipment changes. Children younger than 6 months of age should have their oxygen percentage increased by 10%-20% for the procedure.

b. Adjust the inspiratory flow

With TPTV-type ventilators, increasing the flow increases the tidal volume until the pressure limit is reached. Increasing the tidal volume should result in an increased PaO_2 and is likely to reduce the $PaCO_2$. If the pressure limit is reached, the delivered tidal volume is held in the lungs for the duration of the inspiratory time. This acts as an inflation hold and should also increase the PaO_2. The mean airway pressure ($\overline{Paw}$) is raised by holding the tidal volume in the lungs. (See Fig. 16-8 for the pressure waveforms seen during low-flow and high-flow conditions.) Under high-flow conditions, the pressure waveform takes on a characteristic square shape (square wave) because the pressure limit is reached. This pattern of ventilation is currently widely used with these types of patients.

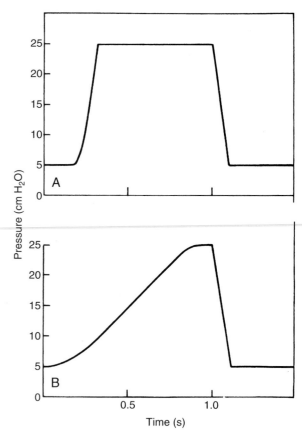

Figure 16-8 Comparison of pressure–time curves showing influence of inspiratory flow when the pressure limit is set at 25 cm water. **A,** Curve at high flow rate. Pressure limit is reached very early in the inspiratory time with resulting square-wave flow pattern. **B,** Curve at low flow rate. Pressure limit is not reached until inspiratory time is almost 1 second. (From Chatburn RL, Lough MD. Mechanical ventilation. In Lough MD, Doershuk CF, Stern RC, editors: Pediatric respiratory therapy, ed 3, St Louis, 1985, Mosby.)

Often, decreasing the flow on a TPTV-type ventilator will result in a smaller tidal volume. This will probably result in a decreased PaO_2 and increased $PaCO_2$.

c. Adjust the inspiratory time

As with increasing the flow, increasing the inspiratory time increases the tidal volume until the pressure limit is reached. If the pressure limit is reached, any increased inspiratory time acts as inflation hold. This also raises the $\overline{Paw}$ and should result in an increased PaO_2. (See Fig. 16-6 for the pressure waveform change as the inspiratory time is increased.)

Some authors have advocated an increased inspiratory time as an important way to improve oxygenation. This has led to the use of inverse I:E ratios of up to 3:1 (0.33) or 4:1 (0.25) to produce an adequate PaO_2. The inspiratory time should be increased in small time increments and followed in 10-20 minutes with a blood gas to determine if the desired improvement in oxygenation was achieved. Inspiratory time is increased only as long as necessary to result in a satisfactory PaO_2. Great care must be taken to adjust expiratory time, respiratory rate, or both when a prolonged inspiratory time is used. Obviously, expiratory time must be reduced to keep the same rate as the inspiratory time is increased, or the rate must be reduced as the inspiratory time is increased if the expiratory time cannot be reduced. Care must be taken to ensure that the tidal volume is fully exhaled to avoid auto-PEEP.

As the neonate's lung compliance improves, the inspiratory time must be decreased for two reasons. First, the alveolar pressure is more readily transmitted throughout the lungs and may decrease venous return to the heart. That results in a decreased cardiac output. Second, the more normal lungs are more prone to barotrauma or volutrauma. The inspiratory time should be decreased in small time increments and followed with a set of blood gases to be sure that the neonate is not hypoxemic.

d. Perform lung recruitment maneuvers (code: IIIC7) [difficulty: R, Ap, An]

Positive end-expiratory pressure, like CPAP, is often needed in neonates with RDS to restore their normal lung volume. PEEP increases the patient's FRC by preventing a complete exhalation to the baseline (atmospheric) pressure. Because PEEP increases the FRC, it is more effective at increasing the PaO_2 than is increasing the tidal volume, increasing the inflation hold, or an inverse I:E ratio. See Table 16-1 for the recommended guidelines for arterial blood gas values in neonates. If the patient needs more than 50% oxygen to keep the desired PaO_2, PEEP should be started; unless there is a contraindication to its use. Often, the proper level of therapeutic PEEP can result in an acceptable PaO_2 with no more than 50% oxygen being inhaled.

As discussed in regard to CPAP therapy, PEEP is usually started out at 4-5 cm water. A blood gas is then checked

and, if necessary, more PEEP is added in 1-2 cm water increments. It is rare for more than 8-10 cm water of PEEP to be needed. Another blood gas should be checked to assess the PaO_2 after every addition of pressure. PEEP has the greatest impact on raising the $\overline{Paw}$ of all the options presented here. For that reason, excessive PEEP may cause a decreased venous return to the heart and decreased cardiac output. It also may cause barotrauma resulting in pulmonary interstitial emphysema (PIE), pneumothorax, or pneumomediastinum. Care must be taken to carefully evaluate the patient after each increase in PEEP. Watch for a sudden deterioration in the patient's condition as a sign of a pulmonary air leak. As the patient's PaO_2 improves, the PEEP level should be reduced in steps of about 1-2 cm water. As always, recheck the blood gases with each adjustment.

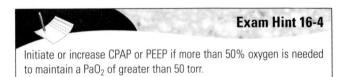

Exam Hint 16-4

Initiate or increase CPAP or PEEP if more than 50% oxygen is needed to maintain a PaO_2 of greater than 50 torr.

e. Adjust the pressure limit

With TPTV mechanical ventilation, in order to deliver a larger tidal volume, it is necessary to increase the pressure limit when it is reached by the PIP. It is also necessary to raise the pressure limit to restore the original tidal volume after the addition of PEEP. This is because the original tidal volume is reduced when PEEP is added and the PIP reaches the pressure limit. This is shown in Figure 16-9. To restore the original tidal volume, the pressure limit (and PIP) must be increased by the same amount as the added PEEP. This maintains the original ventilating pressure. It is important to remember that as PEEP is reduced, the pressure limit must also be reduced by the same amount. This maintains the original ventilating pressure and tidal volume.

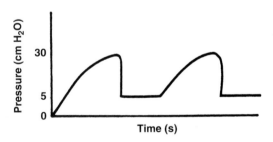

Figure 16-9 Pressure–time curve during TPTV ventilation showing effect of addition of PEEP on tidal volume. Initially, tidal volume is delivered by a pressure difference of 30 cm water (difference between 0 and 30 cm water pressure). With the addition of 5 cm water PEEP, the pressure difference is reduced to 25 cm water (difference between 5 and 30 cm water pressure). This results in less tidal volume being delivered. (From Burgess WR, Chernik V: Respiratory therapy in newborn infants and children, ed 2, New York, 1986, Thieme.)

This adjustment is not needed when the Pressure Control mode is used. With PC, the set pressure level will automatically adjust as the PEEP is increased (or decreased). So, the ventilating pressure and tidal volume should be unchanged.

f. Adjust the respiratory rate

With conventional ventilation, increasing the ventilator respiratory rate increases the minute volume and probably raises the PaO_2 and lowers the $PaCO_2$. Patients with stiff lungs and short time constants of ventilation often respond well to an increased respiratory rate. To that end, some authors advocate using a rate of up to 150/min on a conventional time-triggered, pressure-limited, time-cycled mechanical ventilator, if necessary. With recovery, the rate should be reduced to avoid hyperventilating the patient. (It should be noted that the FDA has set the upper rate limit of 150/min on a conventional ventilator.) A rate of greater than 150/min is termed *high-frequency ventilation* (HFV) and requires a special ventilator.

g. Initiate and adjust high-frequency ventilation (code: IIIC4c) [difficulty: R, Ap, An]

High-frequency ventilation involves the use of a ventilator respiratory rate that is much greater than commonly needed. The FDA defines HFV as a rate of more than 150/min. Because of this FDA definition of HFV, conventional neonatal TPTV ventilators are not considered high-frequency ventilators. Several manufacturers have developed ventilators capable of rates significantly greater than 150/min. One of these must be used when HFV is indicated. The FDA has also set some guidelines for the appropriate use of HFV. Box 16-5 lists the clinical indications for HFV. The most commonly encountered problem is with a premature neonate with infant RDS, a homogeneous lung disease causing low compliance. If the RDS patient is failing despite optimal conventional mechanical ventilation and has a Paw of greater than 15 cm water, high-frequency ventilation is indicated.

Despite the FDA guidelines, many respiratory therapists consider a rate of greater than 40/min on a neonatal patient to be HFV. When a conventional TPTV ventilator is used to deliver a respiratory rate of up to 150/min, the term *high-frequency positive-pressure ventilation* is used. Experience has shown that many RDS infants can be successfully managed with a conventional TPTV ventilator set to deliver a small tidal volume at a rate between 40 and 150/min. However, when these methods fail, true HFV is needed.

Ventilator manufacturers have developed two different technologies for delivering FDA-defined HFV. The first is called *high-frequency jet ventilation* (HFJV). With HFJV, a jet ventilator (Bunnell Life Pulse high-frequency jet ventilator) rapidly sends small jets of gas down the patient's special endotracheal tube. These gas jets entrain additional gas into the tube that comes from a

---

Box 16-5　Common Clinical Indications for the Use of High-Frequency Ventilation in Infants and Children

Severe hypoxemia and hypercarbia unresponsive to conventional ventilation techniques
　Infant respiratory distress syndrome (RDS)
　Acute respiratory distress syndrome (ARDS)
　Pneumonia
　Aspiration syndromes
　Pulmonary hemorrhage
Conventional ventilation with a persistent pulmonary air leak
　Pneumothorax
　Bronchopleural fistula
　Pulmonary interstitial emphysema (PIE)
　Pneumomediastinum
　Pneumoperitoneum
Persistent pulmonary hypertension of the newborn (PPHN)
Pulmonary hypoplasia
Bronchoscopy, laryngoscopy, or tracheal surgery

---

traditional ventilator. The traditional ventilator is set to deliver additional tidal volume breaths at a low rate (usually ≤10/min). The two combined volumes of gas make up the patient's tidal volume. The patient exhales passively because of normal lung recoil. The second method is called *high-frequency oscillation* (HFO) or *high-frequency oscillatory ventilation* (HFOV). With HFO, a pumping device (piston, diaphragm, or sound speaker) actively pushes a small tidal volume into the patient from a continuous flow of gas (called bias flow) passing through the circuit and by the endotracheal tube. HFO technology (SensorMedics Model 3100A high-frequency oscillator) can deliver very high rates because the patient actively exhales the delivered tidal volume. This active exhalation is created by the back stroke of the pumping device that pulls the tidal volume out of the patient's airways and lungs. See Table 16-2 for a comparison of HFV methods and characteristics.

Initial HFV settings depend on the patient's diagnosis, clinical situation, current conventional ventilator settings, and type of high-frequency ventilator to be used. Generally speaking, the initial HFV settings include a tidal volume large enough to see chest movement and a continuation of the patient's original Paw PEEP level, and oxygen percentage. The I:E ratio should be set at 1:2 and the high-frequency rate should be between 10 and 15 Hz, depending on the infant's body weight. (A Hertz is defined as 1 respiratory cycle/s; 60 respiratory cycles/min. For example, a rate of 600/min is 10/s or 10 Hz.) After the patient is stabilized on HFV, arterial blood gases should be drawn and analyzed, vital signs assessed, and a chest radiograph obtained. In a patient without a pulmonary air leak, a chest radiograph finding of lung expansion to T-8 to T-9 on the right hemidiaphragm, without

TABLE 16-2	High-Frequency Ventilation Features and Characteristics		
	HFPPV	**HFJV**	**HFO**
Rate	60-150/min (1-2.5 Hz)	240-660/min (4-10 Hz)	300-3000/min (5-50 Hz)
V_T	3.5 mL/kg (>dead space)	2.5 mL/kg (approx. dead space)	1.3 mL/kg (<dead space)
I:E ratio	1:3 to 1:2	1:3 to 1:2	1:3 to 1:2
Technical application	Conventional ventilator	Special ventilator	Special ventilator
F_IO_2	0.21-1.0	0.21-1.0	0.21-1.0
PEEP	0-20	0-20	0-20
Expiration	Passive	Passive	Active
Gas movement	Bulk flow	Bulk flow	*See below

HFJV, high-frequency jet ventilation; HFO, high-frequency oscillation; HFPPV, high-frequency positive-pressure ventilation. Hz (Hertz) = 1 respiratory cycle/s.
*There are several theories on how gas movement occurs with HFO. See a dedicated mechanical ventilation textbook for a discussion on them.

intercostal bulging, is believed to show the best lung volume. Once established, the HFV rate is seldom changed. Adjustments in tidal volume are made by increasing or decreasing what is referred to as either drive pressure (with HFJV) or amplitude (with HFO). Increasing drive pressure/amplitude increases the tidal volume and decreases the carbon dioxide level. The patient's oxygenation should also improve as the $\overline{Paw}$ is increased. Decreasing drive pressure/amplitude decreases the tidal volume and increases the carbon dioxide level. If the patient's oxygenation should decrease too much, additional therapeutic PEEP may be needed. See Table 15-3 in Chapter 15 for high-frequency ventilation guidelines with infant and adult patients. See Figure 16-10 for a protocol on initiation and adjustment of HFO. Figure 16-11 shows a protocol for weaning from HFO.

Exam Hint 16-5

If a patient with RDS is failing with conventional mechanical ventilation, high-frequency ventilation is indicated.

h. Recommend the instillation of exogenous surfactant (code: IIIE4k) [difficulty: R, Ap]

The primary problem with a premature neonate with RDS is the lack of surfactant, a phospholipid, to reduce the surface tension in the alveoli. In 1991 the FDA approved the use of exogenous surfactant that can be directly instilled into the lungs of RDS neonates. Surfaxin (a synthetic product), Survanta and Infasurf (both bovine lung extract), and Curosurf (a pig lung extract) have been successfully used clinically. See Chapter 9 for more information. These drugs have proven very beneficial to premature neonates with inadequate natural surfactant. After the drug is administered, the patient's lung compliance improves dramatically. When this improvement occurs, be prepared to rapidly reduce the ventilator-delivered oxygen

percentage, rate, pressure limit, and PEEP. The PIP will need to be reduced to keep the same tidal volume. Failure to reduce PIP and PEEP could result in too large a tidal volume and FRC that could cause pulmonary barotrauma. After surfactant has been administered, many, but not all, patients can be supported on nasal CPAP. However, close monitoring is essential and some neonates will continue to need ventilatory support.

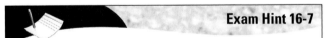

Exam Hint 16-6

Recent exams have included a question about the application or modification of HFV. Know that increasing the amplitude results in a larger tidal volume and a reduction in the patient's $PaCO_2$. Increasing the amplitude should also improve oxygenation. Reducing the amplitude would have the opposite effect.

Exam Hint 16-7

Recent exams have included a question about exogenous surfactant being indicated in a neonate with RDS.

3. Patients with increased airway resistance and normal lung compliance

Although meconium aspiration syndrome (MAS) is a commonly seen cause of increased airway resistance, it is also seen in infants with excessive airway secretions or bronchospasm. These neonates usually have normal lung compliance and their clinical problem is getting enough air into and out of the lungs. The meconium or other obstruction causes uneven airflow and results in hypoxemia, air trapping, auto-PEEP, and an increased risk of barotrauma or volutrauma. Because of these issues, there are two key clinical goals. The first is to minimize turbulence during inspiration by reducing the inspiratory flow

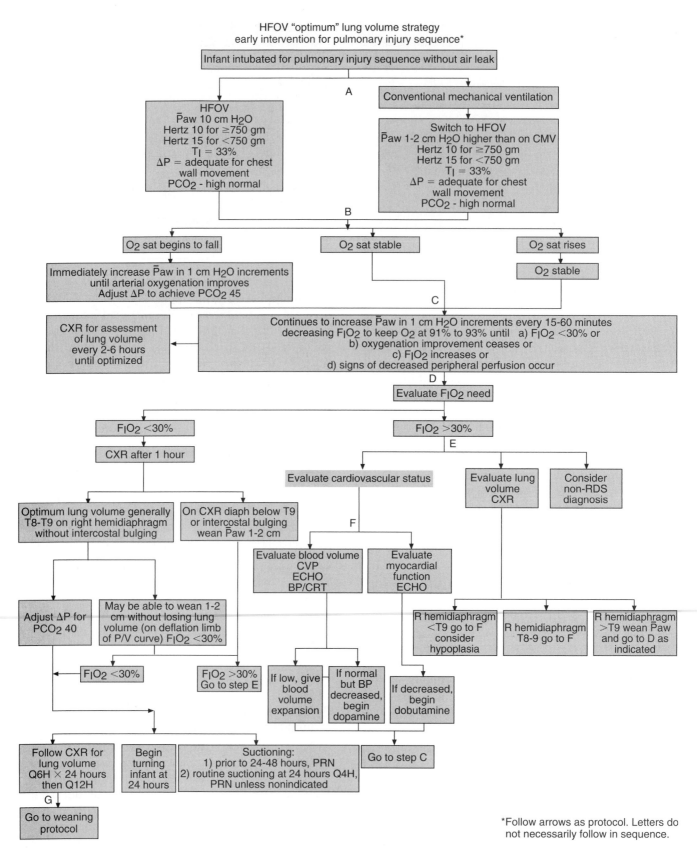

Figure 16-10 Optimum lung volume high-frequency oscillatory ventilation (HFOV) strategy flowchart. (From Minton S, Gerstmann D, Stoddard R: Cardiopul Rev, Yorba Linda, CA, 1995, CareFusion, formerly SensorMedics Corp.)

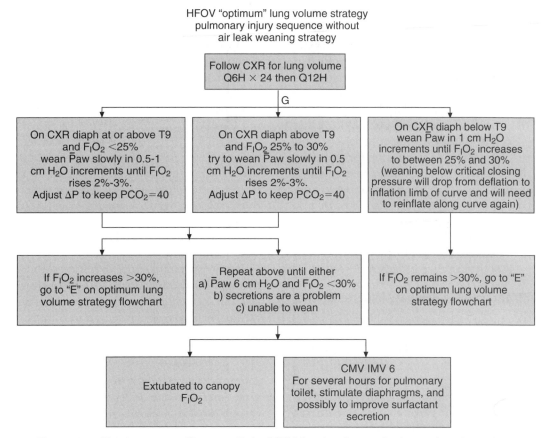

Figure 16-11 High-frequency oscillatory ventilation (HFOV) flowchart for weaning from optimum lung volume strategy. (From Minton S, Gerstmann D, Stoddard R: Cardiopul Rev, Yorba Linda, CA, 1995, CareFusion, formerly SensorMedics Corp.)

rate as much as possible. The second is to give a long enough expiratory time to prevent air trapping. Common recommendations for the ventilator settings are listed in Box 16-6. As discussed earlier, blood gases, vital signs, and so forth must be monitored after the infant is placed on the ventilator. Listen to the breath sounds to detect the end of exhalation and a pause before the start of the next inspiration. This is to ensure that the exhalation has been complete and there is no air trapping that would lead to auto-PEEP. Any further adjustments can then be determined and evaluated by another set of blood gases and vital signs.

Look again at the issue of time constants of ventilation to better understand the various options for adjusting the ventilator. As an example, for a mechanically ventilated neonate with meconium aspiration, the time constant is calculated as follows:

$$T_c = \text{compliance (0.005 L/cm water)} \times \text{resistance}$$
$$\text{(150 cm water/L/s because the infant is intubated}$$
$$\text{and has an obstructive problem.)}$$

Simplify as follows:

$$T_c = 0.005 \times 150 \text{ seconds}$$
$$= 0.75 \text{ second}$$

Box 16-6   Common Mechanical Ventilator Parameters for Neonates with Increased Airway Resistance and Normal Lung Compliance

Delivered tidal volume: 6-8 mL/kg
Pressure limit: less than 20 cm water
Frequency: 20-40/min
I:E ratio: 1:3 to 1:10
Inspiratory time (T_I): between 0.4 and 0.7 second (this may need to be increased)
Expiratory time (T_E): 0.5-1.0 second (this may need to be increased)
PEEP: 4-6 cm water if needed.
Inspiratory flow: sufficient to see the chest move and hear bilateral breath sounds during the inspiration; 5-8 L/min commonly used.
Oxygen percentage: 40% (this may need to be increased to keep the SpO_2 greater than 92%)

(Compare this with a T_c of 0.15 for a normal, spontaneously breathing neonate and a T_c of 0.1 for a ventilated infant with RDS.)

This relatively long time constant means that the tidal volume and peak inspiratory pressure are slowly delivered to the alveoli. There is little chance of causing barotrauma or volutrauma from high ventilating pressures; however, it takes a fairly long inspiratory time to deliver an adequate tidal volume. Care must be taken to provide enough expiratory time for the tidal volume to be exhaled completely. Briefly then, the challenge is to deliver an adequate tidal volume to maintain acceptable blood gases at a rate slow enough to prevent air trapping on exhalation.

In general, the inspiratory flow and rate are kept low, inspiratory and expiratory times are kept relatively long, and the I:E ratio should favor a long time for complete exhalation. Furthermore, it is important to frequently suction the airway to remove meconium or secretions. Postural drainage and percussion are also provided to mobilize the secretions so that they can be suctioned out. Usually these procedures and the natural breakdown of meconium result in reduced airway resistance within a few days. Ventilatory support can then be lessened.

4. Patients with persistent pulmonary hypertension of the newborn

Persistent pulmonary hypertension of the newborn (PPHN) is also referred to as persistent pulmonary hypertension (PPH), persistent pulmonary circulation (PFC), or persistence of the fetal circulation. Infants with PPHN present clinically with an elevated pulmonary artery pressure and a right-to-left shunt through a patent ductus arteriosus or the foramen ovale. Therefore, their oxygenation fluctuates greatly. The problem may be seen right after birth or up to 24 hours later. PPHN seems to result from fetal hypoxemia and acidosis. These, in turn, are caused by or associated with maternal drug addiction, infection, preeclampsia, abruptio placenta, postterm gestation, oligohydramnios, and meconium staining or aspiration.

a. Diagnosis of PPHN

The following four tests are performed to help confirm the diagnosis:

1. Hyperoxia test

This is the first test and is done after an arterial blood gas has shown a low PaO_2. The test involves having the patient inspire 100% oxygen for about 10 minutes and obtaining a second arterial blood gas. If the PaO_2 does not improve to more than 50 torr, a fixed right-to-left shunt is proven. The shunt may be from PPHN or a cyanotic heart defect. If the PaO_2 increases above 100 torr, the neonate probably has parenchymal lung disease and should be treated accordingly.

2. Preductal and postductal arterial blood sampling

Simultaneously draw and then analyze (1) a blood gas sample from the right radial or brachial artery to check the preductal PaO_2 and (2) a blood gas sample from the left brachial, left radial, either femoral artery, or the umbilical artery catheter to check the postductal PaO_2.

Compare the results. A drop in saturation from preductal to postductal blood of greater than 10% or a drop in PaO_2 of greater than 15-20 torr indicates shunting. For example, a preductal PaO_2 of 70 torr and a postductal PaO_2 of 45 torr indicates significant shunting. This same test may be performed noninvasively with either transcutaneous oxygen monitoring or pulse oximetry monitoring. The $PtcO_2$ monitors should be placed over the right upper chest for preductal blood and left upper chest, abdomen, or either thigh for postductal blood. Pulse oximetry monitors should be placed on the right hand for preductal blood and left hand or either foot for postductal blood. Again, a greater than 15-20 torr drop in preductal to postductal $PtcO_2$ or a greater than 10% drop in saturation in preductal to postductal SpO_2 confirms a significant shunt.

It is important to note that if the neonate has a shunt through the foramen ovale instead of the ductus arteriosus, this test will be negative. The preductal and postductal oxygen levels will be the same. Shunting through the foramen ovale is seen in as many as 50% of PPHN babies.

3. Hyperoxia–hyperventilation test

The infant is manually ventilated with 100% oxygen at a rate and pressure adequate to significantly reduce the carbon dioxide level. When this "critical $PaCO_2$" (usually between 20 and 30 torr) is reached, the pulmonary artery pressure drops, the lungs are better perfused, and the PaO_2 improves. Although the patient's color will probably change from cyanotic to pink and the $PtcO_2$ and SpO_2 values will improve, the test is confirmed by a postductal PaO_2 of greater than 80 torr. The critical $PaCO_2$ value, ventilation rate, and manometer pressure on the manual ventilator should be recorded. These values can be used later to set the mechanical ventilator parameters.

4. Doppler echocardiography

This procedure can be used to identify an intracardiac shunt through the foramen ovale, a shunt through a patent ductus arteriosus, or evidence of increased right-ventricular pressure as a sign of pulmonary hypertension.

b. Mechanical ventilation

Any infant who shows signs of PPHN, such as positive results to any of these tests or the need for more than 70% oxygen to prevent hypoxemia, should be mechanically ventilated and considered for hyperventilation therapy. The goal is to reduce pulmonary artery hypertension and thus reduce shunting and improve the PaO_2. This is accomplished by hyperventilating the patient to his or her critical $PaCO_2$. Box 16-7 lists common ventilator parameters used to treat PPHN. Once the proper ventilator settings are found and the blood gas goals are met, the patient is maintained at this level for one or more days. It is often necessary to pharmacologically paralyze the infant with pancuronium bromide (Pavulon)

Box 16-7   Common Mechanical Ventilator Parameters to Treat a Neonate with PPHN

Delivered tidal volume: 6-8 mL/kg initially; 8-10 mL/kg may be needed to hyperventilate the neonate

Pressure limit: 20-25 cm water; use as little pressure as possible but be prepared to increase up to 35 cm water to deliver an adequate tidal volume

Frequency: 40-80/min may be needed to decrease the $PaCO_2$ to the critical level of probably between 20 and 30 mm Hg; a rate of up to 150/min has been used

I:E ratio: 1:2 (this depends on the respiratory rate needed to decrease the carbon dioxide level)

Inspiratory time (T_I): between 0.3 and 0.5 second (this must be decreased at higher respiratory rates)

Expiratory time (T_E): at least 0.5 second (this must be decreased at higher respiratory rates)

PEEP: none if possible to minimize the $\overline{P}aw$ and prevent crushing of the pulmonary capillary bed; 4-5 cm water may be used if needed

Inspiratory flow: sufficient to see the chest move and hear bilateral breath sounds during the inspiration; 5-8 L/min commonly used initially; flow must be increased at higher respiratory rates

Oxygen percentage: up to 70%-100% to keep the postductal PaO_2 greater than 55 torr and ideally between 115 and 120 torr

---

or a similar drug to ensure that the patient's breathing is synchronized with the ventilator. This is especially important when high ventilator rates are needed. After about 24 hours, the ventilator is adjusted to increase the $PaCO_2$ by 1-2 torr. If the peak inspiratory pressure is greater than 45 cm water, it should be reduced first. A blood gas is drawn to see if the PaO_2 is stable and if the $PaCO_2$ increased the desired small amount. If this first reduction in support is tolerated, it may be slowly followed by further reductions. Each step back from hyperventilation should be small so that the $PaCO_2$ increases only by 1-2 mm Hg each time.

As this happens, the patient should be supported in every other way. The medication tolazoline (Priscoline) is a pulmonary vasodilator that has proven to be successful in about one of six neonates with PPHN. Watch for signs of pulmonary barotrauma or bronchopulmonary dysplasia (BPD) from the high peak pressures and oxygen percentages required with these patients.

c. Pulmonary vasodilators

1. Recommend pulmonary vasodilators (code: IIIE4a) [difficulty: R, Ap]

See Chapter 9 for the full discussion of the various pulmonary vasodilators. This discussion will be limited to briefly presenting inhaled nitric oxide (INO) gas. The FDA has approved INO for use as a pulmonary artery vasodilator in neonates with PPHN and increased pulmonary vascular resistance. Inhaled NO has not been approved for adult patients. Some reports of off-label nitric oxide use in patients with hypoxic respiratory failure have shown promising results. However, INO has not benefitted patients with acute respiratory distress syndrome.

2. Administer inhaled nitric oxide (code: IIID4) [difficulty: R, Ap]

The FDA has approved the use of INOmax (0.8% nitric oxide and 99.2% nitrogen) to deliver inhaled nitric oxide to these patients. The currently recommended initial dose of INO to treat PPHN is 20 parts per million (ppm). The possible range for delivered NO is 2-80 ppm. Be prepared to increase the level of NO as needed, to reverse the pulmonary hypertension. When the patient improves, the NO level will need to be decreased. This usually is done by cutting the NO level in half, assessing the patient, and cutting the NO level in half again, etc., as tolerated. For example, cut the dose from 20 to 10 ppm, then 10 to 5 ppm, etc.

To deliver the needed concentrations of nitric oxide and supplemental oxygen, the INOvent delivery system is needed. It is used to set the desired mix of INOmax to the newborn's ventilator and to monitor the levels of NO, nitrogen dioxide (NO_2), and oxygen delivered. The equipment is discussed below in Module D.

Because NO is chemically changed in the body to toxic NO_2 and nitric acid, it is important to closely monitor the level of nitrogen dioxide. Low levels of NO_2 can cause a pneumonitis, and higher levels can cause pulmonary edema. The patient's methemoglobin (MetHb) level also should be monitored, as NO can cause an elevated level. Methemoglobinemia is defined as >7% MetHb. Be prepared to decrease the level of INO to reduce the amount of toxic NO_2 and normalize an elevated MetHb level.

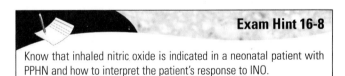

Exam Hint 16-8

Know that inhaled nitric oxide is indicated in a neonatal patient with PPHN and how to interpret the patient's response to INO.

5. Patients with bronchopulmonary dysplasia

The neonate who develops bronchopulmonary dysplasia (BPD) is usually born prematurely with a low birth weight. He or she is a survivor of RDS but has suffered serious chronic lung damage in the process. It is controversial whether high peak pressures, high $\overline{P}aw$, high inspired oxygen percentages, or a combination of these factors is the main cause of BPD. It is important to try to minimize all of them so that new lung tissue can grow to replace lung tissue that has been damaged. It is important to try to wean these infants as quickly as possible to avoid further ventilator-induced damage. If acceptable blood gases can

---

Box 16-8   Common Mechanical Ventilator Parameters for Neonates with BPD

Delivered tidal volume: 6-8 mL/kg

Pressure limit: as low as possible and not to exceed 25 cm water

Frequency: 20-40/min; keep as low as possible to maintain the $PaCO_2$ between 35 and 45 torr; some authors report accepting a $PaCO_2$ as high as 55-65 torr to minimize the need to increase peak and mean pressures

I:E ratio: 1:2 to 1:4

Inspiratory time (T_I): between 0.3 and 0.7 second

Expiratory time (T_E): at least 0.5 second to allow for a complete exhalation

PEEP: no more than 4-6 cm water

Inspiratory flow: sufficient to see the chest move and hear bilateral breath sounds during the inspiration; 5-8 L/min commonly used initially

Oxygen percentage: as low as possible to keep the PaO_2 between 55 and 65 torr; some authors report accepting a PaO_2 as low as 35 torr to minimize the need to increase peak and mean pressures; it must be noted that a PaO_2 below 55 torr increases the risk of pulmonary hypertension

---

be maintained with a ventilator rate of less than 15/min, the infant may be extubated. Nasal CPAP may be used to help maintain the PaO_2. See Box 16-8 for the commonly recommended ventilator settings for a BPD patient.

A number of medications are used to help optimize the patient's pulmonary function. Methylxanthines such as aminophylline or caffeine are beneficial as respiratory stimulants. There is further evidence that they help to strengthen the diaphragm and decrease muscle fatigue. The diuretic furosemide (Lasix) has been widely reported to improve lung compliance and airway resistance by decreasing any pulmonary edema fluid. Remember that patients receiving furosemide must be given a potassium chloride supplement to replace what is lost through the kidneys. Some authors have reported the use of corticosteroids to be helpful in weaning because of increased pulmonary compliance. This possible advantage must be balanced against the known problems associated with the prolonged use of the medication. Finally, a dietary supplement of vitamin E may increase lung healing. It is hoped that the use of surfactant replacement therapy early in the treatment of the RDS neonate will reduce the incidence of BPD.

6. Patient–ventilator monitoring

a. Utilize ventilator graphics (e.g., waveforms, scales) to support oxygenation and ventilation (code: IIIC6) [difficulty: R, Ap, An]

A patient who has been intubated and placed on a modern mechanical ventilator with a microprocessor and graphics software can have ventilator flow, volume, and pressure waveforms visualized on the monitor. Usually these parameters can be individually selected and paired up for comparison (such as pressure vs volume) or compared versus time (such as volume vs time). Select the parameters

that best provide the data to help explain the patient's situation. Some units allow the information to be stored in memory or printed out. Compare current information with any past data.

Because not every ventilator can provide waveform information, the correct unit must be selected for the patient. For example, the Drager Babylog 8000 has the monitor and graphics software built into the unit. Follow the ventilator manufacturer's guidelines to direct the unit to create the desired flow, volume, or pressure waveforms.

Ventilator flow, volume, and pressure waveforms offer much clinically useful information. For example, expiratory flow can be monitored to look for air trapping and auto-PEEP. As discussed earlier, this is a concern if the neonate has obstructive airway disease or if a high respiratory rate is being used. Volume can be monitored as an indicator of improving or worsening lung compliance. Pressure can also be monitored as it relates to improving or worsening lung compliance. Less pressure is needed to deliver the desired tidal volume if the patient's lung compliance is improving. Conversely, more pressure is needed to deliver the desired tidal volume if the patient's lung compliance is worsening. Chapter 15 and this chapter include examples of waveform tracings.

As discussed earlier, be prepared to make adjustments in the ventilator as indicated by graphics. For example, if air trapping and auto-PEEP are observed, be prepared to increase the expiratory time, decrease the inspiratory time, or decrease the tidal volume to ensure that there is a complete exhalation.

b. Mean airway pressure

Mean airway pressure ($\overline{P}aw$, MAP, $\overline{Paw}$) is the average pressure over an entire breathing cycle. A number of current neonatal and adult ventilators are able to calculate the value. $\overline{P}aw$ is influenced by both the patient's C_{LT} and his or her R_{aw}. If the ventilator settings are unchanged, a decrease in compliance or an increase in resistance will result in an increase in the $\overline{P}aw$. This is because in a neonatal ventilator, the pressure limit is reached earlier and held for the duration of the inspiratory time. Conversely, if the patient's compliance increases or the resistance decreases, the $\overline{P}aw$ will decrease. It is important to further evaluate the patient when a change in $\overline{P}aw$ is noticed. This is because the new pressure by itself does not show you whether there has been a change in compliance, resistance, or both. Any treatments that improve lung compliance and reduce airway resistance are shown by a reduced $\overline{P}aw$.

In general, an increase in $\overline{P}aw$ increases the patient's oxygenation. This is because the alveoli are kept open longer, allowing more time for diffusion and preventing alveolar collapse. If alveolar ventilation is improved, the $PaCO_2$ will also be reduced. There is clinical evidence that a $\overline{P}aw$ of 12 or more cm water

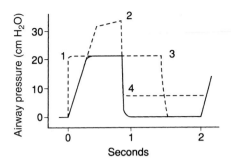

Figure 16-12 Pressure–time tracings showing four different ventilator settings that can be used to increase mean airway pressure. Trace 1, inspiratory flow is increased. Trace 2, pressure limit is increased. Trace 3, inspiratory time is increased. This also changes the I:E ratio by reducing expiratory time if the rate is kept the same. Trace 4, PEEP is added. (Redrawn from Harris TR: Physiologic principles. Goldsmith JP, Karotkin EH, editors: Assisted ventilation of the neonate, Philadelphia, 1981, Saunders.)

is associated with an increased risk of pulmonary barotrauma and decreased cardiac output. This is especially true if PEEP is increased to raise the $\overline{P}aw$. Watch the patient closely whenever a ventilator change is made that increases the $\overline{P}aw$. A sudden deterioration in cardiopulmonary function may be caused by a pneumothorax. A reduction in urine output, an increased heart rate, and decreased blood pressure are often seen when the cardiac output is reduced. The $\overline{P}aw$ should be reduced if either of these situations is observed. To prevent these complications, it is necessary to reduce the $\overline{P}aw$ whenever the patient's compliance improves.

Usually the $\overline{P}aw$ is the result of the patient's lung compliance and airway resistance and the various ventilator settings. The initial $\overline{P}aw$ should be considered along with the ventilator settings when interpreting the first set of arterial blood gases. Based on the blood gas results, ventilator adjustments may be needed. Note the $\overline{P}aw$ at each adjustment.

A number of ventilator control adjustments influence the patient's $\overline{P}aw$. (Fig. 16-12 shows several examples of airway pressure tracings based on ventilator control changes.) If the patient's compliance and resistance are stable, the $\overline{P}aw$ will be *increased* by the following: (1) an increased inspiratory flow, (2) an increased pressure limit (assuming the pressure limit has been previously reached), (3) an increase in PEEP, (4) an increased inspiratory time (assuming no change in ventilator rate and a decreased expiratory time), and (5) a decreased expiratory time (assuming an increased ventilator rate). These ventilator adjustments should result in an increased PaO_2 and possibly a decreased $PaCO_2$. Measure blood gases to be sure of the patient's response.

If the patient's compliance and resistance are stable, the $\overline{P}aw$ will be *decreased* by the following:

- A decreased inspiratory flow
- A decreased pressure limit (assuming the pressure limit has been previously reached)

- A decrease in PEEP
- A decreased inspiratory time (assuming no change in ventilator rate and an increased expiratory time)
- An increased expiratory time (assuming a decreased ventilator rate)

These ventilator adjustments may result in a decreased PaO_2 and possibly an increased $PaCO_2$. Measure blood gases to be sure of the patient's response.

It should be noted that of all the various controls that have an influence on the $\overline{P}aw$, PEEP has the greatest impact. There is usually a one-for-one relationship between the addition or removal of PEEP and the resulting $\overline{P}aw$. For example, the $\overline{P}aw$ is 10 cm water when 5 cm water of PEEP is added. The resulting $\overline{P}aw$ is seen to become 15 cm water. If 2 cm of PEEP is removed, the $\overline{P}aw$ will drop to 13 cm water.

MODULE D

CPAP and mechanical ventilation equipment

1. Continuous positive airway pressure devices

a. Assemble the necessary equipment (code: IIA2) [difficulty: R, Ap, An]

Nasal CPAP devices are widely used with neonates who are born prematurely and have RDS. Their immature lungs lack sufficient surfactant and need the continuous positive airway pressure to keep the alveoli open. Often, after the instillation of surfactant, nasal CPAP meets the patient's needs so that endotracheal intubation and mechanical ventilation can be avoided. Nasal CPAP works with neonates because they are obligate nose breathers.

There are three different patient interface devices for administering nasal CPAP. Nasal prongs (binasal prongs; Fig. 16-2, A) are most commonly used and fit into both nostrils. The prongs come in different diameters so that the proper size can be found to fit snugly the internal diameter of the infant's nares and not leak. Avoid nasal prongs that are too large because they can cause skin erosion or excessively dilate the nares. The second choice is a nasal mask as shown in Figure 16-2, B. They come in a variety of sizes to fit without a leak or cause skin erosion. The third, and least used option, is a nasopharyngeal (NP) tube. The NP tube is actually an endotracheal tube that has been cut shorter (see Fig. 16-2, C). Select a tube that is the largest that can be easily inserted into the patient. An advantage of an NP tube is that it provides a route for a suction catheter to remove oral secretions or for deep tracheal suctioning. Any of these patient interface devices must be held in place. There are a variety of tubing systems and soft caps and straps can be used. Pick the one that fits properly to avoid slipping or excess pressure. See Figure 16-3 for an example.

Nasal CPAP is associated with the hazards of gastric distension and reflux aspiration. These occur when the airway pressure forces air into the stomach. A gastric tube is usually inserted to vent the air out (see Fig. 16-3).

CPAP can be provided by one of three systems: a free-standing or manufactured bubble CPAP system (see Fig. 16-4), a fluidic-type CPAP system, or a mechanical ventilator (Fig. 16-13). A bubble or fluidic-type CPAP system can be used when the neonate is stable and not at risk for apnea. However, if the patient's breathing is unstable, an endotracheal tube and mechanical ventilator should be used. All currently available neonatal ventilators offer a CPAP mode. This allows the practitioner to easily switch the intubated neonate from IMV to CPAP without the need to set up new equipment.

b. Troubleshoot any problems with the equipment (code: IIA2) [difficulty: R, Ap, An]

A sudden drop in the CPAP level to zero indicates a disconnection at the patient or somewhere in the breathing circuit. Check all connections and reassemble the break. The patient may need to be manually ventilated while the problem is corrected.

If the CPAP level drops more than 2 cm of water pressure during an inspiration, the flow is inadequate and should be increased. Flow is also inadequate if the patient shows an increased use of accessory muscles of respiration or appears to have an increased work of breathing. Too high a flow is seen by an inadvertently high level of CPAP or the appearance that the patient is having a difficult time exhaling. Mucous plugging is a common problem with small-diameter airway tubes. A plugged tube may result in a backup of gas and can increase CPAP; however, depending on the CPAP system, there may be no change in pressure. Careful patient monitoring is important. Watch for a decrease in oxygenation, an increase in the respiratory rate, or retractions as signs of airway obstruction. Suction to clear out the mucous plug or remove the tube and place a new one.

2. Continuous positive airway pressure circuit

a. Assemble the necessary equipment (code: IIA14) [difficulty: R, Ap]

Follow the manufacturer's instructions for assembly of the CPAP device and CPAP circuit. See Figures 16-4 and 16-13 as well as the illustration of the CPAP circuit in Chapter 15 for the usual component pieces and assembly guidance. The general discussion and an illustration related to CPAP systems is presented in Chapter 15. Free-standing neonatal systems are similar to those used with adults. Humidification options are similar to those for mechanical ventilation. A heated cascade-type or wick-type humidifier can be used to provide moisture to the inhaled gas.

b. Troubleshoot any problems with the equipment (code: IIA14) [difficulty: R, Ap]

The previous discussion about putting together and fixing problems with the CPAP device applies to the CPAP circuit. CPAP circuits should not be changed routinely for infection control purposes. Current guidelines recommend that they be changed only when visibly soiled (sputum or blood).

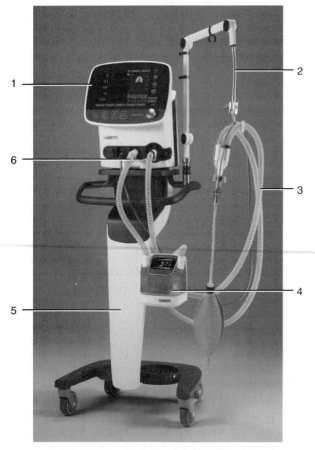

Figure 16-13 Hamilton-C3 ventilator prepared for patient care. This is an example of a pneumatic ventilator that provides only pressure-cycled ventilation. Key features include: (1) graphical user interface for setting ventilator parameters and alarms and viewing graphic images; (2) adjustable support arm for the patient circuit; (3) inspiratory and expiratory limbs of the patient circuit and wye (Y) connector; (4) humidifier included within the inspiratory limb of the circuit; (5) trolley for moving the ventilator; and (6) ventilator connection ports for the inspiratory limb and expiratory limb of the circuit. In addition, a water trap, temperature probe, and oxygen analyzer can be added to the inspiratory limb of the circuit. (Courtesy of Hamilton Medical AG, Bonaduz, Switzerland.)

Exam Hint 16-9

A variable CPAP level indicates insufficient flow or a leak. A sudden drop in CPAP level to zero indicates a disconnection within the circuit or at the patient connection.

---

3. Traditional mechanical ventilators

As discussed in Chapter 15, the literature produced by the manufacturers and the descriptions used in many standard texts break the various ventilators into more categories than used by the NBRC. To avoid confusion, this text uses the NBRC's more simplified terminology.

A *pneumatically powered ventilator* is defined here as powered by compressed gas. It may be electrically controlled with electrical alarm systems. *Fluidic ventilators* are defined here as being pneumatically powered and partially or completely controlled by fluidic methods. Fluidic controls make use of compressed gas for cycling and other ventilator functions. Both of these types of neonatal ventilators use compressed air and oxygen that go to an air-oxygen mixer (blender) to determine the inspired oxygen. The gas then goes to a flowmeter with which the continuous flow per minute through the ventilator circuit is set. Depending on the ventilator, either compressed air or oxygen is used to drive the other control functions in fluidic ventilators.

An *electrically powered ventilator* is defined here as being electrically powered and controlled. Compressed air and oxygen go to a blender in which the inspired oxygen is set. A *microprocessor ventilator* is defined here as being controlled by a microprocessor; it may be pneumatically or electrically powered. These ventilators offer the greatest number of patient care features. All of these types of ventilators are limited to the 150 breaths/min maximum rate set by the FDA. CPAP can be delivered through the types of ventilators described previously, through manufactured CPAP-only units, or through a freestanding, assembled component system.

a. Assemble the necessary equipment (code: IIA8) [difficulty: R, Ap, An]

In addition to the selected ventilator, a humidifier and a patient breathing circuit will need to be connected. Figure 16-13 shows the Hamilton-C3, a typical pneumatically powered ventilator set up with its accessory items. It can be used to deliver pressure-controlled breaths to neonatal, pediatric, or adult patients. Figure 16-14 shows the Servo-i, an electrically powered, microprocessor-type ventilator, without its patient circuit. It can be used to deliver pressure-controlled, volume-controlled, or dual-control mode breaths to all patient populations. In addition, this ventilator offers the neurally adjusted ventilatory assist (NAVA) option for sensing a neonate's breathing efforts. NAVA employs a special esophageal catheter that is able to detect the electrical signal when the diaphragm contracts at the start of a breath. This signal is sent to the Servo-i, which then triggers a breath.

b. Troubleshoot any problems with the equipment (code: IIA8) [difficulty: R, Ap, An]

It is beyond the scope of this text to discuss in detail the functions of pneumatic and other ventilators. However, a respiratory therapist should be aware of commonly found problems. With a pneumatic-type ventilator, make sure that the air and oxygen high-pressure hoses are screwed tightly into the air-oxygen blender. A gas leak is heard as a whistling or hissing sound. If either gas source is cut off to the blender, its alarm will sound. Fluidic-type ventilators are prone to the same kind of

problems with leaking high-pressure air and oxygen hoses as pneumatic ventilators. In addition, they are very sensitive to obstructions. Make sure that all inlet filters are intact and free of debris. With an electrically powered or microprocessor-type ventilator, make sure that the electrical power source is secure. Do not use a unit that does not power up or operate properly. Microprocessor ventilators typically come with self-diagnostic software. If a problem is detected, the unit will display it on the monitor. There is little to repair with these units at the bedside. Occasionally a computer chip must be replaced.

4. Traditional ventilator circuit

a. Assemble the necessary equipment (code: IIA14) [difficulty: R, Ap]

Conventional neonatal ventilators use a patient circuit that has all of the standard features of an adult circuit as discussed in Chapter 15. Commonly, disposable single-patient-use corrugated plastic circuits are used. They are inexpensive and meet the needs of most patients. An obvious difference is the smaller diameter so that there is less compressible volume. Be aware that corrugated circuits have a relatively high internal resistance and compressible volume. The corrugations lead to gas turbulence that increases as the flow is raised. If this is a clinical concern, a smooth-bore circuit can be used to minimize gas turbulence. See Figure 16-13 for the typical patient circuit and humidifier. Patient tidal volume gas exits the ventilator and passes through a short length of large-bore tubing to enter the humidifier. The warmed and humidified gas enters another, longer length of large-bore tubing to go to the patient wye (Y). The Y is connected to the patient's endotracheal or tracheostomy tube to deliver the tidal volume gas. Expiratory gas goes through a long length of large-bore tubing to return to the expiratory valve on the ventilator. Additional items that can be added into the patient circuit include an oxygen analyzer, exhaled carbon dioxide analyzer for capnometry, temperature probe, and water traps. Condensation is drained out into water traps that are placed at low points in the natural draping of the inspiratory and possibly expiratory limbs of the circuit. If excessive moisture is a problem or if the gas temperature must be maintained within a narrow range, a heated-wire circuit may be used. These types of circuits are built with a heated wire either loosely threaded through the lumen or coiled within the tubing itself. They are integrated with the humidification system and a servo unit for automatic temperature regulation. Because of the added wiring, these disposable circuits are considerably more expensive than the simple circuits used with most patients. An HME is usually used only with children because the tidal volume must be greater than the dead space of the HME. If an HME is used for passive humidification, it is added between the patient's endotracheal tube and the Y of the ventilator circuit.

b. Troubleshoot any problems with the equipment (code: IIA14) [difficulty: R, Ap]

When the circuit tubing is warmed, it becomes more stretchable. This stretch results in more tidal volume lost to the circuit instead of being delivered to the patient. If a heated-wire circuit is added, it is important to use it only with the servo-controlled humidifier for which it is designed. Mixing circuits and humidifiers can lead to either overheating or underheating problems.

Furthermore, do not cover a heated-wire circuit with a blanket. The circuit should not be allowed to touch the patient to avoid burns. If the patient is inside an incubator with a radiant warmer, the circuit's temperature probe must be kept outside.

An added neonatal circuit feature is a third small-bore tubing for measuring the proximal airway pressure. The tube runs from the patient Y to the proximal airway pressure nipple on the ventilator. Make sure that all the

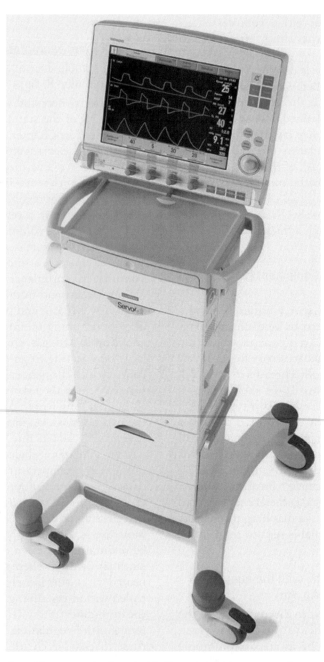

Figure 16-14 The Servo-i is an example of an electrically powered microprocessor-type ventilator. It can provide all pressure ventilation, volume ventilation, and dual-control ventilator modes to all patient populations. In addition, it offers neurally adjusted ventilatory assist (NAVA) to better synchronize neonatal patient breathing efforts with the ventilator. See Figure 16-13 for the features of the patient care circuit that would need to be added to the ventilator. (Courtesy of Maquet, Inc., Bridgewater, NJ.)

connections are tight to prevent gas leaks. If the tidal volume is not being delivered, look for a leak in the circuit or a disconnection from the patient. Water traps must be periodically emptied.

Ventilator circuits should not be changed routinely for infection control purposes. Current guidelines recommend that they be changed only when visibly soiled. An HME may be used for at least 48 hours. Change it whenever it is visibly soiled or contains sputum or blood.

5. High-frequency ventilators

a. Assemble the necessary equipment (code: IIA8) [difficulty: R, Ap, An]

All high-frequency ventilators are capable of delivering a respiratory rate of more than 150/min. The Bunnell Life Pulse high-frequency ventilator provides high-frequency jet ventilation. Figure 16-15 shows the ventilator and its special circuit attached to a special triple-lumen endotracheal tube. *Note:* As of the time of printing, the manufacturer of the Hi-Lo jet tube has stopped production. It is not known if another manufacturer will begin production. Currently, the patient with a standard endotracheal

tube will need to have the adapter replaced with the Bunnell LifePort endotracheal tube adapter (Fig. 16-16).

The following are needed for proper assembly of an HFJV: (1) a pressurized oxygen source, (2) a pressurized air source, (3) an air–oxygen proportioner (blender), (4) an injector line to add the jet volume to the long catheter on the adapter, and (5) a water supply for the unit's humidification system. Most infants who receive HFJV have previously been receiving conventional mechanical ventilation and will continue to do so. The conventional ventilator is attached by its circuit to the large port on the endotracheal tube adapter. This ventilator is typically operated in the SIMV or CPAP mode and must be fully functional.

The SensorMedics 3100A high-frequency oscillatory ventilator is an HFO ventilator. Figure 16-17 shows the ventilator and its special circuit. An HFO ventilator needs the following basic accessories for assembly: (1) a pressurized oxygen source, (2) a pressurized air source, (3) an air–oxygen proportioner (blender), and (4) a pass-over- or cascade-type humidifier, and (5) a low-compliance patient circuit with water trap designed specifically for the ventilator. If desired, a heated-wire circuit with water trap is available. The circuit is attached to a standard endotracheal tube.

b. Troubleshoot any problems with the equipment (code: IIA8) [difficulty: R, Ap, An]

Make sure that gas sources are stable, all tubing connections are tight, and humidification systems are functioning

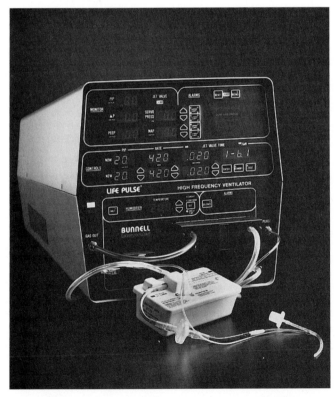

Figure 16-15 The Bunnell Life Pulse high-frequency jet ventilator with its ventilator circuit of small-bore tubing attached to a triple-lumen endotracheal tube. *Note:* As of the time of printing, the manufacturer of the Hi-Lo jet tube has stopped production. It is not known if another manufacturer will begin production. See Figure 15-26 in Chapter 15 for the special adapter that must be used with a standard endotracheal tube to provide HFJV. (Courtesy of Bunnell, Inc., Salt Lake City, UT.)

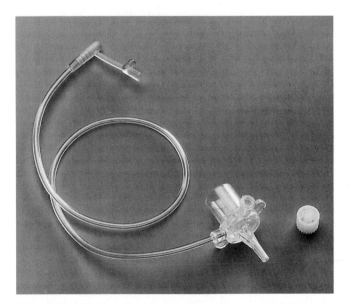

Figure 16-16 The Bunnell LifePort endotracheal tube adapter. When the patient has a conventional endotracheal tube, and the Bunnell jet ventilator will be used, this adapter is substituted for the standard adapter on the endotracheal tube. The jet ventilator is connected to the long catheter. A conventional ventilator is connected to the large port on the adapter. The cap has been removed from the small side port. A small-bore catheter is used to connect this port to the Bunnell jet ventilator to monitor the proximal airway pressure. (Courtesy of Bunnell, Inc., Salt Lake City, UT.)

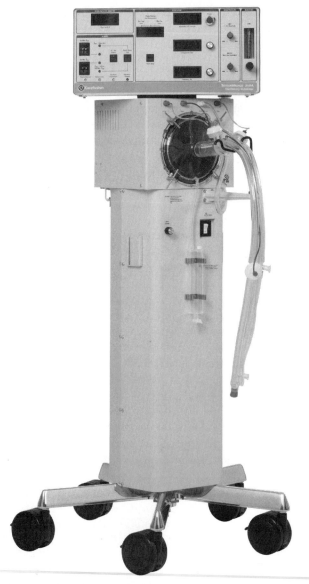

Figure 16-17 The SensorMedics Model 3100A high-frequency oscillator with its special patient circuit. (Courtesy of CareFusion, Inc., San Diego, CA.)

properly. Because the patient's tidal volume is very small, it cannot be accurately measured. Any leaks will result in an undetectable loss of delivered tidal volume.

6. High-frequency ventilator circuit

a. Assemble the necessary equipment (code: IIA14) [difficulty: R, Ap]

See the above description and Figures 16-15 and 16-16 for the Bunnell and Figure 16-17 for the SensorMedics circuits.

b. Troubleshoot any problems with the equipment (code: IIA14) [difficulty: R, Ap]

A leak in the circuit will result in the airway pressure and tidal volume decreasing. Make sure that all connections are tight.

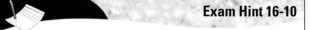

7. Humidification equipment

a. Assemble the necessary equipment (code: IIA3) [difficulty: R, Ap]

The general discussion of humidification equipment was presented in Chapters 8 and 15. See Figure 16-4 for the humidifier setup for CPAP and Figure 16-13 for the humidifier setup for a ventilator. Both heated humidifiers and HMEs are used with pediatric patients. Heated pass-over-type humidifier systems are preferred for neonates. A water trap should be placed in the inspiratory limb of the patient circuit to drain any condensation.

b. Troubleshoot any problems with the equipment (code: IIA3) [difficulty: R, Ap]

Again, see Chapters 8 and 15 for assembly and troubleshooting of humidification systems. With a cascade-type or pass-over-type humidifier, the gas temperature is usually maintained close to the neonate's body temperature to maintain a neutral thermal environment. Make sure that the water level is kept in the recommended range to properly humidify the gas. Regularly empty any condensation from the water trap.

8. Nitric oxide (NO) delivery devices

a. Assemble the necessary equipment (code: IIA18) [difficulty: R, Ap, An]

Inhaled nitric oxide (INO) is used to treat a neonate with PPHN of the newborn. It is currently available for delivery through three different systems: INOvent (GE Healthcare, Waukesha, WI), INOmax DS (Ikaria, Clinton, NJ), and AeroNox (International Biomedical, Austin, TX). Although inhaled nitric oxide can be delivered to the patient by way of nasal prongs, manual resuscitation bag, or a CPAP system, most patients receive it through their mechanical ventilator. Figure 16-18 shows the INOvent system that is designed to be used in tandem with a ventilator. The components of an INO and ventilator system include:

1. Nitric oxide gas analyzer that includes high- and low-concentration alarms.
2. Nitrogen dioxide analyzer with high and low alarms.
3. Oxygen analyzer with high and low alarms.
4. Manual resuscitation bag with NO as a backup ventilation system, if needed.

A small-bore tube delivers the nitric oxide from the reservoir into the inspiratory limb of the patient's ventilator circuit before the humidifier. The NO, nitrogen

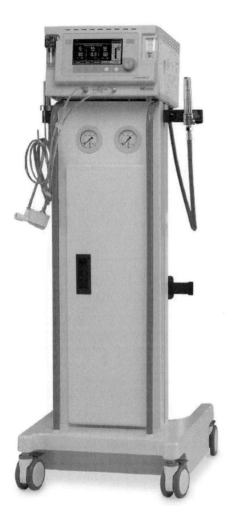

Figure 16-18 The Datex-Ohmeda INOvent is used to deliver and monitor inhaled nitric oxide (INO). (Courtesy of GE Healthcare, Waukesha, WI.)

dioxide, and oxygen analyzers are added into the inspiratory limb of the circuit after the injection point and before the humidifier.

b. Troubleshoot any problems with the equipment (code: IIA18) [difficulty: R, Ap, An]

Make sure that all connections are tight. A leak will result in a drop in the tidal volume and alter the desired NO concentration. Be prepared to manually ventilate the patient with added NO if the ventilator should fail.

9. Perform quality control procedures for mechanical ventilators (code: IIC5) [difficulty: R, Ap]

Follow the manufacturer's guidelines for quality control procedures on mechanical ventilators. The microprocessor ventilators usually have a software package that performs self-diagnostic tests on the unit. If a problem is found, it is displayed on the monitor. Obviously the ventilator should deliver the volume, flow, and pressure that are set on the control. Do not use a ventilator that fails a quality control check.

MODULE E

Respiratory care plan

1. Determine a patient's pathophysiologic state (code: IIIF1) [difficulty: R, Ap, An]

Refer to Chapter 1 or earlier in this chapter for a detailed discussion on neonatal assessment. A brief discussion of pulmonary conditions requiring mechanical ventilation was presented earlier in this chapter.

2. Recommend starting a treatment based on the patient's response (code: IIIE2a) [difficulty: R, Ap, An]

Specific recommendations for ventilatory support for the various pulmonary conditions were given earlier in the chapter.

3. Recommend a change in the therapeutic plan if indicated (code: IIIF2) [difficulty: R, Ap, An]

In many cases, TPTV mechanical ventilation with the IMV mode is utilized. An infant who is attempting to exhale when the IMV breath is being delivered is said to be "bucking" or "fighting" the ventilator. This problem is almost unavoidable because the IMV breaths are difficult to synchronize on the majority of neonatal ventilators. If the asynchrony between the infant's efforts and the ventilator is too great, there is an increased risk of hypoxemia and barotrauma or volutrauma. Carefully evaluate the patient to determine if the patient is breathing rapidly because of pain or improper adjustment of the ventilator. Make sure that the flow, rate, pressure limit, and so forth are correctly set for the patient's condition.

As discussed earlier, the ventilator must be adjusted to maintain desired arterial blood gas goals. It may be necessary to change from CPAP to conventional ventilation modes to high-frequency ventilation as the patient's condition changes.

4. Medications to improve patient tolerance of mechanical ventilation

a. Recommend sedatives and hypnotics (code: IIIE4g) [difficulty: R, Ap]

See below.

b. Recommend analgesics (code: IIIE4h) [difficulty: R, Ap]

See below.

c. Recommend neuromuscular blocking agents (code: IIIE4i) [difficulty: R, Ap]

Sedation or paralysis should be considered only after all other causes of asynchrony have been ruled out. In many cases, when the ventilator is appropriately adjusted, the patient breathes in synchrony with it. If this cannot be achieved, sedation or paralysis must be considered.

Antianxiety agents are not typically used with neonates. Morphine sulfate or other opiates are typically used for pain, but other less powerful medications may also be tried. If the patient must be paralyzed, pancuronium (Pavulon), atracurium (Tracrium), and vecuronium (Norcuron) are commonly used. Remember that these paralyzing agents have no effect on the patient's ability to feel pain or to be afraid of what is happening. Pain medications must be given as necessary.

5. Recommend a treatment be terminated (code: IIIE1) [difficulty: R, Ap, An]

See below.

6. Recommend discontinuing a treatment based on the patient's response (code: IIIE2h) [difficulty: R, Ap, An]

Be prepared to stop a particular treatment or change a ventilator parameter if the patient has an adverse reaction to it. Physical assessment is vitally important because a neonate or small child cannot communicate how he or she feels about the care being provided.

7. Recommend the treatment of a pneumothorax (code: IIIE2b) [difficulty: R, Ap, An]

A chest radiograph and physical examination of the neonate will reveal if abnormal air or fluid is found around the lung(s) or heart. When transillumination of the chest is performed, any free air around the lung will be identified through the chest wall as a halo of light with a nonuniform shape. A nontension pneumothorax of greater than 10% is often also treated by inserting a pleural chest tube. If a patient has a tension pneumothorax, a pleural chest tube *must* be inserted to remove the air and relieve the pressure within the chest. A pleural chest tube is also placed to remove blood or other fluid from the pleural space. Chapter 18 has specific information that relates to treating a pneumothorax.

A pneumomediastinum, pneumopericardium, or pneumoperitoneum that puts the patient at risk must also be treated. A chest tube is then inserted into the area where the abnormal air is found. The same chest tube also removes any abnormal collection of fluid. A chest tube is usually placed behind the heart to remove any blood that should leak out after open-heart surgery.

If a neonate is being ventilated on a constant-volume ventilator, the amount of air that is lost through the pleural chest tube can be calculated. This is done by subtracting the measured exhaled volume from the measured inhaled volume. For example:

Inspired tidal volume =   40 mL
Exhaled tidal volume = −30 mL
10 mL of tidal volume
is lost through the
pleural chest tube

It is not possible to measure tidal volume when the neonate is ventilated by any other means. In a case like this, it is possible only to make a qualitative judgment on pleural air leak. In other words, if air is seen to bubble out through the pleural drainage system, an air leak is present. When the air stops bubbling, the pleural tear has healed. See Chapter 18 for a complete discussion on pleural drainage systems.

8. Liberate the patient from mechanical ventilation (weaning)

a. Evaluate data in the patient record about trends in weaning parameters (code: IA13d) [difficulty: R, Ap]

See below.

b. Recommend liberating from mechanical ventilation (code: IIIE2f) [difficulty: R, Ap, An]

As the neonate's condition improves, weaning must be considered. Indications of improvement include acceptable blood gas results, improved chest radiograph, and stable vital signs.

c. Liberate (wean) the patient from mechanical ventilation (code: IIIC8) [difficulty: R, Ap, An]

Specific steps in increasing ventilator support were discussed earlier for each type of common pathologic condition and the various modes of ventilation. In general, ventilator support should be reduced in a manner opposite that in which it was increased. Remember to evaluate the patient's arterial blood gas values and vital signs before and after making a change in the ventilator parameters. If the patient's condition deteriorates, the ventilator setting(s) should be placed as before. General steps in weaning ventilator support in a patient receiving traditional TPTV include the following:

1. Reduce the oxygen percentage in 2% to 5% steps down to 40% or less, while meeting the oxygenation goal (see Table 16-1).
2. Once the patient is receiving 40% or less oxygen, the PEEP level can be decreased in 1-2 cm water increments. The goal is a PEEP level of 3-4 cm water while meeting the oxygenation goal.
3. Next, peak inspiratory pressure can be reduced in 1-2 cm water increments. The goal is a PIP of 15-18 cm water. The patient's arterial blood gas goals must be met (see Table 16-1).
4. The ventilator rate can now be reduced in steps of 1-5 breaths per minute. The patient's spontaneous breathing rate should increase as the ventilator rate is reduced. The goal is a ventilator rate of less than 10/min. Arterial blood gas goals must continue to be met.
5. Depending on the patient's tolerance of the above steps, the patient may be maintained on CPAP or given a spontaneous breathing trial.

9. Extubation

a. Recommend extubation (code: IIIE2g) [difficulty: R, Ap, An]

If the patient is stable with low-pressure CPAP or a spontaneous breathing trial of 30-120 min, and the endotracheal tube is not needed for a suctioning route, the endotracheal tube can be removed.

b. Perform extubation (code: IIIA8) [difficulty: R, Ap, An]

The following additional steps are generally taken to ensure an appropriate, safe extubation:

1. Feedings should be withheld for several hours to reduce the risk of aspiration.
2. Perform an endotracheal tube "leak test" by delivering a mandatory breath and auscultating a leak at the neonate's larynx. An audible leak indicates the absence of laryngeal edema. If a leak cannot be heard, the neonate should be given a treatment of aerosolized racemic epinephrine to reduce the edema. Do not extubate a patient with laryngeal edema because it is likely that the endotracheal tube will need to be reinserted.
3. Hyperoxygenate the neonate.
4. Suction the trachea and the oral pharynx.
5. Deliver a large tidal volume breath and remove the endotracheal tube when the lungs are full.
6. Suction the mouth as needed.
7. Provide supplemental oxygen by face mask or nasal cannula.
8. Follow-up on arterial blood gases and frequent monitoring of vital signs and breath sounds should be done after extubation.
9. Be prepared to reintubate if the patient's condition deteriorates or a suctioning route is needed.

10. Assist the physician in the withdrawal of life support (code: IIIH10) [difficulty: R, Ap]

Because a mechanical ventilator is providing a vital life support function, removing it would be done only if the patient is legally brain dead. This issue is discussed in Chapter 18.

If the life-support measures are to be stopped, the physician will usually take the patient off of the ventilator. The respiratory therapist will be called upon to turn off the alarms and turn off the ventilator. If permitted by hospital policy, the physician may write an order for the respiratory therapist to discontinue the ventilator. However, the therapist has the right to refuse to perform this task based on his or her philosophical or religious beliefs. It is very important that counseling be available and encouraged for family members and health care team members to help them cope with the passing of the patient.

BIBLIOGRAPHY

AARC clinical practice guideline: application of continuous positive airway pressure to neonates via nasal prongs or nasopharyngeal tube, *Respir Care* 39:817, 1994.

AARC clinical practice guideline: application of continuous positive airway pressure to neonates via nasal prongs, nasopharyngeal tube, or nasal mask—2004 revision and update, *Respir Care* 49(9):1100, 2004.

AARC clinical practice guideline: care of the circuit and its relation to ventilator-associated pneumonia, *Respir Care* 48:869, 2003.

AARC clinical practice guideline: endotracheal suctioning of mechanically ventilated patients with artificial airways, *Respir Care* 55(6):758-764, 2010.

AARC clinical practice guideline: evidence-based guidelines for weaning and discontinuing ventilatory support, *Respir Care* 47:69, 2002.

AARC clinical practice guideline: humidification during invasive and noninvasive mechanical ventilation, *Respir Care* 57:782-788, 2012.

AARC clinical practice guideline: humidification during mechanical ventilation, *Respir Care* 37:887, 1992.

AARC clinical practice guideline: neonatal time-triggered, pressure-limited, time-cycled, mechanical ventilation, *Respir Care* 39:808, 1994a (Retired).

AARC clinical practice guideline: patient-ventilator system checks, *Respir Care* 37:882, 1992a (Retired).

AARC clinical practice guideline: removal of the endotracheal tube—2007 revision & update, *Respir Care* 52:81, 2007.

AARC clinical practice guideline: ventilator circuit changes, *Respir Care* 39:797, 1994b.

AARC clinical practice guideline: evidence-based clinical practice guideline: inhaled nitric oxide for neonates with acute hypoxic respiratory failure, *Respir Care* 58(12):1717-1745, 2010a.

AARC clinical practice guideline: surfactant replacement therapy, *Respir Care* 58(2):367-375, 2013.

AARC clinical practice guideline: long-term invasive mechanical ventilation in the home—2007 revision & update, *Respir Care* 52(1):1056-1062, 2007a.

Aloan CA, Hill TV: *Respiratory care of the newborn and child*, ed 2, Philadelphia, 1997, Lippincott-Raven.

Avery ME, Tooley WH, Keller JB, Hurd SS, Bryan MH, Cotton RB, et al.: Is chronic lung disease in low birth weight infants preventable? A survey of eight centers, *Pediatrics* 79(1):26-30, 1987.

Barnhart SL, Czervinske MP: *Perinatal and pediatric respiratory care*, Philadelphia, 1995, Saunders.

Betis P, Thompson J: Neonatal and pediatric respiratory care. In Wilkins RL, Stoller JK, Kacmarek RM, editors: *Egan's fundamentals of respiratory care*, ed 9, St Louis, 2009, Mosby.

Boros SJ, Matalon SV, Ewald R, et al.: The effect of independent variations in inspiratory-expiratory ratio and end expiratory pressure during mechanical ventilation in hyaline membrane disease: the significance of mean airway pressure, *J Pediatr* 91:794, 1977.

Branson RD, Hess DR, Chatburn RL: *Respiratory care equipment*, ed 2, Philadelphia, 1999, Lippincott Williams & Wilkins.

Brown MK, DiBlasi RM: Mechanical ventilation of the premature neonate, *Respir Care* 56:1298–1313, 2011.

Burgess WR, Chernick V: *Respiratory therapy in newborn infants and children*, ed 2, New York, 1986, Thieme.

Cairo JM: *Mosby's respiratory care equipment*, ed 9, St Louis, 2014, Mosby.

Cairo JM, Pilbeam SP: *Mosby's respiratory care equipment*, ed 8, St Louis, 2009, Mosby.

Carlo WA, Martin RJ: Principles of neonatal assisted ventilation, *Pediatr Clin North Am* 33:221, 1986.

Cavanagh K: High frequency ventilation of infants: an analysis of the literature, *Respir Care* 35:815, 1990.

Chang DW: *Clinical application of mechanical ventilation*, ed 2, Albany, NY, 2001, Delmar.

Chatburn RL: High frequency ventilation: a report on a state of the art symposium, *Respir Care* 29:839, 1984.

Chatburn RL: Principles and practice of neonatal and pediatric mechanical ventilation, *Respir Care* 36:569, 1991.

Chatburn RL, Lough MD: Mechanical ventilation. In Lough MD, Doershuk CF, Stern RC, editors: *Pediatric respiratory therapy*, ed 3, St Louis, 1985, Mosby.

Chatburn RL, Waldemar AC, Lough MD: Clinical algorithm for pressure-limited ventilation of neonates with respiratory distress syndrome, *Respir Care* 28:1579, 1983.

Coghill CH, et al.: Neonatal and pediatric high-frequency ventilation: principles and practice, *Respir Care* 36:596, 1991.

DiBlasi RM: Nasal continuous positive airway pressure (CPAP) for the respiratory care of the newborn, *Respir Care* 54:1209–1235, 2009.

DiBlasi RM: Neonatal noninvasive ventilation techniques: do we really need to intubate? *Respir Care* 56:1273–1297, 2011.

DiBlasi RM: Neonatal and pediatric mechanical ventilation. In Cairo JM, editor: *Pilbeam's mechanical ventilation*, ed 5, St Louis, 2012, Mosby.

Donn SM, Boon W: Mechanical ventilation of the neonate: should we target volume or pressure? *Respir Care* 54:1236–1243, 2009.

Elias S, Sviri S, Orenbuch-Harroch E, Fellig Y, Ben-Yehuda A, Fridlender ZG, et al.: Sildenafil to facilitate weaning from inhaled nitric oxide and mechanical ventilation in a patient with severe secondary pulmonary hypertension and a patent foramen ovale, *Respir Care* 56(10):1611–1613, 2011.

Gagnon C, Simoes J: The management of the mechanically ventilated infant receiving pancuronium bromide (Pavulon), *Neonatal Netw* 4(3):20–24, 1985.

Goldberg RN, Bancalari E: Bronchopulmonary dysplasia: clinical presentation and the role of mechanical ventilation, *Respir Care* 31:591, 1986.

Goldberg RN, Bancalari E: Therapeutic approaches to the infant with bronchopulmonary dysplasia, *Respir Care* 36:613, 1991.

Goldsmith JP, Karotkin EH: *Assisted ventilation of the neonate*, ed 2, Philadelphia, 1996, Saunders.

Hess DR, Kacmarek RM: *Essentials of mechanical ventilation*, New York, 1996, McGraw-Hill.

Hess DR, MacIntyre NR, Mishoe SC, Galvin WF, Adams AB, editors: *Respiratory care principles and practice*, ed 2, Burlington, MA, 2012, Jones & Bartlett Learning.

HIFI Study Group: High-frequency oscillatory ventilation compared with conventional mechanical ventilation in the treatment of respiratory failure in preterm infants, *N Engl J Med* 320:88, 1989.

Jobe A: Surfactant treatment for respiratory distress syndrome, *Respir Care* 31:467, 1986.

Kacmarek RM, Stoller JK, Heuer AJ, editors: *Egan's fundamentals of respiratory care*, ed 10, St Louis, 2013, Mosby.

Kneyber MCJ, van Heerde M, Markhorst DG: Reflections on pediatric high-frequency oscillatory ventilation from a physiologic perspective, *Resp Care* 57(9):1496–1504, 2012.

Koff PB, Eitzman DV, Neu J: *Neonatal and pediatric respiratory care*, ed 2, St Louis, 1993, Mosby.

MacIntyre NR, Branson RD: *Mechanical ventilation*, ed 2, Philadelphia, 2009, Saunders.

Milner AD, Hoskyns EW: High frequency positive pressure ventilation in neonates, *Arch Dis Child* 64:1, 1989.

Miyagawa CI: Sedation of the mechanically ventilated patient in the Intensive Care Unit *Respir Care* 32:792, 1987.

Nicks JJ, Becker MA: High-frequency ventilation of the newborn: past, present, and future, *Respir Ther* 4(4), 1991.

Oishi P, Datar SA, Fineman JR: Advances in the management of pediatric pulmonary hypertension, *Respir Ther* 56:1314–1340, 2011.

Pilbeam SP, Cairo JM: *Mechanical ventilation: physiological and clinical applications*, ed 4, St Louis, 2006, Mosby.

Schmidt JM: Nitric oxide therapy in neonates: adding to the arsenal, *Respir Ther* 7:37, 1994.

Siobal MS: Pulmonary vasodilators, *Respir Care* 52(7):885–899, 2007.

Siobal MS, Hess DR: Are inhaled vasodilators useful in acute lung injury and acute respiratory distress syndrome? *Respir Care* 55(2):144–161, 2010.

Smith I: The impact of surfactant on neonatal Intensive Care Unit management, *Respir Ther* 4(4):22–26, 1991.

Spear ML, Spitzer AR, Fox WW: Hyperventilation therapy for persistent pulmonary hypertension of the newborn, *Neonat Intensive Care: Perinatol/Neonatol* 9:27, 1985.

Tobin MJ: What should the clinician do when a patient "fights the ventilator"? *Respir Care* 36:395, 1991.

Walsh BK, Czervinske MP, DiBlasii RM, editors: *Perinatal and pediatric respiratory care*, ed 3, St Louis, 2010, Saunders.

Whitaker K: *Comprehensive perinatal and pediatric respiratory care*, ed 3, Albany, NY, 2001, Delmar.

Whitaker KB, Trujillo LM: Neonatal mechanical ventilation. In Chang DW, editor: *Clinical application of mechanical ventilation*, ed 4, Clifton Park, NY, 2014, Delmar.

White GC: *Equipment theory for respiratory care*, ed 4, Albany, NY, 2005, Delmar.

Wyka KA, Mathews PJ, Rutkowski J: *Foundations of respiratory care*, ed 2, Clifton Park, NY, 2012, Delmar.

1. In a neonate less than 72 hours old and with pulmonary problems, the PaO_2 should be kept in what range?
   A. 40-45 torr
   B. 45-50 torr
   C. 60-70 torr
   D. 80-90 torr

2. If a respiratory therapist observes that a neonatal patient has apnea spells leading to bradycardia, what should be recommended?
   A. Start CPAP.
   B. Start mechanical ventilation.
   C. Start an aerosolized bronchodilator.
   D. Give endotracheal surfactant.

3. An actively moving neonate is receiving 7 cm water CPAP by nasal prongs with 40% oxygen at a flow of 4 L/min. It is noticed that the CPAP pressure is variable between 4 and 7 cm water. What is the most likely cause of this?
   A. The patient is taking more shallow breaths.
   B. The patient's breathing rate has decreased.
   C. There is a leak when the neonate turns its head.
   D. Someone has accidentally changed the oxygen percentage.

4. A respiratory therapist is taking care of a newborn who has aspirated meconium. Which of the following ventilator settings should be recommended?
   A. I:E of 2:1
   B. I:E of 1:1
   C. I:E of 1:2
   D. I:E of 1:4

5. A premature neonate with a low Apgar score is demonstrating hypoxemia, intercostal retractions, and expiratory grunting noises. What is the best way to correct these problems?
   A. Nebulize albuterol.
   B. Suction the neonate.
   C. Instill surfactant into the airway.
   D. Give supplemental oxygen.

6. A neonatal patient with pneumonia needs regular suctioning. The respiratory therapist notices that the patient's ventilator circuit has blood-streaked sputum in it. What should be done?
   A. Put in an HME.
   B. Change the circuit.
   C. Flush out the sputum with normal saline.
   D. Put in a closed-airway suctioning system.

7. A 28-week gestational age neonate has the following arterial blood gas values while breathing 60% oxygen in an oxyhood: PaO_2 48 torr, $PaCO_2$ 45 torr, and pH 7.35. What should be done in this situation?
   A. Increase the oxygen to 70%.
   B. Begin mechanical ventilation.

   C. Intubate and begin CPAP at 4 cm water.
   D. Begin nasal CPAP at 4 cm water.

8. A hypoxic newborn has been diagnosed with PPHN and is receiving 80% oxygen. What should be recommended to improve the newborn's condition?
   A. Inhaled nitric oxide.
   B. Instill surfactant.
   C. Decrease the oxygen percentage to 70%.
   D. Inhaled 80/20 mix of heliox.

9. If CPAP is administered through an endotracheal tube, the child should be extubated when the CPAP pressure is:
   A. 0-2 cm water
   B. 2-4 cm water
   C. 4-6 cm water
   D. 6-8 cm water

10. The time to switch a patient from CPAP to mechanical ventilation is indicated by:
    1. CPAP of 8-10 cm water with a resulting PaO_2 of less than 50 torr
    2. F_IO_2 of 0.8 or more resulting in a PaO_2 of less than 50 torr
    3. $PaCO_2$ of greater than 60 torr
    A. 1 only
    B. 2 only
    C. 1 and 2 only
    D. 1, 2, and 3

11. Identify the rationale for the use of pressure-limiting or square-wave ventilation in a patient with RDS.
    1. It increases the $PaCO_2$.
    2. It limits the peak pressure.
    3. It decreases the PaO_2.
    4. It increases the patient's oxygenation.
    5. The tidal volume is held for a period of time.
    A. 1 and 3 only
    B. 1, 2, and 3 only
    C. 1, 2, and 4 only
    D. 2, 4, and 5 only

12. Hyperventilation is recommended in which of the following types of patients?
    A. Meconium aspiration
    B. PPHN
    C. RDS
    D. Infant with normal lung compliance

13. A neonate has meconium aspiration syndrome. Increasing the pressure limit on the ventilator increases the patient's risk of:
    A. Retinopathy of prematurity
    B. Oxygen toxicity
    C. Pneumothorax
    D. Tracheoesophageal fistula

14. Given the following choices, which should a respiratory therapist select to increase the PaO_2 in a neonate with pneumonia who is supported on a standard pressure-limited-type ventilator?
    1. **Increase inspiratory time.**
    2. **Increase the pressure limit if it is reached.**
    3. **Decrease flow.**
    4. **Increase PEEP.**
    5. **Decrease the IMV rate.**
    A. 1 and 5 only
    B. 2 and 3 only
    C. 3 and 4 only
    D. 1, 2, and 4 only

15. With TPTV ventilation, if PEEP is increased without increasing the pressure limit by the same amount, the patient's:
    A. Minute volume will increase.
    B. Tidal volume will decrease.
    C. $PaCO_2$ will decrease.
    D. Tidal volume will increase.

16. All of the following are indications for HFV EXCEPT:
    A. Cleft palate before surgical correction
    B. PPHN
    C. RDS unresponsive to conventional ventilation
    D. Mechanical ventilation patient with unresolved pneumothorax

17. HFOV is being used with a neonate with RDS. The following settings are in use: 50% oxygen, rate 700/min, amplitude 10 cm water, and 4 cm water PEEP. The patient's $PaCO_2$ is 52 torr. What should be recommended to correct the carbon dioxide level?
    A. Increase the amplitude.
    B. Decrease the amplitude.
    C. Increase the PEEP level.
    D. Increase the inspiratory time.

18. A premature newborn is becoming progressively more hypoxic and tachypneic despite being in an oxyhood with 50% oxygen. The decision is made to begin CPAP. What initial pressure should the respiratory therapist recommend?
    A. 0-2 cm water
    B. 2-3 cm water
    C. 4-5 cm water
    D. 6-8 cm water

19. A neonate with PPHN is being mechanically ventilated and has responded favorably to 10 ppm of INO and surgical correction of a patent ductus arteriosus. What should be done now?
    A. Wean from the ventilator.
    B. Initiate CPAP.
    C. Decrease the inhaled nitric oxide to 5 ppm.
    D. Discontinue the inhaled nitric oxide.

20. A patient with RDS has been receiving CPAP at 8 cm water and 60% oxygen. The following arterial blood gases are found: PaO_2 48 torr, $PaCO_2$ 58 torr, and pH 7.23. What should be done now?
    A. Initiate volume-cycled ventilation.
    B. Increase CPAP to 10 cm water.
    C. Increase the inspired oxygen to 70%.
    D. Begin high-frequency ventilation.

17 Home Care and Pulmonary Rehabilitation

Note: It can be anticipated that the Therapist Multiple-Choice Examination (TMC) will include an *average of 4 of 140 actual questions* (3% of the exam) on home care, apnea monitoring, and pulmonary rehabilitation. (This is based on the question mix typically found on the National Board of Respiratory Care's (NBRC's) previous Entry Level Examinations and Written Registry Examinations.)

Remember that the TMC version you take will include 20 additional questions being evaluated for possible inclusion in other versions of the TMC. So, there will be a total of 160 questions taken. There is no way to differentiate between the 140 actual questions and the 20 questions being evaluated for future use. Please go to the Introduction for detailed information on the TMC and the Clinical Simulation Examination.

MODULE A

Patient and family education

1. Interview the patient to assess learning needs (code: IB1g) [difficulty: R, Ap]

See Chapter 1 for the general discussion on interviewing the patient to determine learning needs and the possible teaching/learning processes that are best suited to the patient.

2. Initiate and conduct patient and family education about smoking cessation (code: III I3) [difficulty: ELE: R, Ap; WRE: An]

Absolute proof exists that smoking causes emphysema, chronic bronchitis, lung cancer, and heart disease. These conditions occur in the smoker who directly inhales the smoke as well as anyone who inhales secondhand smoke. Most often this affects the nonsmoking spouse and children. Asthmatic patients often find that their bronchospasm is worsened when they inhale tobacco smoke. Obviously it is important that any patient with a smoking-related cardiopulmonary disease cease smoking. The patient's family must also stop smoking. Continued exposure to tobacco smoke harms the patient.

Because nicotine is highly addictive, many patients will need multiple quitting attempts before finally becoming tobacco free. (*Note:* The NBRC has specified smoking cessation. However, all types of tobacco use (chewing tobacco) and nicotine use (e-cigarettes) are dangerous and users should be helped to quit.) The respiratory therapist must make every effort to help his or her smoking patients to quit. When a patient makes a statement about wanting to quit smoking, the following "Five A's" should be carried out:

1. *Ask* the patient about his or her past and current use of tobacco.
2. *Advise* the patient about the health benefits of quitting.
3. *Assess* the patient's willingness to attempt to quit at this time.
4. *Assist* in the quit attempt by discussing helpful medications and counseling.
5. *Arrange* for a follow-up meeting with the respiratory therapist or physician to begin the quitting process.

Even if the patient is not currently interested in quitting smoking, the following "Five R's" should be presented:

1. *Relevance:* Talk with the patient about the relevance of quitting smoking and improving his or her health.
2. *Risks:* Talk with the patient about the risks of smoking.
3. *Rewards:* Talk with the patient about the health and financial rewards of quitting smoking.
4. *Roadblocks:* Ask the patient about any roadblocks or barriers to him or her quitting smoking.
5. *Repeat:* Whenever you visit the patient, repeat your motivational presentation on quitting smoking.

Many patients find that they cannot stop smoking without having nicotine withdrawal symptoms such as agitation and craving for a cigarette. To aid in smoking cessation, it is often helpful to meet with a group of people who also are trying to stop. This group support helps the patient feel less alone in his or her efforts to stop smoking. Tobacco quit-line counseling can help the patient who does not have a social support group. The patient's physician also must be involved in this process.

If the patient has been unable to stop smoking because of withdrawal symptoms, it is likely that he or she is addicted to nicotine. In this situation, nicotine replacement therapy (NRT) allows for a gradual withdrawal that greatly aids in smoking cessation. Although no smoking cessation plan works in every case, the highest percentage of patients are able to stop smoking if they have a combination of psychological support and a gradual reduction in nicotine intake.

Several well-established nicotine replacement and reduction systems currently exist. All of the following are available without prescription. The Commit lozenge is held in the mouth to release a controlled amount of nicotine. Nicotine polacrilex (Nicorette) is a gum that is chewed by the patient to release a dose of nicotine. The Nicotrol inhaler allows the user to inhale nicotine through a device shaped like a cigarette. Nicotine transdermal patches are another nicotine reduction system. ProStep, Nicoderm, and Habitrol are three brands of patches that, when placed onto the skin, allow a set amount of nicotine to be absorbed. With these systems, the patient starts with a relatively high dose of the drug and, over a period of weeks, transitions through a series of patches with less and less nicotine. A nasal spray is also available that allows the nicotine to be absorbed through the nasal mucosa. With any of these NRT products, the goal is to meet the patient's need for nicotine so that cravings will be eliminated and he or she will stop smoking. Over time, the patient will reduce his or her nicotine dose to zero. Patients should not smoke while using one of these systems. Patients who continue to smoke run the risk of a nicotine overdose. Risks include vivid dreams, insomnia, hypertension, dysrhythmias, and angina. NRT is contraindicated in a patient who has had a myocardial infarction within the past 6 weeks.

Another option involves the patient taking a prescription medication to change how the brain reacts to nicotine. Zyban (bupropion SR or XL) alters the brain's chemistry so that nicotine craving is reduced. It was originally found helpful in the care of patients with depression. Chantix (varenicline) is incorporated into the nicotine receptors of the brain. As a result, nicotine withdrawal cravings are reduced and if the patient "cheats" by smoking, there is no nicotine stimulating effect. Chantix has been shown to have the highest cessation success rate of all the NRT products.

Some patients experience problems with nicotine replacement and reduction systems. The transdermal patch can cause skin irritation. If this happens, the patch should be moved to another site. Some patients report insomnia or strange dreams while wearing a nicotine patch at night. Patients with this problem should remove the patch before sleeping.

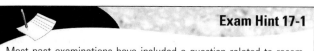

Exam Hint 17-1

Most past examinations have included a question related to recommending a nicotine replacement system to a patient wishing to stop smoking or the possible side effects of the nicotine system.

3. Apply evidence-based or clinical practice guidelines (code: III F3) [difficulty: R, Ap]

Several organizations have released clinical practice guidelines to help in the diagnosis and management of chronic obstructive pulmonary disease (COPD) and asthma and best practices for pulmonary rehabilitation and smoking cessation. Although it is beyond the scope of this book to present them all in detail, their key findings are included here and in other chapters. See each chapter's bibliography for a listing. The American Association for Respiratory Care has included many of these guidelines on its Web site at http://www.aarc.org. Click on Resources and then Clinical Practice Guidelines.

The respiratory therapist should have a solid understanding of the pathophysiology of the commonly found cardiopulmonary and cardiovascular conditions. These include, but are not limited to, asthma, emphysema, chronic bronchitis, pneumonia, pulmonary fibrosis, cystic fibrosis, right and left heart failure, stroke, and neuromuscular diseases. Be prepared to teach the patient and family about the patient's disease, its cause, and its medical management.

4. Initiate and conduct patient and family education about asthma (code: III I5a) [difficulty: R, Ap]

The National Asthma Education and Prevention Program released a comprehensive document in 2007 that recommends the following components of an asthma education program:

1. The patient should have an active partnership with the caregivers (physician, respiratory therapist, nurse) to develop a written action plan for the patient. If the patient is a child, the parent(s) will need to be involved in developing the action plan.
2. The caregivers and patient should regularly review the action plan and how well it is working for the patient.
3. The following should be taught and regularly reinforced to the patient:
   a. Basic facts about asthma as a chronic condition.
   b. Ways to prevent or limit the patient's exposure to known asthma triggers.
   c. Defining well-controlled asthma.
   d. Identifying the patient's current level of asthma control.
   e. The role of the patient's asthma medications.
   f. How to use the inhaled medication devices (small-volume inhaler, dry powder inhaler, metered-dose inhaler, valved holding chamber).
   g. Self-monitoring, including use of a peak flowmeter.
   h. How to respond to signs and symptoms of worsening asthma.
   i. When and where to get help for worsening asthma.

5. Initiate and conduct patient and family education about home care and equipment (code: III I2) [difficulty: R, Ap]

Home care equipment is essentially the same as that found in any hospital. The same types of equipment problems can occur in the patient's home as in the hospital. Those who wish to learn more about specific brands of home care equipment are referred to the books that discuss respiratory care equipment or the manufacturer's literature. Review, if necessary, the respiratory care procedures presented in this or other respiratory care books because they can be performed in the home care setting as well as in the hospital.

Exam Hint 17-2

Past examinations have included a question related to home respiratory care equipment. Examples include (1) recommendation of the use of an oxygen-conserving nasal cannula and oxygen concentrator for the economic delivery of low-flow oxygen, (2) recommendation of the maintenance of an oxygen concentrator (cleaning its filters), (3) changing to a backup source of oxygen (switching to an oxygen cylinder) when an oxygen concentrator fails, and (4) provision of telephone instructions to a home care patient whose nasal cannula has no flow. This includes having the patient place the cannula under water to check for bubbling, tightening all tubing connections, confirming that gas is flowing from the oxygen concentrator, or replacing a defective cannula.

---

6. Initiate and conduct patient and family education about safety and infection control (code: III I1) [difficulty: R, Ap]

The following aspects of the patient's home environment should be evaluated. Patient and family teaching would be individualized as needed.

- Does the patient live alone or have a spouse or companion to help provide care? Make sure that telephone numbers to relatives, helpful neighbors, the patient's physician, ambulance service, local hospital, pharmacy, and any other support services are posted by each telephone.
- Ensure that all respiratory care equipment is cleaned (see Chapter 2 for suggestions on methods of disinfection) and functioning properly. The patient should demonstrate his or her ability to disassemble, clean, and reassemble any respiratory care equipment such as a small-volume nebulizer.
- Check that home oxygen systems are working properly. If the patient has an oxygen concentrator, confirm that the filters are cleaned and that the alarms are set and working. Typical alarms include (1) power failure, (2) high pressure, (3) low pressure, and (4) low oxygen concentration. (See Chapter 6 for more information on oxygen concentrators.) Ensure that an oxygen cylinder, regulator, and oxygen delivery system are working properly as a backup system if the oxygen concentrator fails.
- Have the patient centrally locate all necessary items for daily living. The patient should avoid unnecessary stair climbing. It might be recommended that the patient convert the living room, if it is located near the kitchen and bathroom, into a bedroom. Clothing can

be modified with Velcro fasteners, snaps, or zippers if the patient cannot use buttons easily. Shoes can be put on more easily with a long-handled shoehorn. Avoid shoes with laces. A long-handled comb or brush makes grooming easier.

- The kitchen should be modified so that all commonly used equipment is on the counter. Everyday dishes, utensils, and foods should be placed so that they can be easily within an arm's reach in cabinets and drawers. The patient should not have to bend over, stoop down, or climb onto a footstool to get anything that is needed.
- The bathroom may need handholds added to the walls by the toilet and shower or tub for extra security when using these facilities. A shower chair can be added so that the patient can sit while bathing. A hand-held shower head might make bathing easier.
- Check the home for airborne irritants. Smoking by the patient or anyone else in the home must be stopped. The patient should avoid contact with other forms of indoor pollution such as aerosol sprays, paints, varnishes, and dust. A high-efficiency particulate air (HEPA) filtration system is best for removing indoor airborne pollutants and irritants. Indoor kerosene-fueled space heaters should not be used because they release carbon monoxide.
- The patient should avoid contact with any known allergens, people who smoke, or substances that have resulted in a bad reaction.

MODULE B

Home sleep apnea management

1. Initiate and conduct patient and family education about sleep disorders (code: III I5c) [difficulty: R, Ap]

See Chapter 18 for the discussion on sleep-disordered breathing. This includes a description of a cardiopulmonary sleep study; the three main types of sleep apnea and their treatment, including continuous positive airway pressure (CPAP) or noninvasive positive pressure ventilation (NPPV) titration during sleep; and overnight pulse oximetry. The patient and the patient's family must be educated about the type of sleep apnea that he or she has and the treatment plan to correct the apnea. If CPAP or NPPV equipment has been ordered for the patient with obstructive or mixed sleep apnea, he or she must understand how to operate it. The patient must be able to demonstrate how to disassemble, clean, reassemble, and adjust the equipment.

2. Perform apnea monitoring (code: IC18) [difficulty: R, Ap]

Apnea monitoring is indicated in an infant who has documented periods of apnea of prematurity resulting from an immature central nervous system. This condition is most commonly seen in infants younger than 35 weeks' gestational age. The usual monitoring guidelines include apneic periods that last longer than 20 seconds and are associated with bradycardia with a heart rate of less than 100 beats/min. Hypoxemia is often demonstrated by cyanosis, pallor, or documented desaturation through pulse oximetry. In addition, the infant may show marked limpness, choking, or gagging. Other conditions such as intracranial hemorrhage, patent ductus arteriosus, upper airway obstruction, hypermagnesemia, infection, and maternal narcotic agents should be ruled out before apnea of prematurity is confirmed. If this is the infant's problem, it is usually outgrown by the time the infant is 40 weeks' postconceptional age. Home apnea monitoring is not indicated in normal infants, in preterm infants without symptoms of apnea, or to test for sudden infant death syndrome (SIDS). See Box 17-1 for guidelines on starting and stopping home apnea monitoring.

Apnea monitors currently in use sense respiratory efforts through the changing electrical impedance measured through the chest wall as the infant breathes. Impedance is resistance to the flow of electricity through the skin and other organs. The monitor transmits a small, constant electrical current that results in a voltage across the two electrodes on the infant's chest. As the infant breathes and the chest wall expands and contracts, a resulting change in voltage occurs. This fluctuation is measured and interpreted as inhalation and exhalation. Similarly, smaller voltage changes are measured with each heartbeat. This is measured and interpreted as the heart rate.

The following are desirable features on a home apnea monitor: (1) ability to store and display events for later analysis, (2) identification of breathing patterns and apnea periods, (3) identification of heart rate patterns, (4) estimation of tidal volume, and (5) identification of hypoxemia by pulse oximetry. Assembling a home apnea monitor involves placing the electrodes properly on the infant's chest, turning on the monitor, and setting the proper high and low limits for the alarms.

Two electrodes are usually placed where the greatest amount of movement occurs during breathing. Most often, this is on the infant's upper chest between the nipples and the armpits (Fig. 17-1). With older infants, the electrodes might have to be placed on the sides over the lower ribs. Occasionally one electrode is placed on the chest and the other on the infant's abdomen. Some monitoring systems require that a Velcro belt be placed around the infant over the electrodes to secure their positions. (Obviously this works only if both electrodes are on the chest.) Other systems employ electrodes with an adhesive. In either case, for best results, the infant's chest should be washed with mild soap and water and dried before the electrodes are placed. This results in the best electrical conduction. Do not use baby oils, lotions, or powders over the electrode sites. Attach the lead wires to the electrodes. These connect to the patient cable that is then connected to the monitor. Occasionally static electricity causes some

---

BOX 17-1   Guidelines for Starting and Stopping Home Apnea Monitoring

Indications to Start Home Apnea Monitoring

Infant has experienced one or more apparent life-threatening apnea events.
Infant is preterm and symptomatic of apnea.
Infant is a sibling of two or more SIDS victims.
Infant has central nervous system-based hypoventilation.

Indications to Stop Home Apnea Monitoring

Two to three months have passed without a significant number of alarms.
Two to three months have passed without an apnea episode.
Infant can tolerate stress of illnesses (e.g., nasopharyngitis) or immunizations (e.g., diphtheria–pertussis–tetanus) without apnea episodes.

SIDS, sudden infant death syndrome.

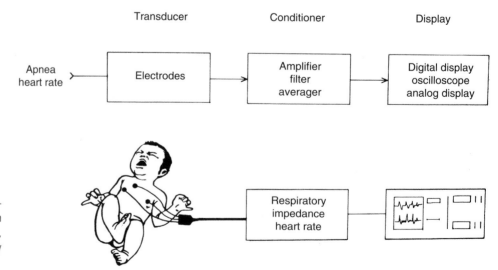

Figure 17-1 Block diagram for impedance apnea and heart rate monitor. (From Lough MD. In Lough MD, Williams TJ, Rawson JE, editors: Newborn respiratory care, St Louis, 1979, Mosby.)

interference with the signal. A third chest electrode is then added to act as a ground wire.

The monitor should be plugged into a working electrical outlet and turned on. Set the unit to charge the internal battery so that it can be made portable for later use. Confirm that the infant's respiratory and heart rates are being sensed and displayed. If pulse oximetry is a feature on the unit, the probe should be properly placed on the infant, and an SpO_2 value should be displayed. Set the high and low alarm values according to the physician's orders or established protocols. For example:

1. Set the apnea alarm to trigger after 20 seconds.
2. Set the low heart rate alarm to trigger if the heart rate is less than 100 beats/min.
3. If available, set the pulse oximeter alarm to trigger if the SpO_2 value decreases to less than 90%.
4. If available, set the high heart rate alarm to trigger if the heart rate is greater than 150 beats/min.

Multiple alarms provide for a greater margin of patient safety. They also indicate what physiologically deteriorates first in the infant. These backup alarm systems are important because the apnea monitor senses chest wall movement, not air movement. It is possible for the infant to have an upper airway obstruction and continue to make breathing attempts; therefore the apnea monitor will not alarm because the chest wall is moving. The bradycardia or desaturation alarms will signal that the infant is in trouble.

It is critically important that the parents (or parent) know about the infant's medical condition. They need to understand how the monitor functions and what to do if the alarms sound. They should demonstrate their knowledge of the monitor's functions and be given written instructions about the monitor. The parents should not be more than 10 seconds away from the infant at any time, which means that the infant will not be apneic for more than 30 seconds (20-second alarm delay and 10 seconds for the parents to respond). The parents must know how to give tactile stimulation to the infant, use the manual resuscitator, call for emergency help, and perform infant cardiopulmonary resuscitation.

3. Evaluate the results of apnea monitoring (code: ID17) [difficulty: R, Ap, An]

Alarm situations fall into two basic categories: patient alarms and equipment alarms. Patient alarms mean that the infant is apneic, has a heart rate below or above an acceptable level, or has desaturated. One, any two, or all three alarms may be triggered. Other than the audible alarm, a visual alarm flashes to show the problem(s), and the recording device keeps track of the events. The parents should be instructed to care for the infant first, and then, when the infant is back to normal, the alarms can be reset.

Three types of equipment alarms are found: electrode or lead problem, low battery, or monitor failure. The unit should have different visual and audible alarms for equipment failure so that the family does not mistakenly believe that the infant is in trouble. An electrode or lead problem alarm usually occurs because the electrode fell off of the infant or the lead became disconnected. The family should be taught how to fix these types of problems. A low battery alarm indicates that time is limited for the monitor to function on battery power. The family should be instructed to plug the monitor into a functioning electrical outlet, and the unit should be set to recharge the battery. A monitor failure alarm indicates a serious internal problem with the monitor. It is not functioning properly and should not be used. The family should be instructed to observe the infant continuously and call the home care company for a replacement monitor.

Apnea monitors in current use record and store the alarm situations discussed previously. The information can usually be downloaded into a computer for a visual display of breathing and heart-rate patterns, equipment problems, and the dates and times of their occurrences. The therapist or physician should review all these data to determine what kinds of problems the patient experienced.

MODULE C

Pulmonary rehabilitation

1. Initiate and conduct patient and family education about COPD (code: III I5b) [difficulty: R, Ap]

The patient with COPD should have an educational plan tailored to his or her individual needs. The primary goal of the plan is help the patient achieve the highest possible level of self-care and independent function. To help with this, the Lung Information Needs Questionnaire (LINQ) can be taken by the patient. The LINQ evaluates the patient's knowledge of the following six areas: disease knowledge, medicine, self-management, smoking, exercise, and diet. The patient's educational plan can be focused on any weak areas. Overall, the components of a COPD educational program typically include the following:

a. Basic facts about COPD as a chronic condition.
b. Explaining the patient's condition.
c. Breathing retraining and dyspnea control.
d. Energy-conservation techniques.
e. The role of the patient's COPD medications.
f. How to use the inhaled medication devices (small-volume inhaler, dry powder inhaler, metered-dose inhaler, valved holding chamber).
g. Oxygen therapy and equipment.
h. Exercise training (discussed below in detail).
i. Psychosocial support.
j. Early recognition of an exacerbation and how to respond.
k. When and where to get help for an exacerbation.

2. Six-minute walk test

A timed walk test has become a widely used standard for measuring a patient's success in a pulmonary rehabilitation program. The usual timed walk test involves having the patient walk as far as possible in 6 minutes. An alternative is to have the patient walk as far as possible in 12 minutes. In either timed walk test, the distance covered is the key outcome measured.

a. Review data in the patient record about 6-minute walk test results (code: IA7) [difficulty: R, Ap]

A 6-minute walk procedure involves the therapist having a patient walk as far as possible in 6 minutes and noting the distance covered. Ideally, this is done by having the patient walk back and forth on a 30-meter (100 feet) long unobstructed and uninterrupted hallway. Although not ideal, the patient could also walk on a treadmill. If the patient has had a previous 6-minute walk, it is especially important to make note of the distance walked, the patient's subjective tolerance of the procedure, and vital signs and pulse oximeter values before, during, and after the walk.

A timed walk test is easy to perform, is generally well tolerated, and directly relates to pulmonary rehabilitation activities. See the discussion on stress testing in Chapter 18 for information on evaluating a patient before a walk test and contraindications to exercise testing that may apply to a patient performing a timed walk.

b. Perform a 6-minute walk test (code: IC8) [difficulty: R, Ap]

See Box 17-2 for a recommended 6-minute walk protocol. Ideally, repeated tests should be performed at the same time each day and at least 2 hours after a meal. Basic equipment for the walk test includes a straight hallway that is marked at intervals for distance, a stopwatch, and a pulse oximeter. Record the temperature in the hallway. Be aware of two outside factors that can alter a patient's performance. First, the so-called practice or learning effect can alter performance. The practice effect means that with repeated attempts, the patient will probably walk farther each time. Therefore the patient should perform at least two 6-minute timed walks that are measured and reported. The patient may rest for about 15 minutes between each walk test. Second, because positive encouragement can boost the patient's walking distance, the respiratory therapist is not to verbally (or nonverbally) encourage the patient to speed up. Only standardized, scripted words are allowed in order to treat all patients the same.

BOX 17-2   Suggested Protocol for a 6-Minute Timed Walk Test

1. *Pretest activities:* Have the patient take all normal preexercise medications, such as an inhaled bronchodilator. If the patient has been prescribed supplemental oxygen, such as a nasal cannula and portable oxygen system, it should be used during the test. Measure the patient's vital signs, pulse oximeter value, and peak flow value (if indicated). Have the patient rank his or her dyspnea (shortness of breath) on the 10-point Borg Scale.* Record this information.

2. Instruct the patient about the timed test, including: "The test involves you walking as far as you can, back and forth in this hallway, for 6 minutes. I'll be checking your oxygen level (with a pulse oximeter) and asking you how you are doing. If you need to rest you can; but, try to walk as far as possible. I'll periodically tell you how much time is left. When I tell you the test is finished, stand where you are. There will then be a 15-minute rest period. You will then repeat the test. If possible, after another 15-minute rest period, I would like you to repeat the test a third time." Ask the patient to repeat back to you the key points of the test so that you know he or she understands the procedure.

3. Place the patient at the starting point. Make sure that both you and the patient are ready to begin.

4. Tell the patient to start walking and start the stopwatch. During the first timed walk, keep pace with the patient to monitor the pulse oximeter value and evaluate the patient's overall appearance.

5. At 30-second intervals, offer the patient words of encouragement, such as the following: "You're doing fine." "Keep up the good work."

6. Tell the patient when 2 and 4 minutes have lapsed. At 6 minutes, tell the patient to stop.

7. In general, stop the test at any time if the patient's pulse oximeter reading drops below 88% saturation or 4% below the starting value. (The physician may set specific criteria for stopping the test.) If ordered, supplemental oxygen may be started or increased to maintain the desired oxygen saturation.

8. Immediately after the test:
   a. Check the patient's vital signs and pulse oximeter value.
   b. Ask the patient to rate his or her dyspnea on the 10-point Borg Scale.
   c. Ask the patient what limited his or her walking distance, for example, shortness of breath, wheezing, leg or chest pain.

9. Document the test results. Make note of the above items. Record the distance walked. If the patient stopped to rest, note when it occurred and how long the patient needed to rest.

10. Tell the patient to rest for 15 minutes and that the test will be repeated.

11. Repeat the above steps for the second 6-minute walk test. If possible, the test should be repeated a third time. *Note:* If the patient did not desaturate during the first timed walk, it may not be necessary to accompany the patient and monitor pulse oximetry values during the second and third walks.

12. Forward all information to the physician for a formal interpretation.

---

*The 10-point Borg Scale allows the patient to assign a numeric value of 1 to 10 to his or her feeling of dyspnea. A large poster of the Borg Scale is placed so the patient can easily see it during the walk test. Before and after the test, the patient is asked to rate his or her dyspnea. For example, a score of 1 indicates very slight dyspnea, 5 is severe dyspnea, and 10 is maximal dyspnea.

c. Evaluate the results of a 6-minute walk test (code: ID7) [difficulty: R, Ap, An]

Research has shown that patients participating in a pulmonary rehabilitation program will usually show an increase in their timed walk distance. The following indicates that the patient is making progress:

- The patient has an increase in the 6-minute walk distance.
- The patient subjectively feels that he or she is doing as well as can be expected. The patient is motivated to try new things.
- Symptoms are reduced or at least under control.
- Cardiopulmonary function tests and blood gases show improvement. Even a slowing in the patient's former rapid rate of decline is a good sign.

The following indicate that the patient's health is deteriorating:

- The patient's 6-minute walk distance has decreased.
- He or she subjectively feels worse. The patient is afraid to try new things.
- Symptoms are worse. The patient feels dyspneic at less exertion than previously.
- The sputum has changed. It may be thick and harder to expectorate or have changed color to yellow or green. The patient may be expectorating more than before, or less, if there is decreased movement of secretions.
- Cardiopulmonary function tests and blood gases are worse. The patient may need more supplemental oxygen, an increase in aerosolized bronchodilator medication, or other cardiopulmonary medications.

Exam Hint 17-3

Increased distance covered in the 6-minute walk would indicate that the patient's pulmonary rehabilitation program is effective.

3. Initiate and conduct patient and family education about pulmonary rehabilitation (code: III I4) [difficulty: R, Ap]

As part of a pulmonary rehabilitation program, a patient who has been diagnosed with COPD needs to be educated about the disease and how to manage it (discussed above). A critical component of the pulmonary rehabilitation program is a graded exercise program. The patient with pulmonary disease who is inactive because of his or her condition experiences a slow deterioration in overall body function. It is well known that physical activity is important for general health. Box 17-3 lists the effects of inactivity.

A graded exercise program is an individually structured sequence of events that is designed to safely increase the patient's exercise tolerance. In 2006, the American Thoracic Society and the European Respiratory Society adopted the following definition:

BOX 17-3   Effects of Inactivity

Metabolism
Decreased metabolic rate, decreased protein catabolism, negative nitrogen balance, decubitus ulcers, imbalance of cellular electrolyte levels, and gastrointestinal hypomotility.

Psychosocial
Decreased learning ability, decreased motivation to learn, decreased retention of new material, decreased problem-solving ability, exaggerated or inappropriate emotional reactions, perceptual and motor changes, and increased somatic concerns.

Respiratory System
Decreased movement of secretions, decreased use of respiratory muscles, and development of microatelectasis and infection.

Muscular System
Loss of normal muscle tone, decreased muscle efficiency, increased local muscle oxygen consumption, rapid onset of fatigue, and contracture.

Cardiopulmonary System
Decreased cardiac output, venous stasis, thromboembolism, and pulmonary emboli.

Skeletal System
Osteoporosis, reabsorption of calcium from the bone, and increased incidence of compression fractures.

From May DF: Rehabilitation and continuity of care in pulmonary disease, St Louis, 1991, Mosby.

Pulmonary rehabilitation is an evidence-based, multidisciplinary, and comprehensive intervention for patients with chronic respiratory diseases who are symptomatic and often have decreased daily life activities. Integrated into the individualized treatment of the patient, pulmonary rehabilitation is designed to reduce symptoms, optimize functional status, increase participation, and reduce health care costs by stabilizing or reversing manifestations of the disease.

a. General considerations in a graded exercise program

The patient's physical condition must be evaluated before designing an exercise program. In addition to COPD, the patient may have other conditions that further limit his or her ability to safely participate in a rehabilitation program. See Box 17-4 for the suggested assessment parameters. If the patient is too ill or too limited in ability, he or she should not be placed into a rehabilitation program.

Although the patient's physical condition is the most important factor to evaluate from a safety point of view, other aspects of the patient's life also must be reviewed. These include a nutritional evaluation, a psychosocial evaluation, and a vocational evaluation. Because these areas are beyond the scope of practice of most respiratory therapists, the physician must refer the patient to other experts. In addition, any patient who is still smoking must be enrolled in a smoking cessation program.

BOX 17-4   Patient Evaluation Before Starting a Pulmonary Rehabilitation Program

History
Complete physical examination
Chest radiograph
Resting diagnostic electrocardiogram
Complete blood count
Serum electrolytes
Urinalysis
Arterial blood gases
Theophylline level
Sputum analysis
Pulmonary function tests
    Spirometry
    Lung volume study
    Diffusion capacity
    Before and after bronchodilator study
Pulmonary stress test including
    Electrocardiogram
    Blood pressure
    Heart rate
    Respiratory rate
    Pulse oximetry
    Maximum ventilation
    Oxygen consumption
    Carbon dioxide production
    Respiratory quotient

See Chapter 4 for information on pulmonary function testing and Chapter 18 for information on cardiopulmonary stress testing.

Similar to preparing a patient for home care, all aspects of the patient's physical condition information must be evaluated. Each patient must have an individualized program and be physically and emotionally prepared to begin the rehabilitation program. As discussed next, the patient is placed into either an open- or a closed-end program format. The starting and ending points of the program are determined based on the patient's physical condition, heart rate target, and stress test results.

The remainder of this discussion focuses on how to start a patient in a graded exercise program and how to monitor the patient's progress. (Note that the education of the patient about normal and abnormal lung function, respiratory care procedures, and medications, for example, is addressed in earlier sections of this book and in other textbooks dedicated solely to pulmonary rehabilitation.)

b. Benefits of an exercise program

The benefits of the exercise program must be stressed to the patient to gain his or her acceptance of it. If the patient does not believe that the program will make his or her life better, he or she will not follow it. In 1981 the American Thoracic Society Executive Committee adopted the following as principal objectives of pulmonary rehabilitation:

- To control and alleviate as much as possible the symptoms and pathologic complications of respiratory ailments
- To teach the patient how to achieve optimal capability for carrying out his or her activities of daily living (ADLs)

Most authors agree with the following general therapeutic goals:

- The primary goal is to increase the patient's functional ability as much as possible. This can best be accomplished by determining what the patient wants to be able to do with his or her life on a daily basis. From this list of ADLs, a series of short- and long-term goals can be developed. One of the primary short-term goals should be that the patient feels better. He or she should be able to control or reduce any symptoms. This alone improves the patient's quality of life. Make sure that the patient's goals are realistic and can be reached. The family must be involved with any major decision-making. Often it is helpful to break a large goal down into several smaller tasks so that the patient and family receive frequent positive feedback.
- Improve the patient's self-image. This should occur after the first goal is reached. The patient should experience less anxiety and depression and also feel better about himself or herself.
- Increase the patient's ability to exercise. This may depend on the level of the patient's disability. In general, the worse the patient's lung disease, the less able the patient is to increase his or her exercise level.
- Decrease the frequency and length of any hospitalizations.
- Prolong the patient's life by the proper use of oxygen and other respiratory care modalities.

Note that the benefits did not list an improvement in the patient's cardiopulmonary condition. Numerous studies have documented that pathologic changes seen in COPD do not improve despite the patient being in a rehabilitation program. It is important that the therapist correct any misunderstanding of this.

Exam Hint 17-4

Past examinations have included one or two questions related to identifying the goals or benefits, or both, of a pulmonary rehabilitation program.

c. Individualized graded exercise program

The program format and features may vary considerably. Minimally, the patient's physician should specify four parts to the exercise prescription: mode, intensity, duration, and frequency. The following program formats and suggestions are typical of what might be ordered.

d. Program format

There are two basic types of formats. Each has its own advantages and disadvantages depending on the limitations and preferences of the patient. The *open-end format* allows the patient to enter and progress through the program at his or her own pace. Because each patient's goals are individualized, the time of their accomplishment is relatively unimportant as long as progress is being made. The program facilitator (often a respiratory therapist) acts as a coordinator. This may include ensuring that educational materials are available for the patient, exercise equipment is available, and the patient's questions are answered. The patient may stay in the program until the last goal is achieved. The advantages of this program are that it is self-directed and can be adjusted if the patient has a schedule conflict. The disadvantage of this program is that no group support or involvement with other people who have COPD is included.

The *closed-end format* involves the program facilitator setting up a formal schedule of educational topics and exercise sessions. These group events commonly last from 1 to 3 hours and may occur from one to three times per week. The whole program can vary in length from 8 to 16 weeks, depending on the content. These events are attended by a group of patients who share a common problem and have common goals to address. One major advantage of this program is that most patients do better when they have peers to ask for emotional support. The facilitator will probably find that it is easier to schedule speakers when an established time frame can be set. The disadvantages of this program relate to the loss of individual goals and attention. If a patient misses a session, he or she will have to wait for the topic to be repeated at the next program. If the group is too large, the facilitator may not have time to help a patient with an individual goal.

e. Strength training

Many patients are so weak from years of relative inactivity that they must regain muscle strength before pursuing increased endurance. The specific muscle groups that need strengthening can be determined by physical examination. In general, the large muscle groups of the legs and arms and inspiratory muscles must be strengthened.

Before beginning strength training, the patient must perform calisthenics for about 10 minutes as a "warm-up." It is important to stretch the muscles and joints and increase circulation before starting more vigorous activity. See Figure 17-2, groups 1 to 7, for a series of progressively more demanding calisthenic exercises. All patients should at least be able to perform the calisthenics shown in groups 1 and 2 for a warm-up. The patient must focus on breath control (pursed-lip breathing) during the warm-up period to avoid dyspnea.

Arm and leg strengthening can be done in a variety of ways for about 10 minutes. Typically, a 1- or 2-lb weight is used. Barbell weights can be held as the arms are moved to the back, front, sides, and overhead to strengthen the arms, shoulders, and chest and back muscles. Ankle weights can be worn. The legs are then moved to the back, front, and sides; the legs can be lifted with the knees bent, or the initial calisthenics can be repeated with added weight. The abdominal muscles can be strengthened by having the patient lie on his or her back and placing a 2-lb weight on the abdomen. The patient then concentrates on maintaining breath control against the added weight.

Inspiratory muscle strengthening is done in two ways. First, the patient is told to take in a deep sigh and hold it for a brief time. This both stretches the rib cage and increases the workload of the primary and secondary inspiratory muscles. The deep sigh should be repeated several times. Second, the patient uses a specific inspiratory muscle training device. The PFLEX device is popular because it is inexpensive and can be gradually adjusted to increase the workload as the patient improves. Review the discussion in Chapter 7 and see Figure 7-1.

Finally, the patient should spend about 10 minutes in "cool-down" activities. This may involve more light calisthenics or slow walking. The cool-down period allows the body to return to a slower metabolic rate while still maintaining good circulation to the arms and legs. This helps to eliminate any lactic acid that might have accumulated in the muscles during the more vigorous exercise. Increased lactic acid may cause some muscle aches after exercise. Inform the patient that some muscle soreness may be felt the next day. It can be relieved by taking an anti-inflammatory medication such as aspirin if the physician approves. See Box 17-5 for specific guidelines for a strength training program.

It is helpful, but not necessary, for the patient to have access to professional body building equipment found in many gymnasiums. In addition, a physical therapist is helpful in designing a training program.

f. Endurance training

Endurance training is designed to improve the patient's stamina to perform essential ADLs. It accomplishes this by improving the functioning of the patient's cardio-pulmonary and cardiovascular systems. When these systems perform better, they can meet the patient's need for increased oxygen delivery to and carbon dioxide removal from exercising muscles.

Endurance training must be preceded by the patient performing calisthenics for about 10 minutes as a warm-up. Just as in strength training, it is important to stretch the muscles and joints and increase circulation before starting more vigorous activity. See Figure 17-2, groups 1 through 7, for a series of progressively more demanding calisthenic exercises. All patients should be able to at least perform the calisthenics shown in groups 1 and 2 for a warm-up.

Patients who can perform the activities shown in groups 3 and 4 gain some endurance training as well. Some very debilitated patients may not be able to perform at this higher level. Some less debilitated patients will eventually be able to advance to the highest levels. The patient must focus on breath control (pursed-lip breathing) during the warm-up period to avoid dyspnea.

The actual endurance exercise that is selected must meet the patient's needs. He or she can walk, use a treadmill,

Group 1 Exercises

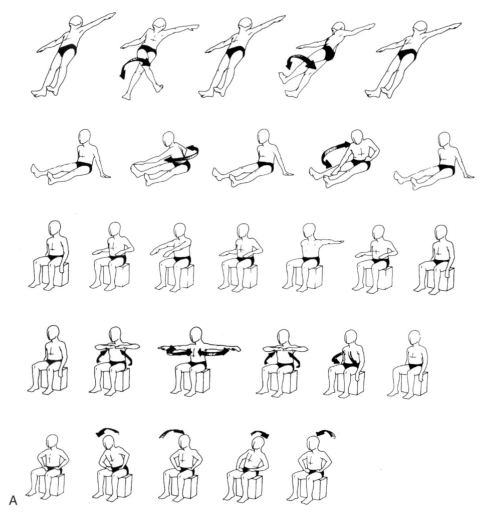

Figure 17-2 Modified calisthenic exercises. In all groups, the figure to the left is the starting point. The figures to the right show the sequence of steps in the exercise. The patient can adjust the pace of exercises to either increase or decrease the energy that is expended. In general, most patients choose 10 to 15 repetitions per minute. Exercises shown in groups 1 and 2 are useful during the warm-up period of either a strength or an endurance program. Exercises shown in groups 3 and 4 are more demanding and can be used for muscle reconditioning by many patients in an endurance program. The most demanding exercises are those shown in groups 5 through 7. Patients with only moderate disability may be able to progress to this level for further muscle conditioning. (From May DF: Rehabilitation and continuity of care in pulmonary disease, St Louis, 1991, Mosby.)

ride a bicycle ergometer, swim, or do a combination of these. The method that is selected must be both practical and fun for the patient. For this reason, walking is usually the main activity; however, the upper body should not be ignored. An arm ergometer, rowing machine, or barbell weights can be used for upper-body endurance.

A key concept of the endurance program is that the patient must exercise at a level great enough to increase the heart rate to a predetermined level. The increased heart rate (HR) reflects the increased metabolic rate and work being performed by the patient. The target heart rate must be maintained for 20-30 minutes to have any muscle training effect. Exercising at a lower heart (and metabolic) rate is not as beneficial. Exercising at a higher heart rate may be dangerous to the patient. The Karvonen formula is used to determine the target HR for endurance training:

$$\text{Target heart rate (HR)} = (\%\text{ intensity [maximum HR} - \text{resting HR])} + \text{resting HR}$$

In which:

Target HR = the target HR for the exercise period

% intensity = 60% to 80%

Group 2 Exercises

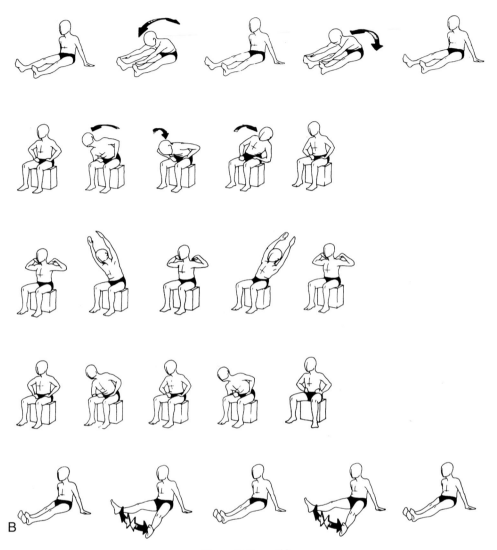

Figure 17-2, cont'd

Continued

Maximum HR is determined by either of the following formulas:

a. Maximum HR = 220 − age of the patient
b. Maximum HR = 210 − (age of the patient × 0.65)

EXAMPLE

Determine the target HR for a 50-year-old patient (of either gender) who is enrolled in an endurance training program. The patient has a resting HR of 80 beats/min. The patient's maximum heart rate is 170 (220 − 50 for the patient's age = 170).

Target HR = (% intensity [maximum HR − resting HR]) + resting HR

$$Lowest\ target\ HR = (0.60\ [170-80]) + 80$$
$$= (0.60\ [90]) + 80$$
$$= (54) + 80$$
$$= 134\ beats/min$$

$$Highest\ target\ HR = (0.80\ [170-80]) + 80$$
$$= (0.80\ [90]) + 80$$
$$= (72) + 80$$
$$= 152\ beats/min$$

The range of target heart rates for this patient is 134-152 beats/min. The patient must monitor his or her HR during the exercise period to make sure that it stays within this range. This is most easily accomplished by feeling the radial or carotid pulse and counting heartbeats for a 15-second period and then multiplying by 4 to find the HR for 1 minute.

Finally, as in strength training, the patient should spend about 10 minutes in cool-down activities. This may involve light calisthenics or slow walking. As discussed earlier, the cool-down period allows the body to return to a slower metabolic rate while still maintaining good circulation to the arms and legs. This helps to eliminate any

Group 3 Exercises

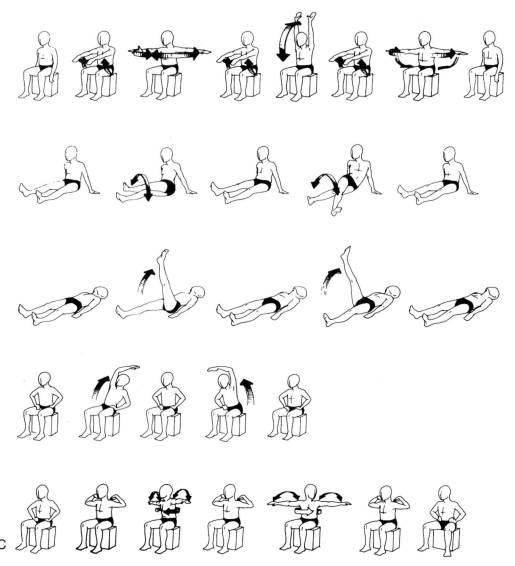

Figure 17-2, cont'd

lactic acid that may have built up in the muscles during the endurance exercise. See Box 17-5 for specific guidelines for an endurance training program.

MODULE D

Respiratory care plan

1. Determine a patient's pathophysiologic state (code: IIIF1) [difficulty: R, Ap, An]

The respiratory therapist should have a solid understanding of the pathophysiology of commonly found cardiopulmonary and cardiovascular conditions. These include, but are not limited to, asthma, emphysema, chronic bronchitis, pneumonia, pulmonary fibrosis, cystic fibrosis, right and left heart failure, stroke, and neuromuscular disease. The scope of this text prevents a full discussion of these conditions; the reader is referred to the many excellent pathology textbooks that are available.

In addition, review the information presented in Chapters 1, 3, 4, and 5. These chapters discuss bedside patient assessment, blood gas interpretation, pulmonary function testing, and hemodynamic monitoring that the NBRC has determined to be testable. Be prepared to evaluate areas such as vital signs, breath sounds, blood gas values, pulmonary function results,

Group 4 Exercises

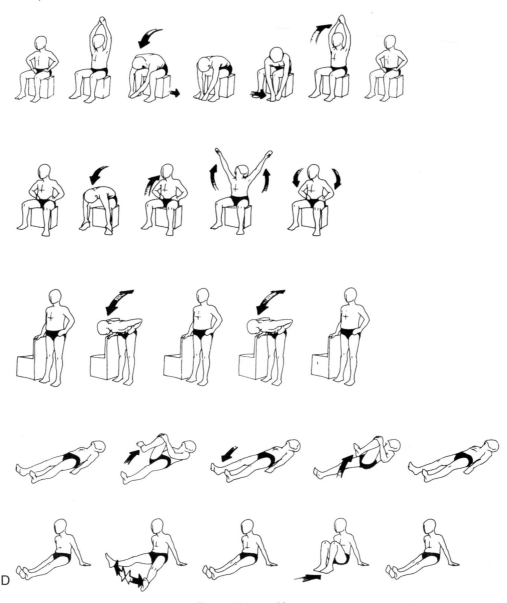

Figure 17-2, cont'd

Continued

and cardiac study results to determine the patient's condition.

2. Recommend starting a treatment based on the patient's response (code: IIIE2a) [difficulty: R, Ap, An]

The patient's physical condition must be evaluated before a home care or rehabilitation program is designed. In addition to the patient's primary cardiopulmonary diagnosis, the patient may have other conditions that further limit his or her ability to safely participate. For example, diabetes and kidney failure are common maladies seen in patients with lung or heart disease. If the patient is too ill or too limited in ability,

he or she should not be placed into a home care or rehabilitation program.

Determination of the patient's ideal therapeutic goals is best accomplished with a team approach. The patient's physician, nurse, and respiratory therapist should work together. The first consideration should be the patient's diagnosis. Then, it should be determined whether the patient's condition is permanent, improving, or worsening. Objective information such as arterial blood gas results, pulmonary function testing results, chest X-ray film findings, sputum production, and vital signs must be evaluated. The patient's physical capabilities should be considered when establishing therapeutic goals. The therapist must also evaluate the patient's mental state. Is

Group 5 Exercises

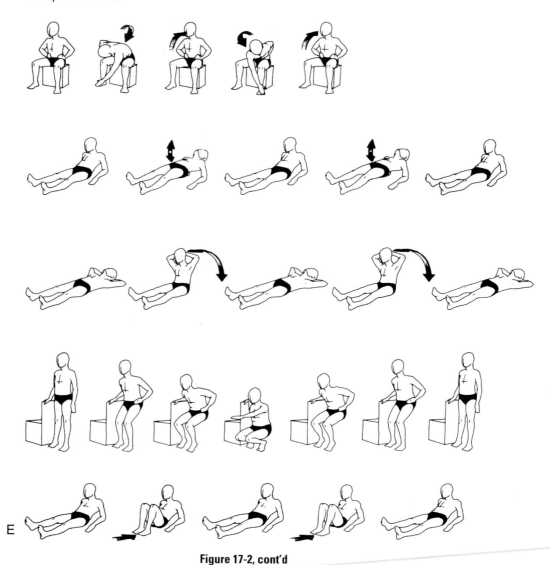

Figure 17-2, cont'd

the patient emotionally prepared to return home and be taught about self-care or start a rehabilitation program? The therapeutic goals for each patient must be individualized. If the patient is not physically or emotionally ready to take care of himself or herself, the family or a paid care provider is needed. Following are common therapeutic goals:

- The primary goal is to improve the patient's functional ability as much as possible. This can best be accomplished by determining the patient's life goals. From this, a list of attainable short- and long-term goals can be developed. One of the primary short-term goals should be that the patient feels better. He or she should be able to control or reduce any symptoms. Make sure that the patient's goals are realistic and can be reached. The family needs to be involved with any major decision-making. Often, it is helpful to break a large goal down into several smaller tasks. In this way,

the patient and family receive frequent positive feedback.
- Improve the patient's self-image. This should follow when the first goal is reached.
- Enhance the patient's ability to exercise. How this is approached may depend on the level of the patient's disability. In general, the worse the patient's lung disease, the less able the patient is to increase his or her exercise level.
- Decrease the frequency and length of any hospitalizations.
- Prolong the patient's life through the proper use of O_2 and other respiratory care modalities.

3. Recommend a change in the therapeutic plan if indicated (code: IIIF2) [difficulty: R, Ap, An]

Be prepared to evaluate the patient's condition and make suggestions for changing goals and methods. The

Group 6 Exercises

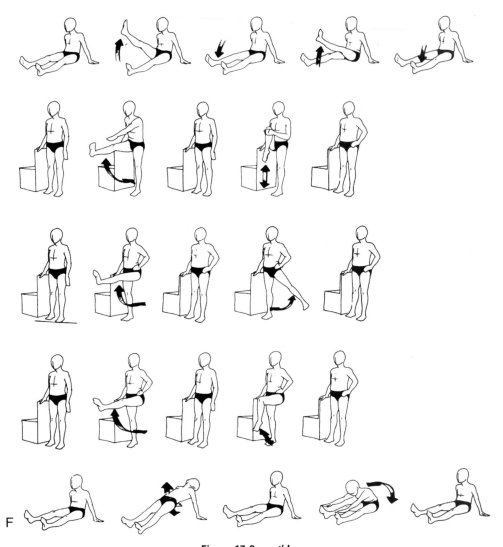

Figure 17-2, cont'd

Continued

therapist must have a thorough understanding of the patient's condition and individual goals to evaluate the progress. Objectively consider the patient's physical, emotional, and social condition. The therapist must also listen to the patient's subjective opinion about his or her situation. Be prepared to make recommendations to the patient and attending physician for modifying the goals according to the patient's changing condition.

The following signs indicate that the patient is stable or making progress:

- The patient subjectively feels that he or she is doing as well as can be expected. The patient is motivated to try new things.
- Symptoms are reduced or at least under control.
- Cardiopulmonary function tests and blood gases show improvement. Even a slowing in the patient's formerly rapid rate of decline is a good sign.

- The patient reports an increase in the distance that can be walked at his or her own pace.
- The patient has an increase in the 6-minute walking distance.

The following indicate that the patient's health is deteriorating:

- He or she subjectively feels worse. The patient is afraid to try new things.
- Symptoms are worse. The patient feels dyspnea at less exertion than before.
- The sputum has changed. It could be thick and harder to expectorate or could have changed color to yellow or green. The patient may be expectorating more than before, or less, if there is decreased movement of secretions.
- Cardiopulmonary function tests and blood gases are worse. The patient may need increased O_2, more

Group 7 Exercises

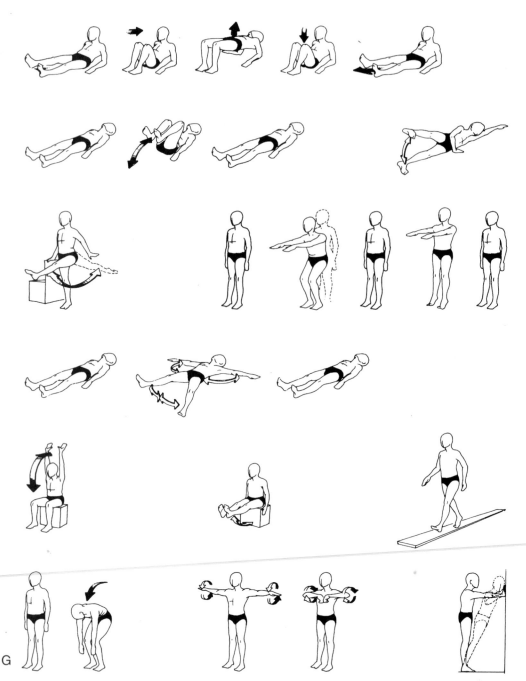

Figure 17-2, cont'd

aerosolized bronchodilator, or other cardiopulmonary medications.
- The patient cannot walk or perform as much work as before without worsening of symptoms.

4. Recommend a treatment be terminated (code: IIIE1) [difficulty: R, Ap, An]

The respiratory therapist should know the complications and hazards of any patient care activity that is performed. These were discussed in the previous chapters. Be prepared to stop the treatment or procedure if the patient has an adverse reaction to it. Additionally, be prepared to recommend to the physician that the treatment or procedure be discontinued if it is likely to result in additional adverse reactions.

5. Recommend discontinuing a treatment based on the patient's response (code: IIIE2h) [difficulty: R, Ap, An]

Be prepared to recommend that a treatment or procedure be discontinued. See the previous chapters for discussion on when respiratory care procedures should be discontinued.

| BOX 17-5 | Guidelines for Strength and Endurance Training |

Strength Training

This involves a low number of repetitions of a high-intensity activity, such as lifting weights.

A warm-up period involving calisthenics should be carried out for about 10 minutes.

The following strengthening program should last about 10 minutes:

Three sets of 10-15 repetitions of an activity should be performed.

Each set is followed by a rest period of a few minutes.

The patient should work at 85%-90% of the maximum capacity of the muscles being exercised.

Follow with a cool-down period involving calisthenics for about 10 minutes.

The patient should exercise every other day (for example, Monday, Wednesday, and Friday).

This program may precede or be done simultaneously with an endurance program.

It takes 4-8 weeks for improved strength to be realized.

Endurance Training

This involves a high number of repetitions of a relatively low-intensity activity, such as walking.

A warm-up period involving calisthenics should be carried out for about 10 minutes.

The patient should do the following:

Exercise continuously for about 20-30 minutes.

Exercise at a level that results in the target heart rate being maintained.

Follow with a cool-down period involving calisthenics for about 10 minutes.

The patient should exercise every other day (for example, Tuesday, Thursday, and Saturday).

This program may follow or be done simultaneously with a strength program.

It takes 4-8 weeks for improved endurance to be realized.

Modified from May DF: Rehabilitation and continuity of care in pulmonary disease, St Louis, 1991, Mosby.

BIBLIOGRAPHY

Almeida FG, Victor EG, Rizzo JA: Hallway versus treadmill 6-minute-walk tests in patients with chronic obstructive pulmonary disease, *Respir Care* 54(12):1712–1716, 2009.

American Association for Respiratory Care: clinical practice guideline: discharge planning for the respiratory care patient, *Respir Care* 40:1308, 1995 (Retired).

American Association for Respiratory Care: clinical practice guideline: suctioning the patient in the home, *Respir Care* 44:99, 1999 (Retired).

American Association for Respiratory Care: clinical practice guideline: exercise testing for evaluation of hypoxemia and/or desaturation: 2001 revision & update, *Respir Care* 44:514, 2001 (Retired).

American Association for Respiratory Care: clinical practice guideline: pulmonary rehabilitation, *Respir Care* 47(5):617, 2002 (Retired).

American Association for Respiratory Care: clinical practice guideline: oxygen therapy in the home or alternate site health care facility—2007 revision & update, *Respir Care* 52(1):1063–1068, 2007a.

American Association for Respiratory Care: clinical practice guideline: long-term invasive ventilation in the home - 2007 revision & update, *Respir Care* 52(1):1056–1062, 2007b.

American Association for Respiratory Care: clinical practice guideline: providing patient and caregiver training 2010, *Respir Care* 55(6):765–769, 2010.

Bell CW, Blodgett D, Goike C, et al.: *Home care and rehabilitation in respiratory medicine*, Philadelphia, 1984, Lippincott.

Cairo JM: Assessment of pulmonary function. In Cairo JM, editor: *Mosby's respiratory care equipment*, ed 9, St Louis, 2014, Mosby.

Carlin BW: Pulmonary rehabilitation and chronic lung disease: opportunities for the respiratory therapist, *Respir Care* 54(8):1091–1099, 2009.

Christopher KL: At-home administration of oxygen. In Kacmarek RM, Stoller JK, editors: *Current respiratory care*, Toronto, 1988, BC Decker.

Cohn RC: Pediatric asthma disease management, *AARC Times* 37(4):10–12, 2013.

Connors G, Hilling L, editors: *American Association of Cardiovascular and Pulmonary Rehabilitation: guidelines for pulmonary rehabilitation programs*, Champaign, IL, 1993, Human Kinetics.

Des Jardins T, Burton GG: *Clinical manifestations and assessment of respiratory disease*, ed 6, St Louis, 2011, Mosby.

Diaz-Guzman E, Dweik RA, Stoller JK: Obstructive lung disease: chronic obstructive pulmonary disease (COPD), asthma, related diseases. In Kacmarek RM, Stoller JK, Heuer AJ, editors: *Egan's fundamentals of respiratory care*, ed 10, St Louis, 2013, Mosby.

Farzan S, Farzan D: *A concise handbook of respiratory disease*, ed 4, Stamford, CT, 1997, Appleton & Lange.

Fiore MC, Jaen CR, Baker TB, Bailey WC, Benowitz N, Curry SJ, et al.: *Clinical practice guideline: treating tobacco use and dependence: 2008 update*, U.S. Department of Health and Human Services, 2008.

Galvin WF: Patient education. In Hess DR, MacIntyre NR, Mishoe SC, Galvin WF, Adams AB, editors: *Respiratory care principles and practices*, ed 2, Burlington, MA, 2012, Jones & Bartlett Learning.

Gardner DD: Patient education and health promotion. In Kacmarek RM, Stoller JK, Heuer AJ, editors: *Egan's fundamentals of respiratory care*, ed 10, St Louis, 2013, Mosby.

Gilmartin M: Transition from the Intensive Care Unit to home: patient selection and discharge planning, *Respir Care* 39:456, 1994.

Global Initiative for Asthma (GINA). Available at www.ginaasthma.org

Global initiative for chronic obstructive lung disease (GOLD): pocket guide to COPD diagnosis, management, and prevention, 2014, Author. Available at www.goldcopd.org

Goodfellow LT, Waugh JB: Tobacco treatment and prevention: what works and why, *Respir Care* 54(8):1082–1090, 2009.

Heffner JE: Chronic obstructive pulmonary disease. In Hess DR, MacIntyre NR, Mishoe SC, Galvin WF, Adams AB, editors: *Respiratory care principles and practices*, ed 2, Burlington, MA, 2012, Jones & Bartlett Learning.

Heuer AJ: Respiratory care in alternative sites. In Kacmarek RM, Stoller JK, Heuer AJ, editors: *Egan's fundamentals of respiratory care*, ed 10, St Louis, 2013, Mosby.

Hodgkin JE: Home care and pulmonary rehabilitation. In Kacmarek RM, Stoller JK, editors: *Current respiratory care*, Toronto, 1988, BC Decker.

Hodgkin JE, Celli BR, Connors GL: *Pulmonary rehabilitation: guides to success*, ed 3, Philadelphia, 2000, Lippincott Williams & Wilkins.

Hodgkin JE, Connors GA: Pulmonary rehabilitation. In Burton GG, Hodgkin JE, Ward JJ, editors: *Respiratory care: a guide to clinical practice*, ed 4, Philadelphia, 1997, Lippincott Williams & Wilkins.

Holden DA, Stelmach KD, Curtis PS, et al.: The impact of a rehabilitation program on functional status of patients with chronic lung disease, *Respir Care* 35:332, 1990.

Jones MA: Asthma self-management patient education, *Respir Care* 53(6):778–786, 2008.

Jones PW: Measurement of breathlessness. In Hughes JMB, Pride NB, editors: *Lung function tests: physiological principles and clinical applications*, London, 2000, Saunders.

King A, McCoy R: Home respiratory care. In Hess DR, MacIntyre NR, Mishoe SC, Galvin WF, Adams AB, editors: *Respiratory care principles and practices*, ed 2, Burlington, MA, 2012, Jones & Bartlett Learning.

Kwiatkowski CA, Tougher-Decker R, O'Sullivan-Maillet J: Nutritional aspects of health and disease. In Scanlan CL, Wilkins RL, Stoller JK, editors: *Egan's fundamentals of respiratory care*, ed 7, St Louis, 1999, Mosby.

Lewis ML, Hagarty EM, Lawlor B: Home respiratory care. In Fink JB, Hunt GE, editors: *Clinical practice in respiratory care*, Philadelphia, 1999, Lippincott Williams & Wilkins.

Lucas J, Golish JA, Sleeper G, et al.: *Home respiratory care*, Norwalk, CT, 1988, Appleton & Lange.

Ludwig B: Airflow limitation diseases. In Wyka KA, Mathews PJ, Rutkowski J, editors: *Foundations of respiratory care*, ed 2, Clifton Park, NY, 2012, Delmar.

MacIntyre NR: Pulmonary rehabilitation. In Hess DR, MacIntyre NR, Mishoe SC, Galvin WF, Adams AB, editors: *Respiratory care principles and practices*, ed 2, Burlington, MA, 2012, Jones & Bartlett Learning.

May DF: *Rehabilitation and continuity of care in pulmonary disease*, St Louis, 1991, Mosby.

McInturff SL, O'Donohue WJ Jr: Respiratory care in the home and alternate sites. In Burton GG, Hodgkin JE, Ward JJ, editors: *Respiratory care: a guide to clinical practice*, ed 4, Philadelphia, 1997, JB Lippincott.

Mulligan SC, Masterson JG, Devane JG, Kelly JG: Clinical and pharmacokinetic properties of a transdermal nicotine patch, *Clin Pharmacol Ther* 47(3):331–337, 1990.

Myers TR: Guidelines for asthma management: a review and comparison of 5 current guidelines, *Respir Care* 53(6):751–769, 2008.

Myers TR, Op't Holt T: Asthma. In Hess DR, MacIntyre NR, Mishoe SC, Galvin WF, Adams AB, editors: *Respiratory care principles and practices*, ed 2, Burlington, MA, 2012, Jones & Bartlett Learning.

National Heart, Lung, and Blood Institute, National Asthma Education and Prevention Program, Expert Panel 3: *Guidelines for the diagnosis and management of asthma*, U.S. Department of Health and Human Services, National Institutes of Health, 2007.

Nett LM: The physician's role in smoking cessation, *Chest Suppl* 97(2):28s, 1990.

Nici L, Donner C, Wouters E, Zuwallack R, Ambrosino N, Bourbeau J, et al.: American Thoracic Society, European Respiratory Society: ATS/ERS statement on pulmonary rehabilitation, *Am J Respir Critical Care Med* 173(12):1390–1413, 2006.

Petty TL: Pulmonary rehabilitation, *Basics Respir Dis*, 1975.

Petty TL: Pulmonary rehabilitation: better living with new technology, *Respir Care* 30:98, 1985.

Petty TL, Nett LM: *Enjoying life with emphysema*, Philadelphia, 1987, Lea & Febiger.

Pulmonary rehabilitation: official American Thoracic Society statement, *Am Rev Respir Dis* 124:663, 1981.

Rennard SI, Daughton D: Transdermal nicotine for smoking cessation, *Respir Care* 38:290, 1993.

Ries AL: Pulmonary rehabilitation: summary of an evidence-based guideline, *Respir Care* 53(9):1203–1207, 2008.

Ries AL, Bauldoff GS, Carlin BW, Casaburi R, Emery CF, Mahler DA, et al.: Pulmonary rehabilitation: joint ACCP/AACVPR evidence-based clinical practice guidelines, *Chest* 131(5):4S–42S, 2007.

Sobush D, Dunning M, McDonald K: Exercise prescription components for respiratory muscle training: past, present, and future, *Respir Care* 30:34, 1985.

Taylor C, Lillis C, LeMond P: *Fundamentals of nursing: the art and science of nursing care*, ed 2, Philadelphia, 1993, JB Lippincott.

Varcelotti Watkins GA: Fundamentals of patient education. In Wyka KA, Mathews PJ, Rutkowski J, editors: *Foundations of respiratory care*, ed 2, Clifton Park, NY, 2012, Delmar.

Vosmus R: Educating the elderly with asthma, *AARC Times* 37(4):10–12, 2013.

White GC: *Equipment theory for respiratory care*, ed 4, Albany, NY, 2005, Delmar.

Wilkins RL, Dexter JR: *Respiratory disease: a case study approach to patient care*, ed 2, Philadelphia, 1998, FA Davis.

Wyka KA: Pulmonary rehabilitation. In Wyka KA, Mathews PJ, Rutkowski J, editors: *Foundations of respiratory care*, ed 2, Clifton Park, NY, 2012, Delmar.

Wyka KA: Cardiopulmonary rehabilitation. In Kacmarek RM, Stoller JK, Heuer AJ, editors: *Egan's fundamentals of respiratory care*, ed 10, St Louis, 2013, Mosby.

Wyka KS, Gourley DA: Respiratory home care. In Wyka KA, Mathews PJ, Rutkowski J, editors: *Foundations of respiratory care*, ed 2, Clifton Park, NY, 2012, Delmar.

ZuWallack RL: The roles of bronchodilators, supplemental oxygen, and ventilatory assistance in the pulmonary rehabilitation of patients with chronic obstructive pulmonary disease, *Respir Care* 53(9):1190–1195, 2008.

1. After instructing a home care patient on the use of a small-volume nebulizer, the respiratory therapist wants to be sure that the patient understands how to fill and clean it. How can this be confirmed?
   1. **Have the patient demonstrate how to use the nebulizer.**
   2. **Have the patient's caregiver demonstrate use of the nebulizer to you.**
   3. **Have the patient answer your questions about the nebulizer.**
   4. **Have the patient show you how the equipment is cleaned.**
   A. 1 and 2 only
   B. 3 and 4 only
   C. 1, 3, and 4 only
   D. 2, 3, and 4 only

2. A patient with COPD is starting a pulmonary rehabilitation program and taking a first 6-minute walk test. If the patient should desaturate, at what pulse oximeter reading would supplemental oxygen be indicated?
   A. <96%
   B. <92%
   C. <88%
   D. <84%

3. A female home care patient tells you that she cannot feel any O_2 coming to her nasal cannula from the O_2 concentrator. All of the following could be done EXCEPT:
   A. Refill the humidifier bottle with sterile water.
   B. Place the cannula prongs under water to see if there is any bubbling of gas.
   C. Tighten all the equipment connections.
   D. Switch the patient to her tank of O_2.

4. On surveying a male patient's home, a respiratory therapist notices that four steps lead to the front door. The patient's bedroom is upstairs, and his wife smokes about one pack of cigarettes a day. All of the following could be recommended EXCEPT:
   A. The patient's wife should stop smoking.
   B. The patient should use a cane when climbing stairs.
   C. The patient's bedroom should be moved downstairs.
   D. A ramp should be added to facilitate entering through the front door.

5. When first visiting a home care patient's house, the respiratory therapist should evaluate all of the following to attempt to eliminate risks associated with the patient's performance of daily activities:
   1. **Bathroom facilities**
   2. **Television and remote control for operation**
   3. **Kitchen facilities**
   4. **Properly cleaned HEPA filtration system**
   A. 1 and 2 only
   B. 1 and 3 only

C. 2, 3, and 4 only
D. 1, 2, 3, 4

6. In attempts to determine the daily exercise tolerance of a male COPD patient, all of the following questions might be asked EXCEPT:
   A. How far can you walk your pet dog around the yard?
   B. Are you able to shave every day?
   C. Is your wife or a relative able to drive you to the grocery store?
   D. How many flights of stairs can you climb before you have to stop?

7. The main goal of a pulmonary rehabilitation program should be to:
   A. Reduce the amount of sputum coughed out every day.
   B. Return the patient to his or her highest possible level of functioning.
   C. Reduce the amount of supplemental O_2 needed.
   D. Increase the patient's appetite to achieve weight gain.

8. A female patient and her husband are both smokers. The patient is about to be discharged after treatment for bronchitis. Which of the following should be recommended?
   1. **She should stop smoking.**
   2. **She should see her physician to get help to stop smoking.**
   3. **Her husband should stop smoking.**
   4. **She should switch to her husband's brand of cigarettes.**
   A. 1 and 2 only
   B. 3 only
   C. 1, 2, and 3 only
   D. 1, 2, 3, 4

9. The therapeutic goals of a rehabilitation program include all the following EXCEPT:
   A. Decrease hospitalizations.
   B. Reverse lung disease.
   C. Increasing the patient's energy level.
   D. Increasing the patient's ability to perform daily tasks.

10. A male home care patient calls to say that he cannot feel any oxygen coming out of the nasal cannula. The oxygen concentrator is making odd cycling noises. What should the respiratory therapist recommend?
    A. Reset the circuit breaker on the concentrator and call back in an hour.
    B. Switch the cannula to a liquid oxygen system at a higher flow rate than the concentrator.
    C. Switch the cannula to an oxygen cylinder at the same flow rate as the concentrator.
    D. Disassemble the concentrator, and clean out the air filter.

11. An open-end format exercise program should be recommended to a patient who has an unpredictable work and social schedule because of the following:
    1. Members of the exercise group can offer support to each other.
    2. It is self-directed by the patient.
    3. The facilitator can easily plan group activities.
    4. The patient can adjust the schedule of activities if necessary.
    A. 2 only
    B. 1 and 3 only
    C. 2 and 4 only
    D. 2 and 3 only

12. All of the following are indications for monitoring infant apnea at home EXCEPT:
    A. Surgically repaired cleft palate
    B. Apnea periods lasting 25 seconds
    C. Two older siblings who died of SIDS
    D. Premature infant with hospital apnea periods

13. The components of a strength training program include
    1. Cool-down period
    2. Strengthening exercises performed daily
    3. Warm-up period
    4. Strengthening exercises performed every other day
    5. Exercises performed for 20-30 minutes continuously
    A. 1 and 2 only
    B. 3, 4, and 5 only
    C. 2, 3, and 5 only
    D. 1, 3, and 4 only

14. A respiratory therapist is supervising a female patient who is participating in an endurance training rehabilitation program. Her target heart rate is between 130 and 150 beats/min. She is exercising on a bicycle ergometer, and her heart rate is 167 beats/min. What would the patient be advised to do?
    A. Exercise only until she begins to perspire.
    B. Continue exercising if she feels that she can handle the workload.
    C. Exercise a maximum of 10 minutes each day.
    D. Slow down on the ergometer until her heart rate decreases to the target level.

15. Home apnea monitoring for an infant can usually be discontinued when all the following conditions exist EXCEPT:
    A. Thirty days have passed without the infant having an apnea episode.
    B. The infant received a diphtheria–pertussis–tetanus immunization without any consequences.
    C. Three months have passed without any alarms sounding.
    D. Two months have passed without an apnea episode.

16. A pulmonary rehabilitation patient is ordered to perform a 6-minute walk to improve endurance. The patient should be instructed to:
    A. Ride a bicycle ergometer for 6 minutes, and note the distance pedaled.
    B. Walk as quickly as possible for 3 minutes, and double the distance covered.
    C. Walk as far as possible in 6 minutes, and note the distance.
    D. Walk as far as possible in 1 minute, and multiply the distance by 6.

17. The respiratory therapist is working with a group of COPD patients who need to begin a pulmonary rehabilitation program. A closed-end program would be best for the group for all of the following reasons EXCEPT:
    A. Group members can offer emotional support to each other.
    B. The program facilitator can direct group activities.
    C. Learning activities can be optimally sequenced.
    D. Each patient can easily adjust activities if a scheduling conflict arises.

18. A COPD patient who is trying to quit smoking is using a nicotine patch. The patient complains of skin irritation on the arm where the patch is placed and difficulty sleeping. The respiratory therapist should recommend the following:
    1. Apply a topical cortisone cream to the irritated skin.
    2. Move the patch to another area.
    3. Take a sleeping pill.
    4. Remove the patch before going to bed.
    5. Drink a beer or a glass of wine before going to bed.
    A. 4 and 5 only
    B. 2 and 4 only
    C. 1, 3, and 4 only
    D. 1, 2, 4, and 5 only

19. A patient receiving public aid is being discharged. The physician has ordered 2 L/min of home oxygen as needed for shortness of breath. Which of the following should be set up in the home?
    A. A bank of H tanks and simple oxygen mask
    B. Liquid oxygen system with air entrainment mask
    C. Oxygen concentrator with oxygen-conserving cannula
    D. A portable, shoulder-bag oxygen tank and a regular nasal cannula

20. A 50-year-old patient with COPD is a participant in an exercise program. Which of the following are expected benefits of the program?
    1. Improved pulmonary function studies
    2. Fewer hospitalizations
    3. More exercise tolerance
    4. Reversal of lung disease
    A. 1 and 2 only
    B. 2 and 3 only

C. 1, 2, and 3 only

D. 1, 2, 3, 4

21. A 12-year-old male patient with asthma needs to be educated about his condition and its management. What should be included?

    1. Use of his metered-dose inhaler.

    2. Energy-conservation techniques.

    3. Use of his peak flowmeter.

    4. Current level of his asthma control.

    5. Oxygen therapy equipment.

A. 1 and 4 only

B. 1, 3, and 4 only

C. 2, 4, and 5 only

D. 1, 2, 3, 4, 5

18

Special Procedures

Note: It can be anticipated that the Therapist Multiple-Choice Examination (TMC) will include an *average of 5 of 140 actual questions* (4% of the exam) on special procedures. (This is based on the question mix typically found on the National Board of Respiratory Care's previous Entry Level Examinations and Written Registry Examinations.)

Remember that the TMC version you take will include 20 additional questions being evaluated for possible inclusion in other versions of the TMC. So, there will be a total of 160 questions taken. There is no way to differentiate between the 140 actual questions and the 20 questions being evaluated for future use. Please go to the Introduction for detailed information on the Therapist Multiple-Choice Examination and the Clinical Simulation Examination.

MODULE A

Provide respiratory care techniques in high-risk situations.

1. Provide care during cardiopulmonary emergencies (code: IIIG1a) [difficulty: R, Ap, An]

a. Tension pneumothorax

See the discussion later in this chapter. A patient may have developed a tension pneumothorax as the result of a traumatic situation, or one may develop during transportation.

b. Cardiac arrest

See Chapter 11 for the discussion. A patient may go into cardiac arrest as the result of a traumatic situation, or one may develop during transportation.

c. Obstructed or lost airway

See the discussion in Chapter 12. A patient may have an obstructed airway as the result of a traumatic situation, or one may develop during transportation.

2. Participate in patient transport within the hospital (code: IIIG2b) [difficulty: R, Ap, An]

See below.

3. Participate in land or air patient transport between hospitals (code: IIIG2a) [difficulty: R, Ap, An]

Be prepared to perform, during patient transport, all the respiratory care practices and procedures that have been

described in this and other texts. It is extremely important that all equipment and supplies be accounted for before leaving the patient's room for the next location. This is especially true if the patient is being moved to another hospital. Obviously, once interhospital transport is under way it is not possible to obtain an item that was forgotten. To help ensure that this does not happen, it is wise to have a checklist of everything that may be needed. In addition, all equipment must be checked for proper function. Calculate the duration of the oxygen cylinders at expected liter flows. Make sure that batteries and light bulbs work and have spare batteries and light bulbs.

If mechanical ventilation will be needed, select a unit that is lightweight and portable and has solid-state circuitry. For intrahospital transport, many respiratory care departments use pneumatically powered units. Typically, for interhospital transport, an electrically powered unit is selected. Make sure that it can be powered by both alternating current (AC) and direct current (DC) from batteries. If the ventilator will be used in a helicopter or unpressurized cabin fixed-wing aircraft, it must be able to deliver intermittent mandatory ventilation (IMV)/ synchronous intermittent mandatory ventilation (SIMV) mode through a demand valve rather than through a reservoir system. The ventilator controls and positive end-expiratory pressure (PEEP) should not be adversely affected by changes in atmospheric pressure during ascent and landing. Be prepared to provide ventilatory support with a bag/mask system if the mechanical ventilator should fail.

4. Participate in the medical emergency team/rapid response team (code: IIIG1c) [difficulty: R, Ap, An]

Respiratory therapists need to be prepared to respond to individual emergency cases such as a cardiopulmonary resuscitation (CPR) or a trauma victim. In addition, there are three mass casualty disaster scenarios that would require respiratory therapists to help care for a large number of casualties. These could be accidental or terrorism incidents.

The first is airborne chemical exposure to the lungs and skin. This could include lung-damaging agents (e.g., ammonia, chlorine, and phosgene gases); blistering agents of the skin, eyes, and mucous membranes (e.g., sulfur mustard [mustard gas] and phosgene); blood agents that block oxygen's metabolism (e.g., hydrogen cyanide and cyanogen chloride); and nerve agents that block the breakdown of acetylcholine (e.g., organophosphate pesticides). In all cases, the first action is to remove the victim from the toxic area. First responders must wear a hazardous materials suit to protect themselves before entering the toxic area to remove any victims. Once a victim is taken to a safe area, specific treatment is based upon the type of chemical exposure. Then the victim will receive other supportive measures such as supplemental oxygen, airway management, and mechanical ventilation.

Second is exposure to airborne infectious agents such as the viruses that cause avian flu and severe acute respiratory syndrome (SARS) or the spores that cause anthrax. In these cases the victim must be treated by caregivers who are wearing personal protective devices such as an N95 mask or a powered air protection respirator (PAPR). See Chapter 2 for the guidelines on airborne infection control precautions.

The third scenario would be trauma, from explosion, gunfire, or train wreck, for example. The most severely injured victims would have trauma to the head, neck, chest, and/or abdomen. Many would require intubation and mechanical ventilation. Airway management and intubation are covered in this chapter and Chapter 12; mechanical ventilation is covered in Chapters 15 and 16.

5. Participate in disaster management (code: IIIG1b) [difficulty: R, Ap]

Respiratory therapists are an important group of health care professionals who respond to local emergencies and take part in mass casualty/disaster planning. They should be part of a hospital's disaster management team. The local hospital is linked to a regional disaster management team that further connects to the state system and finally the national system. Currently, in anticipation of a catastrophe that could overwhelm a local or regional medical system, the federal government has established the Strategic National Stockpile (SNS). If there should be a locally overwhelming need for supplies or equipment, the state government would submit a request to the appropriate division of the Centers for Disease Control and Prevention. The following items can be dispatched by the SNS and received within 1 day:

- Mechanical ventilators (for example, Impact Uni-Vent Eagle 754) and ancillary supplies for pediatric or adult patients
- Intubation supplies
- Oxygen masks and nasal cannulas
- Suction machines and suction catheters
- Medications used to help manage ventilated patients: sedatives, analgesics, and neuromuscular blockers

Other respiratory-care-related supplies and oxygen supply systems must be provided locally. Be prepared to perform any and all respiratory care practices and procedures listed in this book or in other respiratory care textbooks.

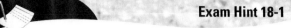

Exam Hint 18-1

Usually one question on the examination deals with the effects of increased altitude when flying in an unpressurized helicopter or airplane. Remember that as altitude increases, barometric pressure (P_B) decreases. Decreased barometric pressure directly leads to a decrease in the alveolar pressure of oxygen (PAO_2), which results in a decrease in the patient's arterial pressure of oxygen (PaO_2). In addition, as barometric pressure decreases at increased altitude, gases within the patient (stomach and intestine, pneumothorax, and lung) expand. The air within the endotracheal tube cuff expands, and the delivered tidal volume increases. This requires adjustments in the ventilator settings. Later, when the aircraft descends to land, the increased barometric pressure results in a decrease in the cuff volume, the tidal volume, and the patient's internal gas volumes. Be prepared to adjust the ventilator again.

MODULE B

Assist the physician/provider with patient care and related procedures.

1. Assist with moderate (conscious) sedation (code: IIIH7) [difficulty: R, Ap]

The phrase moderate (or conscious) sedation refers to the administration of a sedative agent(s) to calm a patient during a medical procedure (for example, cardioversion or bronchoscopy) but not cause the patient to lose consciousness. The sedated patient must be able to cooperate, follow commands, and communicate during the procedure. For safety reasons, the patient must also be able to protect his or her own airway and breathe adequately. Typically the patient has no memory of the procedure after it is completed.

Medications in the benzodiazepine group are preferred for conscious sedation and given intravenously. Currently midazolam (Versed) is preferred but diazepam (Valium) is also commonly used. When the patient's procedure is completed, these medications can be reversed by intravenous flumazenil (Romazicon). Another option is to intravenously administer the narcotic agent fentanyl (Duragesic, Sublimaze) for rapid sedation. After the procedure is completed, naloxone (Narcan) is given intravenously to reverse the effects of fentanyl. The physician performing the procedure may prefer to use a mix or "cocktail" of reduced doses of several sedating medications to achieve the same clinical effect. There is more discussion of these and other sedative agents in Chapter 9, Pharmacology.

The respiratory therapist must be prepared for the possibility of the patient being overdosed with a sedative agent. This could result in a decreased respiratory rate and tidal volume or apnea. Safety guidelines require either a nurse or a respiratory therapist to be solely responsible for monitoring the patient's breathing, pulse oximetry values, heart rate, blood pressure, and electrocardiogram. If the patient's breathing is compromised, the therapist must be prepared to open the airway, administer supplemental oxygen, or begin bag/mask ventilation if needed.

2. Assist with the insertion of venous or arterial catheters (code: IIIH6) [difficulty: R, Ap]

Chapter 5, Advanced Cardiopulmonary Monitoring, contains discussions on preparation, care, and maintenance of central venous, arterial, and pulmonary artery lines. Review the chapter if needed.

The most widely used arterial line insertion site is the radial artery in the patient's nondominant hand. The procedure for inserting a radial arterial line is very similar to the procedure for drawing a blood sample from the radial artery. See Chapter 3 to review the procedure. As presented in Chapter 5, the necessary fluid infusion system and pressure monitoring system must be assembled and working properly. A significant difference is the use of a needle with covering catheter, rather than a needle and syringe, to puncture the artery (Fig. 18-1). As the needle and catheter enter the artery, bright red blood will pulse out. In rapid succession, withdraw the needle and advance the catheter into the artery (Fig. 18-2). Place a gloved fingertip over the proximal hub of the catheter to stop the bleeding. Next, screw the prepared three-way stopcock and high-pressure tubing to the hub of the catheter. Flush some heparinized saline solution through the arterial catheter to prevent any blood from clotting. Make sure the automatic drip system and arterial pressure monitoring system are working properly. The patient's blood pressure should be displayed on the monitor (see Figs. 5-28 and 5-29 in Chapter 5).

Each hospital or physician may have a prescribed way that the catheter insertion procedure is performed. The general steps are listed here:

1. Inform the patient of the procedure and have the patient sign the medical release form if time permits.
2. Have a sedative or pain-relieving agent administered if needed.
3. If necessary, shave body hair from the insertion site.
4. Don a sterile mask, cap, gown, and gloves according to protocol.
5. Disinfect the insertion site with a Betadine (iodine)-soaked sterile 4 × 4-in gauze pad. Place the pad at the center of the insertion site, and move it in a widening spiral away from the center. This step should be repeated with a second gauze pad. Let the Betadine dry.
6. Protect the area around the insertion site with a sterile fenestrated surgical drape.
7. Prepare the sterile field where the catheter, scalpel, supplies, and so forth will be placed. Have a local anesthetic such as Xylocaine (lidocaine) available in a syringe with needle. The physician will inject this into the insertion site.
8. Assist the physician into his or her sterile mask, cap, gown, and gloves.
9. Obtain the properly sized catheter for the procedure or patient.
10. Assist the physician with the procedure as needed. This may include connecting the catheter to the tubing system, flushing the catheter and tubing system, and inflating the balloon on a pulmonary artery catheter.

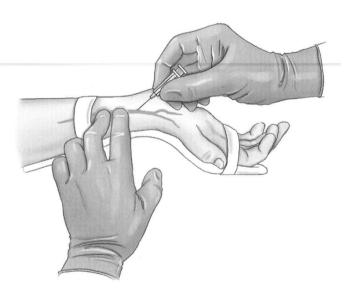

Figure 18-1 Proper positioning of the patient's hand enables the physician to insert a needle and covering catheter into the radial artery for the continuous measurement of blood pressure or arterial blood sampling. Steps in the cannulation procedure are very similar to those described in Chapter 3 and shown in Figure 18-2.

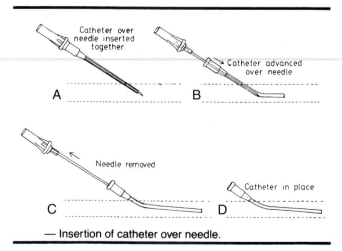

— **Insertion of catheter over needle.**

Figure 18-2 Steps in the procedure for the percutaneous insertion of an arterial catheter (cannula). Once the needle and catheter are inserted into the artery, the needle is withdrawn and the flexible catheter (cannula) is advanced into the artery. The proximal end of the catheter is connected to a tubing circuit and pressure transducer as shown in Figures 5-28 and 5-29. (From Oblouk Darovic G: Hemodynamic monitoring, Philadelphia, 1987, Saunders.)

11. Make any adjustments in the patient's respiratory care equipment as needed.
12. Dispose of any used supplies and so forth after the procedure is completed.
13. Tend to the patient's comfort.

3. Assist with cardioversion (code: IIIH8) [difficulty: R, Ap]

Cardioversion (or countershock) refers to deliberately sending a DC electrical shock through the patient's heart. Its purpose is to suppress an abnormal heartbeat so that the normal pacemaker at the sinoatrial (SA) node assumes control. This is accomplished if a great enough electrical current is sent through the chest wall to cause the depolarization of a critical mass of myocardial cells. After this, the SA node should take over as the pacemaker, provided that the heart muscle is oxygenated and not too acidotic. Two different types of cardioversion exist: defibrillation (also called unsynchronized cardioversion) and synchronized cardioversion. Both were introduced in Chapter 11 for the treatment of specific dysrhythmias.

Defibrillation is performed in an emergency situation (see Fig. 11-27 in Chapter 11). Patients who need to be defibrillated include those who have ventricular tachycardia or ventricular flutter (see Figs. 11-24 and 11-25 in Chapter 11) when they are pulseless, unresponsive, or hypotensive or patients with ventricular fibrillation (see Fig. 11-26 in Chapter 11). Because the fastest possible action is needed, no attempt is made to synchronize the defibrillation shock with the heart's rhythm. While CPR is being performed, the defibrillator unit is prepared. The defibrillating paddles or pads (large positive and negative electrodes) are placed on the patient's right anterior and left lateral chest wall. The physician or other qualified person (respiratory therapist, registered nurse, or paramedic) performing the defibrillation should call out, "Stand clear." All other medical personnel should stand back from the patient and the bed and not touch anything that is electrically grounded. When the buttons on the paddles are pushed, the shock is administered. If it is successful, the patient's heartbeat returns to normal sinus rhythm. If the initial shock is unsuccessful, CPR is continued. The defibrillator is then recharged for another attempt as quickly as possible. Box 18-1 shows the sequence of increasingly more powerful countershocks that can be given.

Synchronized cardioversion is similar in some ways to defibrillation. An electrical shock is sent by two paddles or pads through the heart to suppress supraventricular tachycardia (including atrial tachycardia, atrial flutter, and atrial fibrillation) or monomorphic ventricular tachycardia with pulses (see Figs. 11-11, 11-12, and 11-13 in Chapter 11) so that the SA node assumes control. Its major difference from defibrillation is that the electrical shock is administered automatically by the defibrillator after an R wave is recognized by the electrocardiogram

(ECG) monitor (see Fig. 11-2 in Chapter 11). The ECG electrodes must be in place and the best lead (often lead II) selected to show a clear, strong, upright R wave. The defibrillator unit is programmed for synchronized cardioversion. The physician holds the paddles on the patient's right anterior and left lateral chest wall. When the discharge buttons are pushed on the paddles, the shock is sent after the next R wave is identified by the ECG monitor.

Cardioversion is not considered an emergency; however, it is performed as quickly as possible so that the patient does not stay in the abnormal rhythm any longer than necessary. Synchronized cardioversion is performed only if medical treatment with antiarrhythmia drugs or a vagal nerve stimulation maneuver (like carotid artery massage) has no effect. Because these patients are usually conscious, they should be sedated with diazepam (Valium), midazolam (Versed), or a similar medication. Patients

---

BOX 18-1 Wattage Used in Synchronized Cardioversion and Defibrillation

Child
Synchronized Cardioversion of Supraventricular Tachycardia and Monomorphic Ventricular Tachycardia with Pulses
Monophasic or biphasic defibrillator: 0.5-1.0 J (watt-seconds)/kg.
Stepwise increases in energy up to 2.0 J/kg should be used if the initial shock fails to convert the rhythm.

Defibrillation
Biphasic defibrillator: 2.0-4.0 J/kg.
Stepwise increases in energy from 4.0 to 10.0 J/kg should be used if the initial shock fails to convert the rhythm.

Adult
Synchronized Cardioversion of Supraventricular Tachycardia
Atrial fibrillation
Biphasic defibrillator: 120-200 J.
Stepwise increases in energy should be used if the initial shock fails to convert the rhythm.

Atrial flutter and atrial tachycardia
Biphasic defibrillator: 50-100 J.
Stepwise increases in energy should be used if the initial shock fails to convert the rhythm.

Synchronized Cardioversion of Monomorphic Ventricular Tachycardia with Pulses
Monophasic or biphasic defibrillator: 100 J.
Stepwise increases in energy should be used if the initial shock fails to convert the rhythm.

Defibrillation
Biphasic defibrillator: 120-200 J.
Stepwise increases in energy up to 360 J should be used if the initial shock fails to convert the rhythm.
Monophasic defibrillator: 360 J for initial and subsequent shocks.

J, joules; 1 joule = 1 watt-second of power.

who are hypotensive or already unconscious should not be sedated.

The respiratory therapist's role in cardioversion may include the following:

- Making sure that the ECG electrodes are properly positioned for either monitoring or diagnosing the rhythm, as the physician requires
- Making sure that the ECG monitor and electrocardiograph are working properly
- Making sure that the ECG lead that results in a strong R wave is selected; usually the R wave is upright in lead II
- Charging the defibrillator to the power level ordered by the physician
- Adding the electrode cream to the electrode paddles to decrease the skin's resistance to electricity
- Being prepared to keep a patent airway, perform bag/mask ventilation with oxygen, perform endotracheal intubation, or begin chest compressions, if necessary

4. Bronchoscopy

Bronchoscopy is a procedure that involves looking directly into the patient's tracheobronchial airways. The physician can perform a number of diagnostic and therapeutic tasks under direct vision. (See Box 18-2 for uses, limitations, and risks of bronchoscopy.)

a. Recommend a bronchoscopy procedure (code: IE4) [difficulty: R, Ap, An]

See Box 18-2 for a list of therapeutic and diagnostic uses for rigid and flexible fiberoptic bronchoscopy (FFB). Be prepared to make a recommendation based upon a patient's history and clinical presentation.

b. Recommend a bronchoalveolar lavage procedure (code: IE5) [difficulty: R, Ap, An]

A bronchoalveolar lavage (BAL; also called bronchopulmonary lavage) is a diagnostic procedure most commonly performed if lung cancer or infection is suspected

---

BOX 18-2 Uses, Limitations, and Risks of Bronchoscopy

Rigid Bronchoscopy

Diagnostic use
Biopsy of tumors within the main airway.

Therapeutic Uses
Treatment of massive hemoptysis by cold-saline lavage or placement of a Fogarty catheter to occlude the airway.
Removal of a foreign body from infants and small children.
Aspiration of inspissated secretions and mucous plugs.

Limitations
Cannot be used for observing or treating problems beyond the left or right mainstem bronchus.
Cannot be used on patients with disease or trauma of the cervical spine who cannot hyperextend their neck.
Cannot be used on patients with disease or trauma of the jaw who cannot open their mouth wide enough to pass the tube.

Fiberoptic Bronchoscopy

Diagnostic Uses
Search for the origin of a positive sputum cytologic result
Evaluate lung lesions and perform transbronchial biopsy of lung tissue (should be done only under fluoroscopic control).
Stage lung cancer preoperatively.
Investigate unexplained hemoptysis, unexplained cough, localized wheeze, or stridor.
Search for the cause of unexplained paralysis of a vocal cord or hemidiaphragm.
Search for the cause of superior vena cava syndrome, chylothorax, or unexplained pleural effusion.
Assess airway patency and investigate suspected bronchial tear or other injury after thoracic trauma.
Investigate a suspected tracheoesophageal fistula.
Investigate problems related to an endotracheal tube such as tracheal damage, airway obstruction, or tube placement.

Obtain mucus for identification of pathogens.
Investigate suspected injury secondary to inhaled superheated gas and smoke from an enclosed fire.
Investigate suspected injury secondary to the aspiration of gastric contents.
Perform bronchoalveolar lavage.

Therapeutic Uses
Remove secretions or mucous plugs that cannot be cleared by other methods.
Remove small foreign bodies.
Remove abnormal endobronchial tissue or foreign material by forceps or laser techniques.
Aid in managing a difficult airway: percutaneous tracheostomy, selective intubation of the right or left mainstem bronchus.
Aid in dilating an airway: placement or assessment of an airway stent, airway balloon dilation.
Endobronchial toilet in ventilator-associated pneumonia.

Increased Risks Related to Rigid or Fiberoptic Bronchoscopy
Recent myocardial infarction or unstable angina.
Unstable cardiac arrhythmia.
Partial tracheal obstruction.
Unstable bronchial asthma.
Severe hypoxemia.
Hypercarbia.
Pulmonary hypertension (risk of hemorrhage after biopsy).
Bleeding disorder (risk of hemorrhage after biopsy).
Lung abscess (airway may be flooded with purulent material).
Pulmonary infection from contaminated equipment.
Pneumothorax from transbronchial biopsy.
Respiratory failure requiring mechanical ventilation of the patient.

and expectorated sputum specimens are inconclusive. BAL has also been used in a patient with alveolar proteinosis to help in the removal of obstructing materials. The BAL procedure involves introducing sterile saline through the open channel of a flexible fiberoptic bronchoscope into a specific segment or bronchus. The fluid and any loose alveolar cells or bacteria are then suctioned out through the bronchoscope. The removed materials are sent to the laboratory for cytologic and microbiologic studies.

c. Assist with the bronchoscopy procedure (code: IIIH2) [difficulty: R, Ap]

Typical duties of the respiratory therapist during bronchoscopy may include the following:

1. Inform the patient of the procedure. Have the patient sign the medical release form if not already done. Ask the patient if he or she has eaten within the past 6 hours (If the patient has recently eaten, the procedure will have to be rescheduled.)
2. Have a sedative such as midazolam (Versed) or diazepam (Valium) administered for conscious sedation, if needed.
3. Nebulize a topical anesthetic, such as 4% lidocaine (Xylocaine), to the airway.
4. Check the fiberoptic unit for proper function: working light source, working thumb control to flexible tip, working adjustable eyepiece focus, and patency of the suction and biopsy channel.
5. Check the functioning of the biopsy brush and forceps.
6. Set up and monitor the patient's ECG.
7. Monitor the patient's vital signs.
8. Place a pulse oximeter and capnometer on the patient and monitor.
9. Administer oxygen via a nasal catheter or the suction and biopsy channel on the unit.
10. Collect all suctioned material or other specimens for culture and sensitivity.
11. Perform biopsies and brushings for cytology.
12. Operate any photographic equipment.
13. If the patient is being mechanically ventilated during fiberoptic bronchoscopy, perform the following:
    - Place a bronchoscopy adapter between the endotracheal tube and Y of the circuit. This keeps a seal around the bronchoscopy tube to minimize any decrease in tidal volume.
    - Place a bite block into the patient's mouth so that the endotracheal tube and fiberoptic catheter cannot be bitten.
    - Watch for an increase in the peak pressure from the increased resistance to airflow caused by the bronchoscopy tube.
    - Be prepared to make adjustments in inspired oxygen, respiratory rate, flow, and set tidal volume if there is a leak.
    - Be prepared to switch from volume ventilation to high-frequency jet ventilation if the patient cannot be ventilated conventionally.
14. Assess the patient after the procedure:
    - Check vital signs and auscultate breath sounds every 15 minutes for 1 hour, then every 2 hours for 4 hours, and then as ordered.
    - Monitor cough for hemoptysis, especially after a biopsy procedure.
    - Perform chest radiograph 1 hour after a transbronchial biopsy, to rule out a pneumothorax.
    - Suction secretions if needed.
    - Provide for pain relief if needed.
15. Use a glutaraldehyde disinfecting solution (Cidex) on the equipment between patient procedures.

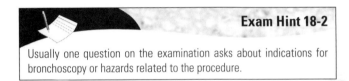

Exam Hint 18-2

Usually one question on the examination asks about indications for bronchoscopy or hazards related to the procedure.

d. Bronchoscopy equipment

1. Assemble bronchoscopes and light sources (code: IIA23) [difficulty: R, Ap]

The rigid bronchoscope is a straight, hollow, stainless-steel tube (Fig. 18-3). It has a distal light source so that the airway can be seen and a side port for providing oxygen or mechanical ventilation to the patient. The right and left mainstem bronchi can be observed by passing a mirror through the main channel. A hook or net can be passed through the main channel into the trachea or either bronchus to remove a foreign body. The rigid bronchoscope is preferred for the treatment of massive hemoptysis or to remove a foreign body.

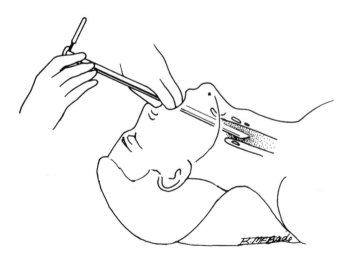

Figure 18-3 A rigid-tube bronchoscope being inserted into a patient's trachea. Note how the head and neck must be hyperextended. (From Simmons KF: Airway care. In Scanlan CL, Spearman CB, Sheldon RL, editors: Egan's fundamentals of respiratory care, ed 5, St Louis, 1990, Mosby.)

FFB uses a smaller-diameter flexible tube with two sets of fiberoptic bundles that shine light into the airway and allow viewing of the airway. It has gained wide popularity because it is better tolerated by the patient and allows for better visualization and collection of specimens from smaller bronchi (Figs. 18-4 and 18-5). The adult bronchoscopy tube has an approximately 5- to 6-mm outer diameter (OD), and the pediatric tube has an about 3-mm OD. The small diameter and ability to guide the catheter allow the operator to look into the bronchus to each lung segment (segmental bronchi). The fiberoptic bronchoscope is preferred over the rigid one when the patient is being mechanically ventilated or has disease or trauma to the skull, jaw, or cervical spine. As shown in Figure 18-4, a photo connection allows the assistant either to take still photographs of pulmonary anatomy or to videotape the entire procedure.

A limitation of the pediatric unit is that there is no channel outlet for suctioning purposes. This is because of its small size. If a patient has an obstructing bronchial tumor, a special laser fiberoptic bronchoscope is used to burn part of the tumor. This enables the patient to breathe more easily, but this procedure is not a cure for the cancer.

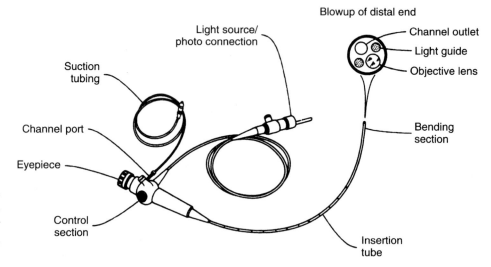

Figure 18-4 A flexible fiberoptic bronchoscope with its components and special features. (From Kacmarek RM, Stoller JK, Heuer AJ: Egan's fundamentals of respiratory care, ed 10, St Louis, 2013, Mosby.)

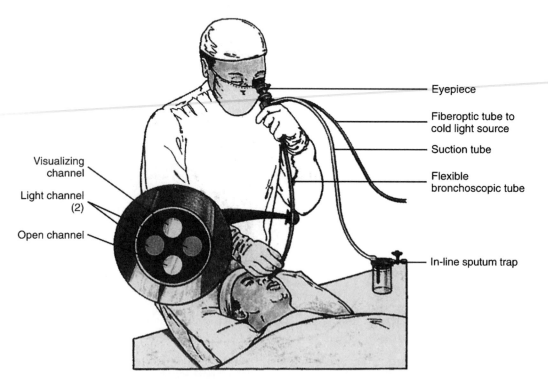

Figure 18-5 A flexible fiberoptic bronchoscopy procedure being performed on a patient. (From Wilson SF, Thompson JM: Respiratory disorders, St Louis, 1990, Mosby.)

The fiberoptic bronchoscope is preassembled (see Fig. 18-4 for its primary features). If photographing or videotaping is planned, the camera must be attached at the photo connection. Have a central or portable suctioning system set up with suction tubing. In addition, the following steps must be used to check for proper functioning:

1. Make sure the light source shines through to the distal end of the bronchoscope.
2. Look through the eyepiece. Point the distal end of the bronchoscope at a close object, and adjust the lens to bring it into focus.
3. Adjust the thumb control to bend the distal tip.
4. Pass biopsy forceps or brush through the channel port to the outlet.
5. Make sure the suction tubing connects to the channel port.

2. Troubleshoot any problems with the equipment (code: IIA23) [difficulty: R, Ap]

If the light source does not work, you must check the manufacturer's equipment manual to help determine if the problem could be something simple such as a burned-out light bulb or a more serious problem. Similarly, problems with the camera equipment can be resolved by checking the manufacturer's equipment manual.

Failure to pass a biopsy forceps or brush through the channel port probably means that an obstruction such as dried blood or tissue is present. Try applying suction through the channel port to clear out the debris. It also may be helpful to squirt sterile distilled water from a syringe through the channel. Try suctioning again or pushing the biopsy forceps through the channel. If alternating suction, instilling water, and pushing the forceps through the channel do not dislodge the debris, the unit cannot be used. Try soaking the bronchoscope in water to soften the debris before repeating these processes. If the channel cannot be cleared, the unit must be sent back to the manufacturer for repairs.

5. Thoracentesis

a. Recommend a thoracentesis (code: IE14) [difficulty: R, Ap]

Thoracentesis (also called thoracocentesis) is the surgical puncture of the chest wall and pleural space with a needle to aspirate pleural fluid for therapeutic or diagnostic purposes. Thoracentesis is performed as a therapeutic procedure to remove air or fluid that has accumulated in the pleural space and is causing the patient pain, dyspnea, hypoxemia, or a combination of these symptoms. Thoracentesis also is performed as a diagnostic procedure to obtain a fluid sample for analysis to diagnose the cause of a pleural effusion. Pleural fluid may be a transudate that results from congestive heart failure, cirrhosis, nephrotic syndrome, or hypoproteinemia. Pleural fluid may also be an exudate that results most often from inflammatory, infectious, or neoplastic diseases of the pleura or lung. Other causes of an exudate include pulmonary infarction, chest trauma, drug hypersensitivity, and collagen vascular disease.

Percutaneous aspiration of pleural tissue or lung tissue involves a cutting needle being inserted through the chest wall into the target tissue(s) and the tissue sample being removed. The general procedure for a needle aspiration is described in the preceding section with the thoracentesis procedure.

A pleural biopsy is indicated when exudative fluid is found during a thoracentesis procedure. The cause could be from an infection, including tuberculosis, or a lung tumor. Additionally, a pleural biopsy is indicated when a chest radiograph shows a pleural tumor or unexplained pleural thickening. A cutting needle is inserted into the parietal pleura to withdraw a specimen for analysis.

A lung biopsy is indicated when a chest radiograph or a computed tomography (CT) scan indicates pulmonary parenchymal disease. A tissue sample is needed to determine if the cause is lung cancer, granuloma, infection, or sarcoidosis. A cutting needle is inserted through the parietal and visceral pleura to withdraw a specimen of suspicious lung tissue for analysis.

b. Assist with a thoracentesis procedure (code: IIIH3) [difficulty: R, Ap]

The respiratory therapist may be responsible for preparing the patient, disinfecting the puncture site, setting up the sterile field, and preparing the equipment and supplies. Each hospital or physician may have a prescribed way of doing this. If the patient had a previous thoracentesis procedure, review the patient's chart for information on the nature of the removed fluid. Be prepared to compare the previously removed fluid with the fluid being removed at this time. The general steps listed here apply to a thoracentesis procedure and a percutaneous needle biopsy of the pleura and lung (described below):

1. Inform the patient of the procedure. Have him or her sign the medical release form if not already done.
2. Have a sedative or pain-relieving agent administered if needed.
3. Position the patient sitting on the side of the bed and leaning on the over-bed table as shown in Figure 18-6. Alternatively, the patient may straddle a chair and rest his or her arms and head on the back of the chair. The patient who cannot sit up is positioned on his or her side with the unaffected lung down on the bed.
4. If necessary, shave the insertion site clear of body hair.
5. Put on a sterile mask, cap, gown, and gloves according to protocol.
6. Disinfect the insertion site with a Betadine (iodine)-soaked sterile 4 × 4-in gauze pad. Place the pad at the center of the insertion site, and move it in a widening spiral away from the center. This step should be repeated with a second gauze pad. Let the Betadine dry.

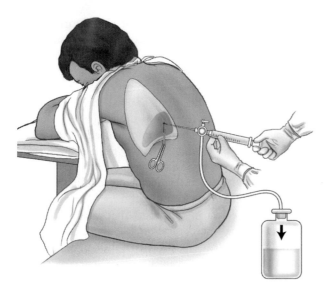

Figure 18-6 Technique for thoracentesis. The patient sits up and leans on the over-bed table. The pleural fluid is withdrawn through the needle by the syringe and then directed into the collection jar.

7. Protect around the insertion site with a sterile fenestrated surgical drape.
8. Prepare the sterile field with needed supplies such as 1% Xylocaine and a variety of needles and syringes. *Note:* A Curity thoracentesis tray or other prepackaged tray will contain the supplies that will most commonly be used.
9. Assist the physician into his or her sterile mask, cap, gown, and gloves.
10. Assist the physician with the procedure as described in the steps below.
11. Make any adjustments in the patient's respiratory care equipment as needed.
12. Dispose of any used supplies and so forth after the procedure is completed.
13. Tend to the patient's comfort.

General steps in the removal of pleural fluid:
1. Check the patient's chest radiograph for the location of the pleural fluid (or targeted tissue for a needle biopsy) and its relationship to the ribs and other tissues.
2. Inform the patient not to move or cough during the procedure so that accidental needle damage to the pleura or lung can be avoided.
3. The physician will anesthetize the thoracentesis site as shown in Figure 18-7, A and B.
4. The physician will insert a large-gauge needle (often 16 gauge) with attached 50-mL syringe into the pleural fluid (see Fig. 18-7, C). (A cutting needle is used during a needle aspiration of pleural or lung tissue.)
5. The sample is then aspirated. If there is more than 50 mL of pleural fluid, the two-way valve or three-way stopcock, rubber hose, and collection tube are assembled to remove the fluid (see Fig. 18-6).
6. The needle is removed and a bandage is placed over the puncture site.

7. Place the patient with the unaffected side down on the bed for 1 hour.
8. Observe the patient for dizziness and cyanosis. Frequently check the patient's pulse oximeter valve. Assess the patient's vital signs according to hospital policy. Auscultate frequently for diminished breath sounds over the affected lung as a sign of pneumothorax. The physician should order a chest radiograph to check for pneumothorax. (See Box 18-3 for the commonly seen complications of a thoracentesis or needle biopsy.)
9. Evaluate the gross appearance of the fluid that has been removed. A *transudate* is found when the fluid is clear, serous, or light yellow. It contains few cells of any kind. This is most commonly found in patients with congestive heart failure and pulmonary edema. A *chylothorax* is found when the fluid is opalescent or pearly white in color. Chyle is lymphatic fluid that drains into the pleural cavity when the thoracic duct is blocked. This could be caused by injury to the neck or a tumor that invades the thoracic duct. A *hemothorax* is found when the pleural fluid is bloody (sanguineous or serosanguineous). Chest wall injury or puncture is the usual cause. An *empyema* is found when the fluid is thick and puslike with a foul odor. The patient usually has a bacterial infection of the lung and/or pleura, and infected fluid has entered the pleural space. In all cases, the collected pleural fluid sample should be sent to the laboratory for detailed analysis.
10. Send the collected sample to the laboratory for analysis. Common tests include total protein, cytology, glucose content, hematocrit, and tumor markers.

6. Management of a pneumothorax

a. Evaluate data in the patient record about chest tubes (code: IA3) [difficulty: R, Ap]

A chest tube (also called tube thoracostomy) may be inserted into either one or both pleural spaces around the lungs, the mediastinal space, or the pericardial space around the heart. This procedure is indicated when air or fluid, or both, in any of these spaces interferes with normal lung or heart function. Box 18-4 lists the indications for the insertion of a chest tube.

The record should state the following: (1) location of the chest tube(s), (2) function of the tube(s) and vacuum system, (3) type of fluid and how much fluid has drained from the patient's chest, and (4) if any air is leaking from the pleural space. The record should also state the changes in any of the above.

b. Treat a tension pneumothorax (code: IIIG1a) [difficulty: R, Ap, An]

In an emergency when the patient has a tension pneumothorax and rapidly worsening vital signs, the trapped pleural air must be rapidly removed from the chest. This

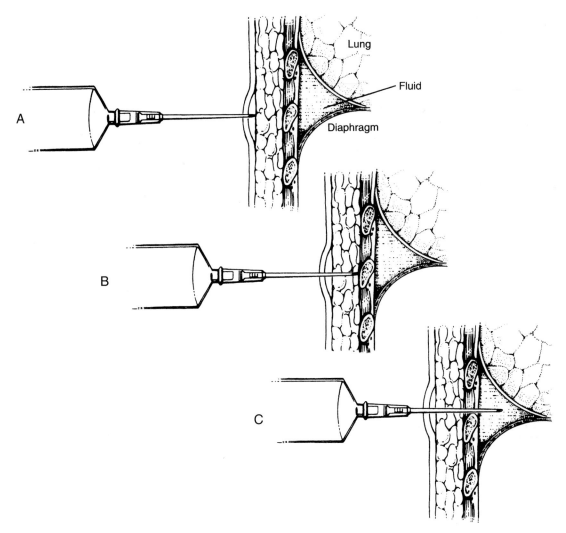

Figure 18-7 Anesthetizing the needle insertion site and performing a thoracentesis. **A,** A 25-gauge needle is used to inject Xylocaine into the thoracentesis puncture site until the skin is raised. **B,** A 22-gauge needle is used to inject Xylocaine into the periosteum of the rib and surrounding tissues. The properly anesthetized patient should feel no pain during the thoracentesis. **C,** A 22- or larger-gauge aspirating needle is pushed through the numbed tissues, over the top edge of the rib, and into the pleural space. The fluid sample can now be aspirated. (From Martin L: Pulmonary physiology in clinical practice: the essentials for patient care and evaluation, St Louis, 1987, Mosby.)

is done by inserting a large-bore needle (in an adult, insert a 14- to 16-gauge needle that is at least 4.5 cm long) through the second or third intercostal space in the midclavicular line of the affected lung. Place the needle over the top of the rib to avoid injury to the blood vessels and nerves below the ribs. The intrapleural air leaves the chest, allowing the lung to expand. A pleural chest tube is then inserted for a long-term solution to the problem. If necessary, review the discussion in Chapters 1 and 15 on the signs and symptoms of a pneumothorax.

In addition to chest tube insertion, the patient is often given 100% oxygen by a nonrebreather mask for two reasons. The first is to treat the patient for hypoxemia. Second, if pure oxygen enters the pleural space through a tear in lung tissue, it will be quickly absorbed into the blood.

This allows the lung to expand faster than if the patient was breathing a lower percentage of oxygen.

c. Assist with chest tube insertion (code: IIIH5) [difficulty: R, Ap]

General steps in inserting a pleural chest tube include:

1. Check the patient's chest radiograph for the location of the air or fluid in the pleural space and its relation to the ribs and other tissues.
2. Prepare the patient as described for the thoracentesis procedure. The patient is usually positioned to lie on his or her back or with the lung of the unaffected side down on the bed.
3. The physician anesthetizes the tube insertion site as shown in Figure 18-7, A and B.

BOX 18-3   Common Complications of Thoracentesis

Complication	Rate of Occurrence
Pneumothorax	3%-30%
Reexpansion pulmonary edema	0.2%-14%
Vasovagal reaction causing unstable vital signs	<3%
Hemothorax	<1%
Pneumohemothorax	<1%
Retained intrapulmonary catheter fragments	<1%
Splenic laceration	<1%

Other reported complications without data on frequency:

Intercostal artery laceration

Infection at puncture site

Subcutaneous emphysema

Air embolism

Modified from Yacovone ML, Kartan R, Bautista M: Intercostal artery laceration following thoracentesis. Respir Care, 55: 1495, 2010.

BOX 18-4   Indications for the Insertion of a Chest Tube

Pleural Space (see Fig. 18-8, D)
Tension pneumothorax
Greater than a 10%-20% simple pneumothorax
Hemothorax
Empyema
Pleural effusion
Chylothorax

Mediastinal Space
Free air
Free blood or other fluid

Pericardial Space (see Fig. 18-9)
Cardiac tamponade
Pneumopericardium
Open-heart surgery

---

4. The physician creates an opening into the patient's chest wall to place the chest tube (see Fig. 18-8). A tube to remove *air* is placed into one of two places and then advanced toward the apex of the lung. With a midclavicular approach, the tube is placed over the top edge of a rib into the second to fourth intercostal space. With a midaxillary approach (preferred site), the tube is placed over the top edge of a rib into the fourth to sixth intercostal space. A tube to remove *fluid* is placed over the top edge of the rib into the sixth to eighth intercostal space. It is inserted at the midaxillary line and advanced toward the posterior base of the lung. Mediastinal or pericardial tubes are placed via an opening below the xiphoid process and positioned posterior to the heart (Fig. 18-9). This is most commonly done during open heart surgery.

5. The tube is secured by sutures and covered with a sterile 4 × 4-in gauze pad and tape.

6. The other end of the tube is connected to the drainage system (discussed later).

7. Place the patient with his or her back against the bed or with the unaffected side down on the bed. The physician may want the head of the bed elevated or flat.

8. Observe the patient for dizziness, cyanosis, and changes in heart rate and respiratory rate. (See Box 18-3 for the most commonly seen complications.)

Exam Hint 18-3

Every past examination has included at least one question that relates to identifying a patient having a tension pneumothorax, requiring the insertion of a large-bore needle or a pleural chest tube. Know the indications of a tension pneumothorax, including sudden deterioration of vital signs and hypoxemia, decreased breath sounds over the affected lung, decreased chest wall movement over the affected lung, hyperresonant percussion noted over the affected lung, and shift of the mediastinal structures away from the affected lung. See Figure 1-5 in Chapter 1 for a chest radiograph showing a pneumothorax.

---

d. Pleural drainage devices

1. Assemble a pleural drainage system (code: IIA20) [difficulty: R, Ap, An]

Modern drainage systems consist of either three or four chambers or sections designed to regulate the vacuum level, hold any drained fluids, prevent any outside air from entering the patient's thorax, and act as a pressure-relief valve in case the vacuum regulator should fail. Argyle and Pleur-evac are two well-known manufacturers. The systems for draining the pleural space are discussed here, but the principles are the same for draining the mediastinal and pericardial spaces.

Refer to Figure 18-10 for the assembly and operation of the three-chamber drainage system. The four-chamber drainage system is shown in Figure 18-11 and is discussed concurrently.

a. Vacuum level

The operation of the wall and central vacuum systems was discussed in Chapter 13. It is common practice to set a partial vacuum of −15 to −20 cm H_2O pressure to the pleural space.

b. Suction control

The suction control chamber is dry when the unit is unpacked. Follow the manufacturer's instructions for adding the correct amount of water. The proper water level is generally 15-20 cm high and results in that level of vacuum being applied to the patient's pleural space.

It is normal to have room air drawn into the opening on top and bubbling through the water column. This corresponds to bottle or chamber C in Figure 18-11. The constant air bubbling causes the water level to gradually decrease from evaporation. Water must be added occasionally.

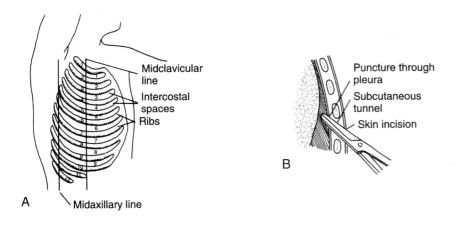

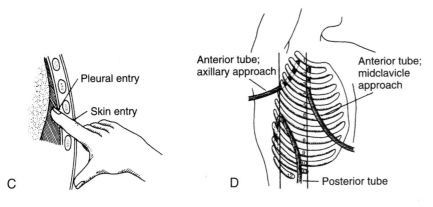

Figure 18-8 Technique for inserting a pleural chest tube. **A,** Anatomic landmarks. **B,** Dissecting through the tissues with a hemostat. **C,** Using a finger to widen the opening and ensure that the lung has not been punctured. **D,** Proper tube placement. Air is removed by a tube that is placed toward the apex of the lung. Fluid is removed by a tube placed toward the posterior base of the lung.

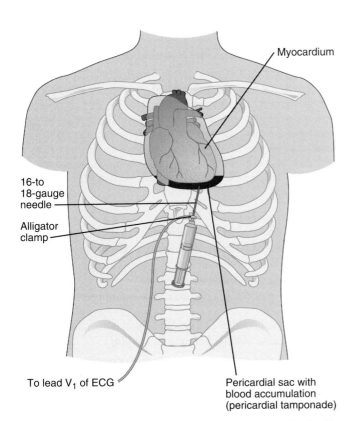

Figure 18-9 Pericardiocentesis procedure. (From Black JM, Hawks JH: Medical-surgical nursing, clinical management for positive outcomes, ed 8, St Louis, 2009, Saunders.)

c. Water seal

The water-seal chamber, which corresponds to chamber B in Figure 18-11, is a safety feature. It is dry when unpacked. Follow the manufacturer's directions regarding the amount of water to add. Typically, the water-seal tube should be filled with about 2 cm of water through which any patient air can bubble. As indicated by the arrows, it is designed to permit air to leave the patient's chest cavity. (Air also will be seen bubbling when fluid enters the drainage collection chamber and displaces some of its air.) However, room air cannot be drawn "backward" through the water to enter the chest if the vacuum fails or is disconnected.

The water-seal chamber must be checked regularly to see if any air is bubbling through from the patient's chest. If so, the patient has an active air leak. If the chest tube has been placed into the pleural space, it shows that the patient has an unhealed pneumothorax or bronchopleural fistula. If the chest tube has been placed into the mediastinum or pericardium, it indicates that air is leaking through a tear in the lung structures to these areas. When the air leak stops, it indicates that the tissues have healed over the tear.

d. Drainage collection

The drainage collection chamber, which corresponds to bottle or chamber A in Figure 18-11, is designed to hold any fluid that is removed from the pleural space. It is divided into several sections that are demarcated for volume measurement. The volume that has accumulated in the

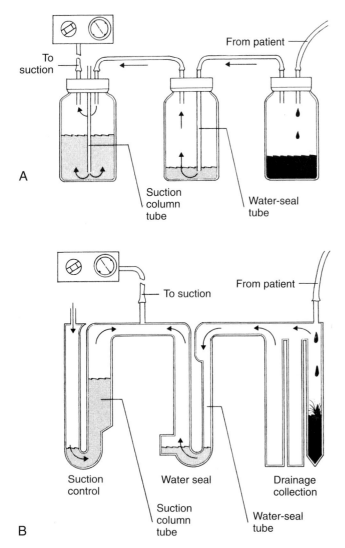

Figure 18-10 Three-chamber pleural drainage systems. **A,** Homemade three-chamber drainage system. The depth at which the suction column tube is placed under water determines the level of vacuum that will be applied against the patient's pleural space. **B,** Schematic drawing of a modern manufactured three-chamber drainage system. (From Shapiro BA, Kacmarek RM, Cane RD, et al.: Clinical application of respiratory care, ed 4, St Louis, 1991, Mosby-Year Book. Used by permission.)

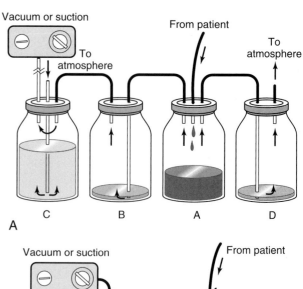

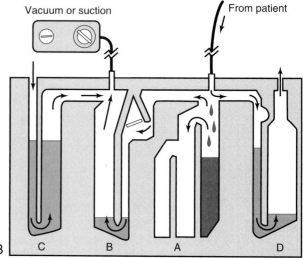

Figure 18-11 Four-chamber pleural drainage systems. **A,** Homemade four-chamber drainage system. The depth at which the suction column tube in chamber C is placed under water determines the level of vacuum that will be applied against the patient's pleural space. **B,** Schematic drawing of a modern manufactured four-chamber drainage system. The fourth chamber acts to vent high-pressure air if the vacuum should be turned off or malfunction. (Modified from Pilbeam SP, Deshpande VM: Chest tubes and pleural drainage, Curr Rev Respir Ther 5:151, 1983. Used by permission.)

chamber should be recorded each hour. A sudden, significant increase in the amount of drainage should be called to the physician's attention. This is especially important if the patient is losing blood. Note the color of the drainage. Blood is obviously red, chyle is white, pus from an empyema is yellow or green, and pleural effusion fluid is a straw-yellow color. The whole drainage system must be replaced when the drainage collection chamber becomes filled.

e. Pressure-relief valve on the four-chamber system

This additional chamber is a safety feature and is seen on four-chamber systems such as those shown in Figure 18-11, chamber D. Its purpose is to act as an escape route for any gas leaking from the patient if the vacuum system is accidentally turned off or disconnected. Without

the relief valve, air pressure from a pneumothorax might increase to a dangerous level. Instead, the air and pressure are released. In three-chamber systems, the pressure has to build up to the point at which water in the suction control chamber "geysers" out before the pressure is relieved.

2. Troubleshoot any problems with the equipment (code: IIA20) [difficulty: R, Ap, An]

A number of problems can occur with chest drainage systems. The practitioner must understand how the systems are designed to work and how to recognize and correct any problems. See Table 18-1 for examples of problems and their correction. Figure 18-12 lists important considerations when assessing the patient who is connected to a chest drainage system.

| TABLE 18-1 | Troubleshooting Problems with Chest Drainage Systems |

Problem	Corrective Action
Drainage system is cracked open or drainage tubing is permanently disconnected from the drainage system	If the patient has a leaking pneumothorax: Leave the tube open to room air so the pleural air can be vented out. As quickly as possible, place the distal end of the tubing into a glass of water to create a water seal. If the patient does not have a leaking pneumothorax, clamp the distal end of the tube to prevent room air from being drawn into the pleural space. In either case, attach the tube to a new drainage system as soon as possible.
No bubbling through the suction control chamber	Increase the vacuum pressure. Correct any leak in the system.
Water is spouting out of the suction control chamber (three-bottle system)	Turn on the vacuum. Remove obstruction inside tubing between vacuum and drainage system.
Air leaks through the water-seal chamber	Check the patient for a pneumothorax; report a new air leak to the physician. Check for a hole in the drainage tube, a loose connection between the tube and the drainage system, or a fenestration in the tubing that has pulled out of the chest wall.
Fluid has filled a dependent loop in the tubing	Drape the tubing so there are no loops or kinks.
No change in drainage	Check for loops or kinks in tube. Carefully milk the tube to remove any clots. Do not rapidly strip the chest tube.
Drainage collection chamber is full	Prepare another unit, clamp the tube while making the exchange, and unclamp the tube after the new unit is functioning.

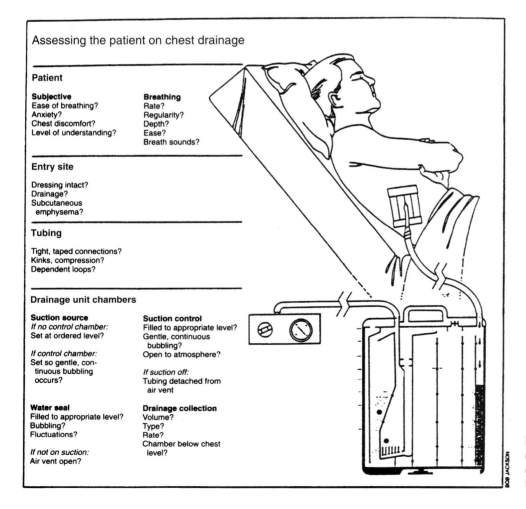

Assessing the patient on chest drainage

Patient

Subjective
Ease of breathing?
Anxiety?
Chest discomfort?
Level of understanding?

Breathing
Rate?
Regularity?
Depth?
Ease?
Breath sounds?

Entry site

Dressing intact?
Drainage?
Subcutaneous
  emphysema?

Tubing

Tight, taped connections?
Kinks, compression?
Dependent loops?

Drainage unit chambers

Suction source
If no control chamber:
Set at ordered level?

If control chamber:
Set so gentle, con-
  tinuous bubbling
  occurs?

Water seal
Filled to appropriate level?
Bubbling?
Fluctuations?

If not on suction:
Air vent open?

Suction control
Filled to appropriate level?
Gentle, continuous
  bubbling?
Open to atmosphere?

If suction off:
Tubing detached from
  air vent

Drainage collection
Volume?
Type?
Rate?
Chamber below chest
  level?

Figure 18-12 Assessing the patient's chest drainage. (From Erickson RA: Chest drainage, II, Nursing 89 19[6]:47-49, 1989. Used by permission.)

Exam Hint 18-4

Remember that a pleural drainage system is operating properly when air leaking from a pneumothorax is seen bubbling through the water seal. Most examinations have a question concerning this or some other aspect of managing a patient with a pleural drainage system.

7. Assist with an intubation (code: IIIH1) [difficulty: R, Ap]

The procedure for a therapist (or physician) performing oral endotracheal intubation was discussed in Chapter 12. The following discussions are limited to assisting an anesthesiologist or other trained physician in performing a nasal endotracheal intubation. Most commonly, the respiratory therapist is the assistant. This procedure is usually carried out only on spontaneously breathing patients. See Box 18-5 for indications and contraindications and Box 18-6 for complications of nasal endotracheal intubation. Two different procedures are used for passing an endotracheal tube by the nasal route: blind nasotracheal intubation and direct vision nasotracheal intubation.

a. Blind nasotracheal intubation

With blind nasotracheal intubation the skilled physician inserts the endotracheal tube through the nasal passage and into the trachea based solely on knowledge of airway anatomy. The procedure is usually limited to adult patients. An infant's or small child's anterior and cephalad larynx placement compared to an adult's larynx makes the procedure almost always unsuccessful. The respiratory therapist should be prepared to assist in blind nasotracheal intubation by positioning the patient properly in a sitting or supine position, providing supplemental oxygen or manual ventilation to the patient, selecting the proper endotracheal tube, making sure the cuff properly inflates and deflates, and securing the tube. Often, the physician orders spraying 1% phenylephrine or 0.25% racemic epinephrine into the patient's nares. These medications constrict the blood vessels. This dilates the nasal passages, makes intubation easier, and also reduces the risk of bleeding. Often, 2%-4% lidocaine (Xylocaine) is sprayed into the nares for its local anesthetic effect. The distal end of the endotracheal tube is usually also covered with a sterile, water-soluble lubricant for easier insertion (K-Y Brand Jelly), or lidocaine ointment can be used to lubricate the tube and numb the nasal passage.

This procedure is done without the aid of a laryngoscope and blade to visualize the patient's anatomy and expose the trachea. However, other supplies will be needed. See Box 12-4 in Chapter 12 for a general list of equipment needed for intubation. Because blind nasotracheal intubation can be challenging, several different devices can aid in this intubation procedure. The physician may choose to place a so-called trigger tube (see Fig. 12-29 in Chapter 12) into the patient. This special endotracheal tube has a wire placed into it along the inside curve to the tip.

BOX 18-5   Indications and Contraindications for Nasal Endotracheal Intubation

General Indications for Endotracheal Intubation
- Provide a secure, patent airway
- Provide a route for mechanical ventilation
- Prevent aspiration of stomach or mouth contents
- Provide a route for suctioning the lungs
- General anesthesia

Indications for Nasal Intubation
- Patient has a cervical spine abnormality or injury
- Use of muscle relaxants may cause a complete loss of the airway
- Limited movement of the cervical spine or mandible
- Lower facial injury or surgery

Contraindications for Nasal Intubation
- Basilar skull fracture
- Nasal tumors
- Nasal fracture
- Deviated nasal septum
- Severe coagulation disorder

BOX 18-6   Complications of Nasal Endotracheal Intubation

General Complications
- Reflex laryngospasm
- Perforation of the esophagus or pharynx
- Esophageal intubation
- Bronchial intubation
- Reflex bradycardia
- Tachycardia or other arrhythmias from hypoxemia
- Hypotension
- Bronchospasm
- Aspiration of tooth, blood, gastric contents, laryngoscope bulb
- Laceration of pharynx or larynx
- Nosocomial infection
- Vocal cord injury
- Laryngeal or tracheal injury from the tube or excessive cuff pressure
- Mucosal bleeding
- Trauma to the larynx during an attempted blind intubation
- Sinusitis

Complications After Extubation
- Reflex laryngospasm
- Aspiration of stomach contents or oral secretions
- Sore throat
- Hoarseness
- Laryngeal edema (postintubation croup)

The wire is pulled when the tube is near the larynx to bend the tip more anteriorly and aim it into the trachea. A flexible lighted stylet can be passed through the tube so that the light source is at the distal tip. The light shines through the skin over the larynx. When this is seen, the tube is advanced and the stylet is removed. A fiberoptic

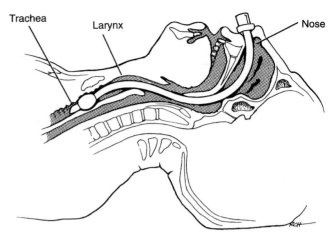

Figure 18-14 Properly placed nasotracheal tube. (From Shapiro BA, Kacmarek RM, Cane RD: Clinical application of respiratory care, ed 4, St Louis, 1991, Mosby.)

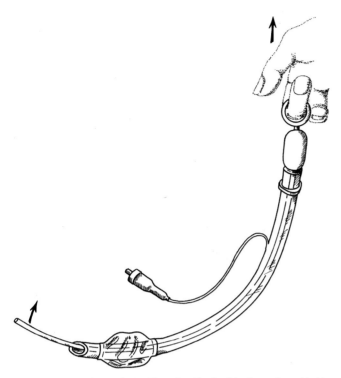

Figure 18-13 An intubation guide stylet. The flexible tip can be guided by pulling or pushing on a ring attached to a wire running to the distal end. Once the end of the guide is directed into the trachea, the endotracheal tube is slipped over it. After the intubation the guide is withdrawn. (Modified from Heffner JE: Managing difficult intubations in critically ill patients, Respir Management 19[3], 1989.)

bronchoscope (see Fig. 12-35 in Chapter 12) can be placed through the tube and guided into the patient's trachea. The tube is then advanced and the bronchoscope removed. Another choice is the intubation guide. This is a stylet with a flexible tip that can be bent through a proximal handle (performed by the physician) (Fig. 18-13). The intubation guide is passed through and beyond the distal end of the endotracheal tube. When the guide is in the oropharynx, the tip can be bent in an anterior direction and directed into the trachea. The tube is then advanced over the guide and into the trachea. The guide is then removed.

The general steps in the unaided blind nasal intubation procedure are listed here:

1. Place the patient in the sniffing position. Apply supplemental oxygen by mask and monitor the patient's vital signs and pulse oximeter value.
2. Select the nasal passage that is the most open by feeling which one has the most airflow.
3. Select the proper endotracheal tube by size and style and check its cuff. See Table 12-1 in Chapter 12 for the proper tube size based on the age of the patient. It may be necessary to place a smaller than ideal size tube because the nasal passage is smaller than the oral passage. The tube should be very flexible and have a bevel that opens to the nasal septum of the selected naris. This is to minimize trauma as the tube is inserted.

4. Estimate the depth the tube will be advanced from the external naris to enter the larynx. In an adult male, this will be to about the 28-cm line on the tube. In adult females, this will be to about the 26-cm line on the tube. In other cases, this will be from the external naris to the earlobe.
5. As described above, prepare the nasal passage and endotracheal tube for the insertion.
6. Remove the supplemental oxygen and monitor the patient.
7. Gently advance the tube through the medial turbinate. The angle of approach may be adjusted, but the tube should not be forced.
8. Advance the tube to less than the predetermined depth in step 4. With one ear positioned at the end of the tube, listen and feel for air movement on exhalation. On inspiration, carefully advance the tube through the oropharynx and into the larynx.
9. A cough with expiratory airflow through the tube usually confirms its placement into the trachea. The cuff needs to be past the vocal cords (Fig. 18-14). If there is no cough or airflow, the tube has probably entered the esophagus. Withdraw the tube until airflow can be heard and felt. Reposition the patient's head and neck and advance the tube on inspiration again. Confirm the tube is properly placed into the trachea.
10. Inflate the cuff to a safe pressure. Apply supplemental oxygen to the endotracheal tube.
11. Auscultate for equal, bilateral breath sounds to confirm the tube is within the trachea. Secure the endotracheal tube. Check vital signs and the pulse oximeter reading.
12. Order a chest radiograph to confirm the position of the endotracheal tube.

See Chapter 12 for the discussion of oral endotracheal intubation. That discussion adds detail on checking the cuff pressure and confirming the endotracheal tube is properly inserted into the trachea.

b. Direct-vision nasotracheal intubation

The respiratory therapist assists in direct-vision nasotracheal intubation by positioning the patient properly, providing supplemental oxygen or manual ventilation to the patient, obtaining the endotracheal tube, ensuring that the cuff properly inflates and deflates, and securing the tube. Often 1% phenylephrine or 0.25% racemic epinephrine is sprayed into the nares. These medications constrict the blood vessels. This dilates the nasal passages, makes intubation easier, and also reduces the risk of bleeding. Often 2%-4% lidocaine (Xylocaine) is sprayed into the nares for its local anesthetic effect. A sterile, water-soluble lubricant (K-Y Brand Jelly) is added to the distal end of the tube for easier insertion. Alternatively, lidocaine ointment can be used to lubricate the tube and numb the nasal passage.

This procedure is different from blind nasotracheal intubation in that intubation equipment is used to visualize the patient's anatomy and see the glottis. See Box 12-4 in Chapter 12 for a general list of equipment needed for intubation. A Magill forceps is needed but a hard stylet is not. Prepare a laryngoscope handle and the physician's choice of either a straight or a curved blade (see Figs 12-33 and 12-34 in Chapter 12). The general steps in the procedure are listed here:

1. Place the patient in the sniffing position. Apply supplemental oxygen by mask and monitor the patient's vital signs and pulse oximeter value.
2. Select the nasal passage that is the most open by feeling which one has the most airflow. Select the proper endotracheal tube by size and style and check its cuff. See Table 12-1 in Chapter 12 for the proper tube size based on the age of the patient. It may be necessary to place a smaller than ideal size tube because the nasal passage is smaller than the oral passage. The tube should be very flexible and have a bevel that opens to the nasal septum of the selected naris. This is to minimize trauma as the tube is inserted.
3. Estimate the depth the tube will be advanced from the external naris to enter the larynx. In an adult male this will be approximately to the 28-cm line on the tube. In adult females this will be to about the 26-cm line on the tube. In other cases this will be from the external naris to the earlobe.
4. As described previously, prepare the nasal passage and tube for the insertion.
5. Remove the supplemental oxygen and monitor the patient.
6. Gently advance the tube through the medial turbinate. The angle of approach may be adjusted but the tube should not be forced.
7. Advance the tube to less than the predetermined depth in step 4. Look into the patient's mouth for the tip of the tube in the oropharynx. If necessary, advance the tube so that the cuff is completely visible.
8. Grasp the laryngoscope handle with the left hand and carefully advance the laryngoscope blade along the

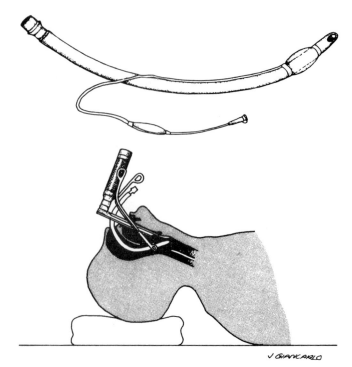

Figure 18-15 Direct-vision nasotracheal intubation. Note that the Magill forceps and laryngoscope and blade are both used. The Magill forceps is used to grasp the tip of the endotracheal tube and pull it anterior into the trachea. (From Shapiro BA, Kacmarek RM, Cane RD: Clinical application of respiratory care, ed 4, St Louis, 1991, Mosby.)

right side of the patient's mouth. Move the tongue to the left side (see Fig. 12-39 in Chapter 12).

9. Advance the blade under the epiglottis and lift at a 45-degree angle toward the patient's chest. To avoid injury to the patient's front teeth, DO NOT pull back on the handle and blade (see Fig. 12-40 in Chapter 12).
10. Observe the patient's open larynx (see Fig. 12-41 in Chapter 12). Hold the Magill forceps with the right hand. Grasp the endotracheal tube proximal to the cuff to avoid damaging it (Fig. 18-15).
11. When the patient inhales, use the Magill forceps to pull the tip of the endotracheal tube between the vocal cords and into the larynx. The respiratory therapist may need to push on the end of the endotracheal tube to help advance it. The cuff needs to be inserted past the vocal cords (see Fig. 18-14).
12. Carefully remove the laryngoscope blade and Magill forceps.
13. Inflate the cuff to a safe pressure. Apply supplemental oxygen to the endotracheal tube.
14. Auscultate for equal, bilateral breath sounds to confirm the tube is within the trachea. Secure the endotracheal tube. Check vital signs and pulse oximeter reading.
15. Order a chest radiograph to confirm the position of the endotracheal tube. See the complete discussion in Chapter 12 about confirming the location of the tube.

Be aware that nasal intubation can be difficult in some patients. It may be necessary to perform oral intubation or

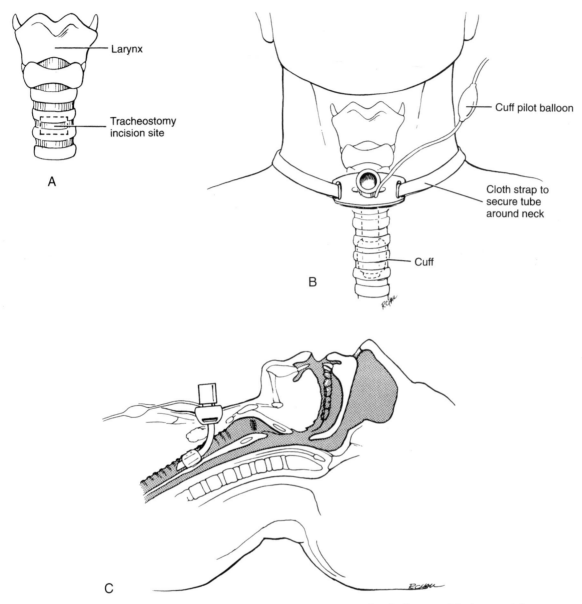

Figure 18-16 Anatomy of the larynx and insertion of a tracheostomy tube. **A,** Close-up of the larynx and the tracheostomy incision site. **B,** Anterior cutaway view of the tracheostomy tube after its insertion. **C,** Lateral cutaway view of the tracheostomy tube after its insertion. (From Eubanks DH, Bone RC: Comprehensive respiratory care: a learning system, ed 2, St Louis, 1990, Mosby.)

perform a tracheostomy to ensure a safe airway. See Chapter 12 for the discussion of oral endotracheal intubation. That discussion adds detail on checking the cuff pressure and confirming the endotracheal tube is properly inserted into the trachea.

8. Assist with a tracheostomy procedure (code: IIIH4) [difficulty: R, Ap]

A tracheostomy is a surgical opening in the anterior tracheal wall. The opening is usually placed below the cricoid cartilage and through the second, third, or fourth ring of tracheal cartilage (Fig. 18-16, A). The term tracheotomy

is used to describe the surgical procedure itself (the two terms are often used interchangeably).

Historically, most tracheostomy procedures were performed in the operating room under sterile conditions. When the respiratory therapist is called to assist at the bedside, it is usually because of a patient emergency. The emergency situation commonly involves an upper airway obstruction, such as that caused by facial trauma, or a surgical patient in which an endotracheal tube cannot be placed by either the oral or the nasal route. Because of time constraints, the full sterile technique may be bypassed in favor of a clean technique. The physician's preference and the situation itself dictate how the procedure is performed. The respiratory therapist also may be called to assist in the procedure when the patient is already intubated. Usually this involves an unstable patient who requires long-term mechanical ventilation. Because of the patient's critical condition, the physician makes the decision to perform the tracheostomy at the bedside rather than in the operating room. The respiratory therapist may be responsible for positioning the patient properly, providing supplemental oxygen or ventilation to the patient, monitoring the patient, obtaining the tracheostomy tube, ensuring that the cuff properly inflates and deflates, and securing the tube. In addition, the respiratory therapist or nurse will be responsible for preparing the patient, disinfecting the tracheostomy site, and setting up the sterile field around the site as well as the equipment and supplies needed for the procedure. Each hospital or physician may have a prescribed way in which this is done. The general steps in the surgical tracheostomy procedure and the percutaneous dilational tracheostomy procedures are listed here:

1. Inform the patient of the procedure, and have him or her sign the medical release form.
2. Have a sedative or pain-relieving agent administered if needed.
3. If necessary, trim or shave the insertion site clear of body hair.
4. Put on a sterile mask, cap, gown, and gloves according to protocol.
5. Disinfect the insertion site with an iodine (Betadine)-soaked sterile 4 × 4-in gauze pad. Place the pad at the center of the insertion site, and move it in a widening spiral away from the center. This step should be repeated with a second sterile gauze pad. Let the iodine dry.
6. Protect the area around the insertion site with a sterile fenestrated surgical drape.
7. Prepare the sterile field with the tracheostomy tube, scalpel, supplies, and so forth. Have a local anesthetic such as lidocaine (Xylocaine) available in a syringe with needle. The physician injects this into the insertion site.
8. Assist the physician into his or her sterile mask, cap, gown, and gloves.
9. Get the proper size tracheostomy tube (see Table 12-1 in Chapter 12). Make sure the cuff inflates and deflates properly.
10. Assist the physician with the procedure as needed.
    - Open *surgical tracheostomy (ST)*: If the patient is already intubated, withdraw the endotracheal tube after the tracheostomy opening has been created and the physician is ready to place the tracheostomy tube into the opening.
    - *Percutaneous dilatory tracheostomy (PDT)*: If the patient is already intubated, withdraw the endotracheal tube but keep the tip within the larynx.

Temporarily adjust the ventilator settings if there is a significant leak. A flexible fiberoptic bronchoscope may be inserted through the endotracheal tube to visualize the trachea during the PDT procedure. The physician will insert a large-gauge needle between the first and the second or between the second and the third tracheal rings to create an opening into the trachea. The physician can then select from two methods to enlarge the initial opening. In the first, a guidewire is inserted through the needle into the trachea. The needle is removed and a series of rapidly increasing diameter dilators are passed over the guidewire. In the second method, a single dilator of gradually increasing diameter is slid over the guidewire into the trachea (Fig. 18-17). (Examples of the single, tapered dilator are Ciaglia Blue Rhino, Balloon Ciaglia Blue Rhino, Percu-Twist, and T-Dagger.) With either method, a stoma large enough to accept the tracheostomy tube has to be created.

11. Insert the tracheostomy tube into the tracheal opening. Inflate the cuff to a safe pressure. Make any adjustments in the patient's respiratory care equipment as needed, such as modifying the oxygen percentage, changing the oxygen delivery apparatus, or adjusting the mechanical ventilator settings.
12. Auscultate for equal, bilateral breath sounds to confirm the tube is within the trachea. Secure the tracheostomy tube. Check vital signs and pulse oximeter reading.
13. Order a chest radiograph to confirm the position of the endotracheal tube.
14. Dispose of any used supplies and so forth after the procedure is completed.
15. Tend to the patient's comfort. A pain-relieving medication may be needed.

See Chapter 12 for further discussion on the indications for the various airway routes and when to routinely change a tracheostomy tube. Table 18-2 lists the common complications of a tracheostomy.

9. Assist with the withdrawal of life support (code: IIIH10) [difficulty: R, Ap]

The decision to withdraw life support (also called terminal weaning) usually involves the discontinuation of mechanical ventilation and/or the removal of an endotracheal tube. Because this will result in the death of the patient, great care must be taken to ensure that this is what the patient and family want. In most instances, the patient has an advance directive (see Chapter 1) stating that if he or she is hopelessly and terminally ill, life-support equipment should not be started. Or, if already on life-support equipment with no hope of recovery, the support should be stopped. Often, this declaration by the patient will help family members to accept the death of their loved one.

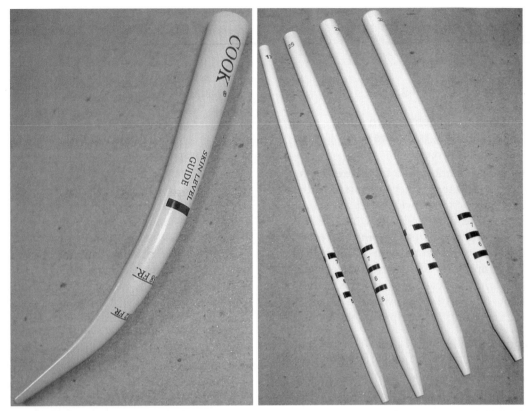

Figure 18-17 Devices for percutaneous dilatory tracheostomy (PDT). The photo on the left shows a tapered dilator, which is inserted as deeply as needed to create the opening for the tracheostomy tube. The photo on the right shows a series of dilators. Initially a small dilator is inserted. Progressively larger dilators are then inserted to create the necessary opening for the tracheostomy tube. (From Cairo JM: Mosby's respiratory care equipment, ed. 9, St Louis, 2014, Mosby.)

TABLE 18-2	Common Complications of a Tracheostomy	
Complications	**Approximate Time of Onset**
Surgical Tracheostomy	
Bleeding	During and after surgery for up to 24 hours; if possible, do not replace the first tube for 2-3 days
Pneumothorax	During the procedure
Infection of the stoma or lungs	Usually seen after second day
Subcutaneous or mediastinal emphysema	May be seen during the procedure or at any later time
Percutaneous Dilatory Tracheostomy	
Fracture of tracheal ring	During the procedure
Pneumothorax	During the procedure
Posterior tracheal wall injury	During the procedure
Tracheoesophageal fistula	During the procedure

In other instances, the patient has been medically shown to be brain dead. Depending on state law and medical practice, this may involve any of the following: (1) two physicians independently perform a neurological exam that shows no brain activity, (2) two electroencephalogram (EEG) tests are performed 24 hours apart and show no brain activity, (3) the patient has a positive apnea test (usually defined as showing a total lack of breathing efforts under conditions of normal oxygenation and elevated carbon dioxide level for approximately 8-10 minutes). The physician and medical team can use this information to help the family accept that their loved one will never recover.

If the patient has previously declared that his or her organs and tissues may be harvested for transplant into other patients, the patient can be supported while those arrangements are being made. When ready, the transplant team will take the patient to the operating room for the harvesting. After that has been accomplished, life-support measures are stopped in the operating room.

If the life-support measures will be stopped at the bedside, the physician will usually take the patient off of the ventilator. The respiratory therapist will be called upon to turn off the alarms and turn off the ventilator. If permitted by hospital policy, the physician may write an order for the respiratory therapist to discontinue the ventilator. However, the therapist has the right to refuse to perform this task based on his or her philosophical or religious beliefs. It is very important that counseling be available and encouraged for family members and health care team members to help them cope with the passing of the patient.

MODULE C

Cardiopulmonary stress testing and oxygen titration with exercise

1. Cardiopulmonary stress testing

a. Evaluate data in the patient record about cardiopulmonary stress testing results (code: IA8) [difficulty: R, Ap]

Cardiopulmonary stress testing (also called exercise testing) is performed to determine a patient's limits to exercise. The limiting factors to exercise provide much information about a patient's medical condition. Box 18-7 lists the indications for stress testing. Before starting a stress test, review the patient's chart for information on any previous stress testing. It is important to know the type of testing that was performed, how the patient tolerated it, and what caused the patient to stop the test. Review the physician's evaluation of the test results and the patient's diagnosis.

b. Evaluate data in the patient record about metabolic study results (code: IA11) [difficulty: R, Ap]

1. Metabolic equivalent of basal metabolic rate

A person who is sleeping or totally relaxed is consuming the minimum number of calories and the least amount of oxygen to stay alive. The minimum amount of carbon dioxide is being produced as a waste product of metabolism. He or she is said to be at basal metabolic rate (BMR) of energy expenditure. At BMR a person consumes about 3.5 mL of oxygen/kg of body weight/min. Multiplying this value by the person's body weight produces the metabolic equivalent of basal metabolic rate for oxygen, or MET, as it is abbreviated. The average adult at BMR consumes the energy equivalent of 1 MET of about 250 mL of oxygen/min

and produces about 200 mL of carbon dioxide/min. Obviously, the more active a person is the more calories and oxygen are consumed and the more carbon dioxide is produced. Often a person's exercise limit is quantified in terms of how many METs he or she can perform. For example, light household cleaning might be 2 METs of exercise, whereas competitive swimming might be 8-10 METs of exercise.

2. Respiratory quotient and respiratory exchange ratio

Respiratory quotient (RQ) is the ratio, at the cellular level, of the amount of carbon dioxide produced in 1 minute to the amount of oxygen consumed in 1 minute. It must be readily apparent that it is impossible to directly measure the RQ because it studies cellular metabolism; however, the same gases can be easily measured in the lungs.

A metabolic study is performed to evaluate a patient's oxygen consumption in 1 minute (VO_2) and carbon dioxide production in 1 minute (VCO_2) for the assessment of a patient's metabolism at rest or during exercise, or as part of a general nutritional assessment. The bedside testing procedure is called *indirect calorimetry* and involves collecting the patient's exhaled gases to send them through a rapid O_2 analyzer and CO_2 analyzer. In a normal, healthy person the cellular metabolic processes, lung function, and cardiovascular function are working properly. As can be seen in Figure 18-18, this results in a cellular RQ of 0.80 and a resulting respiratory exchange ratio (R) measured at the lung of 0.80. This indicates normal oxygen consumption and carbon dioxide production. The calculation is shown in the equation below.

Sick patients will often have an R value of greater than 0.80. This can be the result of the patient's diet. However, in many sick patients, the high R value is because of the inability of the lungs to remove carbon dioxide (many chronic obstructive pulmonary disease [COPD] patients) or insufficient oxygen delivery to the tissues. Tissue hypoxia results in anaerobic metabolism with resulting lactic acid production. This lactic acid, in turn, converts to excessive carbon dioxide. Even a healthy person can have an increased R value during heavy exercise with a stress test.

The respiratory exchange ratio (R or RER) is the ratio, at the alveolar level, of the amount of carbon dioxide produced in 1 minute to the amount of oxygen consumed in 1 minute. The volume of these two gases is determined through indirect calorimetry, as discussed previously. Using the oxygen consumption and carbon dioxide volumes discussed earlier, the R (or RQ) of a resting adult would be calculated as:

$$R = \frac{\dot{V}CO_2}{\dot{V}O_2} = \frac{200 \text{ mL } CO_2}{250 \text{ mL } O_2} = 0.80$$

The R value (and RQ) of 0.80 remains quite steady during light to moderate exercise (see Fig. 18-18).

BOX 18-7   Indications for Stress Testing

Evaluation of nonspecific dyspnea on exertion.

Evaluation of the patient's ventilatory response to increased work.

Evaluation of the patient's need for supplemental oxygen.

Serial testing of the patient to help in evaluating the response to therapy, medication, smoking cessation, or a rehabilitation program.

To determine the presence and/or nature of ventilatory limits to exercise, such as decreased flows, increased or decreased lung volumes, and/or decreased diffusing capacity.

To determine the presence and/or nature of cardiovascular limits to exercise, such as heart rate, cardiac output, arrhythmias, blood pressure, and/or angina pectoris.

To determine the presence and/or nature of muscular limits to exercise such as general deconditioning or decreased local perfusion.

Preoperative assessment for a lung resection or transplantation.

Assessment for the degree of impairment for disability evaluation.

Assessment of an apparently healthy adult more than 40 years of age before starting a vigorous exercise program.

A normal, healthy person can quite easily increase the amount of oxygen consumed and eliminate the extra carbon dioxide produced during exercise. This is what is seen during aerobic metabolism when all body systems are functioning smoothly. It is only during heavy exercise that the body has difficulty coping and must eventually stop.

3. Maximum oxygen consumption and maximum carbon dioxide production

The maximum oxygen consumption ($\dot{V}O_{2max}$) is the highest oxygen consumption attainable by a person. Men have a greater capacity for oxygen consumption than women, and both genders have a natural decline with age. The oxygen consumption at less than a maximum level is recorded as the volume in milliliters of oxygen used in 1 minute and abbreviated as $\dot{V}O_2$. The maximum carbon dioxide production ($\dot{V}CO_{2max}$) is the highest carbon dioxide production attainable by a person. The carbon dioxide production at less than a maximum level is recorded as the volume in milliliters of CO_2 produced in 1 minute and abbreviated as $\dot{V}CO_2$. Healthy, athletic people can increase their $\dot{V}O_2$ and $\dot{V}CO_2$ values by 8-10 times their basal metabolic rate.

4. Anaerobic threshold

Anaerobic threshold (AT) is the highest oxygen consumption during exercise above which a sustained lactic acidosis occurs. When an exercising patient hits the anaerobic threshold, he or she will demonstrate a sudden increase in respiratory rate and tidal volume (minute volume). This is an attempt by the patient to exhale the sudden excess of carbon dioxide produced as a result of anaerobic metabolism—the inability to get enough oxygen to the exercising muscles.

If the patient's oxygen consumption and carbon dioxide production values are graphed during heavy exercise when AT is reached, it will be seen that the patient has a respiratory exchange ratio of 1.0. This indicates equal values for both gases. An R value of 1.0 is reached in most people during heavy exercise at about 50%-60% of the $\dot{V}O_{2max}$. At this exercise level insufficient oxygen reaches the muscles, resulting in the formation of lactic acid. This then converts to additional carbon dioxide until the level

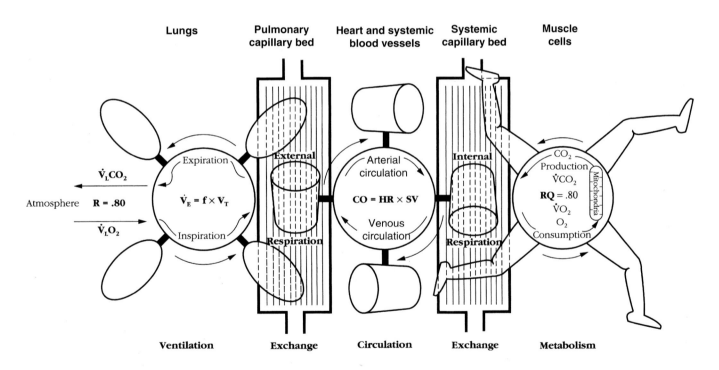

Figure 18-18 Representation of the interconnected relationships between the pulmonary system, the cardiovascular system, and the tissues of the body to show the processes of oxygen delivery and consumption and carbon dioxide production and exhalation. Note how the relationship of oxygen consumption and carbon dioxide production in the mitochondria of the cells results in an respiratory quotient (RQ) of 0.80 and the intake of oxygen and exhalation of carbon dioxide by the lungs result in a matching respiratory exchange ratio (R) of 0.80. This allows indirect calorimetry to be used to evaluate a patient's metabolism at rest and during exercise to assess the pulmonary system, cardiovascular system, and muscle function.

of CO_2 production equals (or exceeds) the level of oxygen consumption. Most healthy people can continue to exercise vigorously for a short time with an R value of 1.1-1.2 until they must stop. Elderly persons or patients with cardiopulmonary disease are rarely intentionally stressed to the anaerobic threshold.

5. Maximum heart rate

The maximum heart rate (HR_{max}) is the highest heart rate that a person should be able to achieve. Either of the following prediction equations for maximum heart rate in beats per minute can be used (the standard deviation for these formulas is ±10 to 15 beats/min):

$$HR_{max} \text{ for males and females} = 210 - (0.65 \times \text{age in years})$$

or

$$HR_{max} \text{ for males and females} = 220 - (\text{age in years})$$

Because it is obviously hazardous to exercise anyone to their maximum heart rate for a prolonged time, a lower target heart rate is usually calculated. Initially, a target heart rate of 60%-70% of maximum is often used. Later, as the patient becomes better conditioned, the target heart rate may be raised.

There are many other concepts and formulas that may be studied by the student who wishes to learn more and become more skilled in performing and interpreting stress tests.

c. Assist a physician/provider in performing cardiopulmonary stress testing (code: IIIH9) [difficulty: R, Ap]

Cardiopulmonary stress testing is the intentional exercising of the patient to the point of exhaustion or physiologic deterioration, when the test must be stopped because the patient cannot continue. Because of this, the procedure is inherently risky to the patient. It is imperative that the patient be carefully evaluated before, during, and after the procedure. An informed consent statement must be signed by the patient before beginning the test. A physician should be present during the test along with the therapist and possibly a nurse.

Despite the risks involved in the procedure, a stress test is an important diagnostic or clinical evaluation tool for many patients (Table 18-3). Box 18-8 lists the steps in the patient workup before testing can be safely performed. Box 18-9 lists the contraindications for stress testing. Patients with any of these problems are too ill to be jeopardized by the procedure. Equipment and protocol considerations follow:

1. Exercise equipment

Whether the patient is exercising on a treadmill or a bicycle, it is very informative to perform indirect calorimetry by analyzing the patient's exhaled gases for oxygen and carbon dioxide. There are two different types of systems

TABLE 18-3	Exercise Intolerance: Differentiating Between Heart Disease, Lung Disease, and Deconditioned Muscles		
Parameter	**Heart Disease**	**Lung Disease**	**Deconditioned Muscles**
$\dot{V}O_{2max}$	D*	D	D
Heart rate reserve	D	I	I
Breathing reserve	N	D	N
Exercise PaO_2 or SpO_2	N	D	N
$\dot{V}O_2$ at anaerobic threshold	D	N	D
$\dot{V}O_2$/heart rate	D	N	N
Exercise $P(A-a)O_2$	N	I	N
Exercise V_D/V_T	N	I	N
Exercise electrocardiogram	Abnormal	Normal	Normal
Common chief complaint	Chest pain	Dyspnea	Leg fatigue or cramps
		Bronchospasm	

Based on a table in Sue D: Exercise testing and the patient with cardiopulmonary disease. In Goldman AL, editor: Problems in pulmonary disease, 2(1), 1986.
*Abbreviations: D, decreased; I, increased; N, normal.

BOX 18-8 Patient Evaluation Before Stress Testing

History of acute or chronic illness leading to the need for stress testing.
General physical exam.
Resting 12-lead electrocardiogram to exclude unexpected cardiac disease.
Chest radiograph.
Laboratory studies for complete blood count and levels of serum electrolytes.
Spirometry with measurement of flows, all lung volumes and capacities, and maximum voluntary ventilation.
Carbon monoxide diffusing capacity.
Pulse oximetry or arterial blood gases for PaO_2 measurement.
Before and after bronchodilator spirometry studies if the patient is using an inhaled β_2-adrenergic medication or has a history of exercise-induced asthma.

---

for this. One utilizes a mixing chamber from which the patient's gases are periodically analyzed. The other is a breath-by-breath system that samples and analyzes each exhaled breath (Fig. 18-19). The measured patient parameters in both systems usually include the following: (1) fraction of exhaled oxygen (F_EO_2), (2) fraction of exhaled carbon dioxide (F_ECO_2), (3) respiratory rate, (4) exhaled gas temperature, (5) exhaled volume, and (6) time from the start of the test.

a. Treadmill

The treadmill is a motorized continuously looped belt combined with a ramp. The belt's speed may be adjusted

BOX 18-9   Contraindications for Stress Testing

Arterial Blood Gases
PaO_2 less than 50 mm Hg when breathing room air.
SpO_2 less than 85% when breathing room air.

Pulmonary
Severe pulmonary hypertension.
Recent pulmonary embolism.
Untreated or unstable asthma.
$FEV_{1.0}$ less than 30% of predicted.

Cardiovascular
Myocardial infarction within the past 4 weeks.
Dissecting thoracic or abdominal aortic aneurysm.
Dissecting ventricular aneurysm.
Thrombophlebitis.
Systemic embolism.
Uncontrolled hypertension.
Unstable angina pectoris.
Second-degree or third-degree heart block.
Atrial arrhythmias with a rapid ventricular response.
Frequent premature ventricular contractions or other life-threatening ventricular arrhythmias.
Congestive heart failure with pulmonary edema.
Severe aortic stenosis.
Acute pericarditis.
Resting diastolic blood pressure greater than 110 mm Hg or resting systolic blood pressure greater than 200 mm Hg.
Neuromuscular disorders that prevent or limit the testing.
Orthopedic disorders that prevent or limit the testing.

from the stopped position to 1.5-10 miles per hour (great enough to exhaust a trained runner). The ramp may be adjusted from flat (0% grade) to sloped (30% grade) (great enough to require the patient to run to keep from falling off the back of the treadmill). There is a railing for the patient to hold if necessary. Commonly there is also an emergency button that the patient can hit to stop the unit. Adjunct equipment is nearby for monitoring the electrocardiogram, exhaled gases, and so forth (Fig. 18-20). The treadmill has an advantage over the bicycle ergometer in that it trains the patient's muscles that are needed for walking. This is an important practical consideration for most patients. However, it is more difficult to quantify the exercise test results from a treadmill compared to a bicycle because the patient's stride and mechanics of walking vary as the speed increases.

b. Bicycle ergometer

The bicycle ergometer is a stationary bicycle with seat, handle bars, and electronics for calculating distance, effort, and so forth. The electromechanical units as shown in Figure 18-21 have electronic brakes to increase the patient's workload. Although less practical in training muscles for everyday tasks such as walking, the ergometer allows for easier workload adjustments and calculation of the exercise test results. Other exercise methods such as an arm ergometer or a rowing machine are rarely performed on patients.

2. Exercise protocols

There are a number of exercise protocols that may be followed. Basically they fall into one of the two following test categories and may be performed on either a treadmill or a bicycle ergometer.

a. Progressive multistage test

This test is designed to examine the effects of rapidly increasing workloads on the cardiopulmonary system. A steady state may or may not be reached because the goals are to trend the measured exercise parameters and find the maximum workload. The following parameters are measured: maximum oxygen consumption, maximum carbon dioxide production, maximum minute ventilation, and maximum heart rate. This is a less exhausting test than the steady state and may be repeated if necessary. This test may be used for its own purposes or to establish maximum workloads before having the patient perform the steady-state test.

Patients with known or suspected cardiac disease use a version of the progressive multistage test called the modified Bruce protocol. Its goal is to rapidly increase the patient's workload until a target heart rate of 85% of predicted is reached. To accomplish this, the speed and angle of the treadmill are increased every 3 minutes until the target heart rate is reached or the patient feels the need to stop.

b. Steady-state test

This test is designed to measure cardiopulmonary parameters under steady metabolic conditions. Commonly these levels are 50% and 75% of the predicted maximum oxygen consumption. The following parameters are measured: oxygen consumption, carbon dioxide production, minute ventilation, and heart rate. This is a more exhausting test than the progressive multistage test because it takes longer. It usually is not repeated the same day.

3. General steps in the procedure

1. Explain the procedure to the patient. Answer any questions. Show the patient how to stop the test in case of an emergency. Develop a hand signal system so that the patient can approve an increase in workload (thumb up) or warn you of the need to stop the test (thumb down).
2. Set up the following monitoring equipment on the patient:
   - Electrocardiogram with chest leads placed as usual and limb leads moved to the shoulder areas and lower abdominal areas
   - Pulse oximeter monitor for SpO_2 or (rarely) arterial line for monitoring PaO_2, other blood gas values, and continuous blood pressure
   - Arm cuff and sphygmomanometer for automatic or manual blood pressure monitoring if an arterial line is not inserted
   - Mouthpiece with one-way valves or head hood to gather exhaled gases for analysis

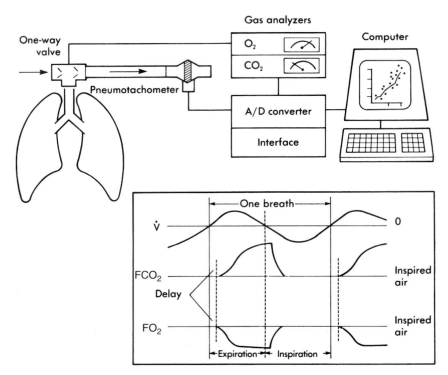

Figure 18-19 Schematic drawing of a breath-by-breath system for gas analysis during exercise testing. Gas is taken continuously from the sampling port. The gas sample in combination with the pneumotachometer information is integrated by the computer to yield data on average mixes of sealed oxygen (F_EO_2) and carbon dioxide (F_ECO_2), respiratory rate, tidal volume, minute volume, $\dot{V}O_2$, $\dot{V}CO_2$, and respiratory quotient. The inset shows a single breath. During inspiration, the oxygen percentage increases and carbon dioxide percentage decreases. During expiration, the oxygen percentage decreases and carbon dioxide percentage increases. There is an unavoidable delay as the gas flows to the analyzer to determine the gas concentrations and send the data to the computer for display. The information that is displayed will still be on a breath-by-breath basis but not synchronized with the patient's real-time breathing efforts. (From Mottram CD: Ruppel's manual of pulmonary function testing, ed 10, St Louis, 2013, Mosby.)

3. Have the patient breathe normally through the system and take a set of baseline parameters. Tell the patient to warm up on the equipment by exercising at a low level (approximately 25% of $\dot{V}O_{2max}$). Take a set of parameters. *Note:* Steps 4, 5, and 6 are for the steady-state test. With the progressive multistage test, the patient will exercise at a given level for only a few minutes before moving to a higher work level.

4. Begin the test by having the patient exercise at a predetermined moderate level (approximately 50% of $\dot{V}O_{2max}$) for 5-8 minutes. Take a set of parameters in the last 1-2 minutes.

5. Increase the workload (approximately 75% of $\dot{V}O_{2max}$) and have the patient exercise at this level for 5-8 minutes. Take a set of parameters in the last 1-2 minutes. Alternatively, the patient may be given a short rest period or low exercise period between the steps of increased workload.

6. Repeat step 5, if necessary, at a higher workload until the patient is exhausted or cannot continue because of one of the conditions listed in Box 18-10.

7. Have the patient exercise at a low level for several minutes during a cool down/recovery period. It is important to monitor the patient during the recovery period because a sudden drop in blood pressure and fainting are known to occur if exercise should stop too quickly. Note how long it takes for the patient to return to baseline conditions.

d. Interpret the results of cardiopulmonary stress testing (code: ID21) [difficulty: R, Ap, An]

1. *In a healthy person the following physiologic changes can be expected*

   a. *Tidal volume, respiratory rate, and minute volume*

All patients will find the combination of tidal volume and respiratory rate that allows the most efficient ventilation. Patients with normal, healthy lungs will increase their tidal volume to about 60% of their vital capacity. They will then increase the respiratory rate to produce the maximum ventilation possible. Patients with obstructive airways disease are flow-limited and cannot increase their respiratory rate adequately. They attempt to raise their tidal volume to increase their minute volume but

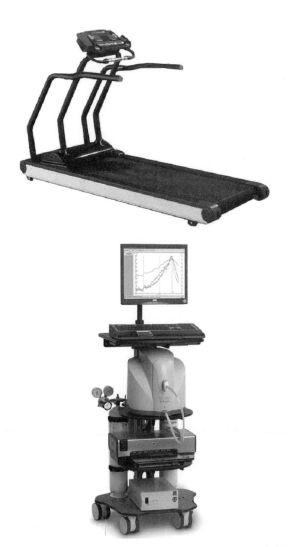

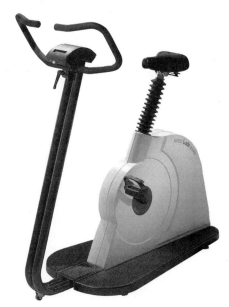

Figure 18-21 An electromechanical bicycle ergometer with controls for electronic braking, pedaling resistance, test timer, meters for pedaling frequency in revolutions per minute (RPM), and external workload in watts. (Courtesy of Medical Graphics Inc., St Paul, Minn. In Mottram CD: Ruppel's manual of pulmonary function testing, ed 10, St Louis, 2013, Mosby.)

BOX 18-10 Indications for Stopping a Stress Test

Arterial Blood Gases
PaO_2 decreasing to less than 55 mm Hg.
Acidosis with or without a rise in the $PaCO_2$ level.
SpO_2 less than 83% or <4% less than the baseline value.

Pulmonary
Exercise-induced bronchospasm.
Severe dyspnea.

Cardiovascular
20 mm Hg fall in systolic blood pressure below the baseline value.
Systolic blood pressure greater than 250 mm Hg.
Diastolic blood pressure greater than 120 mm Hg.
Onset of angina pectoris.
Frequent premature ventricular contractions (PVCs).
Ventricular tachycardia.
ST segment depression or elevation of more than 1 mm.
Onset of second-degree or third-degree heart block.
Onset of left or right bundle branch block.

Equipment
Monitoring equipment failure.
Unavailability of CPR equipment and defibrillator.

Miscellaneous
Request by patient, light-headedness, mental confusion, or headache.
Muscle cramping.
Nausea or vomiting.
Sweating and pallor.
Cyanosis.
Exercise electrocardiogram.
Heart disease.
Bronchospasm.
Deconditioned muscles.

Figure 18-20 Exercise equipment usually consists of a treadmill *(top)* and indirect calorimeter (also called a metabolic cart; *bottom*) for analysis of exhaled oxygen and carbon dioxide. The operator can control the treadmill's speed and angle of incline to vary the amount of work the patient performs. During the exercise test, the indirect calorimeter measures the patient's respiratory rate, tidal volume, and exhaled gas concentrations. (Courtesy of Medical Graphics, Inc., St Paul, Minnesota. In Mottram CD: Ruppel's manual of pulmonary function testing, ed 10, St Louis, 2013, Mosby.)

must stop exercising earlier than predicted. Patients with restrictive lung disease cannot increase their tidal volume as expected. Instead, they increase their respiratory rate to raise their minute volume. They too must stop exercising earlier than predicted.

b. Heart rate, stroke volume, and cardiac output

At low and moderate workloads, the stroke volume increases from about 80 to 110 mL in healthy adults. Increases in heart rate account for the rest of the increase in cardiac output from low to heavy exercise. The heart rate increases are almost parallel with the increases in $\dot{V}O_2$ values (Fig. 18-22). A patient with a diseased left ventricle or heart block would be unable to increase cardiac output sufficiently when exercising and must stop earlier than predicted.

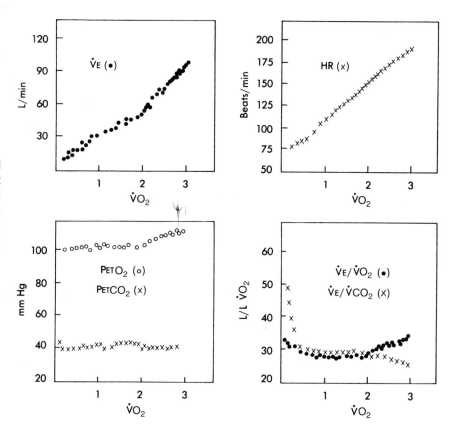

Figure 18-22 Exercise data showing 30-second averages from a normal, healthy adult subject. Heart rate increases linearly as workload is increased and is not the limiting factor in this exercise test. The other three graphic displays show that the anaerobic threshold (AT) occurs at 2 L/min of $\dot{V}O_2$. The following key points should be noted. First, minute volume ($\dot{V}_E$) increases sharply at AT. Second, end-tidal carbon dioxide ($P_{ET}CO_2$) and the ventilatory equivalent for carbon dioxide ($\dot{V}_E/\dot{V}CO_2$) both decrease at the AT, which shows hyperventilation in response to the disproportionate increase in CO_2 production secondary to lactic acid formation. Third, end-tidal oxygen ($P_{ET}O_2$) and the ventilatory equivalent for oxygen ($\dot{V}_E/\dot{V}O_2$) both increase at the AT secondary to hyperventilation. (From Mottram CD: Ruppel's manual of pulmonary function testing, ed 10, St Louis, 2013, Mosby.)

c. Oxygen consumption, carbon dioxide production, and respiratory quotient

Both oxygen consumption and carbon dioxide production will increase linearly with low and moderate exercise. The respiratory quotient will remain at approximately 0.80 or increase slightly. As the subject exercises at levels closer and closer to the $\dot{V}O_{2max}$, the muscles are progressively starved for oxygen. This results in local anaerobic metabolism with lactic acid production. Lactic acid in turn converts to carbon dioxide. Because of this added CO_2, the respiratory center is stimulated to increase ventilation even more than expected. Eventually this fails to keep up with the increased production and the CO_2 level increases. The anaerobic threshold is identified when oxygen consumption equals carbon dioxide production and the respiratory quotient reaches 1.0.

d. Blood gases and pH

PaO_2, $PaCO_2$, and pH will remain stable in the normal ranges during low and moderate exercise. The cardiopulmonary system is able to deliver adequate oxygen to the tissues and remove sufficient carbon dioxide to keep the body functioning properly. However, at high levels of work, a lactic acid buildup occurs and a progressive metabolic acidosis is seen. This forces the patient to decrease the exercise level. Some may need to stop. Patients with cardiopulmonary disease will not be able to exercise heavily because they can provide only very limited increases of oxygen to the muscles or eliminate the extra carbon dioxide produced during even moderate exercise. Figure 18-22

shows the parameter changes seen as a healthy individual exercises from a low to a maximal level.

2. Limitations caused by abnormal physiology

Patients who are forced to stop exercising at a lower than predicted workload will probably fall into one of the following three broad categories. Box 18-10 lists conditions that would require that the stress test be stopped. Table 18-3 lists parameters that will help in differentiating between deconditioned muscles, pulmonary limitations, or cardiac limitations as the reason that exercise had to be stopped.

a. Deconditioned muscles

Normal, healthy people are quite commonly seen in this category. They are deconditioned from lack of exercise. These people are able to do quite well in a training program if there are no underlying cardiopulmonary limitations.

b. Pulmonary limitations

As discussed earlier, patients with obstructive airways disease or restrictive lung disease have limited ventilatory reserve. This limits their exercise tolerance even if they have a normal cardiovascular system. If the limitation is due to bronchospasm, this may be treated by inhaling a bronchodilator before exercising. These patients may also be able to increase their exercise tolerance if given supplemental oxygen to prevent desaturation.

c. Cardiovascular limitations

Patients with a damaged or diseased left ventricle, heart block, exercise-induced angina because of coronary artery disease, hypertension, and so forth are unable to exercise to expected levels. Medical or surgical intervention may enable them to increase their work level.

2. Oxygen titration

a. Perform oxygen titration with exercise (code: IC9) [difficulty: R, Ap]

Oxygen titration with exercise involves determining the amount of supplemental oxygen needed by a patient with cardiopulmonary disease to keep the SpO_2 value at no less than 93% during an exercise period. Many of the principal considerations for this procedure are the same as those discussed for the 6-minute walk exercise in Chapter 17 and earlier in this module. See Box 18-7 for the patient indications for this procedure. Patient evaluation before testing is presented in Box 18-8, and contraindications for testing are listed in Box 18-9.

The patient's history will indicate whether he or she is hypoxemic at rest or becomes so during exercise. Therefore, the patient's oxygen level must be monitored, along with the vital signs and electrocardiogram, during the oxygen titration with exercise procedure. Minimally, continuous pulse oximetry must be done. However, it is preferred to have arterial blood gas samples taken at rest and during peak exercise. Although single samples can be taken, it is preferable to place an arterial catheter into the radial artery. The respiratory therapist's duties will probably include monitoring the patient, changing the oxygen flow (probably by nasal cannula), and adjusting the exercise equipment.

The physician will determine the patient's exercise workload at a given oxygen flow or percentage. It is preferable to measure the workload and heart rate (as a percentage of predicted) at each supplemental oxygen level. At each workload level, make note of the patient's inspired oxygen flow or percentage, vital signs, and pulse oximeter reading. Ideally, obtain an arterial blood gas sample at the peak workload level. The overall goal of the procedure is to keep the patient's $SpO_2 \geq 93\%$ at an increased exercise level.

b. Evaluate the results of oxygen titration with exercise (code: ID8) [difficulty: R, Ap, An]

When the physician or patient decides to stop the procedure, there must be a record of the workload level, inspired oxygen flow or percentage, vital signs, and pulse oximeter reading. An arterial blood gas sample should be taken to send to the laboratory for analysis. Note the reason that the test was stopped. See Box 18-10 for indications for stopping an exercise test.

Based on the physician's interpretation of the data, a plan will be developed so that the patient can safely exercise with a prescribed amount of supplemental oxygen. The patient will need to be instructed about the meaning of the test results, the exercise plan, and how to assess his or her response during exercise. This may be done as part of a pulmonary rehabilitation program.

MODULE D

Sleep-disordered breathing

1. Recommend sleep studies (code: IE13) [difficulty: R, Ap]

Apnea is the cessation of breathing for 10 seconds or longer. Sleep apnea is diagnosed when a patient experiences at least 30 apneic periods during 6 hours of sleep. In addition, the patient will probably have episodes of hypopnea. These harmful, and potentially fatal, problems that lead to repeated episodes of hypoxemia must be diagnosed and treated.

A sleep apnea study (cardiopulmonary sleep study or polysomnography) is performed to determine whether the patient has sleep-disordered breathing. Furthermore, it can help to determine the type of disorder and monitor the patient's response to treatment. Box 18-11 lists the indications for a polysomnography sleep study.

2. Evaluate data in the patient record on sleep study results (code: IA12) [difficulty: R, Ap]

The following procedures are usually performed before the sleep study:
1. History of the problem from the viewpoint of both the patient and the patient's bed partner
2. Physical examination, including neck, upper airway, blood pressure, heart rate, and respiratory rate and pattern
3. Arterial blood gas (ABG) results or pulse oximetry results
4. Hemoglobin level
5. Thyroid function

BOX 18-11   Indications for a Cardiopulmonary Sleep Study

Patient with COPD whose awake PaO_2 is <55 torr but who has pulmonary hypertension, right heart failure (cor pulmonale), or polycythemia.

Patient whose awake PaO_2 is <55 torr without continuous supplemental oxygen and who must have the proper oxygen flow rate set for sleeping at night; overnight sleep ear oximetry should be performed.

Patient with restrictive ventilatory impairment secondary to chest wall or neuromuscular disturbances who also has chronic hypoventilation, polycythemia, pulmonary hypertension, disturbed sleep, morning headaches, or daytime somnolence and fatigue.

Patient with awake $PaCO_2$ <45 torr who also has polycythemia, pulmonary hypertension, disturbed sleep, morning headaches, or daytime somnolence and fatigue.

Patient with snoring, obesity, and other symptoms indicating disturbed sleep pattern.

Patient with excessive daytime sleepiness or sleep-maintenance insomnia.

Patient with nocturnal cyclic bradytachyarrhythmias, atrioventricular conduction abnormalities while asleep, or increased abnormal ventricular beats compared with those when awake.

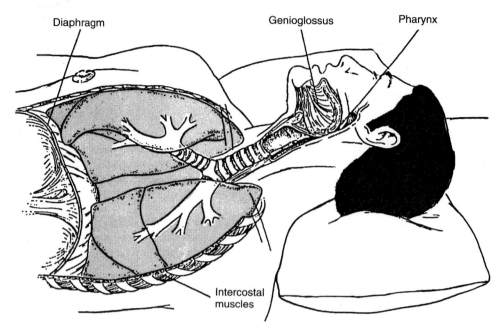

Figure 18-23 Obstructive sleep apnea. These patients often obstruct when lying supine and the genioglossus muscle of the tongue fails to oppose the negative force on the airway during an inspiration. (From Des Jardins TL, Burton GG: Clinical manifestations of respiratory disease, ed 2, St Louis, 1990, Mosby.)

6. Chest and upper airway radiograph examinations; may include a computed axial tomographic scan of the upper airway if obstructive sleep apnea is suspected
7. ECG

The following physiologic parameters are usually measured during a polysomnography sleep study:

- Pulse oximetry for O_2 saturation. An ear or bridge-of-nose oximetry probe is recommended. Finger oximetry is not recommended because the unit may fall off during patient movement.
- Sleep stages through an EEG of brain wave activity and an electro-oculographic recording of eye movements.
- Inspiratory and expiratory airflow by nasal thermistor, pneumotachograph, or end-tidal CO_2 analyzer.
- Inspiratory and expiratory effort by respiratory inductive plethysmography. (Some may prefer to have the patient swallow a transducer to measure esophageal pressure changes.) This is to look for paradoxical thoracoabdominal movements during obstructive apnea episodes.
- Body position related to normal and abnormal breathing patterns.
- Periodic arm and leg movements.
- ECG for monitoring heart rate and arrhythmias.

During polysomnography, the EEG tracing should confirm that the apneic periods occur during both of the major sleep stages. The first stage is called *non-rapid eye movement* (non-REM) sleep and starts soon after the person loses consciousness. The second stage is called *rapid eye movement* (REM) sleep and follows the non-REM stage. Normally people cycle through both stages about every 1-1.5 hours during the night. This normal cycle of sleep is important for both mental and physical health. People with disturbed sleep do not dream as they should and are not physically rested when they awaken. Whether the patient was evaluated by overnight pulse oximetry (OPO)

or polysomnography, the results lead to one of the following classifications for sleep apnea.

a. Obstructive sleep apnea

Obstructive sleep apnea (OSA) results when the patient's upper airway is obstructed despite continued breathing efforts (Figs. 18-23 and 18-24). Patients with this problem often exhibit the following symptoms: loud snoring (reported by the bed partner), morning headache, excessive daytime sleepiness, depression or other personality changes, decreased intellectual ability, sexual dysfunction, bed-wetting (nocturnal enuresis), or abnormal limb movements during sleep.

Obstructive sleep apnea is associated with the following: middle-aged men, obesity, short neck, hypothyroidism, testosterone administration, myotonic dystrophy, temporomandibular joint disease, narrowed upper airway from excessive pharyngeal tissue, enlarged tongue (macroglossia), enlarged tonsils or adenoids, deviated nasal septum, recessed jaw (micrognathia), goiter, laryngeal stenosis or web, or pharyngeal neoplasm. Management of patients with obstructive sleep apnea may include any of the following:

- Losing weight
- Sleeping on either side or the abdomen; do not sleep in the supine position
- Wearing a continuous positive airway pressure (CPAP), noninvasive positive pressure ventilation (NPPV), or bilevel ventilation mask
- Performing surgery to open the airway: mandibular advancement, palatopharyngoplasty, or tracheostomy
- Taking protriptyline (Triptil, Vivactil) to decrease REM sleep (when most obstructive episodes occur)
- Having the patient wear a tongue-retaining device to prevent it from obstructing the pharynx

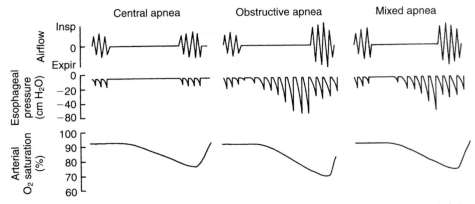

Figure 18-24 Typical patterns of airflow, esophageal pressure (or respiratory inductive plethysmography) showing respiratory effort, and arterial oxygen saturation produced by central, obstructive, and mixed sleep apnea. Central apnea shows a lack of respiratory effort resulting in no airflow. Obstructive apnea shows a continued respiratory effort but no airflow because of the airway obstruction. Mixed apnea begins with an initial lack of respiratory effort (central apnea). Later, breathing efforts are made but there is no airflow because of the airway obstruction (obstructive apnea). Arterial desaturation results from all three types of apnea. When the desaturation becomes great enough and the carbon dioxide level high enough, the patient (normally) awakens enough to breathe again. (From Des Jardins TL, Burton GG: Clinical manifestations and assessment of respiratory disease, ed 5, St Louis, 2006, Mosby.)

- Having the patient wear a neck collar to keep the head and neck aligned with the body

b. Central sleep apnea

Central sleep apnea is diagnosed when the respiratory center of the medulla fails to signal the respiratory muscles for breathing to occur. The patient makes no respiratory effort, and no air movement occurs (see Fig. 18-24). Patients with this problem often exhibit normal weight, mild snoring, insomnia, and lesser levels of daytime sleepiness, depression, or sexual dysfunction than found in the obstructive sleep apnea patient.

Central sleep apnea is associated with primary alveolar (idiopathic) hypoventilation (Ondine's curse), muscular dystrophy, bilateral cervical cordotomy, bulbar poliomyelitis, encephalitis, brain-stem infarction or neoplasm, spinal surgery, or hypothyroidism. Management of patients with central sleep apnea may include the following:

- Variable positive airway pressure (VPAP) technology, which monitors the patient's breathing and increases or decreases tidal volume and rate support as needed
- Negative pressure ventilation (see Fig. 15-24 in Chapter 15)
- Intubation or tracheostomy and positive pressure ventilation if the patient has acute ventilatory failure
- Phrenic nerve pacemaker

c. Mixed sleep apnea

Mixed sleep apnea is diagnosed when the patient shows evidence of both central and obstructive apnea. The patient usually first stops all breathing efforts (central apnea). After some time, the patient makes attempts to breathe but cannot because the upper airway is blocked (obstructive apnea) (see Fig. 18-24). Patients with mixed sleep apnea may show a variety of symptoms and traits from those listed earlier. Clinical management may include any of the treatments mentioned that prove to be effective. This includes the patient using a CPAP or NPPV system to correct the obstructive sleep apnea.

Whatever the cause of the sleep apnea, it must be treated. If the apnea is left to continue its pathologic course, a number of problems may develop, such as pulmonary hypertension, cor pulmonale, polycythemia, cardiac arrhythmias, and even unexplained nocturnal death. At the very least, the patient's personal, family, and social life will suffer.

3. Perform CPAP/noninvasive positive pressure ventilation (NPPV) titration during sleep (code: IC19) [difficulty: R, Ap]

See below.

4. Initiate and adjust mask or nasal CPAP (code: IIIC3) [difficulty: R, Ap, An]

CPAP and NPPV have become essential components of the treatment plan for obstructive sleep apnea. The positive upper airway pressure generated by CPAP or NPPV will act as a "splint" to keep the soft tissues of the upper airway from blocking the oropharynx (see Fig. 18-23). Part of the CPAP or NPPV titration process involves finding a mask or other appliance that fits the patient properly. The appliance should fit the patient's face tight enough to prevent air leaks but without causing skin irritation. See Figures 15-22 and 15-23 and the related discussion in Chapter 15 on CPAP and NPPV masks.

The goal of CPAP titration is to find the proper pressure to eliminate obstructive sleep apnea episodes.

Remember that CPAP supports only the soft tissues of the oropharynx. It does not support tidal volume breathing. Before starting the CPAP titration process, the patient must be assessed, have the CPAP system put on, and fall asleep. When the respiratory therapist recognizes an apnea episode, the CPAP system is activated. The CPAP pressure is gradually increased from zero until the apnea episodes are eliminated over the sleep period. Most adults will need between 7 and 12 cm H_2O pressure of CPAP to eliminate obstructive apnea. The newest generation of CPAP devices is autotitrating and will adjust the CPAP level as needed to maintain an open upper airway. The patient is assessed throughout the polysomnography sleep study.

NPPV is also called bilevel positive airway pressure because it involves using a lower pressure and a higher pressure to support the patient's breathing. The goal of NPPV is to find the proper pressure to eliminate obstructive sleep apnea episodes and to support tidal volume breathing. As stated previously, the patient is assessed, has the NPPV system put on, and falls asleep. During NPPV titration, the lower pressure (known as expiratory positive-pressure airway pressure [EPAP]) acts like CPAP to open the soft tissues of the airway. The higher pressure (known as inspiratory positive-pressure airway pressure [IPAP]) is set to help deliver a tidal volume. When the respiratory therapist recognizes an apnea episode, the NPPV system is activated. Both EPAP and IPAP are gradually increased from zero until the apnea episodes are eliminated over the sleep period. Most adults will need between 7.5 and 12.5 cm H_2O pressure of EPAP to eliminate obstructive apnea. The IPAP is then gradually increased until arousals, hypopnea, and snoring are eliminated. The patient is assessed throughout the polysomnography sleep study.

5. Evaluate the results of CPAP/NPPV titration during sleep (code: ID18) [difficulty: R, Ap, An]

When the proper level of CPAP or NPPV is determined, the following benefits should be found:

- There should be no apneic episodes.
- There should be fewer hypopneic episodes.
- There should be no paradoxical thoracoabdominal movements.
- There should be no snoring.
- The patient's sleeping pattern should return to normal.

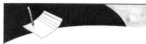

Exam Hint 18-5

There is often a question about the use of CPAP to treat obstructive sleep apnea.

6. Overnight pulse oximetry

a. Perform overnight pulse oximetry (code: IC18) [difficulty: R, Ap]

Because of the cost involved in a polysomnography study, overnight pulse oximetry (OPO) has been studied as a less expensive way to determine desaturation from sleep apnea. OPO can be performed in the patient's home or in the hospital setting. The respiratory therapist may be responsible for preparing the patient and setting up the equipment and supplies. Each hospital or physician may have a prescribed procedure. The general steps are listed here:

1. Inform the patient of the procedure, and have him or her sign the medical release form.
2. Attach the pulse oximeter, ECG leads, and other monitoring equipment to the patient.
3. Calibrate the equipment, and make sure it is working properly.
4. Record the patient's parameters during the course of a 6-hour or longer sleep period. The patient also may be recorded by videotape and audiotape during the sleep period.
5. Make any adjustments in the patient's respiratory care equipment as needed.
6. Dispose of any used supplies after the procedure is completed.
7. Tend to the patient's comfort.

b. Evaluate the results of overnight pulse oximetry (code: ID17) [difficulty: R, Ap, An]

Apnea is the cessation of breathing for 10 seconds or longer. Sleep apnea is diagnosed when a patient experiences at least 30 apneic periods during 6 hours of sleep. Numerous studies have shown that OPO can be used to screen patients with moderate to severe sleep apnea. These patients will have experienced at least 10 apnea episodes per hour in which their SpO_2 levels decreased at least 4% from baseline to less than 90%. In cases in which the OPO results are difficult to interpret, polysomnography is needed. If the patient is found to have obstructive sleep apnea, a CPAP or NPPV system will be needed to help correct the problem.

Exam Hint 18-6

Know how to differentiate between the clinical signs of obstructive and central sleep apnea. Usually a question is asked about identifying whether a patient has obstructive sleep apnea. The key is to recognize that the patient will not be moving any air despite making breathing efforts. Nasal CPAP should be used to treat the patient's condition.

MODULE E

Respiratory care plan

1. Determine a patient's pathophysiologic state (code: IIIF1) [difficulty: R, Ap, An]

See the previous topics for discussion of the patient's disease state.

2. Recommend starting a treatment based on the patient's response (code: IIIE2a) [difficulty: R, Ap, An]

See the previous topics for their indications.

3. Recommend a change in the therapeutic plan if indicated (code: IIIF2) [difficulty: R, Ap, An]

See the previous topics for discussion on changing therapy as needed.

4. Recommend a treatment or procedure be terminated (code: IIIE1) [difficulty: R, Ap, An]

Patient safety should always be an important consideration during the treatment or procedure. Specific concerns were discussed with each of the topics in this chapter. Be prepared to stop the treatment or procedure if the patient has an adverse reaction to it. In addition, be prepared to recommend to the physician that the treatment or procedure be discontinued if it is likely to result in additional adverse reactions.

5. Recommend discontinuing a treatment based on the patient's response (code: IIIE2h) [difficulty: R, Ap, An]

There are typically three reasons for a patient's treatment to be discontinued. First, the patient has recovered and no longer needs the treatment or procedure. It is expensive and wasteful to perform unnecessary treatments. Second, the patient has had an adverse reaction and is likely to have an adverse reaction every time the treatment or procedure is repeated. Third, the patient's condition is terminal, and the patient or responsible family member wants all treatment to be stopped.

BIBLIOGRAPHY

American Heart Association guidelines for CPR & ECC, Part 6. Electrical therapies, *Circulation* 122:S639, 2010.

AARC clinical practice guideline: management of airway emergencies, *Respir Care* 40:749, 1995 (Retired).

AARC clinical practice guideline: polysomnography, *Respir Care* 40:1236, 1995.

AARC clinical practice guideline: exercise testing for evaluation of hypoxemia and/or desaturation: 2001 revision & update, *Respir Care* 46:514, 2001 (Retired).

AARC clinical practice guideline: in-hospital transport of the mechanically ventilated patient: 2002 revision and update, *Respir Care* 47(6):721, 2002.

AARC clinical practice guideline: bronchoscopy assisting—2007 revision & update, *Respir Care* 52:74, 2007.

Altobelli N: Airway management. In Kacmarek RM, Stoller JK, Heuer AJ, editors: *Egan's fundamentals of respiratory care*, ed 10, St Louis, 2013, Mosby.

Anderson HL, Bartlett RH: Respiratory care of the surgical patient. In Burton GG, Hodgkin JE, Ward JJ, editors: *Respiratory care: a guide to clinical practice*, ed 3, Philadelphia, 1991, JB Lippincott.

Antonescu-Turco A, Parthasarathy S: CPAP and bi-level PAP therapy: new and established roles, *Respir Care* 55(9):1216–1229, 2010.

Arand DL, Bonnet: Sleep-disordered breathing. In Burton GC, Hodgkin JE, Ward JJ, editors: *Respiratory care: a guide to clinical practice*, ed 4, Philadelphia, 1997, Lippincott-Raven.

ATS/ACCP statement on cardiopulmonary exercise testing, *Am J Crit Care Med* 167(2):211–277, 2003.

Barnes TA, editor: *Core textbook of respiratory care practice*, ed 2, St Louis, 1994, Mosby.

Barnes TA: Emergency cardiovascular life support. In Kacmarek RM, Stoller JK, Heuer AJ, editors: *Egan's fundamentals of respiratory care*, ed 10, St Louis, 2013, Mosby.

Branson RD, Gomaa D, Rodriquez D: Management of the artificial airway, *Respir Care* 59(6):974–990, 2014.

Branson RD, Hess DR, Chatburn RL, editors: *Respiratory care equipment*, ed 2, Philadelphia, 1999, Lippincott Williams & Wilkins.

Brown-Saltzman K, Upadhya D, Larner L, Wenger NS: An intervention to improve respiratory therapists' comfort with end-of-life care, *Respir Care* 55(7):858–865, 2010.

Brutinel WM, Cortese DA: Fiberoptic bronchoscopy. In Burton GC, Hodgkin JE, Ward JJ, editors: *Respiratory care: a guide to clinical practice*, ed 4, Philadelphia, 1997, Lippincott-Raven.

Byhahn C, Wilke JH, Halbig S, Lischke V, Westphal K: Percutaneous tracheostomy: ciaglia blue rhino versus basic ciaglia technique of percutaneous dilational tracheostomy, *Anesth Analg* 91(4):882–886, 2000.

Cairo JM: Sleep diagnostics. In Cairo JM, Pilbeam SP, editors: *Mosby's respiratory care equipment*, ed 8, St Louis, 2009, Mosby.

Chadha TS, Schneider AW, Tobin MJ, et al.: Noninvasive monitoring of breathing patterns during wakefulness and sleep, *Respir Ther* 27–40, May/June 1985.

Chaudhary BA, Taft A, Mishoe SC: Obstructive sleep apnea. In Hess DR, MacIntyre NR, Mishoe SC, Galvin WF, Adams AB, editors: *Respiratory care principles and practice*, ed 2, Burlington, MA, 2012, Jones & Bartlett Learning.

Chaudhary BA, Whiddon S, Mishoe SC: Polysomnography. In Hess DR, MacIntyre NR, Mishoe SC, Galvin WF, Adams AB, editors: *Respiratory care principles and practice*, ed 2, Burlington, MA, 2012, Jones & Bartlett Learning.

Chavis AD, Grum CM: Fiberoptic bronchoscopy with mechanical ventilation, *Choices Respir Manage* 21:4, 1991.

Chavis AD, Grum CM: Pulmonary procedures during mechanical ventilation, *Choices Respir Manage* 21:29, 1991.

Cheung NH, Napolitano LM: Tracheostomy: epidemiology, indications, timing, technique, and outcomes, *Respir Care* 59(6):895–919, 2014.

Chipman DW, English P: Neonatal and pediatric respiratory care. In Kacmarek RM, Stoller JK, Heuer AJ, editors: *Egan's fundamentals of respiratory care*, ed 10, St Louis, 2013, Mosby.

Collins SR: Direct and indirect laryngoscopy: equipment and techniques, *Respir Care* 59(6):850–864, 2014.

Collins SR, Blank RS: Fiberoptic intubation: an overview and update, *Respir Care* 59(6):865–880, 2014.

Coppolo DP, Brienza LT, Pratt DS, May JJ: A role for the respiratory therapist in flexible fiberoptic bronchoscopy, *Respir Care* 30:323, 1985.

Curity thoracentesis tray package insert, Kendall Hospital Products, Boston, MA.

Davies JD, May RA, Bortner PL: Airway management. In Hess DR, MacIntyre NR, Mishoe SC, Galvin WF, Adams AB, editors: *Respiratory care principles and practice*, ed 2, Burlington, MA, 2012, Jones & Bartlett Learning.

Decker MJ, Smith BL, Strohl KP: Center-based vs patient-based diagnosis and therapy of sleep-related respiratory disorders and role of the respiratory care practitioner, *Respir Care* 39(4):390–400, 1994.

Deshpande VM, Pilbeam SP, Dixon RJ: *A comprehensive review in respiratory care*, East Norwalk, CT, 1988, Appleton & Lange.

Des Jardins TL, Burton GG: *Clinical manifestations and assessment of respiratory disease*, ed 6, St Louis, 2011, Mosby.

Downey III R, Dexter JR: Assessment of sleep and breathing. In Wilkins RL, Krider SJ, Sheldon RL, editors: *Clinical assessment in respiratory care*, ed 3, St Louis, 1995, Mosby.

Durbin CG, Bell CT, Shilling AM: Elective intubation, *Respir Care* 59(6):825–849, 2014.

Epstein LJ, Dorlac GR: Cost-effectiveness analysis of nocturnal oximetry as a method of screening for sleep apnea-hypoventilation syndrome, *Chest* 113:97, 1998.

Erickson RS: Mastering the ins and outs of chest drainage: I, *Nursing* 19:37, 1989.

Erickson RS: Mastering the ins and outs of chest drainage: II, *Nursing* 19:47, 1989.

Eubanks DH, Bone RC: *Comprehensive respiratory care: a learning system*, ed 2, St Louis, 1990, Mosby.

Fischback F: *A manual of laboratory & diagnostic tests*, ed 6, Philadelphia, 2000, Lippincott Williams & Wilkins.

Gardenhire DS: *Rau's respiratory care pharmacology*, ed 8, St Louis, 2012, Mosby.

Garay SM: Therapeutic options for obstructive sleep apnea, *Respir Management* 17(4):11–17, 1987.

Guidelines for fiberoptic bronchoscopy, *ATS News* 12:14, 1986.

Haas CF, Eakin RM, Konkle MA, Blank R: Endotracheal tubes: old and new, *Respir Care* 59(6):933–955, 2014.

Hefflinger RG: Neuromuscular, sedative, anesthetic, and analgesic agents. In Colbert BJ, Kennedy BJ, editors: *Integrated cardiopulmonary pharmacology*, ed 2, Upper Saddle River, NJ, 2008, Pearson Prentice Hall.

Henry NR, Marshall SG: Apnea testing: the effects of insufflation catheter size and flow on pressure and volume in a test lung, *Respir Care* 59(3):406–410, 2014.

Hess DR, Altobelli NP: Tracheostomy tubes, *Respir Care* 59(6):956–973, 2014.

Heuer AJ: Respiratory care in alternative settings. In Kacmarek RM, Stoller JK, Heuer AJ, editors: *Egan's fundamentals of respiratory care*, ed 10, St Louis, 2013, Mosby.

Howard TP: Foreign body extraction by means of combined rigid and flexible bronchoscopy: a case report, *Respir Care* 33:786, 1988.

Indications and standards for cardiopulmonary sleep studies, *Am Rev Respir Dis* 139:559–568, 1989.

Jacobs IN, Pettignano MM, Pettignano R: Airway managment. In Walsh BK, Czervinske MP, DiBlasi RM, editors: *Perinatal and pediatric respiratory care*, ed 3, St Louis, 2010, Saunders.

Johnson MD: Noninvasive monitoring. In Aloan CA, Hill TV, editors: *Respiratory care of the newborn and child*, ed 2, Philadelphia, 1997, Lippincott-Raven.

Kacmarek RM: Discontinuing ventilatory support. In Kacmarek RM, Stoller JK, Heuer AJ, editors: *Egan's fundamentals of respiratory care*, ed 10, St Louis, 2013, Mosby.

Kalavantavanich K, Schramm CM: Pediatric flexible bronchoscopy. In Walsh BK, Czervinske MP, DiBlasi RM, editors: *Perinatal and pediatric respiratory care*, ed 3, St Louis, 2010, Saunders.

Kendall Hospital Products, Curity thoracentesis tray (package insert), Boston, MA.

Khoury JB, Radtke RA: Sleep assessment. In Hess DR, MacIntyre NR, Mishoe SC, et al.: *Respiratory care principles and practices*, Philadelphia, 2002, Saunders.

Lee EJ, Strollo PJ: Disorders of sleep. In Kacmarek RM, Stoller JK, Heuer AJ, editors: *Egan's fundamentals of respiratory care*, ed 10, St Louis, 2013, Mosby.

Lewis CA, Eaton TE, Fergusson W, Whyte KF, Garrett GE, Kolbe J: Home overnight pulse oximetry in patients with COPD: more than one recording may be needed, *Chest* 123:1127, 2003.

Lewis RM: Airway care. In Fink JB, Hunt GE, editors: *Clinical practice in respiratory care*, Philadelphia, 1999, Lippincott Williams & Wilkins.

Littlewood K, Durbin CG: Evidence-based airway management, *Respir Care* 46(12):1392–1403, 2001.

Lough MD: Newborn respiratory care procedures. In Lough MD, Williams TJ, Rawson JE, editors: *Newborn respiratory care*, St Louis, 1979, Mosby.

Ludwig B: Atelectasis: pleural disorders and lung cancer. In Wyka KA, Mathews PJ, Rutkowski J, editors: *Foundations of respiratory care*, ed 2, Clifton Park, NY, 2012, Delmar.

MacIntyre NR: Cardiopulmonary exercise assessment. In Hess DR, MacIntyre NR, Mishoe SC, Galvin WF, Adams AB, editors: *Respiratory care principles and practice*, ed 2, Burlington, MA, 2012, Jones & Bartlett Learning.

Madama VC: *Pulmonary function testing and cardiopulmonary stress testing*, ed 2, Albany, 1998, Delmar.

Malitino EM: Strategic national stockpile: overview and ventilator assets, *Respir Care* 53:91, 2008.

Masini DE: Ethics of healthcare delivery. In Hess DR, MacIntyre NR, Mishoe SC, Galvin WF, Adams AB, editors: *Respiratory care principles and practice*, ed 2, Burlington, MA, 2012, Jones & Bartlett Learning.

Mathewson HS: Drug therapy for obstructive sleep apnea, *Respir Care* 31(8):717–719, 1986.

McIntyre D: Airway management. In Wyka KA, Mathews PJ, Rutkowski J, editors: *Foundations of respiratory care*, ed 2, Clifton Park, NY, 2012, Delmar.

Mims BC: You can manage chest tubes confidently, *RN* 48:39, 1985.

Mishoe SC: The diagnosis and treatment of sleep apnea syndrome, *Respir Care* 32(3):183–201, 1987.

Mottram CD: Cardiopulmonary exercise testing. In Mottram CD, editor: *Ruppel's manual of pulmonary function testing*, ed 10, St Louis, 2013, Mosby.

Muskat PC: Mass casualty chemical exposure and implications for respiratory failure, *Respir Care* 53:58, 2008.

Netzer N, Eliasson AH, Netzer C, Kristo DA: Overnight pulse oximetry for sleep-disordered breathing in adults, *Chest* 120:625–633, 2001.

Pacheco-Lopez PC, Berkow LC, Hillel AT, Akst LM: Complications of airway management, *Respir Care* 59(6):1006–1021, 2014.

Peters RM: Chest trauma. In Moser KM, Spragg RG, editors: *Respiratory emergencies*, ed 2, St Louis, 1982, Mosby.

Phillipson EA: Breathing disorders during sleep, *Basics Respir Dis* 7(3):1–6, 1979.

Plevak DJ, Ward JJ: Airway management. In Burton GC, Hodgkin JE, Ward JJ, editors: *Respiratory care: a guide to clinical practice*, ed 4, Philadelphia, 1997, Lippincott-Raven.

Podnos SD, Chappell TR: Hemoptysis: a clinical update, *Respir Care* 30(11):977-985, 1985.

Rapaport DM: Techniques for administering nasal CPAP, *Respir Management* 17(4):17-21, 1987.

Robinson BRH, Branson RD: Trauma. In Hess DR, MacIntyre NR, Mishoe SC, Galvin WF, Adams AB, editors: *Respiratory care principles and practice*, ed 2, Burlington, MA, 2012, Jones & Bartlett Learning.

Sachs S: Fiberoptic bronchoscopy. In Hess DR, MacIntyre NR, Mishoe SC, et al.: *Respiratory care principles and practices*, Philadelphia, 2002, Saunders.

Scott JB, Gentile MA, Bennett SN, Couture M, MacIntyre NR: Apnea testing during brain death assessment: a review of clinical practice and published literature, *Respir Care* 58(3):532-538, 2013.

Shapiro BA, Kacmarek RM, Cane RD, et al.: *Clinical application of respiratory care*, ed 4, St Louis, 1991, Mosby.

Shilling AM, Durbin CG: Airway management devices and advanced cardiac life support. In Cairo JM, editor: *Mosby's respiratory care equipment*, ed 9, St Louis, 2014, Mosby.

Sitler G: Transport of infants and children. In Walsh BK, Czervinske MP, DiBlasi RM, editors: *Perinatal and pediatric respiratory care*, ed 3, St Louis, 2010, Saunders.

Smalling T, Valente J: Examining laser surgery, *J Respir Care Pract* 11:93, 1998.

Stillwell PC: Disorders of the pleura. In Walsh BK, Czervinske MP, DiBlasi RM, editors: *Perinatal and pediatric respiratory care*, ed 3, St Louis, 2010, Saunders.

Strange C: Pleural diseases. In Kacmarek RM, Stoller JK, Heuer AJ, editors: *Egan's fundamentals of respiratory care*, ed 10, St Louis, 2013, Mosby.

Treece AE, Wahidi MM, Shofer L: Interventional pulmonary procedures. In Hess DR, MacIntyre NR, Mishoe SC, Galvin WF, Adams AB, editors: *Respiratory care principles and practice*, ed 2, Burlington, MA, 2012, Jones & Bartlett Learning.

Truog RD, Campbell ML, Curtis JR, Haas CE, Luce JM, Rubenfeld GD, et al.: Recommendations for end-of-life care in the Intensive Care Unit: a consensus statement by the American college of critical care medicine, *Crit Care Med* 36(11):953-963, 2008.

Whitaker K: *Comprehensive perinatal and pediatric respiratory care*, ed 2, Albany, NY, 1997, Delmar.

Whitman RA: Polysomnography and other tests of sleep disorders. In Wyka KA, Mathews PJ, Rutkowski J, editors: *Foundations of respiratory care*, ed 2, Clifton Park, NY, 2012, Delmar.

Whitman RA, Holland SA: Pulmonary function testing. In Wyka KA, Mathews PJ, Rutkowski J, editors: *Foundations of respiratory care*, ed 2, Clifton Park, NY, 2012, Delmar.

Williams SF, Thompson JM: *Respiratory disorders*, St Louis, 1990, Mosby.

Wyka KA: Cardiopulmonary rehabilitation. In Kacmarek RM, Stoller JK, Heuer AJ, editors: *Egan's fundamentals of respiratory care*, ed 10, St Louis, 2013, Mosby.

Yacovone ML, Kartan R, Bautista M: Intercostal artery laceration following thoracentesis, *Respir Care* 55:1495, 2010.

Yu P: Sudden infant death syndrome and pediatric sleep disorders. In Walsh BK, Czervinske MP, DiBlasi RM, editors: *Perinatal and pediatric respiratory care*, ed 3, St Louis, 2010, Saunders.

SELF-STUDY QUESTIONS

See Appendix for answers.

1. Which of the following should the respiratory therapist evaluate to determine whether a patient's chest tube is functioning properly and removing pleural air?
   A. Fluid is present in the collection chamber.
   B. The vacuum level is set at −15 cm H_2O.
   C. Air is bubbling in the water-seal chamber.
   D. Air is bubbling in the suction control chamber.

2. A patient is being mechanically ventilated when the nurse calls the respiratory therapist to evaluate the patient's condition. It is discovered that the patient's breath sounds are absent over the left lung field, the left-sided percussion note is hyperresonant, and peak airway pressures have increased from 40 to 65 cm H_2O. What would be recommended?
   A. Place a pleural chest tube into the right side.
   B. Increase the V_T to better inflate the atelectatic left lung.
   C. Change the mode to Synchronous Intermittent Mechanical Ventilation from Assist/Control.
   D. Place a pleural chest tube into the left side.

3. A respiratory therapist notices that air is bubbling through the water seal of the patient's pleural drainage system when she coughs. What does this indicate?
   A. The vacuum has to be increased.
   B. Air is still leaking through a tear in the lung.
   C. The proper level of vacuum has been set.
   D. There is a leak in the system.

4. After a sleep study has been performed, a patient is given a diagnosis of obstructive sleep apnea. The patient's physician asks the respiratory therapist for advice. What should be recommended?
   A. The patient should use nasal CPAP when sleeping.
   B. The patient should sleep with an oropharyngeal airway.
   C. The patient should always sleep on the back.
   D. A tracheostomy should be performed.

5. An adult patient with obstructive sleep apnea and frequent pulse oximetry desaturations is fitted with a nasal CPAP system. A pressure of 7 cm H_2O is set. After the CPAP system is set up, the patient's SpO_2 value stays above 90%. How should the results be interpreted?
   A. The CPAP system has corrected the patient's problem.
   B. Greater CPAP pressure is needed.
   C. Improved gas flow is needed through the CPAP system.
   D. The delivered oxygen percentage should be increased.

6. A mechanically ventilated patient is going to have a flexible fiberoptic bronchoscopy performed. How might this affect the ventilator's function?
   1. The V_T must be monitored for a leak.
   2. The inspiratory flow resistance will increase.
   3. The inspiratory pressure will decrease.
   4. The inspiratory pressure will increase.
   A. 1 and 2 only
   B. 3 only
   C. 2 and 3 only
   D. 1, 2, and 4 only

7. During the transport of your patient with a pneumothorax, the chest tube drainage system is pulled off of the drainage tubing and cracked open. The best response is to:
   A. Clamp the tube near the patient's chest at once.
   B. Hold the distal end of the tubing a few centimeters below the surface of a bottle of sterile water or saline.
   C. Leave the tube open to the atmosphere.
   D. Have the patient perform the Valsalva maneuver until a new system can be set up.

8. When preparing to assist the physician with the cardioversion of a patient, which of the following must be checked?
   1. **A strong R wave should be seen on the ECG monitor.**
   2. **The charge level should be set as ordered.**
   3. **The electric paddles should be kept clean for the best possible conduction.**
   4. **Ensure that the ECG electrodes are attached properly.**
   A. 1 and 3 only
   B. 1, 2, and 4 only
   C. 3 and 4 only
   D. 1, 2, 3, 4

9. A 6-year-old patient has aspirated a tooth that was dislodged during a sporting event. The chest radiograph film shows the tooth to be lodged in the right mainstem bronchus; the neck radiograph film is normal. What should be recommended as the best way to quickly remove the tooth?
   A. Flexible fiberoptic bronchoscopy (FFB)
   B. Positive expiratory pressure breathing (PEP)
   C. Rigid-tube bronchoscopy
   D. Postural drainage therapy (PDT)

10. A patient is referred for a sleep study. The attending physician wants to know which parameters are measured during the study. All of the following should be measured EXCEPT:
    A. SpO_2
    B. ECG
    C. Inspiratory and expiratory breathing efforts
    D. ABG values

11. A patient is performing an exercise test and has the following signs and symptoms: systolic blood pressure of 260 mm Hg, cyanosis, headache, and dizziness. Which of the following should be recommended?
    A. Continue until the respiratory exchange ratio reaches 1.1.
    B. Stop the test at this time.
    C. Continue until the patient complains of shortness of breath.
    D. Continue the test at a lower work level.

12. A patient is performing a stress test. Which of the following respiratory exchange ratio values would confirm that the patient has reached the anaerobic threshold?
    A. 0.8
    B. 0.9
    C. 1.0
    D. 1.1

13. A respiratory therapist is assisting a physician with a surgical tracheostomy procedure on a patient with an oral endotracheal tube. When should the endotracheal tube be withdrawn?
    A. After the tracheostomy tube has been inserted
    B. After the cuff of the tracheostomy tube has been inflated
    C. As the tip of the tracheostomy tube is placed into the stoma
    D. Before the stoma is made

14. A respiratory therapist is assisting a physician in a percutaneous dilation tracheostomy (PDT) procedure. What are the most common complications to watch for?
    1. **Bleeding at the insertion site**
    2. **Tracheal ring fracture**
    3. **Pneumothorax**
    4. **Tracheoesophageal fistula**
    A. 2 only
    B. 1 and 3 only
    C. 2, 3, and 4 only
    D. 1, 2, and 3 only

15. All the following should be done when preparing to helicopter transport an adult patient requiring mechanical ventilation EXCEPT:
    A. Select a heated cascade-type humidification system.
    B. Calculate the duration of the oxygen cylinder that will be used.
    C. Select a ventilator that uses a demand-valve IMV system rather than one with an external-reservoir IMV system.
    D. Select a lightweight and portable ventilator.

16. A 60-year-old patient with a smoking history and recurrent bouts of left lung pneumonia has a persistent chest radiograph shadow in the left lower lobe area. Despite 2 days of postural drainage with percussion and incentive spirometry, the haziness has not cleared. What should be recommended next?
    A. Nebulize a bronchodilator medication.
    B. Perform rigid-tube bronchoscopy.

C. Perform flexible fiberoptic bronchoscopy.

D. Nebulize hypertonic saline to induce a cough.

17. Which of the following conditions is first treated by placing a large-bore needle at the midclavicular line through the second or third intercostal space?

A. 5% pneumothorax

B. Pleural effusion

C. Hemothorax

D. Tension pneumothorax

18. A patient was found to have a $\dot{V}O_2$ value of 2000 mL and a $\dot{V}CO_2$ value of 1700 mL during an exercise test. Calculate the patient's respiratory exchange ratio.

A. 0.85

B. 1.18

C. 2000

D. 3700

19. An intubated patient receiving mechanical ventilation will be transported from Chicago to Denver by an airplane with an unpressurized cabin. A pressure-cycled transport ventilator will be used. What should be monitored during the flight?

1. **Increased cuff volume**

2. **Decreased tidal volume**

3. **Hypoxemia**

4. **Increased tidal volume**

5. **Fluid retention**

A. 2 and 3 only

B. 1 and 4 only

C. 1, 3, and 4 only

D. 2, 3, and 5 only

20. A mechanically ventilated patient is having a central venous line inserted by the subclavian vein route. The patient coughs vigorously. Within 1 minute the peak pressure on the ventilator increases significantly, and the SpO_2 value is progressively decreasing. Chest percussion demonstrates a hyperresonant sound over the right side of the chest, and breath sounds are diminished on the right side. What is the most important thing to do at this time?

A. Complete the insertion of the central venous pressure (CVP) line.

B. Insert a pleural chest tube on the right side.

C. Get a chest radiograph.

D. Compare the peak and plateau pressures on the ventilator.

21. A conscious adult patient with atrial fibrillation is being prepared for synchronous cardioversion with a biphasic defibrillator. Which of the following should be recommended?

1. **Administer midazolam (Versed) before starting.**

2. **Administer flumazenil (Romazicon) before starting.**

3. **Charge the defibrillator to 120 J.**

4. **Charge the defibrillator to 360 J.**

5. **Set the ECG machine to lead II.**

6. **Have a manual resuscitation bag on standby.**

A. 2 and 3 only

B. 1, 2, and 4 only

C. 1, 3, and 5 only

D. 1, 3, 5, and 6 only

22. All of the following may be done by a respiratory therapist during a surgical tracheostomy procedure EXCEPT:

A. Insert the tracheostomy tube into the new stoma.

B. Disinfect the surgical site.

C. Check for proper functioning of the tracheostomy tube.

D. Withdraw the endotracheal tube when ordered.

23. A respiratory therapist is assisting an anesthesiologist in the direct-vision nasotracheal intubation of a patient. All of the following equipment will be needed EXCEPT:

A. Magill forceps

B. Laryngoscope handle with blade

C. Sterile, water-soluble lubricant

D. Lubricated hard stylet

24. Calculate the maximum heart rate for a 55-year-old female who is about to undergo a stress test.

A. 55 beats/min

B. 174 beats/min

C. 265 beats/min

D. 275 beats/min

25. What would be expected of a patient's ventilation efforts during light exercise that progresses to moderate exercise?

A. It decreases as $\dot{V}O_2$ increases.

B. It decreases as carbon dioxide production increases.

C. It increases as workload levels increase.

D. It remains constant in normal subjects as workload levels increase.

26. While performing a sleep study, the respiratory therapist notices the following: the respiratory inductive plethysmography reading indicates chest and abdominal movement, the nasal thermistor shows no air movement, and the patient's pulse oximeter value drops to 85%. After 35 seconds, the patient snores loudly, rolls on the side, and resumes normal breathing. What best describes the patient's problem?

A. Central sleep apnea

B. Airway obstruction

C. Cheyne-Stokes respiration

D. Hyperventilation

27. A respiratory therapist is assisting a physician performing a thoracentesis on a mechanically ventilated patient. The patient cannot sit up on the edge of the bed because of weakness. Which position should be recommended for the procedure?

A. Lying with the abnormal side down on the bed

B. Lying face down on the bed

C. Supine on the bed with the head down 30 degrees

D. Lying with the normal side down on the bed

28. After undergoing a thoracentesis in which 1400 mL of straw-colored yellow fluid was removed, the patient complains of shortness of breath and has increased heart and respiratory rates. What should the assisting respiratory therapist recommend to further evaluate the patient's reaction to the procedure?
    1. Measure the pulse oximeter value.
    2. Obtain a chest radiograph.
    3. Send the fluid to the laboratory for analysis.
    4. Remove additional fluid.
    A. 1 only
    B. 3 only
    C. 1 and 2 only
    D. 3 and 4 only

29. A respiratory therapist is about to assist in the bronchoscopy of a patient with COPD and suspected lung cancer. The patient is quite nervous before the procedure and conscious sedation will be done. All of the following drugs could be used to help in managing her sedation EXCEPT:
    A. Diazepam (Valium)
    B. Fluticasone (Flovent)
    C. Flumazenil (Romazicon)
    D. Midazolam (Versed)

30. A 40-year-old unconscious patient is in the Intensive Care Unit for treatment of congestive heart failure. You will be assisting the physician with the insertion of an arterial catheter. Which of the following medications would be appropriate for the procedure?
    1. Naloxone (Narcan)
    2. Fentanyl (Sublimaze)
    3. Iodine (Betadine)
    4. Lidocaine (Xylocaine)
    A. 3 and 4 only
    B. 1 and 2 only
    C. 2, 3, and 4 only
    D. 1, 2, 3, 4

Answer Key for the Self-Study Questions

Chapter 1

1. **A.** Negative results for creatine kinase, troponin I, and troponin T would rule out a myocardial infarction. Negative results for brain natriuretic peptide would rule out congestive heart failure. None of these tests is a marker for pneumonia. So, by the process of elimination, the patient's dyspnea has to be caused by a worsening of his COPD.

2. **C.** Bronchial breath sounds are not normal in the right lower lobe and indicate consolidation of the alveoli. Neither pneumothorax nor pleural effusion can be identified by bronchial breath sounds.

3. **B.** The patient's signs and symptoms best fit those of a right-sided pneumothorax. Although it is possible for a patient to break a bone while lifting weights, this would not produce shortness of breath, a hyperresonant percussion note on the right side, and a tracheal shift to the left. An acute myocardial infarction could cause a sudden chest pain and shortness of breath but would not cause a hyperresonant percussion note on the right side or a tracheal shift to the left.

4. **D.** The patient's history of injury and crepitus indicates air under the skin. The air under her skin would have to come from a pneumothorax.

5. **A.** All of the patient's symptoms point to a bacterial pneumonia problem. The other options may have some but not all of the noted symptoms.

6. **C.** The patient is reacting with anger to his diagnosis of cancer. He should be evaluated for emotional state. The other problems should not cause anger.

7. **C.** The correct two questions relate to the patient's level of consciousness and understanding. The first question about the "day" relates to the patient's understanding of *time*. The third question about "where you are" relates to the patient's understanding of *place*. The fifth question about the "president" relates to the patient's understanding of *person*.

8. **C.** Orthopnea relates to the patient's inability to lie down and breathe comfortably. Extra pillows are needed to raise the head and body. The other questions relate to other areas of assessment.

9. **A.** An infant's chest is basically round in dimension.

10. **B.** Diminished breath sounds mean that less air than normal is entering an area. A tracheal shift to the side of the diminished breath sound indicates less air in the lung. Both of these point to atelectasis.

11. **B.** Left-sided pneumonia and pneumothorax both result in decreased movement on that side. Emphysema and congestive heart failure would not cause a one-sided change in movement. Right-sided pneumonia would result in less movement on the right side.

12. **C.** Inspiratory stridor is the only listed breath sound that can be heard with the unaided ear. It is a respiratory emergency.

13. **D.** Only Cheyne-Stokes respiration fits the description. Review Figures 1-24 and 1-25.

14. **B.** The high air pressure found with a tension pneumothorax causes the mediastinal contents to be shifted to the opposite side and the diaphragm on the affected side to be depressed. These drastic changes can cause the patient's vital signs to deteriorate rapidly.

15. **A.** A pleural friction rub is identified as a localized area of abnormal grating breath sound; it is often localized to an area of pain on breathing.

16. **B.** Fluid overload causes the jugular veins to be distended. Dehydration may result in the jugular veins being flat. Emphysema and hypertension should not have any effect on the jugular veins.

17. **C.** Tactile fremitus would be reduced in pneumothorax and COPD because the lung is overinflated. A pleural effusion would block and decrease the sounds coming from the lung.

18. **C.** It is appropriate to ask about advance directives, such as a DNR order, for a patient with a fatal illness. Eating and bowel habits are not essential to know at this time. He will be given new orders for medications during his stay in the hospital, so it does not matter if he brought his medications with him.

19. **A.** It is important to assess the patient's level of pain from the broken ankle. Severe pain should be managed with increased medication. The other issues are less important to assess unless there is an apparent problem.

20. **B.** All listed conditions except bilateral lower lobe pneumonia would shift the mediastinum. Because bilateral lower lobe pneumonia affects both lungs, the mediastinum would stay centered properly.

21. **A.** It is most likely that a patient with respiratory distress would show an *increased* respiratory rate.

22. **B.** Patients with emphysema usually have chest radiograph findings of increased AP diameter, depressed

hemidiaphragms, and widened intercostal spaces. These are the result of enlarged lungs caused by air trapping. If the patient had pulmonary fibrosis, the lungs would be small rather than enlarged. A person is supposed to take a large breath before a chest radiograph. The findings are not consistent with an enlarged heart seen with left-ventricular failure.

23. **C.** Severe vomiting and diarrhea can result in significant loss of fluids and electrolytes. Her cardiac problems are likely to be the result of this. If an electrolyte abnormality is found, it must be promptly corrected by intravenous replacement. A urinalysis will be helpful for the evaluation of the patient's kidneys but is not needed at this time. An arterial blood gas analysis will be helpful to determine whether the patient's acid–base balance is altered. However, it is not needed at this time, because it will not guide the patient's clinical management. A complete blood count will not reveal any information that will guide the patient's care related to her cardiac arrhythmia.

24. **B.** The patient's history plus recent illness and worsening symptoms indicate a pulmonary infection. It is important to get a sputum sample for a culture-and-sensitivity study to determine the infectious organism and the antibiotic to fight it. Although the patient's illness may make him hypoxic, no information suggests that he has a home oxygen concentrator. A 6-minute walk test would cause unnecessary stress on the patient at this time. It will surely make him feel more short of breath. Although it may be interesting to know the position of the patient's hemidiaphragms, this will not help him with the current problem. This procedure can be done later if indicated.

25. **D.** A normal term newborn should have a respiratory rate of 30-60 beats/min. All of the other listed vital signs are normal for a term newborn.

26. **D.** An Apgar score of 8 (of a maximum of 10) indicates that the newborn is in good condition and can be given to its mother. Review Table 1-17 for the scoring of the five Apgar signs. Because the newborn is in good condition, there is no need to give it or the mother oxygen or to begin bag/mask rescue breathing.

27. **A.** Laryngotracheobronchitis (croup) is a swelling of the mucous membrane below the vocal cords (subglottic area). This is often identified by a narrowing of the dark air column below the vocal cords. This pointed narrowing is sometimes referred to as the steeple sign. If the patient had aspirated a coin, a solid shape would be seen. In addition, the patient with an aspiration problem has a history of a sudden problem, not one of being sick for 2 days. Epiglottitis is a swelling of the airway above the vocal cords (supraglottic area). Tonsillitis is a swelling of the soft tissue above the vocal cords. In both cases the upper airway radiograph shows haziness in the throat area with a normal tracheal air column.

28. **D.** The young, healthy heart usually responds to a fluid-overload situation by increasing its rate (tachycardia). The excessive intravenous fluid tends to leak out of the capillaries into the tissues in the dependent parts of the body, such as the feet and lower legs. The kidneys quickly put out the extra fluids, and a low urine specific gravity is found. It is highly unlikely that the heart will slow (bradycardia) in a fluid-overload situation. Rather than a high urine specific gravity, indicating low urine output, the kidneys put out extra fluid, resulting in a low urine specific gravity.

29. **D.** A right-sided hemothorax pushes the mediastinum to the left side. A left-sided tension pneumothorax pushes the mediastinum to the right side. Left lower-lobe atelectasis pulls the mediastinum to the left side. Fibrosis of the left lung pulls the mediastinum to the left side. Review Figure 1-8 if needed. If a patient has bilateral lower-lobe pneumonia, both lungs are affected; therefore no shifting of the lungs or the mediastinum would be seen.

30. **C.** An increased C:T ratio (greater than 50%) indicates an enlarged heart and is abnormal. The patient should be evaluated for left-ventricular failure. An athletic heart is not significantly enlarged compared with a normal-sized heart. What makes it athletic is that it can pump more effectively with a higher than normal stroke volume. A left pleural effusion is identified by an obscured left costophrenic angle; a pleural air/fluid level may be seen. A left-middle-lobe infiltrate will have a distinctive shadow over the affected lung area, not the heart.

31. **A.** It is highly unlikely that a patient with ARDS, which results in small, stiff lungs and significant hypoxemia, would be breathing with a normal respiratory rate. A patient with these serious problems will probably show nasal flaring (to reduce airway resistance), intercostal retractions (because of the stiff lungs), and use of accessory muscles of inspiration (to assist the diaphragm in breathing).

32. **B.** The PA position has the radiographs penetrating from the back to the front of the patient. Because the heart is located behind the sternum, less distortion of its actual size appears on the radiograph. With the AP position, the radiographs penetrate from the front to the back of the patient. This results in the heart's shadow being abnormally enlarged on the film. The lateral and oblique chest radiograph views are indicated to help find the location of a tumor or other lung lesion. These views are not that useful in evaluating a patient with COPD and left-ventricular failure.

33. **D.** It is best to obtain a chest radiograph. The film will show whether the endotracheal tube is within the trachea (or esophagus or a mainstem bronchus) and where the tip of the tube is located within the trachea.

Hearing stomach sounds during ventilation confirms that the endotracheal tube is in the esophagus. Absent stomach sounds does not help to determine if the tube is in the trachea or a bronchus. Breath sounds also must be auscultated to confirm whether the tube is located within the trachea or a mainstem bronchus. Palpation of the larynx can be used during the initial intubation to confirm that the endotracheal tube has entered the trachea. It cannot be used to determine tube tip location within the trachea. Percussion of the patient's chest will not help determine endotracheal tube location. Abnormal sounds can be from a variety of problems.

34. **A.** Both the blunting of the left costophrenic angle and the air/fluid level with a meniscus are consistent with a left pleural effusion (fluid in the intrapleural space). The patient's history also confirms this problem. Pulmonary edema or pneumonia of the left lung is seen on the radiograph film as a distinctive shadow within the lung field, not around it. Occasionally a pulmonary embolism results in a fluid leak within the lung and a localized shadow within the lung field, not around it.

35. **C.** Transillumination is an easy test for a pneumothorax in a newborn, because the chest wall is relatively thin. If a pneumothorax is present, a "halo" of light shines through the chest wall where the lung is collapsed. Abnormal arterial blood gas results will not be specific to a pneumothorax in this patient. An Apgar score is performed only shortly after a baby has been born to determine how it tolerated the birthing process. A thoracentesis would be performed to remove fluid from around the lung, which has not been shown.

36. **B.** See Table 1-17 for the five Apgar signs and how they are scored. In this example, all five signs would be rated at 1 point each, for a total score of 5 points.

37. **A.** Potassium is the most important electrolyte to monitor for several reasons. First, it affects the functioning of the heart's conduction system. Second, the serum level is relatively low compared with those of the other electrolytes. Third, potassium, in addition to sodium chloride, tends to be lost through the kidneys when a diuretic medication is given. In general, when a patient is given a diuretic medication, all of the serum electrolyte values should be closely watched. Be prepared to recommend the replacement of electrolytes as needed.

38. **C.** A score of 5 indicates moderate respiratory distress. With the Silverman score a score of 0 is normal and a score of 10 indicates severe respiratory distress. See Figure 1-38 for more details.

Chapter 2

1. **B.** A glutaraldehyde solution soak for 10 hours is the only way listed to sterilize plastic equipment without damaging it. Putting plastic equipment into a steam autoclave causes it to melt and be destroyed. Pasteurization or soaking the equipment in an alcohol solution disinfects but does not sterilize the equipment as needed.

2. **A.** A hot water wash with detergent will remove secretions and other debris from the equipment. Soaking the equipment in white vinegar (acetic acid) will kill many of the microorganisms commonly found on home care equipment. The heat generated in an oven under the broiler will melt plastic used in a small-volume nebulizer and other respiratory care equipment. Rinsing the equipment in salt water will not make a significant difference in killing microorganisms. In addition, the dried salt crystals may plug up the capillary tube of a nebulizer.

3. **D.** Steam autoclaving is the only method listed that is acceptable for sterilizing the bacteria filter of a ventilator. Glutaraldehyde solutions will damage the filter medium and will make the filter useless.

4. **C.** The equipment must be resterilized because living spores of *Bacillus subtilis* indicate that the sterilization process was not successful. Other microbes also may have survived. Because of this concern, the equipment should not be used. Aeration of the equipment will not sterilize it, and 70% alcohol will not remove the spores from the equipment or sterilize it.

5. **A.** Acetic acid is found in white vinegar and can be used at home as a low-level disinfectant. It is inexpensive and available in any grocery store. Acid glutaraldehyde and ethylene oxide systems are too expensive to use in a home. Warm, soapy water can be used to clean secretions from equipment but does not disinfect it.

6. **C.** Pasteurization is the least expensive way to disinfect large amounts of the plastic equipment used in respiratory care departments. Steam autoclave and dry heat are used to sterilize, not disinfect, equipment. In addition, the high temperatures used with these methods melt the plastic tubing and oxygen masks. Seventy percent ethyl alcohol is used only to wipe off the surfaces of large equipment items for disinfection.

7. **B.** Ethylene oxide gas should be used on an IPPB machine because it sterilizes the unit without causing any damage. Pasteurization and glutaraldehyde involve solutions that damage the internal structures of any IPPB machine. The heat of steam autoclaving melts any plastic or rubber components of the unit and seriously damages the machine.

8. **D.** It is recommended that patients with cardiopulmonary conditions, such as COPD, get an influenza vaccination each fall. In patients with preexisting conditions, the flu can be a very serious illness. Routine vaccination is also recommended for those older than 50 years of age. The flu is a seasonal problem through the fall and winter months. So, the vaccination should be given in September or October. There

is no indication that the patient has been exposed to tuberculosis or has a throat infection.

9. **A.** Poor hand-washing technique is the most common cause of *E coli*, *Staphylococcus aureus*, and *Streptococcus* bacterial infections. The fact that all infected patients have *E coli* infection points to a single person as the cause. In this case, it most likely would be the home respiratory therapist. It is very unlikely that the infections would result from poor manufacturing processes. These equipment and supply items are produced and sterilized under very demanding standards. If the patients' family members were the cause of the infections, it is likely that a variety of bacterial infections would be present—not just one.

10. **A.** Patients who are coughing should be sitting at least 3 feet away from anyone else to help prevent the spread of infection by droplets. In addition, coughing people should wear a surgical-type mask and should use facial tissues to cough into and to blow their nose. Used tissues should be disposed of safely.

11. **C.** An N-95 or higher face mask is worn by all caregivers who work with the patient to protect them from infected droplets. Airborne and Contact Precautions are used to minimize contact with infected droplets and surfaces in the patient's room. The patient needs to wear an N-95 mask only when transported outside of his or her room. The patient's room must have negative airflow compared with the hallway to prevent contaminated droplets from leaving.

12. **B.** The Pneumovax vaccination is recommended for anyone older than 50 years of age and for anyone with a chronic cardiopulmonary disease. No current vaccination against SARS is available. A patient who needs continuous oxygen therapy should not be removing her nasal cannula for an hour at a time. In addition, glutaraldehyde is not typically used in the home care setting. This patient should not need a booster Pneumovax vaccination until she is 65 years of age.

13. **B.** A patient who is only suspected of having SARS is placed under Standard and Droplet Precautions until the disease is confirmed or ruled out. If SARS is confirmed, Airborne and Contact Precautions are added.

14. **A.** An alcohol solution may be wiped onto the surface of any equipment item that will not be damaged by the solution. The glutaraldehyde solutions are used for high-level disinfection or sterilization by immersion for a prolonged time. Ethylene oxide gas is used for sterilization.

15. **C.** Infants need to be 6 months of age or older to receive the influenza vaccination. All health care workers should be vaccinated because of their high risk of contact with infected patients. Children and adults with chronic cardiopulmonary diseases should be vaccinated to prevent an exacerbation of their condition. Routine vaccination is recommended for everyone 50 years of age and older.

16. **B.** First, an enzymatic detergent is used to remove any organic matter from the exterior of the bronchoscope. After that, the unit is immersed in a glutaraldehyde solution for high-level disinfection. An iodine solution is used only for surface cleaning and low-level disinfection. A hot water wash (pasteurization) is not appropriate for a bronchoscope.

17. **A.** The CDC requires that bleach (a chlorine solution) be used for the surface disinfection of any equipment with a blood splash. Alcohol can be used for the surface low-level disinfection of any equipment without a blood splash. A pulse oximeter would be damaged by soaking in a glutaraldehyde solution. It is not necessary to sterilize a pulse oximeter for a surface blood splash. In addition, ethylene oxide could damage the unit.

Chapter 3

1. **B.** A modified Allen test is used to determine whether adequate perfusion exists through the ulnar artery in case the radial artery should become occluded. This would ensure that the hand is still well perfused. The Allen test is used to determine adequate perfusion through the radial artery. Adequate arm blood pressure does not ensure adequate perfusion of the hand, should the radial artery become blocked. Pressing on the nail bed to make it blanch and then releasing the pressure to check on reperfusion is only a general indicator of peripheral perfusion. It does not confirm adequate circulation through either the radial or the ulnar arteries.

2. **A.** When there is the possibility that a patient has carbon monoxide poisoning, blood gas analysis should be performed through a CO oximeter or hemoximeter to check for COHb. The other three choices cannot measure COHb level. Additionally, pulse oximetry and $PtCO_2$ monitoring do not give CO_2 or pH values.

3. **C.** The described test and its results are of a positive modified Allen test. This positive result means that the patient has adequate ulnar circulation.

4. **C.** When a blood sample is not quickly cooled in ice water, the living tissue will continue to consume O_2 and produce CO_2. The increased CO_2 level will decrease the pH value.

5. **D.** All of the listed conditions would warrant a blood gas analysis because they all deal with significant oxygenation and/or CO_2 removal issues.

6. **C.** Standard Precautions necessitate that gloves be worn on both hands when blood may be contacted by either hand. Additionally, the eyes should be protected from possible blood splashes.

7. **B.** A PaO_2 value of <72 torr indicates mild hypoxemia. Review Table 3-3 for the categories of hypoxemia.

8. **B.** Shapiro and associates (1994) have stated that an acute rise in CO_2 of 20 mm Hg results in a drop in pH of 0.10 unit. So, an acute rise in CO_2 of 10 mm Hg would result in a drop in pH of 0.05 unit.

9. **D.** A PaO_2 value of less than 80 torr is uncorrected hypoxemia. A compensated respiratory acidosis is indicated by the increased $PaCO_2$ value coupled with an increased bicarbonate level and increased base excess found with a normal pH. (Review Tables 3-3 and 3-8.)

10. **B.** A PaO_2 value greater than 80 torr with supplemental O_2 is corrected hypoxemia. An uncompensated metabolic acidosis is indicated by the normal $PaCO_2$ value coupled with decreased bicarbonate concentration and decreased base excess found with an acidotic pH. (Review Tables 3-3 and 3-8.)

11. **C.** Normal oxygenation is indicated because the patient's PaO_2 level is elevated as a result of hyperventilation ($PaCO_2$ value of 20 torr). An uncompensated respiratory alkalosis is indicated by the low $PaCO_2$ value coupled with normal bicarbonate concentration and normal base excess found with an alkalotic pH. (Review Tables 3-2 and 3-8.)

12. **A.** A PaO_2 level of less than 80 torr is uncorrected hypoxemia. A combined metabolic and respiratory acidosis is indicated by the increased $PaCO_2$ value coupled with decreased bicarbonate level and decreased base excess found with an acidotic pH. (Review Tables 3-3 and 3-8.)

13. **C.** A PaO_2 value of less than 80 torr is uncorrected hypoxemia. A compensated respiratory alkalosis is indicated by the decreased $PaCO_2$ value coupled with decreased bicarbonate concentration and decreased base excess found with a normal pH. (Review Tables 3-3 and 3-8.)

14. **C.** An $S\bar{v}O_2$ value of 75% is normal and correlates with normal tissue oxygenation. A $P\bar{v}O_2$ value of 30 torr indicates tissue hypoxia. Normal ABG values do not necessarily correspond to normal tissue oxygenation values. (See Table 3-11.)

15. **B.** Two SDs are considered "in control" with a blood gas analyzer. (See Fig. 3-8.)

16. **C.** The patient's $PaCO_2$ value best correlates with her ventilatory status and level of fatigue. The other tests are of value but give less direct evidence of her ability to breathe effectively.

17. **B.** The results of an ABG measurement inform you of the patient's oxygenation status and $PaCO_2$ level. Pulse oximetry gives information only on oxygenation status. Pulmonary function tests do not give any information on the patient's PaO_2 and $PaCO_2$ levels. Additionally, a full set of pulmonary function tests can be very tiring for the patient.

18. **C.** Some pulse oximeters obtain inaccurate readings through the skin of darkly pigmented patients. Blocking outside light with an opaque wrap or moving the probe to a lightly pigmented area such as a fingertip (without nail polish) often results in accurate readings. (See Table 3-12.)

19. **A.** The patient's approximate $PaCO_2$ value of 54 torr is found by dividing the $PtcCO_2$ value of 63 torr by the correlation factor of 1.4. (See an example calculation in the text.)

20. **C.** The patient's PAO_2 value (pressure of alveolar oxygen) can be calculated as follows:

$$PAO_2 = \left(\left[P_B - P_{H_2O} \right] F_IO_2 \right) - \frac{PaCO_2}{0.8}$$
$$= \left([750 - 54] \, 0.5 \right) - \frac{36}{0.8}$$
$$= \left([696] \, 0.5 \right) - 45$$
$$= (348) - 45$$
$$= 303 \text{ torr}$$

21. **C.** The patient's $P(A-a)O_2$ value (difference between alveolar pressure and arterial pressure of oxygen) can be calculated as follows:

$$\text{The patient's } PAO_2 = 303 \text{ torr}$$
$$\text{The patient's } PaO_2 = \frac{-60 \text{ torr}}{243 \text{ torr}}$$

22. **D.** The normal $P(A-a)O_2$ difference should be no more than 25 torr for a healthy person of this age. The patient's difference of 243 torr is far greater than normal for any patient. (See Fig. 3-21.) There is no indication that the blood gas analyzer needs recalibration. This equation is not used to evaluate ventilation.

23. **C.** The $P(A-a)O_2$ value should be 15 torr or less in a normal person because of good matching of ventilation and perfusion. Therefore this patient's alveolar-arterial difference is increased. Review the example calculations in this chapter.

24. **A.** The sudden increase in the $PtcO_2$ value can be explained by the electrode being pulled loose from the skin, allowing room air to contact it. If the patient's oxygen percentage was decreased (less than 21% in room air), there would be a decrease in the $PtcO_2$ value. If the patient's pulmonary condition suddenly improved, her $PtcCO_2$ value would probably also have changed. If the patient was hyperventilating to raise her oxygen value, her carbon dioxide value would have decreased.

25. **D.** The results of the modified Allen test performed on the patient's right wrist are abnormal. It took 25 seconds for the return of adequate circulation through the ulnar artery. No arterial blood sample should be taken from the right radial artery because of poor collateral circulation through the ulnar artery (see Fig. 3-2). Check the circulation on the patient's left wrist by doing a modified Allen test on it. Draw from the left radial artery if the test result is normal (less than 15 seconds for the return of circulation). The Allen test is a test of circulation through the radial artery, whereas the modified Allen test is a test of circulation through the ulnar artery.

26. **D.** The best way to assess the oxygenation status of a patient with carbon monoxide poisoning is to run an ABG sample through the CO oximeter. The

CO oximeter is the only device that can accurately differentiate between carboxyhemoglobin and oxyhemoglobin (as well as other types of hemoglobin) and measure the amounts of each. Therefore it gives an accurate SaO_2 value. The first-generation pulse oximeter device is unable to distinguish between carboxyhemoglobin and oxyhemoglobin. This provides a false high value for SaO_2. The transcutaneous oxygen probe can be used to give an approximate tissue oxygen value. However, it is not the clinically accepted way to evaluate a patient with CO poisoning. Running an ABG sample through a standard blood gas analyzer results in measurements of oxygen and carbon dioxide concentrations and of pH. However, the SaO_2 value is calculated from the PaO_2 value. This can result in a falsely high value for the calculated SaO_2 level if the patient is receiving supplemental oxygen and has an elevated PaO_2 value (measured from the blood plasma).

27. **D.** A PaO_2 level of less than 80 torr is uncorrected hypoxemia. A compensated respiratory acidosis is indicated by the increased $PaCO_2$ value coupled with an increased bicarbonate level and increased base excess found with a normal pH. (Review Tables 3-3 and 3-8.)

28. **D.** A normal $P\overline{v}O_2$ value of 40 torr with supplemental oxygen indicates corrected hypoxemia. Normal acid–base balance is shown by the normal mixed venous carbon dioxide and pH. (Review Table 3-11.)

29. **C.** A PaO_2 value of less than 80 mm Hg is uncorrected hypoxemia. A compensated respiratory alkalosis is indicated by the decreased $PaCO_2$ value coupled with a decreased bicarbonate level and decreased base excess found with a normal pH. (Review Tables 3-3 and 3-8.)

30. **B.** A $P\overline{v}O_2$ value of 25 torr is quite low. A $P\overline{v}O_2$ value of 40 torr is normal, and a value below 30 torr usually indicates tissue hypoxemia. An $S\overline{v}O_2$ value of 80% is above the normal value of 75% and indicates above-normal tissue oxygenation. Although a PaO_2 value of 55 torr and an SaO_2 value of 88% are below normal, they do not necessarily indicate tissue hypoxemia. Many patients with chronic lung disease live acceptable lives with values in this range. (Review Table 3-11.)

31. **B.** Because the $PtcCO_2$ has rapidly changed from the normal range of 45 mm Hg to the current very low value of 5 torr, the only possible explanation has to be a leak of room air under the electrode. Check the adhesive ring. If loose, seal the ring on the skin and look for a rise in the carbon dioxide level. If the patient had a patent ductus arteriosus, a decrease in the $PtcO_2$ value would be found over the patient's left chest area and body. An increased temperature inside the incubator would have no effect on the $PtcCO_2$ value. Even if the patient's cardiopulmonary condition had improved, a neonate would not spontaneously hyperventilate to a $PtcCO_2$ value of 5 torr.

32. **C.** Recheck the blood gas analyzer for a problem with the PO_2 electrode. A calculation of the patient's PAO_2 level shows that the maximum PaO_2 value the patient can have is 127 torr. Until an accurate PaO_2 value can be determined, no change should be seen in the patient's inspired oxygen percentage. Although no reason exists to doubt the pH and $PaCO_2$ values, no decision to maintain the patient on his or her present ventilator settings can be made until a correct PaO_2 value is obtained. No indication exists to hyperventilate this drug-overdose patient. Do not confuse this case with hyperventilation of a patient with a head injury and increased intracranial pressure.

33. **A.** An arterialized capillary blood gas sample will provide pH and carbon dioxide values that are close to those found in an arterial sample. Oxygenation cannot be reliably evaluated through a capillary sample.

34. **B.** The approximate difference between the arterial and the central venous carbon dioxide levels should be about 6 torr. This patient's larger than expected difference could be the result of low cardiac output and decreased peripheral circulation. As the blood passes through the body more slowly, there is more time for carbon dioxide to accumulate, resulting in the high $PcvCO_2$. There is no reason to believe that there was a preanalytic error with either blood gas sample. Because the patient's $PaCO_2$ is in the normal range of 43 torr, he or she is not being hyperventilated or in ventilator failure.

35. **D.** With the P:F ratio, the PaO_2 of 85 torr is divided by the oxygen percentage as a whole number (or, in an alternate equation version, by the F_1O_2 as a decimal fraction of 0.50). So, the equation is set up as follows:

$$\frac{PaO_2}{O_2\,\%} = \frac{85}{50} = 1.7$$

36. **C.** The lateral area of the heel is the preferred puncture site. (See Fig. 3-4.) A fingertip, toe tip, or earlobe could be used if the lateral heel puncture was unsuccessful.

Chapter 4

1. **D.** The MEP test is a measure of expiratory muscle strength. A value of +40 cm H_2O usually indicates enough strength for spontaneous breathing and the ability to cough effectively. The pressure should be sustained for a short time to ensure that the measurement is accurate.

2. **C.** African Americans have been shown to have an FVC that is 10%-15% less than age- and height-matched Caucasians. Review the FVC discussion.

3. **D.** Review Figure 4-7 for volumes and capacities. The total lung capacity can be found by adding the residual volume and VC together. See Figure 4-7 for the other combinations of volumes and capacities that can be added together to find TLC.

4. **A.** Flow at the midpoint of expiration normally is less than flow at the midpoint of inspiration, because the small airways are beginning to close at the halfway point of an expiratory effort. A flow-volume loop test cannot measure lung diffusion or RV to calculate the FRC.

5. **D.** A progressively declining VC and MIP indicate that the patient is getting weaker and her condition is getting worse. If her condition were improving, these tests would show increasing values. It is up to the respiratory therapist to ensure that the patient is performing the tests properly. If done properly, the test results will be valid. The MIP test is not used to help in the diagnosis of asthma, because it measures strength, not flow.

6. **C.** A differential-pressure pneumotachometer is portable enough to be taken to a patient's bedside. It can be used to determine a patient's V_T, FVC, and peak flow. A Stead-Wells water-seal spirometer is not typically moved, because it is large, and the water will be splashed about while it is moving. The device can be used for all three listed tests when done in the pulmonary function laboratory. A maximum inspiratory pressure manometer is used for the MIP test. It may be reconfigured for a MEP test but cannot measure any gas flows. A body plethysmograph is far too large to move to a patient's bedside. However, it can be used for all three listed tests when they are done in the pulmonary function laboratory.

7. **C.** A known volume of air is pumped into and out of the circuit and pneumotachometer to check its accuracy and identify any leakage. CO_2 buildup is not a problem with the FVC test, because the patient does not rebreathe his or her own gas for very long. A gas analyzer and kymograph are not used with an FVC test on a pneumotachometer.

8. **A.** A bronchoprovocation study would be the best test for a patient with an unclear history or signs and symptoms of asthma. If the patient has any airway hypersensitivity, this test will cause a measurable decrease in expiratory flow. The other three tests can be used in the diagnosis of asthma but are not as specific to asthma as a bronchoprovocation study.

9. **C.** Emphysema is the only condition listed in which the lung compliance would be increased. Normal compliance is 0.1 L (100 mL)/cm H_2O.

10. **C.** Review the calculation shown in Exam Hint 4-1.

11. **C.** It has been determined that blowing out from TLC results in the greatest expiratory force. This is the recommended procedure.

12. **B.** V_T is estimated as 3-4 mL/lb (or 7-9 mL/kg) of ideal body weight, which results in a range of about 300-400 mL.

13. **A.** Alveolar ventilation is estimated by subtracting the patient's ideal body weight in pounds (170) from the V_T (580 mL).

14. **D.** The patient exhaled a normal percentage of his or her VC in 1 second. The other conditions would all result in a low value. Review the normal values discussed earlier in the chapter.

15. **B.** The FVC is the largest capacity that can be measured by spirometry.

16. **A.** The V_T would be seen as the repeated smallest volumes.

17. **D.** The IRV is found from the end of a V_T inspiration to the TLC. It represents the additional volume that can be inhaled after a normal V_T. Review Figure 4-7 if needed. Do not be confused by VC efforts that look "upside down" compared with others. Review the various volume–time curve tracings in the chapter for extra practice determining volumes. Volume No. 2 is the ERV. Volume No. 3 is the VC. Volume No. 4 is the ERV and V_T combined. Volume No. 1 is the V_T.

18. **B.** The ERV represents the volume of air that can be exhaled after a normal V_T is exhaled. Review Figure 4-7 if needed. Do not be confused by VC efforts that look "upside down" compared with others. Review the various volume–time curve tracings in the chapter for extra practice determining volumes. Volume No. 1 is the V_T. Volume No. 3 is the VC. Volume No. 4 is the ERV and V_T combined.

19. **D.** The VC is made up of these three volumes. The VC can also be found by adding the IC and ERV. Review Figure 4-7 if needed.

20. **C.** PF is directly related to height and indirectly related to age. When done properly, the PF will be seen at the start of an FVC effort, because that is when air is emptied from the upper airway.

21. **D.** Inconsistent high and low pressures are most likely the result of inconsistent effort. A leak would result in a consistently low value. A patient should have a consistent value starting from either the RV or the FRC.

22. **C.** See the following equation.

$$\text{Percentage of change} = \frac{\text{After drug airflow} - \text{Before drug airflow}}{\text{Before drug airflow}} \times 100$$

$$\text{Percentage of change} = \frac{9.4 \text{ L/min} - 7.5 \text{ L/min}}{7.5 \text{ L/min}} \times 100$$

$$= \frac{1.9}{7.5} \times 100$$

$$= 0.25 \times 100$$

$$= 25\%$$

23. **D.** All of the data in the table indicate severe obstructive lung disease. The TLC and RV are both greater than 120% of predicted, indicating significant air trapping. All three flow measurements are far lower than predicted. If the patient had restrictive lung disease, the TLC and RV values would be smaller than predicted.

24. **C.** Patients with severe air trapping, as found with emphysema, take much longer than normal to "wash" the nitrogen out of their lungs. Often the test must be prolonged for several minutes past the usual 7-minute duration to eliminate enough nitrogen to complete

the test. The nitrogen washout test requires the patient to breathe in 100% oxygen to displace the resident nitrogen found in the lungs. The respiratory exchange ratio has to do with oxygen consumption and carbon dioxide production; it has nothing to do with nitrogen elimination. Nitrogen is not active in metabolism. The normal amount of nitrogen found in the body is not significantly affected by the nitrogen washout test.

25. **B.** The lung diffusion test would be most affected in that the CO in the cigarette smoke would bind to the hemoglobin of the patient's blood. This results in a lower than true test result. The other tests are not affected by CO.

26. **B.** All patient flows, volumes, and capacities must be mathematically converted from ATPS to BTPS conditions. This results in the exhaled flows or volumes measured at room temperature being adjusted for the expansion of gas found at the patient's body temperature. STPD conditions are used only with diffusing capacity tests. Atmospheric temperature, pressure, dry (ATPD) is not used for reporting any pulmonary function results.

27. **C.** It is necessary to place a carbon dioxide absorber in the PFT system when the patient has to breathe on a closed system for an extended period. Without one, the patient will rebreathe his or her own exhaled carbon dioxide. If too much water is around the spirometer bell, some splashing may occur. However, too much water will not cause the patient to feel short of breath. If nose clips were left off the patient, he or she may breathe through the nose instead of the mouth. This will not cause a feeling of shortness of breath.

28. **D.** A body plethysmography test for TLC will be the most accurate for a patient with severe emphysema, because it can measure the volume of *all* gas within the chest. This includes gas in damaged parts of the lungs that do not ultimately connect to larger airways and the outside atmosphere. The 7-minute nitrogen washout test and helium dilution test measure only the gas in areas of the lungs that connect to the larger airways and outside atmosphere. This may result in an undermeasurement of the patient's true lung volumes. The single-breath nitrogen washout test is not used to measure the TLC. It is used to assess the evenness of inspiratory and expiratory gas flow.

29. **B.** Patients with uncontrolled asthma will have increased airway inflammation. This causes an increase in eNO. The exhaled nitric oxide analyzer can measure this level so that the physician is more aware of the patient's condition. To a lesser extent, patients with an exacerbation of their COPD will also have an increase in eNO. This technology has not been shown to be beneficial in patients with ARDS or asbestos exposure.

30. **B.** Because the FVC test lasts for only a few seconds, the patient will not rebreathe significant amounts of carbon dioxide; therefore a carbon dioxide absorber

is not needed. In addition, in some pulmonary function systems, a carbon dioxide absorber slows the flow of exhaled gas and results in lower reported FVC values than are actually present. The PFT circuit must be airtight to prevent any leakage and resulting lower volumes and flows. Volume calibration is done by pumping a known volume (3 L) into and out of the spirometer. Any leak will result in a lower than expected volume being found. The kymograph should have its speed settings checked to make sure that the timing of the test is accurate.

31. **D.** All listed items must be avoided to ensure an accurate FVC test. Coughing causes variable flows and cuts off the full FVC volume. A leak results in a loss of volume. A weak patient effort results in a slower expiratory flow than the patient can optimally provide. When tests are done properly, they show consistent results. Excessive variability shows inconsistent patient effort.

32. **C.** A diffusion study measures carbon monoxide diffusion to evaluate oxygen diffusion across the alveolar–capillary membrane. It is not helpful in the diagnosis of asthma. The other three listed tests can be very useful in diagnosing asthma. With a before and after bronchodilator study, a patient with asthma who is responsive to inhaled bronchodilator medications shows improved flows after inhaling the medication. A patient with an asthma problem often reveals a distinctive flow–volume loop tracing (see Fig. 4-12). A bronchoprovocation test usually produces a decreased expiratory flow in a patient with asthma.

33. **C.** Spirometry before and after inhalation of a beta-agonist bronchodilator (albuterol) is the best test to differentiate between asthma and emphysema. Most patients with asthma have some reversibility of the bronchospasm. Their spirometry should show improved expiratory flows after inhalation of a beta-agonist. Patients with emphysema have very little, if any, improvement in expiratory flows after the inhalation of this class of medication. This is because their alveoli, not the airways, are damaged. The other three listed tests may not show significant differences between patients with asthma and those with emphysema.

34. **D.** Tracing D shows a severe "scoop" during the expiratory part of the patient effort after the peak flow. This dramatic decrease in expiratory flow is characteristic of severe small-airway obstruction. Tracing A shows a less severe decrease in expiratory flow after the peak flow. Tracing B shows a severely reduced peak flow that is characteristic of a fixed extrathoracic obstruction. Tracing C shows a normal flow–volume loop. Review Figure 4-12 if needed for a comparison of different flow–volume loops.

35. **B.** Tracing B shows a severely reduced peak flow that is characteristic of a fixed extrathoracic obstruction.

This might be caused by a laryngeal tumor, paralyzed vocal cord, or other upper airway problem. Tracing D shows a severe "scoop" during the expiratory part of the patient effort after the peak flow. This dramatic decrease in expiratory flow is characteristic of severe small-airway obstruction. Tracing A shows a less severe decrease in expiratory flow after the peak flow. Tracing C shows a normal flow–volume loop. Review Figure 4-12 if needed for a comparison of different flow–volume loops.

36. **A.** Tracing C shows an increased peak flow compared with tracing A and correction of the expiratory "scoop" seen in tracing A. In addition, the inspiratory flow on tracing C is greater than that on tracing A. All of these changes show significant improvement, indicating that the patient's condition is treatable. The patient's effort or lack of effort cannot be determined by looking at the two tracings. Tracing C is normal and does not justify another bronchodilator treatment.

37. **C.** The patient's value is increased, because the upper end of normal is 25 ppb. This would indicate increased airway inflammation, possibly from asthma. The analyzer should be calibrated before use, but there is no indication that this was not done or that the equipment is not functioning properly. The eNO test should always be performed first in a sequence. If other tests are performed first, the patient's eNO will be artificially increased.

38. **A.** The patient's eCO level should be checked to make sure he or she has not been smoking. This is because smoking increases the carboxyhemoglobin level and will result in an inaccurate lung diffusion test. Although the other three exhaled gases are measured in other clinical situations, they are not needed for a lung diffusion test.

39. **D.** The Wright respirometer's vanes and gears can be distorted and damaged by the high gas flow from an FVC effort. The patient breathes slowly with the other three tests.

Chapter 5

1. **A.** The pulmonary artery catheter first enters the RA of the heart. It then follows the flow of blood through the heart by entering the RV. Next the catheter enters the pulmonary artery and the PAP is recorded. When the balloon at the tip of the catheter advances as far into the pulmonary artery as it can, it "wedges" in place. The resulting pressure is called the PCWP.

2. **C.** Stroke volume is the blood volume pumped by each ventricle with each heartbeat and has a range of 50-120 mL in the adult. The CI is an indicator of the adequacy of perfusion of the body's tissues. Cardiac output is the output of blood for 1 minute. Afterload is the resistance to flow. It is caused by the level of tone in the blood vessels and the viscosity of the blood. (See Box 5-2.)

3. **C.** This problem requires the calculation of the decimal fraction or percentage of dead space. To do so, place the patient's arterial and end-tidal carbon dioxide values into this formula:

$$V_D/V_T = \frac{(PaCO_2 - P_{\overline{E}}CO_2)}{PaCO_2}$$

In which:

V_D/V_T or V_D = the patient's physiologic dead space
$PaCO_2$ = the patient's arterial carbon dioxide pressure
$P_{\overline{E}}CO_2$ = the patient's average exhaled carbon dioxide pressure
Calculate the V_D/V_T as follows:

$$V_D/V_T = \frac{(53-20)}{53}$$
$$= \frac{33}{53} = 0.62$$

The patient's V_D/V_T or V_D fraction can be recorded as 0.62 or 62%. (Note that this equation must be used when the patient's tidal volume is not known.)

4. **B.** This problem requires the calculation of the patient's dead space volume. To do so, place the patient's arterial and end-tidal carbon dioxide values into this formula:

$$V_D = \frac{(PaCO_2 - P_{\overline{E}}CO_2)}{PaCO_2} \times \overline{V}_E$$

In which:

V_D = the patient's physiologic dead space
$\overline{V}_E$ = the average exhaled tidal volume
$PaCO_2$ = the patient's arterial carbon dioxide pressure
$P_{\overline{E}}CO_2$ = the patient's average exhaled carbon dioxide pressure

Calculate the V_D as follows:

$$V_D = \frac{(43-22)}{43}$$
$$= \frac{21}{43} \times 650 = 0.49 \times 650 \text{ mL} = 319 \text{ mL}$$

The patient's physiologic V_D volume equals 319 mL. (Note that this equation must be used when the patient's tidal volume is known.)

5. **A.** A normal adult's SVR has a range of 900-1400 dyn/s/cm^{-5}. This patient's SVR value of 600 dyn/s/cm^{-5} is well below normal. This may result from vasodilation or hypovolemia. All of the other values are within normal range. (See Box 5-2.)

6. **B.** If excessive fluid is given to a patient with congestive heart failure, the fluid is likely to accumulate in the pulmonary vessels because the left ventricle cannot pump effectively. This increased fluid will increase the pulmonary capillary wedge pressure. The patient should be monitored for pulmonary edema. If the patient develops pulmonary edema, a chest

radiograph will show increased, rather than decreased, lung markings and haziness in the lungs. The patient's PaO_2 level can be expected to decrease rather than increase if pulmonary edema develops. If fluid builds up from the left ventricle into the pulmonary vessels, the pulmonary artery pressure will increase along with the pulmonary capillary wedge pressure.

7. **D.** The patient's history and current situation suggest that a pulmonary embolism has developed. The V_D/V_T test should be performed to determine whether the patient's dead space has increased. If it has, this will match the clinical suspicion of a pulmonary embolism. It is doubtful that the patient's lung compliance will change if a pulmonary embolism occurred. There is no specific change in the electrocardiogram that corresponds to a pulmonary embolism or other sudden cause of shortness of breath. Chest radiograph changes are unlikely to be seen soon after a pulmonary embolism has occurred.

8. **A.** A capnograph is zero calibrated on room air because it contains only a trace of carbon dioxide. A capnograph cannot measure oxygen percentage or anesthetic gases. Either 5% or 10% carbon dioxide is often used for the second point (high point) in two-point calibration of the capnograph.

9. **A.** A PCWP level of 2 mm Hg is very low and would indicate that the patient is hypovolemic. (See Box 5-2.) A PCWP of 8 mm Hg is normal. In general, a PCWP of greater than 8 mm Hg would indicate that the patient has some degree of fluid overload (hypervolemia) or has left-ventricular failure. A PCWP of 24 mm Hg is significantly higher than normal.

10. **B.** The normal PAP level is about 25/10 mm Hg. The normal PCWP value is about 8 mm Hg. A PAP value of 35/15 mm Hg would be elevated. Normal arterial blood pressure is about 120/80 mm Hg. (Review the values in Box 5-2.)

11. **C.** Carbon dioxide absorbs infrared light at a specific wavelength. The higher the carbon dioxide level, the greater the absorption. See Chapter 3 for a discussion of blood gas analysis, the Clark and Severinghaus electrodes, and a CO oximeter.

12. **D.** The difference between the PAP diastolic pressure of 12 mm Hg and the PCWP pressure of 8 mm Hg is 4 mm Hg.

13. **D.** The patient's estimated $PaCO_2$ value is 34 torr. It is found by adding the $PetCO_2$ value of 30 torr and the $P(a-et)CO_2$ gradient value of 4 torr. Review the math examples in the chapter, if necessary.

14. **B.** Patients with COPD have significant ventilation-to-perfusion mismatches. This results in increased dead space ventilation and shunt-like effects. The COPD patient would not be expected to have normal or decreased dead space.

15. **C.** An $S\bar{v}O_2$ level of 75% would be normal and indicate normal tissue oxygenation. Values of less than 75%

saturation would indicate tissue hypoxia. A saturation of 90% is far higher than that needed in venous blood.

16. **B.** When ventilation and perfusion match well, as in a normal person, the gradient between the arterial carbon dioxide level and the exhaled carbon dioxide level is 2-3 torr with a range between 1 and 5 torr. A carbon dioxide level of less than this would indicate either no alveolar ventilation or no production of CO_2. Gradients of greater than 5 torr have been found in patients with significant ventilation/perfusion mismatching.

17. **A.** The patient's blood pressure of 115/78 mm Hg is within normal limits for an adult. Blood pressure cannot be used as an indicator of an intracranial bleed. (See Box 5-2 and review Chapter 1, if necessary.)

18. **D.** The patient should be kept on 28% oxygen because the pulmonary vascular resistance decreased from 9 to 5 mm Hg/L/min and the PaO_2 increased from 57 to 63 torr when the patient was increased from 24% oxygen. The patient is not hypoxemic; there is no indication for beginning mechanical ventilation. A bronchodilating agent such as albuterol may help the patient's breathing somewhat, but it is not effective at reducing pulmonary vascular resistance.

19. **C.** The patient's pulmonary vascular resistance can be determined by calculating the PAd–PCWP as follows:

$$
\begin{array}{ll}
\text{PAd} & 20 \text{ mm Hg} \\
\text{PCWP} & \underline{-9 \text{ mm Hg}} \\
& 11 \text{ mm Hg}
\end{array}
$$

Because a normal PAd–PCWP gradient is no more than 5 mm Hg, this patient's value of 11 mm Hg indicates increased pulmonary vascular resistance. Even though the patient's PAP is elevated at 35/20 mm Hg, that pressure alone does not provide enough information to determine that the patient has right-ventricular failure/cor pulmonale. An increased right-ventricular pressure in a patient with COPD indicates right-ventricular failure/cor pulmonale. Because the patient has a normal PCWP of 9 mm Hg, she does not have left-ventricular failure. This problem is identified by an increased PCWP. This same normal PCWP of 9 mm Hg indicates normal blood volume. Hypovolemia is identified by a PCWP that is less than 4 mm Hg.

20. **A.** If a clot is at the tip of the catheter it will prevent the patient's blood pressure from being transmitted back to the transducer for measurement. By withdrawing the clot, the lumen of the catheter will be open and the blood pressure can be measured. If an air bubble is in the arterial line, the measured blood pressure will be less than actual. This is because the patient's blood pressure will partially collapse the gas bubble (Boyle's law) and transmit a lower pressure to the transducer. Withdrawing the air bubble allows the patient's blood pressure to be accurately transmitted to the transducer. If the ventilator's peak pressure is too high, the patient's cardiac output will be reduced.

This will result in a drop in blood pressure that will be measured equally on both arms. There is no evidence that the patient has a ventricular septal defect. Even if a septal defect were present, the blood pressure would be the same in both arms.

21. **B.** There are two significant changes in the patient's parameters that indicate that the patient has a pulmonary embolism. First, the patient's pulmonary vascular resistance has almost tripled in 2 hours. Second, the patient's PAd–PCWP difference has increased significantly.

	9:00 AM	**11:00 AM**
PAd	10 mm Hg	21 mm Hg
PCWP	–8 mm Hg	–10 mm Hg
	2 mm Hg (Normal)	11 mm Hg (Increased)

The fact that both of these parameters have quickly increased significantly, combined with the sudden drop in the patient's oxygen level, indicates that a pulmonary embolism has developed. Because the patient's PCWP remains normal at 8 and 10 mm Hg, pulmonary edema is not supported as a diagnosis. Pulmonary edema results in an increased PCWP. Pneumonia will result in hypoxemia. However, the other parameters do not match this diagnosis. Cardiac tamponade will decrease the patient's cardiac output but will not increase pulmonary vascular resistance or PCWP.

22. **A.** The increase in the patient's $P_{ET}CO_2$ level from 33 to 41 torr indicates that alveolar ventilation has decreased. There are no data that correlate with pulmonary edema (such as an increased pulmonary capillary wedge pressure). If the patient were hyperventilating, the $P_{ET}CO_2$ level would have decreased instead of increased. Also, the $PaCO_2$ value would have decreased. There are no data that correlate with an increased cardiac output (such as a decreased difference between the oxygen content of arterial blood and the oxygen content of venous blood).

23. **D.** It is necessary to zero the transducer by exposing it to local barometric pressure. Adjust the transducer so that it reads zero when exposed to room barometric pressure. The patient must lie flat in bed with the transducer at midchest level to give accurate blood pressure readings. If the patient sits up, the blood pressure will read low. If the patient's head is lower than his or her body, the blood pressure will read too high. Saline must fill the pressure tubing, transducer dome, and arterial catheter so that the patient's blood pressure is measured accurately. If air fills the transducer dome, it will be variably compressed based on the patient's systolic and diastolic blood pressure changes. This is the result of Boyle's law and results in a lower-than-actual blood pressure being measured.

24. **A.** The patient's history of vomiting and diarrhea would lead to a loss of body fluids. Hypovolemia correlates with tachycardia and all of the patient's low blood pressure values. High ventilating pressures can result in a drop in the cardiac output. This can cause the systemic blood pressure to drop, but is unlikely to result in all of the hemodynamic values being low. In addition, there is no information given that relates to the patient's ventilating pressures. There is no mention of the patient's breath sounds showing bronchospasm. Even if bronchospasm was present, it would not cause all of the low hemodynamic values. If the balloon on the catheter ruptured, there would be a small volume of gas released into the pulmonary circulation. This would act as a small gas embolism. Although not good for the patient, this small gas embolism is unlikely to cause a drop in all of the hemodynamic pressures.

25. **C.** A pressure transducer for blood pressure monitoring should be zero calibrated at the patient's midchest level. This will result in accurate blood pressure measurements. If the patient is below the level of the transducer, the measured blood pressure will be less than actual. Conversely, if the patient is above the level of the transducer, the measured blood pressure will be greater than actual. If an air bubble or clot was in the arterial catheter, the problem would not be resolved when the patient's position was changed. Although postural drainage positions can cause a decrease in blood pressure, this does not always occur or fit the circumstances in this situation.

26. **C.** The low PCWP value of 3 torr indicates hypovolemia. The best treatment would be to administer intravenous fluids. Other clues to hypovolemia include the high electrolyte values from dehydration. Review these values in Chapter 1, if necessary. Giving a diuretic would make the situation worse. More O_2 is not needed because the patient is not hypoxemic. It is doubtful that giving a chronotropic agent (such as atropine) to increase the heart rate would be very helpful to increase the low PCWP.

27. **A.** After treatment, the patient's $P\overline{v}O_2$ value has increased from 35 to 41 torr. This improvement is now within the normal range and would indicate that the patient has normal tissue oxygenation. If the patient had worsening heart failure or decreased tissue perfusion, the $P\overline{v}O_2$ value would have decreased to less than the original value of 35 torr.

28. **D.** If the patient has a ventricular septal defect, the oxygen level gradient from the right atrium to the right ventricle will be increased. This is because high-oxygen blood from the left ventricle will leak through the defect into the right ventricle. Capnography and dead space values will not specifically indicate a hole in the ventricular septum. It is insufficient to check only the $P\overline{v}O_2$ value from the pulmonary artery. This value will not provide a comparison with the oxygen value before the right ventricle.

29. **D.** A triple-lumen ScvO$_2$ CVP catheter is the only catheter that will provide the needed information. The CVP pressure will indicate fluid balance. The ScvO$_2$ level will indicate the patient's central venous oxygen saturation, which correlates with the patient's oxygen consumption.

30. **B.** Mrs. Decker should have an arterial line placed because of her diagnosis of sepsis and her unstable blood pressure. Mr. Boone's blood pressure is stable within the normal range. Mrs. Dylan's blood pressure is returning to normal as her dehydration is corrected. Although Mr. Zawinal's blood pressure is slightly elevated, it is stable and he does not have a condition prone to hemodynamic instability.

31. **A.** Although not as accurate a measurement as mixed venous oxygen saturation (SvO$_2$%) at evaluating tissue oxygenation, an ScvO$_2$ value of 60% very likely indicates tissue hypoxia. The usual clinical goal is to keep the patient's ScvO$_2$ level ≥70%. The decreasing ScvO$_2$ value could indicate decreased cardiac output, not increased. There is no correlation between ScvO$_2$ level and pulmonary vascular resistance.

Chapter 6

1. **B.** See the sample H-tank duration calculation given earlier in the chapter. Common calculation errors include using the E-tank factor and failing to convert from minutes to hours by dividing by 60.

2. **B.** A patient with COPD who is hypercarbic and is breathing on hypoxic drive should be given supplemental O$_2$ with great care. Too much O$_2$ will result in too high an arterial O$_2$ level and will blunt the hypoxic drive. Hypoventilation will result in a rising CO$_2$ level. Pulmonary edema from O$_2$ toxicity would necessitate a high percentage of O$_2$ for an extended period. ROP is seen only in premature infants. Hyperventilation is not caused by breathing of supplemental O$_2$.

3. **C.** In addition to the special high-flow nasal cannula, a blender with high-pressure air and oxygen sources and humidifier will be needed. Sterile water is needed rather than sterile saline.

4. **D.** The reservoir tubing holds O$_2$ from which the patient can inspire. Losing the reservoir results in inhalation of room air and a decrease in the overall O$_2$ percentage. When set up properly, any exhaled CO$_2$ is blown clear from the reservoir tubing before the next inspiration.

5. **C.** There is no condition called O$_2$-induced hyperventilation. Do not confuse this with O$_2$-induced hypoventilation, which needs to be monitored in some patients with COPD. See the rationale for question 2.

6. **D.** Because the face tent is open on top and O$_2$ is heavier than room air, the O$_2$ in the face tent tends to "pour" out if the patient lies supine. When all is set up properly, CO$_2$ should not build up in a face tent, no matter the patient's position. A face tent should not influence a patient's V$_T$. Lying supine may result in decreased V$_T$.

7. **D.** The three listed items are all important for minimizing hypoxemia during a treatment or procedure. Increasing the O$_2$ by 20% will help to minimize hypoxemia, but it is appropriate to raise the percentage much higher.

8. **A.** Many patients who do not tolerate a face mask find an HFNC acceptable. The HFNC is able to deliver the same high oxygen percentage as a nonrebreathing mask. It is unlikely that the anxious patient will tolerate any type of face mask. None of the other masks provide as high an oxygen percentage as the nonrebreathing mask or HFNC.

9. **D.** When properly operating, a partial-rebreathing mask's reservoir bag should not collapse during inspiration. Raise the O$_2$ flow so that the bag stays at least two-thirds full during inspiration. Hypoxic patients usually breathe in at whatever pattern and rate is most efficient for them. It may be counterproductive to try to have the patient breathe differently. A standard, low-flow nasal cannula cannot deliver as high an O$_2$ percentage as can be delivered by the partial-rebreathing mask.

10. **B.** The reservoir membrane is defective, so the cannula should be replaced. The O$_2$ flow should not be increased because this would give the patient more O$_2$ than is intended. Decreasing (or increasing) the O$_2$ flow will not unstick a defective reservoir membrane. Changing to an air entrainment mask would be a possible remedy if a replacement cannula did not exist.

11. **B.** An air entrainment mask (high-flow delivery system) is designed to provide enough flow of the prescribed O$_2$ percentage (fixed concentration) at any patient rate, V$_T$, and so forth. The other three devices do not provide enough flow to deliver a consistent, known O$_2$ percentage.

12. **A.** A properly fitting nonrebreathing mask with enough flow to keep the reservoir bag inflated will deliver the highest O$_2$ percentage of all available devices.

13. **C.** A Bourdon flowmeter is the only unit that will accurately indicate the flow when it is laid horizontally. The others read accurately only in a vertical position.

14. **D.** Review the information on pinholes in Table 6-3.

15. **B.** Review the sample E-tank duration calculation in this chapter. Common calculation errors include using the H-tank factor and failure to convert from minutes to hours by dividing by 60.

16. **C.** Covering the air entrainment ports on an air entrainment mask will result in the patient receiving a higher O$_2$ percentage than desired. In addition, the total flow will be decreased.

17. **D.** Because a major obstruction exists in the transtracheal oxygen catheter, it must be replaced. But first,

the patient must switch her oxygen delivery system to a nasal cannula. Attempts to force out the obstruction by doubling the oxygen flow or forcing the saline or cleaning rod through the catheter can result in injury to the trachea.

18. **D.** The patient's current blood gases show unacceptable hypoxemia with a PaO_2 of 47 torr and an SaO_2 of 80%. Increasing the patient from 2 to 3 L/min through the transtracheal oxygen catheter should help to correct the situation. The patient should be monitored for a possible increasing carbon dioxide level as well as an improving oxygen level. Changing the patient to 24% oxygen by an air entrainment mask probably will not change his actual inspired oxygen percentage. In addition, there is no indication that the transtracheal oxygen catheter has failed. The patient's ventilation is stable, with no indication that bilevel mask ventilation is needed. Changing the patient to a nonrebreathing mask with 10 L/min of oxygen is potentially dangerous. This much oxygen may blunt his hypoxic drive to breathe.

19. **A.** Adding 100 mL of aerosol tubing as a reservoir will help to maintain the patient's inspired O_2 percentage. No clear reason exists for changing the patient's O_2 percentage by protocol, and no physician order exists to do so. Changing the flow probably will not stabilize the patient's O_2 percentage without the added reservoir tubing. A comatose patient will not follow instructions to "not breathe so deeply."

20. **D.** A high-flow nasal cannula should be able to provide enough oxygen to the patient to correct her hypoxemia. In addition, she should keep it on because it will not make her feel claustrophobic. A traditional nasal cannula is not run at over 6 L/min of oxygen. It could be dangerous to sedate a hypoxic patient. It is likely that the CPAP mask also will make her feel claustrophobic.

21. **C.** A nonrebreathing mask with reservoir bag is the best way to deliver heliox because it will provide all of the patient's inspiratory flow needs. A partial-rebreathing mask with reservoir bag is not a sealed system. Room air will be entrained, which will reduce the patient's helium and oxygen percentages. A heliox mix can be given by a high-flow nasal cannula. However, the patient would have to cooperate to use a handheld small-volume nebulizer. There is no indication at this time that mechanical ventilation is needed. In addition, several technical challenges are associated with providing heliox through most mechanical ventilators.

22. **A.** At a flow of 1 L/min, a molecular sieve oxygen concentrator delivers at least 90% oxygen to the patient. A portable LOX system is not needed if the patient is not actively and frequently mobile. A semipermeable-membrane oxygen concentrator delivers only about 40% oxygen to the patient. A piston compressor

is useful for delivering pressurized air to power a small-volume nebulizer. However, it does not deliver more than 21% oxygen (room air) to the patient.

23. **D.** A polarographic oxygen analyzer does not have a gas sampling capillary tube; the paramagnetic type does. The other four listed problems can cause a polarographic analyzer to fail. The probe has a membrane through which oxygen diffuses. It must not be torn and must not have water, blood, or mucus covering it. An adequate amount of electrolyte solution must be present within the probe for the oxygen-related chemical reaction to take place. A functional battery is needed to drive the chemical reaction within the electrolyte solution.

24. **D.** A properly applied and used nonrebreathing mask should deliver at least 60% O_2. CPAP is not indicated in a patient with CO poisoning and more than 40% O_2 should be delivered. A simple mask or 50% oxygen air entrainment nebulizer does not deliver as much O_2 as is provided by a nonrebreathing mask.

25. **B.** Carbogen will help to keep an open patent ductus arteriosus to maintain system circulation. Nitric oxide is indicated for pulmonary hypertension, not for HLHS. It would be dangerous to close the patent ductus arteriosus in this patient. Heliox is indicated for airway obstruction, not for HLHS.

26. **D.** A Thorpe-type flowmeter will read accurately if backpressure is placed upon the exit of gas. Thus, the flowmeter will read less flow than zero, as the outlet is partially and then completely blocked.

27. **C.** The patient's ABG results show her PaO_2 to be 84 torr. This is too high for many patients with COPD. It is likely that her hypoxic drive to breathe has become blunted. This has resulted in her hypoventilating, with an increasing carbon dioxide level and secondary drowsiness. Although it is not possible to know the patient's inspired oxygen percentage with a 6 L/min nasal cannula, this flow has resulted in a PaO_2 that is too high. It is best to switch her to an air entrainment mask so that a known low oxygen percentage (24%) can be administered. Then, she should be monitored closely for returning alertness, and another ABG sample should be obtained. This should be evaluated for a lower, but safe, PaO_2 and a lower $PaCO_2$. The patient should not be left on her present oxygen flow through the nasal cannula because of her unnecessarily high oxygen level, hypoventilation, increasing carbon dioxide level, and secondary drowsiness. Changing her from a cannula to a simple face mask at the same oxygen flow will not correct these problems. She needs to be awakened because her drowsiness is not the result of simple fatigue.

28. **A.** It is likely that the biopsy site has developed some edema, which is causing the shortness of breath and "tight" throat feeling. Giving the patient 80% helium and 20% oxygen should help to ease the patient's shortness of

breath because helium is less dense than nitrogen. Commonly, a patient's head is put down 30 degrees when the patient's blood pressure is low; this is unlikely to ease a feeling of shortness of breath. Carbogen (carbon dioxide and oxygen mix) stimulates the breathing center of the brain but will not relieve the patient's shortness of breath caused by laryngeal edema. The 7-minute helium dilution test is performed in the pulmonary function laboratory to measure the patient's residual volume. It is not intended to relieve the patient's feeling of shortness of breath from laryngeal edema.

29. **B.** The significant discrepancy between the pulse oximeter reading and the CO oximeter can be explained only by the patient's having CO poisoning. In this situation, only the CO oximeter reading will be accurate. A CO oximeter reading of 73% indicates severe hypoxemia. Therefore the patient should be changed to a nonrebreathing mask with enough flow to keep the reservoir bag inflated. This maximizes the inspired oxygen percentage to the patient. Maintaining the simple oxygen mask at the present flow or decreasing the oxygen flow to the simple oxygen mask to 4 L/min will worsen rather than improve the patient's condition. Nothing indicates that the CO oximeter is malfunctioning and should be recalibrated.

30. **C.** Because the reservoir bag has collapsed, the flow of heliox must be increased. Ideally, the reservoir bag should not collapse by more than one-third on inspiration. Decreasing the flow of gas to the patient will worsen the problem of shortness of breath, not improve it. When the gas flow to the mask is inadequate, it does not matter what oxygen percentage the patient gets. There is no need to increase the patient to 40% oxygen. By doing so the helium percentage will drop and could decrease it beneficial effects.

31. **B.** Setting 4.4 L/min on the oxygen flowmeter will deliver 7 L/min of a 70/30 heliox mix. See Exam Hint 6-6 for the heliox factors and an example of how to make this calculation.

32. **B.** INO_{max} is indicated to dilate the pulmonary vascular bed of a newborn with PPHN. When the pulmonary vascular bed dilates, more blood flows through the lungs, and oxygenation should improve. Instillation of intratracheal surfactant is indicated only in a newborn with infant respiratory distress syndrome (RDS). Surfactant therapy is not indicated in PPHN. Although PEEP increases the functional residual capacity of an infant with RDS and improves oxygenation, PEEP must be used with great care, if at all, in a newborn with PPHN. PEEP at 10 cm water may overexpand the alveoli of a newborn with PPHN and prevent blood from flowing through the capillary bed. Oxygenation will worsen rather than improve. Carbogen (carbon dioxide and oxygen mix) may be harmful to a newborn with PPHN, because an increased carbon dioxide level further constricts the newborn's

pulmonary vascular bed. Carbogen is indicated in a newborn with HLHS.

33. **A.** Heliox therapy should be helpful in reducing the patient's work of breathing. This should allow more time for the corticosteroid and aminophylline medications to begin working. Nitric oxide is a pulmonary vasodilator and is not indicated for status asthmaticus. Review Box 6-1 if needed. It is not necessary at this time to go against a patient's wishes and begin mechanical ventilation without first trying heliox therapy. Absolutely no reason justifies allowing this patient to die of status asthmaticus! It should not be fatal if managed appropriately and aggressively.

34. **B.** Because the patient's PVR is now in the normal range, the concentration of nitric oxide can be slowly reduced. The patient's PVR then should be reassessed. It is more prudent to wean off the NO level rather than to discontinue the gas in one step. There is no need to increase the NO to 30 ppm because the patient's PVR is in the normal range. It also is possible that this level of NO could be toxic. Carbogen is not indicated for pulmonary hypertension.

35. **C.** The heliox factor for a 70% helium/30% oxygen mix is 1.6. To calculate the total flow of this heliox mix through an oxygen flowmeter, the following calculation is made: 8 L/min of gas observed on the oxygen flowmeter × 1.6 = 12.8 (13) L/min actual heliox gas flow. See Exam Hint 6-6 for the heliox factors and an example of how to make this calculation.

36. **A.** A portable liquid oxygen system should have a long enough duration to provide her with oxygen for the trip. An E tank of oxygen could be awkward to take on the trip. It would be challenging to prestage oxygen tanks at various stores. The patient should not decrease her oxygen flow just to increase the duration of the E tank.

Chapter 7

1. **C.** Switching the patient from a flow-oriented to a volume-oriented incentive spirometer lets her see the results of her breathing efforts. This should help to motivate her to keep trying.

2. **D.** IS is the most reasonable treatment for atelectasis at this time. The other three options are more equipment and labor intensive and therefore are more expensive. IPPB would be needed only if the patient could not perform IS. CPAP and PEP therapy would not be appropriate.

3. **D.** An initial IS goal of twice the V_T is widely accepted as a starting volume. As the patient improves, the IS goal should be increased toward the predicted IC. A bedside IC and VC may be less than those measured under laboratory conditions.

4. **A.** A so-called "chicken breath" (see Fig. 7-1) can be added to a huff cough or midinspiratory cough to help

a patient with small-airways disease increase expiratory airflow. Because there is less airway pressure generated during a huff or midinspiratory cough, the small airways are more likely to stay open. A quad cough and lateral chest compression cough are needed only with a neuromuscular/neurological disease patient who lacks the muscle strength to cough effectively. A postoperative abdominal or thoracic surgery patient may need to "splint" the wound with a pillow to reduce the pain when coughing.

5. **D.** Tingling fingers and dizziness are signs of acute hyperventilation. Relaxing and breathing normally will restore the CO_2 level.

6. **A.** A pinched breathing tube would prevent a patient from inspiring through the IS unit. Flow-oriented units do not operate by setting flow resistance. Only volume-oriented IS units have a bellows.

7. **C.** Multiply the volume in 1 second by the number of seconds that the ball is elevated to calculate the inhaled volume (900 mL/s × 1.5 s = 1350 mL).

8. **D.** Because the patient is comfortable breathing at the current resistance level, it is reasonable to have him work a little harder by breathing through the next smallest hole.

9. **C.** An assisted inspiration, in which the respiratory therapist delivers a large tidal volume with a manual resuscitation bag, will help to open up atelectatic areas. In addition, when the patient coughs out this large tidal volume, his secretions should be mobilized. A quad cough, in which the respiratory therapist applies gentle pressure to the epigastric area, will increase the expiratory volume and airflow to help mobilize secretions. Together, these two procedures should help to open up areas of atelectasis and expel secretions. IS will not be useful because the patient cannot inspire a large breath. IPPB will make the patient inspire a large breath but will not help to mobilize his secretions.

10. **A.** IS is the simplest and least expensive way to correct a limited case of atelectasis. PEP therapy is indicated when a patient has difficulty mobilizing secretions. Nasotracheal suctioning is limited to unconscious, uncooperative patients who cannot cough out their secretions. IPPB would be needed only if the patient could not adequately perform IS. It is not needed yet.

11. **B.** It is very doubtful if the patient could perform an effective IS treatment. A properly performed IPPB treatment (nose clips and mouth seal may be needed) should deliver a large enough breath to help treat his atelectasis. There is no clinical indication that PEP therapy or postural drainage therapy is needed at this time to help in mobilizing secretions.

12. **C.** Pursed-lip breathing should help the patient regain control over his breathing and be able to calm down. The patient should not be encouraged or allowed to change his own oxygen flow. This is potentially dangerous. The PFLEX unit is indicated only to help strengthen inspiratory muscles. It will not help to reduce dyspnea. The variable backpressure created by blowing through the Flutter valve unit will help only to mobilize secretions. It will not help to reduce dyspnea.

13. **B.** If the patient inhales at a slower rate, she should be able to hold the IC longer. If her IC target is appropriate, she will not be able to inhale an additional 500 mL. There is no advantage to having her exhale faster. There is no therapeutic reason to lower her target volume by 100 mL and raise her respiratory rate to 25 times/min. IS is most effective at treating atelectasis when the IC is inhaled slowly and sustained for several seconds.

14. **C.** It is best to increase her goal by 500 mL because she can easily reach her current volume goal. Doubling her volume goal is too large of a step. It is best to increase volume goals gradually as the patient improves, so that progress can be seen. Switching to a flow-oriented device with the same volume goal provides no benefit. The patient seems to be doing well with the self-directed protocol. So, there is no reason to change to IPPB at this time.

15. **C.** A patient with COPD should not attempt a normal cough because the high lung pressure generated would cause the airways to collapse. This could lead to air trapping.

16. **C.** Vesicular (normal) breath sounds indicate normal lung expansion with no atelectasis.

17. **A.** The PFLEX unit (and other similar units from other manufacturers) is designed specifically to help strengthen the inspiratory muscles. Maximal inspiratory pressure and maximal expiratory pressure are bedside spirometry tests to measure a patient's respiratory accessory muscle strength. Neither is intended to exercise the patient's muscles to increase strength over time. Trendelenburg positioning is used in some surgical procedures and in some postural drainage positions. Although the patient may have to work harder to breathe with his or her head down, this position is not used to increase respiratory muscle strength.

Chapter 8

1. **C.** The patient's signs and symptoms indicate hyperventilation. The easiest way to correct this situation is to have the patient breathe more slowly (and/or less deeply). If the patient continues to breathe in the same pattern, the hyperventilation will continue. Although albuterol may cause tachycardia, it is unlikely to cause dizziness and tingling fingers in the patient. If the patient is advised to breathe deeper and faster, the hyperventilation will get worse.

2. **A.** Adding 100 mL of aerosol tubing as a reservoir will help to increase the amount of inhaled medication

and maintain the patient's inspired O_2 percentage. Increasing the flow of oxygen will make the nebulizer dispense the medication more quickly and waste more of it. Decreasing the oxygen flow may result in the nebulizer not working properly and could decrease the patient's O_2 percentage. If the patient were told not to breathe deeply, less medication would be inhaled into the lungs.

3. **D.** An MDI with VHC is the only practical way to deliver this type of medication to a small child. In addition, a face mask will probably need to be attached to the VHC. A DPI necessitates an inspiratory flow that is too high for a small child. Holding chambers are not used with a DPI. Some small children may be able to use an SVN with mouthpiece. However, the MDI with VHC and face mask is the better choice.

4. **A.** Hypertonic saline (1.8%-10%) is the most widely used liquid for an initial induced sputum procedure. If the patient finds it too irritating, normal saline (0.9% saline) or hypotonic saline (0.45% saline) may be used. Distilled water is never used.

5. **B.** Upper (larger) airway deposition is enhanced by V_T breathing at a normal speed and in a normal pattern. A slowly inhaled IC would increase the change of deposition of medication in smaller airways, not larger airways.

6. **C.** An ultrasonic nebulizer generates the greatest quantity of aerosol particles from among the listed choices. An aerosol mask is appropriate for an adult. A hand-held nebulizer used every 4 hours does not deliver enough aerosol fast enough to help the patient, as the ultrasonic nebulizer would. A mist tent is not appropriate for an adult. A cascade-type humidifier does not deliver an aerosol that meets the patient's needs.

7. **D.** A pass-over-type humidifier that is heated to near body temperature will provide almost 100% of the patient's body humidity needs. All the other devices are much cooler than body temperature and provide a lower humidity level.

8. **C.** The small, uniform droplet size produced by the ultrasonic unit is a reason for its use. It should not be used to nebulize all medications because vibrations of the ultrasonic unit may break down the drug.

9. **C.** An unheated bubble-type humidifier delivers humidity at room temperature or cooler. All of the other units deliver humidity or aerosol at a warmer temperature.

10. **D.** The absolute humidity of 44 mg/L is found in the airways of a person at normal body temperature.

11. **A.** Condensation will occur because the saturated air is heated to above room temperature and will cool down as it goes through the tubing. The air will stay saturated with water vapor despite the cooling.

12. **C.** Backpressure on the humidifier will make the pop-off valve whistle. Pinched tubing could cause this. The

delivered O_2 flow does not affect the pop-off valve. If a leak occurs between the reservoir jar and the top of the humidifier, the gas will not leak out of the pop-off valve.

13. **B.** An infant with laryngotracheobronchitis (or croup) usually is best managed with a *cool*, bland aerosol. This helps to reduce swelling in the large airways. Body-temperature aerosol is delivered to a patient with a tracheostomy or thick (viscous) secretions to minimize the patient's humidity deficit. A hypothermic patient is given body temperature or warmer aerosol to speed up warming.

14. **D.** A nebulizer will fail because of too little water in the reservoir, a clogged jet, or a clogged capillary line to the reservoir. Air entrainment nebulizers do not have one-way valves. O_2 flows down a capillary tube in a bubble-type humidifier.

15. **D.** Particles in the 1- to 3-μm range will penetrate to the alveoli. All other sizes will affect the airways.

16. **C.** Low water level in the couplant chamber will cause the light to flash. No other indicators help with troubleshooting.

17. **C.** Wastewater should be emptied out of the tubing to prevent contamination. The water level in the reservoir jar has nothing to do with water in the tubing.

18. **D.** The three listed criteria all indicate that the patient's inhaled air is saturated completely with water vapor at body temperature.

19. **B.** The best way for the patient to deposit an aerosol in small airways and alveoli is to slowly inhale an IC with a breath-hold when the lungs are full. A rapidly inhaled V_T tends to deposit aerosol in the larger airways.

20. **D.** Any of the following will result in delivery of less or no aerosol: (1) if the nebulizer is not tightly screwed into the DISS connector on the flowmeter, the gas will leak and will not go through the nebulizer; (2) if the nebulizer jet is obstructed, no aerosol will be created; (3) if the water level is below the refill line on the nebulizer's reservoir jar, no water will be drawn up the capillary tube to the jet and baffle; therefore no aerosol will be created; or (4) if the capillary tube is obstructed, the water in the reservoir jar will not be drawn up to the jet and baffle. However, if the water level is *above* the refill line on the nebulizer's reservoir jar water, water will be drawn up the capillary tube to the jet and baffle. Aerosol will be generated if everything else is functioning normally.

21. **A.** It is likely that a patient who has chronic bronchitis is always producing secretions. So, it is important to know if the volume has gone up or down recently. If the volume of secretions has gone down or the secretions are thicker, aerosol therapy may be helpful. Because the patient probably is taking pulmonary-related medications, it is important to know whether

they are helping his breathing. If his medications are not effective, the physician should evaluate the patient and consider a change. Hours of sleep at night and exercise tolerance are important to know but do not relate directly to secretions and the need for aerosol therapy.

22. **C.** A vibrating-mesh nebulizer is electrically powered by batteries or AC/DC current. The other three types of nebulizers require a compressed gas source. This would make them less than ideal when traveling frequently.

23. **C.** It is likely that this dehydrated patient also has dried secretions. When continuous aerosol therapy was started, her secretions absorbed the aerosol and swelled in size. The swollen secretions could block small airways, resulting in shortness of breath and crackles for breath sounds. Intravenous fluids should reduce her dehydration. Even if she were more dehydrated, this would not cause her new signs and symptoms. Although it is possible that her influenza may be getting worse, it is unlikely to result in these new signs and symptoms. Normal saline is a bland aerosol that should not cause any allergic reactions such as the ones the patient is demonstrating.

24. **A.** A heated humidifier is the best device for humidifying the airway of a patient receiving invasive mechanical ventilation. This will ensure that every breath is warmed and humidified. An HME may be used in some patients who will require invasive mechanical ventilation for only a relatively short time. It is not acceptable to provide only intermittent nebulized bland aerosol. The patient will be breathing dry gas between these treatments.

25. **C.** Severe coughing and wheezing so quickly after the DPI medication is taken indicate an adverse reaction. Treatment should be stopped. The physician should be contacted about the possible need for an inhaled bronchodilator medication. Because it is possible that the rapidly inhaled breath triggered the cough and wheezing, the patient should not do it again. Breathing slowly through the DPI will not aerosolize the medication powder. No order states that more than the ordered dose of corticosteroid should be given. In addition, a corticosteroid is a controller-type medication and will not help a person with acute bronchospasm.

26. **B.** Most patients receiving noninvasive ventilation (NIV) find it more comfortable when they receive humidification. Because of this they are more likely to keep the NIV mask on. So, a wick-type (heated) humidifier is the best choice. A large-volume nebulizer would provide an aerosol rather than humidity. An HME is not recommended for NIV.

27. **A.** Humidity deficit will be *decreased* by aerosol therapy. Some patients with hypersensitive airways could have bronchospasm after inhaling a bland aerosol. Infants can become fluid overloaded with prolonged aerosol therapy. Dried secretions can absorb water and can swell up to block small airways.

28. **D.** A lung abscess is a serious infection. If the patient has this problem, the secretions would have a foul odor, would contain cellular debris, and would have a dark yellow or green color. If the secretions were collected and saved, they would settle out into three layers, as is shown in Figure 1-26. Review Table 1-12 and related discussion in Chapter 1, if needed. Specific gravity is performed on a urine specimen, not on secretions. Although some blood may be evident in secretions, a platelet count is not performed on a secretion sample.

Chapter 9

1. **A.** Lasix is a diuretic and is known to cause patients to urinate large amounts of potassium. The loss of potassium can result in cardiac arrhythmia. Giving more Lasix could worsen the loss of potassium. No indication is given that the patient has a life-threatening arrhythmia that needs to be defibrillated. There is no indication to give epinephrine.

2. **C.** Caffeine citrate (Cafcit) is known to be a respiratory center stimulant in infants and will stimulate breathing. This should help to prevent the apnea spells. Xylocaine is a local anesthetic agent. It is used to numb an injury or to stop cardiac arrhythmias, such as premature ventricular contractions. Prostigmin is used to reverse the paralyzing effects of nondepolarizing neuromuscular blocking agents such as Pavulon. Albuterol is a short-acting beta-adrenergic bronchodilator. It does not stimulate breathing.

3. **A.** Morphine is indicated to relieve severe, acute pain. In addition to controlling the pain, morphine will sedate the patient. Advil is not effective against severe pain. Anectine is a paralyzing medication. Atrovent is a parasympatholytic (anticholinergic) medication.

4. **C.** QVAR is an inhaled corticosteroid that is widely used to treat asthma. Narcan is a reversing agent for morphine and related opium-based drugs. Prostigmin is a reversing agent for nondepolarizing neuromuscular blocking agents. Solu-Medrol is a steroid taken by pill or intravenously for systemic effects.

5. **B.** Combivent Respimat combines a sympathomimetic (albuterol) agent and an anticholinergic (ipratropium) agent for effective bronchodilation. Vanceril is an inhaled corticosteroid medication and Singulair is a leukotriene blocker. Atrovent is an anticholinergic agent and Intal is a mast cell stabilizer. Serevent is a long-duration sympathomimetic agent and fluticasone is an inhaled corticosteroid.

6. **A.** MicroNefrin will stimulate the α-receptors in the mucous membrane of the patient's airway to cause vasoconstriction and reduce edema. Mucomyst is a mucolytic. Xopenex and Isoetharine HCl are beta-adrenergic agents with no α-receptor effect.

7. **D.** All four of these medication classes can be helpful to a patient with COPD. The inhaled corticosteroid will help to reduce airway inflammation and will increase the effectiveness of the beta-agonist drugs. The long-acting beta-agonist and anticholinergic will provide sustained bronchodilation. The short-acting beta-agonist is used as a rescue bronchodilation medication if needed.

8. **C.** The physician should be contacted because 5 mL is too large a dose of Proventil. A respiratory therapist should know not to give this large a dose even if the order is written. A respiratory therapist should not alter a written order from a physician or presume to know what a physician might want to do.

9. **C.** Pulmozyme is indicated in patients with cystic fibrosis who have pulmonary infection and thick secretions. A normal saline solution is not the most effective option for liquefying secretions. Mucomyst has no effect against purulent secretions with bacterial DNA. In addition, Mucomyst is not currently recommended by aerosol or tracheal instillation in this patient with cystic fibrosis.

10. **B.** Review the first two drug dosage calculations shown in Module C to see how to set up this problem.

11. **C.** It is commonly accepted that an aerosolized bronchodilator treatment should be stopped if the patient's pulse rate increases by 20% or more (from 85 to $\geq$102 beats/min).

12. **D.** Tremor, headache, nervousness and irritability, and tachycardia are all known possible adverse effects.

13. **A.** Brovana is a long-duration medication indicated in stable patients with bronchospasm. The other medications are all sympathomimetic bronchodilators with a shorter duration of action.

14. **B.** Hypertonic (10%) saline is commonly used to induce a sputum sample in patients with tuberculosis. Pulmozyme is indicated in patients with cystic fibrosis who have purulent secretions. Mucomyst is no longer recommended because of likely complications such as bronchospasm. Isoniazid is the most widely used antibiotic against TB.

15. **A.** Xopenex is a fast-acting sympathomimetic bronchodilator that should help to prevent a bronchospasm reaction from Mucomyst. Sterile water and normal saline are not bronchodilators and can cause bronchospasm in some asthmatic patients. Nembutal is a barbiturate.

16. **D.** Aminophylline is recognized as a medication that may be beneficial to a patient with status asthmaticus after inhaled bronchodilators and corticosteroids have been given. If a fast-onset beta-agonist bronchodilator such as albuterol (in Combivent Respimat) has not been effective, it is doubtful if Proventil (more albuterol) or Brethaire would be effective. Foradil is a long-acting beta-agonist bronchodilator that is not given for a fast effect.

17. **B.** Although adrenaline is an ultrashort-acting beta-agonist bronchodilator, it is not used to prevent or treat an asthma attack. It is used in a CPR effort to increase the patient's heart rate and blood pressure. Intal, Accolate, and Zyflo are all used as prophylactic agents to prevent an asthma attack. Intal stabilizes mast cells to prevent the release of leukotriene agents. Accolate and Zyflo block the effect of released leukotriene agents.

18. **C.** Treatment should be stopped because the patient's heart rate has increased by more than 20%. Monitor the patient's heart rate to find out if it returns to normal; chart the results. Only the physician can order a change in type of medication or medication amount. Only the physician can terminate treatment. Adding more saline to the medication will dilute the mixture but not reduce the amount of medication the patient receives. The same adverse reaction will probably happen again.

19. **D.** Decreasing the dose of Proventil is reasonable because it may be causing the patient's heart rate to increase. Adding saline will not reduce the total amount of medication that the patient will receive. There is no need to stop the treatment at this point based on the 15% increase in her heart rate.

20. **D.** Romazicon reverses a barbiturate medication, and Narcan reverses a narcotic medication in the patient. After the sedation is reversed, the patient should breathe spontaneously. Intropin is used to raise blood pressure. Anectine is a depolarizing neuromuscular blocking agent. Valium is a barbiturate.

21. **A.** Review the third and fourth drug dosage calculations shown earlier in the chapter to see how to set up this problem (Module C).

22. **A.** The patient's treatment can be continued because his heart rate has not increased by at least 20% from the baseline. The therapist cannot change a medication or decrease a medication amount without the physician's approval.

23. **B.** Ampicillin is used against gram-positive bacteria. Virazole is used against RSV. Garamycin and TOBI are used against gram-negative bacterial pneumonia.

24. **A.** Virazole has been approved by the FDA for the treatment of RSV. NebuPent is nebulized and Bactrim is given systemically to treat *P. carinii*. Garamycin is used against gram-positive bacteria.

25. **A.** Flumazenil (Romazicon) is used to reverse the effects of the benzodiazepine-type sedative agents (Valium, Versed). There is no indication that the patient had been given a sedative. The other three drugs (Survanta, Infasurf, Curosurf) are used in surfactant replacement therapy in neonates with RDS.

26. **B.** The patient's continued wheezing justifies more medication. The small increase in heart rate does not justify stopping the treatment. Ventolin will not be any more effective than Xopenex. Aminophylline

is not indicated at this time. First, find out if more Xopenex causes bronchodilation.

27. **C.** A patient with status asthmaticus should be admitted to the Intensive Care Unit (ICU) for expert care. An intravenous corticosteroid will reduce her airway inflammation. Xopenex is a fast-onset bronchodilator that is indicated for continuous nebulization. Continuous ECG monitoring should be performed to observe tachycardia or arrhythmia. Continuous pulse oximetry should be performed to monitor oxygen level. Serevent is a slow-onset, long-duration bronchodilator that is indicated in stable patients with asthma.

28. **D.** A sedative agent will have a calming effect on a patient anxious about being unable to move or communicate while paralyzed on the ventilator. A sedative will not control pain or sustain a pharmacologic paralysis. Although a high enough dose of a sedative will put a patient to sleep and therefore prevent "fighting" the ventilator, that is not its primary purpose. In addition, if the patient is pharmacologically paralyzed, no need exists for any other medication to control the patient's breathing efforts.

29. **A.** Epinephrine has vasoconstricting properties (as well as properties causing bronchodilation and tachycardia) and should help to stop bleeding at the biopsy site. Intravenous heparin is contraindicated because it increases clotting time and will probably increase the bleeding. Albuterol (Proventil) is a very effective bronchodilator but has no effect on peripheral blood vessels. Lidocaine (Xylocaine) is used to stop cardiac arrhythmias but has no effect on peripheral blood vessels.

30. **B.** Hypertonic (1.8%-10%) saline has been shown to be an effective mucolytic in patients with cystic fibrosis. Acetylcysteine (Mucomyst) is no longer recommended for cystic fibrosis patients because of possible complications from long-term use. Serevent is a long-acting bronchodilator and not a mucolytic. Normal (0.9%) saline will not be as effective a mucolytic as hypertonic saline.

31. **D.** Increasing the dose of albuterol should improve the patient's bronchodilation and result in an improved peak flow. Because the patient's peak flow is only 65% of personal best, the albuterol dose should not be maintained or decreased. Adding an intravenous corticosteroid to the patient's medications would require the home care patient to travel to the physician's office for injections. This is not a practical solution. In addition, no clear indication exists that intravenous corticosteroids are needed at this time.

32. **B.** INO$_{max}$ is a very effective pulmonary vasodilator in neonatal patients. Surfaxin is a type of synthetic surfactant used in neonates with RDS. Anoro combines a long-acting anticholinergic drug and an ultralong-acting beta-agonist drug. It has been approved only for the treatment of COPD.

33. **A.** Flumazenil (Romazicon) is used to reverse the effects of benzodiazepine-type sedative agents (Versed, Valium). Rather than calming a patient, flumazenil is used to reverse the effects of oversedation. Pancuronium bromide (Pavulon) and succinylcholine (Anectine) are medications used to paralyze a patient. This will certainly result in the patient's breathing being controlled by the ventilator. Morphine sulfate (Duramorph) is given to control pain and will have a secondary benefit of sedating the patient if enough is given.

34. **A.** Adrenaline will cause vasoconstriction of the systemic blood vessels to raise the patient's blood pressure. In addition, the laryngeal blood vessels will constrict and reduce the airway swelling. Adrenaline is also a bronchodilator. Advil has some anti-inflammatory properties but will not have any effect on the patient's low blood pressure. Nebulized racemic epinephrine (Nephron) is useful with upper airway edema but will not have enough systemic effect to raise the blood pressure significantly. Narcan is a reversing agent for the narcotic-type analgesics.

35. **D.** Tobramycin (TOBI) has been approved by the FDA to prevent the development of *P. aeruginosa* pneumonia in cystic fibrosis patients. Pentamidine (Pentam or NebuPent) has been approved by the FDA to prevent the development of *P. carinii* pneumonia, not *P. aeruginosa* pneumonia. Isoniazid (INH) is used to prevent or treat a TB infection.

36. **B.** Ribavirin (Vibrazole) is given to stop the reproduction of RSV. It is given by the SPAG II nebulizer. Racemic epinephrine (MicroNefrin) is a vasoconstricting drug and is given by SVN to shrink edematous mucous membranes of the upper airway. Intratracheal beractant (Survanta) is given to a premature neonate with RDS. It would not be needed in this older patient who has recovered from the condition. Cromolyn sodium (Intal) is given by SVN to prevent the onset of asthma. It is not effective against RSV.

37. **B.** NebuPent is given by SVN once every 4 weeks as a preventative agent for *P. carinii* pneumonia. Bactrim is the preferred medication to treat an actual *P. carinii* pneumonia infection. TOBI is given by SVN to treat a cystic fibrosis patient with *P. aeruginosa* pneumonia. Relenza is given to treat influenza, a viral infection.

38. **A.** The potassium level of 3.1 mEq/L is lower than normal. Her PVCs could be caused by the hypokalemia. She should be given intravenous potassium to raise her K$^+$ level into the normal range. Giving more diuretic medication and restricting her potassium could be dangerous. It would be best to continue 40% oxygen until her lung function has further improved.

39. **B.** Breo combines a corticosteroid (fluticasone) and ultralong-acting beta-agonist (vilanterol) that needs

to be taken only once a day. Spiriva is an ultralong-acting anticholinergic that needs to be taken only once a day. These two drugs include all three classes of bronchodilator medications with the longest duration available. (In addition, the patient should also have available a short-acting beta-adrenergic "rescue" medication such as albuterol.) Combivent Respimat combines a short-acting anticholinergic (ipratropium) and short-acting beta-agonist (albuterol) that has a duration of only 4-6 hours. Dulera combines an inhaled corticosteroid (mometasone) and beta-agonist bronchodilator (formoterol) that has a duration of 12 hours. Anoro combines an anticholinergic (umeclidinium) and beta-agonist (vilanterol) with 24 hours duration.

Chapter 10

1. **C.** PEP therapy has been shown to help in mobilizing secretions. In addition, some PEP units can be coupled with an SVN to more efficiently deliver the medication. Incentive spirometry does not help with secretion mobilization or medication delivery. IPPB *may* help with medication delivery if the patient cannot properly perform the SVN treatment. However, no indication of this problem exists. The benefits of improperly positioning a patient for PDT are questionable. (See Box 10-5.)

2. **D.** Manual percussion should be performed with a cupped hand and relaxed wrist and elbow joints.

3. **C.** Vibration should be performed only on expiration. Most people cannot vibrate at a faster rate than about 3 cycles/s.

4. **C.** There is no reason that a bedridden patient with a small vital capacity cannot have CPT. Head-down positions place a patient with a recent stroke or known increased intracranial pressure at risk for further brain damage. A patient who has just eaten should not be placed in a head-down position because of the risk of vomiting. (See Box 10-2.)

5. **A.** Regular turning is an easy and inexpensive way for the patient to alter his breathing pattern and to move the V_T into different lung segments. This helps to prevent atelectasis. PEP and IPPB may be needed, but only after regular turning has been shown to be ineffective. CPAP is not indicated for the treatment of simple atelectasis from inactivity.

6. **D.** The lateral basal, superior, and posterior basal segments are all located in the right lower lobe where the infiltrates are located. The apical segment is located in the upper lobe, and the medial segment is located in the middle lobe. (Review Figs. 10-6, 7, and 9.)

7. **C.** A bedside spirometer is not needed because the patient's exhaled volume does not need to be measured. In addition, a spirometer cannot be connected to the unit for volume measurement. All of the other listed items are needed. The variable orifice resistor is needed to set the level of expiratory resistance. A pressure manometer is needed to determine that the expiratory pressure is kept in the 10- to 20-cm water range. An SVN with reservoir is needed to deliver the albuterol. (See Fig. 10-21, A.)

8. **B.** Many references indicate that percussion and vibration are beneficial in mobilizing large quantities of secretions. Review Box 10-2 for contraindications for percussion and vibration.

9. **A.** Review Figure 10-8 for the recommended position to drain the anterior basal segment of the right lower lobe.

10. **A.** When the patient exhales through a larger hole, the pressure should decrease and the expiratory time should shorten. Review Box 10-9 for the steps to be followed in the PEP therapy procedure. Having the patient exhale faster or exhale through a smaller hole increases the pressure and expiratory time. A bronchodilator medication has not been ordered for the patient.

11. **C.** Because an empyema is a collection of pus in the pleural cavity, it cannot be drained through postural drainage. The other options are all indications for postural drainage. See Box 10-1 for the indications.

12. **C.** Neither manual nor mechanical percussion or vibration should be performed over female breast tissue. (See Box 10-2.)

13. **B.** It is likely that the patient coughed secretions into the unit. Check for an obstruction. If one is present, it must be removed. A cotton swab or warm running water should remove any secretions. The patient blows out (does not breathe in) through the Flutter valve. It is not an incentive spirometer device. Removing the steel ball from the device will prevent it from working as intended. If the patient blows out hard, the obstruction may be blown deeper into the unit.

14. **A.** Hypoxemia is the only possibility for the problem from among those listed. A full stomach does not cause vagal stimulation that results in PVCs. The patient's symptoms of SOB and PVCs do not correspond with increased intracranial pressure or increased venous return to the heart.

15. **A.** Switching to an electrically powered percussor is the only workable option from among those provided. A pneumatically powered percussor does not have batteries or an electrical cord. The way that the percussor gradually lost function indicates that the tank did not have any compressed O_2 with which to run the unit.

16. **D.** Try another type of pad on the percussor to determine whether it is more comfortable for the patient. A flat one is probably best for the lower back. The patient is not having a reaction to the head-down position and does not need to sit up. No indication exists that the patient is hypoxic. Increasing the speed on the percussor is likely to increase the skin irritation.

17. **C.** A properly trained caregiver can perform CPT on an infant. As the child grows older, he or she can take a more active role in the therapy. Often a child of about 4 years can learn OPEP therapy. By the age of 6, ACBT can be taught. A child will usually have to be about 10-12 years of age to learn IPV and AD because of their complexity.

18. **B.** By changing the expiratory resistance to a larger diameter orifice, the patient will be able to exhale more quickly. Telling the patient to blow out harder will increase the pressure within the system. This could increase the patient's discomfort. Changing the expiratory resistance to a smaller-diameter orifice will further increase the expiratory time, not decrease it. Although a PEP system can have oxygen added to it to power the nebulizer, no mention of one is made in the question. In addition, the use of supplemental oxygen to a nebulizer does not have any effect on the expiratory time of the patient. (See Fig. 10-21, A.)

19. **A.** All available IPV machines include an SVN so that a medication can be delivered with the IPV breaths. The initial settings for an IPV treatment should include a low pressure (and low rate). As the patient gains comfort with the treatment, the pressure and rate can be increased as tolerated.

20. **D.** The patient should sit up because tachycardia and dyspnea are definite indications of intolerance of the head-down position. It could be dangerous for the patient to continue in the head-down position for even 5 more minutes. The treatment should be stopped, and the patient should sit up rather than being turned to the other side. Give the patient supplemental oxygen only if it is determined that the patient is hypoxic after the patient sits up. (See Box 10-3.)

21. **A.** It is reasonable to increase the PEP level from 5 to 10 cm water. Have the patient try this moderately increased pressure for several minutes, and evaluate the effectiveness of the patient's cough effort. The PEP level should not be increased to 15 cm water unless 10 cm water has been shown to be ineffective. Incentive spirometry is indicated for atelectasis or the prevention of atelectasis. It is not indicated for secretion clearance, as is PEP therapy. It is too early in the treatment to determine that PEP therapy should be discontinued.

22. **A.** To drain the lateral basal segment of the left lower lobe, the patient must be placed with the right side down on the bed and the head of the bed dropped 30 degrees. The other positions will not properly drain the left lower lobe. Review the postural drainage positions if needed. (See Fig. 10-7.)

23. **A.** Review Figure 10-11 for the proper position to drain the superior and inferior lingula segments.

24. **D.** The Flutter is designed to cause rapid airway vibrations. These vibrations result in a rapid variation in airway pressure. This results in the airways rapidly dilating and then contracting to their resting diameter. These changes seem to loosen secretions so that they can be expectorated more easily by the patient. Neither increased transpleural pressure nor increased intrapleural pressure has any effect on the mobilization of secretions.

25. **B.** PEP therapy will increase end-expiratory lung pressure. This should increase alveolar volume and prevent the development of atelectasis. Blow bottles are no longer in use because they have been shown to be ineffective in the management of atelectasis. A mechanical chest percussor can be used with CPT to help mobilize secretions. However, it does not have any benefit in preventing atelectasis. Inspiratory muscle training is beneficial in patients with chronic obstructive lung disease because they are usually deconditioned. This should be part of a general conditioning program. However, inspiratory muscle training has no direct effect on atelectasis and should not be confused with use of an incentive spirometer. (See Box 10-5.)

26. **A.** The patient must sit up straight because the vest is ridged. To work best, it should have even contact with the patient's entire chest wall. This would not happen if the patient were lying on a side. It is best to have the patient start at the lowest rate and pressure to gain confidence in the unit and not risk injury. The HFCWO unit does not have a nebulizer.

27. **B.** The position described would be used to drain secretions from the patient's posterior segment of the right upper lobe. See Figure 1-16 for the area of consolidation, Figure 10-5 for all lung segments, and Figure 10-12 for the postural drainage position.

28. **C.** Hemoptysis indicates pulmonary trauma. The treatment should be stopped and the physician notified. No further treatment should be done until after the patient is assessed and it is found safe to proceed with the treatment. (See Box 10-3.)

29. **D.** According to the AARC *Clinical Practice Guideline* (1991), CPT (postural drainage, percussion, and vibration) should be discontinued when the patient is able to expectorate secretions without other assistance. Continuing the treatment and adding procedures are not necessary and may unnecessarily add to the patient's costs.

30. **D.** CPAP is indicated to increase a patient's functional residual capacity to improve oxygenation. It has no effect on secretions. OPEP therapy, the Quake, and HFCWO have all been shown to be effective at mobilizing secretions. (See Box 10-5.)

31. **B.** The Acapella unit is inexpensive and easy for most patients to learn to use. HFCWO and IPV are expensive and complicated technologies. ACBT is not a form of high-frequency airway oscillation.

32. **C.** MIE is indicated in a patient with a neuromuscular condition or spinal cord injury who has a peak cough

flow (peak flow) of <270 L/min (<4.5 L/s). A patient using HFCWO or PEP should be able to perform a normal cough to clear secretions. CPT should not be performed on a patient with an unstable spinal cord injury. Further injury could be caused by changing the drainage positions.

Chapter 11

1. **B.** See Figure 11-22 for a tracing and explanation of a PVC.

2. **B.** Current CPR guidelines state that effective ventilation can be achieved by an endotracheal tube, mouth-to-valve resuscitator, or manual resuscitator. A pneumatic (demand-valve) resuscitator is not recommended for use because it is difficult to control the delivered tidal volume and air tends to be forced into the patient's stomach.

3. **A.** ECG monitoring is justified because the patient's signs and symptoms could indicate a cardiac problem. An exercise program is not indicated in this situation and could be dangerous for the patient. A peak flow test is not indicated now and would not help with the diagnosis of exercise-induced asthma. It is best to wait at least 10 minutes after putting O_2 on a patient before drawing an ABG sample to check on the patient's O_2 level. Even if the ABG sample shows hypoxemia, there is no indication of the cause.

4. **B.** Defibrillation is indicated if the patient has VT and is without pulse or blood pressure. The patient should then be evaluated for full CPR efforts. The other options would delay effective treatment.

5. **C.** See Figure 11-22 for a tracing of a PVC and explanation. *Unifocal* means that all of the PVCs originate from a single area. *Multifocal* means that PVCs originate from more than one area.

6. **C.** A portable defibrillator must be with the patient in case it is needed. The other items are useful for monitoring but offer no way to treat a life-threatening arrhythmia.

7. **A.** Direct instillation into the patient's airways and lungs offers the fastest way to administer the medications when an IV line is not available.

8. **D.** Defibrillation should be performed as quickly as possible when a patient is in ventricular fibrillation. Figure 11-26 shows another example. All of the other options delay effective treatment.

9. **C.** Reversing the arm electrodes results in the heart's electrical signal being received by the ECG machine in the opposite direction of normal. This results in reversal of the ECG signal. A loose electrode or shivering would cause different types of artifacts. Miscalibration would not cause inversion of the QRS complex.

10. **A.** Blood flow through the coronary arteries can be performed only during a left-heart catheterization procedure. Right-heart catheterization evaluates the valves and functioning of the right side of the heart.

A stress echocardiogram is helpful to evaluate the pumping ability of the left ventricle but does not evaluate the coronary arteries. A 12-lead ECG is diagnostic for a heart attack but does not directly evaluate the condition of the coronary arteries.

11. **C.** An echocardiogram is indicated to evaluate the functioning of the mitral valve (and other heart valves) and blood flow through it. If there is a leak through the mitral valve, the echocardiogram will detect the blood flow. Because the mitral valve is on the left side of the heart, a right-heart catheterization could not detect any problem with it. A PA chest radiograph will indicate the size of the heart but is not able to detect any valve problems. A stress test will evaluate the patient's ability to exercise. But, any limitation cannot be specified to the mitral or any other heart valve.

12. **A.** The CK-MB and troponin I tests are specific for an MI. If the patient has had an MI, these two values will be elevated. The D-dimer test is diagnostic for a pulmonary embolism. It would be elevated with a PE but normal with an MI. The BUN (blood urea nitrogen) test is done to evaluate kidney function. The LDL (low density lipoprotein) test is one of several tests done to evaluate a patient's cholesterol values. A high LDL value is a risk factor for heart disease but is not specific for an MI.

13. **B.** A mouth-to-valve device allows for quick ventilations without the risk of an infection being spread from the patient to the rescuer. Mouth-to-mouth ventilation should be avoided if possible in this situation. The other options would unnecessarily delay ventilations.

14. **D.** All are correct except that the air/O_2 intake valve should not open when the resuscitation bag is squeezed. This allows the gas to escape rather than be directed to the patient.

15. **D.** The femoral site is recommended because it is a large artery that should be relatively easy to hit and is away from the patient's chest during compressions.

16. **C.** It is easy and quick to check the valve for proper position. Fix the valve if necessary, and attempt to ventilate the patient again. Because the patient's pulse has not yet been checked, there is no indication that chest compressions are needed. Getting a lateral neck radiograph will greatly delay (probably fatally) ventilating the patient. There is not yet an indication that the patient needs abdominal thrusts to clear an airway obstruction. If the patient cannot be ventilated by the fixed mouth-to-valve resuscitation device, check for an obvious obstruction in the mouth or throat. Reposition the head, and attempt to ventilate again. If the patient still cannot be ventilated, then perform abdominal thrusts.

17. **D.** See the text listing in Module C of the identifying traits of NSR. See Figure 11-2 showing a tracing of NSR and Table 11-1.

18. **D.** Sinus arrhythmia is shown in Figure 11-8. Review the associated discussion if needed. In a patient receiving mechanical ventilation and PEEP, it is possible to put too much pressure on the heart, which reduces venous return. If the returning blood volume is decreased, the cardiac output also will decrease. The patient should be monitored and key people informed. It is too early to decide whether the PEEP level is too high and should be reduced. The physician should be consulted before making any change. Atropine will increase the patient's heart rate and is not indicated in this situation. No indication suggests that the patient has an arrhythmia that requires synchronized cardioversion.

19. **A.** ECG monitoring will not provide any useful information about peripheral perfusion. The patient could have a normal heart rhythm and have altered perfusion. Electrolyte disturbances, especially the potassium (K^+) level, can alter the heart's electrical conduction system. It is wise to monitor a patient with a known history of arrhythmias in case they return. Fast or excessive infusion of potassium can lead to serious arrhythmias that justify ECG monitoring.

20. **B.** The rhythm strip shows two identical premature ventricular contractions (unifocal PVCs). This, combined with the patient's history of sudden chest pain and shortness of breath, suggests a heart problem. A 12-lead ECG is indicated for the physician to be able to determine the patient's cardiac condition. Oxygen is indicated for the shortness of breath. In addition, the oxygen will help the heart if it is hypoxic. The patient's condition is not life threatening, and no need is seen for either synchronized cardioversion or defibrillation. A cardiac catheterization procedure is needed to identify any coronary artery blockages before angioplasty is indicated.

21. **D.** Current ACLS guidelines state that atropine, epinephrine (both for bradycardia), and lidocaine (to suppress ventricular arrhythmias) can be given via the endotracheal tube during a CPR attempt if the patient does not have a functioning IV line. Potassium chloride can be given only intravenously.

22. **A.** The rhythm strip shows ventricular fibrillation. The best way to treat this dangerous arrhythmia is to defibrillate the patient immediately. All of the other listed options are reasonable in a CPR attempt when appropriate. However, they are all secondary to treating the patient's ventricular fibrillation.

23. **C.** Interpretation of the patient's ABG results shows hyperventilation with a metabolic acidosis. Intravenous sodium bicarbonate should be given to correct the patient's acidosis. It is appropriate to keep the patient's PaO_2 at 210 torr during the CPR attempt to try to oxygenate the brain. Decreasing the respiratory rate or adding mechanical dead space to the manual resuscitator will increase the patient's carbon dioxide and further reduce the pH. If necessary, review ABG interpretation in Chapter 3.

24. **B.** Current ACLS guidelines state that atropine, epinephrine, and lidocaine can be given via the endotracheal tube during a CPR attempt if the patient does not have a functioning IV line. Intraosseous (within the bone) injection of CPR drugs is approved for neonatal resuscitation attempts. Intracardiac injection of CPR drugs is no longer performed. Only Narcan can be given by the nasal route.

25. **A.** The patient's symptoms indicate a cardiac problem. It is wise to begin ECG monitoring quickly in case the patient has an arrhythmia. An ABG sample can be drawn after ECG monitoring has been started. A chest radiograph also can be done after ECG monitoring has been started. A capnometer value to check the patient's exhaled carbon dioxide value is not indicated at this time.

26. **C.** Pulseless ventricular tachycardia is a life-threatening arrhythmia. (See Fig. 11-24.) If the rate is so fast that a pulse cannot be felt, the cardiac output and blood pressure will be very low. The patient must be defibrillated as soon as possible to restore NSR. Second-degree heart block is treated with drugs or a pacemaker to speed the heart rate. Atrial flutter and sinus tachycardia are fast, but not life-threatening arrhythmias that are first treated with medications to slow the heart rate.

27. **B.** Intravenous naloxone (Narcan) can be given to reverse the sedating effect of the anesthetic drugs that passed from the mother to the infant. Epinephrine and atropine are cardiac stimulants, not breathing stimulants. Bag/mask ventilation may be needed but will not get the sedated infant to breathe by itself.

28. **D.** Giving intravenous epinephrine should increase the patient's heart rate and blood pressure. Lidocaine is given to suppress PVCs. Although the patient is bradycardic and hypotensive, chest compressions are not yet indicated. Because the patient is already being ventilated with supplemental oxygen, endotracheal intubation will not provide any significant improvement.

Chapter 12

1. **C.** Common problems with intubation equipment include a loose or burned-out light bulb in the laryngoscope blade or depleted batteries in the handle. Replacing the blade with one that is larger or smaller than appropriate would make the intubation procedure more difficult and dangerous. A plastic handle cannot be used with a stainless-steel blade.

2. **D.** An oropharyngeal airway is indicated to open the airway of an unconscious patient, protect the airway of a patient with seizures, and prevent an oral endotracheal tube from being bitten. A patient with a tracheostomy does not need an oral airway because he or she is not breathing through the mouth.

An oropharyngeal airway probably should not be inserted into the mouth of a patient with a traumatic jaw injury because of the risk of further injury.

3. **C.** A cuff pressure of up to 30 cm H_2O should be safe for a patient with a normal blood pressure. A cuff pressure of greater than 30 cm H_2O (>22 mm Hg) is likely to place the patient at risk for damage to the mucous membrane of the trachea.

4. **A.** A fenestrated laryngectomy tube will enable him to have esophageal speech through the voice prosthesis. The other tubes will provide only an open airway.

5. **A.** If the tip of the tracheostomy tube has been placed into the subcutaneous tissues, the patient will not be able to ventilate at all. The tube must be immediately withdrawn. Because the tracheotomy site is below the larynx, it does not matter if the patient has closed her epiglottis over the trachea. She still can breathe through the tracheostomy tube. It is unlikely that the new cuff requires any more air than the previous one. Even if this were the case, the patient should still be able to breathe through the tube. It should not be possible to place a tracheostomy tube into a patient's esophagus.

6. **D.** A 9.0-mm-ID oral endotracheal tube is appropriate for a large adult male. Also, the oral tube is more appropriate than a nasal tube in an emergency situation. (See Table 12-1.)

7. **B.** To reduce the risk of ventilator-associated/health care-associated pneumonia, it is recommended to keep the cuff pressure at least 15 mm Hg. A cuff pressure of 10 mm Hg many not be high enough to prevent supraglottic secretions from leaking past the cuff and into the lungs. A cuff pressure of 30 cm water (22 mm Hg) is probably higher than necessary to seal the airway. There is no indication that a larger tube is needed.

8. **B.** A tracheostomy tube is indicated in a patient with trauma to the nose and mouth and an upper airway obstruction. All of the other airway devices would pass through the upper airway.

9. **B.** A 2.5-mm-ID tube would be most appropriate for this size neonate. See Table 12-1 for a listing of tube sizes for the weight or age of the patient.

10. **C.** An adult woman normally has a 7.5 (or 8.0)-mm-ID endotracheal tube inserted. Review Table 12-1 for the recommended sizes of endotracheal and tracheostomy tubes for patients of all sizes.

11. **C.** A disposable colorimetric CO_2 detector would be easy to use and give an immediate indication if the tube were removed from the trachea. A capnography device is expensive and is not designed for easy use in a transport situation. Pulse oximetry will give information on O_2 saturation, not on CO_2 removal from the lungs. An ECG will not give immediate feedback on the patient's condition related to the tube. If the patient were accidentally extubated, both the pulse oximeter and the ECG devices would eventually give information indicating that the patient is in trouble. However, this information is not specific to the patient who has been extubated.

12. **B.** Bowel sounds should not be affected by the placement of a tracheostomy tube. It is highly unlikely that the tracheostomy tube would be accidentally placed into the esophagus, which can happen during the placement of an endotracheal tube. All other items should be monitored.

13. **A.** Placement of the endotracheal tube into the right mainstem bronchus would result in the absence of breath sounds over the left lung. Placement of the tube into the left mainstem bronchus would result in the absence of breath sounds over the right lung. Placement of the tube into the esophagus would result in the absence of breath sounds over both lungs. A right pneumothorax could result in absent breath sounds over the right lung, not over the left lung.

14. **C.** Everything listed, except the Magill forceps, would be needed. These forceps are used only during a nasal intubation procedure. (Review Box 12-4.)

15. **A.** A patient should be extubated when the lungs are full so that the greatest volume of air can be coughed out. This should clear any secretions in the airways. All of the other options would result in less volume in the patient's lungs for coughing.

16. **B.** The tracheostomy tube should be removed quickly if there is evidence that the tube is blocked. In addition, the tracheostomy tube should be replaced with a new one so that a secure airway is maintained.

17. **B.** Right bronchial intubation is indicated by the presence of the patient's breath sounds on the right side but diminished sounds on the left side. There is no direct evidence of a left-sided pneumothorax. The exhaled CO_2 monitor is functioning properly because it is supposed to change color (from dark purple to yellow when exposed to exhaled carbon dioxide) during the breathing cycle. Even a small tidal volume should deliver equal air to both lungs and result in equal breath sounds over both lungs.

18. **A.** A double-lumen tube is indicated because she can receive independent lung ventilation through it. This mode of ventilation would allow her lung with atelectasis to be ventilated differently from her normal lung. None of the other tubes offer this option.

19. **C.** A wire-reinforced (armored) tube would prevent her from biting and collapsing the tube during a seizure. None of the other tubes offer this security.

20. **D.** Substituting a fenestrated tracheostomy tube for the single-cannula tube allows her to breathe spontaneously through the upper airway when the inner cannula is removed. This allows her to talk, which can have a very positive emotional impact on the patient. It is probably going too far to remove the tracheostomy tube when she is off of the ventilator. This

necessitates removing the tube, covering the stoma, and reinserting the tube later in the day. This can lead to damage to the tracheal tissue. In addition, if the patient's condition suddenly deteriorates while the tracheostomy tube is removed, there is no secure airway. Although a speaking-type tracheostomy tube allows her to speak while on the ventilator, it does not enable her to breathe through her upper airway when she is off of the ventilator as a fenestrated tube allows. Replacing the current 7.5-mm-ID tracheostomy tube with one that is 6.0-mm ID greatly increases the patient's work of breathing. This can fatigue the patient and delay her recovery.

21. **B.** A nasopharyngeal airway can be inserted to protect the nasal passage from damage by the suction catheter. An oropharyngeal airway should be used only in unconscious patients and does not protect the nasal passage. There was no mention of the patient having a tracheostomy.

22. **D.** It is best to remove the speaking valve to determine if that is the cause of the dyspnea. If the patient can now breathe comfortably, attach a new speaking valve to the button. If the patient still cannot breathe comfortably, remove the tracheostomy button and reassess the patient.

23. **B.** A laryngeal mask airway is commonly used in the operating room to provide a secure airway without an endotracheal tube. The Combitube is an emergency airway and is not employed in the operating room. Oropharyngeal and nasopharyngeal airways do not provide a secure airway. There is no indication for two nasopharyngeal airways to be used at once.

24. **A.** It could be challenging to place an oral endotracheal tube because the patient has a neck brace. Because of the neck injury, her head cannot be hyperextended. An anesthesiologist would need to be called to perform the intubation. A nasopharyngeal airway, oropharyngeal airway, or LMA can be easily inserted into the patient without the need to hyperextend her neck.

25. **C.** A tracheoesophageal fistula is a risk related to high cuff pressure; it would take several days to develop. The other complications would occur during placement of the tube. (See Box 12-6 for a more complete list of complications.)

26. **D.** In an emergency situation it is fastest and easiest to place an oral endotracheal tube into most patients. A safe and secure airway can usually be ensured within 20-30 seconds. An oropharyngeal airway only keeps the tongue from blocking the back of the throat. It does not provide a safe, secure airway. Hyperextending the patient's neck into the sniff position opens the airway but does not secure it from possible dangers such as vomiting and aspiration. Placing a nasal endotracheal tube requires an anesthesiologist and special equipment. This delay is unnecessary when oral endotracheal intubation can be done by a trained respiratory therapist.

27. **B.** A patient with a cervical spine injury should *not* have his or her neck hyperextended, as is needed during an oral intubation procedure. (See Box 12-5.)

28. **A.** A mild case of stridor is first treated by nebulizing with the vasoconstrictor medication racemic epinephrine. This usually results in enough constriction of the throat's mucous membrane blood vessels to dilate the airway and correct the stridor. If this does not work, the patient may need to be intubated. A cricothyrotomy is done only to create an emergency airway opening if the patient's upper airway is obstructed by a foreign body or trauma. A tracheostomy is performed only if a long-term surgical airway opening is needed. This patient certainly does not need either of the last two solutions to his or her problem.

29. **C.** Because the cuff pressure is so high on the small tracheostomy tube, it is best to replace the tube with one that has an 8.5-mm ID. This is the correct size for an adult man. Increasing the tidal volume by 100 mL may deliver a larger tidal volume or it may just increase the leak around the tracheostomy tube. The actual problem is a tube that is too small for the patient's trachea. It is unsafe to increase the cuff pressure to seal the trachea and stop the tidal volume leak. Although the increased pressure overinflates the cuff to stop the leak, the circulation to the patient's tracheal mucosa is blocked and the mucosa can die. It is unsafe to deflate the cuff enough to reduce the cuff pressure to 20 mm Hg because the patient's tidal volume leak can worsen. (See Table 12-1.)

30. **B.** An adult patient usually has the proximal end of the tube at the 23- to 25-cm mark at the teeth for a midtracheal tube tip position. This, and the observation that the left side of the patient's chest is not moving as much as the right side, indicates that the tube has been pushed down into the right mainstem bronchus. The best thing to do is reposition the tube by suctioning the patient's airways and throat, deflating the cuff, withdrawing the tube about 4 cm, and reinflating the cuff. Of course, check for bilateral breath sounds, confirm a safe cuff pressure, and get a chest radiograph to complete the procedure. There is nothing to be gained by checking the abdominal radiograph because signs of vomiting and aspiration are not seen on it. Pneumonitis can be seen on a chest radiograph but not on an abdominal radiograph because an abdominal radiograph does not include the chest. Checking the patient's end-tidal carbon dioxide level demonstrates exhaled CO_2. However, this is not specific enough for this situation because the right lung can release carbon dioxide even if the left lung is not ventilated. Delivering a larger tidal volume breath does not inflate the left lung any better

because the endotracheal tube has been pushed down the right mainstem bronchus.

31. **D.** All of the listed procedures can be used to confirm that the endotracheal tube is located within the trachea. Clinical experience has shown that the greater the number of positive indicators, the more likely it is that the tube is properly located.

32. **C.** The patient should be reintubated because of the serious nature of the inspiratory stridor that is unresponsive to the inhaled vasoconstricting drug (racemic epinephrine), the low SpO₂ value, and the combative nature of the patient. An ABG value is not necessary because the SpO₂ value of 80% confirms hypoxemia. Getting the ABG sample and waiting for the results only delay the necessary intubation. Increasing the patient to 50% oxygen helps relieve the hypoxemia. However, once the patient is intubated and can breathe adequately, the SpO₂ value should increase to a safe level on the previous 40% oxygen. It could be very dangerous to administer a sedative medication to this patient. Sedating the patient further reduces the patient's ability to breathe through the narrowed airway.

33. **C.** A lateral neck radiograph film will probably not show the location of the distal tip of the tube. A chest radiograph should always be taken to confirm the location of the tube in the trachea. The presence of bilateral or at least right upper lobe breath sounds indicates proper tube placement.

34. **D.** A cuff pressure of 35 mm Hg will cut off venous and arterial blood flow to the tracheal soft tissues. This would result in tracheal wall damage and possibly tracheomalacia, tracheoesophageal fistula, and innominant artery erosion and bleeding. The tracheostomy tube does not pass between the vocal cords and will not injure them.

35. **D.** A properly inserted Combitube will usually be inserted into the esophagus. When the cuff is inflated the patient cannot vomit and the airway is maintained open. While the trachea is occasionally intubated with a Combitube, it is unintentional, and the patient can still vomit. However, because the trachea is intubated the patient cannot aspirate and the airway is secure. (See Box 12-2.)

36. **B.** A nasopharyngeal airway can be easily inserted to push the tongue forward and open the airway. Prone positioning may cause the tongue to move forward and open the airway. More aggressive and invasive procedures, such as placing a tracheostomy button (or tube) or endotracheal intubation, should be used only if the first two options do not work.

37. **A.** A 7.0-mm nasotracheal tube would provide a secure airway and is the appropriate size for an adult female. Because of the nasal route, the tube should be smaller than that chosen for the oral intubation route. The Berman oropharyngeal airway device will support the tongue but does not provide a secure airway. The remaining two endotracheal tubes are too large for the patient whether an oral or nasal intubation is performed. (See Table 12-1.)

38. **A.** With a fenestrated tracheostomy tube, when the inner cannula is removed and the cuff deflated, the patient can breathe through her natural upper airway and speak. At night, the inner cannula can be reinserted and the cuff inflated so that mechanical ventilation can be provided. It is impractical and possibly hazardous to switch a tracheostomy tube and tracheostomy button into and out of the patient twice a day. If the patient had an uncuffed tracheostomy tube, there would be a significant leak when she is put back onto the ventilator to sleep. It would be *fatal* to put the obturator into the tracheostomy tube without deflating the cuff. The patient's airway would be completely obstructed.

39. **A.** When the Combitube is placed into the esophagus, a gastric tube can be inserted into the stomach to empty it. The patient's lungs can be ventilated whether the tube is placed into the esophagus (as intended) or the trachea. Neither the Combitube nor the LMA can be placed by the nasal route. Unlike the LMA, the Combitube is not available in small pediatric sizes. (See Boxes 12-1 and 12-2.)

Chapter 13

1. **D.** A Lukens trap is used during a suctioning procedure to get a sputum sample from a patient who cannot cough productively.

2. **D.** A closed-system suction catheter allows the patient to be ventilated and keep the PEEP level while suctioning is performed. This should help to prevent hypoxemia. Changing to a smaller- or larger-diameter open-airway suction catheter will not significantly improve the patient's situation. When the patient is taken off of the ventilator and suctioned, she will become hypoxemic. Additional PEEP will not prevent hypoxemia when the patient is taken off the ventilator.

3. **B.** It is commonly accepted that a suction catheter's OD should not be greater than one-half (50%) the ID of the endotracheal tube. This ensures that the patient has room to breathe around the catheter. See Table 13-1 for the recommended suction catheter for a given endotracheal and tracheostomy tube.

4. **C.** Increasing the vacuum pressure from −60 to −80 mm Hg will result in the secretions being removed more quickly. The whole suctioning procedure usually is limited to 15 seconds. Suctioning for 20 seconds will remove more secretions but is also likely to cause hypoxemia. Suctioning more frequently will not prove effective if the suctioning level is too low at −60 mm Hg. A hospital's central vacuum system is more powerful than a portable one and will suction more effectively.

5. **A.** All patients should be preoxygenated before suctioning and given added O_2 after suctioning to quickly restore the presuctioning O_2 level. One hundred percent O_2 should be given unless there is a reason to give less.

6. **D.** Hyperextending the patient's head and neck (sniff position) helps open the airway so that the catheter can be inserted more easily into the trachea. Placing the patient in the semi-Fowler's position helps the individual to take a deeper breath as needed.

7. **A.** The full (maximum) vacuum level is too great to be safely applied to a patient's airway. See the text for recommended maximum negative pressure ranges.

8. **B.** A suction catheter with a Coudé tip may help guide the catheter either to the left or to the right mainstem bronchus. In adults, a straight catheter has a tendency to go down the right mainstem bronchus because it comes off of the trachea at the carina at a more acute angle than the left mainstem bronchus. (In newborns, no significant difference exists in the angles of the mainstem bronchi from the trachea.) The diameter of the catheter used with an adult should be no more than one-half the ID of the endotracheal tube. Any adult-size suction catheter is long enough to suction adequately. Increasing the time of suctioning puts the patient at risk for hypoxemia.

9. **D.** The best course always is to replace a broken or defective piece of equipment.

10. **C.** Failure to have vacuum at the tip of the catheter can be caused by the vacuum regulator not being turned on, an obstruction of the catheter or rubber vacuum tubing, or a leak anywhere in the system. If all connections are airtight and the vacuum is turned on, suction should be felt at the tip of the catheter.

11. **A.** More frequent suctioning is needed if the patient has more secretions. Suctioning for longer periods puts the patient at risk for hypoxemia. No indication exists (e.g., hypoxemia or therapeutic PEEP) that a closed-airway suction catheter is needed or would be more effective than a standard catheter. Nebulized atropine in a large enough dose reduces secretion production. However, a dose large enough to do this also is likely to cause tachycardia. Atropine is rarely given to control secretions other than in the operating room. A physician's order is needed to give this medication.

12. **D.** All of the listed options can occur when saline is instilled into the trachea. In addition, the patient could have dyspnea, tachycardia, and an increased intracranial pressure. Saline should be instilled only when necessary to lubricate the suction catheter or to help in the removal of thick secretions.

13. **A.** The most reasonable course is to reduce the vacuum level slightly and assess how easily the secretions can be removed. Suctioning frequency should not be reduced unless fewer secretions are produced. The vacuum level does not need to be increased.

14. **B.** Because the patient is having an adverse reaction to the suctioning procedure, the suctioning time should be shortened. Changing to a catheter with a larger diameter increases the risk of trauma to the mucous membrane of the nasal passage. Inserting an oropharyngeal airway before suctioning may stimulate the gag reflex in a conscious patient. In addition, the airway may block the suction catheter, preventing it from passing through the patient's oropharynx to the larynx and trachea. Squirting 5 mL of saline down the suction catheter into the patient's trachea will probably trigger coughing. This could worsen the patient's distress with the whole procedure.

15. **D.** To seal the system and determine the set vacuum pressure, check the manometer while pinching off the connecting tubing. The system is not sealed off if the therapist just occludes the catheter tip; the thumb control valve is still open. Setting the vacuum control to maximum without sealing off the system allows air to leak, and the pressure cannot be measured. The system is not sealed off if the therapist just closes the thumb control valve on the catheter; the catheter tip opening is still open.

16. **A.** The only way to obtain an uncontaminated sputum sample is to place a Lukens trap between the suction catheter and the vacuum tubing. This way, the patient's secretions are collected in the Lukens trap after they have passed through the sterile suction catheter. Suctioning the patient's oropharynx with a sterile Yankauer suction catheter provides an oral sample, not a tracheal sample. The patient's mouth probably contains microorganisms in addition to those causing the pneumonia. Placing a Lukens trap between the vacuum tubing and the collection bottle would provide a contaminated sample, because unlike a suction catheter, the vacuum tubing is not sterile. The Lukens trap is designed to hold secretions and prevent them from becoming contaminated. It is not designed to hold a suction catheter.

17. **A.** Shallow suctioning would be appropriate because the patient has clear breath sounds and no history of significant secretions. Deep suctioning with a standard or Coudé tip catheter is not likely to remove any secretions and may traumatize the patient's airway. Saline is not needed because the patient does not have thick (viscous) secretions.

18. **D.** Suctioning removes secretions, as intended, as well as air (and its contained O_2) from the airways and lungs. This causes a transient drop in the patient's O_2 level. Vagal stimulation has no connection to hypoxic drive.

19. **D.** It is recommended when suctioning an infant to limit the OD of the catheter to no more than 70% the ID of the endotracheal or tracheostomy tube. This allows the patient to breathe spontaneously around the catheter during the procedure. A smaller catheter

may be used but will not remove as many secretions with each suctioning effort. This may result in the need to suction more frequently. Too frequent suctioning can result in a greater risk of trauma to the mucous membrane, hypoxemia, and vagal stimulation. A larger suction catheter prevents the patient from breathing around it. See Table 13-1 for recommended catheter sizes.

20. **B.** Lubricating the tip of the catheter with sterile, water-soluble lubricating jelly helps the catheter to slide more easily through the patient's nasal passage. This should help to minimize the risk of trauma. Neither water nor saline is a good lubricant, because these drip off the catheter. A suction catheter should be flexible, not firm.

21. **D.** Suctioning is a *sterile* procedure. A clean-gloved hand is not sterile. The contaminated catheter should be replaced with a sterile one.

22. **A.** Suctioning of blood indicates that airway trauma has occurred. It is best to stop suctioning and monitor the patient. Apply suction only when there is a clear indication of retained secretions or blood. Tissue trauma can happen with a closed-airway suctioning system the same as with open-airway suctioning. There is no indication, such as thick secretions, for a saline lavage. There is no indication to change from an oral to a nasal route for the endotracheal tube. The tissue trauma is in the trachea or mainstem bronchi, not the upper airway.

23. **B.** If the Yankauer suctioning device hits the back of the patient's throat, gagging, retching, and vomiting can be induced. Bradycardia should not happen, because vagal stimulation does not occur with oropharyngeal suctioning. Hypoxemia should not occur, because oropharyngeal suctioning does not remove air (and oxygen) from the patient's lungs. Oropharyngeal stimulation should not produce any adrenergic stimulation or tachycardia.

24. **C.** Change to a 10-Fr catheter, because the 14-Fr catheter is too large for the endotracheal tube. (See Table 13-1 for the catheter and tube combinations that should be used.) A physician's order is needed to administer 10 cm H_2O PEEP. There is no indication that the patient is having any difficulties other than bradycardia during the suctioning procedure. Suctioning should be done as often as needed and not be limited to twice per shift. The patient experiences bradycardia whenever she is suctioned because the catheter is too large. No indication is found that a catheter with a Coudé tip is needed to guide the catheter down the left (or right) mainstem bronchus. (See Table 13-1 for recommended catheter sizes.)

25. **C.** Because the patient experiences repeated serious hazards, suctioning should be discontinued. Switching to closed-airway suctioning may prevent hypoxemia and allow suctioning to be resumed. Because PEEP can

have serious side effects, it should not be increased just for suctioning purposes. Because removing the patient from ventilatory support is the cause of the hypoxemia and related problems, shortening the duration of suctioning may lessen the hypoxemia. Increasing the frequency of suctioning exposes the patient to more frequent hypoxic episodes. It is safer to discontinue the suctioning procedure until a closed-airway suction system can be set up and used. Increasing the oxygen level from 80% to 100% is unlikely to prevent hypoxemia during suctioning. Again, it is safer to discontinue the suctioning procedure until a closed-airway suction system can be set up and used.

26. **C.** The greatest amount of negative pressure that can safely applied in any clinical situation is −150 mm Hg. Any greater negative pressure has been shown to cause airway tissue trauma, hypoxemia, and atelectasis. In general, use the least amount of suctioning pressure that effectively removes the patient's secretions.

Chapter 14

1. **C.** The sensitivity control determines how much effort (negative pressure) the patient has to generate to trigger a breath. Pressure, flow, and terminal flow will adjust the functioning of the IPPB unit after the breath is started.

2. **C.** Terminal flow on a Bennett PR-2 unit is adjusted to attain additional flow at the end of an inspiratory effort. This added flow compensates for a small leak and cycles the unit to exhalation. Pressure, flow, and expiratory retard will adjust the functioning of the IPPB unit after the breath is started.

3. **D.** Pure O_2 is most clearly indicated in a patient with pulmonary edema and signs of hypoxemia. Room air (21% O_2) would not be very helpful. Intermediate levels of supplemental O_2 (40% or 80%) would be helpful but not as effective as pure O_2.

4. **D.** A cooperative patient with atelectasis should first be treated with a less expensive method such as IS. IPPB would be indicated in the other types of patients.

5. **B.** A face mask would allow a treatment to be given without injury to the lip ulcers. A mouthpiece cannot be held by a comatose patient. A Bennett seal would injure the lip ulcers. Intubation is unnecessarily invasive and risky.

6. **B.** A small negative pressure of −1 cm H_2O would not make the patient work harder than necessary to turn on the unit. A pressure of 0 cm H_2O would result in the self-cycling of the unit when ambient (room) barometric pressure is reached.

7. **A.** When the air-mix knob on a Bird unit is pushed in, only pure source gas (100% O_2) is given to the patient. Because no room air is entrained with the source gas, the overall total gas flow is decreased.

8. **B.** Adding expiratory retard adds some backpressure to the patient's airways and allows for a more

complete exhalation. Increasing inspiratory flow increases turbulence, and increasing system pressure increases V_T. Neither of these will help the patient's problem of air trapping. There is no indication that the patient is hypoxic and needs 100% oxygen.

9. **B.** A loose nebulizer medication jar would result in a hissing sound from the leaking air and a prolonged inspiratory time. If any of the hoses are misconnected, the IPPB machine will fail to function properly but the described problems would not be found. A missing bacteria filter does not cause any hissing sound or prolong the inspiratory time.

10. **C.** The patient's signs and symptoms indicate a pneumothorax. Treatment should be stopped, the patient evaluated, and the physician notified.

11. **A.** Pneumothorax or expectoration of blood indicates a serious patient problem. Treatment should be stopped, the patient evaluated, and help sought. It may be necessary to use a Bennett seal or face mask to get an airtight seal if the patient cannot seal his or her lips. The treatment can then be continued. If the patient feels faint or dizzy, he or she may be hyperventilating. Have the patient pause the treatment until the faintness or dizziness stops. Then begin again with a slower breathing rate.

12. **D.** Because the patient is calmer now, it is best to reduce the flow from the IPPB machine. This allows the delivered V_T and medication to be more equally delivered to all areas of the lungs. There is no need at this time to deliver a larger V_T. The goal is to deliver medication effectively to the lungs. Machine sensitivity is not a problem at this time.

13. **B.** The 1993 *AARC Clinical Practice Guideline* states that an IPPB-assisted breath should be at least 25% greater than the patient's spontaneous V_T. Considering the patient's condition, this would result in an initial IPPB breath goal of at least 450 mL (350 mL spontaneous $V_T \times 1.25$ = 438 mL). The V_T can be increased later, as tolerated.

14. **A.** The 2003 *AARC Clinical Practice Guideline* states that an FVC <70% of predicted is an indication for IPPB when another form of therapy has been unsuccessful. It is doubtful that IS would be effective in an unconscious, uncooperative patient. There is no indication of the need for nasotracheal suctioning, such as retained secretions. There is no indication of the need for a Flutter treatment, such as retained secretions.

15. **C.** Expiratory retard cap setting 3 is best because the patient's V_T is adequate, wheezing is found only in the bases, and the patient is comfortable with the breath. The smaller settings (1 and 2) resulted in too long of an exhalation for patient comfort. With the largest setting (4) the patient's V_T decreased, wheezing was heard in all lobes, and the patient's lungs felt full.

16. **C.** Increasing the flow of gas to the patient will result in a smoother delivery of V_T to the patient. This will be seen as a gradual, steady increase in the pressure. Increasing the target pressure will only deliver a larger V_T. It will not meet the patient's need for a faster breath. Increasing the sensitivity setting lets the patient start a breath easier but does not deliver a faster breath. If the patient inhales more quickly, she will increase her work of breathing even more. If her breathing pattern is to be coached, she should be told to inhale more slowly.

17. **A.** The best way to deliver a larger V_T is to deliver more pressure to the lungs. Decreasing the flow will only deliver the gas more slowly to the preset pressure. Less flow will not increase the V_T. Expiratory retard is added only if the patient has a problem with air trapping on exhalation. It will help with the exhalation of the delivered V_T but will not increase the size of the delivered V_T. If the patient inhales more forcefully, he or she will only increase the work of breathing because the flow will be inadequate.

18. **C.** The 2003 *AARC Clinical Practice Guideline* was used to determine this patient's minimum IPPB-delivered V_T. Steps in the calculation include:
    1. Convert the patient's body weight in pounds (lb) to kilograms (kg):

       $$\frac{180 \text{ lb}}{2.2 \text{ lb/kg}} = 81.82 \text{ kg} \quad (\text{use 82 kg for this calculation})$$

    2. Calculate the patient's predicted inspiratory capacity:

       Predicted IC = 50 mL × kg of ideal body weight

       Therefore, predicted IC = 50 mL × 82 kg = 4100 mL

    3. Calculate the patient's minimum IPPB-assisted V_T goal:

       Minimum IPPB goal = 0.33 × predicted IC
       = 0.33 × 4100 mL = 1353 mL

    Therefore a 1400-mL tidal volume is the best answer.

Chapter 15

1. **A.** In a patient with ARDS, one of the clinical goals is to keep the plateau pressure (P_{plat}) less than 30 cm water to reduce the risk of barotrauma. The best way to reduce this risk of ventilator-induced lung injury (VILI) is to decrease the V_T. To maintain the same minute volume and acceptable blood gas values, the respiratory rate must be increased. Increasing the V_T would increase the risk of VILI. Without refractory hypoxemia, there is no indication to increase PEEP at this time.

2. **B.** The initial V_T for this patient on an older ventilator is 10 mL/kg. This would result in a set, uncorrected V_T of 800 mL (10 mL × 80 kg). Because some volume will be lost owing to compressed volume (compressed gas and circuit stretch), the actual V_T will be smaller than 800 mL and probably within the now recommended range of 6-8 mL/kg.

3. **C.** The goals of a lung recruitment maneuver are to find the opening pressure of the alveoli (the lower

inflection point) and the maximum stretch of the alveoli (the upper inflection point). Once these two points are determined, the PEEP level and V_T delivery pressure should stay between them. See Figure 15-16.

4. **C.** The V_T, dead space, and shunt are acceptable. However, the VC and maximum inspiratory pressure are low and do not indicate successful weaning.

5. **C.** SIMV would be the safest weaning method for this patient with an acceptable V_T but inadequate VC or maximum inspiratory pressure. The ventilator will still provide intermittent deep breaths and alarms for safety. T-piece weaning offers no alarms, and the patient is not ready for extubation. PCV is not a weaning method.

6. **D.** SIMV offers intermittent deep breaths while allowing the patient to breathe spontaneously. PS should be used to overcome the airway resistance caused by the small endotracheal tube. PEEP is not needed to maintain her FRC and oxygenation. MMV is a weaning technique used with a patient with an unstable drive to breathe.

7. **D.** The information given indicates that the patient is tiring. Waiting another hour to reevaluate will only put him at risk for exhaustion. Decreasing the CPAP causes a lower FRC and less oxygenation. Raising the CPAP level may increase FRC and oxygenation but does not help the patient's fatigue and work of breathing.

8. **B.** A heated wick-type humidifier will do the best job of providing 100% relative humidity to the patient. Neither instilling a few milliliters of saline nor switching to a cool pass-over-type humidifier would do a good a job of adding moisture to the patient's secretions. HME devices can be heated only by the patient's warm exhaled gas.

9. **A.** The PC, A/C mode will deliver a V_T at a lower peak pressure. The patient should be able to ventilate without further injury to her lung. APRV has been used successfully in some patients with ARDS who have not responded to VC ventilation. It may be needed if the patient first fails with the PC, A/C mode. CPAP will not ventilate the patient at all. This patient needs a fully supporting mode of ventilation. Sedation will not lower the high delivered ventilator pressures.

10. **B.** The pressure sensitivity control should be set so that the patient can easily trigger an inhalation with a slightly negative pressure. A pressure of 0 cm H_2O or in the positive range will result in self-cycling of the ventilator to inspiration. A pressure of −5 cm H_2O will make the patient work more than necessary to trigger a breath.

11. **D.** The patient should be told of any significant change in the ventilator unless there is a clinical reason not to. Sigh breaths are not used with SIMV because the mandatory breaths should be large enough to serve as a sigh. Mechanical dead space should be removed because it could result in CO_2 retention during the patient's spontaneous breaths. The sensitivity control should function so that the patient can trigger the synchronous machine breaths. SIMV is not a reason to add PEEP.

12. **D.** Too much PEEP will overstretch the lungs and result in decreased compliance. The overstretched lung areas compress their pulmonary capillaries, which causes blood to be diverted to other lung areas. This is likely to increase shunting. If the level of PEEP is too great, the lungs will compress the heart. This will reduce venous return to the heart. As a result, the cardiac output will drop, as will the blood pressure. (See Box 15-3.)

13. **A.** According to the current VAP guidelines, a circuit that is visibly soiled with blood or secretions should be replaced. Flushing is not adequate to remove any residual blood as a bacterial growth medium. Coughing is normally not a reason to sedate a patient. A nebulized local anesthetic such as lidocaine will block pain in the airways. But, the aerosol will not reach the neck tissues to block their pain.

14. **B.** A fouled, obstructed HME needs to be replaced. When the HME is replaced with a new one, the peak pressure will drop to normal and the alarm will stop. A medication treatment should not be stopped because the patient has secretions. Suctioning should be done only if the patient cannot cough out the secretions.

15. **C.** Disconnecting the tubing to the external exhalation valve will cause it to fail, which causes the machine V_T to bypass the patient. A self-cycling ventilator would deliver the V_T to the patient. If the inspiratory and expiratory limbs of the circuit were reversed, no volume would be delivered and the peak pressure alarm would sound. Even if the spirometer were out of calibration, the V_T would be delivered to the patient, and pressure would build in the system. (See Fig. 15-25, A.)

16. **B.** Expiratory retard is indicated in a condition with air trapping on exhalation, such as asthma. The back-pressure acts as a "splint" to the airways for a complete exhalation. The other three conditions do not cause air trapping within the lungs or interfere with exhalation.

17. **C.** The patient's oxygenation is normal. The other three parameters are not normal and indicate the need for mechanical ventilation. (Review Box 15-1.)

18. **C.** Increasing the IPAP level will lead to an increased V_T. If the IPAP level is decreased, the V_T will also decrease. The EPAP level is similar to CPAP or PEEP in its effect on the patient's FRC. Therefore, EPAP is adjusted only to change the FRC to affect the patient's oxygenation.

19. **C.** Increasing the lower pressure level will increase the CPAP pressure to open the patient's soft throat tissues and stop the snoring. A rate change will not affect the ventilator pressures. Increasing the upper

pressure level will increase the V_T; it will not affect the lower pressure to stop the snoring. Loosening the nasal mask would cause a leak and lower pressures. The snoring would worsen.

20. **A.** Decreasing the mechanical dead space will decrease the patient's CO_2 level. Decreasing the $\dot{V}_E$ will increase the CO_2 level. Neither changing the I:E ratio nor adding PEEP would have any effect on CO_2 elimination.

21. **C.** Retained secretions and bronchospasm are Raw problems and cause only the peak pressure to increase. (See Fig. 15-5.) The other two conditions decrease C_{LT} and make the P_{plat} increase. The peak pressure increases as a result. (See Fig. 15-8.)

22. **B.** PEEP elevates the patient's baseline pressure and raises the $\overline{P}aw$ by the same amount. The other three options would decrease the $\overline{P}aw$ by increasing expiratory time.

23. **A.** The *AARC Clinical Practice Guideline* recommends the use of a heated humidifier warmed to body temperature to help liquefy thick secretions. An HME should be used only if the patient has few secretions. The secretions should not be allowed to dry out. If they did, it would be very difficult to remove them by suctioning.

24. **A.** A spirometer is not needed because the patient's V_T cannot be measured accurately while on the CPAP system. If a spirometer were incorporated into the CPAP system, it would register continuous flow rather than patient volumes. An alarm system is needed for patient safety, and water traps are used to keep the tubing clear. A pressure-generating device must be added to set and maintain the CPAP level. (See Fig. 15-29.)

25. **A.** Auto-PEEP (expiratory air trapping) is identified when the expiratory flow does not return to zero before the next ventilator tidal volume is delivered. The expiratory time should always be long enough for the patient to fully exhale a V_T of any size regardless of the patient's lung compliance or airway resistance. (See Fig. 15-4.)

26. **C.** See the following calculation:

$$\text{Airway resistance (Raw)} = \frac{\text{Peak airway pressure} - \text{Plateau pressure}}{\text{Flow in L/s}}$$
$$= \frac{40 \text{ cm H}_2\text{O} - 20 \text{ cm H}_2\text{O}}{0.75 \text{ L/s}}$$
$$= \frac{20 \text{ cm H}_2\text{O}}{0.75 \text{ L/s}}$$
$$= 27 \text{ cm H}_2\text{O L/s}$$

27. **C.** If the bronchodilator therapy is effectively reversing the patient's bronchospasm, his airway resistance will be decreasing. Bronchodilator therapy will not have any effect on lung compliance. Although breath sounds should reveal less wheezing, each caregiver could interpret breath sounds differently. It is better

to objectively evaluate a patient's airway resistance to determine whether the bronchodilator therapy is effective. Although a chest radiograph will show changes in a patient's lungs, it will not help to assess airway resistance.

28. **B.** If the diuretic medication is benefiting the patient, his lungs will "dry out." This will result in improvement in lung compliance over time. Although a diuretic medication should improve his urine output and cause weight loss, this is not the best way to evaluate his pulmonary status. Pulmonary edema is a lung compliance problem, not an airway resistance problem. If the diuretic medication has improved his urine output and his lungs have dried out, breath sounds should improve. However, this is not the best way to quantitatively evaluate a patient's response to care.

29. **D.** A pressure-cycled transport-type ventilator will be able to provide effective ventilation through the transportation and the cardiac procedure. Manual ventilation is not recommended because, if the therapist should tire, the respiratory rate and tidal volume will decrease. A microprocessor-type ventilator is the most sophisticated and expensive unit available. It probably is not needed for the anticipated short period of time. NIV is done only on a patient without an endotracheal tube. It would not be safe to extubate the patient for NIV and then reintubate the patient after this short medical procedure.

30. **C.** Air trapping and auto-PEEP are corrected by increasing the expiratory time for complete exhalation of the V_T. If the PC mode is used to deliver the same V_T and the other settings are kept the same, the patient still will have air trapping and auto-PEEP. Decreasing the inspiratory flow while keeping the same V_T and rate will result in an even shorter expiratory time. This will result in even more air trapping. It is unlikely that a larger endotracheal tube will help a patient with COPD to exhale more completely.

31. **A.** The use of accessory muscles and ventilator dyssynchrony indicate that the patient needs a faster breath. Increasing the inspiratory flow should help this. There is no indication that her V_T is too large. Too much pain medicine will sedate the patient and could make weaning difficult. Without a set of ABG values, there is no way to assess her oxygenation. The real issue here is the patient's desire for a faster tidal volume.

32. **D.** The difference between the patient's respiratory efforts (24) and total breaths (15) indicates that the ventilator is not sensing all of his efforts. Adjust the sensitivity control on the ventilator so that all of the patient's efforts result in ventilator breaths. The ABG values indicate that the patient is not hypoxemic. So, this cannot be the reason his efforts are not triggering ventilator breaths. Although increasing the flow will deliver a faster V_T, it will not correct the difference between the patient's breathing efforts and the

ventilator sensing those efforts. Increasing the set rate to 15 will only match the current total rate. The patient is making 24 respiratory efforts/min. The real problem is that the ventilator is not sensing all of his breathing efforts.

33. **B.** An initial set V_T of 700 mL is appropriate at almost 10 mL/kg of ideal body weight. Because of compressed volume, the delivered V_T will be less. A V_T of 1000 mL is probably too large at almost 14 mL/kg of ideal body weight. A set V_T of 500 mL is probably too small because less than 7 mL/kg will be delivered. A V_T of 320 mL is certainly too small, with less than 5 mL/kg delivered.

34. **B.** Because children normally breathe faster than adults, a rate of 20/min is appropriate. A rate of 14 would be appropriate for an adult but is too slow for a child. A rate of 50 would be appropriate for a newborn infant and far too fast for a child. An initial rate of 80 is too fast for any patient. (See Table 1-2.)

35. **C.** Decreasing the respiratory rate will allow the patient's carbon dioxide level to rise. This should correct the respiratory alkalosis. Although the patient's PaO_2 is higher than normal, it is not necessary to make a change in the oxygen percentage at this time. In addition, if the patient's carbon dioxide were to increase to the normal level, the PaO_2 would decrease. Increasing the respiratory rate will further decrease the carbon dioxide level. This could produce a dangerous respiratory alkalosis. Although decreasing the V_T will result in a higher $PaCO_2$ level, it is better to decrease the respiratory rate. The patient's V_T of 500 mL is appropriate at about 7 mL/kg of ideal body weight.

36. **A.** The patient should be given 100% oxygen before each suctioning procedure and afterward until he is stable again. Because cardiopulmonary risks are associated with PEEP, it should not be increased and decreased frequently for each suctioning episode. Suctioning should be done as often as necessary. If suctioning is performed less often than needed, secretions will accumulate in the patient's airways. The suction catheter should not be larger than one-half of the inner diameter of the patient's endotracheal tube. A larger catheter will block too much of the endotracheal tube, so that the patient cannot breathe around it.

37. **D.** As the patient recovers, it is appropriate to change to the PS mode to let her do more spontaneous breathing. The APRV mode is sometimes needed in a patient with ARDS when he or she fails with more conventional ventilation. It is not needed as she recovers. There is no need to increase the set rate. The patient is able to trigger additional breaths as she desires and has normal blood gas values. The V_T does not need to be decreased. It is set at about 7 mL/kg.

38. **C.** ATC or PS can be initiated to overcome a patient's increased WOB. In this case, a 7.0-mm-ID endotracheal tube would increase the patient's workload because the tube is too small for an adult. Keeping the ventilator rate at 8/min is just enough to not exhaust the patient. However, it does not really solve the problem of increased WOB through a small endotracheal tube. Increased flow during machine breaths will not decrease the patient's spontaneous WOB. No evidence suggests that the patient has asthma or any condition that would cause bronchospasm.

39. **D.** The patient is exhibiting refractory hypoxemia. The best way to correct this problem is with PEEP therapy to reestablish the patient's FRC. If the patient is hypoxic while getting 70% oxygen, it is doubtful that giving 100% oxygen will make much difference. Increasing the set rate to 18 will only ensure that the patient is hyperventilated. Mechanical dead space will correct the hyperventilation but will not correct the hypoxemia.

40. **D.** Because the patient has normal bedside spirometry values and is awake, she can have weaning procedures started. A T-piece would be appropriate because she can fully support her own breathing. It is overly cautious to wait 4 more hours to reevaluate the patient or change to the SIMV mode. However, it is overly aggressive to extubate the patient without a spontaneous breathing trial. (See Box 15-5.)

41. **D.** ARDS results in stiff lungs that are at risk of volutrauma if too large a V_T is forced into them. PCIRV is used with these patients because the peak pressure is limited to a safe level. The long inspiratory time used with PCIRV helps to oxygenate the patient. Asthma and chronic bronchitis are noted for high airway resistance, not stiffness of the lungs. These patients need a long expiratory time for complete exhalation. PCIRV would probably cause more air trapping because of the long inspiratory time and short expiratory time. A pulmonary contusion is a lung bruise from trauma. It is neither helped nor hindered by PCIRV.

42. **A.** The fluctuating CPAP pressure indicates that the flow is too low for the patient's needs. It should be increased. It could be dangerous to sedate a patient breathing on CPAP. The current low-pressure alarm settings are appropriate.

43. **C.** Pulmonary edema, pneumonia, and ARDS are all conditions in which the lungs become stiff. This results in decreased lung compliance and an increased P_{plat}. The patient's WOB will be increased. Emphysema is caused by loss of connective tissue within the lungs and results in increased lung compliance. As a result, the lungs are overinflated.

44. **A.** MMV is used to provide a secure minimum minute volume to unstable patients. Often, these patients have an unstable respiratory drive because of stroke or brain injury. MMV is a variation on SIMV. It does not allow the patient to trigger each breath as the A/C mode does. MMV is not like CPAP because MMV delivers mandatory V_T breaths.

45. **B.** Near-drowning patients are ventilated traditionally with the A/C or SIMV mode with a constant volume. HFV has been shown effective in ventilating patients with airway procedures such as laryngoscopy and bronchoscopy. HFO has been shown effective in patients with a bronchopleural fistula because the small V_T's and low driving pressures do not force gas out through the lung tear. This allows the tissues to heal.

46. **D.** Review the indications for ventilatory support in Box 15-1. These indications include a rapid, shallow breathing index of more than 105, a $PaCO_2$ of more than 55 torr, and cardiac dysrhythmias. The patient is not dangerously hypoxic with a PaO_2 of 70 torr.

47. **A.** Because the patient's left lung has been removed, he should have a V_T that is about half of normal for two lungs. Giving a normal or larger than normal tidal volume for two lungs is likely to overdistend the patient's one remaining lung. CPAP will not support the patient's breathing and could be dangerous in the immediate postoperative period.

48. **A.** ARDS is characterized by very stiff lungs. A negative-pressure ventilator is unable to generate enough pressure to adequately ventilate any patient with low lung compliance. Also, a negative-pressure ventilator offers very few modes or adjustment options and cannot add PEEP. The other three conditions (neuromuscular defects, kyphoscoliosis, and COPD in acute failure) are not as challenging to ventilate. These patients are not intubated and require assisted ventilation only for a short period. Negative-pressure ventilation has been used successfully with these patients.

49. **B.** See Box 15-3 and Figure 15-20 for information on the evaluation of an optimal PEEP study. As PEEP establishes the patient's FRC, the pulmonary compliance should improve. Ventilation better matches perfusion, so that shunt will decrease and PaO_2 will increase. In addition, the patient's pulmonary vascular resistance (PVR) decreases as the lungs are properly ventilated and blood flow through them is normalized. Set the PEEP level where these four parameters are optimized. If too much PEEP is applied, the lungs will be overstretched. This causes the PVR to increase and cardiac output to decrease as venous return to the lungs and heart is decreased. As a result, the patient's blood pressure decreases and heart rate increases.

50. **C.** Static compliance is calculated as follows:

$$Cst = \frac{\text{Exhaled tidal volume} - \text{Compressed volume}}{\text{Plateau pressure} - \text{PEEP}}$$

In this situation, use the corrected V_T because the compressed volume has already been subtracted from the exhaled V_T. The following equation results:

$$Cst = \frac{600\ mL}{48-12}$$
$$= \frac{600\ mL}{36}$$

$$Cst = 17\ mL/cm\ water$$

51. **D.** Cst is calculated as follows:

$$Cst = \frac{\text{Exhaled tidal volume} - \text{Compressed volume}}{\text{Plateau pressure} - \text{PEEP}}$$

$$\text{Compressed volume} = \text{Compliance factor} \times \text{Plateau pressure}$$
$$(4\ mL/cm\ water \times 25\ cm\ water) = 100\ mL$$

$$Cst = \frac{700\ mL - 100\ mL}{25-6}$$
$$= \frac{600\ mL}{19}$$

$$Cst = 32\ mL/cm\ water$$

52. **B.** Cdyn is calculated as follows:

$$Cdyn = \frac{\text{Exhaled volume} - \text{Compressed volume}}{\text{Peak pressure} - \text{PEEP}}$$

$$\text{Compressed volume} = \text{Compliance factor} \times \text{Peak pressure}$$
$$(4\ mL/cm\ water \times 35\ cm\ water) = 140\ mL$$

$$Cdyn = \frac{700\ mL - 140\ mL}{35-6}$$
$$= \frac{560\ mL}{29}$$

$$Cdyn = 19\ mL/cm\ water$$

53. **A.** HFJV involves the delivery of very small V_T breaths at a very high rate. It is impractical to try to measure these very small tidal volumes. The other three listed items plus a high-pressure air source, suitable patient circuit, and the ventilator itself are needed for HFJV.

54. **C.** An increased airway resistance (caused by bronchospasm or airway secretions) causes the peak pressure to increase. A decrease in lung compliance (caused by pulmonary edema, pneumonia, or pleural effusion) causes the plateau pressure to increase. This, in turn, drives up the peak pressure. Without having both the peak and the plateau pressures, there is no way to know more specifically what has caused the peak pressure to increase. If the lung compliance had increased or the airway resistance had decreased, the peak pressure would have decreased. Review Figures 15-5, 7, 8, 9, 10, and 11 for examples of airway resistance and lung compliance changes.

55. **D.** Therapeutic PEEP increases a patient's FRC. This increased lung volume enables better ventilation and perfusion matching. As a result, intrapulmonary shunting past underventilated alveoli is reduced. Increasing inspiratory time and sigh volume improves alveolar filling and may help to increase oxygenation. However, they do not increase FRC and therefore do not reduce shunting.

56. **A.** A 200-mL air leak through the pleural chest tube would explain the difference in delivered and returned V_T. If the patient had a deflated endotracheal tube cuff, the delivered V_T would be decreased. The

selected ventilator is microprocessor driven and has the ability to monitor itself. A warning of a system failure such as a miscalibrated spirometer would have occurred. No indication is noted that the patient has asthma or any condition causing bronchospasm. This ventilator has the ability to monitor auto-PEEP, and none is indicated.

57. **C.** Recent research has shown that alveolar over-stretching and damage can occur when the P_{plat} is 30 cm water or greater. Therefore the patient should be switched from volume-cycled ventilation (VC) to pressure-cycled ventilation (PC) with a P_{plat} of no higher than 30 cm water. A high peak pressure may be caused by high airway resistance or lung stiffness. Lung compliance is calculated from V_T divided by P_{plat}. There is no direct connection between calculated lung compliance and alveolar overstretching. Both peak pressure and plateau pressure should be monitored. However, the combination has no direct connection to alveolar overstretching.

58. **C.** Interpretation of the patient's ABG results indicates hypercarbia and resulting respiratory acidosis. The best solution is to increase the respiratory rate. There is no urgent need to decrease the patient's 35% oxygen because this is not a toxic amount. Decreasing the patient's minute volume further raises the carbon dioxide level and lowers the pH. There is no indication of air trapping and auto-PEEP. So, there is no need to increase the expiratory time. After another set of ABGs is drawn and analyzed, the rate can be increased if still needed to blow off CO_2.

59. **D.** Atelectasis is best treated by giving the patient a larger sigh volume. This should help to open up alveoli that have collapsed or are prone to collapsing. Changing flow rate, expiratory time, and ventilator frequency has no impact on lung volume.

60. **D.** Permissive hypercapnia involves the gradual increasing of a patient's carbon dioxide level such that the pH does not become overly acidotic. During permissive hypercapnia, the patient's $PaCO_2$ can increase to well above 50 torr, and the pH probably will decrease to below the normal range of 7.35. It may be necessary to give the patient intravenous bicarbonate to keep the pH greater than 7.25.

61. **C.** SIMV allows the patient to breathe spontaneously when she wants to while still receiving support from the ventilator. A low level of PS should help to reduce her added WOB from the small endotracheal tube. Therapeutic PEEP is justified because of her PaO_2 measurement of only 63 torr on 55% oxygen. The A/C mode does not allow her to take any totally spontaneous V_T breaths. In addition, she would benefit from some therapeutic PEEP. High-level PSV does not offer her the "safety net" of support offered by SIMV at this stage of her recovery. Some therapeutic PEEP is needed.

62. **C.** Interpretation of the patient's ABG values shows an increased carbon dioxide level with resulting respiratory acidosis. A SIMV rate of 10/min does not increase the patient's baseline minute volume from the PC rate of 10. Because the patient is apneic, she will not be adding to the minute volume total. The patient's minute volume will be increased by both a higher respiratory rate and a larger V_T. Removing the mechanical dead space will prevent the patient from rebreathing her own carbon dioxide. All three of these options result in a lower $PaCO_2$ and correction of the low pH. Additionally, increasing the V_T probably will increase the PaO_2.

63. **A.** Review Box 15-2 for indications of SIMV tolerance/intolerance if needed. An increased respiratory rate (usually accompanied by a decreasing V_T) indicates that the patient is fatigued and needs more ventilator support. Review the rapid, shallow breathing index calculation shown in Box 15-1 if needed. Stable vital signs and blood gas values indicate good tolerance of the WOB. Lack of accessory muscle use indicates that the diaphragm is strong enough to ventilate the patient. See Box 15-1.

64. **B.** ABG results show adequate oxygenation; therefore the PEEP level can be reduced safely from 10 to 7 cm water. A decrease in SIMV rate from 10 to 3 is too large. A smaller rate decrease from 10 to about 6 is more reasonable at this stage in the patient's recovery. ABG results show adequate ventilation. There is no need to increase the SIMV rate at this time. There is no indication that the patient has an increased airway resistance problem that would justify the addition of PS. Her tracheostomy tube is the appropriate size, and her spontaneous rate and V_T are adequate.

65. **C.** Review Box 15-5 for indications of the ability to wean. Only patients 2 and 3 have all parameters within the normal ranges listed. Patient 1 has a low respiratory rate, V_T, and FEV_1. Patient 4 has a fast respiratory rate, low V_T, and low MIP. Patient 5 has a fast respiratory rate, low FEV_1, and low MIP.

66. **B.** The only patient parameter that has changed significantly is the increase in P peak from 30 to 45 cm water. This can be caused only by an increase in airway resistance. Although several things can cause this (bronchospasm, secretions, biting or kinking of the endotracheal tube), the only option that fits is giving a bronchodilating agent. Increasing PEEP has no effect on airway resistance. A diuretic agent (such as furosemide [Lasix]) would help to eliminate pulmonary edema and lower a patient's plateau pressure (P plateau). However, this value is unchanged, so no worsening is indicated. A paralyzing agent will not affect any of the recorded patient values. See Figure 15-5 for an example of changing peak pressures.

67. **C.** Even though the patient is paralyzed and cannot request a medication for pain relief, the patient can

feel the surgical pain. Paralyzing medications do not block touch (pain) or the other senses. A narcotic medication (morphine) is justified for pain relief. Caffeine does not have a role in the care of a patient who has been paralyzed pharmacologically. A sedative medication may be given to relieve any anxiety the patient may have, but it would not affect the patient's pain. Unfortunately, there is no easy way to tell when the paralyzed patient is awake or sleeping. Regardless, it is important to talk normally to the patient so that he or she knows what medical care is being given.

68. **B.** Increasing the V_T will decrease the patient's $PaCO_2$ toward the goal. Another ABG sample should be taken in about 15 minutes to see if the ordered $PaCO_2$ of 25 torr has been achieved. Adding mechanical dead space will increase, rather than decrease, the patient's carbon dioxide level. Decreasing the oxygen percentage has no effect on the $PaCO_2$. Decreasing the ventilator rate results in a higher rather than lower carbon dioxide level.

69. **D.** The decrease in patient V_T is significant. Probably the patient's lung compliance has worsened. With the PC mode, V_T will decrease with decreased lung compliance. The patient has increased his respiratory rate to make up for the lost minute volume. The best solution is to increase the PC inspiratory pressure to produce the previous V_T of 800 mL. Sedating the patient will result in a dramatic decrease in minute volume with resulting hypercarbia and hypoxia. Increasing the set respiratory rate will deliver a higher minute volume and will relieve the patient of some of the burden of triggering the ventilator. However, it will not correct the main problem—a decreased V_T. There is no indication of increased airway resistance to justify the addition of PS. PS will not deliver a larger V_T.

70. **C.** The flow/time tracing enables any auto-PEEP to be detected. See Figure 15-4 for the graphic. If the expiratory flow does not return to baseline before the next breath is delivered, the patient has auto-PEEP. The Maximum Voluntary Ventilation tracing is done in the pulmonary function laboratory to evaluate a patient's overall breathing ability. It is not useful for detecting auto-PEEP. A flow/volume loop can be done on many microprocessor ventilators and is helpful in evaluating flow at the end of exhalation. However, the flow/time tracing is the best detector of auto-PEEP. A pressure/time tracing (see Fig. 15-5) shows a change in peak pressure but is not helpful in detecting auto-PEEP.

71. **C.** Increasing the IPAP level from 15 to 20 cm H_2O will deliver a larger V_T to the patient. This should correct her feeling of not getting enough air. Increasing the EPAP level will put more pressure on the upper airway to keep it open. However, there is no indication that the patient has an upper airway obstruction (snoring) at the present EPAP level. In addition, increasing the EPAP level, without increasing the IPAP level, will result in delivery of a smaller V_T. When the patient complained that she was not "getting enough air," she was referring to needing a larger V_T. A faster respiratory rate will not give her a larger V_T. There is no indication that the patient is hypoxemic with 30% oxygen. The oxygen percentage should not be increased without knowledge of the patient's oxygenation.

72. **A.** The patient's blood gas results show hypoventilation and his spirometry results got worse after 40 minutes. Mechanical ventilation should be resumed for his safety. Extubation could be dangerous for the patient. He is not strong enough to breathe entirely on his own. PEP therapy is used to help mobilize secretions and will not support his breathing. The weaning trial should be stopped now because the patient is getting worse. He needs additional ventilatory support. (See Box 15-5.)

73. **B.** The patient's carbon dioxide level is too high, causing a respiratory acidosis. The most effective way to increase alveolar ventilation to reduce the $PaCO_2$ is to increase amplitude. Increasing PEEP and changing the I:E ratio to 1:1 will improve oxygenation but will not blow off carbon dioxide.

Chapter 16

1. **C.** A PaO_2 in the range of 60-70 torr is adequate for a newborn infant. Less would result in unnecessary hypoxemia. A higher value is not needed and may increase the risk for retinopathy of prematurity. See Table 16-1 for all blood gas recommendations.

2. **B.** Mechanical ventilation is indicated to support the patient's breathing when prolonged apnea spells lead to bradycardia. CPAP improves oxygenation but does not provide ventilation to support a patient with apnea spells. An aerosolized bronchodilator does not affect a patient in a way that corrects apnea. While endotracheal surfactant can help a neonate with RDS, there is no indication of why the patient is having apnea spells.

3. **C.** A variable CPAP pressure indicates a leak in the system, in this case, most likely with the fit of the CPAP prongs into the neonate's nostrils. A smaller V_T or decreased respiratory rate should not have any effect on the CPAP level. The flow through the system should be the same without regard to the oxygen percentage set on the blender.

4. **D.** When meconium is aspirated, it causes a serious airway obstruction problem. For this reason, additional time is needed for the patient's V_T to be exhaled. Therefore, select the longest expiratory time possible. (See Box 16-6.)

5. **C.** The neonate is premature with signs of RDS. The best way to improve the patient's lung compliance and function is to administer exogenous surfactant. Albuterol has no effect on lung compliance. There are

no signs of secretions that need to be suctioned out. Although supplemental oxygen may help to correct the hypoxemia, it does nothing to correct the fundamental problem caused by RDS.

6. **B.** A ventilator circuit that is visibly soiled should be changed. This is because the blood or sputum in the circuit can act as a medium for bacterial growth. An HME provides passive humidification and is not intended as a place to collect sputum. Saline can be used to help with the suctioning procedure but is not recommended for flushing out sputum from a circuit. A closed-airway suctioning system helps to prevent hypoxemia during suctioning but does not remove sputum from the circuit.

7. **D.** Nasal CPAP at 4 cm water is appropriate. There is no clear indication that the neonate needs to be intubated to provide the end-expiratory pressure. Most premature neonatal patients with moderate hypoxemia respond well to about 4 cm water pressure. Mechanical ventilation would be needed only if the neonate's hypoxemia did not respond to CPAP or if the carbon dioxide value increased significantly. Because the neonate is hypoxic on 60% oxygen, it is doubtful that 70% oxygen would result in a clinically significant improvement.

8. **A.** INO is a pulmonary artery vasodilator in neonatal patients with PPHN. Its use should help to increase blood flow through the lungs and improve oxygenation. Although surfactant is indicated in a neonate with RDS, this patient does not have that problem. Decreasing the oxygen percentage could make the patient more hypoxic and does not help PPHN. Heliox may help reduce the asthmatic patient's work of breathing but does not help PPHN.

9. **B.** Extubation is performed with a CPAP level of 2-4 cm water because this small amount of pressure is typically the minimum used to maintain the neonate's normal FRC. A lower CPAP pressure while intubated would result in too little FRC and possibly hypoxemia. If a higher CPAP level is needed to treat hypoxemia, the patient should not be extubated.

10. **D.** All three listed items are indications to change from CPAP to mechanical ventilation. A neonatal patient who is receiving 8-10 cm water CPAP and 80% oxygen and who is still hypoxemic should have mechanical ventilation started.

11. **D.** Pressure-limited square-wave ventilation is widely accepted as the standard way to ventilate the majority of neonatal patients with RDS because it (1) limits the peak pressure to a predetermined safe level and (2) increases the patient's oxygenation by maintaining the peak pressure during a V_T breath for the duration of the inspiratory time.

12. **B.** It has been clinically shown that hyperventilation of the patient with PPHN causes pulmonary vasodilation. This improves the patient's condition by allowing more blood to pass through the pulmonary circulation to be oxygenated. Hyperventilation has not been shown to improve the other listed conditions.

13. **C.** Increasing the pressure limit on the ventilator increases the patient's V_T. This increased pressure and V_T can increase the risk of lung tissues being torn. This can result in a pneumothorax or other types of barotrauma or volutrauma. Retinopathy of prematurity is a complex condition related to prematurity and frequent swings in the patient's arterial blood oxygen and carbon dioxide levels. Oxygen toxicity is related to the patient inhaling a high percentage of oxygen for a prolonged period of time. A tracheoesophageal fistula can be the result of a developmental defect or caused by tissue damage from an endotracheal tube and nasogastric tube.

14. **D.** Increased inspiratory time keeps the alveoli open longer to improve oxygenation. If the pressure limit is increased, a larger V_T will be delivered and oxygenation will be improved. Additional PEEP increases the patient's FRC and improves oxygenation. If flow is decreased, the tidal volume will be decreased. This results in the oxygen level dropping. Decreasing the ventilator's IMV rate decreases the patient's minute volume. This results in the oxygen level dropping.

15. **B.** With TPTV, the patient's V_T is determined by the difference between the pressure limit and the PEEP level. If the PEEP is increased without increasing the pressure limit, the difference between them decreases and the V_T decreases. Minute volume decreases, not increases, if the difference between the pressure limit and the PEEP level is decreased. The patient's $PaCO_2$ increases, not decreases, if the V_T and minute volume decrease. Tidal volume decreases, not increases, when the difference between pressure limit and PEEP decreases.

16. **A.** An oral or nasal endotracheal tube is inserted into a patient's airway before a cleft palate is surgically repaired; a standard neonatal ventilator is used if needed. There is no special reason to use HFV. Patients with all of the other clinical situations have been shown to benefit from HFV.

17. **A.** With HFO, the amplitude is directly related to the tidal volume. So increasing amplitude will increase the patient's V_T and reduce the $PaCO_2$. Decreasing the amplitude would have the opposite effect. Increasing PEEP would reduce the difference between the PEEP level and the amplitude (peak pressure). This would reduce the patient's tidal volume. The I:E ratio probably has little impact, in this situation, on the patient's carbon dioxide level.

18. **C.** It is common clinical practice to begin CPAP at 4-5 cm water. Less than this is not likely to improve the patient's condition significantly. An initial CPAP of 6-8 cm water may not be needed to improve oxygenation and may result in cardiopulmonary complications. It is safer to start at 4-5 cm water, assess the patient, and determine if more CPAP is needed.

19. **C.** It is appropriate to wean the INO by decreasing the dose by 50%. Next, assess the patient to determine if the INO can be further reduced. The patient should probably not be weaned from the ventilator or changed to CPAP until nitric oxide is no longer needed. Nitric oxide should be weaned down in steps of 50% rather than being abruptly discontinued.

20. **A.** The patient's arterial blood gas results show refractory hypoxemia and hypoventilation with respiratory acidosis. Conventional mechanical ventilation is indicated. This could be with either a volume-cycled ventilator or a pressure-cycled ventilator. Increasing CPAP may help to improve oxygenation but will not correct the hypoventilation. It is doubtful that increasing the oxygen percentage will correct the patient's refractory hypoxemia. HFV is not indicated until after conventional mechanical ventilation has been tried and shown to not be effective.

Chapter 17

1. **C.** The best way to be sure that the patient understands the purpose of the equipment is to ask her questions about it and have her demonstrate its function. Any misunderstandings then can be clarified. In addition, the patient should show that she has the necessary dexterity to operate the equipment.

2. **C.** Current guidelines recommend that supplemental oxygen be used during exercise when a patient's SpO_2 value drops to <88%. Values between 96% and 90% are within the normal range. A value of <84% shows serious hypoxemia. The patient should not be allowed to become this hypoxemic, if possible.

3. **A.** The level of water in the humidifier does not affect the ability of O_2 to flow through the O_2 delivery system. Tightening of all connections and placement of the cannula prongs under water reveal whether gas is flowing through the prongs. If no gas is flowing out from the O_2 concentrator, the nasal cannula should be switched over to the O_2 tank. (See Exam Hint 17-2.)

4. **B.** A cane should not be used without a documented need. The patient's life situation can improve if his spouse stops smoking, he minimizes climbing of stairs, and a front door ramp is added.

5. **B.** Many injuries occur in the bathroom and kitchen when weak patients fall while climbing into showers or tubs or onto chairs to reach high objects.

6. **C.** A patient's exercise tolerance is not evaluated by determining if a relative can drive the patient somewhere. Exercise tolerance can be assessed by determining the patient's ease or difficulty in performing specific tasks.

7. **B.** Restoring the patient to his or her highest possible functional capacity is the main goal of a rehabilitation program. All other goals are secondary to this.

8. **C.** The patient and her husband must both stop smoking. If she is the only one to quit, she will continue to inhale secondhand smoke from her husband. Her physician should be involved in her care to offer medical support and recommend group support.

9. **B.** Research has shown that lung disease cannot be reversed by a patient attending a rehabilitation program. However, a rehabilitation program can be expected to decrease a patient's number of hospitalizations, increase the patient's energy level, and increase the patient's ability to perform ADLs. These are all worthy goals that will improve the quality of the patient's life.

10. **C.** The oxygen concentrator has failed. The patient should switch the cannula to an oxygen cylinder at the same flow rate as the concentrator. This delivers the needed oxygen supply to the patient until the therapist can repair the unit. It is not the patient's responsibility to perform equipment repairs, such as resetting the circuit breaker on the concentrator or disassembling the concentrator to clean the air filter. In addition, the patient should not have to risk discontinuation of ordered oxygen while waiting for an equipment repair or for further assistance. The patient should not be told to increase the flow of oxygen through a liquid oxygen system above that ordered by the physician.

11. **C.** An open-end exercise program offers these two advantages: (1) it is self-directed by the patient and (2) the patient can adjust the schedule of activities if necessary. A closed-end exercise program offers these two advantages: (1) members of the exercise group can offer support to one another and (2) the facilitator can easily plan group activities.

12. **A.** A surgically repaired cleft palate has no connection with infant apnea. Apnea periods lasting 25 seconds, death of two or more older siblings from SIDS, and a premature infant with apnea periods are all serious situations that indicate apnea monitoring. (See Box 17-1.)

13. **D.** These three steps are needed in a strengthening program: (1) warm-up period, (2) strengthening exercises performed every other day, and (3) cool-down period after the strengthening exercises. Strengthening exercises should not be performed daily because the muscles that have been worked need a day to recover before exercising again. Endurance exercises should be performed for 20-30 minutes continuously, *not* strengthening exercises.

14. **D.** It would be safer to have the patient slow down on the ergometer until her heart rate decreases to the target level. The patient's target heart rate range is based on her age and physical conditioning. If the patient exercised only until she began to perspire, she would probably not gain any exercise benefit. As previously stated, the target heart rate range is based on the patient's age and physical conditioning. She should not continue exercising at this elevated heart rate even if she feels that she can handle the workload.

The patient gains little benefit from exercising for a maximum of 10 minutes each day. Current guidelines dictate that a person should exercise for 20 to 30 continuous minutes. (See Box 17-5.)

15. **A.** Current guidelines dictate that an infant must have at least 2-3 months without an apnea episode, *not* 30 days without an apnea episode, to discontinue apnea monitoring. An infant can have apnea monitoring stopped if the other listed options are met. (See Box 17-1.)

16. **C.** A 6-minute walk test requires that the patient walk as far as possible in 6 minutes and note the distance. It is hoped that as the patient's conditioning improves, her distance walked will increase. The patient must walk, rather than ride a bicycle ergometer, for 6 minutes.

17. **D.** It is only in an open-end format rehabilitation program that each patient can easily adjust activities if a scheduling conflict arises. In a closed-end format rehabilitation program, all group members do the same thing at the same time. This way they can offer emotional support to each other, and the program facilitator can direct group activities and optimally sequence learning activities.

18. **B.** Moving the patch to another area of skin allows the irritated area to heal. Removing the patch before going to bed removes the stimulating nicotine that has been preventing sleep. A physician, not a respiratory therapist, should make the recommendation to apply a topical cortisone cream to the irritated skin. Only a physician should make the recommendation that the patient take a sleeping pill. Although a patient may choose to drink a beer or a glass of wine before going to bed to help induce sleep, the respiratory therapist should not make this recommendation. If nicotine is preventing the patient from sleeping at night, it is best to remove the patch. Sleeping pills and alcohol can probably be avoided if the nicotine patch is removed at night.

19. **C.** An oxygen concentrator and oxygen-conserving cannula economically provide the necessary oxygen to the patient. A bank of H tanks is expensive to assemble and takes up more space than a concentrator. In addition, a nasal cannula is preferred over a simple oxygen mask to deliver 2 L/min of oxygen to a patient going home. A liquid oxygen system is more expensive to set up than a concentrator for a patient who will be using the system only during periods of shortness of breath. In addition, an air entrainment mask order must specify the patient's oxygen percentage (e.g., 24%, 28%). A portable oxygen tank does not provide a long enough duration of flow to the cannula if the patient has prolonged shortness of breath. An oxygen-conserving cannula is more economical than a regular cannula. (See Exam Hint 17-2. If necessary, review oxygen delivery systems in Chapter 6.)

20. **B.** Studies have shown that patients who complete a rehabilitation program can expect fewer hospitalizations and more exercise tolerance. Unfortunately, the patient cannot expect to experience clinically significant improvement in pulmonary function studies. This is because the lung damage sustained by COPD patients is not reversible.

21. **B.** Among other things, the asthmatic patient should understand his current level of control, how to use any inhaled medication devices, and how to use a peak flowmeter to assess his condition. A COPD patient should be taught energy-conservation techniques and the proper use of any supplemental oxygen equipment. These are not needed by an asthmatic patient, who is essentially normal between episodes.

Chapter 18

1. **C.** If air is seen to bubble in the water-seal chamber, it is known that vacuum is applied to the drainage system and the patient has pleural air (pneumothorax) that is being removed. The presence of fluid in the collection chamber confirms that the patient has pleural fluid that is being removed. It does not confirm that pleural air is being removed. A vacuum level of −15 cm H_2O is normal and should result in air bubbling in the suction control chamber. However, it does not confirm that pleural air is being removed.

2. **D.** The physical signs indicate that the patient has a left-sided pneumothorax; a pleural chest tube is indicated. Do not place a tube into the right pleural space. Increasing the V_T or changing the mode would not correct the problem.

3. **B.** An air leak through the water seal when the patient coughs indicates that the air is coming from the patient's lung. If a leak exists in the system, air will bubble through the water seal at all times. The vacuum level has no impact on the air leak from the patient.

4. **A.** Nasal CPAP would be indicated for the management of a patient with obstructive sleep apnea. An oropharyngeal airway would be indicated only in an obtunded patient with an obstructed upper airway. For many patients, sleeping on the back worsens the obstruction. A tracheostomy and mechanical ventilation may be indicated in a patient with central sleep apnea if all other efforts have failed.

5. **A.** A normal SpO_2 value indicates that the CPAP system at 7 cm H_2O pressure has corrected the patient's problem. There is no need to raise the CPAP level because the patient's pulse oximetry value is normal. There is no indication of inadequate flow through the CPAP system. There is no need to raise the delivered oxygen percentage because the saturation is within the normal range.

6. **D.** Performing a bronchoscopy on a ventilated patient necessitates the use of a special bronchoscopy adapter

between the endotracheal tube and the circuit. The bronchoscope is placed through the adapter, which may result in a V_T leak. In addition, the bronchoscope partially obstructs the endotracheal tube, which increases resistance and causes inspiratory pressure to increase.

7. **B.** The easiest way to seal the chest tube but allow air leaking from the patient to escape is to place the distal end of the tube under water. Clamping the tube does not allow any pleural air to escape. Leaving the tube open allows pleural air to escape but also allows room air to enter the pleural space. The Valsalva maneuver would require breath-holding by the patient for an extended time and is not practical. (See Table 18-1.)

8. **B.** Cardioversion requires a strong R wave on the ECG monitor, a proper electrical charge level, and proper placement of the ECG leads. The electrode paddles should be well covered with a conducting jelly to maximize the flow of current into the patient without a burn.

9. **C.** Rigid-tube bronchoscopy is preferred in the removal of a large foreign body from a large airway. FFB may be used with a small foreign body or one that is in a smaller airway. Positive expiratory pressure and postural drainage therapy are not likely to dislodge a large foreign body such as a tooth. Postural drainage therapy with percussion may dislodge a foreign body. (See Box 18-2.)

10. **D.** ABGs are not monitored during a sleep study because it is an invasive procedure and the patient would awaken as the blood sample is drawn. The other items are routinely monitored during a sleep study.

11. **B.** The test should be stopped because the patient's signs and symptoms indicate that he is not tolerating the procedure. A healthy person who does not have dangerous signs and symptoms may tolerate an R of 1.1 for a short time; this patient should not be pushed to this point. This patient has several signs and symptoms showing intolerance and does not need to be pushed to complain of shortness of breath. Although the patient may tolerate the stress test at a lower work level, it is safer to stop the test and evaluate the patient.

12. **C.** When indirect calorimetry is used to evaluate a patient's oxygen consumption and carbon dioxide production during an exercise test, the anaerobic threshold is confirmed by an R of 1.0. Before the R value reaches 1.0, the patient will dramatically increase his or her tidal volume and respiratory rate when the tissues are hypoxic and anaerobic metabolism occurs.

13. **C.** The endotracheal tube should be removed from the patient as the tracheostomy tube is to be placed into the stoma. This ensures that the patient has a secure airway throughout the procedure.

14. **C.** Bleeding at the insertion site is a common complication of a surgical tracheostomy. Bleeding is uncommon with a PDT. A tracheal ring may fracture as the

dilator is being inserted through the anterior tracheal wall. If the dilator is misdirected, it can puncture a lung, causing a pneumothorax. If the dilator is pushed in too deeply, it can pierce the posterior tracheal wall and cause a tracheoesophageal fistula.

15. **A.** A heated cascade-type humidification system is inappropriate because the water will splash through the ventilator circuit and into the patient because of the constant motion during transport. A heat and moisture exchanger should be used instead. The oxygen cylinder duration should be calculated to be sure that sufficient oxygen is present for the trip. A demand-valve IMV system should be chosen because it is not affected by altitude changes. A lightweight and portable ventilator is needed because the helicopter has a weight limit for equipment and passengers, and the chosen ventilator should be designed to tolerate the rough motion that can occur during a transport.

16. **C.** An FFB is indicated for two reasons. First, the patient has a history of smoking and recurrent bouts of pneumonia of the left lung. Second, other treatment procedures have failed to produce improvement in the patient's chest radiograph. These facts should make one suspicious of a lung tumor. It is very doubtful that nebulizing a bronchodilator medication or hypertonic saline will make any difference in this patient's condition. No indication of bronchospasm or retained secretions is noted. A rigid-tube bronchoscope cannot be used to visualize the left lower-lobe bronchus because it is not flexible. It can be used only to view the trachea and right and left mainstem bronchi. (See Box 18-2.)

17. **D.** A tension pneumothorax can be immediately treated by placing a large-bore (often 16-gauge) needle through the second or third intercostal space at the midclavicular line on the affected side. Later, a pleural chest tube should be inserted. Although a 5% pneumothorax is abnormal, it is probably not life-threatening. Sometimes the patient is given supplemental oxygen as needed and monitored. The pneumothorax gas may be reabsorbed into the tissues, and no other treatment may be necessary. A pleural effusion or hemothorax requires a thoracentesis procedure to remove the fluid. This would probably be done through the lower area of the patient's back because the fluid is gravity dependent.

18. **A.** The R value is calculated by placing the patient's $\dot{V}O_2$ and $\dot{V}CO_2$ values into the following equation:

$$R = \frac{\dot{V}CO_2}{\dot{V}O_2} = \frac{1700 \text{ mL}}{2000 \text{ mL}} = 0.85$$

19. **C.** According to Boyle's law, pressure and volume are inversely proportional. Therefore as barometric pressure decreases at increased altitude, the volume of gas in the patient's endotracheal tube cuff increases and the tidal volume increases. Despite the increased tidal

volume, the patient is likely to become hypoxic because the alveolar pressure of oxygen (PAO_2) decreases and therefore the PaO_2 decreases as the barometric pressure decreases. The patient's tidal volume should be monitored and adjusted during the flight, and the pulse oximetry value should be monitored to assess for hypoxemia and the need to increase the inspired oxygen percentage. No link exists between fluid retention and change in barometric pressure. (See Exam Hint 18-1.)

20. **B.** All of the stated signs indicate a tension pneumothorax. Because the patient's condition is rapidly deteriorating, it is most important to insert a pleural chest tube on the right side. Because it is very likely that the central venous pressure needle pierced the lung and caused the pneumothorax, the procedure should be stopped at this time. Although a chest radiograph would be indicated if the patient's condition were stable, obtaining one now will unnecessarily delay inserting the needed chest tube. Nothing of clinical value is to be gained at this time by comparing the peak and plateau pressures on the ventilator. They will both increase because of the tension pneumothorax. This information only reinforces the previous signs, and performing this procedure now delays the needed chest tube. (See Exam Hint 18-3.)

21. **D.** Before a conscious patient undergoes a cardioversion procedure, he or she should be given a sedative. The drug midazolam (Versed) is given intravenously for conscious sedation. The proper initial power setting for the first attempt at cardioversion of an adult patient with atrial fibrillation is 120 J (see Box 18-1). Set the ECG machine to lead II so that an upright R wave is detected by the unit. On occasion, the medication midazolam and shock from the cardioversion can cause a patient to stop breathing temporarily. For this reason, the respiratory therapist should have a manual resuscitation bag on standby and be ready to assist the patient's breathing. The drug flumazenil (Romazicon) is given intravenously after the procedure is finished to reverse the sedating effect of the midazolam. A defibrillator charge of 360 J is the maximum used to defibrillate a patient. It is far too high for a first attempt at cardioversion. (See Box 18-1.)

22. **A.** The surgeon should insert the first tracheostomy tube into the stoma in case there is a problem. A respiratory therapist may replace a tracheostomy tube after the stoma is well established. The therapist may assist with the procedure by disinfecting the surgical site, checking the tube cuff, and withdrawing the endotracheal tube when the surgeon has created the stoma and is ready to insert the tracheostomy tube.

23. **D.** A stylet (lubricated or not) is not inserted into an endotracheal tube during a nasotracheal intubation procedure. This is because the tube should be kept flexible to follow the natural contours of the patient's airway anatomy. A stylet makes the endotracheal tube stiff and causes damage to the nasal passage. A Magill forceps is used to lift the tip of the tube for insertion into the trachea. A laryngoscope handle with blade is used as during an oral intubation procedure (see Fig. 18-15). The tip of the endotracheal tube is lubricated so that it slides easily through the patient's nasal passage.

24. **B.** The HR_{max} can be calculated by two different equations. Both are shown below for this 55-year-old patient. The first equation was used for this question.

(1) HR_{max} for males and females $= 210 - (0.65 \times \text{age in years})$
$= 210 - (0.65 \times 55)$
$= 210 - (35.75)$
$= 174.25$

Round off to the nearest whole number for a maximum heart rate of 174 beats/min.

(2) HR_{max} for males and females $= 220 - (\text{age in years})$
$= 220 - (55)$
$= 165$

By this alternate equation the patient's HR_{max} would be 165 beats/min.

25. **C.** Normally, as a person progressively exercises more vigorously, his or her ventilation efforts (larger tidal volume and faster respiratory rate) will increase proportionately. This is because the exercising muscles produce more carbon dioxide and require more oxygen. A decreasing or constant ventilation effort at increasing workload levels would be abnormal. The patient would soon have to stop exercising. Decreasing ventilation when carbon dioxide production increases would result in respiratory acidosis. This would be markedly abnormal and cause the person to quickly stop exercising.

26. **B.** The lack of air movement, and related hypoxemia, while respiratory efforts are being made documents that the patient has an airway obstruction problem. If the patient had central sleep apnea, he would have stopped making breathing efforts during the time when no air was moving. Cheyne-Stokes respiration is identified by cyclical increasing and decreasing of tidal volume breathes. There may or may not be short periods of apnea between the cycles. Hyperventilation can be documented only by a decreased arterial carbon dioxide level.

27. **D.** The normal lung should be down (i.e., in a dependent position) and the problem lung up during a thoracentesis. This will ensure that the good lung receives most of the air and blood for gas exchange.

28. **C.** A pulse oximeter value will quickly tell you the patient's oxygenation status. The chest radiograph will allow you to visualize how much the lung has expanded and if there is still fluid in the pleural space. If there is any more fluid, it should be removed until

the patient's condition has stabilized. Because the pleural fluid must be sent to the laboratory for analysis, the results will not be known for at least a day and do not help with understanding the patient's reaction to the procedure.

29. **B.** Fluticasone (Flovent) is an inhaled corticosteroid. It is not used as a sedating medication. Diazepam (Valium) and midazolam (Versed) are sedatives used in conscious sedation. Flumazenil (Romazicon) would be used as a reversing agent against Valium and Versed when the procedure is completed.

30. **A.** Betadine is a topical antiseptic that is used to clean the puncture site. Xylocaine is a local anesthetic used to numb the puncture site. Sublimaze could be used to sedate the patient if he or she was anxious before the procedure. However, the patient is already unconscious. If Sublimaze were to be used, it would be reversed with Narcan.

Index

Note: Page numbers followed by *b, t,* and *f* indicate boxes, tables, and figures respectively.